MW01596020

Parkinson Disease and Other Movement Disorders

Parkinson Disease and Other Movement Disorders

Motor Behavioural Disorders and Behavioural Motor Disorders

editors

Erik Wolters
Christian Baumann

International Association of Parkinsonism and Related Disorders

VU University Press

Video fragments on Dropbox:
www.dropbox.com/sh/bj1qt1yy1qum2bd/WkT2T1yrP-

First print, January 2014

In the United States and Canada this book is distributed by Independent Publishers Group, Chicago
www.ipg.com

In the United Kingdom this book is distributed by Gazelle Books
www.gazellebooks.com

This book can also be ordered form regular internet stores

VU University Press
De Boelelaan 1105
1081 HV Amsterdam
The Netherlands

www.vuuniversitypress.com
info@vuuitgeverij.nl

© 2014 VU University Press

Video editing: Frans Wolters, Amsterdam
Text editing: Alison Fisher, Amsterdam
Design jacket: Titus Schulz, Arnhem
Design contents: Sjoukje Rienks, Amsterdam
Printing: Wilco, Amersfoort

ISBN   978 90 8659 666 9
NUR   910

Preface

We do not look at things as they are, but as we are.
Wayne W. Dyer

In 'Parkinson Disease and Other Movement Disorders', an up-to-date, multidisciplinary overview of motor and behavioural movement disorders is provided by eminent authors, under the auspices of the International Association of Parkinsonism and Related Disorders (IAPRD), on the occasion of their XXst World Congress on Parkinson's Disease and Related Disorders in Geneva, December 2013.

Following an introduction covering the functional anatomy, physiology and pathology in protein aggregation disorders, this book deals with the aetiology, pathophysiology, diagnostic and differential diagnostic procedures as well as conventional, pharmacological and neurosurgical strategies in movement disorders. Not only motor behavioural disorders are covered, behavioural motor disorders are also dealt with, including psychogenic/psychiatric behavioural motor disorders, impulse control disorders, obsessive-compulsive disorders and the attentional deficit hyperactivity disorder. This book provides extensive visual information with numerous video fragments of these patients via Dropbox, improving its function as a guide to recognize and classify these disorders, and meeting the need for well formulated, generally accepted definitions. 'Parkinson Disease and Other Movement Disorders', provides you with the essential tools to recognize, interpret and understand the clinical manifestations and underlying disorders and to select the best therapeutic strategies. It is an excellent practical source for all medical and allied health professionals involved with movement disorder patients, and for researchers seeking a comprehensive, in-depth, translational overview of the fundamental and clinical aspects of movement disorders. By publishing this textbook, the International Association of Parkinsonism and Related Disorders hopes to contribute to achieving its goals: sharing knowledge and increasing the quality of life of all patients suffering from these invalidating diseases.

The editors want to pay their respect not only to all of the authors but also to the publisher Jan Oegema, the graphic designer Sjoukje Rienks, the language editor Alison Fisher and the editor of the video fragments Frans Wolters for their greatly appreciated endeavours in the production of this book. This publication has been made possible by an unrestricted grant from both Abbvie and the International Association of Parkinsonism and Related Disorders. We truly appreciate their generosity, and hope that this book will help to improve the quality of life of patients around the world suffering from this variety of debilitating, though fascinating, movement disorders.

Erik Ch. Wolters, Christian Baumann
Amsterdam / Zurich, December 2013

Contents

Authors

Angelo Antonini MD, PhD
Dept for Parkinson's disease
IRCSS San Camillo
Venice
Italy

Melissa J. Armstrong, MD
Dept of Neurology
University of Maryland School of Medicine
Baltimore, MD
USA

Julien F. Bally, MD
Dept of Neurology
University Hospital of Geneva
Geneva
Switzerland

Claudio Bassetti, MD
Dept of Neurology
Inselspital
Berne
Switzerland

Christian Baumann, MD
Dept of Neurology
University Hospital
Zurich
Switzerland

Daniela Berg, MD
Hertie-Institute of Clinical Brain Research
and German Center for Neurodegenerative Diseases
Tübingen
Germany

Wilma D.J. van de Berg, MD, PhD
Dept of Anatomy and Neuroscience
Vrije Universiteit Medical Center
Amsterdam
The Netherlands

Thröstur Björgvinsson, PhD, ABPP
Dept of Psychology, McLean Hospital
Dept of Psychiatry, Harvard Medical School
Belmont, MA
USA

Kathrin Brockmann, MD
Hertie-Institute of Clinical Brain Research
and German Center for Neurodegenerative Diseases
Tübingen
Germany

David Brooks, MD, DSc, FRCP, FMedSci
Faculty of Medicine, Centre for Neuroscience
Imperial College
London
United Kingdom

Peter Brown, MD
Dept of Clinical Neurology
John Radcliffe Hospital, University of Oxford
Oxford
United Kingdom

Heidi Cartwright, BSc
Neuroscience Research Australia
University of New South Wales
Randwick
Australia

John N. Caviness, MD
Mayo Clinic Movement Disorders Division
Mayo Clinic College of Medicine
Phoenix, Arizona
USA

Lama Chahin, MD
Dept of Neurology
Perelman School of Medicine
University of Pennsylvania
Philadelphia, PA, USA

K Ray Chaudhuri, DSc, FRCP, MD
Dept of Neurology, Movement Disorders Unit
King's College Hospital
London
United Kingdom

Patrick Cras, MD
Dept of Neurology
University of Antwerp Hospital
Edegem
Belgium

Jesse M. Crosby, PhD
Dept of Psychology, McLean Hospital
Dept of Psychiatry, Harvard Medical School
Belmont, MA
USA

Dirk Dressler, MD, PhD
Dept of Neurology
Hannover Medical School
Hannover
Germany

Mark J. Edwards, MBBS, BSc, PhD
Sobell Dept of Motor Neuroscience and
Movement Disorders
UCL Institute of Neurology
London, United Kingdom

Jan Willem Elting, MD, PhD
Dept of Clinical Neurophysiology
University Medical Centre Groningen
Groningen
The Netherlands

Karen Frei, MD
Dept of Neurology
LLU Medical Center, Loma Linda University
Loma Linda, CA
USA

Andrzej Friedman, MD, PhD, cFANA
Dept of Neurology
Medical University of Warsaw
Warsaw
Poland

Shinsuke Fujioka, MD
Dept of Neurology
Mayo Clinic Florida
Jacksonville, FL
USA

Manfred Gerlach, PhD
Dept of Child and Adolescent Psychiatry,
Psychosomatics and Psychotherapy
University of Wurzburg
Würzburg, Germany

Jay van Gerpen, MD
Dept of Neurology
Mayo Clinic
Jacksonville, Florida
USA

Henk J. Groenewegen, MD, PhD
Dept of Anatomy and Neuroscience
Vrije Universiteit Medical Center
Amsterdam
The Netherlands

Mark Hallett, MD
Human Motor Control Section
NINDS, National Institutes of Health
Bethesda
USA

Glenda Halliday, MD, PhD
Neuroscience Research Australia
University of New South Wales
Randwick
Australia

Andreas Hartmann, MD
Dept of Neurology
Groupe Hospitalier Pitié-Salpêtrière
Paris
France

Rick C. Helmich, MD, PhD
Donders Institute for Brain, Cognition and
Behaviour, Dept of Neurology
Radboud University Medical Centre
Nijmegen, The Netherlands

Dagmar H. Hepp, MD
Dept of Anatomy and Neurosciences
Dept of Neurology, VU Medical Center
Amsterdam
The Netherlands

Franziska Hopfner, MD
Dept of Neurology
University Hospital Schleswig Holstein
Kiel
Germany

Anne-Catherine M. L. Huys, BM/BCh, MRCP
Dept of Neurology
University Hospital of Geneva
Geneva
Switzerland

Hans H. Jung, MD
Dept of Neurology
University Hospital
Zurich
Switzerland

Marina AJ de Koning-Tijssen, MD, PhD
Dept of Neurology
University Medical Centre Groningen
Groningen
The Netherlands

Berry Kremer, MD, PhD
Dept of Neurology
University Medical Centre Groningen
Groningen
The Netherlands

Florian Krismer, MD
Dept of Neurology
Innsbruck Medical University
Innsbruck
Austria

Mónica M. Kurtis, MD
Dept of Neurology, Movement Disorders Unit
Hospital Ruber Internacional
Madrid
Spain

Anthony E. Lang, OC, MD, FRCPC, FAAN,
FCAHS, FRSC
Dept of Medicine, Division of Neurology
Toronto Western Hospital
Toronto, Ontario, Canada

Andrew Lees, MD
The Rita Lila Weston Institute of Neurological Studies
UCL Institute of Neurology
London
United Kingdom

Marie-An de Lettere, MD, PhD
Dept of Neuropsychiatry
Spital Linth
Uznach
Switzerland

Vladimir Litvak, MD
Dept of Clinical Neurology
John Radcliffe Hospital, Oxford University
Oxford
United Kingdom

Francesca Mancini, MD
Dept for Parkinson's Disease
Clinic San Pio X
Milan
Italy

Marc Mahone, MD
Dept of Neuropsychology, Kennedy Krieger Institute
Johns Hopkins University
Baltimore, MD
USA

Pablo Martínez-Martín, MD
Alzheimer Center Reina Sofia Foundation
CIBERNED, Carlos III Institute of Health
Madrid
Spain

Hans de Munter, MD
Dept of HMeNS
University Maastricht
Maastricht
The Netherlands

Karen Murphy, MD
Neuroscience Research Australia
University of New South Wales
Randwick
Australia

Ashwini Oswal, MA, MBBS, MRCP
Dept of Clinical Neurology, John Radcliffe Hospital
University of Oxford
Oxford
United Kingdom

Isabel Parees, MD
Sobell Dept of Motor Neuroscience and
Movement Disorders
UCL Institute of Neurology
London, United Kingdom

Barbara Pickut, MD
Dept of Neurology
University of Antwerp Hospital
Edegem
Belgium

Pierre Pollak, MD
Dept of Neurology
University Hospital of Geneva
Geneva
Switzerland

Ronald B. Postuma, MD, MSc
Dept of Neurology
McGill University, Montreal General Hospital
Montreal, Quebec
Canada

Deepa Pothalil, MD
Dept of Clinical Neurosciences
CHUV-UNIL
Lausanne
Switzerland

Alex Rajput, MD, FRCPC
Division of Neurology
University of Saskatchewan,
Royal University Hospital
Saskatoon, Canada

Carmen Rodríguez-Blázquez, MD
National Center of Epidemiology
CIBERNED Carlos III Institute of Health
Madrid
Spain

Marcel Romanos, MD
Dept of Child and Adolescent Psychiatry,
Psychosomatics and Psychotherapy
University of Wurzburg
Würzburg, Germany

Jan Roth, MD, PhD
Dept of Neurology, Center of Clinical Neuroscience
Charles University
Prague
Czech Republic

Annemieke J.M. Rozemuller, MD, PhD
Netherlands Prion Laboratory,
University Medical Center Utrecht
and Dept of Pathology, VU Medical Center
Amsterdam, The Netherlands

Tom H.J. Ruigrok, PhD
Dept of Neuroscience
Erasmus Medical Center Rotterdam
Rotterdam
The Netherlands

Yanush Sanotsky, MD
Dept of Neurology
Lviv Regional Clinical Hospital
Lviv
Ukraine

Susanne A. Schneider, MD, PhD
Dept of Neurology
University Hospital Schleswig Holstein
Kiel
Germany

Elisaveta Sokolov, MD
Dept of Neurology
King's College Hospital
London
UK

Harry Steinbusch, PhD
Dept of HMeNS
University Maastricht
Maastricht
The Netherlands

Matthew B. Stern, MD
Dept of Neurology, Pennsylvania Hospital
University of Pennsylvania
Philadelphia, PA
USA

Fabrizio Stocchi, MD, PhD
Dept of Neurology
IRCCS San Raffaele
Roma
Italy

Alexander Tarnutzer, MD
Dept of Neurology
University Hospital
Zurich
Switzerland

Daniel Truong, MD
The Parkinson's and Movement Disorder Institute
Orange Coast Memorial Medical Center
Fountain Valley, CA
USA

Francois J.G Vingerhoets, MD, PhD
Dept of Clinical Neurosciences
CHUV-UNIL
Lausanne
Switzerland

Valerie Voon, MD, PhD
Dept of Psychiatry
University of Cambridge
Cambridge
United Kingdom

Daniel Waldvogel, MD
Dept of Neurology
Klinik St. Anna
Luzern
Switzerland

Daniel Weintraub, MD
Perelman School of Medicine
University of Pennsylvania
Philadelphia, PA
USA

Gregor K. Wenning, MD, PhD, MSc
Dept of Neurology, Division of Neurobiology
Innsbruck Medical University
Innsbruck
Austria

Erik Ch. Wolters, MD, PhD
Dept of Neurology, University Hospital Zurich,
Switzerland
and Dept of HMeNS, University Maastricht
Maastricht, The Netherlands

Zbigniew K. Wszolek, MD
Dept of Neurology
Mayo Clinic Florida
Jacksonville, FL
USA

Rodi Zutt, MD
Dept of Neurology
University Medical Centre Groningen
Groningen,
The Netherlands

Abbreviations

A	adenosine	ANT	adenine nucleotide translocator
Aβ	amyloid-β	AOA	ataxia with ocular motor apraxia
A8	retrorubral area	AOAxD	adult-onset Alexander disease
AAA	achalasia-addisonianism-alacrima	AOS	apraxia of speech
AADC	aromatic amino acid decarboxylase	APO-E	apolipoprotein E
ABL	abetalipoproteinaemia	APP	amyloid precursor protein
ACD	alcoholic cerebellar degeneration	ARA	anti-reticulin antibodies
AD	Alzheimer's disease	ARCA	autosomal recessive cerebellar ataxia
ADCA	autosomal dominant cerebellar ataxia	ARHGEF9	collybistin
ADCA-DN	autosomal dominant cerebellar ataxia with deafness and narcolepsy	ARSAC	autosomal recessive spastic ataxia of Charlevoix-Saguenay
ADDS	arm dystonia disability scale	ASD	acid sphingomyelinase deficiency
ADf	autonomic dysfunction	ASM	acid sphingomyelinase
ADHD	attention-deficit hyperactivity disorder	AT	ataxia telangiectasia
		ATLD	ataxia telangiectasia-like disorder
ADIS	anxiety disorder interview schedule	ATP	adenosine triphosphate
ADL	activities of daily living	ATXN	ataxin
ADOAD	autosomal-dominant optic atrophy and deafness	AVED	ataxia with vitamin-E deficiency
		AxD	Alexander disease
AFG	ATPase family gene		
AGA	anti-gliadin antibodies	BABS	Brown assessment of beliefs scale
AIMS	abnormal involuntary movement scale	BAEP	brainstem auditory evoked potentials
		BARS	Barnes akathisia rating scale
AJ	Ashkenazı Jews	BART	balloon analogue risk task
AI ADIN	alacrima–achalasia–adrenal insufficiency neurologic disorder	BAS	Barnes akathisia rating scale
		BDD	body dysmorphic disorder
ALS	amyotrophic lateral sclerosis	BDNF	brain-derived neurotrophic factor
ALSP	adult-onset leukoencephalopathy with axonal spheroids and pigmented glia	BDS	blepharospasm disability scale
		BFC	benign familial chorea
		BHC	benign hereditary chorea
ALS-PDC	amyotrophic lateral sclerosis-parkinsonism-dementia complex	BIBD	basophilic inclusions body disease
		BMAA	β-N-methylamino-l-alanine
AMPA	α-amino-hydroxy-methylisoxazole-propionate	BOLD	blood oxygen level-dependent
		BOSH	behaviour observation scale of Huntington disease
AMRFS	action myoclonus-renal failure syndrome	BP	bereitschaftspotential
ANCL	adult neuronal ceroid-lipofuscinose	BRS	blepharospasm rating scale
ANG	angiogenin	BST	bone marrow stromal cell antigen
ANO	anoctamin	BT	botulinum toxin
ANS	autonomic nervous system	BTP	benign tremulous parkinsonism

bvFTD	behavioural variant frontotemporal dementia	CDSS	cervical dystonia severity scale
		CERAD	consortium to establish a registry for Alzheimer disease
^{11}C-CFT	carbon labelled carbomethoxy-fluorophenyl tropane	CH	cyclohydrolase
		ChA	choreoacanthocytosis
^{11}C-CNS5161	carbon labelled methylguanidine	CHF1512	melevodopa
^{11}C-PK11195	carbon labelled isoquinoline carboxamide	CHMP	charged multivesicular body protein
		CHRNA	nicotinic cholinergic receptor
^{11}C-DTBZ	carbon labelled dihydro-tetra-benazine	CHS	Chediak-Higashi syndrome
		CI	capsula interna
^{11}C-flumazenil	carbon labelled flumazenil	CISI-PD	clinical impression of severity index Parkinson's disease
^{11}C-N-methylpyrrolidon			
	carbon labelled methylpyrrolidon	CJD	Creutzfeldt-Jakob's disease
^{11}C-NMP4A	carbon labelled piperidyl acetate	CK	creatine kinase
^{11}C-nomifensine		CL	carbidopa/levodopa
	carbon labelled nomifensine	CLCN	chloride channel
^{11}C-MP	carbon labelled methylphenidate)	CLD	continuous levodopa delivery
^{11}C-PIB	carbon labelled phenyl-hydroxy-benzothiazole	CLDII	continuous levodopa delivery by intestinal infusion
^{11}C-polymethylpentene		CLN	ceroid-lipofuscinoses
	carbon labelled polymethylpentene	CM	cortical myoclonus
^{11}C-raclopride		CM-Pf	central parafascicular nucleus of the thalamus
	carbon labelled raclopride		
^{11}C-SCH442416		CMT	Charcot-Marie Tooth disease
	carbon labelled pyrazolo-triazolo-pyrimidine	CNS	central nervous system
		CNV	copy number variation
^{11}C-TSMX	carbon labelled dihydro-purine-dione	CoA	coenzyme A
		COMT	catechol-O-methyltransferase
C10orf2	chromosome 10 open reading frame 2 (twinkle)	COQ	coenzyme Q
		COX	cytochrome c oxidase
C19orf	chromosome 19 open reading frame	CP	cerulopasmin
CAA	cerebral amyloid angiopathy	CPAP	continuous positive airway pressure
CACNA	P/Q type voltage-dependent calcium channel alpha	CPEO	chronic progressive external ophthalmoplegia
CADASIL	cerebral arteriopathy with subcortical infarcts and leukoencephalopathy	CRPS	complex regional pain syndrome
		CS	conditional stimulus
CANVAS	cerebellar ataxia, neuropathy, vestibular areflexia syndrome	CSAI	continuous apomorphine infusion
		CSF	cerebrospinal fluid
CBD	[pathological] corticobasal degeneration	CSF	colony-stimulating factor
		CST	card sorting test
CBS	[clinical] corticobasal syndrome	CSTC	cortico-striatal-thalamo-cortical circuit
CD	cervical dystonia		
CDD	continuous dopaminergic delivery	CSWS	continuous spike waves during sleep
CDS	continuous dopamine receptor stimulation	CTT	classical test theory
		CTX	cerebrotendinous xanthomatosis

CUPS	clinically uncertain parkinsonian syndrome	DRD	dopa-responsive dystonia
CYP	cytochrome P450	DRPLA	dentatorubro-pallidoluysian atrophy
		DS	global dystonia rating scale
D	dopamine receptor	DSM	diagnostic and statistical manual of mental disorders
DA	dopamine agonist	DT	dystonic tremor
Da T	dopamine transporter	DTBZ	dihydrotetrabenazine
DAWS	dopamine withdrawal symptoms	DTI	diffusion tensor imaging
DBN	downbeat nystagmus	DYT	dystonia
DBS	deep brain stimulation		
DBS-CI	deep brain stimulation of capsula interna	EA	episodic ataxia
		ECOG	electrocortigraphy
DBS-CM-Pf	deep brain stimulation of the thalamic central parafascicular nucleus	ECT	electroconvulsive therapy
		ED	erectile dysfunction
		EDS	excessive daytime sleepiness
DBS-GPi	deep brain stimulation of the pallidal globe, pars interna	EEG	electroencephalography
		EFHC	myoclonin
DBS-NA	deep brain stimulation of the nucleus accumbens	EFNS	European federation of neurological societies
DBS-PSA	deep brain stimulation of the posterior subthalamic area	EGF	epidermal growth factor
		EIF	eukaryotic translation initiation factor
DBS-STN	deep brain stimulation of the subthalamic nucleus	EMA	anti-endomysial antibodies
DBS-Tcm	deep brain stimulation of the thalamic centromedian nucleus	EMA	European medical authority
		EMG	electromyography
DBS-Til	deep brain stimulation of the thalamic intralaminary nucleus	EOAD	early-onset Alzheimer's disease
		EOCA	early onset cerebellar ataxia
DBS-Tmn	deep brain stimulation of the thalamic median nucleus	EP	evoked potential
		EPM	essential palatal myoclonus
DBS Vim	deep brain stimulation of the thalamic ventral intermediate nucleus	EPM	progressive myoclonus epilepsy
		EPS	extra pyramidal syndrome
DBS-VLp	deep brain stimulation of the thalamic ventrolateral posterior nucleus	ER	extended release
		ERD	event-related desynchronisation
DCTN	dynactin	ERP	exposure and response prevention
DDS	dopamine dysregulation syndrome	ERS	event-related synchronisation
DG	deoxyglucose	ESRS	extrapyramidal symptoms rating scale
DIP	drug-induced parkinsonism		
DIREQT	duodopa infusion randomized efficacy and quality of life trial	ESS	Epworth sleepiness scale
		ESSTS	European society for the study of Tourette syndrome
DLB	dementia with Lewy bodies		
dmX	dorsal motor nucleus of the vagus nerve	ET	essential tremor
		ETM	essential tremor
DNMT	DNA methyl transferase		
DOPS	dihydroxy-phenylserine	18F-DTBZ	fluoro-dihydro-tetrabenazine
DR	dopamine receptor	18F-DOPA	fluoro-phenylalanine

18F-FDG	fluoro-deoxyglucose		GCI	glial cytoplasmic inclusion
18F-FP-CIT	fluoro-propyl-carbomethoxy-iodophenyl nortropane		GD	Gaucher disease
			GDNF	glia cell-derived neurotrophic factor
5-FU	5-fluorouracil		GDS	global dystonia severity rating scale
F	fluor		GEN	gaze-evoked nystagmus
FA	fractional anisotropy		GFAP	glial fibrillary acidic protein
FAM	frequency of abnormal movements		GLB	β-galactosidase
FBS	frontal behavioural spatial syndrome		GLR	glycine receptor
FCMTE	familial cortical myoclonic tremor with epilepsy		Gly2019Ser	leucine-rich repeat kinase 2
			GlyR	glycine receptor
FDA	federal drug administration		GM	monosialic ganglioside
FDG	fluorodeoxyglucose		GOSR	golgi SNAP receptor complex
FGF	fibroblast growth factor		GPe	pallidal globe external segment
FM scale	Fahn-Marsden dystonia rating scale		GPHN	gephyrin
FMR	fragile-X mental retardation		GPi	pallidal globe internal segment
fMRI	functional magnetic resonance imaging		GSD	Gerstmann-Straussler disease
			GSS	Gerstmann Sträussler Scheinker's disease
FMRS	fragile-X mental retardation syndrome			
			GTP	guanosine triphosphate
FOG	freezing of gait		GTS	Gilles de la Tourette syndrome
FRDA	Friedreich's ataxia		GWAS	genome-wide association studies
FSS	fatigue severity scale			
FTD	frontotemporal dementia		5-HIAA	5-hydroxyindoleacetic acid
FTDL	frontotemporal lobar degeneration		5-HT	serotonin
FTDP	fronto-temporal dementia-parkinsonism		H&E	haematoxylin & eosin
			H&Y	Hoehn and Yahr staging scale
FTG	finely tuned gamma		Hcy	homocysteine
FTL	ferritin light chain		HD	Huntington disease
FTLD	frontotemporal lobar degeneration		HD-ADL	Huntington's disease activities of daily living scale
FUS	fused in sarcoma			
FXN	fraxatin		HDC	Huntington disease phenocopies
FXTAS	fragile X-tremor ataxia syndrome		HDC	L-histidine decarboxylase
			HDL	Huntington's disease-like
GABA	gamma-amino-butyric acid		HDLS	hereditary diffuse leukoencephalo-pathy with spheroids
GABRA	gamma-aminobutyric acid type A receptor			
			HDP	Huntington disease phenocopies
GABRB	gamma-aminobutyric acid type B receptors		HDRS	Hamilton depression rating scale
			HFE	hemochromatosis
GAD	glutamic acid decarboxylase		HH	hereditary hemochromatosis
GAK	cyclin G associated kinase		HLA	human leucocyte antigen
GBA	glucocerebrosidase		HMDPC	hypermanganesemia with dystonia, polycythemia, and cirrhosis
GBA	glucosylceramidase			
GBS	Guillain Barré syndrome		HPBH4A	hyperphenylalaninemia with BH4-deficiency type A
GCase	glucocerebrosidase			
GCH1	GTP cyclohydrolase 1		HPX	hyperekplexia

HRT	habit reversal training	JHD	Juvenile Huntington disease
HSP	hereditary spastic paraplegia	JHRLSS	Johns Hopkins restless legs syndrome severity scale
HTT (Htt)	huntingtin		
HUGO	human genome organization	JME	juvenile myoclonus epilepsy
HVA	homovanillic acid	JNCL	juvenile neuronal ceroid-lipofus-cinose
^{123}I-E-IAFCT	iodium labelled altropane	JPH	junctophilins
^{123}I-β-CIT	iodium labelled carbo-methoxy-iodophenyl nortropane	KCNA	potassium voltage-gated channel
^{123}I-FP-CIT	iodium labelled fluoropropyl-carbomethoxy-iodophenyl nortropane	KIAA0196	spatacsin
		KIF5A	kinesin heavy chain
		KMnO4	potassium permanganate
^{123}I-IBZM	iodium labelled iodobenzamide	KRS	Kufor-Rakeb syndrome
^{123}I- MIBG	iodium labelled meta-iodobenzyl-guanidine	KSS	Kearns Sayre syndrome
IBGC	idiopathic basal ganglia calcification	LB	Lewy bodies
IBMPDB	inclusion body myopathy related to Paget disease of bone	LC	locus ceruleus
		LC	levodopa/carbidopa
IBMPFD	inclusion body myopathy related to frontotemporal dementia	LC	lute carrier
		LCE	levodopa/carbidopa/entacapone
ICARS	international cooperative ataxia rating scale	LCIG	levodopa-carbidopa intestinal gel
		L-DOPA	levodopa
ICD	impulse control disorders	LDRS	leg dystonia disability scale
ICD-10	international classification of diseases, 10th edition	LEDD	levodopa-dose equivalent daily dose
		LFP	local field potential
ICSD	international classification of sleep disorders	LHON	Leber's hereditary optic neuropathy
		LID	levodopa-induced dyskinesias
iLBD	incidental Lewy body disease	LINCL	late-infantile neuronal ceroid-lipofuscinose
ILOCA	idiopathic late onset cerebellar ataxia		
INAD	infantile neuroaxonal dystrophy	LINGO	leucine-rich repeat and Ig domain containing nogo receptor interacting protein
INCL	infantile neuronal ceroid-lipofus-cinoses		
IOSCA	infantile onset spinocerebellar ataxia	LMN	lower motor neuron
IR	immediate release formulation	LN	Lewy neurites
iRBD	idiopathic rem sleep behavioural disorder	LOTS	late-onset Tay-Sachs disease
		LRRK	leucine-rich repeat kinase
IRLS	international restless legs syndrome study group	LS	Leigh syndrome
		LTD	long-term depression
IRT	item response theory	LTP	long-term potential
ISAPD	intermediate scale for assessment of Parkinson's disease	LTT	latent trait theories
		LYST	lysosomal trafficking regulator
ITB	intrathecal baclofen therapy		
ITPR	inositol trisphosphate receptor	M1	primary motor cortex
		MAO	monoamine oxidase
JBTS	Joubert syndrome	MAO-B	monoamine oxidase-B

MAPT	microtubule-associated protein tau	MSA-C	multiple system atrophy, cerebellar type
MCI	mild cognitive impairment		
MCP	mitochondriopathies	MSA-P	multiple system atrophy, parkinsonian type
MD	mediodorsal nucleus		
MD	myoclonus dystonia	MSS	Marinesco-Sjögren syndrome
MDMA	methylene-dioxymethamphetamine (ecstasy)	MT scale	Martí & Tolosa Scale
		MTCYB	mitochondrial cytochrome b
MDpl	mediodorsal nucleus paralamellar part	mtDNA	mitochondrial DNA
		mTOR	mechanistic target of rapamycin
MDRS	Mattis dementia rating scale	MTS	Mohr-Tranebjaerg syndrome
MDS	movement disorder society	MTTK	mitochondrially encoded tRNA lysine
MECP	methyl-cytosine–guanine-binding protein		
		NA	neuroacanthocytosis
MEG	magnetoencephalography	NA	nucleus accumbens
MELAS	myopathy, encephalopathy, lactate acidosis and stroke-like episode	NAA	N-acetyl-aspartate
		NAC	non-Aβ component of AD amyloid
MEP	motor evoked potential	NADH	ubiquinone oxidoreductase
MERFF	myoclonic epilepsy and ragged red fibers	NADH	nicotinamide adenine dinucleotide dehydrogenase, ubiquinone
mGLU	metabotropic glutamate	NAM	negative allosteric modulators
mGLUr	metabotropic glutamate receptor	naPPA	non-fluent/agrammatic variant of primary progressive aphasia
MGUS	monoclonal gammopathy of undetermined significance	NARP	neuropathy ataxia and retinitis pigmentosa
MHPG	methoxy-hydroxy-phenylglycol		
MIBG	meta-iodobenzylguanidine	NBIA	neurodegeneration with brain iron accumulation
MILS	maternally inherited Leigh syndrome		
MIRAS	mitochondrial autosomal recessive ataxia syndrome	NBM	nucleus basalis of Meynert
		NBS	Nijmegen breakage syndrome
MJD	Machado Joseph disease	NCI	neuronal cytoplasm inclusions
MLS	McLeod syndrome	NCL	neuronal ceroid-lipofuscinoses
MM	mitochondrial myopathies	nDNA	nuclear DNA
MMSE	mini-mental-state-examination	NDUFV	ubiquinone flavoprotein,
MNS	malignant neuroleptic syndrome	NF	neurotrophic factor
MP	methylphenidate	NFLE	nocturnal frontal lobe epilepsy
MPAN	mitochondrial protein-associated neurodegeneration	NFP	neuroferritinopathy
		NgR	nogo receptor
MPTP	methyl-phenyl-tetrahydropyridine	NGS	next generation sequencing
MRC	motor response complications	NIA-AA	national institute on ageing-Alzheimer's association
MRC	mitochondrial respiratory chain		
MRI	magnetic resonance imaging	NIFID	neuronal intermediate filament inclusion disease
mRNA	messenger RNAs		
MRS	magnetic resonance spectroscopy	NINDS	national institute of neurological disorders and stroke
MRX	X-linked mental retardation		
MS	multiple sclerosis	NINDS-SPSP	NINDS research criteria for the clinical diagnosis of PSP
MSA	multiple system atrophy		

NJ	non-Jewish	PC	Purkinje cell
NMDA	N-methyl-D-aspartate, glutamate, ecstasy	PCA	posterior cortical atrophy
		PCQ	patient card questionnaire
NMDAR	glutamate receptor	PD	Parkinson's disease
NMP	N-methylpyrrolidon	PDB	Paget disease of bone
NMS	non-motor symptoms	PDD	Parkinson's disease-related dementia
NMSQuest	non motor symptoms questionnaire	PDGF	platelet-derived growth factor
NMSS	non motor symptom scale	PD-MCI	Parkinson's disease-related mild cognitive impairment
NNI	neuronal nuclear inclusions		
NNIPPS	natural history and neuroprotection in Parkinson plus syndromes scale	PDQ	Parkinson's disease questionnaire
		PDRP	PD related profile
NP031112	tideglusib	PDSS	Parkinson's disease sleep scale
NPC	Niemann-Pick type C disease	PDSS-2	Parkinson's disease revised sleep scale
NPD	Niemann-Pick disease	PDYN	prodynorphin
NPH	normal pressure hydrocephalus	PEO	progressive external ophthalmoplegia
NPI	neuropsychiatric inventory	PERM	progressive encephalomyelitis with rigidity
NREM	non-rapid eye movement		
NTRK	neurotrophic tyrosine kinase	PET	positron emission tomography
		PFC	prefrontal cortex
6-OHDA	6 hydroxy-dopamine	PG	pathological gambling
OBQ	obsessive beliefs questionnaire	PGRN	progranulin
OCD	obsessive-compulsive disorders	PINK	phosphatase and tensin homologue-induced putative kinase
OCI-R	obsessive-compulsive inventory-revised		
		PKAN	pantothenate kinase-associated neurodegeneration
OCPD	obsessive-compulsive personality disorder		
		PKCγ	protein kinase C gamma
ODRS	oromandibular dystonia rating scale	PKDYS	infantile parkinsonism-dystonia
ODT	orally disintegrating tablet	PL	phospholipase
OFD	oral-facial-digital syndrome	PLAN	phospholipase 2G6-associated neurodegeneration
OH	orthostatic hypotension		
O-LD	oral levodopa	PLMS	periodic limb movements during sleep
OMIM	online Mendelian inheritance in man		
OMS	opsoclonus myoclonus syndrome	PM	palatal myoclonus
ON	olivary nucleus	PMA	progressive myoclonus ataxia
OPA	optic atrophy	PMD	psychogenic movement disorders
OPCA	olivopontocerebellar atrophy	PME	progressive myoclonic epilepsy
OPT	oculopalatal tremor	PMP	polymethylpentene
OT	orthostatic tremor	PN	polyneuropathy
OT-AT	orthostatic and action tremor	PNFA	progressive non-fluent aphasia
OXPHOS	oxidative phosphorylation	PNN	pedunculopontine nucleus
		PNS	peripheral nervous system
PAF	pure autonomic failure	POLD	pigmented orthochromatic leukodystrophy
PANDAS	streptococcal-associated autoimmune neuropsychiatric disorders		
		POLG	polymerase gamma
PANK	pantothenate kinase	PPA	primary progressive aphasia

PPM-X	neonatal pyramidal signs, parkinsonism and macroorchidism	RBD	rapid eye movement sleep behaviour disorder
PPN	pedunculopontine nucleus	RC	respiratory chain
PPT	palmitoyl-protein thioesterase	RDysRS	Rush dyskinesia rating scale
PQ	wearing-off questionnaire (32 items)	REM	rapid eye movement
PRKCG	protein kinase C gamma	RLS	restless legs syndrome
PRKN	parkin	RMT	Rasch measurement theory
PRKRA	protein kinase, interferon-inducible, double-stranded RNA-dependent activator	RN	raphe nuclei
		ROS	reactive oxygen species
		RRA	retro-rubral area
PRNP	prion protein	RSGE	rating scale for gait evaluation
PrP	prion protein	rTMS	repetitive transcranial magnetic stimulation
PRRT	proline-rich transmembrane protein		
PS	Perry syndrome	RTT	Rett syndrome
PSEN	presenilin		
PSG	polysomnogram	SACS	sacsin
PSP	progressive supranuclear palsy, classical Richardson's syndrome	SANDO	sensory axonal neuropathy with dysarthria and ophthalmoparesis
PSP-CBS	PSP, corticobasal type	SAOA	sporadic adult-onset ataxia
PSP-P	PSP, parkinsonistic type	SARA	scale for the assessment and rating of ataxia
PSP-PAGF	PSP with pure akinesia and freezing-of-gait		
		SAS	Simpson-Angus Scale
PSP-PNFA	PSP with progressive non-fluent aphasia	SC	Sydenham's chorea
		SCA	spinocerebellar ataxia
PSPRS	progressive supranuclear palsy rating scale	SCAN	spinocerebellar ataxia with axonal neuropathy
PSPS	progressive supranuclear palsy syndrome	SCAR	spinocerebellar ataxia, recessive
		SCI	structured clinical interview
PT	psychogenic tremor	sCJD	sporadic Creutzfeldt-Jakob disease
PT	palatal tremor	SCL6A5	glycineT2
PTEN	phosphatase and tensin homologue	SCLC	small cell lung cancer
PTS	pyruvoyl-tetrahydropterin synthetase	SCOPA	scales for outcomes in Parkinson's disease
PWT	primary writing tremor		
PWT-A	primary task-specific writing tremor	SCOPA-AUT	scale for outcomes in PD autonomic dysfunctions
PWT-B	primary position-sensitive writing tremor		
		SCOPA-Motor	scales for outcomes in PD motor parkinsonism
QoL	quality of life	SCS	spino-cerebellar ataxia
QQ	wearing-off questionnaires (19 items)	SDMT	symbol digit modalities test
QUIP	questionnaire for impulsive-compulsive disorders	SDS	detergent to lyse cells and release soluble proteins
		SDS	Shy-Dräger syndrome
R	repeats	SEM	standard error of measurement
R2*	susceptibility imaging	SEP	somatosensory evoked potential
		SES	Schwab and England scale

SETX	senataxin	TAF	TATA box-binding protein-associated factor
SIT	Stroop interference test		
SLC	solute carrier	TAN	tonically active neuron
SLE	systemic lupus erythematosus	TARDBP	transactive response DNA-binding protein
SMA	spinal muscular atrophy		
SMA	supplementary motor area	TAWD	tremor associated with dystonia
SN	nigral substance	TBP	TATA box-binding protein
SNARE	soluble N-ethylmaleimide-sensitive-factor attachment protein receptor	TBS	transcranial magnetic brain stimulation
SNCA	α-synuclein	TCI	temperament and character inventory
SND	striatonigral degeneration		
SNP	single-nucleotide polymorphism	Tcm	thalamus centromedian nucleus
SNpc	nigral substance, pars compacta	TCS	transcranial sonography
SNRI	serotonin-norepinephrine reuptake inhibitor	TH	tyrosine hydroxylase
		THAP	thanatos-associated domain-containing apoptosis-associated protein
SP	spastic paraplegia		
SPAX	spastic ataxia		
SPECT	single photon emission computed tomography	THD	tyrosine hydroxylase deficiency
		Tin	thalamic intralaminary nucleus
SPET	single-photon emission tomography	TK2	mitochondrial thymidine kinase 2
SPG	spastic paraplegia	Tmn	thalamic median nucleus
SPM	symptomatic palatal myoclonus	TMS	transcranial magnetic stimulation
SPR	sepiapterin reductase	TNFα	tumor necrosis factor-α
SPS	stiff person syndrome	TPJ	temporoparietal junction
SPSP	society for progressive supranuclear palsy	TPPWG	Tourette practice parameter work group
SPT	spectrin	TRIG	tremor investigation group
SREAT	steroid-responsive encephalopathy associated with autoimmune thyroiditis	TRS	torticollis rating scale
		TS	Tourette syndrome
		TS	tic syndrome
		TS	transcranial sonography
SRI	serotonin reuptake inhibitor	TSE	transmissible spongiform encephalopathies
SSEP	somatosensory evoked potential		
SSRI	selective serotonin reuptake inhibitor	TSGS	Tourette syndrome global scale
STN	subthalamic nucleus	TSPO	translocator protein
STRIDE-PD	stalevo reduction in dyskinesia evaluation in Parkinson disease	TWSTRS	Toronto Western spasmodic torticollis rating scale
STRS	spasmodic torticollis rating scale		
STSSS	Shapiro Tourette syndrome severity scale	UDRS	unified dystonia rating scale
SUDS	subjective units of distress	UDysRS	unified dyskinesia rating scale
SWEDD	scan without evidence of dopaminergic deficit	UE	upper extremity
		UHDRS	unified Huntington's disease rating scale
T1WI	T1-weighted imaging	UKPDSBB	UK Parkinson's disease society brain bank
T2WI	T2-weighted imaging		

UL	Unverricht Lundberg	VP	vascular parkinsonism
UMRS	unified myoclonus rating scale	VP	ventral pallidum
UMSARS	unified multiple system atrophy rating scale	VPS	vacuolar protein sorting
		VTA	ventral tegmental area
UPDRS	unified Parkinson's disease rating scale		
		WCRS	writer's cramp rating scale
UPS	ubiquitin-proteasome system	WD	Wilson's hepatolenticular degeneration, Wilson's disease
UR	unconditioned response		
US	unconditional stimulus	WE	Wernicke encephalopathy
USCRS	UFMG Sydenham's chorea rating scale	WHIGET	Washington Heights-Inwood genetic study of essential tremor rating scale
		WOPQ	wearing-off patient questionnaire
VA (Tva)	ventral anterior nucleus of the thalamus	WOQ	wearing-off questionnaires
		WOQQ	wearing-off quick questionnaire
VAMP	vesicle-associated membrane proteins	WPW	Wolff-Parkinson-White syndrome
		WSS	Woodhouse-Sakati Syndrome
VBM	voxel-based morphometry		
VCP	valosin-containing protein	XLSA/A	X-linked sideroblastic anemia with ataxia
VED	vitamin E deficiency		
Vim	ventral intermediate thalamic nucleus	XPDS	x-linked parkinsonism with spasticity
VLa	anterior ventrolateral thalamic nucleus	Y-BOCS	Yale-Brown obsessive compulsive scale
vLOFA	very late-onset Friedreich ataxia	YGTSS	Yale global tic severity scale
VLp	posterior ventrolateral thalamic nucleus	ZI	zona incerta
VMAT	vesicle monoamine transporter		
VOR	vestibulo-ocular reflex		

Motor Behavioural Disorders and Behavioural Motor Disorders

Erik Wolters & Christian Baumann

Behaviour is considered the response to internal and external stimuli. Both the basal ganglia as well as the cerebellum process internal (homeostatic) and external (environmental) information in order to orchestrate adequately adapted behaviour, and send this processed information via the thalamus back to the cortex for final execution. Based on this information, the basal ganglia arrange for the appropriate selection of behavioural fragments (response selection) out of the available pool of learned standard behaviours, and define their magnitude, while the cerebellum deals with the exact timing and coordination of different body parts. Traditionally, therefore, disorders of the basal ganglia and/or the cerebellum (but not cortical or neuromuscular disorders), leading to hypokinesia (scarcity of movements), hyperkinesia (excess of movements) and/or dyskinesia (abnormal executed movements) in the presence of clear consciousness, are listed as movement disorders and will be discussed after a basic introduction in three different sections. Abnormal movements during disturbed consciousness, such as epileptic disorders, and also motor abnormalities induced by upper and lower motoneuron diseases, neuromuscular diseases and/or arthrogenic disorders, with normal basal ganglia and cerebellar functions, are not part of this group of disorders and will not be dealt with in this book.

The basal ganglia have long been associated with sensorimotor functions only. In the last few decades, it has become generally accepted that thanks to their functional-anatomical organization, they arrange a wide array of functions ranging from pure sensorimotor to cognitive-executive and emotional-motivational behaviours. This allows them to produce the most appropriate response for each particular context, and to suppress inadequate behaviour.

Thus, we interpret the variety of symptoms caused by an inadequate response selection of not only motor but also cognitive and emotional/motivational (affective) responses to internal and external stimuli as manifestations of movement disorders. In this book, we deal with motor behavioural disorders (see Figure 1) as well as behavioural motor disorders (see Figure 2), such as psychogenic and/or psychiatric movement disorders, stereotyped behaviours, chorea and attention-deficit hyperactivity disorders, and behavioural abnormalities within the obsessive-compulsive disorder spectrum.

Dyskinesias may manifest as syndromatic and/or symptomatic, and the recognition and categorization of these manifestations form a complex process. Generally accepted definitions are essential, not only for this recognition and categorization, but also for selecting the appropriate therapeutic strategies and developing clinical pharmacological research. This textbook hopes to provide you with the proper tools. To complete this introduction, a short definition will be given of the most important dyskinetic symptoms, as well as their phenomenological classification.

Dyskinesia

In daily clinical practice, the term dyskinesia is used in particular to refer to iatrogenic (dopamine agonist- or antagonist-induced) cho-

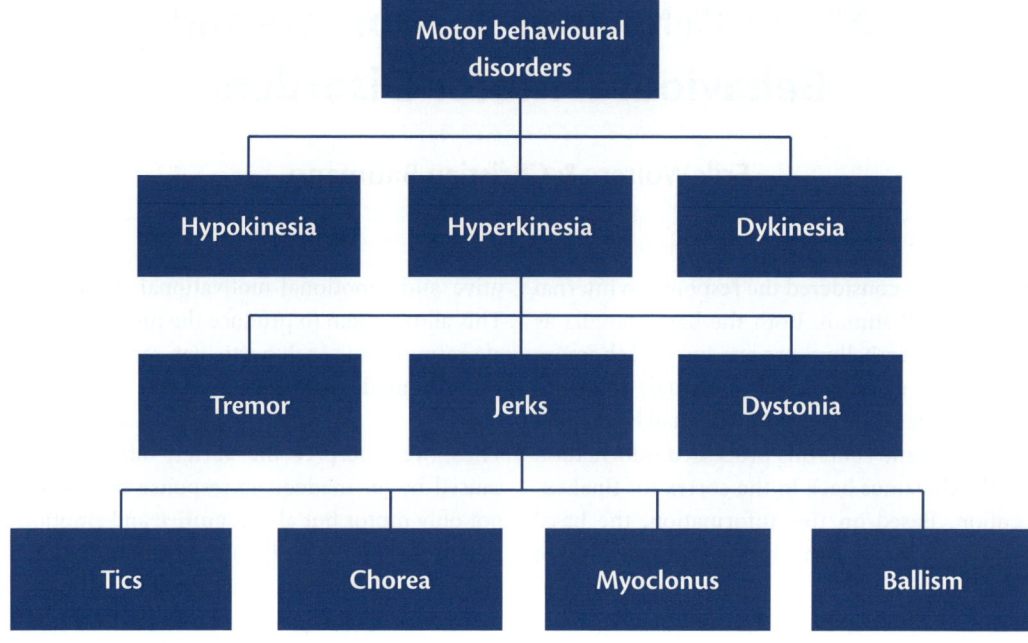

Figure 1
Phenomenology of motor behavioural disorders.

rea-like and dystonic movements. It is actually the general term for all consistent or episodic involuntary movement disorders in full consciousness, comprising basal ganglia dysfunction-induced slowing down of movements (bradykinesia), scarcity of spontaneous movements (akinesia), and/or excess of spontaneous movements: tremor, chorea, tic, myoclonus, ballism, and dystonia (hyperkinesia), as well as cerebellar dysfunction-induced executional failures (ataxia).

Tremor

A tremor is a rhythmic, involuntary, sinusoidal, oscillatory, alternating movement of one or more body parts, particularly the limbs, but also including the head, chin and soft palate, with a relatively fixed frequency and amplitude that occurs over an extended period of time. Tremors can be classified on the basis of their clinical characteristics (isometric tremor, resting tremor, postural tremor, kinetic tremor), their origin (cerebellar, extrapyramidal) or their pathophys-

iological mechanism (physiological, essential, iatrogenic).

Chorea

Chorea is a state of excessive, spontaneous movements, irregularly timed, non-repetitive, randomly distributed and abrupt in character, which might primarily occur in some genetic disorders and secondary to various (para)infectious, auto-immune and structural conditions and some toxic, iatrogenic and metabolic encephalopathies. These movements may vary in severity from restlessness with mild, intermittent exaggeration of gestures and expression, fidgeting movements of the hands, unstable dance-like gait to a continuous flow of disabling, violent movements.

Ballism

Ballism is defined as a movement disorder characterized by involuntary, forceful, flinging, high-amplitude 'throwing' movements. Ballism is often accompanied by choreatic movements, the latter being more distal, while ballism describes

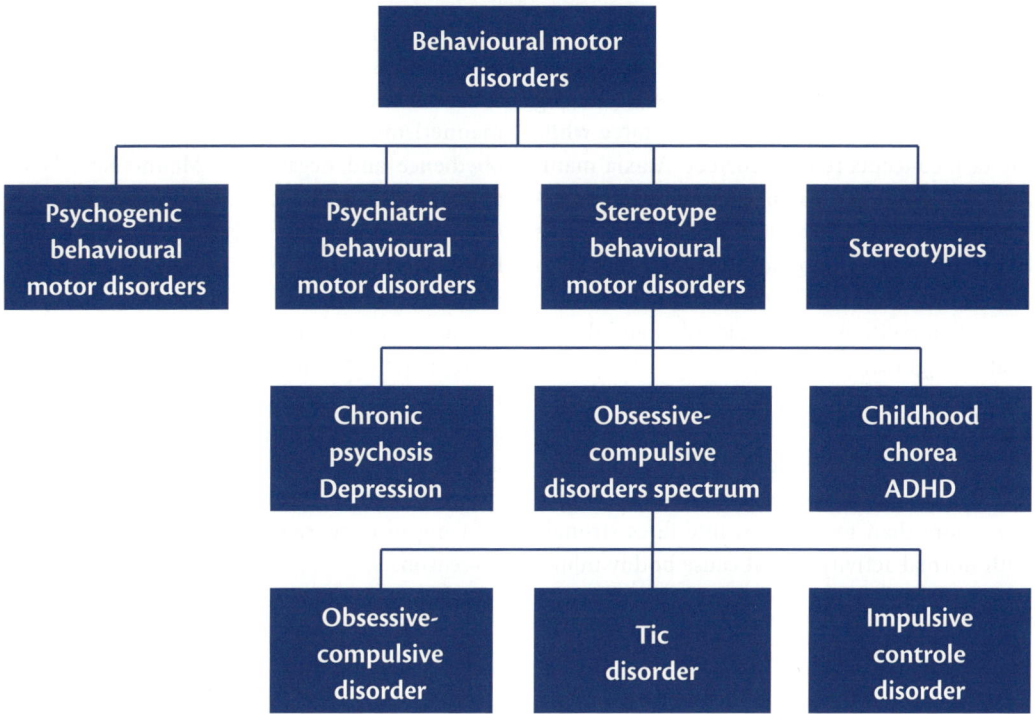

Figure 2
Phenomenology of behavioural motor disorders.

predominantly proximal movements. With time, the proximal ballistic movements may become less pronounced and the distal choreatic movements predominate. Ballism typically increases with action and is absent during sleep.

Myoclonus

Myoclonus is a sudden, brief, involuntary jerk of a muscle or a group of muscles, consistent in time and space, which might be caused by muscle contraction (positive myoclonus) or by interruptions of tonic muscle activity (negative myoclonus). These movements can be focal or multifocal, though they are mostly restricted to one area of the body (eye, hand, palate), sometimes persisting for some time (for instance in action myoclonus), making it difficult to distinguish them from tremor.

Tics

Tics are repetitive, not rhythmical, spasmodic or twitching, simple or complex movements, mainly occurring at irregular intervals and inconsistent in space. They primarily affect muscles (or groups of muscles) in the face and neck, though they may spread all over the body. They normally can be voluntarily suppressed; this suppression though only lasts a short time.

Dystonia

Dystonia is a neurological condition which produces sustained or intermittent muscle contractions, affecting one or more muscles (focal, segmental, or generalized), and causing abnormal, often repetitive (dystonic tremor) or persistent (dystonic posturing) movements.

Ataxia

Ataxia is a dysmetric motor behaviour caused by defect coordination of the muscles during movements in time, direction, and force while the task concepts remain correct. Ataxia manifests with impaired balance and lack of coordination due to problems of stance and gait (wide base, imbalance), limb movements, speech (cerebellar dysarthria) and eye movements (saccadic smooth pursuit, dysmetric saccades, and downbeat nystagmus).

Stereotypy

Stereotypy is a repetitive or ritualistic, non-functional movement, posture or utterance, which lasts more than four weeks, interferes strongly with normal activity, might cause bodily injury, and is not necessarily due to a medical condition or substance. Stereotypies, mostly the result of abnormal operant conditioning, include mannerisms, echopraxia, mitgehen, automatic obedience and negativism. Mannerisms (such as rocking, head banging, whistling, humming and/or grimacing or repeatingly running one's hand through one's hair) suggest social significance and include goal-directed activities, but are out of context or odd in appearance. Echopraxia is the imitation of another person's movements. Mitgehen is moving a limb in response to light pressure despite being told not to do so, automatic obedience is carrying out commands in a robot-like fashion, and negativism is refusing to cooperate with simple requests for no reason.

PART I

Basic Introduction

1

Physiology of Behaviour

Mark Hallett

To paraphrase the Wikipedia definition, *behaviour* is the range of actions made by organisms; it is the 'response of the organism to various stimuli or inputs, whether internal or external, conscious or subconscious, overt or covert, and voluntary or involuntary'. This is certainly a topic that should interest movement disorder specialists. There is another subspeciality field of neurology called behavioural neurology, which, however, deals mainly with cognitive function such as memory and language. Movement disorders seem wedged in between neuromuscular and behavioural neurology. The field of movement disorders began with a focus on disorders stemming from the basal ganglia, not muscle or cortex, but as the field has matured it has expanded on both ends, including added interest now in behaviour as we try to understand more aspects of our complex patients.

Basic principles

Movement generation

Movement occurs as a result of muscle contraction, and muscle is controlled by the alpha motoneurons in the spinal cord. Alpha motoneurons are influenced by both segmental and suprasegmental input, with the most important suprasegmental signals coming via the corticospinal and reticulospinal tracts. It is likely that the corticospinal tract conveys the most important information with the reticulospinal system generally playing a supportive role. The corticospinal tract originates most importantly from the primary motor cortex (M1), but has contributions from some premotor areas as well. Input to the corticospinal tract from sensory cortex may largely modulate sensory input. M1 itself receives input from cortical and subcortical structures. Subcortically, the two major systems are the basal ganglia and the cerebellum. Both derive much of their input from the cortex and send processed information back to the cortex via the thalamus. While these two systems have been thought to be largely separate, recent evidence shows clear connections between them (1). In general, the basal ganglia system supports features of movement concerning which movements to make and the magnitude of contraction while the cerebellar system supports features of movement dealing with the detailed timing and coordination of the different body parts (see also chapters 2 and 3) (2).

M1 also receives much cortico-cortical input coming from the entire cortical mantle (Fig. 1.1). In general terms, the posterior part of the brain is the sensory portion receiving visual, somatosensory and auditory information. This information is integrated in multisensory regions in the parietal lobe and is the source of external triggering of movement. The parietal to premotor pathways have been the object of intense study in recent decades, and highly specific connections have been identified to which specific functions can be attached (3). For example, the reach and grasp components of a reach-to-grasp movement have separate parietal premotor pathways (4). Again, in general, the front part of the

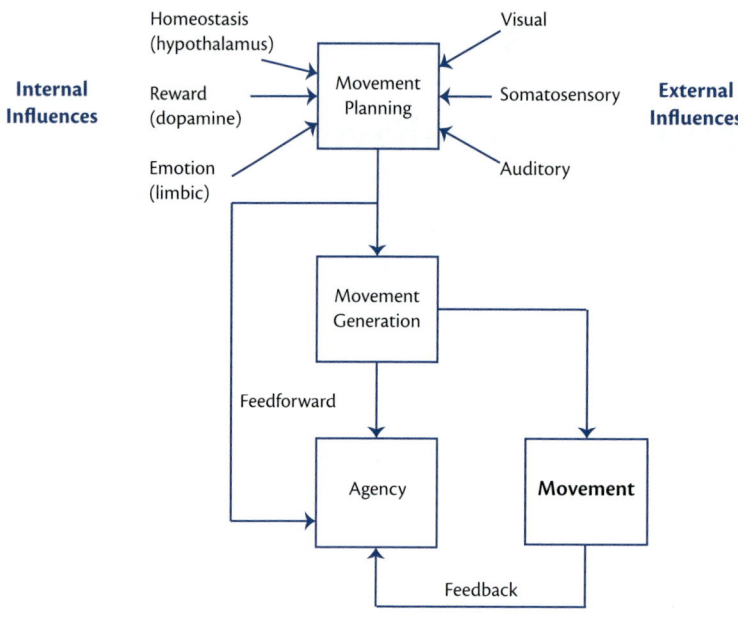

Figure 1.1
Scheme for the generation of behaviour. Movement is planned under internal and external influences and then generated. Feedforward signals indicate that a movement is being initiated and feedback signals detect that a movement has occurred. See more detail in the text.

In essence, behaviour is constantly influenced by all environmental (external) stimuli and multiple forces from frontal (internal) drives. The more information available about all these factors, the more behaviour can be probabilistically predicted. It is ordinarily a difficult calculation, which also is influenced by neural noise. However, in some circumstances individual factors are so strong, that prediction would be fairly certain. If someone is hungry and is presented with a pizza, it is very likely that he would eat it. If someone had immense pleasure from cocaine and was offered it again, he might take it again even though cognitively he knows that this will only make the situation worse in the long run.

brain receives and integrates information about the body and is considered the source of internal triggering. Internal input includes homeostatic drive from regions such as the hypothalamus and includes factors such as hunger and thirst. Other internal input is limbic and includes factors such as vigilance, fear, anxiety and sex. Another critical internal input is reward, seeking of pleasure, and this appears largely mediated by mesolimbic dopaminergic function. If a past behaviour produced reward, the brain wants to do it again. Facilitation of behaviour by repeated reward is called *operant conditioning*.

Both the external and internal inputs are integrated in mesial frontal areas such as the cingulate and pre-supplementary motor area as well as the premotor areas directly (5). Strong inputs come from the mesial frontal areas to the premotor and motor cortex. What the motor cortex will produce, as behaviour, at any one time, is the consequence of the integration of all these factors.

Consciousness and voluntariness

From all we know about the brain, it is constantly in action, and it appears that many different things are being processed simultaneously. For example, it was already pointed out that there are multiple external and internal inputs that are continuously coming. Additionally, many different thought processes can be going on simultaneously. If you are asked a question, such as someone's name and cannot immediately think of it, you can go on and think about something else, and, often, sooner or later, the name will 'pop into your head'. This is likely the product of ongoing searching. If given a difficult decision, you might say, 'I will think about it and let you know later.' Even if you do not devote considerable time thinking about it at a conscious level, you will be able to come to the decision. Much of all this brain activity is unconscious. Only one thing at a time, or rarely two things, will bubble up into consciousness. And the stream of consciousness does not always flow smoothly; the topic may change quickly and not always logically from one to the next. What is in consciousness must be in some way what is important at the time, and is a result of the process called attention. Attention can be bottom up or top down. A strong external stimulus will usually bottom up into consciousness regardless of what else is going on. However, if a soldier is paying top down attention to fighting with an enemy, he might not notice that he has been shot in the leg. The individual elements of consciousness are called *qualia*, and one quale, relevant for movement disorders and other reasons, is voluntariness (6). Much of the time, it would be fair to say that persons are not thinking about whether a movement is voluntary or not. Things happen. For most movement, people generally think that they are the 'agent' of the movement, that is, they willed the movement and it occurred. This is the sense of agency or, specifically, *self-agency*. Self-agency presumably requires both a sense of willing, a feedforward signal, and the sense that the willed movement occurred, a feedback signal. If willing precedes the specific action that was willed, then the quale of agency can be created (see Figure 1.1). The sense of agency utilizes a brain network with a prominent role for the temporoparietal junction (TPJ) (7). Presumably this feedforward-feedback process is happening all the time, but does not create a quale since it is so routine. However, if the process does not work correctly, for example, a movement occurs for which there is no feedforward signal, that might bubble up to consciousness as a surprise, generating the quale of an involuntary movement. Whether movements are voluntary or involuntary is often a concern to the patient and to the movement disorder neurologist.

Behavioural movement disorders

Many of the patients seen by movement disorder neurologists have some behavioural aspects and some are even 'primarily' behavioural. Several features are easier to explain than others, and some examples will be given here to illuminate general as well as specific issues. These disorders overlap to some extent to the '*disorders of volition*' (see Table 1.1) (6,8).

Table 1.1
Some disorders of volition.

Disorder	Clinical features
Tic	Movements are often considered voluntary, but the patients cannot not do them, and often say that they let the movements happen.
Psychogenic movement disorder	Movements look like normal movements and share much of the normal voluntary movement physiology, but the patients believe them to be involuntary.
Huntington's chorea	Early in the disease, patients believe that the movements are voluntary.
Anosognosia	Patients may believe that they have moved when they have not.
Alien hand	Unwanted movements/postures arise without the sense that they are willed.
Schizophrenia	In patients with passivity phenomena, the movements may look normal and even goal-directed, but the patient feels as if he is being externally controlled.

Behavioural abnormalities due to parietal-premotor disorders (apraxia and task-specific disorders)

There are many types of apraxia; the one most commonly recognized is *ideomotor apraxia* in which there appears to be the loss of a motor memory for a skilled movement (9). The patient seems to understand what movement is to be made, there is no responsible deficit of language, and the motor machinery is in good enough shape to make the movement, but the proper sequence of actions is not generated. Bedside testing is generally done with external movements, either asking someone to make a particular movement (such as 'show me how you would use a hammer') or to mimic the examiner making a novel movement. However, such patients often cannot make the complex movement even in the natural context and might be impaired in activities of daily living. Such an apraxia, for example, is characteristic in patients with corticobasal syndrome (see chapter 21).

Patients with focal hand dystonia commonly begin with a derangement of just a single task, such as only writing or only playing the piano. Other tasks are done normally. When attempting the task, the motor coordination falls apart and a dystonic spasm intervenes. This is referred to as *task specificity*. It is similar to ideomotor apraxia in that there is a failure of a learned motor program. There is good evidence that skilled movements are stored in the brain in the parietal area or, perhaps more accurately, in parietal-premotor networks, mainly in the left hemisphere, for both right or left hand movements (10). Basic observations as to how movements are learned in human studies show that activity in parietal-premotor pathways increases as movements are learned. As the movements are learned to the point of automaticity, the activity declines but the connectivity in the network becomes stronger (11). In praxis movements, such as handwriting (12), the activation of left-sided parietal-premotor pathways can be identified with both neuroimaging and EEG studies (see Figure 1.2). So, in apraxia there appears to be a general failure of the parietal-premotor pathway. Lesions of the parietal area are common causes of the disorder, but premotor lesions can also be responsible as well as 'pure disconnections' between the two areas. In writer's cramp, we identified that

Right side transitive movement	Left side transitive movement

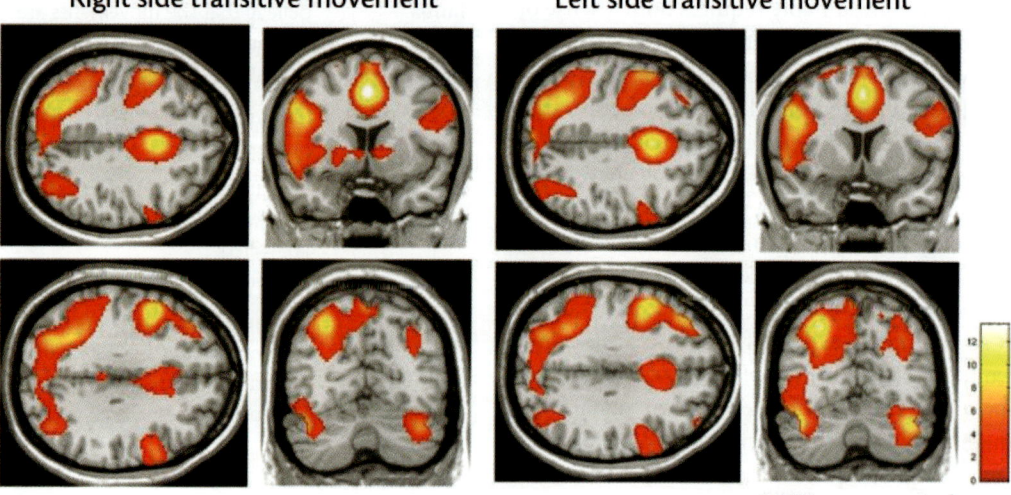

p < 0,001, uncorrected

Figure 1.2
fMRI from normal subjects making transitive movements (mimicked movements that employ a tool) with right and left hands. Axial and coronal sections are shown. There are prominent activations in parietal, premotor and supplementary motor cortex, more on the left side even with left sided movement. Modified from Bohlhalter et al.(10) with permission.

the specific writing parietal-premotor connection is hypoactive, but why this is accompanied by dystonic spasm is not understood.

Behavioural abnormalities due to paralimbic disorders (tics)

Tics are on the border between voluntary and involuntary movements. Most adults who have tics say, if pressed, that they are voluntary movements made to reduce an inner psychic tension or a sensory feeling. When the movement is made, the person feels temporarily better, but then the tension or sensation begins rising again. However, the movements are done so automatically that ordinarily there is no sense of willing or even that the tic occurred. Children with tics have a more difficult time explaining the nature of their movements, but will generally say that they are involuntary. When a movement leads to a good feeling, it can be considered rewarding, and it is possible that tics are perpetuated in part due to operant conditioning. Thus, a tic could be thought of as an undesirable habit (13).

The sensory feeling that provokes the tic is called a sensory tic, and little work has been done to understand it. Patients feel that they are particularly sensitive to sensory stimuli; they become very annoyed, for example, with tags on shirts. However, the psychophysics of their sensory perception, including thresholds, is normal, suggesting a possible failure of habituation (14). The urge to tic is similar to normal urges such as the urge to scratch an itch or the urge to blink when trying to keep the eyelids open. fMRI studies of the urge to blink show that the anterior insula is particularly active (15,16). Using an event-related design with fMRI, it has been demonstrated that the anterior insula and the anterior cingulate are active prior to tics (see Figure 1.3) (17). Additionally, comparing the resting brain activity while awake, with tics occurring, and asleep, when tics are rare, there is also increased activity of the anterior insula and cingulate (18). Hence, the urge to tic may well arise in these structures.

There is an EEG signature, called the *Bereitschaftspotential* or BP, that can be identified in the 1.5 sec or so prior to a voluntary movement (19,20). It is a slowly rising negativity that begins fairly symmetrically around the vertex, and as the movement approaches the negativity rises a bit faster and, at least for right-sided dominant

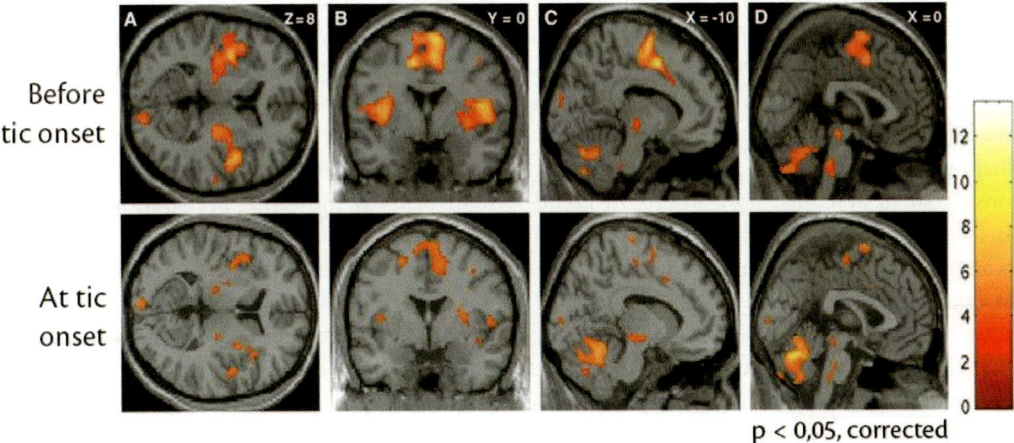

p < 0,05, corrected

Figure 1.3
fMRI of axial (A), coronal (B) and sagittal (C and D) views in event-related design of spontaneous tics. The upper row shows significant activations (P < 0.05, corrected for multiple comparisons) of paralimbic areas (anterior cingulate cortex and insular region bilaterally) before tic onset; these activations were much less prominent at tic onset (lower row). From Bohlhalter et al.(16) with permission.

hand movements, the potential peaks more over the left sensorimotor cortex. The early part of the potential, BP1, arises from the supplementary motor area (SMA) and the lateral premotor cortex, both parts of area 6. The later part of the potential, BP2, emphasizes more the premotor cortex and the primary motor cortex (M1). With tics, there is either no BP at all or just a BP2. This suggests that tics originate with only minimal involvement of area 6. Perhaps the anterior insula and anterior cingulate access the motor cortex directly.

Behavioural abnormalities due to the loss of 'self-agency' (psychogenic movement disorders)

Psychogenic movement disorders or functional movement disorders come in many varieties, both positive and negative. Virtually any organic movement disorder can be mimicked. The negative disorders of weakness and paralysis are common, but typically present to neurologists, for example, seeing strokes, neuromuscular disease or multiple sclerosis. At the other extreme, paroxysmal hyperkinetic psychogenic movements are often categorized as psychogenic non-epileptic seizures. The underlying aetiology for such disorders is complex and multifactorial, and requires considering a biopsychosocial model, including genetic factors, stress responsivity, childhood trauma, and the current social structure (21-23).

The psychiatric aetiology is most commonly considered to be conversion, where, in Freudian terms, a psychological symptom is converted to a somatic symptom. This is an unconscious process and the movement is not voluntary. Alternate etiologies are factitious and malingering, where the movement is voluntary but the patient says that they are involuntary. At present, we have no clinical or laboratory way of separating these entities, except by secret surveillance. For the rest of this discussion, the aetiology will be assumed to be conversion.

Psychogenic movements appear to utilize brain mechanisms very close to those used by ordinarily voluntary movements (24). In psychogenic paralysis, transcranial magnetic stimulation (TMS) of the motor cortex produces normal motor evoked potentials (MEPs), indicating a normal motor cortex and pathway all the way to the muscle. The MEPs when imagining movement of a body part should enhance, but in psychogenic paralysis, the MEPs are reduced, suggesting an inhibitory influence on M1. fMRI of psychogenic paralysis when apparently trying to move the paretic limb shows activity changes in frontal lobe areas. Perhaps, the inhibition comes from the frontal lobe.

In psychogenic tremor, one important observation is the tremor can be *entrained* by voluntary rhythmic movement of another body part. This suggests that the psychogenic tremor generator is likely shared with the voluntary generator. Similarly, psychogenic tremor is typically synchronous in different limbs, different from organic tremors such as seen in Parkinson's disease (PD) and essential tremor.

Psychogenic myoclonus has an EMG pattern similar to quick voluntary movements in terms of EMG burst length and antagonist muscle relationships. When stimulus-induced, it behaves like a normal reaction time movement in terms of mean latency and variability of latency, unlike organic myoclonus where the latency is very short with little variability. Importantly, there is often a typical BP preceding the psychogenic myoclonus, indicating preparation for movement in area 6 (see Figure 1.4).

While the origin of psychogenic movements is obscure, there is fMRI evidence in several circumstances of a hyperactive limbic system. The passive response of the right amygdala is increased to emotional faces, and several structures in the limbic system are hyperactive even with voluntary movements (25,26). Another relevant fMRI observation is that the right temporoparietal junction (TPJ) is hypoactive with psychogenic tremor compared to voluntarily

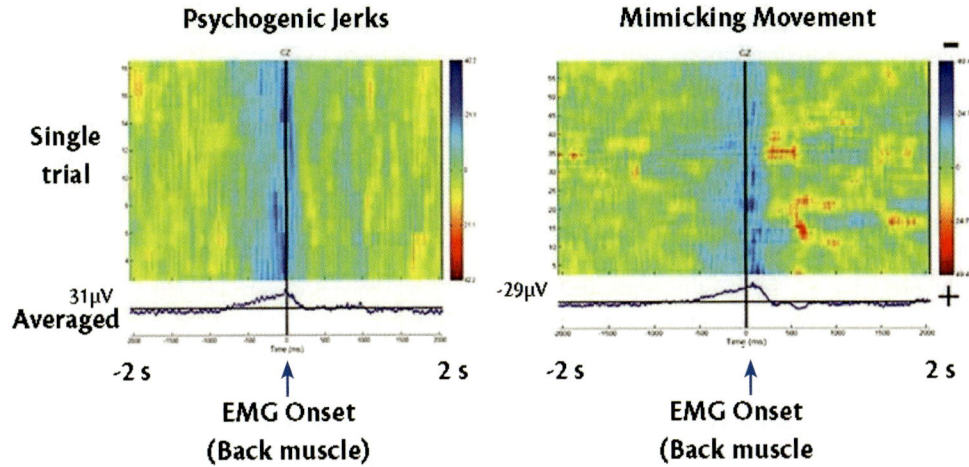

Figure 1.4
EEGs associated with psychogenic jerks of trunk and self-initiated movements mimicking the jerks, arranged time-locked to the EMG discharge. Fifty traces of individual EEG records are shown on the top panel (Single trial) and averaged waveforms are shown on the bottom (Averaged). In single trials, blue and red colors indicate surface-negative and surface-positive, respectively. Note slowly rising surface-negative potential preceding both the psychogenic jerks and the mimicking jerks. Data recorded by Dr. Zoltan Mari in the Human Motor Control Section, NINDS. From Shibasaki 2012 (19) with permission.

mimicked tremor (27). As noted, earlier, the TPJ is implicated in the sense of agency, and therefore, this hypoactivity might explain the loss of self-agency for the movements. It can be speculated that the lack of the normal feedforward signal from the aberrant movement intention may explain the abnormal TPJ activity.

If stress is one of the responsible factors in psychogenic movements, abnormal signals from the limbic system can well be understood as the prime mover. A further question that typically arises is why different persons have different types of movement disorders. One possible explanation for this is that the brain often mimics what it knows. If a person knows someone with a stroke, he might have paralysis. If another person has a relative with PD, she might have a tremor. Some subjects even mimic themselves. This is most common with psychogenic non-epileptic seizures, where many of these patients also have organic seizures. Mimicry is a major function of the brain which aids in the process of motor learning and which also may be responsible for

empathy (28). I feel your pain. The mirror neurons, those motor neurons that show responses when seeing specific movements, as well as when making those same movements, may be the underlying substrate for the mimicry (29).

Behavioural abnormalities due to reduced internal triggering (akinesia, hypokinesia, bradykinesia)

Slowness of movement, or bradykinesia, is one of the major features of PD. In general terms, the explanation fits well into the scheme of behaviour put forward here. The basal ganglia support mainly the front half of the brain, and it is the front half where internal triggering of movement is generated. Hence, patients find it difficult to initiate movement (akinesia), and end up making slow (bradykinetic) and small (hypokinetic) movements. Patients have to compensate for this difficulty by paying more attention to movements requiring more cortical resources. Externally triggered movements are much better since these appear to require less basal ganglia support. External triggering underlies the phenomenon of paradoxical kinesia (30).

Another feature of the slowness in PD is the *sequence effect*, where repetitive movements get gradually slower or smaller. The sequence effect is easily seen with handwriting which gradually becomes more micrographic through the sentence. Additionally, the sequence effect commonly precedes a gait-freezing episode. This feature may be specific to PD; at least, it is not seen in progressive supranuclear palsy (31). The pathophysiol--89ogy of this behaviour is not known. It is not responsive to dopamine (32) and hence can be a significant clinical problem even when the PD is generally responsive to oral therapy.

Behavioural abnormalities due to abnormal operant conditioning (impulse control disorders)

PD patients may show a variety of abnormal behaviours, which will be discussed in chapter 39 in this book. Such behaviours include pathological gambling, pathological shopping and punding (33). These are all repetitive activities, which, similar to other forms of addiction, the patient continues to do even though recognizing that it might not be the best thing to do. These behaviours are related to abnormal dopamine functioning and operant conditioning creating undesirable habits.

This work was supported by the NINDS Intramural Research Program.

References

1 Bostan AC, Dum RP, Strick PL. The basal ganglia communicate with the cerebellum. Proc Natl Acad Sci U S A. 2010;107:8452-8456.

2 Fahn S, Jankovic J, Hallett M. Principles and Practice of Movement Disorders. Second ed. Philadelphia: Elsevier Saunders; 2011.

3 Rizzolatti G, Luppino G, Matelli M. The organization of the cortical motor system: new concepts. Electroencephalogr Clin Neurophysiol. 1998;106:283-96.

4 Cavina-Pratesi C, Monaco S, Fattori P, et al. Functional magnetic resonance imaging reveals the neural substrates of arm transport and grip formation in reach-to-grasp actions in humans. J Neurosci. 2010;30:10306-10323.

5 Paus T. Primate anterior cingulate cortex: where motor control, drive and cognition interface. Nat Rev Neurosci. 2001;2:417-424.

6 Hallett M. Volitional control of movement: The physiology of free will. Clin Neurophysiol. 2007;118:1179-1192.

7 Nahab FB, Kundu P, Gallea C, et al. The neural processes underlying self-agency. Cereb Cortex. 2011;21:48-55.

8 Kranick SM, Hallett M. Neurology of Volition. Exp Brain Res. 2013;(in press).

9 Wheaton LA, Hallett M. Ideomotor apraxia: A review. J Neurol Sci. 2007;26:1-10.

10 Bohlhalter S, Hattori N, Wheaton L, et al. Gesture subtype-dependent left lateralization of praxis planning: an event-related fMRI study. Cereb Cortex. 2009;19:1256-1262.

11 Wu T, Chan P, Hallett M. Modifications of the interactions in the motor networks when a movement becomes automatic. J Physiol. 2008;586:4295-4304.

12 Horovitz SG, Gallea C, Najee-Ullah MA, Hallett M. Functional anatomy of writing with the dominant hand. PLoS One 2013;8(7):e67931.

13 Graybiel AM. Habits, rituals, and the evaluative brain. Annu Rev Neurosci. 2008;31:359-387.

14 Belluscio BA, Jin L, Watters V, Lee TH, Hallett M. Sensory sensitivity to external stimuli in Tourette syndrome patients. Mov Disord. 2011;26:2538-2543.

15 Berman BD, Horovitz SG, Morel B, Hallett M. Neural correlates of blink suppression and the buildup of a natural bodily urge. Neuroimage. 2012;59:1441-1450.

16 Lerner A, Bagic A, Hanakawa T, et al. Involvement of insula and cingulate cortices in control and suppression of natural urges. Cereb Cortex. 2009;19:218-223.

17 Bohlhalter S, Goldfine A, Matteson S, et al. Neural correlates of tic generation in Tourette syndrome:

an event-related functional MRI study. Brain. 2006;129:2029-2037.

18 Lerner A, Bagic A, Boudreau EA, et al. Neuroimaging of neuronal circuits involved in tic generation in patients with Tourette syndrome. Neurology. 2007;68:1979-1987.

19 Shibasaki H, Hallett M. What is the Bereitschaftspotential? Clin Neurophysiol. 2006;117:2341-2356.

20 Shibasaki H. Cortical activities associated with voluntary movements and involuntary movements. Clin Neurophysiol. 2012;123:229-243.

21 Czarnecki K, Hallett M. Functional (psychogenic) movement disorders. Curr Opin Neurol. 2012;25:507-512.

22 Kranick SM, Gorrindo T, Hallett M. Psychogenic movement disorders and motor conversion: a roadmap for collaboration between neurology and psychiatry. Psychosomatics. 2011;52:109-116.

23 Hallett M, Lang AE, Jankovic J, et al., eds. Psychogenic Movement Disorders and Other Conversion Disorders. Cambridge: Cambridge University Press; 2011.

24 Hallett M. Physiology of psychogenic movement disorders. J Clin Neurosci. 2010;17:959-965.

25 Voon V, Brezing C, Gallea C, et al. Emotional stimuli and motor conversion disorder. Brain. 2010;133:1526-1536.

26 Voon V, Brezing C, Gallea C, Hallett M. Aberrant supplementary motor complex and limbic activity during motor preparation in motor conversion disorder. Mov Disord. 2011;26:2396-2403.

27 Voon V, Gallea C, Hattori N, Bruno M, Ekanayake V, Hallett M. The involuntary nature of conversion disorder. Neurology. 2010;74:223-228.

28 Baird AD, Scheffer IE, Wilson SJ. Mirror neuron system involvement in empathy: a critical look at the evidence. Social neuroscience. 2011;6:327-35.

29 Rizzolatti G, Sinigaglia C. The functional role of the parieto-frontal mirror circuit: interpretations and misinterpretations. Nat Rev Neurosci. 2010;11:264-74.

30 Hallett M. Bradykinesia: why do Parkinson's patients have it and what trouble does it cause? Mov Disord. 2011;26:1579-1581.

31 Ling H, Massey LA, Lees AJ, Brown P, Day BL. Hypokinesia without decrement distinguishes progressive supranuclear palsy from Parkinson's disease. Brain. 2012;135:1141-1153.

32 Kang SY, Wasaka T, Shamim EA, et al. Characteristics of the sequence effect in Parkinson's disease. Mov Disord. 2010;25:2148-55.

33 Voon V, Mehta AR, Hallett M. Impulse control disorders in Parkinson's disease: recent advances. Curr Opin Neurol. 2011;24:324-30.

2

Basal Ganglia

Henk J. Groenewegen

The basal ganglia consist of a number of large nuclei in the forebrain and midbrain that are extensively connected to different parts of the cerebral cortex, various thalamic nuclei and specific mesencephalic structures. They receive information from virtually all parts of the cerebral cortex and project via partially closed loops back to the prefrontal and premotor cortices. With the expansion of the neocortex in the course of evolution, the basal ganglia have become increasingly involved in processing highly associated cortical information in order to contribute to the complex process of planning and selecting movements and behaviour. Via the midline and intralaminar thalamus, a phylogenetically older system of projections ascending from brainstem structures like the superior colliculus and pedunculopontine nucleus provides the basal ganglia with relatively unprocessed signals containing external (visual, auditory, somatosensory, etc.) and internal (viscerosensory, homeostatic, etc.) information. The output of the basal ganglia likewise has dual characteristics. An 'ascending' component, which in humans is the most extensive by far, consists of basal ganglia projections, via medial and ventral thalamic nuclei, to the premotor and prefrontal cortical areas in the frontal lobe, thus closing the so-called basal ganglia-thalamocortical circuits. This arrangement in cortical-subcortical loops forms the neuronal basis for the influence of the basal ganglia on sensorimotor, cognitive and executive behavioural and emotional-motivational functions. A 'descending' component consists of basal ganglia projections directed to mesence-

phalic structures that, in turn, give rise to fibers that descend further to motor output structures in the lower brainstem and spinal cord, as well as to fibers that ascend to forebrain structures. These projections form the neuronal basis for the influence of the basal ganglia on posture and balance as well as on muscle tone.

The basal ganglia have long been associated almost exclusively with sensorimotor functions, and in line with that concept, dysfunctions of these structures were related primarily to neurological diseases, in particular movement disorders. However, it is now generally accepted that the basal ganglia also play an important role in cognitive and affective behavioural functions. Thus, basal ganglia dysfunctions appear to be associated also with a number of neuropsychiatric disorders. This chapter summarizes the functional-anatomical organization of the connections of the basal ganglia with the thalamo-cortical systems and brainstem. From this overview, it will indeed be clear that this connectional organization forms the neural basis for such a wide array of functions in which the basal ganglia are involved, ranging from pure sensorimotor to cognitive-executive and emotional-motivational behaviours. Across this broad array of motor and behavioural functions, the mechanism by which the basal ganglia contribute to these functions is through 'response selection'. Such a mechanism fits well with the arrangement of the intrinsic connections between the individual basal ganglia nuclei, supporting the selection of appropriate responses in a particular context and, at the same time, the suppression of inadequate responses. A variety of symptoms as part of neurological movement disorders, such as Parkinson's disease, Huntington's disease and dystonia, or neuropsychiatric diseases like obsessive-compulsive disorder, mood disorders and drug addiction, might be interpreted as an inadequate selection of motor, cognitive or affective responses to internal or external stimuli. The present chapter starts with an overview of the architecture of the basal ganglia, followed by a survey of their extrinsic and intrinsic connections. Subsequently, some of the functions and dysfunctions of the basal ganglia will be briefly discussed in the light of their structure and connections.

Components of the basal ganglia

The basal ganglia are a group of strongly interconnected and functionally related nuclei located in the forebrain and midbrain (see Figure 2.1). Four main nuclei comprise the basal ganglia: striatum, pallidum, subthalamic nucleus and substantia nigra. Macroscopically, most of these nuclei consist of a number of large subnuclei (1). Thus, the striatum encompasses the caudate nucleus, putamen and nucleus accumbens; the pallidum is composed of the external and internal segments of the globus pallidus and the ventral pallidum; the substantia nigra consists of a pars reticulata and a pars compacta (the latter containing the dopaminergic neurons). The cytoarchitectonic, chemoarchitectonic and connectional characteristics, as well as some specific topological relationships, all provide the basis for the various ways of 'clustering' these macroscopically recognizable nuclei into the larger functional-anatomical units mentioned above.

Striatum

The striatum is the largest nuclear mass of the basal ganglia. In the human brain the internal capsule divides the striatum into the caudate nucleus and the putamen, located medially and laterally to this fiber bundle, respectively (1).

The caudate nucleus forms the lateral wall of the lateral ventricle and is largest in the frontal lobe where the head of the caudate (caput nucleus caudati) is located (see Figure 2.1A). The caudal extension of the caudate nucleus, becoming increasingly smaller in size in the caudal direction, follows the caudal and subsequently rostrolateral curve of the lateral ventricle into the temporal lobe. The most caudal end of the tail of the caudate nucleus terminates at the level of the caudal amygdala and merges with the central amygdaloid nucleus (1). The putamen is an oval-shaped nucleus located just underneath (is medial to) the insular cortex, separated from this cortical area by the claustrum (see Figure 2.1B-D). Rostrally, the caudate nucleus and putamen form extensive cell bridges since the anterior limb of the internal capsule is merely composed of a number of smaller and larger fascicles (see Figure 2.1A). The posterior limb of the internal capsule forms a more compact mass of white matter, but small cell bridges exist between the caudate nucleus and putamen in these caudal regions also (see Figure 2.1D). At rostral levels, both the caudate nucleus and putamen merge with the more ventrally located nucleus accumbens (see Figure 2.1A). This nucleus is situated deep to the caudal parts of the orbitofrontal cortex and comes close to the surface of the brain at the caudal level of the olfactory trigonum. At its caudal limits the nucleus accumbens abuts the bed nucleus of the stria terminalis and the septal nuclei (2,3).

Pallidum

The pallidum consists of three subnuclei, i.e., the external and internal segments of the globus pallidus and the ventral pallidum (see Figure 2.1C, D). The globus pallidus is located lateral to the internal capsule and medial to the putamen. Both segments of the globus pallidus together with the putamen form the so-called lentiform nucleus (see Figure 2.1C, D). As a result of an increasingly higher concentration of myelinated fibers, the external pallidal segment appears paler than the putamen, and in turn, the inter-

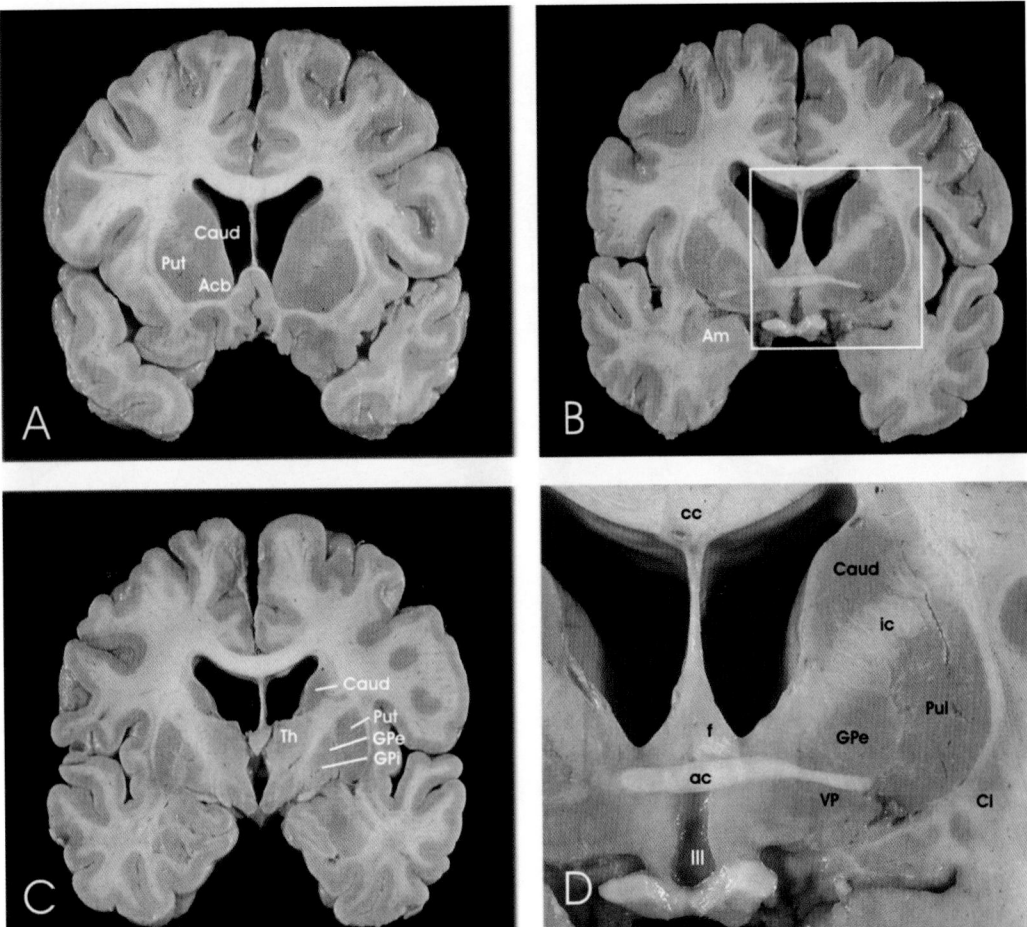

Figure 2.1
Three transverse (frontal) sections through the human forebrain showing different parts of the basal ganglia: A. rostral, C. caudal. D shows a higher magnification of the basal ganglia at the level of the crossing of the anterior commissure (boxed area In B).
Abbreviations: ac, anterior commissure; Acb, nucleus accumbens; Am, amygdala; Caud, caudate nucleus; cc, corpus callosum; Cl, claustrum; f, fornix; GPe, external segment of the globus pallidus; GPi, internal segment of the globus pallidus; ic, internal capsule; Put, putamen; Th, thalamus; VP, ventral pallidum.

nal pallidal segment is paler than the external segment. The ventral pallidum is located underneath the posterior limb of the anterior commissure in an area of the basal forebrain that has long been labelled the substantia innominata (see Figure 2.1D). Following the seminal work of Heimer and colleagues (2-4) the substantia innominata is now known to harbor three main functional-anatomical units: 1. the ventral pallidum; 2. the nucleus basalis of Meijnert that contains the basal forebrain cholinergic neurons projecting to the cerebral cortex; 3. part of the so-called 'extended amygdala', a rostral extension of the central and medial amygdaloid nuclei that rostrally merges with the bed nucleus of the stria terminalis. Macroscopically, the ventral pallidum appears as a ventral extension of the external pallidal segment. However, ventral and medial parts of this nucleus have also internal pallidal characteristics (see below).

Subthalamic nucleus

The subthalamic nucleus is a relatively small, oval-shaped nucleus located at the junction of the diencephalon and mesencephalon (see Figure 2.2A, C). It is located ventral to the thalamus, just underneath the zona incerta and the fields of Forel that contain the fibers from the pallidum to the thalamus (1). The caudomedial half of the subthalamic nucleus abuts the rostro-lateral part of the pars compacta of the substantia nigra.

Substantia nigra

The substantia nigra, located in the rostroventral part of the mesencephalon, dorsal to the cerebral peduncle, consists of a pars reticulata and a pars

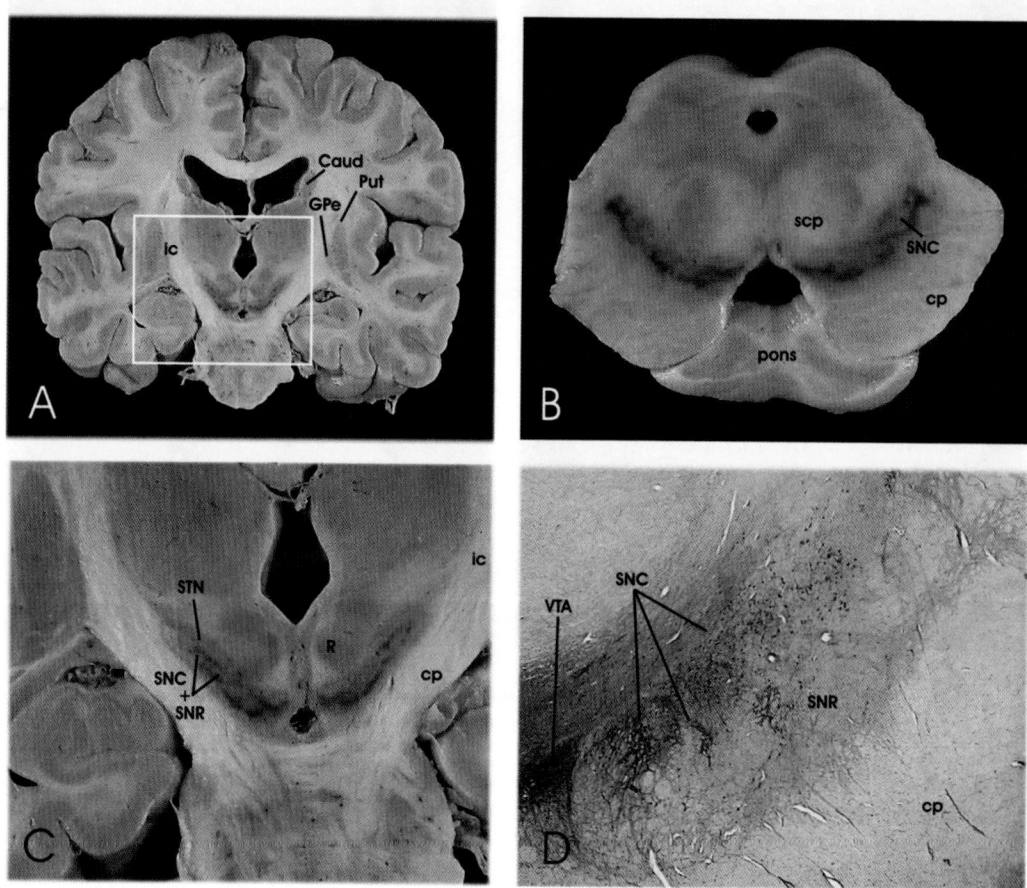

Figure 2.2

A, C. Transverse (frontal) section through the forebrain and brainstem at a level caudal to figure 2.1C. The boxed area in A is shown at higher magnification in C. Note the close topographical relationship between the subthalamic nucleus (STN) and the substantia nigra (SNC + SNR). B. Transverse section through the mesencephalon in which the substantia nigra, pars compacta (SNC) is clearly visible. D. Microscopy section through the ventral part of the mesencephalon, immunohistochemically stained with an antibody against tyrosine hydroxylase (synthesizing enzyme for dopamine). The dark, tyrosine hydroxylase-positive cell bodies form the pars compacta of the substantia nigra (SNC) and the ventral tegmental area (VTA). Note the clustering of tyrosine hydroxylase-positive neurons, in part embedded in the pars reticulata of the substantia nigra (SNR).

Abbreviations: Caud, caudate nucleus; cp, cerebral peduncle; GPe, external segment of the globus pallidus; GPi, internal segment of the globus pallidus; Put, putamen; R, red nucleus; scp, superior cerebellar peduncle; SNC, substantia nigra, pars compacta; SNR, substantia nigra, pars reticulata; STN, subthalamic nucleus; VTA, ventral tegmental area.

compacta (see Figure 2.2A-C). As will be discussed below, the reticular part of the substantia nigra has many characteristics in common with the internal segment of the globus pallidus. The pars compacta consists of densely packed neurons that produce the neurotransmitter dopamine (A9 cell group) and, in the course of life, accumulate the pigment neuromelanin as a metabolite in the metabolic degradation of dopamine. Although in general terms the pars compacta is situated dorsal to the pars reticulata, in the human brain both parts of the substantia nigra are intensely intermingled with numerous clusters of dopaminergic neurons embedded in the reticular part (see Figure 2.2D) (1). Medial to the substantia nigra the ventral tegmental area (VTA) is located, which also contains dopaminergic neurons (A10 cell group) and is connectionally related to ventral parts of the basal ganglia (see Figure 2.2D). In a wide area of the rostral mesencephalon, situated dorsolateral to the substantia nigra, dopaminergic neurons (A8 cell group) are more diffusely located (1). These neurons also have close connectional relationships with other structures of the basal ganglia.

Architecture and fiber connections of the basal ganglia

Considering the basal ganglia as a functional-anatomical entity, this complex as a whole receives 'external' information from virtually all parts of the cerebral cortex, the midline and intralaminar thalamic nuclei, and limbic structures like the amygdala and hippocampus. In addition, serotonergic inputs from the raphe nuclei and cholinergic fibers from the pedunculopontine nucleus reach parts of the basal ganglia (see Figure 2.3) (1). Most of these inputs 'enter' the basal ganglia at the level of the striatum where specific, topographically organized inputs from the cerebral cortex, thalamus and limbic structures strongly converge and are modulated by the dopaminergic and serotonergic systems. Therefore, the striatum may be considered the

main 'input structure' of the basal ganglia (5-8). However, frontal cortical, intralaminar thalamic and brainstem inputs also target the subthalamic nucleus as well as to a lesser degree the pallidum and the substantia nigra. In view of its position in the circuitry of the basal ganglia (see below), the subthalamic nucleus may thus also be considered as an input structure of the basal ganglia (8,9).

The basal ganglia primarily influence the premotor and prefrontal cortices of the frontal lobe, via particular thalamic nuclei. In addition, there are descending projections to the superior colliculus and pedunculopontine nucleus in the mesencephalon. The output from the basal ganglia primarily originates from the internal segment of the globus pallidus, the ventral pallidum and the pars reticulata of the substantia nigra (5-8). These nuclei together may be considered the main 'output structures' of the basal ganglia (see Figure 2.3).

The input and output structures of the basal ganglia are strongly interconnected via different *intrinsic connections* within this nuclear complex (8). As will be discussed below, the intrinsic basal ganglia connections consist of direct connections between the input and output structures of the basal ganglia, as well as an indirect network of connections that modulates the direct pathway (10). An important role in the indirect intrinsic basal ganglia pathways or network is played by the external segment of the globus pallidus and the subthalamic nucleus (8,10,11). Furthermore, dopamine fibers stemming from the substantia nigra pars compacta and the VTA modulate the information transfer via the direct and indirect pathways, primarily at the level of the striatum (8).

Striatum

Cellular composition
Cytoarchitectonically, the striatum appears as a rather homogeneous structure, consisting of two main classes of neurons, i.e. medium-sized,

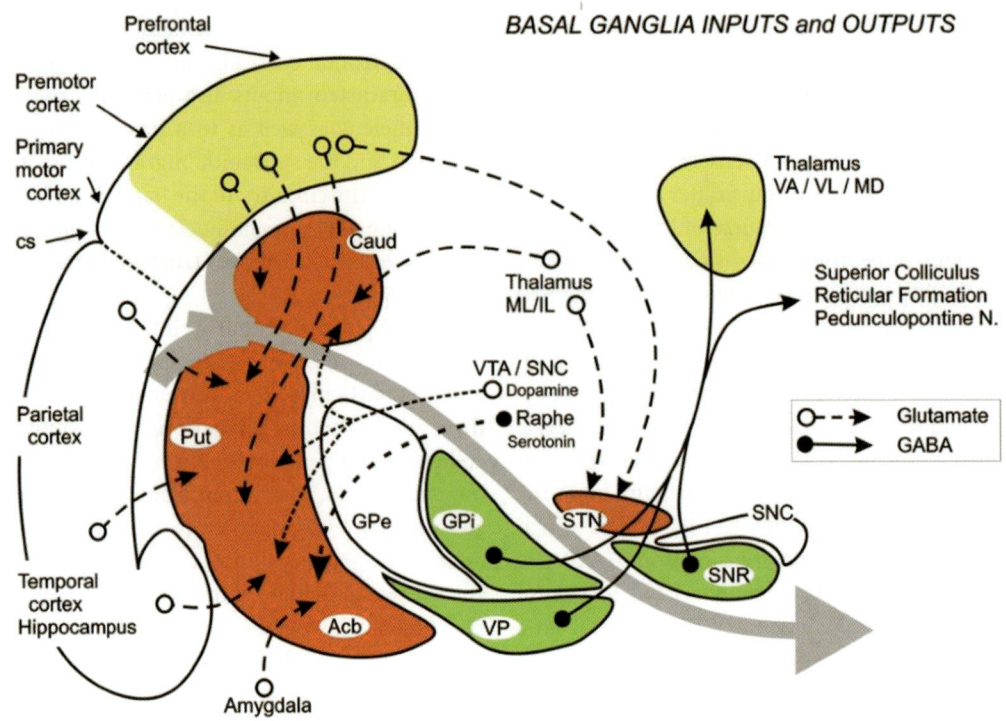

BASAL GANGLIA INPUTS and OUTPUTS

Figure 2.3
Schematic, semi-sagittal representation of the cerebral cortex, the different nuclei of the basal ganglia and the thalamus, illustrating the most important afferent and efferent connections of the basal ganglia. The inputs of the basal ganglia are primarily directed at the striatum and the subthalamic nucleus (basal ganglia input structures). The outputs of the basal ganglia stem from the internal segment of the globus pallidus, the substantia nigra pars reticulata and the ventral pallidum (basal ganglia output structures).
Abbreviations: Acb, nucleus accumbens; Caud, caudate nucleus; GPe, external segment of the globus pallidus; GPi, internal segment of the globus pallidus; MD, mediodorsal thalamic nucleus; ML, midline thalamic nuclei; IL, intralaminar thalamic nuclei; Put, putamen; cs, central sulcus; SNC, substantia nigra, pars compacta; SNR, substantia nigra, pars reticulata; STN, subthalamic nucleus; VA, ventral anterior thalamic nucleus; VL, ventral lateral thalamic nucleus; VTA, ventral tegmental area; VP, ventral pallidum.

densely spiny projection neurons and a heterogeneous group of interneurons (8, 12). The medium-sized spiny projection neurons make up approximately 95-97% of the total population, while the neurochemically and morphologically heterogeneous group of interneurons represents the remaining 3-5% of the neurons (8). The medium-sized spiny projection neurons primarily collect the specific information from the cerebral cortex, thalamus and limbic structures, the heads of their dendritic spines being the main target of such inputs (see Figure 2.4). Dopaminergic terminals tend to terminate on the necks of the spines and are thus in a position to modulate or 'gate' the transfer of information from the spine head to the shaft of the dendrite (13). Cholinergic and GABAergic terminals from striatal interneurons and neighboring medium-sized spiny projection neurons terminate on the shafts of the dendrites (14) (see Figure 2.4). Medium-sized spiny neurons thus integrate the inputs from the various striatal afferents and the intrinsic striatal neurons, and they formulate the striatal output. Several types of striatal interneurons exist: cholinergic interneurons and different GABAergic interneurons including the

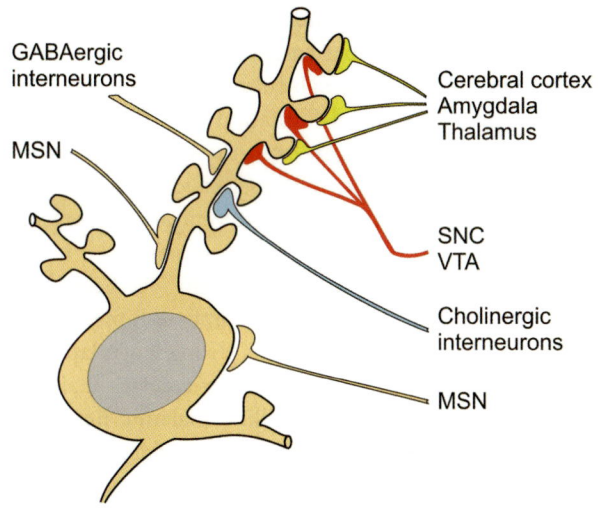

GABAergic
interneurons

MSN

Cerebral cortex
Amygdala
Thalamus

SNC
VTA

Cholinergic
interneurons

MSN

Figure 2.4
Schematic representation of the position of the terminals of different inputs on the dendrites of a medium-sized, densely spiny neuron (MSN) in the striatum. Excitatory inputs from the cerebral cortex, amygdala and thalamus terminate preferentially on the heads of the spines; thalamic inputs have also been described on the shaft of the dendrites. Dopaminergic fibers terminate, in close association with the excitatory terminals, on the necks of the spines or on the shaft of the dendrites. The terminals of GABAergic and cholinergic striatal interneurons, as well as the inhibitory GABAergic terminals of the recurrent collaterals of other medium-sized spiny projection neurons, are positioned on the more proximal parts of the dendrites and also on the cell body.
Abbreviations: SNC, substantia nigra, pars compacta; VTA, ventral tegmental area.

larger, aspiny, fast-spiking neurons that co-express the calcium-binding peptide parvalbumin (10,15). The cholinergic interneurons have been physiologically identified as tonically active neurons, so-called TANs, whose firing is strongly related to the behavioural- or reward-related significance of external stimuli. The electrophysiological activity of dopamine neurons is likewise related to the salience of external stimuli, and the two systems appear to interact strongly at the level of the striatum to govern behavioural responses via the medium-sized spiny projection neurons (15).

The electrophysiological properties of medium-sized spiny projection neurons can be characterized by two states: a down-state with a low resting membrane potential (-80/-90 mV) and an up-state with a membrane potential close to the firing threshold (-55 mV). In the down-state the medium-sized spiny neurons are 'silent'. On the basis of coincident excitatory afferent activity converging on the neurons, for example from different cortical, limbic and thalamic sources, they may be brought to the up-state and be more easily elicited to fire (16). On the basis of their intrinsic electrophysiological properties and the specific arrangement of afferent fibers on their dendrites, the medium-sized spiny projection

neurons may be characterized as 'coincidence detectors' (17).

Organization of afferent striatal connections
Excitatory inputs reach the striatum from all parts of the cerebral cortex (with the exception of the primary visual and auditory areas), the basolateral amygdaloid complex, the midline and intralaminar nuclei of the thalamus and the hippocampus (1,6-8). The topographical and partly somatotopic arrangement of the cortical projections forms the basis for a functional subdivision of the striatum (Figure 2.5). The thalamic and dopaminergic projections to the striatum are also topographically organized. The dorsolateral region of the striatum, including parts (large) of the putamen and parts (smaller) of the caudate nucleus receive fibers from the motor, premotor and somatosensory cortical areas. Therefore, this part of the striatum is considered the sensorimotor striatal area (see Figure 2.5). This sensorimotor striatal area is projected upon by the caudal intralaminar nuclei and the centromedian/parafascicular complex, nuclei of the thalamus that issue fibers also to the sensory and motor cortices (6-8). Dopaminergic fibers to this area of the striatum originate in lateral parts of the substantia nigra pars compacta (18).

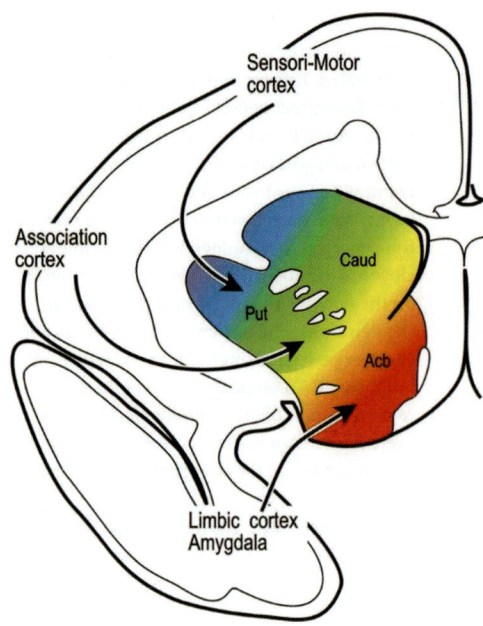

Figure 2.5
Schematic representation of the topographical organization of the projections from functionally different cortical areas to the striatum. Note that the functional division of the striatum, related to the corticostriatal topography, does not follow the boundaries between caudate nucleus and putamen: there is a dorsolateral to ventromedial gradient rather than a mediolateral subdivision.
Abbreviations: Acb, nucleus accumbens; Caud, caudate nucleus; Put, putamen.

The central region of the striatum, including a ventromedial part of the putamen as well as the largest part of the head of the caudate nucleus, receives cortical inputs from associative cortical areas in the frontal (dorsolateral prefrontal and orbitofrontal cortices), parietal and temporal lobes. This part of the striatum can be characterized as the associative or cognitive striatal area (6-8). It receives thalamic inputs from the rostral nuclei of the intralaminar thalamic complex and dopaminergic inputs from the intermediate mediolateral parts of the pars compacta of the substantia nigra (18). Sparse inputs come from the anterior parts of the basolateral amygdaloid complex.

Finally, the ventral parts of the striatum, prominently including the nucleus accumbens, receive input from the medial prefrontal cortex, the parahippocampal cortex in the medial temporal lobe and the subiculum and CA1 region of the hippocampal formation (19). Furthermore, strong inputs stem from the basolateral amygdaloid complex, the most caudal parts of this complex projecting most ventrally and medially in the ventral striatum, in particular to the shell of the nucleus accumbens (see below). In the shell of the nucleus accumbens hippocampal and amygdaloid afferents strongly overlap (19). The ventral striatum further receives thalamic afferents from the midline thalamic nuclei, in particular the paraventricular thalamic nucleus, and dopaminergic inputs from the medial part of the pars compacta of the substantia nigra and the medially adjacent VTA, i.e., the mesolimbic dopamine system (18). Only the caudomedial part of the shell of the nucleus accumbens is the recipient of noradrenergic fibers (20). On the basis of functional characteristics of its afferent fibers, the ventral striatum is considered the 'limbic' or emotional-motivational part of the striatum (see Figure 2.5).

It is of interest to note that the three functionally distinct sectors of the striatum described above receive their arterial blood supply largely from three different, main striatal arteries. The sensorimotor sector is vascularized by the lateral lenticulostriate artery, the associative sector by the medial lenticulostriate artery, and the limbic sector by the recurrent artery of Heubner (21).

Organization of efferent striatal connections
The pallidum and the substantia nigra are the main recipients of striatal efferents. Two levels of organization can be recognized in the striatofugal pathways. First, a topographical organization with the sensorimotor part of the striatum projecting primarily to the dorsolateral parts of the internal and external segments of the globus pallidus and to the ventrolateral parts of the substantia nigra pars reticulata. The associative striatal area sends fibers to more medial parts of both segments of the globus pallidus and to

dorsal and medial parts of the reticular part of the substantia nigra (6-8). Finally, the ventral, limbic striatum projects to the ventral pallidum and the most dorsomedial part of the substantia nigra pars reticulata (19). As will be discussed below, the ventral striatum has a number of additional target areas in the basal forebrain, hypothalamus and mesencephalon outside the pallidum and the substantia nigra.

The second level of organization of the efferent striatal projections is based on the fact that there are two main populations of medium-sized spiny projection neurons. The entire population utilizes γ-aminobutyric acid (GABA) as its neurotransmitter, but it divides into two subgroups of neurons on the basis of the expression of various neuropeptides and dopaminergic receptor subtypes (8). Half of the population expresses the neuropeptides substance P and dynorphin, as well as the dopamine D1 receptor subtype. These neurons project to the internal segment of the globus pallidus and substantia nigra pars reticulata, and in this way form the *direct striatal output pathway* to the output nuclei of the basal ganglia (22-24) (see Figure 2.6). The other half of the population expresses the neuropeptide enkephalin as well as the dopamine D2 receptor subtype. These striatal neurons project preferentially to the external segment of the globus pallidus. The external segment of the globus pallidus projects by way of its GABAergic neurons to the subthalamic nucleus, which, in turn, projects through glutamatergic excitatory fibers to the internal segment of the globus pallidus and the substantia nigra pars reticulata. This multisynaptic pathway from the striatum to the basal ganglia output nuclei is referred to in general as the *indirect striatal output pathway* (22-24) (see Figure 2.6).

Pallidum

The internal and external segments of the globus pallidus have many cellular and electrophysiological characteristics in common, but their afferent and efferent connections differ consid-erably. The cellular density in both segments is rather sparse. Most pallidal neurons are relatively large, with dendrites that form disc-like configurations with a diameter of up to 1 mm. These 'dendritic disks' are oriented perpendicular to the incoming striatal fibers, and in that way these neurons integrate information from a relatively large striatal area. In the external pallidal segment, a population of smaller neurons exists with more randomly extending dendrites (8).

Pallidal neurons are in general tonically active (60-80 s^{-1}). In the external segment of the globus pallidus, a sizable population of neurons exists with lower firing frequencies (10 s^{-1}). The firing frequencies of pallidal neurons have been shown to change in relation to movements of the limbs. However, there is no clear correlation between such changes in firing frequency and particular aspects of the movements, such as strength, orientation or amplitude (25). Changes in firing patterns occur during the *execution* of the movement. A clear role for pallidal neurons in the *initiation* of movements has not been demonstrated. The ventral pallidum has many cytoarchitectonic characteristics in common with the rest of the pallidum. In particular, the subcommissural part that is directly continuous with the external pallidal segment has 'classical' pallidal characteristics with large neurons that are tonically active. The more ventral and medial parts of the ventral pallidum contain somewhat smaller neurons, and there is a greater variety of neuronal types, possibly indicating that these parts of the ventral pallidum form a transition area with other nuclei of the basal forebrain (19,26).

Afferent connections of the different parts of the pallidum

The major input to both the external and internal segments of the globus pallidus is derived from the striatum. The caudate nucleus and putamen project upon the globus pallidus; the nucleus accumbens targets the ventral pallidum. Myelinated striatopallidal fibers converge in

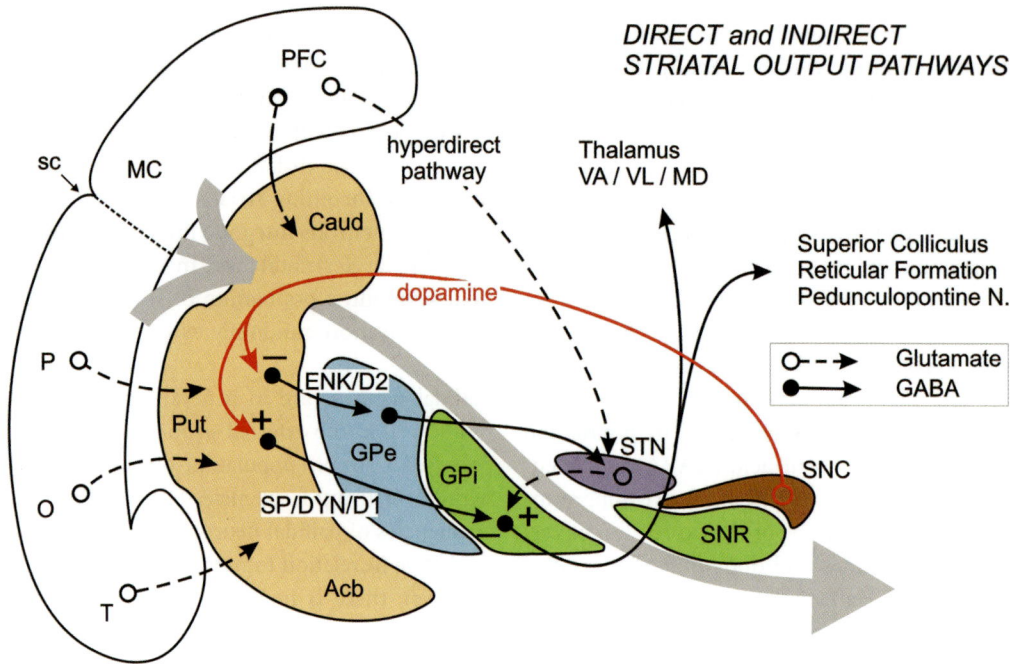

DIRECT and INDIRECT STRIATAL OUTPUT PATHWAYS

Figure 2.6
Direct and indirect striatal output pathways and the influence of dopamine on these routes, represented in a semi-sagittal scheme of the cerebral cortex and the basal ganglia. The direct pathway runs from the striatum to the internal segment of the globus pallidus and the substantia nigra pars reticulata. This pathway contains the peptides substance P (SP) and dynorphin (DYN) as well as the dopamine D1 receptor. The first link in the indirect striatal output pathway consists of the projections from the striatum to the external segment of the globus pallidus. These striatal neurons express the peptide enkephalin (ENK) and the dopamine D2 receptor. The subsequent steps in the indirect route are the pallido-subthalamic and the subthalamo-pallidal projections. Dopamine has opposite effects on the two striatal output routes, stimulating the direct pathway and inhibiting the indirect pathway.
Direct projections from the cerebral cortex to the subthalamic nucleus are being indicated as the 'hyperdirect pathway'.
Abbreviations: Acb, nucleus accumbens; Caud, caudate nucleus; GPe, external segment of the globus pallidus; GPi, internal segment of the globus pallidus; MC, primary motor cortex; MD, mediodorsal thalamic nucleus; O, occipital cortex; P, parietal cortex, PFC, prefrontal cortex; Put, putamen; sc, central sulcus; SNC, substantia nigra, pars compacta; SNR, substantia nigra, pars reticulata; STN, subthalamic nucleus; T, temporal cortex; VA, ventral anterior thalamic nucleus; VL, ventral lateral thalamic nucleus.

small fascicles like the spokes of a wheel onto both pallidal segments (1). There is a rather strict topographical organization in the striato-pallidal projections, maintaining mediolateral, dorsoventral and rostrocaudal coordinates. In this way, the functional subdivision of the striatum, as well as the somatotopic organization of particular parts, is 'imposed' upon the pallidum. While the main orientation of the disc-like dendritic arborizations of the pallidal neurons is perpendicular to the incoming striatal axons,

integration of information travelling through the distinct striatopallidal channels is very likely. As noted above, the striatal input to the two pallidal segments is derived from distinct populations of striatal neurons (see Figure 2.6). The external segment of the globus pallidus receives input from the population of striatal neurons that expresses the opioid peptide enkephalin and the D2 dopamine receptor. The internal pallidal segment is targeted by the striatal medium-sized spiny neurons that express the neuropeptides dynorphin and substance P, as well as the dopamine D1 receptor (8,22,23).

Within the ventral pallidum the segregation between direct and indirect pathways is less clear. The part of the ventral pallidum directly underneath the anterior commissure is rich in substance P-positive fibers and shares the most characteristics with the external pallidal segment. As will be discussed below, this part of the ventral pallidum in association with the shell of the nucleus accumbens takes a somewhat special position in the circuitry of the basal ganglia (19, 26). The more ventral and medial parts of the ventral pallidum contain both substance P- and enkephalin-positive fibers and in this way have characteristics of both the external and internal pallidal segments.

In addition to the GABAergic/peptidergic striatal afferents, the pallidum receives glutamatergic inputs from the subthalamic nucleus. Maintaining a global topographical arrangement, subthalamic projections reach segments of the globus pallidus and the subcommissural ventral pallidum. There is some controversy about how precise this topographical arrangement is (11,27); in view of the role of the subthalamic nucleus in suppressing unwanted outputs of the basal ganglia, a more diffuse distribution of subthalamo-pallidal projections seems likely (28). Finally, dopaminergic and serotonergic inputs also reach the pallidum (5).

Efferent connections of the different parts of the pallidum

Efferent projections of the external segment of the globus pallidus remain within the circuitry of the basal ganglia. Their primary target is the subthalamic nucleus, in this way establishing the second step in the indirect striatal output pathway. The neurons of the external pallidal segment tonically inhibit the subthalamic neurons. Fibers from the external globus pallidus also reach the internal pallidal segment, the substantia nigra pars reticulata, and they establish a feedback projection to the striatum (10).

These pallidostriatal fibers specifically target the fast-firing GABAergic, parvalbumin-positive striatal interneurons. In this way, the pallidostriatal projections play a crucial role in the regulation of the activity of the medium-sized spiny projection neurons of the striatum (10).

Efferent projections of the internal pallidal segment primarily reach the ventral nuclei of the thalamus, in particular the 'oral part' of the ventrolateral nucleus and the parvicellular part of the ventral anterior nucleus (7,11). These thalamic nuclei are reciprocally connected to the motor and premotor cortices and, to a lesser degree, areas of the dorsolateral prefrontal cortex. Descending projections from the internal pallidum reach the caudal mesencephalic areas, including the non-cholinergic part of the pedunculopontine nucleus (also indicated as the 'midbrain extrapyramidal area'; see below). Furthermore, neurons in the medial and ventral margins of the internal segment of the globus pallidus project to the lateral habenula (6,8). The functional significance of this output pathway of the basal ganglia is not well understood. It is of interest, however, that the habenula projects strongly to the midbrain raphe and caudal parts of the periaqueductal grey matter that contain serotonergic and cholinergic neurons, respectively, supplying extensive parts of the forebrain (19).

The projections of the ventral pallidum parallel those of both the external and internal segments of the globus pallidus and, in addition, have a number of extra targets that are not reached by the 'classical' basal ganglia structures (see below). The main termination areas of ventral pallidal efferents include the mediodorsal, ventromedial and reticular thalamic nuclei, as well as the dorsomedial part of the subthalamic nucleus (19). Via the mediodorsal thalamic nucleus, the ventral striatopallidal system influences several different prefrontal cortical areas. The lateral habenula also receives projections from the ventral pallidum, providing an influence of the ventral striatopallidal system on the serotonergic and cholinergic cell groups in the mesencephalon. In addition, the dorsomedial part of the substantia nigra, both the pars reticulata and the pars compacta, and the caudal mesencephalic areas including the pedunculopontine nucleus are reached by ventral pallidal fibers (19).

Subthalamic nucleus

The neurons of the subthalamic nucleus are relatively small and, as indicated above, they are excitatory using glutamate as the neurotransmitter. Afferent projections to the subthalamic nucleus originate in the external globus pallidus as well as the subcommissural part of the ventral pallidum. There is a distinct topographical arrangement in these pallido-subthalamic projections such that the sensorimotor parts of the globus pallidus project most ventrally and laterally, while the more medially located associative parts of the globus pallidus project more medially and dorsally in the subthalamic nucleus. The most dorsomedial parts of the subthalamic nucleus receive inputs from the ventral pallidum. This topographical organization therefore imposes a functional subdivision of the subthalamic nucleus into a sensorimotor, an associative and a limbic sector (11,29). In addition to the pallidal afferents, the subthalamic nucleus also receives inputs from the motor, premotor and prefrontal cortices, as well as from the caudal intralaminar thalamic nuclei, i.e., the centromedian-parafascicular complex (9). Recent findings indicate that the deep layers of the superior colliculus also innervate the subthalamic nucleus (30). Efferent subthalamic projections target the internal globus pallidus, the ventral pallidum and the pars reticulata of the substantia nigra. These subthalamic projections form the second and final step in the indirect striatopallidal output pathway. The subthalamic nucleus in addition projects to the external globus pallidus (11,27).

Substantia nigra pars reticulata

Neurons in the reticular part of the substantia nigra are large, with structural, neurochemical and electrophysiological characteristics that strongly resemble those of pallidal neurons. Like pallidal neurons, the dendritic arborizations of nigral neurons are disk-like in shape. Nigral neurons are tonically active (60-80 s^{-1}) and use GABA as their neurotransmitter (8). While changes of activity patterns of pallidal neurons are related to movements of the limbs, changes in firing patterns of neurons in the reticular part of the substantia nigra are related to eye movements.

Afferent and efferent connections

The main source of afferent fibers to the substantia nigra pars reticulata is formed by the striatum. In particular, striatal neurons of the direct striatal output pathway, i.e. containing the neuropeptides substance P and dynorphin and expressing the dopamine D1 receptor, project to the substantia nigra (8,10). As indicated above, there is a topographical organization in the striatonigral pathways, establishing functionally distinct input-output channels from different parts of the striatum via the substantia nigra to different basal ganglia targets in the thalamus and brainstem (8,31). In addition to striatal afferents, the substantia nigra pars reticulata also receives GABAergic inputs from the different parts of the pallidum and glutamatergic fibers from the subthalamic nucleus. The GABAergic efferent projections of the reticular part of the substantia nigra reach the magnocellular part of the ventral anterior thalamic nucleus (VAmc), the paralamellar part of the mediodorsal nucleus (MDpl) and extensive parts of the intralaminar thalamic nuclei (8). Through these thalamic nuclei, the substantia nigra has an influence on the premotor and prefrontal cortical areas, including the so-called frontal eye field, just anterior to the premotor cortex. The substantia nigra pars reticulata further strongly projects to the deeper layers of the superior colliculus, subserving saccadic eye movements and orienting responses. Nigral fibers are also directed towards more caudal mesencephalic areas including the reticular formation and the pedunculopontine nucleus, in particular its non-cholinergic part (8).

Substantia nigra pars compacta and ventral tegmental area

The pars compacta of the substantia nigra consists of relatively large neurons that produce dopamine as their neurotransmitter; these neurons belong to the so-called A9 dopaminergic cell group (1). As can be appreciated from Figure 2.2D, dopaminergic neurons in the human substantia nigra are organized in clusters that dominate in the dorsal part of the nucleus but are also located more ventrally, embedded in the reticular part of the nigra. Mesencephalic dopaminergic neurons are not restricted to the substantia nigra but are also present in the medially adjacent VTA (A10 cell group), and more dispersed in the mesencephalic reticular formation dorsolateral to the substantia nigra (A8 cell group) (1,8,32).

Nigrostriatal, mesolimbic and mesocortical dopamine systems

The neurons of the substantia nigra pars compacta project primarily to the striatum, forming the nigrostriatal dopamine system. A global medial to lateral topographical organization exits in the nigrostriatal projections such that lateral parts of the substantia nigra pars compacta project to lateral parts of the striatum, in particular the putamen, while progressively more medial parts of the nigra project to more medial striatal areas, progressively involving the caudate nucleus (8,18). The VTA consists of a mixture of dopaminergic and GABAergic neurons, both constituting approximately 50% of the population. Dopaminergic projections from the VTA reach the ventromedial parts of the striatum, including the nucleus accumbens, as well as medial prefrontal cortical areas. The VTA dopaminergic fibers to the striatum are in general referred to as the mesolimbic dopaminergic system, and the dopaminergic VTA-cortical pathway as the mesocortical dopamine system. It must be noted that an important component of the projections from the VTA to the cortex appears to consist of GABAergic fibers (33). Recent studies have in-

dicated that glutamate may be co-expressed in part of the dopaminergic projections from the VTA to the ventral striatum (34). The dopaminergic neurons of the A8 cell group project primarily to ventrolateral parts of the striatum (8).

Afferents of the dopaminergic neurons

Dopaminergic neurons receive inputs from the striatum, in particular from the ventral striatum and striatal neurons in specific compartments of the caudate nucleus and putamen, i.e., the striosome/patch compartment (8). The latter compartments are preferentially innervated by the medial prefrontal cortex, the amygdala and the paraventricular thalamic nucleus (8,35,36). In other words, the GABAergic striatal input to the dopaminergic neurons originates from limbic-innervated parts of the striatum. Other inputs to the dopaminergic neurons originate in different parts of the pallidal complex, the prefrontal cortex, the central amygdaloid nucleus and other basal forebrain structures in the septal-preoptic-hypothalamic continuum (8). At least part of these projections to the dopaminergic neurons may be excitatory. A cholinergic innervation of the nigral dopaminergic neurons originates in the mesencephalic pedunculopontine nucleus (37). Interestingly, it has recently been shown that an excitatory input to the dopaminergic neurons originates in the superior colliculus (38).

Functional aspects

Dopaminergic neurons basically have a low spontaneous electrophysiological activity ($2\ s^{-1}$), while changes in the activity of these neurons is not clearly related to particular aspects of movements or sensory stimulation. The activity of dopaminergic neurons increases, however, in relation to environmental stimuli that are of motivational or instrumental significance in a particular behavioural context, like the presentation of a reward or a specific cue for the guidance of a movement or behavioural act (39,40). Schultz and colleagues (40) have shown in conditioning experiments in primates that, after a period of training, the increased activity of dopaminergic neurons can shift from the moment of the presentation of a reward to the moment at which a conditioned stimulus predicts the upcoming reward. The interpretation of these findings is that dopaminergic neurons signal stimuli (external) that are relevant for the guidance of behaviour in a particular context. It is of interest to note that the dopaminergic afferents in the striatum terminate on the medium-sized spiny neurons, in particular on the necks of the spines, i.e., in a crucial position to modulate the input from cortical, thalamic and limbic structures to these neurons (Figure 2.4). As indicated above, the arrangement of excitatory afferents to the striatal medium-sized spiny neurons may be viewed as perfectly suited for the 'detection' of coincident, contextual stimuli. Dopamine might play an important role in facilitating the behavioural output, which is relevant in a particular context. It has long been an enigma via which route external stimuli reach the dopaminergic neurons since the latencies for changes in firing patterns of the neurons following such salient stimuli is relatively short. The direct, excitatory projections from the superior colliculus, which not only receives retinotopic visual information but also somatosensory and auditory inputs, might play an essential role in this process (38).

Pedunculopontine nucleus – relationships with the basal ganglia?

It has long been known that the pedunculopontine nucleus has strong interactions with several basal ganglia structures. Therefore, it has recently been suggested that this nuclear complex in the caudodorsal part of the mesencephalon could be considered part of the basal ganglia 'family' (37,41). The pedunculopontine nucleus primarily consists of large cholinergic neurons, but an approximately equal number of non-cholinergic neurons may be considered part of this nuclear complex. The latter 50% of the pedunculopontine population constitutes a heterogeneous group of neurons with different neuro-transmitter identities, such as GABA, glutamate and dopamine. The population of non-cholinergic neurons, also indicated as the pars dissipata, is situated medially and slightly dorsally to the population of cholinergic neurons that has been characterized as the pars compacta. Based on structure and connections, the pedunculopontine nucleus has many characteristics in common with the substantia nigra (42). The cholinergic pars compacta of the pedunculopontine nucleus, like the dopaminergic pars compacta of the substantia, has many functional characteristics of the 'ascending reticular activating system'. The cholinergic neurons of the pars compacta project to the thalamus and, in addition, give a strong input to the substantia nigra pars compacta. Moreover, non-cholinergic, glutamate-containing compacta neurons project to the subthalamic nucleus. The non-cholinergic pars dissipata of the pedunculopontine nucleus is strongly interconnected with the striatopallidal system, having reciprocal connections with the internal segment of the globus pallidus, the ventral pallidum and the substantia nigra pars reticulata (37,42). The pedunculopontine nucleus receives inputs not only from basal ganglia structures, but also from sensory-related structures like the superior colliculus and other brainstem nuclei. In addition to the ascending projections, the pedunculopontine nucleus also sends descending projections to caudal brainstem nuclei and the spinal cord (41). Functionally, the pedunculopontine nucleus, through its ascending cholinergic projections to the thalamocortical system, has been demonstrated to be crucial for wakefulness and REM sleep (37,41). Traditionally, the pedunculopontine nucleus has also been associated with locomotion since stimulation of this area in decerebrate animals has been described to elicit patterns of locomotor activity. However, recent evidence suggests the pedunculopontine nucleus to be involved in reinforcement, behavioural learning and the control of action selection rather than simply locomotion (41,42).

Some specific notes on the ventral striatum

As already noted above, the ventral striatum is generally considered that part of the striatum that is connectionally associated with limbic structures such as the amygdala, hippocampus, midline thalamus and certain regions of the prefrontal cortex. Moreover, the ventral striatum is part of the mesolimbic dopamine system since it is strongly innervated by dopaminergic fibers from the VTA (A10 cell group). The term 'ventral striatum' was introduced by Heimer and Wilson (43) in 1975 to differentiate it from the dorsal, sensorimotor-related part of the striatum, i.e., the caudate nucleus and putamen. The recognition of a ventral striatopallidal system, organized in parallel to the 'classic' dorsal striatopallidal system, has had great impact on the functional-anatomical concept of the basal ganglia. In particular, it paved the way for the now generally accepted notion that the basal ganglia are not only involved in sensorimotor functions but also play a role in cognitive and emotional-motivational behavioural functions (44,45).

Dorsal versus ventral striatum

It is important to note that there are no clear-cut boundaries between the dorsal and ventral striatum, either on the basis of a specific set of cortical, thalamic or dopaminergic inputs or based on other structural or functional markers (46). Therefore, in the literature the dorsal and ventral striatum have been virtually equated with the caudate-putamen complex on the one hand and the nucleus accumbens on the other. However, the ventral striatum as defined on the basis of the above-mentioned limbic inputs, as well as on certain cyto- and chemoarchitectonic characteristics, occupies a more extensive striatal area than the nucleus accumbens alone, and extends dorsally and caudally into the ventral parts of the caudate nucleus and putamen, including areas of the caudal putamen dorsal to the amygdala, the so-called amygdalostriatal transition area (46,47). Even though it is important to view the ventral striatum as an integral part of the striatum as a whole, a number of specific characteristics of the ventral striatum, in particular the nucleus accumbens, will be discussed in the following sections since those aspects are important for understanding the functional role of this region of the striatum.

Shell and core of the nucleus accumbens

The basic cytoarchitectonic and chemoarchitectonic features of the dorsal and ventral striatum are very similar. Yet, the ventral striatum contains a greater diversity and a more heterogeneous distribution of neurotransmitters and neuroactive peptides than the dorsal striatum (46). Within the nucleus accumbens, the differential distribution of neuroactive substances, along with the organization of afferent and efferent connections, has led to a distinction between the so-called shell and core subregions (19,26,48). A generally accepted marker for the outer, medially and ventrally located, crescent-shaped shell and the more dorsally and laterally located, inner core subregion is the calcium-binding protein calbindin-D_{28K} which, at least in rats, is dense in the core and virtually absent from the shell (19,26,48,49). Further inhomogeneities exist within shell and core in the distribution of various neurochemical substances and neurotransmitter receptors, including mu-opioid (Figure 2.7A) and dopamine D1 and D2 receptors (50,51). Interestingly, the highest concentration of dopamine D3 receptors in the brain is present in the shell of the nucleus accumbens (52).

Afferent and efferent connectivity of shell and core

As mentioned above, the general pattern of afferent and efferent connections of the ventral striatum is very similar to that of the dorsal striatum. However, remarkable differences exist between the shell and core subregions in their input-output characteristics, although these differences are not absolute (19). Thus, the core subregion receives inputs primarily from the dorsal parts of the medial prefrontal cortex (dorsal prelimbic and anterior cingulate areas), the parahippocampal cortex, the caudal midline and rostral intralaminar thalamic nuclei, and the anterior part of the basolateral amygdaloid nucleus (see Figure 2.7B). In its outputs the core parallels the dorsal striatal projection patterns by sending fibers to the subcommissural part of the ventral pallidum (ventral extension of the external segment of the globus pallidus under- neath the anterior commissure), the medial part of the internal segment of the globus pallidus and the dorsomedial part of the substantia ni- gra pars reticulata (53,54) (see Figure 2.7B). The subcommissural ventral pallidum is in recipro- cal connection with the dorsomedial part of the subthalamic nucleus (55). The medial parts of the internal segment of the globus pallidus and substantia nigra project to the ventromedial and mediodorsal thalamic nuclei. These thalamic nuclei reach the medial and lateral orbital pre-

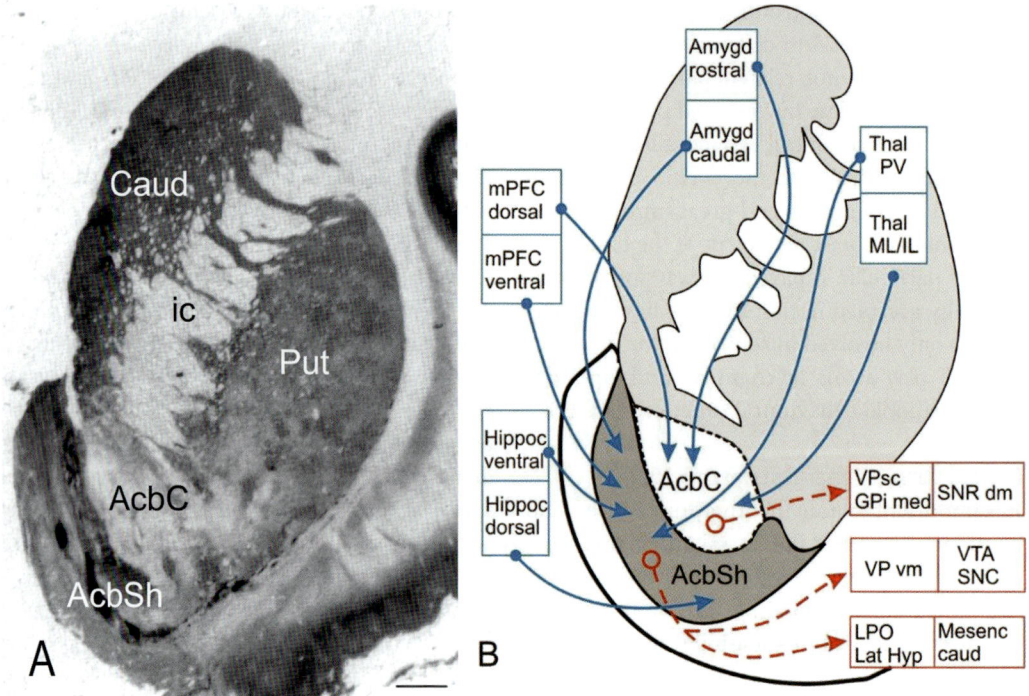

Figure 2.7
A. Frontal section through the rostral part of the human striatum illustrating the pattern of mu-opioid receptor binding (for details see 55). Note the differences in binding between the nucleus accumbens shell (AcbSh) and core (AcbC), and the caudate nucleus (Caud) and putamen (Put). Bar represents 5 mm. Courtesy of Dr. P. Voorn. B. Sche- matic drawing of the inputs and outputs of the shell and core of the nucleus accumbens (see also Fig. 2.1). Dopamin- ergic, serotonergic, and noradrenergic inputs have been omitted from the drawing. Note that virtually all structures project to both shell and core, although via different subdivisions or subnuclei. Note that the indicated projections are based on an extrapolation of experimental data obtained in rodents and sub-human primates.
Abbreviations: AcbC, nucleus accumbens core; AcbSh, nucleus accumbens shell; Caud, caudate nucleus; Amygd, amygdala; Hippoc, hippocampal formation; ic, internal capsule; Lat Hyp, lateral hypothalamus; LPO, lateral preoptic area; Mesenc caud, caudal mesencephalic regions; ML/IL, midline and intralaminar thalamic nuclei; mPFC, medial prefrontal cortex; Put, putamen; PV, paraventricular thalamic nucleus; SNRdm, dorsomedial part of the substantia nigra pars reticulata; Thal, thalamus; VPsc, subcommissural part of the ventral pallidum; VPvm, ventromedial part of the ventral pallidum.

frontal areas that in turn project to the core of the nucleus accumbens, closing one of the 'limbic' basal ganglia-thalamocortical circuits (see below) (19,44,56).

The shell receives inputs from the ventrally located medial prefrontal areas (infralimbic and ventral prelimbic), the midline paraventricular thalamic nucleus, the posterior parts of the basolateral amygdaloid nucleus, and the subiculum and CA1 regions of the hippocampal formation (see Figure 2.7B). Moreover, in addition to dopaminergic and serotonergic inputs from the VTA and dorsal raphe, respectively, the caudomedial shell receives significant numbers of noradrenergic fibers. These latter fibers most likely originate from noradrenergic cell groups in the caudal brainstem (19,20). The outputs of the shell target the ventral and medial parts of the ventral pallidum and adjacent portions of the septal and lateral preoptic areas (see Figure 2.7B). Furthermore, shell fibers reach the lateral hypothalamus as well as dopaminergic cell groups in the VTA and the dorsal tier of the substantia nigra pars compacta. Even more caudally in the mesencephalon, fibers from the shell reach the pedunculopontine nucleus. Via the ventromedial parts of the ventral pallidum, the shell is involved in a re-entrant 'limbic' basal ganglia-thalamocortical circuit that further includes the mediodorsal thalamic nucleus and medial prefrontal areas (see below) (19). Through the projections to the VTA and adjacent substantia nigra pars compacta, the shell appears to be in a position to influence the dopaminergic inputs to more dorsal parts of the striatum. These connections may form one of the neuronal substrates for the integration of activity in various parallel, functionally segregated, basal ganglia-thalamocortical circuits (18,57).

Functional aspects of shell and core

On the basis of the functional characteristics of the inputs to the nucleus accumbens, this part of the ventral striatum may be viewed as a site for the integration of signals with emotional content (amygdala), contextual information (hippocampus), motivational significance (dopaminergic inputs), as well as information about the state of arousal (midline thalamus) and the planning of executive or cognitive activities (prefrontal cortex). The outputs of the accumbens directly, or via ventral pallidal and dopaminergic and non-dopaminergic nigral relays, lead to brain areas involved in basic functions like feeding and drinking behaviour (lateral hypothalamus), motivational behaviour (VTA and nigral dopaminergic neurons), and more complex cognitive and executive functions (via medial thalamic nuclei to the prefrontal cortex). In other words, the concept of Mogenson and colleagues (58) of the nucleus accumbens as a functional interface between the limbic and motor systems is still valid in general terms, but our current understanding is more differentiated. Specifically, the functional differentiation between the shell and core has been worked out in relatively great detail in the past few decades (59). It has been shown that the shell can be distinguished from the core and the rest of the striatum through its involvement in the expression of certain innate, unconditioned behaviours such as feeding or defensive behaviour (59-62). Shell and core subregions both play important, but distinct roles in Pavlovian and instrumental conditioned learning (63-66). Furthermore, the core subregion is preferentially involved in response-reinforcement learning. The shell is not involved as much in motor or response learning per se; rather, it integrates basic biological 'drives' with the viscero-limbic and motor effector systems. The mesolimbic dopamine system at the level of the nucleus accumbens appears to have a role in enhancing the gain by which conditioned stimuli and contexts exert control over behaviour.

Specific information about ventral striatal functioning in the human brain is unfortunately rather scarce. Dysfunctioning of this part of the striatum has been associated with schizophrenia, obsessive-compulsive disorder, depression and drug addiction. Preliminary positive effects of deep brain stimulation in the region of the nucleus accumbens in cases of otherwise intractable obsessive-compulsive behaviour have been reported (67,68). How these effects should be explained is still unclear, and in that light it is difficult to predict whether the ventral striatum will indeed become a surgical or pharmacological target for therapeutic interventions in neuropsychiatric diseases.

Parallel, functionally segregated, basal ganglia thalamocortical circuits

In the previous sections of this chapter, the functional anatomy of the various components of the basal ganglia has been described. Below, we will deal with the circuitry involving the basal ganglia with the cerebral cortex and the thalamus to understand their functional role in the brain better. Concepts about the basal ganglia, their position in the circuitry of the forebrain, and their functions have changed considerably in the past few decades based on detailed neuroanatomical and electrophysiological work. Following the seminal paper by Nauta and Mehler (69) in the mid-1960s, demonstrating that the major output of the basal ganglia is not to the brainstem but to the thalamus and subsequently the cerebral cortex, it became generally accepted that the basal ganglia, via the ventral anterior nucleus of the thalamus, reach the premotor cortex and in this way play a role in the preparatory phases of the initiation of movements. However, at that time the view of the basal ganglia was still very much focused on the caudate-putamen complex, the globus pallidus and the substantia nigra. Functionally, these large structures in the forebrain were largely associated with the motor system. Following the introduction of the concept of the above-mentioned 'ventral striatopallidal system' by Heimer and Wilson (43) in the mid-1970s, it became generally accepted that the basal ganglia are also involved in non-motor, i.e., cognitive and affective (or limbic) functions. Heimer and Wilson (43) emphasized the

parallel nature of the neocortical and allocortical inputs into the dorsal and ventral striatum, respectively. Likewise, the parallel organization of the outputs of the dorsal and ventral striatum to pallidal and, subsequently, thalamic targets was noted by these authors. We may now conclude that Heimer and Wilson (43) formulated the first principles of the parallel nature of basal ganglia-thalamocortical circuits. The full concept of the parallel organization of re-entrant cortical-subcortical circuits was presented in 1986 by Alexander and colleagues (44), who described the parallel organization of several basal ganglia-thalamocortical circuits, mostly based on functional-anatomical studies of the connections of the basal ganglia in non-human primates. This landmark paper by Alexander et al. (44) has dominated the basal ganglia literature in the past two decades. Alexander and coworkers (24,44) hypothesized that functionally different (pre)frontal cortical areas are involved in closed cortico-subcortical loops that successively include discrete, non-overlapping parts of the striatum, the pallidum/ substantia nigra reticulata, the thalamus and the (pre)frontal cortex. The basic design of each circuit is thought to be similar (see Figure 2.8). Thus, each basal ganglia-thalamocortical circuit receives input from several functionally related cortical areas, at the level of a specific part of the striatum (see above). Such connectionally and functionally characterized striatal regions subsequently send projections to distinct parts of the pallidum and/ or the substantia nigra that in turn project to a specific nucleus or its subdivision in the thalamus. Each thalamic (sub)nucleus projects back to the frontal cortical area that feeds into the particular circuit, thereby completing the 'closed loop' portion of the circuit (44,70). In this way, different parts of the basal ganglia are viewed, along with their connected cortical and thalamic areas, as components of a 'family' of basal ganglia-thalamocortical circuits that are organized in a parallel manner and remain largely segregated from one another, both structurally and

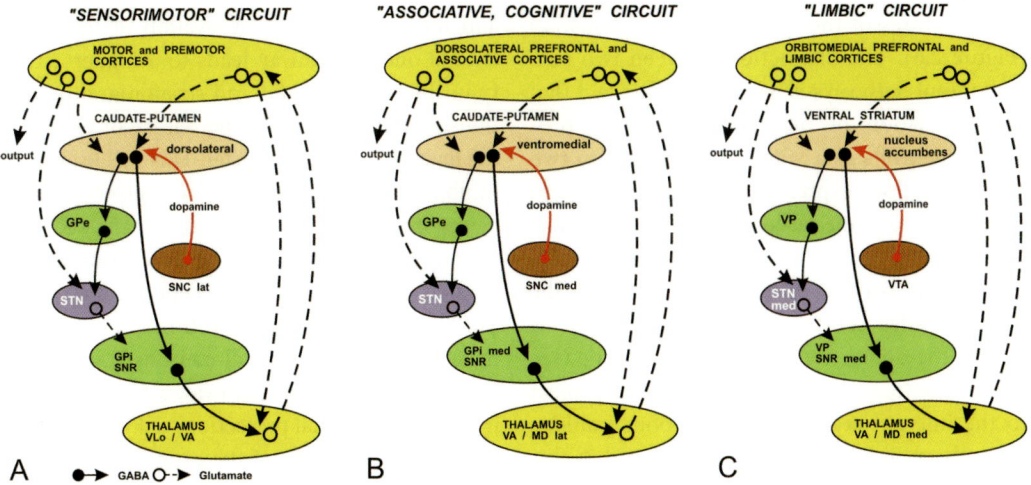

Figure 2.8
Schematic representation of the three main basal ganglia-thalamocortical circuits. As outlined in the text, each of these circuits consists of multiple sub-circuits.
Abbreviations: GPe, external segment of the globus pallidus; GPi, internal segment of the globus pallidus; lat, lateral; med, medial; MD, mediodorsal thalamic nucleus; SNC, substantia nigra, pars compacta; SNR, substantia nigra, pars reticulata; STN, subthalamic nucleus; VA, ventral anterior thalamic nucleus; VLo, ventral lateral thalamic nucleus, pars oralis; VP, ventral pallidum; VTA, ventral tegmental area.

functionally (44, 70). Alexander et al. (44) tentatively identified five circuits: a 'motor circuit' that includes the dorsolateral part of the striatum and the premotor cortices, an 'oculomotor circuit' that involves the dorsomedial part of the striatum and the frontal and supplementary eye fields, two 'prefrontal circuits' that include more central parts of the striatum and the dorsolateral prefrontal and orbitofrontal cortices, and finally, a 'limbic circuit' that involves the ventral striatum and the anterior cingulate and medial prefrontal cortices. Each individual circuit defined by Alexander et al. (44) may consist of several sub-circuits. As demonstrated by Alexander and Crutcher (71), the motor circuit might consist of various sub-circuits that are all concerned with different aspects of movements, for example separate sub-circuits related to the force, direction and speed of arm movements. Another example concerns the limbic circuit that, as we have seen in the preceding paragraphs, consists of distinguishable sub-circuits entertaining the shell and core of the nucleus accumbens, respec-

tively. A most convenient way of representing the parallel, functionally segregated, basal ganglia-thalamocortical loops is by 'clustering' them into three main functional categories, i.e., sensorimotor, cognitive and limbic (Figure 2.8), with the realization that all three main circuits consist of several functionally related sub-circuits. The main thrust of the concept of a parallel organization of cortical basal ganglia-thalamocortical loops is that not only the motor and premotor cortical areas receive basal ganglia inputs, but that *all* prefrontal cortical areas are under the influence of the basal ganglia. Consequently, the basal ganglia are not only concerned with motor functions but also with cognitive, executive and emotional-motivational functions (44,71).

Direct and indirect pathways

As has already been alluded to in the previous sections, the intrinsic basal ganglia connections can be categorized into two pathways connecting either directly or indirectly to the input and output structures of the basal ganglia (8,23,24,72) (Figure 2.6). The distinction between two striatal output pathways is based upon the fact that the population of medium-sized spiny projection neurons as a whole falls apart into two sub-populations expressing different neuropeptides and dopamine receptors and having different projection patterns. The direct striatal output pathway consists of neurons that express the neuropeptides substance P and dynorphin as well as the dopamine D1 receptor subtype (see Figure 2.6) (8,22). These striatal neurons project to the internal segment of the globus pallidus and substantia nigra pars reticulata, and in this way form a direct link between the striatum and the output nuclei of the basal ganglia (see Figure 2.6). The medium-sized spiny projection neurons that form the origin of the multisynaptic, indirect striatal output pathway express the neuropeptide enkephalin as well as the dopamine D2 receptor subtype (see Figure 2.6) (8,22). These striatal neurons project preferentially to the external segment of the globus pallidus. Subsequent steps in the indirect parthway include the projections of the GABAergic neurons of the external segment of the globus pallidus to the subthalamic nucleus. The subthalamic nucleus, in turn, projects through excitatory glutamatergic fibers to the internal segment of the globus pallidus and the substantia nigra pars reticulata (see Figure 2.6). Recent studies have shown that the motor cortex preferentially innervates striatal neurons, giving rise to the indirect pathway, while sensory and limbic cortices predominantly innervate striatal neurons of the direct pathway. Dopaminergic and thalamic inputs are distributed equally over both populations (73). Since the projection neurons in the basal ganglia output structures have the electrophysiological characteristic of being tonically active, they exert a tonic inhibitory influence on their target nuclei in the thalamus and mesencephalon. Activity in the corticostriatal or thalamostriatal pathways has the following differential influence on the output of the basal ganglia through the direct and indirect pathways. Activation of the direct striatal output pathway leads to a higher activity in the striatopallidal and striatonigral projections and an increase in the release of GABA at the level of the output nuclei. This will lead to an inhibition of the tonically active output neurons of the internal globus pallidus and the substantia nigra reticulata, resulting in a disinhibition of their thalamic and mesencephalic target areas (72). Following activation through cortical or thalamic activity of striatal neurons at the origin of the indirect output pathway, a higher activity in the striatopallidal projections will lead to inhibition of the neurons of the external segment of the globus pallidus. Inhibiting these GABAergic neurons leads to a disinhibition of the neurons of the subthalamic nucleus. The resulting increased activity of the excitatory subthalamic projections to the internal segment of the globus pallidus and the substantia nigra pars reticulata leads to a stronger activity of these basal ganglia output neurons and hence an increased inhibition of their target areas in the thalamus and brainstem. If it may be assumed that higher activity in the basal ganglia-thalamocortical circuits is associated with increased motor or cognitive/behavioural output of the brain, we can conclude that the direct striatal output pathway facilitates, while the indirect striatal output pathway suppresses motor, cognitive and emotional behavioural output. This fits very well with the idea that the basal ganglia play a role in selecting appropriate while suppressing unwanted motor or behavioural outputs (e.g. 7,28,74). As has been discussed in relation to the inputs and outputs of the individual basal ganglia nuclei, there are more connections between these structures than summarized above for the indirect pathway. Consequently, Bolam et al. (10) have proposed that rather than an indirect *pathway*, there is an indirect *network* which modulates the output of the basal ganglia via the direct pathway.

The subthalamic nucleus not only receives an inhibitory(tonic) input from the external segment of the globus pallidus, it is also projected upon directly by excitatory cortical and thalamic fibers (9,75) (Figure 2.3). The direct pathway from the cerebral cortex has also been referred to as the 'hyperdirect pathway'. This implies that the cerebral cortex may play an important role through the subthalamic nucleus in a stronger inhibition of the basal ganglia target areas and, thereby, the suppression of motor and cognitive/behavioural outputs.

Via the differential expression of the dopamine D1 and D2 receptor subtypes in the two subpopulations of striatal projection neurons, dopamine has an opposing influence on the two output pathways of the striatum (22). The functional significance of the segregation of dopamine D1 and D2 receptors in the two striatal neuronal populations has been shown by gene regulation studies (8,22). It could thus be demonstrated that the levels of enkephalin and substance P are oppositely regulated by dopamine. Thus, dopamine depletion results in an elevation of enkephalin and a reduction of substance P peptide and mRNA levels in the indirect and direct striatal output pathways, respectively. In contrast, enhanced dopaminergic neurotransmission results in elevated substance P and reduced enkephalin peptide and mRNA levels in the direct and indirect striatal output pathways, respectively. This has been taken as an indication that dopamine stimulates the direct pathway and inhibits the indirect pathway. In other words, higher dopamine concentrations at the striatal level may lead to a decreased inhibition of the basal ganglia target areas and, therefore, a higher activity of the thalamocortical system. Conversely, lower dopamine concentrations at the striatal level may lead to a stronger inhibition of the basal ganglia target areas and, therefore, a lower activity of the thalamocortical system (8). This concurs with the fact that, as in Parkinson's disease, low levels of striatal dopamine are associated with bradykinesia and hypokinesia, whereas high levels of striatal dopamine correlate with a facilitation of movements and cognitive/behavioural acts (24,28).

Subcortical loop systems

As discussed above, the main excitatory afferents of the striatum, like the input structure of the basal ganglia, originate from the cerebral cortex and the midline and intralaminar thalamic nuclei. The cerebral cortex, in particular the premotor and prefrontal cortical areas, forms the main target of the cortical basal ganglia-thalamocortical circuits, and the role of the basal ganglia appears to be to 'assist' the cortex in selecting the appropriate motor or behavioural output of the system (see below). The position and functional significance of the thalamic inputs into the basal ganglia have remained rather elusive up till now. There are strong indications that the thalamostriatal projections play an important role in attentional mechanisms and arousal since these midline and intralaminar nuclei receive most of their inputs from the brainstem (76,77). Interestingly, it has recently been suggested that these thalamic nuclei may form way stations in closed subcortical loops through the basal ganglia that are organized in a parallel fashion similar to the cortical basal ganglia-thalamocortical loops (see Figure 2.9) (78). Like the cortico-subcortical loops involving the basal ganglia, these subcortical loops appear to be designed to assist brainstem sensorimotor structures like the superior colliculus in selecting an appropriate motor output. In brief, it has been postulated that there are at least three closed circuits, which consecutively involve the superficial or deep layers of the superior colliculus, the caudal and rostral intralaminar thalamic nuclei, different parts of the striatum, the substantia nigra pars reticulata and finally, closing the loop, the deep or superficial layers of the superior colliculus (see Figure 2.9) (78). The superior colliculus, in its superficial layers, receives retinotopic visual input, responsive primarily to motion and the appearance or disappearance of objects in the visual field. The deep layers of the superior colliculus are multimodal, receiving tactile and auditory stimuli in addition to visual information. The output of the superior colliculus

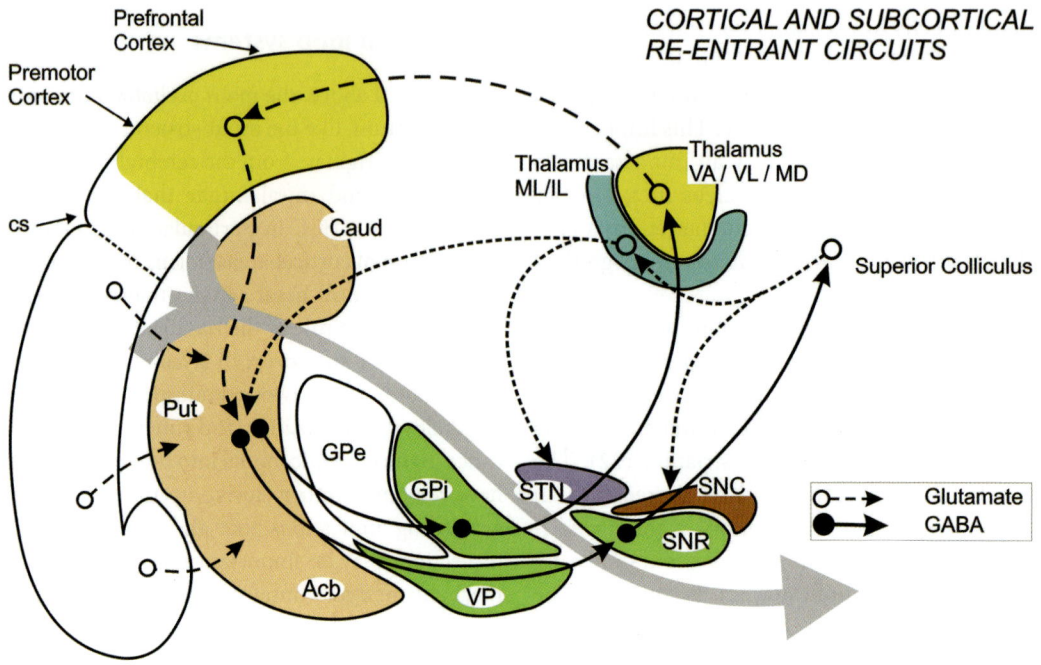

Figure 2.9
Schematic representation of the architecture of a cortical and a subcortical re-entrant circuit involving the basal ganglia. A cortical re-entrant circuit involves the prefrontal or premotor cortex. A subcortical re-entrant circuit originates
and terminates in the superior colliculus and entertains the midline and intralaminar thalamic nuclei that have strong
and topographically organized projections to the striatum. Also indicated are projections from the intralaminar nuclei
to the subtahlamic nucleus and from the superior colliculus to the substantia nigra, pars compacta (cf. text).
Abbreviations (see legend to figure 2.1): Acb, nucleus accumbens; Caud, caudate nucleus; GPe, external segment of
the globus pallidus; GPi, internal segment of the globus pallidus; MD, mediodorsal thalamic nucleus; ML/IL, midline
and intralaminar thalamic nuclei; Put, putamen; SNC, substantia nigra, pars compacta; SNR, substantia nigra, pars
reticulata; STN, subthalamic nucleus; VA, ventral anterior thalamic nucleus; VL, ventral lateral thalamic nucleus.

is to a large degree descending towards the 'gaze
centers' in the brainstem as well as to the ventral,
motor horn of the cervical spinal cord. Through
these outputs, the superior colliculus is responsible for orienting movements of the eyes (gaze) as
well as of the head and/or the body (tectospinal
projections). The superior colliculus is a phylogenetically old brain structure that has connections
via the thalamus with the basal ganglia in lower
vertebrate species also. While the superior colliculus still has a very prominent role in guiding
visuo-motor responses in the primate brain, including the human, the hypothesis is that relatively 'unprocessed' information through subcortical
structures like the superior colliculus may com-

pete or cooperate at the level of the basal ganglia
with 'higher processed' information that arrives
through the corticostriatal pathways in order to
produce an adequate (motor) output. The recognition of these subcortical loops through the
basal ganglia, in addition to or phylogenetically
even preceding the loops that involve the cerebral cortex and the basal ganglia, is important in
view of the relative 'weight' these two families of
circuits may have at the level of the basal ganglia
in determining their output. Future studies may
reveal whether the two loop systems primarily
cooperate or compete in determining the basal
ganglia output (78).

Interactions between basal ganglia-thalamocortical circuits

Whereas the closed nature and the functional segregation of both the cortical basal ganglia-thalamocortical circuits (44) and the subcortical basal ganglia loops (78) have been emphasized, there also appear to be extensive interactions between these circuits. Such interactions seem to be essential for the integration of the parallel processes that take place in the various circuits in order to produce coherent behaviour in which emotional, cognitive and sensorimotor aspects are integrated. In any event, the output of the various parallel basal ganglia-thalamocortical processes can ultimately make use of only a restricted set of effector structures, and interactions in the form of competition or cooperation and selection mechanisms must take place.

Several possibilities for interactions between cortical basal ganglia-thalamocortical circuits have been suggested. For example, Zahm and Brog (26) noted the existence of 'open' components in the loops between the cerebral cortex, the basal ganglia and the thalamus, suggesting a 'spiral' of connections leading from the limbic-innervated part of the basal ganglia via the thalamus to the premotor cortex. In a similar vein, Joel and Weiner (79) described the so-called 'split circuits' that include both 'open' and 'closed' basal ganglia-thalamocortical loops and also have a tendency to lead from limbic to cognitive- and motor-related circuits. Likewise, behavioural studies provide suggestions for interactions between basal ganglia circuits at the functional level (80). For example, information about cues signaling reward processed via the shell of the nucleus accumbens may be crucial for activating circuits involving the accumbens core to guide actions that are instrumental to gaining access to basic supplies, such as water and food (80). Thus, while the shell and core appear to have differential functional roles, as outlined above, these two subregions and their related circuitry are thought to interact with each other.

In the context of the issue of interactions between different parallel basal ganglia-thalamocortical circuits, the role of the ascending dopaminergic system appears to be of great importance. Several studies have demonstrated that the nucleus accumbens shell massively innervates the region of the ventral tegmental area and substantia nigra pars compacta that contains the dopamine neurons innervating the nucleus accumbens core in both rodents and primates (18,81,82). In turn, the nucleus accumbens core innervates the dorsomedial region of the substantia nigra pars reticulata that is overlaid by the dopamine neurons innervating the medial and central portions of the dorsal striatum receiving inputs from the anterior cingulate and prefrontal cortical areas (18,54,82). Accordingly, each striatal domain regulates its own dopamine innervation and, in addition, that of its adjacent domain. Based on such observations, Haber and colleagues (18) proposed that the striato-nigrostriatal pathways form an ascending spiral from the shell to the dorsolateral striatum in each subsequent step involving a laterally adjacent subset of ascending dopaminergic projections to the striatum. These ascending spiraling projections through the dopaminergic system might play a role in the transition of unconditioned behaviours, mediated by the shell of the nucleus accumbens, to conditioned, instrumental behaviours and finally to the formation of habits, mediated by the dorsal striatum. While a gradual shift of the involvement of limbic, cognitive and sensorimotor circuits probably plays an important role in the normal process of behavioural and motor learning, disturbances might lead to maladaptive behaviours like addictive behaviour or to the breakdown of the coherence of normal motor patterns and behaviour such as in Parkinson's disease.

Functional aspects of the basal ganglia

The functions of the basal ganglia are not yet completely understood but, as argued above, they must be considered in the context of their close association with the cerebral cortex, i.e., their inclusion in the basal ganglia-thalamocortical circuitry. In very general terms, it has been suggested that the basal ganglia may play an important role, in close association with the (pre) frontal cortex, in selecting an appropriate motor or behavioural output in a particular context (7,28,59,74,83). The link between 'context' and 'motor or behavioural' output stresses the important aspect of convergence and integration of sensory, motor/behavioural and mnemonic (~ past experience) information in the basal ganglia. This integration of perceptive and executive functions has its neuronal substrate within the basal ganglia most clearly at the level of the striatum where there is a strong convergence of corticostriatal projections originating from various functionally different cortical areas. Yet, as a consequence of the topographical arrangements of the corticostriatal projections (see above), there appear to be different sectors of the striatum that are involved in different functional aspects of the basal ganglia. In the dorsolateral part of the striatum, a convergence of inputs from sensory and motor cortices takes place, leading to an involvement of this part of the striatum in stimulus-response associations. When such stimulus-response associations have been well-established and are sustained even in the absence of continued reinforcement, such contextually elicited motor sequences or behavioural procedures may also be indicated as 'habits'. Habit formation has been attributed to the basal ganglia for many years (84). In the medial and ventral parts of the striatum, inputs from prefrontal cortical areas converge with inputs from the amygdala and hippocampus, representing contextual information and information related to the emotional value of environmental cues, respectively. The medial and ventral portions of the striatum, therefore, are thought to be involved in complex behavioural procedures depending on emotional/motivational and mnemonic aspects (59,83,85). In line with this, the medial and ventral sectors of the striatum have

been indicated to guide behaviour using stimulus-reward associations (86). Dopamine has been shown to play an important role in the establishment and maintenance of the various types of association at the level of the striatum. Despite this variety of basal ganglia functions, the neuronal mechanism of the selection process that leads to the appropriate response to a particular stimulus might be rather universal throughout the striatum.

It may be clear from the foregoing that the basal ganglia are thought to play a major role in the process of selecting the most wanted or appropriate motor or behavioural output in a given situation. However, the question of what the exact neuronal substrate is for the selection process that takes place in the basal ganglia cannot be fully answered at present. The above-described architecture of the intrinsic connections within the circuitry, i.e., the direct and indirect striatal output pathways, may provide some clue. These opposing parallel pathways may play a role in adjusting the magnitude of the inhibitory output of the internal pallidal segment to the thalamus in order to facilitate or suppress the expression of behavioural acts (22,28). Thus, an increased output from the internal segment of the globus pallidus slows or prevents movements, while a decreased output from the internal pallidum facilitates movement. However, although the arrangements of the two intrinsic pathways connecting the input and output structures of the basal ganglia provide some explanation in terms of selection of movements or behavioural acts, more intricate mechanisms are necessary to fully explain the complex repertoire of our behaviour. Various theories have been put forward to provide an explanation for such neuronal mechanisms at the level of the basal ganglia, at either the macrocircuit or the microcircuit (striatal) level (e.g. 28,74,59,87).

An attractive hypothesis for the selection mechanism in the dorsal, motor-related striatum is provided by Mink (28). According to him, the tonically active inhibitory output of the basal ganglia acts as a 'brake' on motor programs that compete with the execution of a desired motor program. Conversely, the disinhibitory output of the basal ganglia acts as an 'acceleration' on the desired motor program (28). Thus, according to this hypothesis, when a desired movement is to be initiated by a certain motor program, the basal ganglia output neurons involved in competing motor programs increase their firing rate, thereby increasing inhibition and applying a 'brake' on those motor programs. The selected movements are in this way enabled, and competing postures and movements are prevented from interfering with the one selected. In the selection hypothesis of Mink, the subthalamic nucleus plays an important role. To be more specific, when a person makes a voluntary movement, that movement is initiated by mechanisms in the prefrontal, premotor, supplementary motor, and primary motor cortices, as well as in the cerebellum. Initially, the cerebral cortical areas send an excitatory signal to the subthalamic nucleus. The subthalamic nucleus projects in turn to the internal segment of the globus pallidus and provides an excitatory drive on the internal pallidal neurons. This increased activity of the internal segment of the globus pallidus causes inhibition at the level of the thalamus and the brainstem. This mechanism may lead to the suppression of the competing thalamocortical and brainstem motor programs. Parallel to this pathway, the cerebral cortical areas send a signal to the striatum. This cortical input is translated by the striatal integrative circuitry into a focused, context-dependent output that inhibits specific neurons in the internal segment of the globus pallidus. The inhibitory striatal input to the internal segment of the globus pallidus is slower but more powerful than the excitatory input from the subthalamic nucleus. This results in a decreased activity of the internal segment of the globus pallidus that in turn selectively disinhibits the desired set of thalamocortical and descending projections in order to express the desired motor program through the brainstem

or spinal cord. The indirect striatal output pathway from the striatum to the internal segment of the globus pallidus via the external segment of the globus pallidus and the subthalamic nucleus results in further focussing of the output. In the most general sense, the concept put forward by Mink (28) provides a selection mechanism for surround inhibition (the 'brake' of competing motor programs) and center excitation (the 'acceleration' of the desired motor program). This general principle of selection of the desired motor program and inhibition of competing programs at the level of the output structures may also be applied to the other functional domains of the basal ganglia.

From a different perspective, Redgrave et al. (74) have hypothesized that the basal ganglia operate as a hierarchical selection device. This hypothesis states that when multiple sensorimotor systems seek simultaneous access to a final common motor path, selections at various functional levels are required. For instance, selections between competing systems to decide the general course of action are an initial requirement. The sensory processing of an unexpected event that is represented by separate cortico-basal ganglia thalamo-cortical loops as well as by loops connecting subcortical sensorimotor structures with the basal ganglia, converge and compete in the ventral limbic domain of the striatum. Then the 'winning' system may selectively prime command systems, at the level of the intermediate or central associative domain of the striatum, capable of specifying appropriate patterns of coordinated behavioural acts in the context of the current aim. Multi-dimensional contextual afferents are likely to originate in the cerebral cortex and limbic structures, such as the hippocampus, amygdala and thalamus. The final choice will be made at the level of the dorsolateral sensorimotor domain of the striatum, where patterns of appropriate motor activity that can deliver the currently selected action will be specified. At this level, motor-related projections from the motor cortex and subcortical sensorimotor structures (e.g. superior colliculus) reach the striatum directly (via the cortex) or indirectly (via the thalamus) and are likely to provide the striatum with a running multi-dimensional record (or motor efference copy) of commands related to ongoing goals, actions and movements (cf. also 88). This 'system-level hypothesis' implies a temporal relationship in striatal activation, with ventral striatal activity preceding dorsal striatal activation, in line with the ascending spiral from ventral to dorsal striatum discussed above.

In the preceding paragraphs, two current hypotheses of selection mechanisms at the circuit level of the basal ganglia-thalamocortical system have been described. Other theories have emphasized the importance of the intrinsic striatal circuitry as a neural basis for selection mechanisms in the basal ganglia. Most of these theories have been based on the assumption that the recurrent collaterals of medium-sized spiny projection neurons contact adjacent projection neurons, leading to lateral inhibitory processes supporting the suppression of competing outputs (e.g. 83,87,89). Along these lines, Pennartz and colleagues (87) launched the 'ensemble hypothesis', which states that the functions of the nucleus accumbens are based on the organization of collections or 'ensembles' of striatal neurons that function as parallel-distributed units with distinct functions in guiding different types of behaviour. Such ensembles are thought to be variably active in different behavioural situations. Which ensembles of neurons become active and provide an output from the nucleus accumbens depends upon the patterns of convergence of active glutamatergic, excitatory inputs of cortical, hippocampal, thalamic and amygdaloid origin, the level of activity of the dopaminergic inputs from the mesencephalon and the intrinsic circuitry of the nucleus accumbens. Lateral inhibitory processes between the different ensembles play an important role in the selection of the particular competing neuronal ensemble(s) that will ultimately provide the appropriate output.

To summarize, the three different basal ganglia domains, i.e., dorsolateral sensorimotor, intermediate or central associative, and ventral limbic, may be viewed as part of three independent, interacting macrocircuits that entertain different parts of the frontal lobe. Within these macrocircuits, smaller (micro)circuits can be recognized that subserve specific functions within the broader domain. Several mechanisms within this (micro)circuitry support a role for the basal ganglia in regulating motor and behavioural functions by selectively promoting desired and suppressing unwanted neuronal programs. The striatum appears to have a specific role in the selection mechanisms that take place in the basal ganglia.

The basal ganglia and movement disorders

The current basal ganglia model, i.e., the organization of the connectional relationships between the basal ganglia and the cerebral cortex in parallel, functionally segregated, cortico-subcortical re-entrant circuits, including the organization in two opposing striatal output pathways within these circuits, has had a great impact on the insight into the pathophysiology of several movement disorders, including most prominently Parkinson's disease. Moreover, this model has formed the rationale for some of the new and successful therapeutic interventions. Paradoxically, the effects of some of the successful new therapies, such as deep brain stimulation in Parkinson's disease, have challenged the validity of the basal ganglia model, and consequently, revisions of the model need to be made (90,91). In spite of its limitations, the basal ganglia model is helpful in explaining the pathophysiological background of at least some symptoms in a number of movement disorders. The clearest aspect concerns the distinction between hypokinetic and hyperkinetic symptoms (Figure 2.10). Taking as a first example Parkinson's disease, the pathophysiological explanation of the bradykinesia and hypokinesia in this disease is as follows. The degeneration of the dopaminergic system, as one of the cardinal neuropathological symptoms of Parkinson's disease, leads to lower levels of dopamine in the striatum in a particular stage of the disease. Motor symptoms occur when approximately 60% of the dopaminergic neurons have degenerated. The effect of the lower striatal dopamine levels has differential effects on the two striatal output pathways. In the direct striatal output pathway, the dopamine D1 receptors lose their stimulatory effect, and the neurons in this pathway become less active. As a result, the output neurons at the level of the internal segment of the globus pallidus and the reticular part of the substantia nigra are less inhibited and become more active. Loss of dopamine at the level of the neurons giving rise to the indirect pathway means a loss of inhibition through the dopamine D2 receptors. These striatal neurons become more active, providing a stronger inhibition of their pallidal target neurons in the external segment of the globus pallidus. Consequently, the tonic inhibition of the subthalamic nucleus by these neurons decreases, and the subthalamic nucleus neurons will therefore provide a stronger excitatory effect on the basal ganglia output neurons. In other words, these pallidal and nigral neurons will be less inhibited by the direct pathway and more strongly excited by the indirect pathway, both mechanisms leading to a higher activity of these neurons and a stronger inhibitory tone of the basal ganglia outputs onto the thalamus and the brainstem (Figure 2.10). The stronger inhibition of the thalamocortical system is most probably associated with the bradykinesia and hypokinesia in Parkinson's disease. The stronger inhibition of mesencephalic structures like the pedunculopontine nucleus and the reticular formation may be associated with rigidity, but the model cannot explain the characteristic parkinsonian tremor.

The pathophysiological mechanisms of some hyperkinetic movement disorders may also be understood on the basis of the basal ganglia model (see Figure 2.10B). For example, a lesion of the subthalamic nucleus of vascular or other origin will result in a decreased excitation of the basal ganglia output neurons and, consequently, a decreased inhibition of the thalamic and mesencephalic targets of the basal ganglia. When lesions involve large parts of or the entire subthalamic nucleus, unwanted movements are expressed in the contralateral half of the body in the form of hemiballism. In pathophysiological terms, a lesion of the subthalamic nucleus releases the 'brake' on the expression of unwanted movements. Another example of a hyperkinetic disorder is Huntington's disease (see Figure 2.10B). In the early phase of Huntington's disease, there is a preferential degeneration of the striatal neurons that express the peptide enkephalin and give rise to the indirect striatal output pathway, while the neurons of the direct pathway that express substance P remain relatively spared (92). The decreased striatal inhibition of the neurons in the external segment of the globus pallidus results in a stronger inhibition of the subthalamic nucleus, which in this way becomes functionally inactive. A decreased excitation from the subthalamic nucleus at the level of the basal ganglia output nuclei consequently leads to a decreased inhibition of the target nuclei of the basal ganglia in the thalamus and the brainstem (see Figure 2.10B). Again, this may be viewed as releasing the 'brake' on the expression of unwanted movements.

The insight into basal ganglia circuitry and the pathophysiological mechanisms of several movement disorders has certainly played an important role in the development of new therapeutic strategies. Following the introduction of the L-dopa therapy for Parkinson's disease in the 1960s, neurosurgical treatment of the disease was considered virtually obsolete. However, it subsequently became clear that L-dopa treatment has its limitations since its effectiveness wears off, and serious side effects develop after long-term treatment. The first step in the revival of neurosurgical interventions in Parkinson's

HYPOKINESIA
PFC
output
MC
sc
Thalamus
VA / VL / MD
Caud
dopamine
Superior Colliculus
Reticular Formation
Pedunculopontine N.
Glutamate
GABA
P
ENK/D2
Put
STN
GPe
GPi
SNC
O
SP/DYN/D1
SNR
T
Acb
A
HYPERKINESIA
PFC
output
MC
sc
Thalamus
VA / VL / MD
Caud
dopamine
Superior Colliculus
Reticular Formation
Pedunculopontine N.
Glutamate
GABA
P
ENK/D2
Put
STN
GPe
GPi
SNC
O
SP/DYN/D1
SNR
T
Acb
B

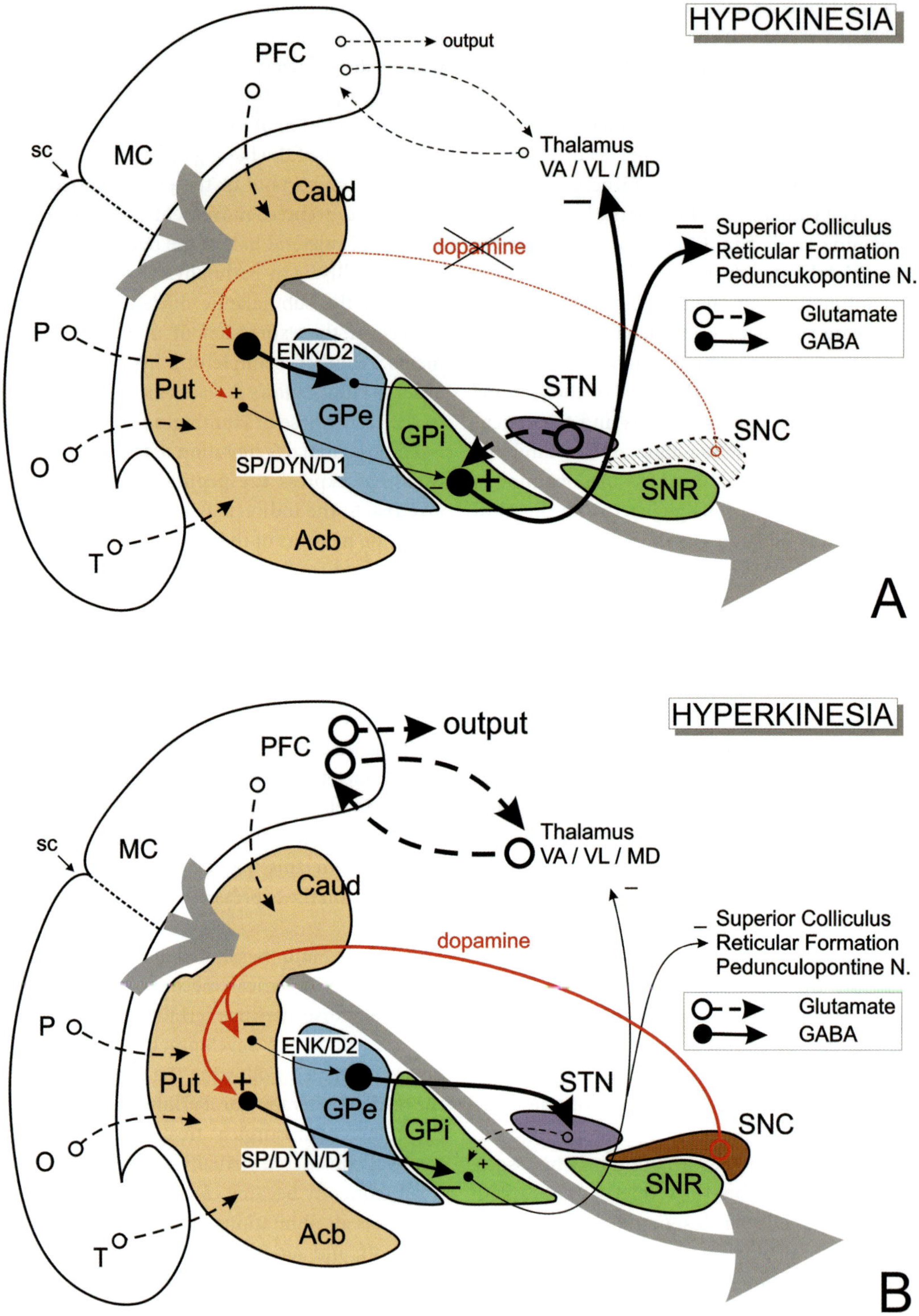

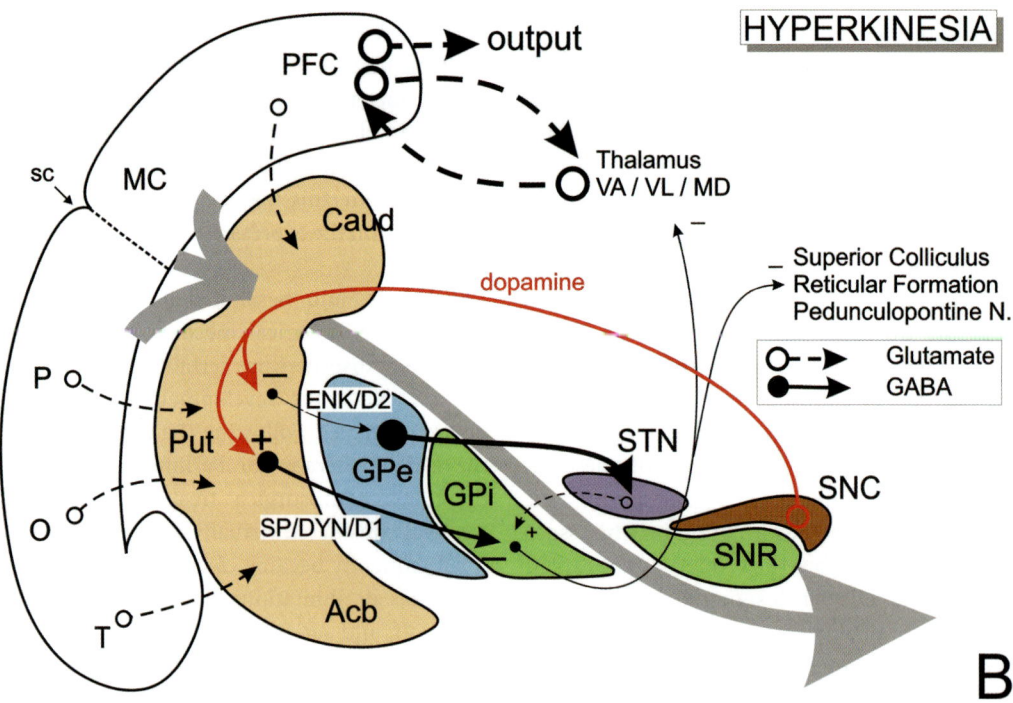

disease was made by Bergman et al. (93), who lesioned the pathologically active subthalamic nucleus in the MPTP primate model of Parkinson's disease and showed a substantial improvement of the parkinsonian symptoms. Subsequently, the neurosurgical approach in Parkinson's disease underwent a revival by employing *lesions* of specific parts of the globus pallidus, mimicking the early approaches in the 1950s and 1960s by Hassler (94), and of the subthalamic nucleus. At present, the lesion technique has been almost completely replaced by deep brain stimulation since this is in principle a reversible approach

that allows stimulation parameters to be adjusted according to the individual effects in the patient. The preferred target for deep brain stimulation in Parkinson's disease patients is now the subthalamic nucleus, although other targets, like the globus pallidus, are still used as well. In addition, new targets are being explored, such as the pedunculopontine nucleus in the brainstem (95). Although stimulation of the subthalamic nucleus has positive effects on bradykinesia and hypokinesia as well as on tremor and rigidity in Parkinson's disease patients, side effects have also been reported. The most prominent ones are the effects of subthalamic stimulation on cognition and affect (96). Such side effects may be explained by the fact that the medial parts of the subthalamic nucleus are involved in associative and limbic circuits rather than sensorimotor circuits (29,55).

Figure 2.10

Schematic representation of the pathophysiological basis of (A) a hypokinetic movement disorder (Parkinson's disease) and (B) a hyperkinetic movement disorder (e.g. early stage of Huntington's disease).

A. Degeneration of the dopaminergic system results in a decreased inhibition at the level of the output structures of the basal ganglia (GPi and SNR) by the direct route and in an increased excitation by the indirect route. Consequently, the target areas of the basal ganglia in the thalamus and the brainstem receive a stronger inhibitory input. Consequently, thalamocortical activity and the cortical output are greatly reduced.

B. In an early stage of Huntington's disease, the striatal neurons giving rise to the indirect output pathway, i.e., the enkephalin-expressing neurons, are more strongly affected than the substance P-expressing neurons (114). Consequently, there is a decreased inhibition of the tonically active neurons of the external segment of the globus pallidus and, subsequently, an increased inhibition of the subthalamic neurons. As a result, the neurons of the internal segment of the globus pallidus and the substantia nigra pars reticulata will be less excited, which leads to a lesser inhibition of the thalamic and brainstem targets of the basal ganglia. As a consequence, thalamocortical activity and cortical output are higher than normal.

Abbreviations: Acb, nucleus accumbens; Caud, caudate nucleus; GPe, external segment of the globus pallidus; GPi, internal segment of the globus pallidus; MC, primary motor cortex; MD, mediodorsal thalamic nucleus; O, occipital cortex; P, parietal cortex, PFC, prefrontal cortex; Put, putamen; sc, central sulcus; SNC, substantia nigra, pars compacta; SNR, substantia nigra, pars reticulata; STN, subthalamic nucleus; T, temporal cortex; VA, ventral anterior thalamic nucleus; VL, ventral lateral thalamic nucleus.

References

1 Nieuwenhuys R, Voogd J, Van Huijzen Chr. The Human Central Nervous System. A Synopis and Atlas. 4th Revised Edition. Heidelberg: Springer-Verlag; 2008.

2 Sakamoto N, Pearson J, Shinoda K, Alheid GF, De Olmos JS. Heimer L. The human basal forebrain. Part I. In: Bloom FE, Björklund A, Hökfelt T, eds. Handbook of Chemical Neuroanatomy, Vol.15. The Primate Nervous System. Part III. Amsterdam, Elsevier; 1999. p. 1-55.

3 Heimer L, de Olmos JS, Alheid GF, Pearson J, Sakamoto N, Shinoda K, Marksteiner J, Switzer III RC. The human basal forebrain. Part II. In Bloom FE, Björklund A, Hökfelt T, eds. Handbook of Chemical Neuroanatomy, Vol.15. The Primate Nervous System. Part III. Amsterdam: Elsevier; 1999. p. 57-226.

4 Heimer L, Harlan RE, Alheid GF, Garcia MM, de Olmos J. Substantia innominata: a notion which impedes clinical-anatomical correlations in neuropsychiatric disorders. Neuroscience 1997;76:957-1006.

5 Parent A, Cote PY, Lavoie B. Chemical anatomy of primate basal ganglia. Prog Neurobiol. 1995;46:131-197.

6   Parent A, Hazrati L-N. Functional anatomy of the basal ganglia. I. The cortico-basal ganglia-thalamo-cortical loop. Brain Res Rev. 1995;20:91-127.

7   Wise SP, Murray EA, Gerfen CR. The frontal cortex-basal ganglia system in primates. Crit Rev Neurobiol. 1996;10:317-356.

8   Gerfen CR. Basal ganglia. In: Paxinos G, ed. The Rat Nervous System. Third Edition. Elsevier: Amsterdam; 2004. p. 455-508.

9   Haynes WIA, Haber SN. The organization of prefrontal-subthalamic inputs in primates provides an anatomical substrate for both functional specificity and integration: implications for basal ganlia models and deep brain stimulation. J Neurosci. 2013;33:4804-4814.

10 Bolam JP, Hanley, JJ, Booth PAC, Bevan MD. Synaptic organisation of the basal ganglia. J Anat. 2000;196:527-542.

11 Parent A, Hazrati L-N. Functional anatomy of the basal ganglia. II. The place of subthalamic nucleus and external pallidum in basal ganglia circuitry. Brain Res Rev. 1995;20:128-154.

12 DiFiglia M, Pasik P, Pasik T. A Golgi study of neuronal types in the neostriatum of monkeys. Brain Res. 1976;114:245-256.

13 Smith AD, Bolam JP. The neural network of the basal ganglia as revealed by the study of synaptic connections of identified neurones. Trends Neurosci. 1990;13:259-265.

14 Tepper JM, Koos T, Wilson CJ (2004) GABAergic microcircuits in the neostriatum. Trends Neurosci. 2004;27:662-669.

15 Cragg SJ. Meaningful silences: how dopamine listens to the Ach pause. Trends Neurosci. 2006;29:125-131.

16 Wilson CJ. The generation of natural firing patterns in neostriatal neurons. Progr Brain Res. 1993;99:277-297.

17 Houk JC. Information processing in modular circuits linking basal ganglia and cerbral cortex. In: Houk JC, Davis JL, Beiser DG, eds. Models of Information Processing in the Basal Ganglia. Cambridge: MIT Press; 1995. p. 3-9.

18 Haber SN, Fudge JL, McFarland NR. Striatoni-grostriatal pathways in primates form an ascending spiral from the shell to the dorsolateral striatum. J Neurosci. 2000;20:2369-2382.

19 Groenewegen HJ, Wright CI, Beijer AVJ. The nucleus accumbens: gateway for limbic structures to reach the motor system? Prog Brain Res. 1996;107:485-511.

20 Berridge CW, Stratford TL, Foote SL, Kelley AE. Distribution of dopamine beta-hydroxylase-like immunoreactive fibers within the shell subregion of the nucleus accumbens. Synapse. 1997;27:230-241.

21 Feekes JA, Cassell MD. The vascular supply of the functional compartments of the human striatum. Brain 2006;129:2189-2201.

22 Gerfen CR, Ssurmeier DJ. Modulation of strital projection systems by dopamine. Annu Rev Neurosci. 2011;34:441-466.

23 Albin RL, Young AB, Penney JB. The functional anatomy of basal ganglia disorders. Trends Neurosci. 1989;12:366-375.

24 DeLong MR. Primate models of movement disorders of basal ganglia origin. Trends Neurosci. 1990;13:281-285.

25 Mink JW, Thach WT. Basal ganglia motor control. II. Late pallidal timing relative to movement onset and inconsistent pallidal coding of movement parameters. J Neurophysiol. 1991;65:301-329.

26 Zahm DS, Brog JS. On the significance of subterritories in the "accumbens" part of the rat ventral striatum. Neuroscience. 1992;50:751-767.

27 Shink E, Bevan MD, Bolam JP, Smith Y. The subthalamic nucleus and the external pallidum: two tightly interconnected structures that control the output of the basal ganglia in the monkey. Neuroscience. 1996;73:335-357.

28 Mink JW. The basal ganglia: focused selection and inhibition of competing motor programs. Prog Neurobiol. 1996;50:381-425.

29 Temel Y, Blokland A, Steinbusch HW, Visser-Vandewalle V. The functional role of the subthalamic nucleus in cognitive and limbic circuits. Prog Neurobiol. 2005;76:393-413.

30 Coizet V, Graham JH, Moss J, Bolam JP, Savasta M, McHaffie JG, Redgrave P, Overton PG. Short-latency visual input to the subthalamic nucleus is provided by the midbrain superior colliculus. J Neurosci. 2009;29:5701-5709.

31 Deniau JM, Chevalier G. The lamellar organization of the rat substantia nigra pars reticulata: distribution of projection neurons. Neuroscience 1992;46:361-377.

32 Domburg PH, ten Donkelaar HJ. The human substantia nigra and ventral tegmental area. A neuroanatomical study with notes on aging and aging diseases. Adv Anat Embryol Cell Biol. 1991;121:1-132.

33 Carr DB, Sesack SR. GABA-containing neurons in the ventral tegmental area project to the prefrontal cortex. Synapse. 2000;38:114-123.

34 Chuhma N, Zhang H, Masson J, Zhuang X, Sulzer D, Hen R, Rayport S. Dopamine neurons mediate fast excitatory signal via their glutamatergic synapses. J Neurosci. 2004;24:972-981.

35 Eblen F, Graybiel AM. Highly restricted origin of prefrontal cortical inputs to striosomes in the macaque monkey. J Neurosci. 1995;15:5999-6013.

36 Berendse HW, Galis-de Graaf Y, Groenewegen HJ. Topographical organization and relationship with ventral striatal compartments of prefrontal corticostriatal projections in the rat. J Comp Neurol. 1992;316:314-347.

37 Mena-Segovia J, Bolam JP, Magill PJ. Pedunculopontine nucleus and basal ganglia: distant relatives or part of the same family? Trends Neurosci. 2004;27:585-588.

38 Comoli E, Coizet V, Boyes J, Bolam JP, Canteras NS, Quirk RH, Overton PG, Redgrave P. A direct projection from superior colliculus to substantia nigra for detecting salient visual signals. Nat Neurosci. 2003;6:974-980.

39 Schultz W, Apicella P, Ljungberg T. Responses of monkey dopamine neurons to reward and conditioned stimuli during successive steps of learning a delayed response task. J Neurosci. 1993;13:900-913.

40 Schultz W, Romo R, Ljungberg T, Mirenowicz J, Hollerman JR, Dickinson A. Reward-related signals carried by dopamine neurons. In: Houk JC, Davis JL, Beiser DG, eds. Models of Information Processing in the Basal Ganglia. Cambridge: MIT Press; 1995. p. 233-248.

41 Benarroch EE. Pedunculopontine nucleus. Functional organization and clinical implications. Neurology 2013;80:1148-1155.

42 Winn P. How to best consider the structure and function of the pedunculopontine tegmental nucleus: evidence from animal studies. J Neurol Sci. 2006;248:234-250.

43 Heimer L, Wilson RD. The subcortical projections of the allocortex: similarities in the neural associations of the hippocampus, the piriform cortex, and the neocortex. In: Santini M, ed. Golgi Centennial Symposium: Perspectives in Neurobiology. New York: Raven Press; 1975. p. 177-193.

44 Alexander GE, DeLong MR, Strick PL. Parallel organization of functionally segregated circuits linking basal ganglia and cortex. Ann Rev Neurosci. 1986;9:357-381.

45 Bornstein AM, Daw ND. Multiplicity of control in the basal ganglia: Computational roles of striatal subregions. Curr Opin Neurobiol. 2011;21:374-380.

46 Voorn P, Vanderschuren LJ, Groenewegen HJ, Robbins TW, Pennartz CM. Putting a spin on the dorsal-ventral divide of the striatum. Trends Neurosci. 2004;27:468-474.

47 Fudge JL, Haber SN. Defining the caudal ventral striatum in primates: cellular and histochemical features. J Neurosci. 2002;22:1078-1082.

48 Zaborszky L, Alheid GF, Beinfeld MC, Eiden LE, Heimer L, Palkovits M. Cholecystokinin innervation of the ventral striatum: a morphological and radioimmunological study. Neuroscience. 1985;4:427-453.

49 Meredith GE, Pattiselanno A, Groenewegen HJ, Haber SN. Shell and core in monkey and human nucleus accumbens identified with antibodies to calbindin-D28k. J Comp Neurol. 1996;365:628-639.

50 Voorn P, Brady LS, Berendse HW, Richfield EK. Densitometrical analysis of opioid receptor ligand binding in the human striatum--I. Distribution of mu opioid receptor defines shell and core of the ventral striatum. Neuroscience. 1996;75:777-792.

51 Berendse HW, Richfield EK. Heterogeneous distribution of dopamine D1 and D2 receptors in the human ventral striatum. Neurosci Lett. 1993;150:75-79.

52 Joyce JN, Gurevich EV. D3 receptors and the actions of neuroleptics in the ventral striatopallidal system of schizophrenics. Ann N Y Acad Sci. 1999;877:595-613.

53 Haber SN, Wolfe DP, Groenewegen HJ. The relationship between ventral striatal efferent fibers and the distribution of peptide-positive woolly fibers in the forebrain of the rhesus monkey. Neuroscience. 1990;39:323-338.

54 Deniau JM, Menetrey A, Thierry AM. Indirect nucleus accumbens input to the prefrontal cortex via the substantia nigra pars reticulata: a combined anatomical and electrophysiological study in the rat. Neuroscience. 1994;61:533-545.

55 Groenewegen HJ, Berendse HW. Connections of the subthalamic nucleus with ventral striatopallidal parts of the basal ganglia in the rat. J Comp Neurol. 1990;294:607-622.

56 Ferry AT, Ongur D, An X, Price JL. Prefrontal cortical projections to the striatum in macaque monkeys: evidence for an organization related to prefrontal networks. J Comp Neurol. 2000;425:447-470.

57 Groenewegen HJ, Van den Heuvel OA, Cath DC, Voorn P, Veltman DJ. Does an imbalance between the dorsal and ventral striatopallidal systems play a role in Tourette's Syndrome? A neuronal circuit approach. Brain Dev.. 2003;25:S3-S14.

58 Mogenson GJ, Jones DL, Yim CY. From motivation to action: functional interface between the limbic system and the motor system. Prog Neurobiol. 1980;14:69-97.

59 Humphries MD, Prescott TJ. The ventral basal ganglia, a selection mechanism at the crossroads of space, strategy, and reward. Prog Neurobiol. 2010;90:385-417.

60 Kelley AE. Ventral striatal control of appetitive motivation: role in ingestive behavior and reward-related learning. Neurosci Biobeh Rev. 2004;27:765-776.

61 Reynolds SM, Berridge KC. Positive and negative motivation in nucleus accumbens shell: bivalent rostrocaudal gradients for GABA-elicited eating, taste "liking"/"disliking" reactions, place preference/avoidance, and fear. J Neurosci. 2002;22:7308-7320.

62 Cardinal RN, Parkinson JA, Hall J, Everitt BJ. Emotion and motivation: the role of the amygdala, ventral striatum, and prefrontal cortex. Neurosci Biobeh Rev. 2002;26:321-352.

63 Parkinson JA, Olmstead MC, Burns LH, Robbins TW, Everitt BJ. Dissociation in effects of lesions of the nucleus accumbens core and shell on appetitive pavlovian approach behavior and the potentiation of conditioned reinforcement and locomotor activity by D-amphetamine. J Neurosci. 1999;19:2401-2411.

64 Corbit LH, Muir JL, Balleine BW. The role of the nucleus accumbens in instrumental conditioning: Evidence of a functional dissociation between accumbens core and shell. J Neurosci. 2001;21:3251-3260.

65 Di Chiara G. Nucleus accumbens shell and core dopamine: differential role in behavior and addiction. Behav Brain Res. 2002;137:75-114.

66 Ito R, Robbins TW, Everitt BJ. Differential control over cocaine-seeking behavior by nucleus accumbens core and shell. Nat Neurosci. 2004;7:389-397.

67 Sturm V, Lenartz D, Koulousakis A, Treuer H, Herholz K, Klein JC, Klosterkotter J. The nucleus accumbens: a target for deep brain stimulation in obsessive-compulsive- and anxiety-disorders. J Chem Neuroanat. 2003;26:293-299.

68 Denys D, Mantione M, Figee M, Van den Munchof P, Koerselman F, Westenberg H, Bosch A, Schuurman R. Deep brain stimulation of the nucleus accumbens for treatment-refractory obsessive-compulsive disorder. Arch Gen Psychiatry 2010;67:1061-1068.

69 Nauta WJH, Mehler WR. Projections of the lentiform nucleus in the monkey. Brain Res. 1966;1:3-42.

70 Groenewegen HJ, Berendse HW, Wolters JG, Lohman AHM. The anatomical relationship of the prefrontal cortex with the striatopallidal system, the thalamus and the amygdala: evidence for a parallel organization. Prog Brain Res. 1990;85:95-118.

71 Alexander GE, Crutcher MD. Functional architecture of basal ganglia circuits: neural substrates of parallel processing. Trends Neurosci. 1990;13:266-271.

72 Chevalier G, Deniau JM. Disinhibition as a basic process in the expression of striatal functions. Trends Neurosci. 1990;13:277-280.

73 Wall NR, De la Parra M, Callaway EM, Kreitzer AC. Differential innervation of direct- and indirect-pathway striatal projection neurons. Neuron 2013;79:1-14.

74 Redgrave P, Prescott TJ, Gurney K. The basal ganglia: a vertebrate solution to the selection problem? Neuroscience. 1999;89:1009-1023.

75 Mouroux M, Hassani OK, Feger J. Electrophysiological and Fos immunohistochemical evidence for the excitatory nature of the parafascicular projection to the globus pallidus. Neuroscience. 1997;81:387-397.

76 Van der Werf YD, Witter MP, Groenewegen HJ. The intralaminar and midline nuclei of the thalamus. Anatomical and functional evidence for participation in processes of arousal and awareness. Brain Res Rev. 2002;39:107-140.

77 Smith Y, Raju DV, Pare JF, Sibide M. The thalamostriatal system: a higly specific network of the basal ganglia circuitry. Trends Neurosci. 2004;27:520-527.

78 McHaffie JG, Stanford TR, Stein BE, Coizet V, Redgrave P. Subcortical loops through the basal ganglia. Trends Neurosci. 2005;28:401-407.

79 Joel D, Weiner I. The organization of the basal ganglia-thalamocortical circuits: Open interconnected rather than closed segregated. Neuroscience. 1994;63:363-379.

80 Corbit LH, Muir JL, Balleine BW. The role of the nucleus accumbens in instrumental conditioning : Evidence for a functional dissociation between accumbens core and shell. J Neurosci. 2001;21:3251-3260.

81 Groenewegen HJ, Berendse HW and Wouterlood FG. Organization of the projections from the ventral striatopallidal system to ventral mesencephalic dopaminergic neurons. In: Percheron G, McKenzie JS, eds. The Basal Ganglia IV. New York: Plenum Press; 1994. p. 81-93.

82 Maurin Y, Banrezes B, Menetrey A, Mailly P, Deniau JM. Three-dimensional distribution of nigrostriatal neurons in the rat: relation to the topography of striatonigral projections. Neuroscience. 1999;91:891-909.

83 Sesack SR, Grace AA. Cortico-basal ganglia reward network: microcircuitry. Neuropsychopharmacology 2010;35:27-47.

84 Packard MG, Knowlton BJ. Learning and memory functions of the Basal Ganglia. Annu Rev Neurosci. 2002;25:563-593.

85 Devan BD, White NM. Parallel information processing in the dorsal striatum: relation to hippocampal function. J Neurosci. 1999;19:2789-2798.

86 Robbins TW, Everitt BJ. Neurobehavioural mechanisms of reward and motivation. Curr Opin Neurobiol. 1996;6:228-236.

87 Pennartz CMA, Groenewegen HJ, Lopes da Silva FH. The nucleus accumbens as a complex of functionally distinct neuronal ensembles: an integration of behavioural, electrophysiological and anatomical data. Progr Neurobiol. 1994;42:719-761.

88 Redgrave P, Gurney K. The short-latency dopamine signal: a rol in discovering novel actions? Nat Rev Neurosci. 2006;7:967-975.

89 Suri RE, Schultz W. Learning of sequential movements by neural network model with dopamine-like reinforcement signal. Exp Brain Res. 1998;121:350-354.

90 Marsden CD, Obeso JA. The functions of the basal ganglia and the paradox of stereotaxic surgery in Parkinson's disease. Brain. 1994;117:877-897.

91 Obeso JA, Rodriguez-Oroz MC, Rodriguez M, Lanciego JL, Artieda J, Gonzalo N, Olanow CW. Pathophysiology of the basal ganglia in Parkinson's disease. Trends Neurosci. 2000;23(S10):8-19.

92 Richfield EK, Maguire-Zeiss KA, Vonkeman HE, Voorn P. Preferential loss of preproenkephalin versus preprotachykinin neurons from the striatum of Huntington's patients. Ann Neurol. 1995;38:852-861.

93 Bergman H, Wichmann T, DeLong MR. Reversal of experimental parkinsonism by lesions of the subthalamic nucleus. Science. 1990;249:1436-1438.

94 Laitinen LV. Ventroposterolateral pallidotomy. Stereotact Funct Neurosurg. 1994;62:41-52.

95 Temel Y, Visser-Vandewalle V. Targets for deep brain stimulation in Parkinson's disease. Expert Opin Ther Targets. 2006;10:355-362.

96 Temel Y, Kessels A, Tan S, Topdag A, Boon P, Visser-Vandewalle V. Behavioural changes after bilateral subthalamic stimulation in advanced Parkinson's disease: a systematic review. Parkinsonism Relat Disord. 2006;12:265-272.

3
Role of the Cerebellum

Tom J.H. Ruigrok

The cerebellum, like the basal ganglia, is specifically involved in the proper execution of movement. However, aspects of movement execution governed by the cerebellum are clearly distinct from those controlled by the basal ganglia. Lesions of the cerebellum, or of its afferent or efferent fibre systems, usually result in more or less specific problems that concern the timely initiation and coordination of composite movements (ataxia), in intention tremors, and in the adaptation and learning of movements. As such, the cerebellum seems particularly critical for the execution of fine and precise movements. Several lines of research show that the cerebellum may also be involved in autonomic, affective and cognitive processes, again like the basal ganglia. Because the movement control by both the basal ganglia and the cerebellum is to a large extent imposed upon the motor and pre-motor cortices and their control over the pyramidal tract, it might be expected that dysfunction of one system will affect the control exerted by the other system. Indeed, the potential interaction between the two systems in clinical manifestations such as tremor has recently received more attention (1,2). Yet as studies dealing with the interactions between both systems are still only beginning (3,4), basal ganglia and cerebellar disorders are usually studied independently of one another. This chapter, therefore, will mostly focus on the main characteristics of the cerebellar anatomy and its function in movement control without implicit reference to the basal ganglia.

Macroscopic anatomy

The cerebellum lies in the posterior fossa of the skull base. Its rostral part forms the roof of the fourth ventricle while its caudal part overhangs the caudal half of the ventricle (see Figure 3.1). It consists of an outwardly positioned cortex, which is characterized by highly structured and organized lobulations due to many transverse fissures. Lobules are further extensively subdivided into folia, resulting in a huge increase of surface area. This remarkable architectonic pattern of the cerebellum can be particularly appreciated when studying the mid-sagittal plane (see Figure 3.1C).

From this plane, the division of the cerebellum into an anterior and larger, posterior lobe by the very deep primary fissure is also quite obvious. Anterior and posterior lobes each consist of essentially five main lobules, which all radiate outward like the spokes of a wheel. Each lobule is subdivided into many folia by multiple, transversally oriented fissures.

From a dorsal and caudal view, the division of the cerebellum by two parasagittal grooves can be clearly recognized. These grooves separate the centrally positioned vermis (worm) from both hemispheres (Figure 3.1A, B). Note that these grooves are less prominent in the anterior lobe. Between the vermis and the hemisphere, a paravermal or intermediate cerebellum is frequently delineated. The complex morphology of the human cerebellum is best understood when following the comparative anatomical description

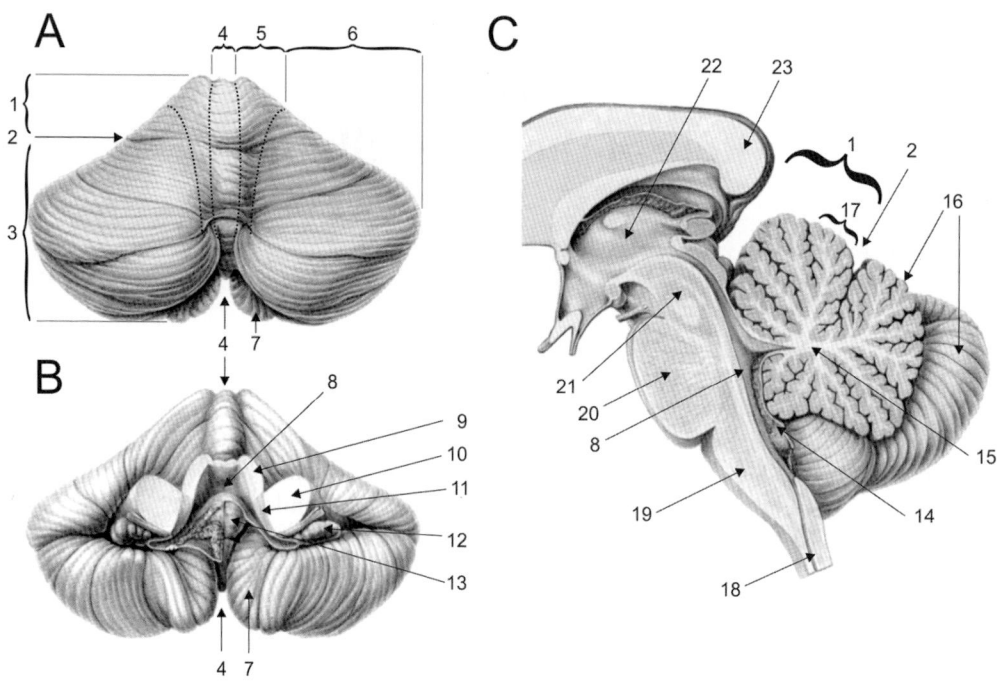

Figure 3.1

Macroscopic views of the human cerebellum. A: dorsal view; B: ventral view with cut cerebellar peduncles; C: midsagittal view and relation with the brainstem. Modified after (101).

1 anterior lobe	8 fourth ventricle	12 flocculus	19 medulla oblongata
2 primary fissure	9 superior cerebellar	13 nodulus	20 pons
3 posterior lobe	peduncle	14 choroid plexus	21 mesencephalon
4 vermis	10 middle cerebellar	15 white matter	22 third ventricle
5 paravermis	peduncle	16 cerebellar folium	23 corpus callosum
6 hemisphere	11 inferior cerebellar	17 cerebellar lobule	
7 tonsilla	peduncle	18 spinal cord	

of the Dutch anatomist Lodewijk Bolk (5). After comparing the cerebella of many mammals, he came to the conclusion that the hemispheral lobules diverge from the vermal ones at two places, thereby forming two laterally protruding loops (see Figure 3.2). The first one, essentially consisting of the hemisphere of lobule VII, includes most of the human superior and inferior semilunar lobules, which in most mammals are referred to as the crura of the ansiform lobule. The hemispheral part of lobule VIII is closely related to the vermal cortex and was named the paramedian lobule by Bolk. It is thought to be homologous to the gracile lobule of the human cerebellum. The second outward loop of the cer-

ebellar cortex begins with the copula pyramidis (hemisphere of the caudal part of lobule VIII) and continues as the dorsal and ventral paraflocculus, which should be homologous to the biventer and tonsillar lobules in man. Finally, the hemisphere of lobule X, the flocculus, is still discontinuous with the vermal nodulus. An excellent and detailed account of the human cerebellar morphology and the homologies between various cerebellar nomenclatures used in the literature has been provided by Schmahman (6); see also (7).

The cerebellar cortex consists of three cytoarchitectonic layers: the most prominent ones are an

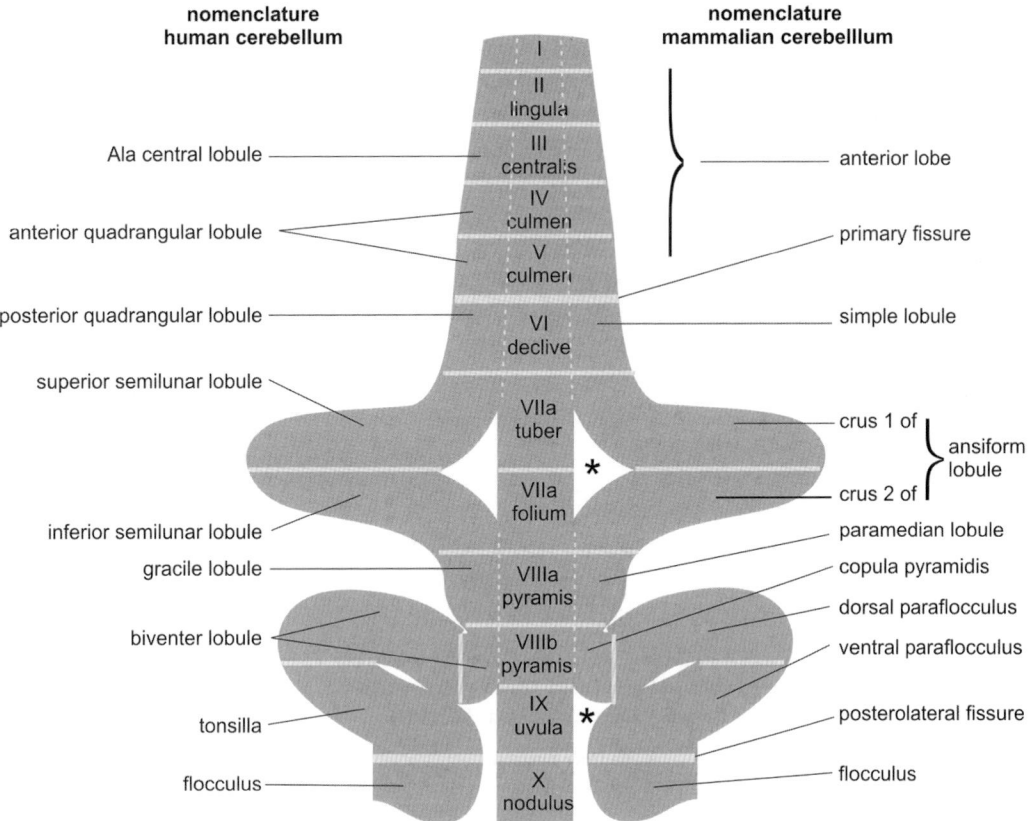

nomenclature human cerebellum

nomenclature mammalian cerebelllum

I

II
lingula

Ala central lobule — III centralis — anterior lobe

IV culmen

anterior quadrangular lobule — V culmen — primary fissure

posterior quadrangular lobule — VI declive — simple lobule

superior semilunar lobule — VIIa tuber — crus 1 of

*

VIIa folium — crus 2 of — ansiform lobule

inferior semilunar lobule — paramedian lobule

gracile lobule — VIIIa pyramis — copula pyramidis

dorsal paraflocculus

biventer lobule — VIIIb pyramis — ventral paraflocculus

tonsilla — IX uvula * — posterolateral fissure

flocculus — X nodulus — flocculus

Figure 3.2
Schematic diagram of the unfolded cerebellar cortex with the conventional human nomenclature of human cerebellar divisions on the left-hand side (102) and the cerebellar nomenclature as based on the comparative anatomy of mammalian cerebella by Bolk on the right-hand side (5). Asterisks denote discontinuity of the cortex between the vermal and hemispheral sheets, which was stressed in the work of Bolk.

outward and relatively cell-poor region, which constitutes the molecular layer, and a very cell-dense granular layer. In between these layers a monolayer with large cells is found, which are the cell bodies of the so-called Purkinje cells (named after their Czech discoverer, Jan Purkyně). Below the granular layer the efferent and afferent fibres of the cortex form the white matter. Deep in the white matter, on either side of the midline, groupings of neurons form the cerebellar nuclei. These nuclei receive the output from the cerebellar cortex and constitute the main source of cerebellar output. They consist of four pairs of nuclei: the medially positioned fastigial nucleus and laterally the conspicuously shaped dentate

nucleus are easily recognized. Two interposed nuclei are located between them, which in man are called the globose and the emboliform nuclei positioned somewhat rostrolateral to it (see Figure 3.3).

The cerebellum communicates with the rest of the nervous system by means of three fibre bundles. The restiform body (inferior cerebellar peduncle) consists of various sources of input originating in the spinal cord and lower brainstem. The brachium pontis (middle cerebellar peduncle) contains cerebellar afferent fibres that originate in the pontine nuclei. Finally, the brachium conjunctivum (superior cerebellar peduncle)

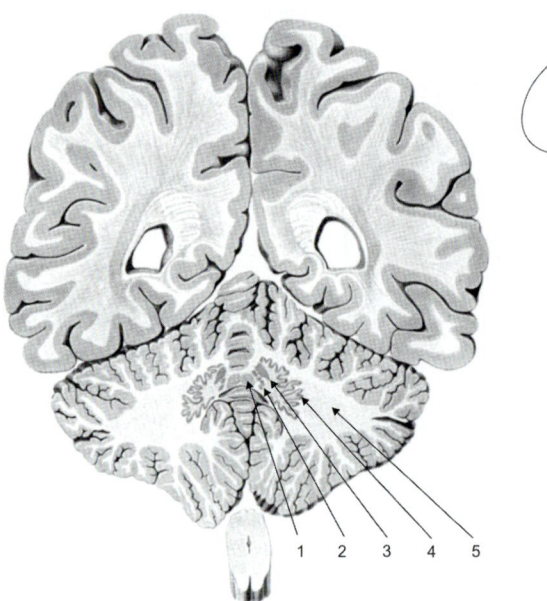

as spinocerebellum, mostly receives input of a somatosensory nature and seems to be involved in controlling and adjusting ongoing movements. Finally, the hemispherical parts of the cerebellum, hugely proliferated in man, are of a much younger phylogenetic date and, due to their close relations with the cerebrum, are referred to as cerebrocerebellum.

Figure 3.3
Coronal slice (see inset) through the posterior part of the cerebrum, the cerebellum and junction between medulla and spinal cord. The cerebellar nuclei are located in the center of the cerebellar white matter. Modified after (101).

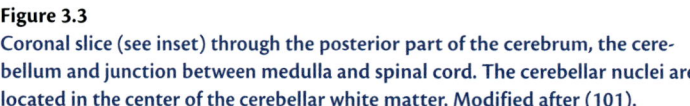

1 fastigial nucleus
2 globose nucleus
3 emboliform nucleus

4 dentate nucleus
5 white matter

Microscopic anatomy

The microscopic anatomy of the cerebellar cortex is very homogenous throughout all cortical regions, thereby contrasting the clear differences noted in the cerebral cortex (i.e. Brodmann's areas). Only five major cell types are found within the three layers of the cerebellar cortex. Purkinje cells provide the output of the cortex and are located in a monolayer; huge numbers of very small granule cells (they constitute the most abundant cell type of the nervous system) are located in the granular layer in which Golgi cells are also found. The molecular layer harbors the stellate and basket cells. Four of the five main cell types, i.e. Purkinje, Golgi, stellate and basket cells, make use of the inhibitory transmitter gamma-aminobutyric acid (GABA); most Golgi cells also use glycine (8). Granule cells are glutamatergic and therefore excite their targets.

encloses the efferent fibres from the cerebellar nuclei towards the brainstem and thalamus (see Figure 3.1B). In addition to the main cerebellar peduncles, there are connections from the fastigial (i.e. the uncinate tract) and vestibulocerebellum that connect more diffusely to the vestibular nuclei, which are found on either side of the fourth ventricle in the dorsal medulla.

The caudal-most vermal and hemispheral lobuli (i.e. the nodulus and flocculus), both located completely under (i.e. ventrally of) the cerebellum due to its strong curvature, are seen as the oldest parts of the cerebellum. Because both parts mostly process vestibular (and to some extent visual) information and their output is specifically directed to the vestibular nuclei, they are collectively known as the vestibulocerebellum. The remaining part of the vermis and the paravermal regions, often referred to

The morphology of and the basic connections between these cell types demonstrate an architectural regularity that was already recognized more than a century ago by Santiago Ramon y Cajal (9). The dendrites of the Purkinje cells show complex branching patterns within the molecular layer reaching the subpial surface. However, the whole dendritic tree is extremely flattened in the parasagittal direction, resulting in a fan-like overall shape. Moreover, they are studded with spines (see Figure 3.4A,B). The spines are contacted by the axons of the granule cells. Their axons travel from the granular layer into the molecular layer where they bifurcate and form the parallel fibres. Each collateral runs in the transverse direction, parallel to the surface and to the direction of the folial fissures for several millimeters, i.e. perpendicular to the orientation of the dendritic tree of the Purkinje cells. This orthogonal arrangement of Purkinje cell dendrites and course of parallel fibres allow a single fibre to reach an optimal number of Purkinje cells. Conversely, individual Purkinje cells will receive input from huge numbers of different granule cells.

The input to the cerebellar cortex essentially consists of two types of afferents, each with a very different origin and mode of distribution. Quantitatively, the most abundant afferent system is formed by the mossy fibre system. Mossy fibres terminate in a characteristic grape-like arrangement of terminal boutons known as mossy fibre rosettes (see Figure 3.4E). These rosettes make excitatory contacts with the claw-like dendrites of the granule cells (see Figure 3.4C). Each granule cell contains three or four of these short dendrites which are each influenced by a single rosette. A single rosette may contact multiple granule cells, however. Mossy fibres find their origin in many areas of the brainstem and spinal cord. In man, the majority are derived from the basal pontine nuclei. A single granule cell can receive input from multiple mossy fibre sources (10).

The second type of afferent originates from the contralateral inferior olive and terminates in a very characteristic 'climbing' pattern within the dendritic tree of Purkinje cells. Every Purkinje cell receives input from only one such climbing fibre, and a single olivary neuron may provide about ten climbing fibres. A climbing fibre makes several hundred synaptic contacts with a single Purkinje cell (see Figure 3.4D). It is evident that the mossy and climbing fibre systems are very differently structured. Information carried by individual mossy fibres, by way of granule cells and their parallel fibres, will diverge over large areas of the cerebellar cortex, while the climbing fibre system is characterized by a converging pattern of organization (see Figure 3.5).

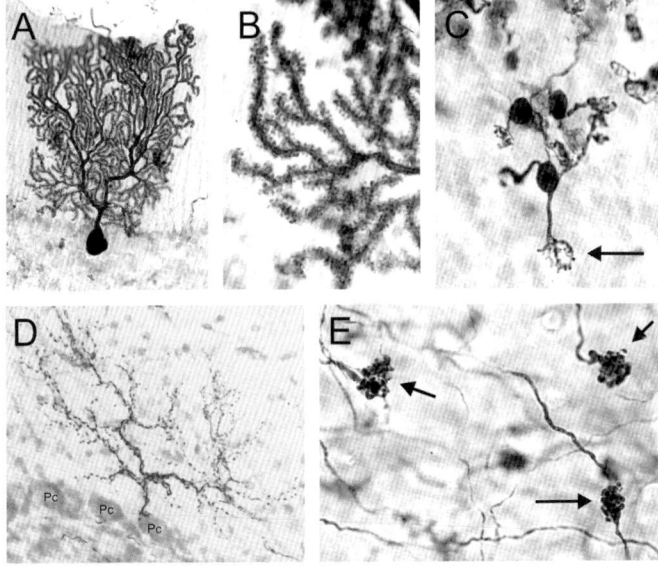

Figure 3.4
Cell and fibre types of the cerebellum, visualized with a neuroanatomical tracer (biotinylated dextran amine). A: Purkinje cell; B: detail of the dendritic tree of a Purkinje cell with its many spines, which receive the parallel fibre synapses; C: granule cells with their characteristic claw-shaped dendrites (arrow), upon which the mossy fibre rosettes terminate; D: climbing fibre terminal upon the dendritic tree of a single Purkinje cell (invisible). The somata of several Purkinje cells are indicated (Pc); E: mossy fibre rosettes in the granular layer (arrows).

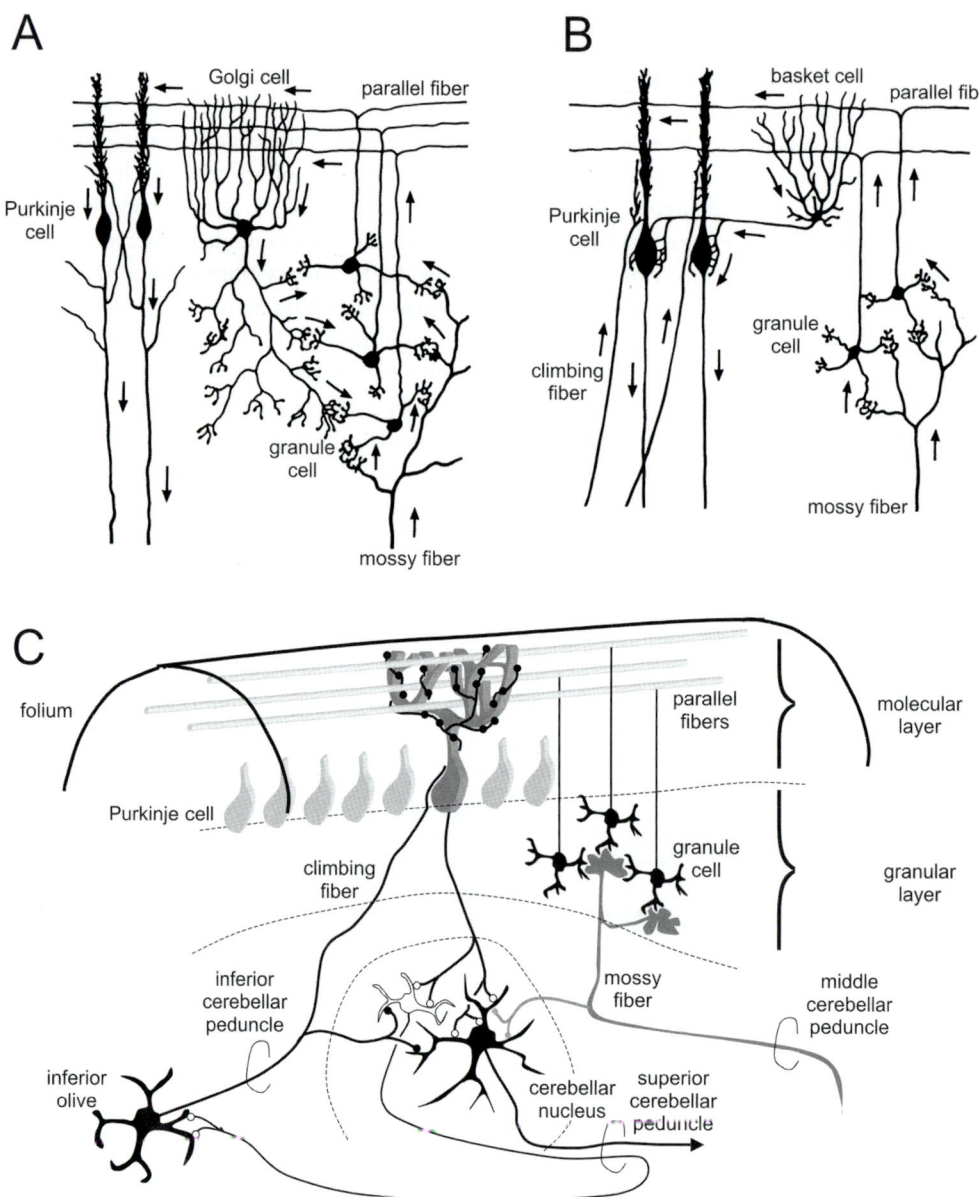

Figure 3.5
Cell types and connections in the cerebellum. A, B: classic drawings after Golgi material by Ramón y Cajal 9. Arrows in A indicate the information route from mossy fibres via granule cells and their parallel fibres to the Purkinje cell and their axons. Golgi cells form an inhibitory feedback loop from the parallel fibres to the granule cells. B: basket cells (like stellate cells, not shown), located in the molecular layer, also receive input from parallel fibres but form an inhibitory feedforward loop because they terminate upon the Purkinje cells. Climbing fibres are also shown in this scheme. C: diagram of the main circuits of the cerebellum. Information reaches the cerebellar cortex via mossy and climbing fibres. Mossy fibre input is distributed via their parallel fibres to many Purkinje cells. Every Purkinje cell receives only a single climbing fibre. Axons of the Purkinje cells make up the cortical output and terminate upon large, excitatory neurons that project to various places in the brainstem and thalamus, but also terminate upon small, GABAergic neurons that provide input to the inferior olive. Climbing and mossy fibres send collaterals to the cerebellar nuclei.

Moreover, the climbing fibre system is essentially arranged in the longitudinal plane, while the mossy fibre/parallel fibre system is predominantly arranged in the transverse plane (see below). The remarkable differences in the organizational principles of the mossy and climbing fibre systems are likely to form the foundation of cerebellar functioning.

The two distinct excitatory circuits that converge upon the Purkinje cells (i.e. mossy fibre-granule cell- Purkinje cell and climbing fibre-Purkinje cell) are curtailed by the inhibitory connections of the stellate, basket and Golgi cells. Stellate and basket cells form GABAergic connections with the dendrites and soma (basket cells) of the Purkinje cells, while the axon of Golgi cells may influence the efficacy of information transfer between the mossy fibre-granule cells. Figures 3.5A and B show diagrams of their basic connections within the cerebellar cortex. The inhibitory interneurons receive input from the parallel fibres, but some types may also be activated by climbing fibres (11-14) (not shown in Figure 3.5).

The output of the cerebellar cortex consists of the axons of the Purkinje cells and reaches the cerebellar nuclei and the vestibular nuclei for the vestibulocerebellum. Part of the lateral vermis of the anterior lobe terminates in the lateral vestibular nucleus (15,16). The cerebellar nuclei receive excitatory input from collaterals of both the mossy fibre and climbing fibre systems (see Figure 3.5C).

Because the intrinsic cortical circuitry is remarkably uniform in its distribution over the cerebellar cortex, it is likely that the specificity of cerebellar functioning depends on the organization of the afferent and efferent connections. Indeed, a strictly zonal pattern is very evident in the axonal projections of the Purkinje cells to the cerebellar nuclei (17). This zonal projection is precisely matched by the organization of climbing fibres to the Purkinje cells (18). Climbing fibres originating from specific homogenous parts of the inferior olive project to Purkinje cells that are arranged in a parasagittally organized strip. The Purkinje cells of such a strip project to a specific part of the cerebellar nuclei. As such, a number of olivo-cortico-nuclear modules have been recognized (19). The connections of the climbing fibres to the cerebellar nuclei and of GABAergic neurons in the cerebellar nuclei to the inferior olive completely adhere to this modular organization (18,20) (see Figure 3.6). The output of every module has a distinct distribution in the brainstem and thalamus by way of the participating part of the cerebellar nucleus (21). Modules may make use of similar information, at least partly, by the distribution of diverging mossy fibres input and the parallel fibres (22).

The modular construction of the cerebellum has been confirmed with physiological techniques that show that in certain regions of the cerebellar cortex, the receptive fields of Purkinje cells, induced by climbing fibres' activity, adhere to the boundaries of the anatomically defined modules (23). In addition, modules are also reflected in differences in the chemical identity within the cerebellar cortex. Zonal compartments based on the presence or absence of specific chemical markers such as 5'-nucleotidase, acetylcholine esterase, and aldolase c (zebrin) have been described and are reported to adhere to the anatomically defined modules (18,24,25).

The harmony in the anatomical, physiological and chemical properties of the Purkinje cells forms the basis of the hypothesis that cerebellar modules constitute the functional or operational units of the cerebellum (19,23,25).

Physiological properties of Purkinje cells

The Purkinje cell is generally considered the pivotal cell type of the cerebellum. Due to its size, the extraordinary geometry of its dendrites that integrate the activity of huge numbers of parallel fibres and that of a single climbing fibre, togeth-

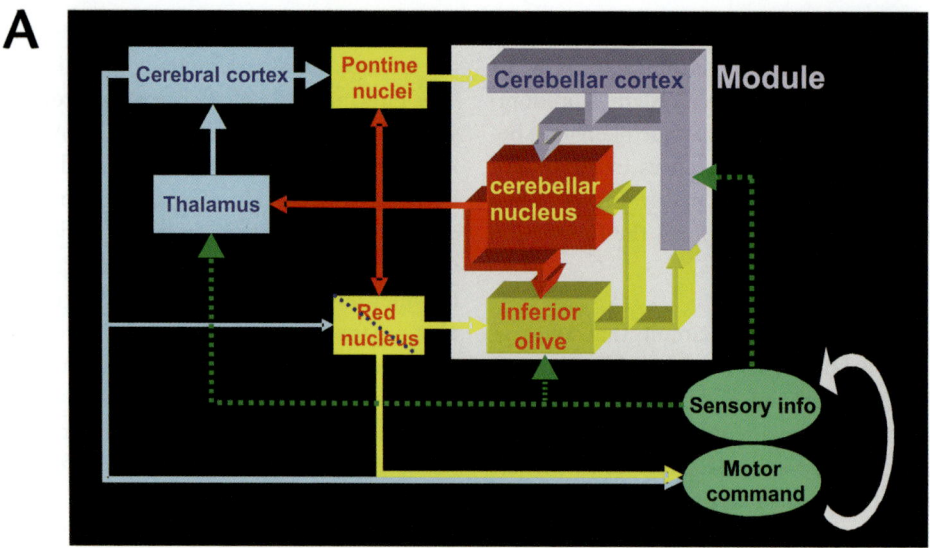

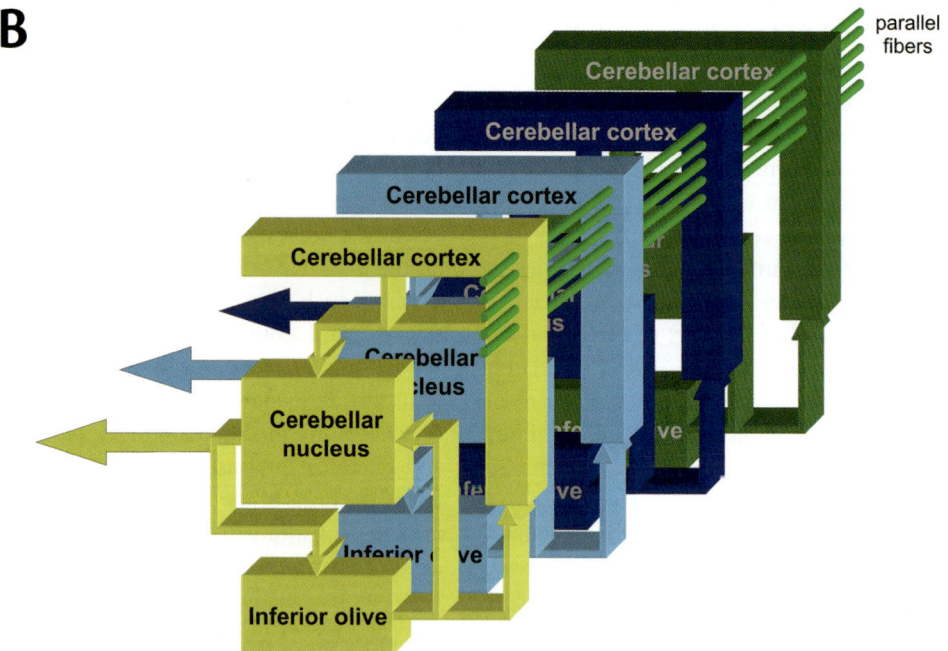

Figure 3.6
Schematic diagrams of the modular principle of cerebellar connections. A: a cerebellar module consists of a longitudinal strip of cortex. Purkinje cells of this strip receive their climbing fibres from a well-defined area of the inferior olive and send their axons to a specific part of the cerebellar nuclei. This modular circuitry is complemented by matching olivo-nuclear and nucleo-olivary connections. The output of such a module is characteristic and may comprise regions of the red nucleus, thalamus and pontine nuclei. B: the cerebellum may be interpreted as consisting of many parasagittally organized modules, each of them with their own characteristic output pattern and, hence, function. Connections between modules are formed by the mossy fibre/parallel fibre system.

er with the fact that they constitute the only efferent cell type of the cerebellar cortex, this has resulted in the view that they are at the center of cerebellar functioning (26,27). Studying the electrophysiology of Purkinje cells, in particular, has proven to be a rewarding topic of research. Their characteristic patterns of activity, which are easily recognized due to the large size of the cell body and the specific geometry of its dendrites, can be examined in anesthetized as well as non-anesthetized animals (11,28-30). However, Purkinje cells can also be studied in *in vitro* systems. They survive and can be studied for relatively long periods of time in cerebellar slices or even in whole brainstem-cerebellum preparations that are kept in oxygenated Ringer baths but are also amenable to culturing for several weeks (31-33). These techniques have enabled the execution and maintenance of intracellular or patch clamp registrations while influencing the extracellular or even intracellular pharmacological conditions of the recorded cell and have resulted in a virtual explosion of literature concerned with the physiology of Purkinje cells.

A key characteristic of Purkinje cell physiology is formed by the observation that its activation in response to parallel fibre activation differs from its activation due to climbing fibre discharges (34,35). The intimate synaptic arrangement of the climbing fibre with the Purkinje cell dendrite warrants that climbing fibre discharges result in a striking response of the postsynaptic membrane. Unfailingly, this will lead to the triggering of a relatively long-lasting dendritic spike, which depends on the opening of specific calcium channels present in the dendritic membrane. This calcium spike will be conducted towards the soma, where it results in the triggering of a short burst of four to six action potentials within a period of 10-15 msec. This burst of activity is very specific to Purkinje cells and is known as the complex spike. Under normal physiological conditions, climbing fibre-triggered complex spikes have an average frequency of 1-2 Hz, and even under specific conditions they will never exceed 8-10 Hz (e.g. see Figure 3.9). Purkinje cell activation by the mossy fibre/parallel fibre system results in the triggering of 'normal'-looking action potentials, known as simple spikes. The frequency of simple spike firing is usually quite high and may even exceed 100 Hz. Recent studies of Purkinje cell cultures have shown that so-called resurgent sodium currents, carried by a specific class of sodium channels, form the basis of these high states of firing. These currents enable Purkinje cells to fire even in the absence of synaptic input, i.e. these channels may cause Purkinje cells to be spontaneously active (36). How synaptic activity by parallel fibres interacts with spike formation due to the resurgent sodium currents is presently unclear. Despite many theories, there is as yet no consensus as to the precise function of either climbing or parallel fibres and the resulting complex and simple spikes. Several attractive possibilities will be discussed below.

Numerous studies have established that climbing fibre activation of Purkinje cells interacts with the effect of parallel fibres in a number of ways. One of the first observations was that the frequency of complex spikes and that of simple spikes are inversely related to each other in most circumstances. A complex spike rate exceeding 2-3 Hz is accompanied by a reduction in simple spike discharges. Reducing complex spike firing increases the simple spike frequency (37,38). This phenomenon explains why lesions of the inferior olive have a dramatic impact on cerebellar functioning. Blocking the climbing fibre-evoked complex spikes results in a dramatic and long-lasting increase of simple spike firing, which can be expected to effectively and fully inhibit any cerebellar output due to their GABAergic terminals to the cerebellar nuclei. It is for this reason that the functional effect of a complete olivary lesion is remarkably similar to that of a complete cerebellectomy (i.e. involving the cerebellar nuclei).

Apart from the virtually instantaneous effect of climbing fibre activity upon the rate of simple spike firing, a long-term effect has also been described which has been specifically implicated in the learning capabilities of the cerebellum. Decades ago, this effect was hypothesized to exist and to form the basis of cerebellar functioning (27,39,40). It was proposed that climbing fibre discharges had an effect on the parallel fibre synapses that discharged simultaneously with the climbing fibre. The synaptic activity of non-synchronously active parallel fibres would be unaltered. Therefore, repeated activation of a climbing fibre with the same combination of parallel fibres would result in a long-term change in behaviour of the Purkinje cell simple spike firing (see below). Indeed, initially with *in vivo* studies (41) and later *in vitro* preparations (42), long-lasting interactions between both types of afferents were described. In more recent years, mostly using *in vitro* techniques, the pharmacological and molecular basis of these interactions have been studied in considerable detail (e.g. 43). Although it was initially suggested that climbing and parallel fibre interaction could only result in a long-term depression (LTD) of the synaptic efficacy of parallel fibre synapses, more recent studies have shown that:

i   the effect of climbing fibre discharges also displays variable and plastic properties (44-46),

ii reducing or blocking climbing fibre discharges may result in a reversal of LTD, ultimately leading to long term potentiation (LTP) of parallel fibre synapses (47), and

iii many substances and processes seem to be able to influence the plastic capabilities of these synapses (e.g. 48).

The plasticity in the synaptic efficacy in the transfer of information to Purkinje cells is seen by many as the most important property of these cells and enables the cerebellum to play its essential role in the learning and automation of movements (49,50). Below we discuss how these LTD and LTP processes may be involved in adapting or learning movements.

Cerebellar information processing

Although LTD/LTP processes are regarded as interesting phenomena and may be seen as keystones of cerebellar functioning, it should be stressed that there is by no means consensus on their role in movement control. Rather, it seems probable that various aspects of cerebellar functioning may be recognized and that these aspects each concern different aspects of motor control (51,52). It is likely that the impact of the cerebellum on non-motor functions will follow similar principles (53). Here, we will briefly discuss some popular theories specifically concerning motor functions.

'Learning' hypothesis

This theory was originally formulated by Marr (40), modified by Albus (39) and subsequently adapted by Ito (27,53) to account for the involvement of the cerebellar flocculus in the adaptation of the vestibulo-ocular reflex (VOR). Vestibular information is continuously being used to control eye position in order to maintain a stabilized position of the visual world. However, adaptation of this reflex pathway is used to correct a wrongly adjusted VOR (e.g. when donning spectacles or as the result of weakening eye muscles). Ito proposed that adaptation of the VOR was initiated by the activity of climbing fibres coding for such a wrongly adjusted VOR (see Figure 3.7). In this situation the vestibularly induced eye movements under- or overcompensate for changes in head position on the retina, i.e. the visual world will shift over the retina, which is known as retinal slip. Retinal slip is recognized by accessory optic nuclei in the brainstem and results in the activation of a specific region of the inferior olive that supplies climbing fibres to the flocculus. Hence, the signal that the olivary neurons send to the floccular Purkinje cells can be regarded as an 'error' signal (i.e. the

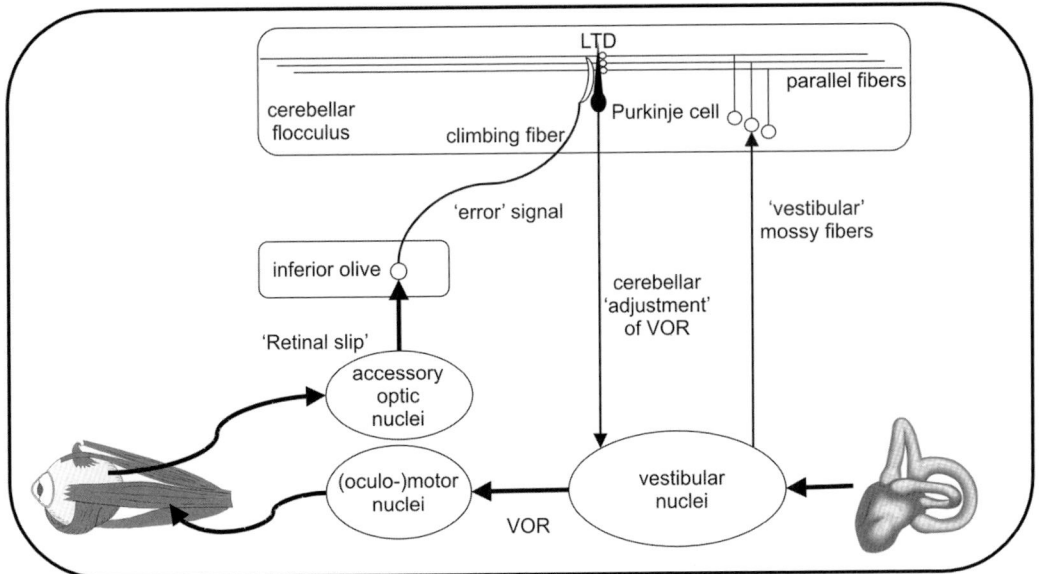

Figure 3.7

Schematic diagram of the basic hypothesis concerning cerebellar adaptation of the vestibulo-ocular reflex (VOR). A wrongly adjusted VOR will result in 'retinal slip', which upon transmission to the inferior olive, will cause climbing fibre-mediated 'error' signals to be sent to the Purkinje cells of the flocculus. These signals will cause long-term changes in the efficacy of the parallel fibre-Purkinje cell synapses (LTD), resulting in an adjustment of the VOR gain.

system notes unintended retinal slip). Increased activity of the climbing fibres will induce subsequent LTD processes that reduce the efficacy of those mossy fibre/parallel fibre synapses that are simultaneously active during this moment of retinal slip. This will result in a diminishing output of the involved Purkinje cells in reaction to a particular vestibular input (that also initiated the VOR). So, in a following identical situation (i.e. movement of the head), the same vestibular input to the vestibular nuclei will be differently modified by Purkinje cell input and will therefore result in an adjusted vestibular output to the oculomotor nuclei. Hence, the gain in the VOR will be changed. Ultimately, this gain will be continuously adjusted and optimized until no retinal slip is detected by the accessory optic system, thereby reducing the number of error signals sent to the flocculus by the inferior olive. Ito suggested that the same principles of operation may also hold true for other parts of the cerebellum.[53] Although the precise formula-

tion of the basic theory has been adjusted and improved numerous times by many groups, the principle of this idea on cerebellar functioning still stands and has received much acclaim. Nevertheless, recent work using genetically modified mice has indicated that, apart from LTD, several additional plasticity mechanisms operating at different levels in the cerebellar circuitry appear to be involved in different learning paradigms (49,54-56).

One of the functions in which Ito's basic theory has also been suggested to play a significant role concerns the cerebellar involvement in associative or classical conditioning. Associative conditioning implies that an unconditional reflex response such as an eye blink (UR: unconditioned response) triggered by an air puff to the cornea (i.e. the unconditional stimulus: US) can also be triggered by an unrelated stimulus such as a tone (conditional stimulus: CS) when this is continuously paired with the US. When a suffi-

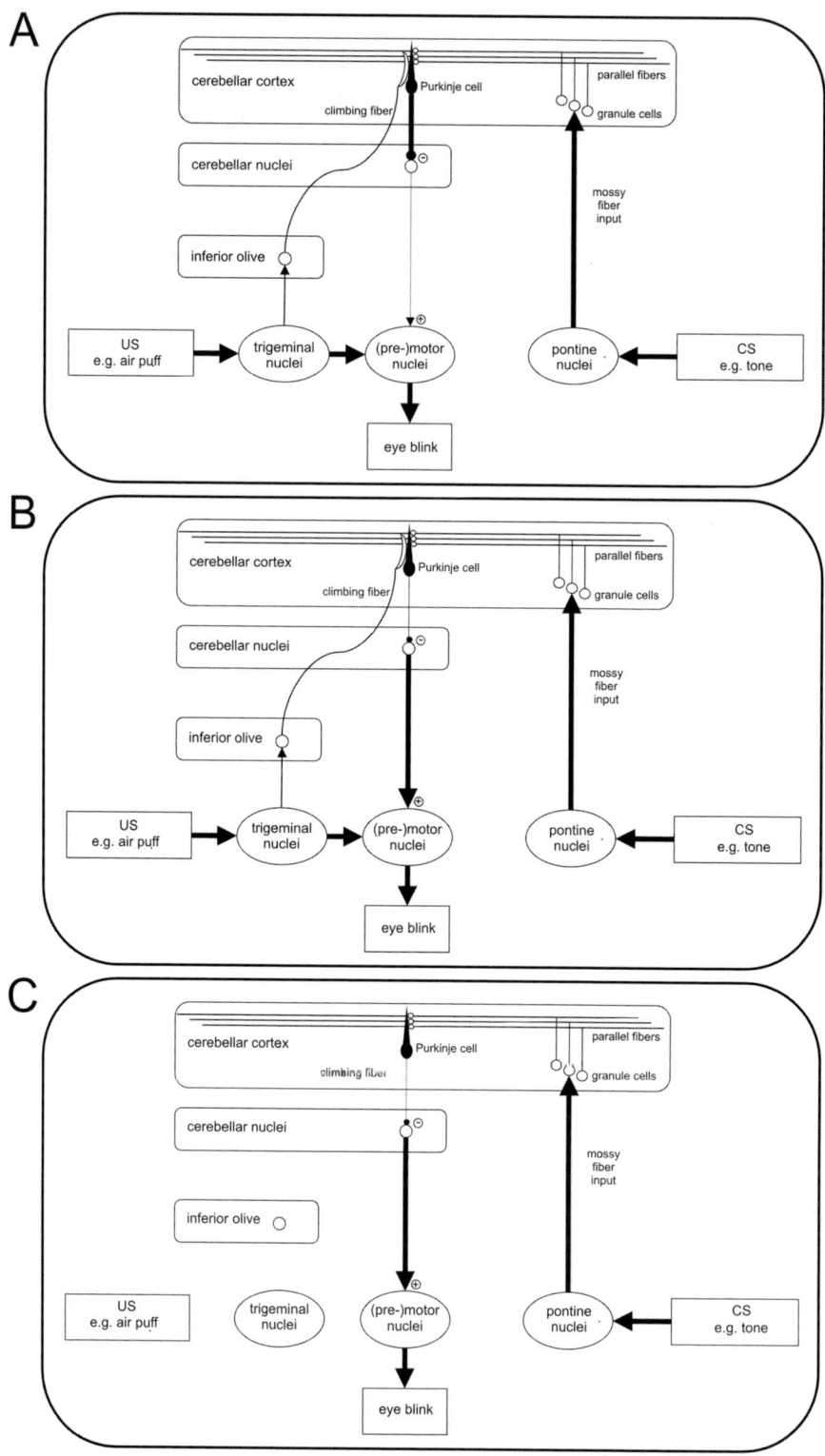

Figure 3.8
Schematic diagram of the hypothesized role of the cerebellum in associative conditioning (simplified after 103).
A: the unconditional stimulus (US), e.g. an air puff, will cause a blink reflex, which is mediated via the somatosensory trigeminal nuclei and the facial motor nucleus. A corollary of the US reaches the cerebellar cortex via the climbing fibre system (inferior olive). A tone, administered simultaneously as a normally neutral, conditional stimulus (CS), will enter the cerebellar cortex by the mossy fibre/parallel fibre system. B: the Purkinje cells that receive (near) simultaneous and repetitive information on the US and CS will, via the LTD process, gradually change their firing frequency derived from a CS alone. The Purkinje cell response to this particular type of input will therefore diminish. This will cause a small category of cerebellar nuclear neurons to be disinhibited, resulting in an increased activity of the pre-motor regions that receive their efferents. It should be noted that the plastic effects of joint climbing fibre and parallel fibre activation may also result in plastic changes in the activity of cerebellar cortical interneurons.
C: eventually the enhanced activity of pre-motor nuclei can trigger a response to the CS only.

cient number of simultaneous presentations of CS (tone) and US (air puff) have been administered, the eye blink can be triggered by the CS alone. Several groups have shown that the cerebellar cortex is critically involved and quite possibly responsible not just for learning, but also for the optimal timing, maintenance and 'unlearning' of the conditioned reflex response (for review, see 57). The hypothesis explaining the cerebellar involvement suggests that the climbing fibre system mediates the US towards the Purkinje cells of a specific 'strip'-like region of the cerebellar cortex (see Figure 3.8). In this specific example, the involved Purkinje cells would project to regions of the cerebellar nuclei that send their axons to pre-motor nuclei, such as the red nucleus, that would be able to control the facial muscles involved in blinking. The CS is mediated to the cerebellum by the mossy fibre system. Due to the strong divergence in the anatomical distribution of mossy fibres amplified by the transverse distribution of parallel fibres, this CS signal will at some point interact with the strip of Purkinje cells activated by the US-mediating climbing fibres. The ensuing plastic processes in this region ultimately ensure that the simple spike activity of these Purkinje cells will start to diminish. As a consequence, the neurons in the cerebellar nuclei that are controlled by these Purkinje cells will be disinhibited, resulting in an enhanced activity that will eventually affect the blink motoneurons (see Figure 3.8). For the resulting plasticity processes, it should

be noted that only the parallel fibres activated by the specific acoustic stimulus will change their synaptic efficacy on the relevant Purkinje cells and/or local inhibitory interneurons and not those that transmit other, e.g. visual, information to these same Purkinje cells. The attractiveness of this hypothesis is related to its wide applicability. Due to the enormous divergence of the mossy fibre/parallel fibre system and the wide convergence of large numbers of parallel fibres to a single Purkinje cells, it can be appreciated that large numbers of Purkinje cells have access to the same type of rather diverse information. However, plasticity processes will only be triggered in those Purkinje cells in which a specific combination of information repetitively coincides with activated climbing fibres. By means of the highly specific and organized projections of Purkinje cells to the cerebellar nuclei, this will result in disinhibition of only a small, selective area of the cerebellar output stations. Recently, Germund Hesslow and his group, in a series of demanding recording experiments in a physiologically relevant setting, quite beautifully provided direct evidence that conjunctive stimulation of mossy fibres and climbing fibres indeed results in the required specific, long-term changes of Purkinje cell activation by mossy fibres (58-60).

In summary, from the anatomy it is clear that the cerebellum should be able to process large amounts of information of a very diverse nature.

By using different access routes to the cerebellar cortex, i.e. climbing and mossy fibre routes, it seems able to correlate the received information in a functionally significant way. It is attractive to speculate that LTD, LTP and other plasticity processes are invaluable in the acquisition and automation (i.e. in the learning) of simple and complex movements. As long as the inferior olive reports error signals, the cerebellar output will be continuously adjusted and optimized, thereby perfecting the execution of ongoing motor programs.

'Timing' hypothesis

Although the induction of long-term changes of synaptic efficacy generated by simultaneous activation of climbing and mossy fibre/parallel fibre systems are amongst the most popular and widely accepted hypotheses on cerebellar functioning, there are many alternative or complementary ideas. In addition, several structural or physiological characteristics of the cerebellar system are not or inadequately explained by the 'learning' hypothesis. For example, it is essential to understand that in the learning hypothesis, the role of the climbing fibres is only seen as a trigger to induce plasticity processes in parallel fibre-Purkinje cell and/or parallel fibre-interneuron synapses. This would be in line with the usually very low firing frequency of olivary cells which, according to many researchers, would rule out that the complex spike that the Purkinje cell discharges in response to a climbing fibre trigger would have a direct and physiologically distinctive influence on postsynaptic structures. Nevertheless, the complex spike does reach the cerebellar nuclei as a high-frequency burst and would seem to be able to induce a specific reaction in these postsynaptic structures. Note that the nuclei also receive the modularly organized collaterals of the climbing fibre system.[20] It was Rodolfo Llinás and colleagues who stressed two important characteristics of olivary physiology which both suggest that the climbing fibre system may have additional, and potentially even more important, roles than inducing parallel fibre plasticity (30,61).

The first characteristic concerns the observation that the firing pattern of olivary neurons reflects a preferred rhythmicity. This seems to be related to their subthreshold oscillations of the membrane potential that have a frequency of 8-10 Hz and results in a propensity of these cells to discharge action potentials specifically during the 'up'- going phase of the membrane potential. In other words, olivary cells discharge preferably at the beat of an intrinsic 10 Hz clock (62). The second characteristic relates to a structural property of olivary neurons. The dendritic spines of olivary neurons are electrotonically coupled to surrounding cells by gap junctions, meaning that changes in the membrane potential that occur in one cell will directly affect the membrane potential of the coupled cells (63). Olivary cells that are coupled in this way will adjust their intrinsic oscillation to each other and, as a result, will have a tendency to fire action potentials in synchrony. Several studies have provided evidence that the strength of the electrotonic coupling may be modified by active synapses that surround the places where gap junctions are found (64,65). Many of these synapses are GABAergic and are derived from the cerebellar nuclei (66), which suggests that the activity of these synapses could dynamically control synchrony levels between changing sets of olivary cells (30,65,67,68).

Several observations suggest that both characteristics of olivary neurons (i.e. their tendency to fire rhythmically and in synchrony) are indeed important and may be used for the actual 'online' control of movements. Under the influence of tremorgenic agents such as the indolamine harmaline (62,69), the depth of the membrane oscillations is increased, resulting in olivary neurons that will discharge action potentials at a frequency of approximately 10 Hz (see Figure 3.9). Moreover, due to the coupling, these action potentials will tend to be highly synchronous.

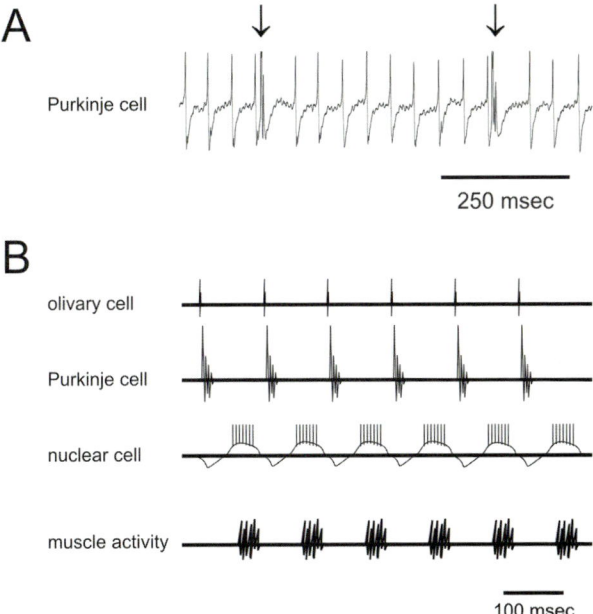

A: extracellular recording of a Purkinje cell. Two types of spikes

Figure 3.9
A: extracellular recording of a Purkinje cell. Two types of spikes are triggered; most spikes are so-called 'simple' spikes and are activated by parallel fibres or spontaneously (36). In addition, two 'complex' spikes are shown (arrows) that result from climbing fibre activation of this Purkinje cell. B: schematic representation of the effect of harmaline. This hallucinatory and tremorgenic substance causes the neurons of the inferior olive to increase their activity to approximately 10 Hz (top trace). The Purkinje cells react with discharging complex spikes in exactly the same frequency (2nd trace). Note that at this level of complex spike firing, the Purkinje cells are not able to discharge simple spikes. The third trace indicates that the neurons of the cerebellar nuclei are hyperpolarized by the 'incoming' complex spikes. However, release from hyperpolarization results in a 'rebound' depolarization, causing the cell to fire a burst of action potentials. Due to the synchrony in the olivary firing, there will also be synchrony in these bursts of activity of the nuclear cells. The output of these cells to pre-motor areas will eventually result in the rhythmical activation of muscles at the same frequency as the olivary discharges.

The rhythmically active climbing fibres will induce the Purkinje cells to discharge complex spikes at the same rate, thereby causing a complete blockage of simple spike firing (see above). The target neurons in the cerebellar nuclei (and those of the vestibular nuclei that are targeted by the Purkinje cells of the vestibulocerebellum) reportedly respond with a short-lasting 'deep' hyperpolarization due to the incoming GABA-

ergic burst of the complex spike. Cerebellar nuclear neurons are known to possess specific calcium conductances which may cause a powerful 'rebound' polarization, i.e. when they are released from inhibition, they are prone to discharge a burst-like pattern of action potentials (69-71). This burst is suddenly terminated upon the 'arrival', after about 100 msec, of a subsequent, synchronously arriving, complex spike volley. Hence, these bursts will also show a 10 Hz pattern, and are translated into a 10 Hz tremor in large parts of the muscular system by means of the projections of the cerebellar nuclei to pre-motor areas in the brainstem (see Figure 3.9B). Under physiologically 'normal' circumstances, the propensity of olivary neurons to discharge rhythmically and in synchrony has been linked to the 10 Hz component of physiological tremor (72). Llinás has also suggested that this idea may be linked to the well-known ultimate reaction time of at least 100 msec when performing voluntary movements (73). The basic 10 Hz frequency would be the internal clock that initiates and organizes muscle activity. In this respect, it is interesting to mention that small amounts of alcohol, which have been shown to have a dampening effect on the oscillatory properties of olivary cells (74), also reduce physiological tremor. Finally, a recent study by Llinás' group showed that the olivary neurons involved in eye muscle coordination by the vestibular system appear to possess rather different characteristics which seem to tie in with the lack of the 10 Hz component of physiological tremor in eye movements (75).

'Optimalization' hypothesis
Another, relatively new and interesting hypothesis on cerebellar functioning has been proposed

by Jim Bower (76). He suggested that the cerebellum does not use the incoming sensory information to coordinate or optimize movements per se, but rather that its goal is to optimize the quality of the sensory input. In this view the executed movements are dedicated to the acquisition of optimal sensory information. He refers to the relatively large areas of cerebellar cortex that receive incoming information of the vibrissae, lips and teeth in the rat, which stand in marked contrast to those of e.g. the hindlimb. He points out that it is hard to imagine why the cerebellar coordination of limb musculature would require a considerably smaller part of the cerebellum than the coordination of vibrissal movements. Bower explains this by assuming that not the movements as such are being coordinated but rather the acquisition of sensory input obtained by the body parts that are moving. For a rat, the mechanical information obtained by the vibrissae will be extremely important in order to be able to respond optimally to environmental clues.

In man, clues have also been obtained that the cerebellum is involved by optimal acquisition of somatosensory input. In a well-known fMRI (functional magnetic resonance imaging) experiment, Bower and colleagues showed that the activity of the cerebellar nuclei drastically increases when subjects are required to provide discriminatory information concerning tactile stimuli that are either actively or passively being perceived by their fingertips (77). The increase in cerebellar activity is hardly seen when similar tactile stimuli are being presented but with-

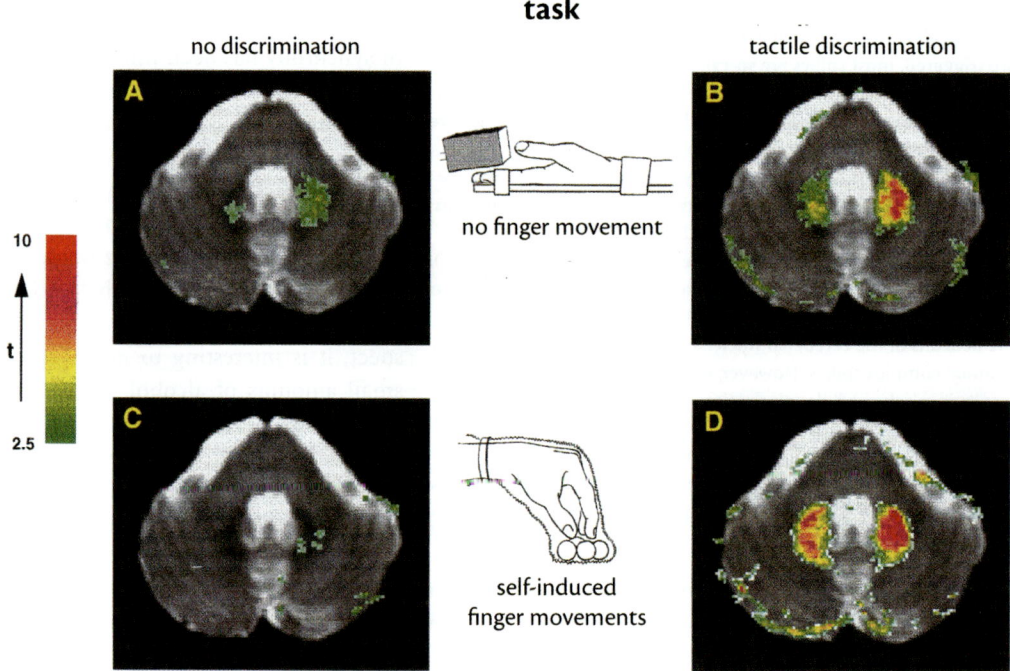

Figure 3.10
Functional magnetic resonance study of cerebellar participation in tactile discrimination tasks. A, B: activity levels in the dentate nuclei resulting from stimulation of the fingers with different grades of sandpaper. In B, the subject was asked to indicate if a fine or coarse grade was used. The fingers did not move in either situation. C, D: activity levels due to self-induced finger movements. Subjects were asked to pick up and drop small objects. In D, they had to indicate whether the objects were large or small. Note that in both discrimination tasks, the activity levels of the dentate nucleus were much higher, providing evidence for cerebellar participation in this type of task. Modified after (77).

out the requirement of making a discriminatory response (see Figure 3.10). Obviously, these and similar tests are also being cited when discussing the potential cerebellar role in cognitive processing of information (see below).

Function and dysfunction of the cerebellum

From the foregoing it will be obvious that our understanding of the way(s) the cerebellum contributes to controlling, coordinating and learning of movements is far from complete or unambiguous. Nevertheless, it appears possible to interpret specific cerebellar deficits in terms of these hypotheses and/or in relation to the functional connectivity of the specific cerebellar regions that are affected. A short account will be given below of the connections and functional role of the vestibulo-, spino- and cerebrocerebellum (see Figure 3.11). However, in the context of this introductory chapter, it is by no means intended to be exhaustive.

The vestibulocerebellum

The vestibulocerebellum (i.e. the nodulus and flocculus) primarily receives its mossy fibre information from the vestibular nuclear complex and even directly from the vestibular organ itself (i.e. semicircular canals, utricule and saccule). Visual information derived from the accessory optic nuclei and information from the vestibular nuclei reach the vestibulocerebellum via climbing fibres from several small olivary subnuclei located caudally in the olivary nuclear complex. The Purkinje cells of the flocculus and nodulus project to the vestibular nuclei, which distribute this information via the medial longitudinal fascicle to the extraocular muscle motor nuclei (abducens, trochlear and oculomotor nuclei) and to the upper cervical cord. In this way, the coordination of head and eyes can be adjusted (see Figure 3.11A). Lesions of the vestibulocerebellum will disrupt this coordination, particularly during self-initiated movements. These patients will have problems with maintaining equilibrium and usually demonstrate a tendency to a wide-based stance. However, when equilibrium is not important in maintaining posture, i.e. when in a prone or supine position with their head resting or firmly supported, the patients are able to execute well-coordinated movements with their limbs.

Within the flocculus of several species of mammals, but also in that of pigeons, several zones or modules have been recognized, each of which could be linked to the control of eye positions in different directions (78-80). It seems attractive to extrapolate this modular control principle to other parts of the cerebellum and their control over skeletal muscles (7,23).

The spinocerebellum

Classically, the spinocerebellum consists of most of the vermis (without the nodulus and lower uvula) and of the paravermis. These areas of the cerebellum mostly receive somatosensory information from the spinal cord and medulla (see Figure 3.11B). Information from the spinal cord arrives either directly by way of the dorsal and ventral spinocerebellar pathways or indirectly via relays in the reticular formation. The spinocerebellum probably also involves those areas that receive rather similarly organized information via the trigeminal nuclei. The dorsal spinocerebellar tract, ascending superficially in the dorsal (posterior) and superficial part of the lateral funiculus, originates in the column of Clarke (posterior thoracic nucleus), which mostly codes for proprioceptive information derived from the hindlimbs. The forelimb equivalent of this type of information reaches the cerebellum via the lateral (external) cuneate nucleus. This information arrives through the inferior cerebellar peduncle. The ventral spinocerebellar tract runs directly anterior to the dorsal tract and relays information that relates to interneuronal processing within the spinal cord. It reaches the cerebellum along the superior peduncle (although their fibres do not mix with the cer-

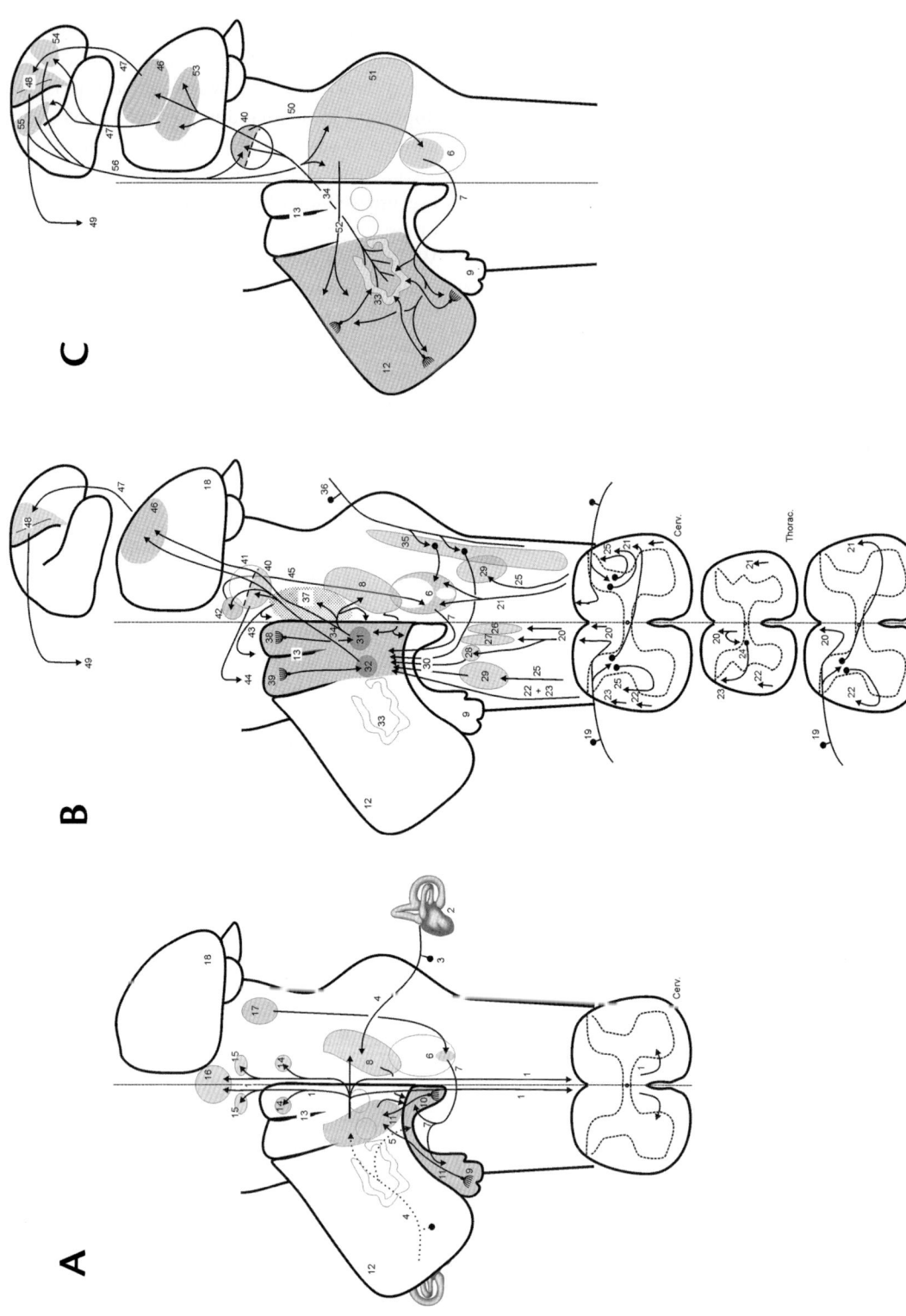

Figure 3.11
Overview of main connections of the vestibulocerebellum (A), spinocerebellum (B) and cerebrocerebellum (C). See text for further details.

1 medial longitudinal fascicle	21 spino-olivary tracts	42 prerubral nuclei
2 vestibular organ	22 ventral spinocerebellar tract	43 reticulospinal tract
3 vestibular ganglion	23 dorsal spinocerebellar tract	44 rubrospinal tract
4 vestibular nerve	24 column of Clarke	45 medial tegmental tract
5 primary vestibulocerebellar fibres	25 spinoreticular tract	46 ventrolateral nucleus of thalamus
6 inferior olive	26 gracile nucleus	47 thalamocortical tract
7 olivocerebellar fibres	27 cuneate nucleus	48 primary and pre-motor cortex
8 vestibular nuclei	28 lateral cuneate nucleus	49 pyramidal tract
9 flocculus	29 lateral reticular nucleus	50 central tegmental tract
10 nodulus	30 inferior cerebellar peduncle	51 basal pontine nuclei
11 corticovestibular fibres	31 fastigial nucleus	52 middle cerebellar peduncle
12 cerebellar hemisphere	32 interposed nuclei	53 interlaminar thalamic nuclei (and others)
13 spinocerebellum	33 dentate nucleus	54 (pre-)frontal associative cortex
14 abducent nucleus	34 superior cerebellar peduncle	55 parietal association cortex
15 trochlear nucleus	35 descending trigeminal nucleus	56 cerebral peduncle
16 oculomotor nucleus	36 trigeminal ganglion	
17 accessory optic nuclei	37 reticular formation	
18 thalamus	38 vermis	
19 spinal ganglion	39 paravermis	
20 dorsal (posterior) columns	40 red nucleus, magnocellular part	
	41 red nucleus, parvicellular part	

ebellar nuclear efferents) (81). Experiments in cats have shown that both spinocerebellar tracts modulate their activity in phase with the stepping rhythm during locomotion. However, in the dorsal tract this modulation disappears after dissection of the dorsal roots or after administration of muscle relaxants. Neurons of origin of the ventral spinocerebellar tract maintain their rhythmic activity under these circumstances. This suggests that the spinocerebellum receives information on the planned movements (via the ventral spinocerebellar tract) as well as on the actually achieved movements (via the dorsal spinocerebellar tract) (82). The spinocerebellum receives additional information from the vestibular nuclear complex, as well as from the cerebral cerebral cortex by way of the pontine nuclei (not shown in Figure 3.11, although see fig. 3.13) (83,84). Climbing fibres of the spinocerebellum are mostly derived from the dorsal and medial accessory olivary subnuclei (18,24).

The somatosensory input is processed in a structured way. In principle, two somatotop-ically organized areas can be discerned in the spinocerebellum. In the lower part of the anterior lobe, information is mostly derived from the ipsilateral hindlimbs, while the ipsilateral upper limbs are represented in the upper parts of the anterior lobe. Somatosensory input from the head is mostly processed in cortical regions surrounding the primary fissure. An additional, but inverted representation is observed in the posterior lobe (85). Mossy and climbing fibres that reach e.g. the posterior somatotopic area often provide collaterals to the same somatotopic regions of the ipsilateral anterior lobe (22,86). Detailed electrophysiological studies in several species have shown that the somatotopy is not absolute because it does not provided a unified representation of the body surface. Rather, it has been demonstrated that the sensory information that reaches the granular layer by way of mossy fibres and carrying information from e.g. the upper lip is directed to multiple, small regions of the cerebellar cortex, which are referred to as 'patches'. Adjacent patches receive information from the same global, but not directly adjacent,

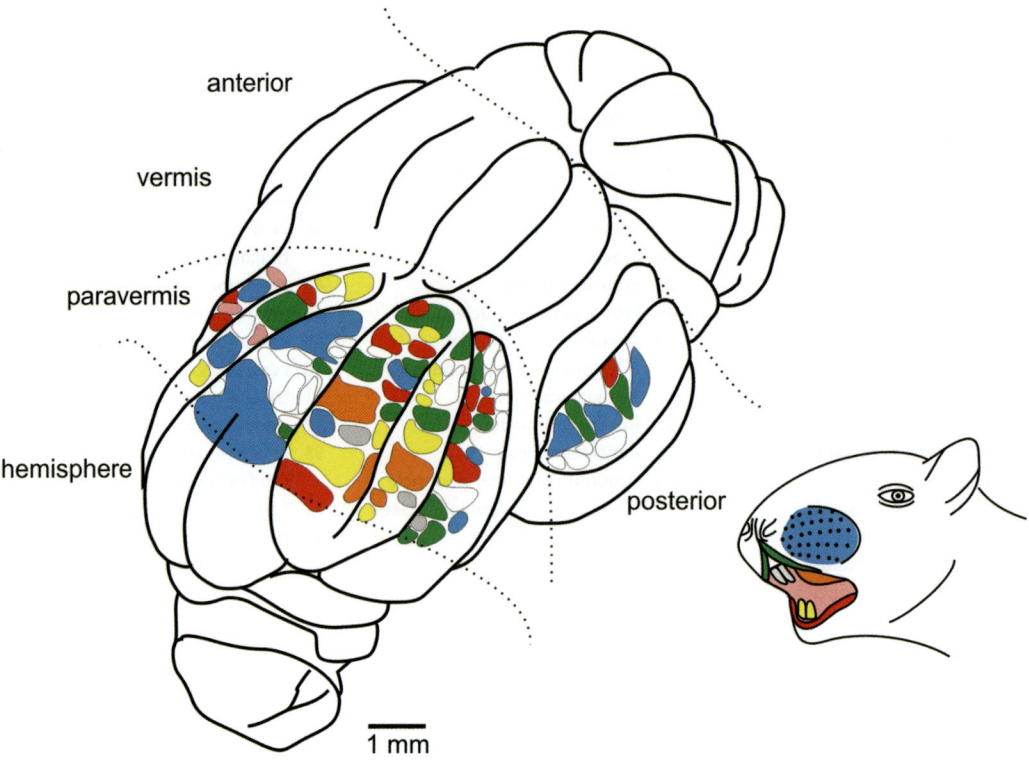

Figure 3.12
Fractionated somatotopy of mossy fibre input to the cerebellar cortex. Distribution over the rat cerebellum of 'patches' of cortex that receive mossy fibre input from a common receptive field. Only patches representing receptive fields of several snout regions of the rat are indicated by different patterning. 'Empty' patches located between coded patches contain mossy fibres from other parts of the body. Note that many patches have the same receptive fields but are bordered by different combinations of patches with other receptive fields. Modified after (87).

body regions (see Figure 3.12). This mode of representation was first described as 'fractionated somatotopy' by Welker and his colleagues (87). The functional implications of this fractionated somatotopy and its relation to the modules (which are mostly based on the anatomical organization of olivocorticonuclear connections) are still not completely understood (22). Somatotopic representations of the body can also be discerned within the cerebellar nuclei and inferior olive. The most readily recognized representations are those in the anterior interposed nucleus (which would be the emboliform nucleus in man) and the dorsal accessory olive (23). Processed information of the spinocerebellar cortex is relayed to the cerebellar nuclei. The

fastigial nucleus receives information from the vermal regions and sends its information to the medullary and pontine reticular formation, vestibular nuclear complex, midbrain and several thalamic nuclei. Through these connections, the fastigial nucleus mostly affects control of the axial musculature (including the extraocular eye muscles). In this respect, there appears to be some overlap with connections that are controlled by the vestibulocerebellum. The Purkinje cells of the lateral part of the vermis specifically direct their axons to the lateral vestibular nucleus, from which the lateral vestibulospinal tract originates. This tract seems to be mostly involved in controlling extensor and posture musculature (51,82,88). The interposed nuclei, which receive their input from the paravermal regions, mostly impact pre-motor areas in the brainstem such as the red nucleus and the ventrolateral nucleus of the thalamus. In this way, the spinocerebellum can influence the activity patterns of the rubrospinal tract and of the pyramidal tract (via the thalamic- primary motor cortex relay, Figure 3.13). The thalamic regions that process cerebellar information also receive information from the basal ganglia to some extent (4). It should be noted that the projections from the cerebellar nuclei are mostly directed to the contralateral brainstem and thalamus. Therefore, due to the subsequent decussation of both the rubrospinal as well as of the pyramidal tracts, motor deficits of a cerebellar lesion will mostly concern the ipsilateral side.

Because Purkinje cells inhibit the more or less continuously firing projection neurons of the cerebellar nuclei, the effect of a cortical lesion will be rather different from that of a cerebellar lesion that involves the nuclei. In the former situation, the activity of the nuclei will increase due to the removal of the inhibiting Purkinje cell influence, thereby resulting in a facilitation in the pre-motor nuclei. In the latter situation, the outgoing activity of the nuclei will be hampered, resulting in a reduction of excitation of these pre-motor nuclei. Although both types of lesion will initially result in inadequately performed movements, it will be obvious that lesions that only involve the cortex tend to have a better prognosis. These lesions generally do not involve the whole cortex, thereby sparing some cortical regions that may also have connections to the same nuclear regions as the lesioned area (e.g. Figure 3.6), thus resulting in potential restoration/improvement of function. For both lesion types, simple movements will tend to show a systematic error by either overshooting or not reaching their intended target (dysmetria). When multi-joint movements are attempted, the error will dramatically increase and may also involve problems with the order of muscle contractions, which will result in ataxic

movement patterns. Self-induced corrections often aggravate the problem. The inability to time activation patterns of agonists and antagonists correctly would seem to form the basis for the characteristic intention tremor often present in cerebellar patients.

The cerebrocerebellum

The cerebellar hemispheres receive most of their mossy fibre inputs via the basal pontine nuclei. In man, the massive cortico-ponto-cerebellar stream of information involves two of the largest fibre tracts in the nervous system. Although the pontine nuclei receive their input from many regions of the cerebral cortex, the most abundant sources lie in the somatosensory, visual and associative visual, auditory, motor and pre-motor cortices (see Figure 3.11C). Additional information reaches the pontine nuclei from many sources in the brainstem (89). The organization of the cortico-ponto-cerebellar connections is very complex and displays both diverging and converging properties that are reminiscent of the fractionated somatotopy of the spinocerebellum (e.g. 83,84,90). The climbing fibres of the cerebrocerebellum are mostly derived from the principal olivary nucleus (24).

The Purkinje cells of the lateral cerebellar parts project to the dentate nucleus, which sends its efferents to many areas of the brainstem and thalamus (21,91). Most projections, however, will reach the small-celled part of the red nucleus and the ventrolateral parts of the thalamus. In man, the red nucleus is virtually exclusively parvocellular. By way of the central tegmental tract, the red nucleus sends its axons to the principal nucleus of the inferior olivary complex. In this way, a conspicuous excitatory dentate-rubro-olivo-cerebellar circuit is formed, which might operate in conjunction with the similarly organized GABAergic projection from the cerebellar nuclei to the olive (65,81,92). The functional implications of these circuits are not fully understood, but it has been speculated that they are indispensable in learning/automating movements, e.g. by functioning as a switching device between the conscious cortical and automated brainstem control of movements (93). The dentato-thalamic connections, like those of the interposed nuclei, may be used to influence activity in the pyramidal tract but are more likely to be involved in planning rather than actual execution of movements (see Figure 3.13). As such, lesions that involve the cerebrocerebellum mostly affect the ability to coordinate phased movements, i.e. the different components of such movements are not executed in the correct order and duration. The inability to execute complex and rhythmic movements seems to relate to a hampered intrinsic sense of timing. This contrasts with lesions of the spinocerebellum where a sense of timing seems to be intact, but prob-

lems are induced by the inability to carry out the actual motor programs.

By virtue of the possibilities of modern brain imaging techniques, many recent studies have implicated that the lateral cerebellum and dentate nucleus are involved in many cognitive tasks such as word-association tasks and tasks requiring spatial awareness and planning (see also Figure 3.10). Indeed, apart from their motor deficits, cerebellar patients may also display difficulties with the execution of specific cognitive tasks such as the Tower of Hanoi task (94). In this respect, it is interesting to note that several studies have provided evidence of dentate projections to thalamic regions that are involved with associative and even emotional parts of the cerebral cortex (95,96).

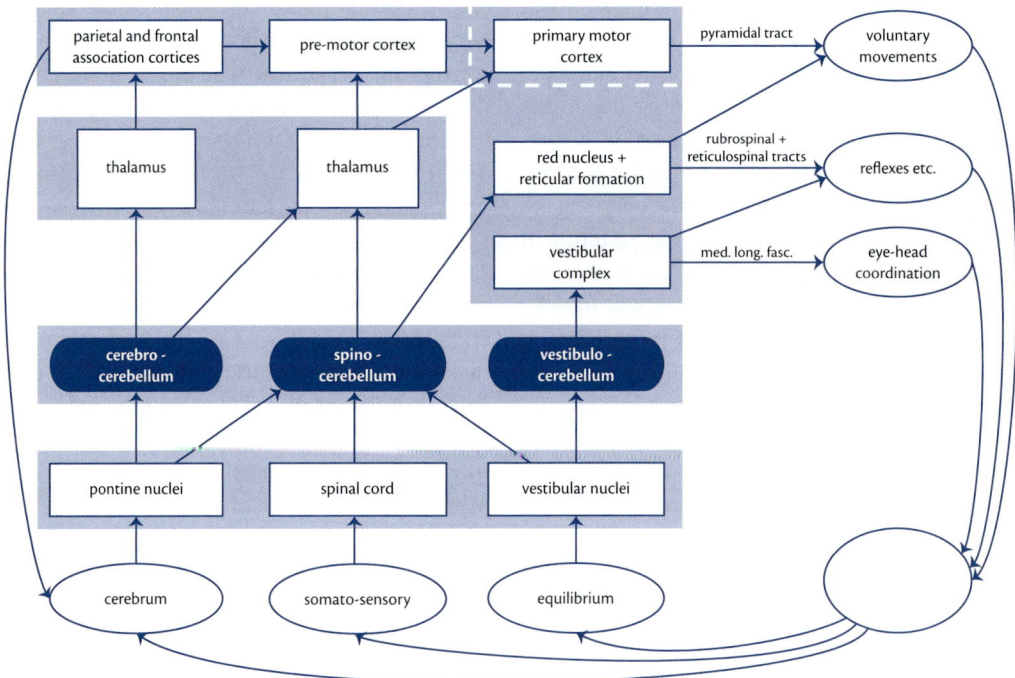

Figure 3.13
Schematic overview of the hierarchy in the organization of cerebellar connections. Many parts of the cerebellum may influence different levels of movement control. The term 'reflexes' in this respect comprises 'unconsciously' executed movements like walking and other rhythmical and automated movements.

Cerebellum and clinical disorders

Despite the recently acquired view that the cerebellum seems to be involved in many brain functions, cerebellar disorders are mostly recognized by the involvement of motor deficits. Handicaps in motor control mainly involve the proper execution of an attempted movement and seem to be caused by the inability to test or compare the actually executed movements with their intended or learned counterparts. It will be evident that proper evaluation of such a comparison requires more than functioning cerebellar circuitry; the systems transmitting the afferent and efferent cerebellar information should be intact. Malfunctioning of any link in this circuitry, consisting of several feedforward as well as feedback connections, will result in ineffective cerebellar control, ultimately leading to the typical cerebellar clinical symptoms. Three symptoms are placed centrally: muscle weakness (hypotonia), ataxia, and tremor (97).

The location of the affected body regions requires some consideration. Unilaterally affected movements usually reflect a cerebellar deficit on the same side. This relation is caused by the twofold decussation of the cerebellar output. First, cerebellar output decussates at the superior cerebellar peduncles (brachium conjunctivum) in the midbrain (98). Subsequently, after one or several synaptic relays, there is another decussation of the corticospinal (and also rubrospinal) tract. Note that the spinocerebellar and spino-reticulo-cerebellar mossy fibre pathways are mostly uncrossed. Lesions of the vestibulocerebellum specifically result in the inability to maintain balance (especially in the absence of visual information) and a deficit in vestibulo-ocular and optokinetic reflexes, which may result in nystagmus. Lesions of the spinocerebellum induce ataxia and intention tremor of the affected body parts. Smaller lesions of the lateral cerebellum may remain unnoticed, while larger lesions may result in widely different complaints involving the inability to carry out or learn complex movements (e.g. speech, writing) and specific cognitive deficits. Indeed, the cerebellar cognitive affective syndrome has recently been recognized as a specific cerebellar disorder (99,100). If the disease process remains confined to selective regions of the cerebellum, many cerebellar symptoms may improve somewhat over time because other cerebellar regions, or even extracerebellar regions, seem to be able to compensate for their dysfunction.

Hypotonia

The sudden removal of cerebellar output in case of, for instance, trauma will diminish the tonic excitatory drive to the pre-motor regions. This will result in a general reduction of activation of the related motoneuron pools, which will be reflected by a reduced muscle tonus (hypotonia). Hypotonia may disappear (partly) after a period of weeks or months, probably through adjustment of the tonic drive to pre-motor regions by other, unaffected, cerebellar or extracerebellar brain regions.

Ataxia

Although ataxia is typical for cerebellar disorders, it is not easily characterized. It usually reflects the inability of a patient to execute voluntary movements in a 'normal' way. Movements, or parts thereof, are not initiated at the correct moment, are not terminated at the appropriate moment, and are not corrected adequately. This results in improperly conducted and dysmetric movements. Because antagonistic and correcting activity is inadequately timed, oscillations will easily occur around the intended target or result in pendular reflexes. Due to dysmetria and failure to time movements, cerebellar patients also encounter problems with the execution of fast rhythmic movements (dysdiadochokinesis). When these disorders concern the mouth, pharynx or larynx musculature, they will result in cerebellar dysarthria that typically involves changes in rhythm and amplitude in combination with a careless or 'slurred' pronunciation.

Intention tremor

This form of tremor is also very characteristic in cerebellar disorders and, as noted earlier, seems to be related to the dysfunction in properly timed components of movements, ultimately reflecting a disturbance in the beat and rhythm of movements, with tremor as a consequence. Increased pendular reflexes (see above) are clearly related to this phenomenon. Cerebellar nystagmus may be seen as a form of intention tremor reflecting dysfunction of the vestibulocerebellum.

References

1 Helmich RC, Hallett M, Deuschl G, Toni I, Bloem BR. Cerebral causes and consequences of parkinsonian resting tremor: a tale of two circuits? Brain 2012;135:3206-3226.

2 Helmich RC, Janssen MJ, Oyen WJ, Bloem BR, Toni I. Pallidal dysfunction drives a cerebellothalamic circuit into Parkinson tremor. Ann Neurol 2011;69:269-281.

3 Bostan AC, Dum RP, Strick PL. The basal ganglia communicate with the cerebellum. Proc Natl Acad Sci USA 2010;107:8452-8456.

4 Hoover JE, Strick PL. The organization of cerebellar and basal ganglia outputs to primary motor cortex as revealed by retrograde transneuronal transport of herpes simplex virus type 1. The Journal of neuroscience : the official journal of the Society for Neuroscience 1999;19:1446-1463.

5 Bolk L. Das cerebellum der Saugetiere. Jena, Germany: Bohn-Fischer; 1906.

6 Schmahmann JD, Doyon J, McDonald D, et al.Three-dimensional MRI atlas of the human cerebellum in proportional stereotaxic space. Neuroimage 1999;10:233-260.

7 Voogd J, Ruigrok TJH. Cerebellum and precerebellar nuclei. In: Mai JK, Paxinos G, editors. The human nervous system, 3rd edition. Amsterdam: Elsevier 2012;471-545.

8 Simat M, Parpan F, Fritschy JM. Heterogeneity of glycinergic and gabaergic interneurons in the granule cell layer of mouse cerebellum. J Comp Neurol 2007;500:71-83.

9 Ramón y Cajal S. Histologie du système nerveux de l'homme et des vertébrés. Azoulay L, translator. Paris: Maloine 1911.

10 Huang CC, Sugino K, Shima Y, et al. Convergence of pontine and proprioceptive streams onto multimodal cerebellar granule cells. eLife 2013;2:e00400.

11 Jorntell H, Ekerot CF. Reciprocal bidirectional plasticity of parallel fiber receptive fields in cerebellar Purkinje cells and their afferent interneurons. Neuron 2002;34:797-806.

12 Mathews PJ, Lee KH, Peng Z, Houser CR, Otis TS. Effects of climbing fiber driven inhibition on Purkinje neuron spiking. J Neurosci 2012;32:17988-17997.

13 Szapiro G, Barbour B. Multiple climbing fibers signal to molecular layer interneurons exclusively via glutamate spillover. Nat Neurosci 2007;10:735-742.

14 Galliano E, Baratella M, Sgritta M, et al. Anatomical investigation of potential contacts between climbing fibers and cerebellar Golgi cells in the mouse. Frontiers in neural circuits 2013;7:59.

15 Voogd J. The human cerebellum. J Chem Neuroanat 2003;26:243-252.

16 Voogd J, Ruigrok TJ. The organization of the corticonuclear and olivocerebellar climbing fiber projections to the rat cerebellar vermis: the congruence of projection zones and the zebrin pattern. J Neurocytol 2004;33:5-21.

17 Voogd J, Glickstein M. The anatomy of the cerebellum. Trends Neurosci. 1998;2:305-371.

18 Pijpers A, Voogd J, Ruigrok TJ. Topography of olivo-cortico-nuclear modules in the intermediate cerebellum of the rat. J Comp Neurol 2005;492:193-213.

19 Ruigrok TJ. Ins and outs of cerebellar modules. Cerebellum 2011;10:464-474.

20 Ruigrok TJH. Cerebellar nuclei: the olivary connection. In: De Zeeuw CI, Strata P, Voogd J, editors. The cerebellum: from structure to control. Progr Brain Res 1997;114:162-197.

21 Teune TM, van der Burg J, van der Moer J, Voogd J, Ruigrok TJH. Topography of cerebellar nuclear projections to the brain stem in the rat. In: Gerrits NM, Ruigrok TJH, De Zeeuw CI, editors. Cerebellar modules: molecules, morphology and function. Volume 124, Progr Brain Res 2000;124:141-172.

22 Pijpers A, Apps R, Pardoe J, Voogd J, Ruigrok TJ. Precise Spatial Relationships between Mossy Fibers and Climbing Fibers in Rat Cerebellar Cortical Zones. J Neurosci 2006;26:12067-12080.

23 Apps R, Garwicz M. Anatomical and physiological foundations of cerebellar information processing. Nat Rev Neurosci 2005;6:297-311.

24 Sugihara I, Shinoda Y. Molecular, topographic, and functional organization of the cerebellar cortex: a study with combined aldolase C and olivocerebellar labeling. J Neurosci 2004;24:8771-8785.

25 Apps R, Hawkes R. Cerebellar cortical organization: a one-map hypothesis. Nat Rev Neurosci 2009;10:670-681.

26 Eccles J, Ito M, Szentagothai J. The cerebellum as a neuronal machine. Springer, Berlin 1967.

27 Ito M. The cerebellum and neural control. New York: Raven press; 1984.

28 Kitazawa S, Kimura T, Yin P-B. Cerebellar complex spikes encode both destinations and errors in arm movements. Nature 1998;392:494-497.

29 Lang EJ. Organization of olivocerebellar activity in the absence of excitatory glutamatergic input. J Neurosci 2001;21:1663-1675.

30 Welsh JP, Lang EJ, Sugihara I, Llinas R. Dynamic organization of motor control within the olivocerebellar system. Nature 1995;374:453-457.

31 Linden DJ. Cerebellar long-term depression as investigated in a cell culture preparation. Behav Brain Sci 1996;19:339.

32 Llinás R, Sugimori M. Electrophysiological properties of in vitro Purkinje cell somata in mammalian cerebellar slices. J Physiol 1980;305:171-195.

33 Llinas R, Yarom Y, Sugimori M. Isolated mammalian brain in vitro: new technique for analysis of electrical activity of neuronal circuit function. Fed Proceed 1981;40:2240-2245.

34 Eccles JC, Llinás R, Sasaki K. The excitatory synaptic action of climbing fibers on the Purkinje cells of the cerebellum. J Physiol 1966;182:268-296.

35 Eccles JC, Llinás R, Sasaki K. Parallel fibre stimulation and the responses induced thereby in the Purkinje cells of the cerebellum. Exp Brain Res 1966;1:17-39.

36 Raman IM, Bean BP. Resurgent sodium current and action potential formation in dissociated cerebellar Purkinje neurons. J Neurosci 1997;17:4517-4526.

37 Badura A, Schonewille M, Voges K, et al. Climbing fiber input shapes reciprocity of Purkinje cell firing. Neuron 2013;78:700-713.

38 Simpson JI, Wylie DR, De Zeeuw CI. On climbing fiber signals and their consequence(s). Behav Brain Sci 1996;19:384-398.

39 Albus JS. A theory on cerebellar function. Math Biosci 1971;10:25-61.

40 Marr D. A theory of cerebellar cortex. J Physiol 1969;202:437-470.

41 Ito M, Sakurai M, Tongroach P. Climbing fibre induced depression of both mossy fibre responsiveness and glutamate sensitivity of cerebellar Purkinje cells. J Physiol 1982;324:113-134.

42 Sakurai M. Synaptic modification of parallel fibre-Purkinje cell transmission in in vitro guinea-pig cerebellar slices. J Physiol 1987;394:463-480.

43 Jorntell H, Hansel C. Synaptic memories upside down: bidirectional plasticity at cerebellar parallel fiber-Purkinje cell synapses. Neuron 2006;52:227-238.

44 Hansel C, Linden DJ. Long-term depression of the cerebellar climbing fiber--Purkinje neuron synapse. Neuron 2000;26:473-482.

45 Bazzigaluppi P, De Gruijl JR, van der Giessen RS, Khosrovani S, De Zeeuw CI, de Jeu MT. Olivary subthreshold oscillations and burst activity revisited. Frontiers in neural circuits 2012;6:91.

46 Mathy A, Ho SS, Davie JT, Duguid IC, Clark BA, Hausser M. Encoding of oscillations by axonal bursts in inferior olive neurons. Neuron 2009;62:388-399.

47 Coesmans M, Weber JT, De Zeeuw CI, Hansel C. Bidirectional parallel fiber plasticity in the cerebellum under climbing fiber control. Neuron 2004;44:691-700.

48 van Beugen BJ, Nagaraja RY, Hansel C. Climbing fiber-evoked endocannabinoid signaling heterosynaptically suppresses presynaptic cerebellar long-term potentiation. J Neurosci 2006;26:8289-8294.

49 Gao Z, van Beugen BJ, De Zeeuw CI. Distributed synergistic plasticity and cerebellar learning. Nature reviews. Neuroscience 2012;13:619-635.

50 Schonewille M, Gao Z, Boele HJ, et al. Reevaluating the role of LTD in cerebellar motor learning. Neuron 2011;70:43-50.

51 Ruigrok TJ, Pijpers A, Goedknegt-Sabel E, Coulon P. Multiple cerebellar zones are involved in the control of individual muscles: a retrograde transneuronal tracing study with rabies virus in the rat. Eur J Neurosci 2008;28:181-200.

52 Pijpers A, Winkelman BH, Bronsing R, Ruigrok TJ. Selective impairment of the cerebellar C1 module involved in rat hind limb control reduces step-dependent modulation of cutaneous reflexes. J Neurosci 2008;28:2179-2189.

53 Ito M. Cerebellar circuitry as a neuronal machine. Progress in neurobiology 2006;78:272-303.

54 Boyden ES, Katoh A, Pyle JL, Chatila TA, Tsien RW, Raymond JL. Selective engagement of plasticity mechanisms for motor memory storage. Neuron 2006;51:823-834.

55 Boyden ES, Katoh A, Raymond JL. Cerebellum-dependent learning: the role of multiple plasticity mechanisms. Annu Rev Neurosci 2004;27:581-609.

56 Wulff P, Schonewille M, Renzi M, et al. Synaptic inhibition of Purkinje cells mediates consolidation of vestibulo-cerebellar motor learning. Nat Neurosci 2009;12:1042-1049.

57 De Zeeuw CI, Yeo CH. Time and tide in cerebellar memory formation. Curr Opin Neurobiol 2005;15:667-674.

58 Jirenhed DA, Bengtsson F, Hesslow G. Acquisition, extinction, and reacquisition of a cerebellar cortical memory trace. J Neurosci 2007;27:2493-2502.

59 Rasmussen A, Jirenhed DA, Zucca R, Johansson F, Svensson P, Hesslow G. Number of spikes in climbing fibers determines the direction of cerebellar learning. The Journal of neuroscience : the official journal of the Society for Neuroscience 2013;33:13436-13440.

60 Jirenhed DA, Hesslow G. Time course of classically conditioned Purkinje cell response is determined by initial part of conditioned stimulus. J Neurosci 2011;31:9070-9074.

61 Llinás R, Welsh JP. On the cerebellum and motor learning. Curr Opin Neurobiol 1993;3:958-965.

62 Llinás R, Yarom Y. Oscillatory properties of guinea-pig inferior olivary neurones and their pharmacological modulation: an in vitro study. J Physiol 1986;376:163-182.

63 Llinás R, Baker R, Sotelo C. Electrotonic coupling between neurons in the cat inferior olive. J Neurophysiol 1974;37:560-571.

64 Lang EJ. GABAergic and glutamatergic modulation of spontaneous and motor-cortex-evoked complex spike activity. J Neurophysiol 2002;87:1993-2008.

65 Bazzigaluppi P, Ruigrok T, Saisan P, De Zeeuw CI, de Jeu M. Properties of the nucleo-olivary pathway: an in vivo whole-cell patch clamp study. PLoS One 2012;7:e46360.

66 De Zeeuw CI, Simpson JI, Hoogenraad CC, Galjart N, Koekkoek SKE, Ruigrok TJH. Microcircuitry and function of the inferior olive. Trends Neurosci 1998;21:391-400.

67 Llinás R, Sasaki K. The functional organization of the olivo-cerebellar system as examined by multiple Purkinje cell recording. Eur. J. Neurosci. 1989;1:587-603.

68 Blenkinsop TA, Lang EJ. Block of inferior olive gap junctional coupling decreases Purkinje cell complex spike synchrony and rhythmicity. J Neurosci 2006;26:1739-1748.

69 Llinás R, Volkind R. The olivo-cerebellar system: functional properties as revealed by harmaline-induced tremor. Exp. Brain Res. 1973;18:69-87.

70 Llinás R, Mühlethaler M. Electrophysiology of guinea pig cerebellar nuclear cells in the in vitro brainstem-cerebellar preparation. J Physiol 1988;404:241-258.

71 Hoebeek FE, Witter L, Ruigrok TJ, De Zeeuw CI. Differential olivo-cerebellar cortical control of rebound activity in the cerebellar nuclei. Proc Natl Acad Sci USA 2011;107:8410-8415.

72 Llinás R. Rebound excitation as the physiological basis for tremor: a biophysical study of the oscillatory properties of mammalian central neurones in vitro. In: Findley LJ, Capildeo R, editors. Movements disorders: tremor. New York: Oxford University Press 1984;165-182.

73 Llinás RR. The noncontinuous nature of movement execution. In: Humphrey DR, Freund H-J, editors.

Motor control: concepts and issues. Chichester: John Wiley & Sons 1991;223-242.

74 Sinton CM, Krosser BI, Walton KD, Llinas RR. The effectiveness of different isomers of octanol as blockers of harmaline-induced tremor. Pflugers Arch 1989;414:31-6.

75 Urbano FJ, Simpson JI, Llinas RR. Somatomotor and oculomotor inferior olivary neurons have distinct electrophysiological phenotypes. Proc Natl Acad Sci USA 2006;103:16550-16555.

76 Bower JM. Perhaps it's time to completely rethink cerebellar function. Behav Brain Sci 1996;19:438.

77 Gao J-H, Parsons L, Bower JM, Xiong J, Li J, Fox PT. Cerebellum implicated in sensory acquisition and discrimination rather than motor control. Science 1996;272:545-547.

78 Voogd J, Wylie DR. Functional and anatomical organization of floccular zones: a preserved feature in vertebrates. J Comp Neurol 2004;470:107-112.

79 van der Steen J, Simpson JI, Tan J. Functional and anatomic organization of three-dimensional eye movements in rabbit cerebellar flocculus. J Neurophysiol 1994;72:31-46.

80 Voogd J, Barmack NH. Oculomotor cerebellum. Prog Brain Res 2006;151:231-268.

81 Voogd J, H.K.P. F, Schoen JHR. Cerebellum and precerebellar nuclei. In: Paxinos G, editor. The human nervous system. New York: Academic Press 1990.

82 Arshavsky YI, Gelfand IM, Orlovsky GN. Cerebellum and rhythmical movements. Braitenberg V, Barlow HB, Bullock TH, Florey E, Grüsser O-J, Peters A, eds. Berlin Heidelberg: Springer-Verlag 1986.

83 Pijpers A, Ruigrok TJ. Organization of pontocerebellar projections to identified climbing fiber zones in the rat. J Comp Neurol 2006;496:513-528.

84 Suzuki L, Coulon P, Sabel-Goedknegt EH, Ruigrok TJ. Organization of cerebral projections to identified cerebellar zones in the posterior cerebellum of the rat. J Neurosci 2012;32:10854-10869.

85 Manni E, Petrosini L. A century of cerebellar somatotopy: a debated representation. Nat Rev Neurosci 2004;5:241-249.

86 Voogd J, Pardoe J, Ruigrok TJ, Apps R. The distribution of climbing and mossy fiber collateral branches from the copula pyramidis and the paramedian lobule: congruence of climbing fiber cortical zones and the pattern of zebrin banding within the rat cerebellum. J Neurosci 2003;23:4645-4456.

87 Welker W. Spatial organization of somatosensory projections to granule cell cerebellar cortex: functional and connectional implications of fractured somatotopy (summary of Wisconsin studies). In: King JS, editor. New concepts in cerebellar neurobiology. New York: Alan R. Liss, Inc 1987;239-280.

88 Ruigrok TJH. Cerebellar influences on descending spinal motor systems. In: Manto M, Gruol JD, Schmahmann N, Koibuchi N, Rossi F, editors. Handbook of the cerebellum and cerebellum disorders. Dordrecht: Springer 2013;497-528.

89 Ruigrok TJH. Precerebellar nuclei and red nucleus. In: Paxinos G, editor. The rat nervous system, third edition. San Diego: Elsevier Academic Press 2004;167-204.

90 Leergaard TB, Lyngstad KA, Thompson JH, et al. Rat somatosensory cerebropontocerebellar pathways: spatial relationships of the somatotopic map of the primary somatosensory cortex are preserved in a three-dimensional clustered pontine map. J Comp Neurol 2000;422:246-266.

91 Chan-Palay V. Cerebellar dentate nucleus: organization, cytology and transmitters. Berlin: Springer-Verlag 1977.

92 Ruigrok TJH, Voogd J. Cerebellar influence on olivary excitability in the cat. Eur . Neurosci 1995;7:679-693.

93 Kennedy PR. Corticospinal, rubrospinal and rubro-olivary projections: a unifying hypothesis. Trends Neurosci 1990;13:474-479.

94 Grafman J, Litvan I, Massaquoi S, Stewart M, Sirigu A, Hallett M. Cognitive planning deficit in patients with cerebellar atrophy. Neurol 1992;42:1493-1496.

95 Kelly RM, Strick PL. Cerebellar loops with motor cortex and prefrontal cortex of a nonhuman primate. J Neurosci 2003;23:8432-8444.

96 Schmahmann JD, Caplan D. Cognition, emotion and the cerebellum. Brain 2006;129:290-292.

97 Thach WT, Bastian AJ. Role of the cerebellum in the control and adaptation of gait in health and disease. Prog Brain Res 2004;143:353-366.

98 Voogd J, van Baarsen K. The Horseshoe-Shaped Commissure of Wernekinck or the Decussation of the Brachium Conjunctivum Methodological Changes in the 1840s. Cerebellum 2013;Epub ahead of print.

99 Schmahmann JD. Disorders of the cerebellum: ataxia, dysmetria of thought, and the cerebellar cognitive affective syndrome. J Neuropsychiat Clin Neurosci 2004;16:367-78.

100 Schmahmann JD, Sherman JC. The cerebellar cognitive affective syndrome. Brain 1998;121:561-579.

101 Nieuwenhuys R, Voogd J, van Huijzen C. The human central nervous system. Berlin, Heidelberg, New York: Springer-Verlag 1981.

102 Jansen J, Brodal A. Das Kleinhirn. Springer, Germany 1958.

103 Yeo CH, Hesslow G. Cerebellum and conditioned responses. Trends Neurosci. 1998;2:322-330.

4

Neuropathology in Movement Disorders

Wilma D.J. van de Berg, Dagmar H. Hepp & Annemieke J.M. Rozemuller

Neurodegenerative disorders, including move-ment disorders, are complex multisystem dis-orders characterized by abnormal protein ag-gregates that accumulate in select regions in the central, peripheral and autonomic nervous system. Alzheimer's disease (AD) and Parkin-son's disease (PD) are the two most common ones. They are associated with the abnormal deposition of proteins, namely amyloid-β (Aβ) and tau in AD and α-synuclein in PD. Fronto-temporal dementia is another heterogeneous group of neurodegenerative disorders with ab-normal protein aggregations such as tau, TAR DNA binding protein-43 (TDP-43) or fused in sarcoma (FUS) protein, while the chaperone protein ubiquitin can always be found in these inclusions. Immunohistochemical methods are currently used as standards to visualize post-mortem the abnormal protein deposits that de-fine the diseases, develop staging schemes and establish correlations between neuropathologi-cal and clinical phenotypes (1-3). Comorbidity is often found in neurodegenerative disorders, and immunohistochemistry with panels of an-tibodies has to be performed to be able to asses the protein aggregation in various regions.

Neuropathological hallmarks in neurodegenerative disorders

The pathological hallmark of PD and a number of other neurodegenerative diseases is the pres-ence of cytoplasmic inclusions, termed Lewy bodies (LBs), and abnormal neuritic deposi-tions, termed Lewy neurites (LNs). The bio-chemical nature of characteristic filaments in LBs was unknown until a genetic and neuro-pathological study in 1997 identified the protein α-synuclein as the central piece in the puzzle of the pathogenesis of PD (4,5). Firstly, a missense mutation in the encoding gene, SNCA, on chro-mosome 4 was found in a family with juvenile PD (4). Secondly, antibodies against α-synucle-in strongly stained filaments of LBs and LNs in sporadic PD and dementia with Lewy bodies (DLB) cases (5). α-Synuclein belongs to a group of natively unfolded proteins that transiently at-tach to lipid membranes, such as vesicles, in ax-ons and presynaptic terminals of neurons. It is involved in the maintenance, storage and regu-lation of dopamine vesicles at synaptic terminals (6). This protein changes its conformation from a soluble α-helical structure into oligomers and finally into insoluble β-sheet configurations for currently unknown reasons and accumulates in the processes and somata of neuronal and glial populations. The structural plasticity of α-synu-clein has raised the question whether α-synucle-in may be a direct consequence of abnormal pro-tein misfolding. The exact mechanisms through which α-synuclein oligomers and aggregates are formed and are toxic to the cell remain elusive (7). The diverse group of neurodegenerative dis-orders that share pathological lesions composed of α-synuclein aggregates, collectively termed synucleinopathies, include not only the Lewy body disorders PD and DLB but also multiple system atrophy (MSA), neuroaxonal dystrophy, motor neuron disease and neurodegeneration with brain iron accumulation (NBIA) (8). Anti-α-synuclein antibodies are nowadays used as diagnostic tools to detect LBs and, especially, LNs in synucleinopathies at postmortem examination. In some parkinsonian disorders, such as most cases of autosomal recessive juvenile parkinsonism with mutations in the PARK2 gene, there is no distinctive histopathological hallmark detected at postmortem examination, only nigrostriatal neuronal loss and gliosis (9,10).

Another protein involved in neurodegenerative diseases is tau, which plays an important role in the pathophysiology of tauopathies, a family of diseases including AD, corticobasal degeneration (CBD), progressive supranuclear palsy (PSP), Pick's disease, frontotemporal dementia and parkinsonism linked to chromosome 17 (FTLD-17T), Guam Parkinson-dementia complex, chronic traumatic encephalopathy (3,11,12), tangle-predominant senile dementia and argyrophilic grain disease (13). Tau proteins belong to the group of microtubule-associated proteins which interact with tubulin, promotes its assembly into microtubules and stabilizes them (14,15). In AD and PD, the protein tau is hyperphosphorylated three- to fourfold. The abnormal hyperphosphorylated tau binds to normal tau, leading to tau oligomerization and neurofibrillary pathology (16). The discovery of mutations in the tau gene in families with FTLD-17T has established that dysfunction of tau proteins can cause an aggregation of hyperphosphorylated tau and neurodegeneration in neurodegenerative diseases (17). Six insoluble tau isoforms exist, differing in an extra insert of the microtubule-binding part and/or an extra small insert in the N-terminal part (14). All six tau isoforms occur in AD, while 4-repeat isoforms occur in CBD and PSP, and 3- and 4-repeat in glia and neurons occur in Pick's disease. Antibodies against isoforms with 3-repeats of the microtubule-binding part and antibodies against the 4-repeat isoforms are used to distinguish between different neurodegenerative diseases with tau accumulation (18).

The neuropathological classification of frontotemporal lobar degeneration (FTLD), another group of neurodegenerative diseases, has been revised recently, emphasizing the recent advances in our understanding of the neuropathological basis of the most prominent immunohistochemical profiles FTLD-TAU, FTLD-TDP and FTLD-FUS (19).

Morphological aspects of some important polyglutamine (polyQ) diseases, particularly CAG trinucleotide repeat diseases such as Huntington's disease and autosomal dominant spinocerebellar ataxias (SCA1, SCA2, SCA3, SCA6, and SCA7), are the presence of neuronal intranuclear aggregates. Huntington's disease is an autosomal dominant inherited neurodegenerative disease, which is caused by a dysfunction of the Huntington gene. The symptoms and neuropathology vary between cases and with disease progression. Neurodegeneration in Huntington's disease is especially marked in the striatum, anterior cingulate gyrus and/or primary motor cortex. An important diagnostic tool for Huntington's disease and some SCA types is the detection of neuronal intranuclear inclusions by applying antibodies against anti-ubiquitin, anti-polyglutamin (1C2) and the ubiquitin-binding protein P62 (20).

Creutzfeldt-Jakob (CJD) and Gerstmann-Straussler-Scheinker's disease (GSSD) are rare, rapidly progressive, fatal, neurodegenerative disorders with several subtypes, all caused by prion accumulation, a misfolded protein encoded on chromosome 20. Parkinsonism and dystonia can be clinical manifestations of these prion disorders if the nigrostriatal circuitry is markedly affected. In those cases, α-synuclein, ubiquitin, tau, and 14-3-3 protein aggregation may coexist with prion protein (PrP) aggregation, leading to mixed pathological features (21).

Macroscopic and microscopic neuropathological hallmarks of above-described neurodegenerative disorders will be discussed in more detail in the following sections.

Neuropathological guidelines in movement disorders

Diagnostic criteria and guidelines have been developed to classify and stage movement disorders and define the protein aggregates (22-24). Systematic assessment of multiple brain regions based on the current diagnostic criteria has to be carried out by an experienced neuropathologist in order to define and categorize the multifocal lesions in the neurodegenerative disorders. Here we provide a practical guide for the dissection of the brain and spinal cord of patients with movement disorders for research purposes.

After measuring the brain weight, the macroscopic appearance of the external aspect of the cerebrum, cerebellum, brainstem and spinal cord is described. Special attention is paid to the presence of atrophy, abnormalities of the cranial nerves and any indications of increased intracranial pressure. The cerebral blood vessels are examined grossly for atherosclerosis and other anomalies. Depending on the clinical diagnosis, either coronal or 'MRI' horizontal thick sections are made. The presence or absence of atrophy of the hippocampus and entorhinal cortex as well as discolouring of the basal ganglia are noted. Infarcts and haemorrhages are recorded. Asymmetry and the degree of pigmentation of the substantia nigra and locus ceruleus must be indicated. The cerebellar hemispheres, vermis and cerebellar nuclei, pons and medulla oblongata are inspected. For the pathological diagnosis of Lewy body disease, tissue blocks of the medulla oblongata, locus ceruleus, pons, midbrain including the substantia nigra, limbic regions and neocortex have to be collected according to a standardized protocol (25). Important parts of the allocortex, such as the amygdala, hippocampus and entorhinal region should be studied in more detail (26). In addition, tissue samples of the basal ganglia, thalamus, cerebellum and olfactory bulb should be collected. The motor cortex must be sampled in FTLD, motor neuron diseases and polyQ diseases. Depending on the clinical data, snap frozen tissue may be collected for biochemical or genetic research. For electron microscopy studies, small pieces must be fixed in glutaraldehyde or osmium tetroxide.

The neuropathological guidelines recommend microscopic evaluation of the neuropathological lesions detected on 6-8-μm-thick sections of a minimum sampling of brain regions (24). If all tissue is collected and stained according to the standardized protocol, the recommended brain regions are evaluated for AD and cerebral amyloid angiopathy (CAA) neuropathological changes. Practical guidelines were recently published by the national institute on ageing-Alzheimer's association (NIA-AA) for obtaining an 'ABC score' for the classification of AD neuropathologic change (24). The classification is based on i) Aβ plaque score, ii) Braak NFT stage, and iii) the consortium to establish a registry for AD (CERAD) neuritic plaque score. A modified version of earlier described phases of Aβ plaque accumulation is recommended that uses a four-point scale (27), and the NFT staging scheme by Braak and Braak (28) is reduced to four stages to improve inter-rater reliability. The CERAD protocol for neuritic plaque is used to characterize the occurrence of phosphorylated tau-immunoreactive dystrophic neurites (24).

The presence of α-synuclein-immunoreactive LBs and LNs is determined in the brainstem, limbic and neocortical brain regions and classified according to a modification of early criteria: none, brainstem-predominant, limbic, neocortical (diffuse), or amygdala-predominant, following the recommendations of the BrainNet Europe criteria (22). Cerebrovascular pathology is common among neurodegenerative disorders, and all infarcts, haemorrhages and microvascular lesions should be assessed in multiple regions and reported, including the location, size and age (29). Recent guidelines for the nomenclature and neuropathologic evaluation of FTLD include major subdivisions designated by the protein abnormality that is most characteristic to the subtype and classification of the distribution pattern of the pathology (2,19).

To assess pathologies, the following staining techniques can be applied: haematoxylin & eosin (H&E), Nissl, silver stainings (Gallyas, the modified Bielschowsky for tangles and neuritic plaques, and methenamine silver for all senile plaques) and myelin stainings (Klüver, PAS-luxol). Immunohistochemistry is indispensable as it plays an important role in the differential diagnosis of movement disorders and enhances the detection of protein inclusions. Antibodies against the following proteins are commonly used: Aβ, neurofilament, glial fibrillary acidic protein (GFAP), iba1 (against microglia), vimentin, the chaperone proteins ubiquitin and P62, α-synuclein, tau (including AT8, 3-repeat antibodies and 4-repeat antibodies), α-crystallin, synaptophysin, antibodies against calcium-binding proteins (calbindin, parvalbumin, calretinin), phosphorylated TDP-43 (pTDP-43), proteins of the ubiquitin-proteasome system (UPS) and FUS. There are also specific antibodies against proteins involved in polyQ diseases, such as anti-ataxin, anti-huntingtin and 1C2. Prion antibodies, such as mab3F4, can be used to exclude rare forms of prion diseases that mimic PSP, DLB or other movement disorders. It is important to note that differences in commercial antibodies and antigen retrieval protocols can influence the results profoundly (30). Therefore, uniform protocols for tissue sampling and histological and immunostaining techniques during routine diagnostics are recommended (28).

Synucleinopathies

Parkinson's disease

Macroscopically, the external surface of the brain of a sporadic Parkinson patient is unremarkable, and atrophy is uncommon. On the cut surface of the midbrain, the pallor of the substantia nigra (see Figure 4.1) and locus ceruleus is evident. The appearance of other nuclei of the basal ganglia is normal, including the globus pallidus, putamen, and caudate nucleus. The currently available pathological criteria for PD require two key histopathological features: neuronal loss in the SNpc at the level of the third cranial nerve and the presence of LB pathology (see Figure 4.2) (31,32).

A standardized assessment of neuronal loss in the substantia nigra is performed using a semi-quantitative staging system (no, mild, moderate and severe neuronal loss) in H&E-stained sections (33). Determining the presence of astrocytosis and extraneuronal neuromelanin can aid in the assessment of neuronal loss. How-

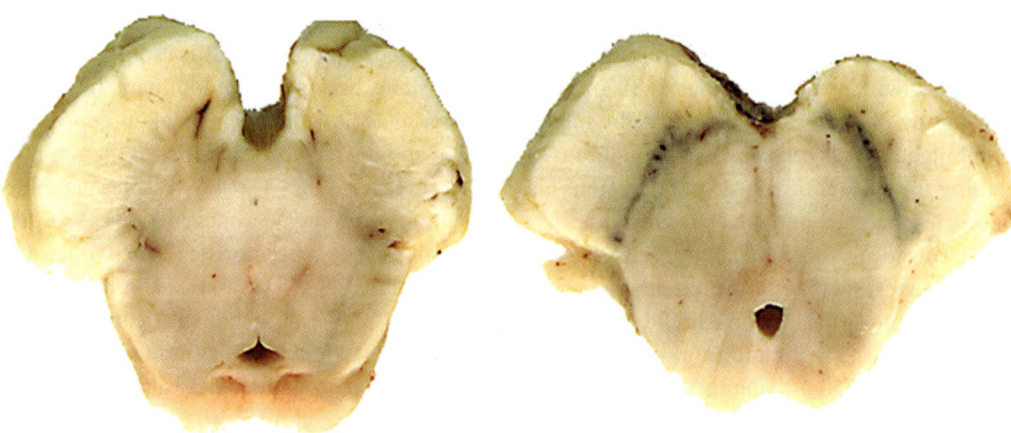

Figure 4.1
Depigmentation of the substantia nigra in Parkinson's disease (mesencephalon, right: control).

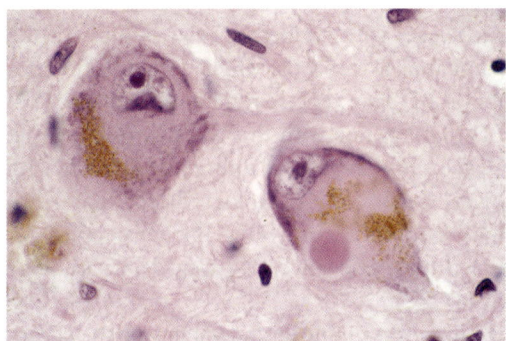

Figure 4.2
Neurons in the substantia nigra showing a typical Lewy body (mesencephalon, haematoxylin & eosin staining).

ever, characterizing PD as a loss of nigrostriatal dopamine overemphasizes a single feature of this multisystem disorder in which many neuronal types in specific regions of the peripheral, autonomic and central nervous system become progressively involved. Current concepts of the neuropathology in PD are changing, and a more widespread distribution of pathology has received increased attention, including noradrenergic, serotonergic and cholinergic output nuclei (34). The presence of α-synuclein pathology in these nuclei and the loss of these neuronal populations contribute to the numerous non-motor symptoms in early stage PD and to clinical heterogeneity. Understanding the susceptibility of dopaminergic as well as non-dopaminergic neurons during the course of the disease may provide important clues for developing neuroprotective strategies to prevent or stop disease progression in PD.

LBs and LNs are made of unbranched α-synuclein filaments with a width of 5-10 nm and a cross-β-sheet structure (35). Ultrastructurally, the halo of classical LBs consists of straight, radially arranged, intermediate filaments associated with a granular, electron-dense coating material and vesicular structures. Nuclear magnetic resonance spectroscopy has indicated that regions of KTKEGV-type repeats and the non-Aβ component of AD amyloid (NAC) of the α-synuclein protein contribute to fibril formation in

LBs (36). In addition, post-translational modifications of α-synuclein, such as hyperphosphorylation, ubiquitination and acetylation, contribute to fibril formation (37). A variety of data suggest that α-synuclein can be secreted in both monomeric and aggregated forms by non-classical exocytic or endocytic pathways. Secreted extracellular α-synuclein may affect neighbouring neurons and glial cells and contribute to the propagation of the disease, acting as a pathogenic 'prion-like' agent in PD (38). The nature and conformations of extracellular α-synuclein pathology and their impact on the neuronal network are still largely unknown.

LBs and LNs are easily visualized by staining for α-synuclein and by ubiquitin, P62 or the Campbell-Switzer silver staining method. Ubiquitin and P62 staining are less specific and sensitive than an α-synuclein staining, however, because they stain corpora amylacea and neurofibrillary tangles along with LBs and LNs. The proposed precursors of LBs and LNs are so-called pale bodies and neurites, which are visible as faintly eosinophilic inclusions displacing neuromelanin in brainstem neurons of the substantia nigra and locus ceruleus. These structures have a similar immunohistohemical profile to LBs and LNs and contain α-synuclein-immunoreactive filaments (39). Because of their close association with true LBs, the presence of pale bodies alone is sufficient reason to look for LBs. Traditionally, two types of LBs are distinguished: a brainstem and cortical type. Brainstem LBs show a classical morphology comprising an acidophilic and argyrophilic core and a pale staining peripheral halo that is strongly immunoreactive for α-synuclein. The cortical type shows a more uniform structure and lacks a halo (40).

Based upon an extensive survey of postmortem human brains of pathologically confirmed PD cases and brain donors of healthy elderly without manifest neurodegenerative disorders, Braak and colleagues were the first to suggest that the α-synuclein pathology progresses in a predictable manner throughout the brain. The pathological process (formation of LBs and LNs) begins at two sites and continues in a topographically predictable sequence in six stages, during which parts of the olfactory, autonomic, limbic and somatomotor systems become progressively involved (41,42). In the first two stages, α-synuclein pathology is confined to the dorsal motor nucleus of the vagus nerve (dmX), anterior olfactory nucleus in the olfactory bulb, and pontine tegmentum (locus ceruleus, caudal raphe nucleus, gigantocellular reticular nucleus). As the disease progresses, other areas, such as the substantia nigra pars compacta, midbrain and basal forebrain (stages 3-4), become affected. In the end-stages 5-6, the pathological process reaches the sensory association cortex, prefrontal cortex and ultimately the entire neocortex. The first two stages may represent the prodromal phase of the disease in which the classical motor symptoms of PD are not yet visible. At stages 3-4, the symptomatic phase of the disease starts. This distribution pattern of α-synuclein pathology in the elderly has largely been confirmed in other cohorts (43,44) and observed in 10-20% of aged healthy cases with no clinical reference to neurological disorders at postmortem examination (45,46). A postmortem study of DelleDonne and colleagues has provided evidence for nigrostriatal dopaminergic cell loss in such cases with incidental Lewy bodies (ILBD) compared to controls, which supports the idea that iLBD may represent the premotor phase of PD (47). In line with this finding, Buchman et al. showed that healthy, unimpaired elderly with nigral Lewy body pathology display parkinsonian symptoms, providing further support for the clinical relevance of α-synuclein pathology in PD (48).

An important issue in understanding the pathological progression in PD is the selective vulnerability of specific anatomical areas and neuronal types. Vulnerable regions include the pigmented parabrachial and paranigral nuclei of the ventral tegmentum, locus ceruleus, reticular formation (especially in the gigantocellular reticular nucleus), dmX and anterior olfactory nucleus (see Figure 4.3) (41).

Neuronal loss and LBs in these brainstem regions are often accompanied by the presence of macrophages (filled with pigment) and gliosis, and α-synuclein-immunoreactive astrocytes are rarely seen. The amygdala undergoes severe pathological changes during the course of PD, and neuronal loss in this area may contribute to olfactory deficits and diminishing facial expression. The most prominent changes in the amygdala occur in the cortical and basolateral nuclei of the amygdala (49). LBs and LNs can also be

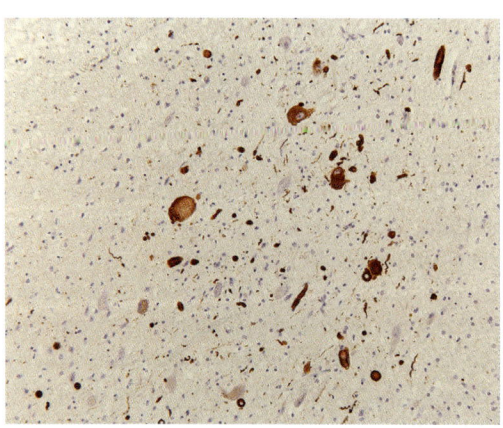
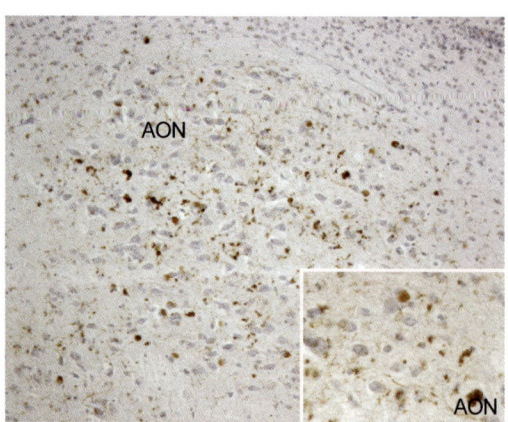

Figure 4.3A/B
Lewy bodies and Lewy neurites in the dorsal vagus nucleus (A) and anterior olfactory nucleus (AON) (B; insert: higher magnification) in Parkinson's disease (α-synuclein staining).

found in the hippocampus and both the transentorhinal and entorhinal regions. They are often present in the magnocellular nuclei of the forebrain (medial septal nucleus, both vertical and horizontal limbs of the diagonal band), the basal nucleus of Meynert, the tuberomammillary nucleus, and the caudal intralaminar, parataenial, cucullar and central lateral nuclei of the thalamus (50). They are also found in areas of the neocortex, especially in the anterior cingulate (see Figure 4.4), insular, and temporal cortices, and less frequently in the occipital cortex. In the spinal cord, parasympathetic and sympathetic neurons exhibit α-synuclein-immunoreactive LB pathology (51). Outside the central nervous system, LBs and LNs may be seen in sympathetic and parasympathetic neurons, as well as in the enteric nervous system (myenteric and submucosal plexuses) (52), cardiac sympathetic nerves (53) and sympathetic trunk (see Figure 4.5), peripheral vagal nerves and submandibular glands, one of the major salivary glands (27).

α-Synuclein-immunoreactive inclusions in astrocytes have also been reported in the brains of advanced sporadic PD patients (54). The topographical distribution pattern of these astrocytes closely resembles that of the intraneuronal LBs and LNs in the brain. The astrocytic α-synuclein-immunoreactive inclusions are mainly observed in the amygdala, thalamus, septum, striatum, claustrum and cerebral cortex (54).

Neuropathological studies have shown that there are multiple factors contributing to the clinical heterogeneity and dementia in PD. These factors include cortical LB load, cortical tau burden and the presence of Aβ plaques in the neocortex (55,56). This does not rule out the possibility that other causes, such as the co-occurrence of argyrophilic grains or multiple infarctions, contribute to dementia or subtype in PD. The early-onset and the tremor-dominant PD subtypes demonstrate similar distribution patterns and severity of α-synuclein pathology throughout the brain (57). Patients in the non-tremor-dominant group display significantly more cortical LB, Aβ plaques load, and cerebral amyloid angiopathy than the early-onset and tremor-dominant subtypes (see Figure 4.6) (58,59). The late-onset PD patients (> 70 years old) reveal many cortical depositions of α-synuclein and Aβ (60).

Tremendous progress has been made in the past 15 years in our understanding of the molecular basis and defining subtypes in PD by genetic discoveries and the recognition of familial forms of PD (61). To date, 17 'PARK' loci and multiple genetic associations have been identified by linkage studies in families affected by PD, genome sequencing and genome-wide association (GWAS) studies (62). Many of the rare genetic forms of PD have a clinical phenotype consistent

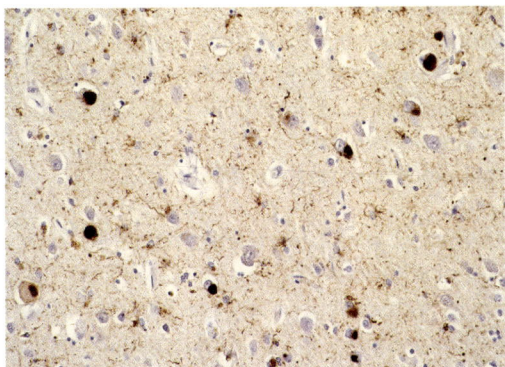

Figure 4.4
Lewy bodies and Lewy neurites in the cingulate gyrus in Parkinson's disease (α-synuclein staining).

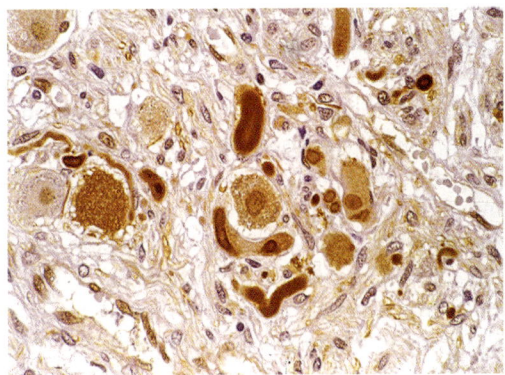

Figure 4.5
Lewy neurites in autonomic ganglia in Parkinson's disease (sympathic trunk, α-synuclein staining).

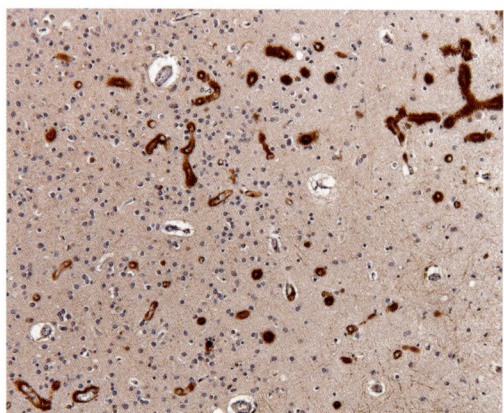

Figure 4.6
Concomitant capillary amyloid angiopathy in occipital region in Parkinson's disease (amyloid-β staining).

with severe parkinsonism, an early age at onset and neuropathological hallmarks resembling typical PD (see Table 4.1). In some genetic forms of PD, e.g. in most cases with Parkin mutations, LBs may be absent, although these cases are clinically indistinguishable from idiopathic PD (9). Three different missense mutations in α-synuclein and duplication/triplication of the SNCA locus have been identified as a cause of PD. At autopsy, patients with SNCA mutations display nigral neuronal loss, as well as widespread brainstem and cortical Lewy bodies. Triplications and duplications display a similar pathology and, in addition, vacuoles in the temporal lobe. The various mutations that have been identified in Parkin and leucine-rich repeat kinase 2 (LRRK2) lead to varying pathology. Mutations in the gene encoding parkin (PARK2) are the most common cause of autosomal recessive, juvenile-onset and young-onset parkinsonism. Parkin mutations are pathologically characterized by severe dopaminergic loss in the substantia nigra pars compacta. Sparse LBs were identified in two cases, but most cases lack LB pathology (63). LRRK2 cases display neuropathological changes ranging from loss of dopaminergic neurons in the substantia nigra pars compacta, LBs in the brainstem, and sometimes plaque and tangle pathology or glial cytoplasmic inclusions reminiscent

of MSA (64,65). Unfortunately, no large autopsy series of genetically defined Parkin and LRRK2 cases have been collected and neuropathologically examined yet. A patient with a heterozygous PTEN-induced kinase 1 (PINK1) mutation from a large Spanish family with six members with parkinsonism revealed dopaminergic loss in the SNpc and LBs and LNs in the reticular nuclei of the brainstem, the substantia nigra pars compacta and Meynert nucleus, while the locus ceruleus and amygdala were spared (66). Histopathological features of 85 kDa calcium-independent phospholipase A2 (PLA2G6) mutations have not been reported yet. Pantothenate kinase-associated neurodegeneration is a progressive movement disorder caused by PANK2 homozygous or heterozygous mutations. Upon postmortem examination, iron deposition, selective neurodegeneration and marked gliosis are observed in the globus pallidus, but α-synuclein pathology is lacking (67). Neuropathological examination of carriers with mutations in the glucocerebrosidase (GBA) gene, which encodes the lysosomal enzyme that is deficient in Gaucher's disease, revealed abundant α-synuclein pathology throughout the brain, especially in the cerebral cortex and hippocampal regions CA2-4. In some GBA-carriers, a more diffuse distribution of LBs was noted, resembling the pattern of LB pathology of DLB. Patients with GBA-associated parkinsonism exhibit varying parkinsonian phenotypes but tend to have an earlier age of onset and show cognitive changes more frequently than patients with parkinsonism without GBA mutations (68). Pathological substrates associated with other mendelian gene mutations have yet to be determined.

Dementia with Lewy bodies (DLB)

As in Parkinson's disease dementia (PDD), there are no characteristic or specific macroscopic abnormalities for DLB. Substantial cortical or subcortical atrophy is usually lacking in the pure forms (85). In the mesencephalon, a variable pallor of the substantia nigra is visible (see

Table 4.1
Mutations identified in genetic forms of Parkinson's disease and the histopathological features observed on postmortem examination (for review see (61)).

Locus/gene	Mutation	Neuropathology	References
PARK1,4/ SNCA	A53T E46K A30P	Neuronal loss in SN, cortical and brainstem LBs, many aSyn-immunoreactive LNs and NFTs, temporal lobe vacuolation, gliosis	(69, 70, 71, 72)
	Triplication/ duplication SNCA	Cortical and brainstem LBs, temporal lobe vacuolation	(73)
PARK2/ PARKIN	Exon4Del Exon4Del	Neuronal loss in SN and locus ceruleus, no LBs or NFTs, slight spongiosis and astrocytic gliosis	(74, 75, 76, 77)
	K211 N Exon4Del		
	Q34fs/Q34fs		
	Exon3Del Exon3Del	Neuronal loss in SN and LC, no LBs, gliosis, αSyn-immunoreactive inclusion in the pedunculopontine nucleus.	(78)
	R275W Pro113fsX51	LBs in SN, LC, nucleus basalis of Meynert and amygdala-parahippocampal region, but not in other limbic or neocortical brain regions. Occasional LBs in dmX. No NFTs.	(9)
	Del1072T Exon7Del	Neuronal loss in SN LBs in the locus ceruleus and SN, reactive gliosis	(79)
PARK6 PINK1	Exon7Del c.1488 g>A	Neuronal loss in the SN, LBs and LNs in the reticular nuclei of the brainstem, SN and nucleus basalis of Meynert	(66)
PARK8/ LRRK2	G2019S	Neuropathology ranging from neuronal loss in SN, with and without widespread LBs and LNs.	(80, 81, 82)
	R1441C	Neuropathology varies from LBs to neuronal loss in SN with ubiquitin-immunoreactive inclusions and severe tau pathology	(64)
	R1441G I2020T	Neuronal loss in the SN without LBs or LNs. aSyn, tau, LRRK2 or ubiquitin inclusions were absent.	(83)
	Y1699C	Varying neuropathological phenotypes. LBs and LNs in the SN, olfactory bulb and neocortex. Severe loss of neurons in SN. Ubiquitin-immunoreactive inclusions and NFT pathology. Occasional Ab deposits in the neocortex and mild Purkinje cell loss.	(81, 64)
PARK14 PLA2G6	R37X c.1078–3C	Range from mild to severe LBs, with NFTs and axonal spheroids	(84)
	T572I, T572I		
PANK2	G521R G521R	No neuronal loss in SN or locus ceruleus. Severe degeneration of globus pallidus. No LBs, ubiquitinated and iron deposits, diffuse NFT pathology	(67)
GBA	N370S, L444P	Abundant LBs in brainstem, cortex and hippocampus	for review see (68)

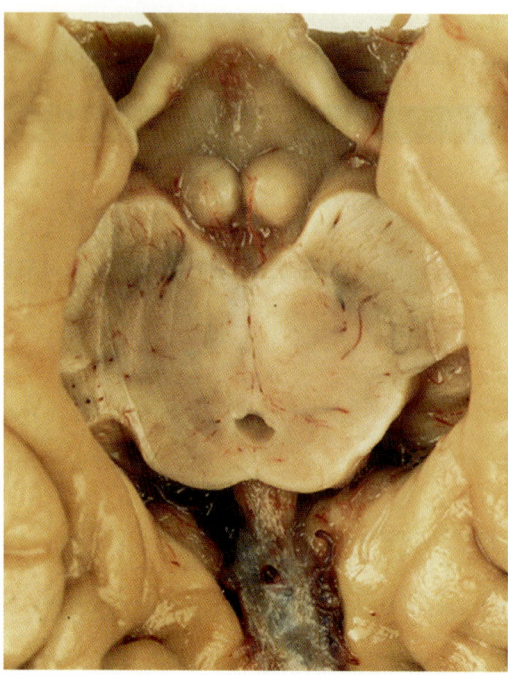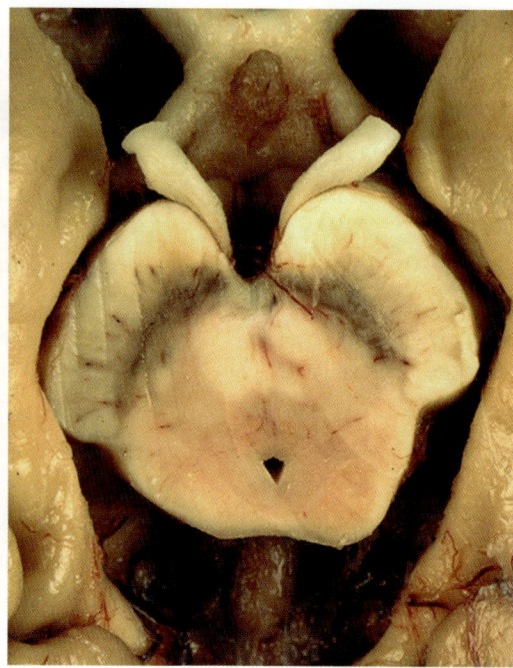

Figure 4.7
Depigmented substantia nigra in dementia with Lewy bodies (mesencephalon, right: control).

Figure 4.7). In contrast, the locus ceruleus is usually depigmented.

The pathological hallmarks of DLB are brainstem- or cortical-type LBs and neuritic degeneration, but there is no accepted 'gold standard' for the pathological diagnosis of DLB (86). In 2005, the DLB consortium formulated consensus pathological guidelines for the diagnoses of DLB with a semiquantitative assessment of LB density in the substantia nigra, locus coerulerus, dmX, nucleus basalis of Meynert, amygdala and five cortical regions (23). These guidelines do not provide a protocol for the diagnosis of DLB, however. The consortium proposed a semiquantitative grading of the severity of Lewy body pathology (0 = none; 1 = mild; 2 = moderate; 3 = severe; 4 = very severe). Depending on the anatomical distribution pattern, three different categories can be assigned: i) brainstem dominant; ii) limbic (or transitional) type; and iii) diffuse neocortical type.

Besides α-synuclein pathology, AD pathology is frequently present in DLB patients, usually in the form of diffuse Aβ plaques or as neuritic plaques. PD, PDD and DLB are pathologically quite similar and difficult to discriminate. However, recent studies indicate some differences can be observed. The load of Aβ plaques in the striatum is higher in DLB, compared to non-demented PD patients (87,88). Striatal Aβ depositions might thus contribute to early dementia within the Lewy body disease spectrum (i.e. PD, PDD and DLB). The DLB consortium recommends an assessment of AD pathology in DLB cases as well, using the NIA-Reagan criteria for neuritic plaques (89), and recently, the consensus criteria for AD changes were recommended. A validation of the neuropathological criteria for DLB by the consortium in prospectively diagnosed cases showed that the diagnostic accuracy of clinically probably DLB can be improved by a modification of the criteria, considering cases with NFT stage VI to be low-likelihood DLB (90).

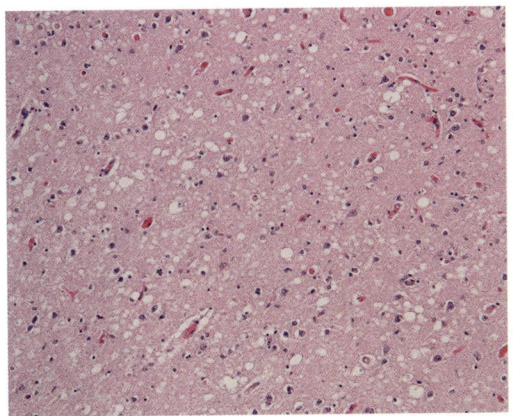

Figure 4.8
Severe spongiosis in the temporal cortex of a patient with rapidly progressive dementia with Lewy bodies (haematoxylin & eosin staining).

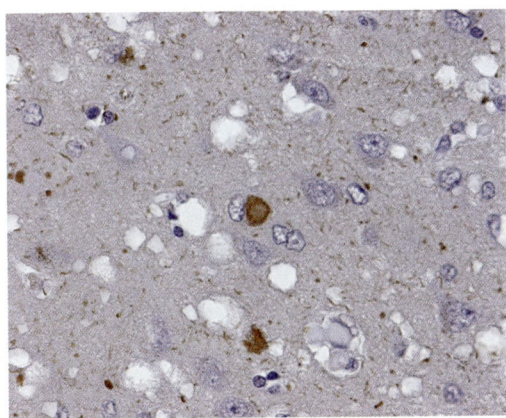

Figure 4.9
Severe spongiosis in the entorhinal cortex of a patient with rapidly progressive dementia with Lewy bodies (α-synuclein staining).

The Braak model of PD, suggesting that the LB pathology starts in the brainstem and advances to the limbic and neocortical areas, might not be applicable to DLB patients. Since the sequence of clinical symptoms is per definition different in DLB, i.e. early dementia and parkinsonism occurring at least one year later, the site of the initial lesions might be different in PD/PDD and DLB (91).

In addition, spongiform changes in the temporal and entorhinal cortex in DLB have been described (see Figure 4.8 and 4.9). Vacuolization seems to be more common in DLB than in AD (92) and is associated with a more rapid disease progression. Vascular pathology is not uncommon in DLB, approximately 30% of the DLB cases show some vascular abnormalities (93). The clinical significance of these vascular abnormalities in DLB is unknown, however.

Multiple system atrophy

MSA is considered an adult-onset, sporadic, progressive neuropathologic entity defined by the selective degeneration of striatonigral and olivopontocerebellar structures and distinctive glial cytoplasmic inclusions (GCIs) predominantly composed of filamentous α-synuclein proteins (94,95). The terminology of the different clinical variants in MSA has changed since the discovery that the underlying pathological hallmark is similar. Historically, the term striatonigral degeneration was used for patients with predominantly parkinsonian features. This type of MSA is now referred to as the MSA-P subtype. Sporadic olivopontocerebellar atrophy was used for those patients with predominant cerebellar ataxia (nowadays referred to as the MSA-C subtype). The term Shy-Dräger syndrome was applied to patients with early prominent autonomic failure. However, since most patients suffer from some degree of autonomic failure, the term Shy-Dräger syndrome is no longer used (95).

The macroscopic appearances in MSA range from normal to focal atrophy of the affected brain regions, which is generally related to the clinical pattern of the disease. On the cut surface, the putamen shows variable atrophy, being most pronounced in patients with MSA-P. There is often a gray-green discoloration of the atrophic putamen, especially its posterior part (se Figure 4.10). The substantia nigra and locus ceruleus are pale as a result of loss of pigment. Atrophy of the cerebellum, cerebellar peduncles, pons (see Figure 4.11), and medulla is most marked in MSA-C.

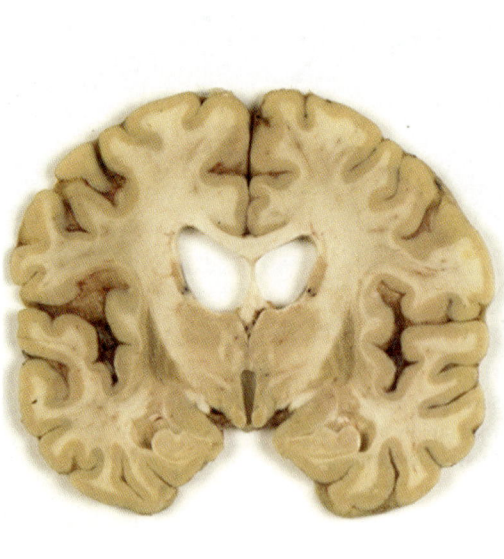
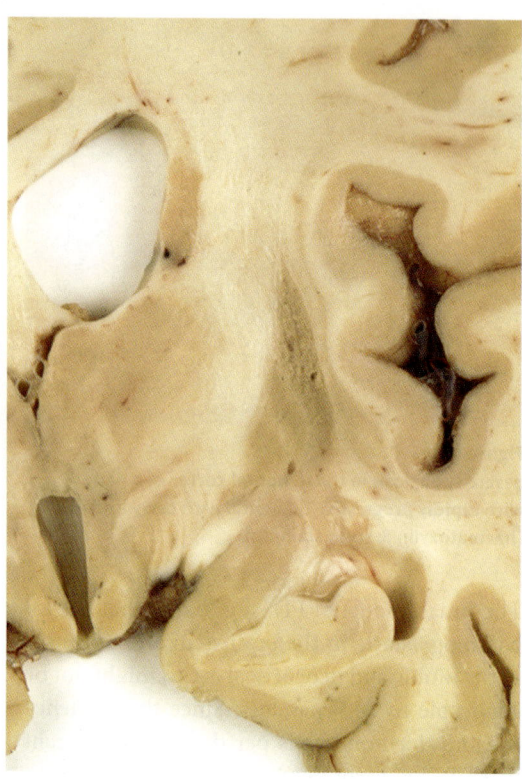

Figure 4.10
Atrophic and discoloured putamen in multiple system atrophy, parkinsonism subtype (MSA-P) (right: detail).

More than 20 years ago, Papp et al. described GCIs in the central nervous sytem of 11 patients with autonomic failure with parkinsonism or cerebellar ataxia or both (96). The GCIs in MSA are partly argyrophilic (first noted with Gallya's silver impregnation), and their shape varies from triangular, sickle, half-moon, oval or conical, to occasionally flame-shaped. They are of variable size, often completely occupying the cytoplasm to displace the nucleus eccentrically. The GCIs as a pathological hallmark of MSA contain many proteins, including predominantly hyperphosphorylated α-synuclein (on serine129 residue), tubulin, ubiquitin, tau (see Figure 4.12), αB-crystallin, DJ-1, LRKK2 and a long list of other proteins demonstrated by immunohistochemical and/or mass spectrometry studies; see for review (97). Ultrastructural studies have shown that GCI constituents of cytoplasmic aggregates include loosely packed

filaments or tubules and straight filaments, consisting of polymerized α-synuclein and other types of filaments. GCIs are observed in all three types of oligodendrocytes: satellite cells adjacent to neurons in the gray matter, in the white matter in the interfascicular variant, and in the perivascular oligodendrocytes of the affected areas (98,99).

The cerebral white matter is affected in an anatomically selective manner, involving the pons, medulla, putamen, substantia nigra, cerebellum and preganglionic autonomic structures (100,101). α-Synuclein-immunoreactive neuronal cytoplasmic inclusions are found in the pons, putamen, subthalamic nucleus, inferior olivary nucleus, and arcuate nuclei. Neuronal intranuclear inclusions are found in the pons, putamen, subthalamic nucleus, inferior olivary nucleus, arcuate nuclei, and motor cortex (102).

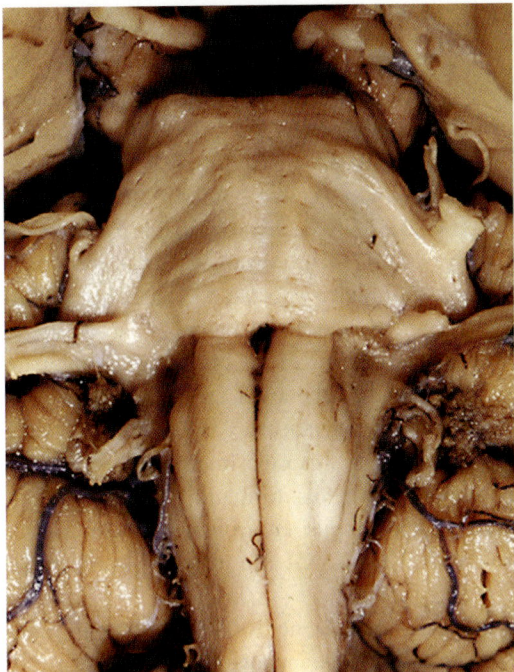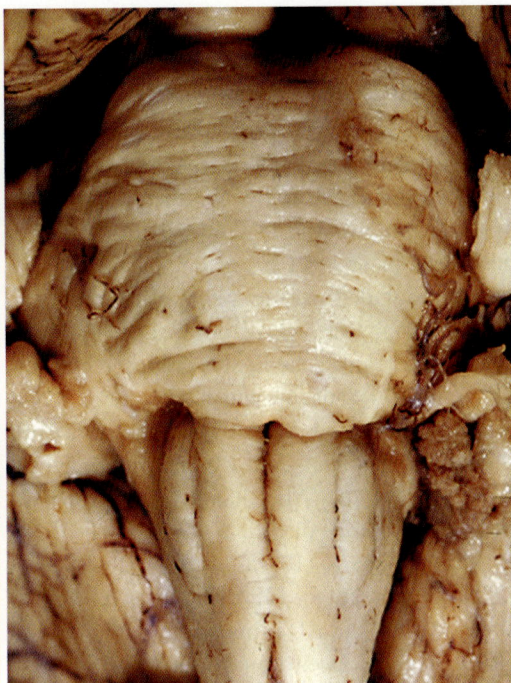

Figure 4.11
Atrophy of pons in multiple system atrophy, cerebellar subtype (MSA-C) (right: control).

Rare ubiquitin-immunoreactive neuronal cytoplasmic inclusions and tau-negative dystrophic neurites have also been described. The pathology in MSA is not only found in the central nervous system, but also in the peripheral system, i.e. demyelination in the nervus suralis, and abnormal EMG in muscles (103,104). Converging data from recent animal, genetic and postmortem studies emphasize a central role of aberrant oligodendroglial α-synuclein accumulation in the pathogenesis of MSA, leading to oligodendroglial dysfunction, early myelin disruption and associated axonal damage, resulting ultimately in neuronal degeneration (97).

In the cerebral cortex, there is neuronal loss in the primary and supplementary motor cortex, with an accompanying increase in glial cells. This neuronal loss occurs in those areas that are also rich in GCIs. Neuronal loss/gliosis is severe in the fifth and sixth layer of the motor cortex and pyramidal tract (100), lateral horn of the spinal cord, striatum (especially dorsolateral zone of the caudal putamen), substantia nigra, inferior olive, pontine nuclei, and cerebellar Purkinje cells, and is less severe in the dentate nucleus, nucleus ambiguus, vestibular nuclei, arcuate nucleus (medulla), dmX, intermediolateral column of the spinal cord, Onuf's nucleus, anterior horn cells, and pyramidal tracts (anterior and lateral corticospinal tracts). The white matter shows demyelination,

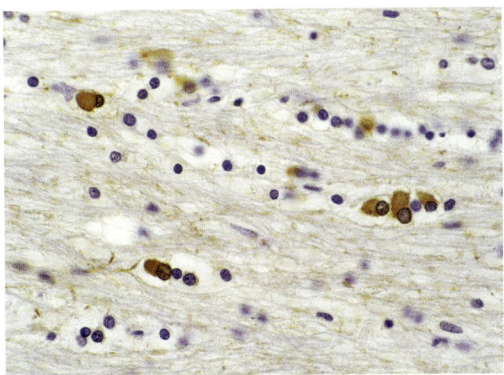

Figure 4.12
Inclusions in oligodendrocytes in multiple system atrophy (white matter, tau (AT8) staining).

especially in affected areas (105). Excessive iron accumulation has been demonstrated, especially in the basal ganglia. The cell types that contain iron pigment include predominantly oligodendroglia and microglia, but neurons and astrocytes are also affected.

Jellinger proposed a staging scheme for the classification of MSA based on the severity of nigrostriatal degeneration and olivopontocerebellar atrophy on a three-point scale (106). In addition, a similar scheme was proposed by Halliday and colleagues in which two major MSA types (MSA-P and MSA-C) are defined, and their overlap is classified (8). The presence of MSA-like pathology in elderly people without neurodegenerative disorders ('incidental MSA') is extremely sparse (107). Therefore, developing a staging protocol for MSA similar to the Braak staging in PD and AD is not feasible.

GCIs have also been found in PSP, CBD, AD, Pick's disease, spinocerebellar ataxia type 1 (SCA1), which is a subgroup of hereditary familial olivopontocerebellar atrophy (spinocerebellar atrophy), and FTLD-17T. In addition, glial inclusions have been described in PD cases (54).

Tauopathies

Progressive supranuclear palsy (PSP)

Apparent macroscopical abnormalities are not always visible, and if so, they are restricted to atrophy of the frontal cortex, midbrain and cerebellum. The midbrain may be shrunken, the substantia nigra can be pale, the red nucleus, globus pallidus and subthalamic nucleus are atrophied and discoloured (108). The pontine tegmentum is occasionally atrophied and the locus ceruleus less pigmented. In the cerebellum, the superior cerebellar peduncles and dentate nuclei are sometimes shrunken, while the hilus appears discoloured. The inner segment of the globus pallidus and the subthalamic nucleus may be atrophied and discoloured. There may be mild dilatation of the third and fourth ventricles and/or aqueduct.

Microscopical abnormalities are related to neuronal inclusions composed of filamentous tau protein, i.e. neurofibrillary tangles with neuronal loss, neuropil threads, and tau inclusion in astrocytes glial cells (so-called 'tufted astrocytes') and oligodendroglia ('coiled bodies') (109-113). The latter glial lesions are distinguishable from the glial cytoplasmic inclusions of MSA based on their immunoreactivity with tau and their morphology. A predominance of 4-repeat tau accumulates is characteristic for PSP (114). These changes are not confined to the areas mentioned above but can extend to the neocortex and subcortical white matter, striatum, capsula interna, substantia innominata, thalamus, formatio reticularis, amygdala, hippocampus, entorhinal cortex, nuclei of NIII, IV, VIII, X, XII and inferior olivary nuclei (see Figure 4.13).

In contrast to AD, neurofibrillary tangles, neuronal loss, gliosis and neuropil threads in PSP

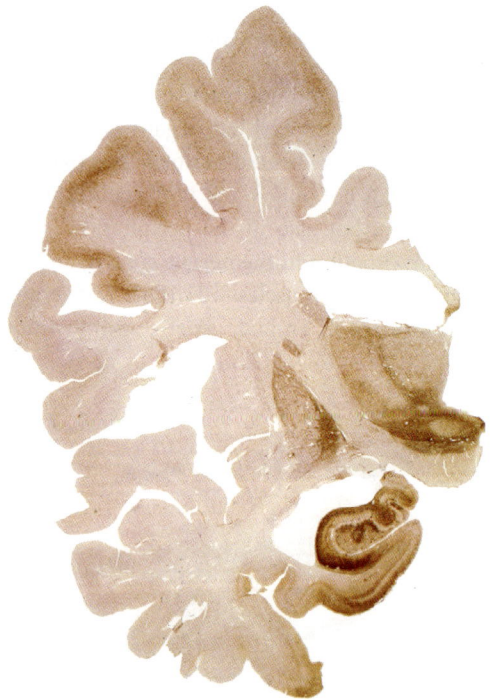

Figure 4.13

Overview of large hemisheric slice with typical distribution pattern of tau in progressive supranuclear palsy (tau (AT8) staining).

are primarily seen in the motor and premotor cortex, including the white matter in these areas (104,115). In the cortex, glial tau is more prominent than tangles (109). The neuropil threads in PSP, demonstrated by the Gallyas stain and tau antibodies, are partly oligodendrocytic (109) in contrast to those seen in AD. They often run along axons extending across grey and white matter. In Gallyas staining, the aggregation pattern, orientation, and appearance of these threads are different from those seen in AD. The density of neuropil threads is highest at the corticomedullary junction and is overall less pronounced than it is in corticobasal degeneration (116). Their distribution overlaps with that of the coiled bodies. Neuropil threads are prominent in the pre- and postcentral gyrus and are also found in the internal capsule, and pencil fibers in the globus pallidus and tegmentum of the midbrain. In the pontine base, coiled bodies and threads are rare in progressive supranuclear palsy, in contrast to the consistent presence of neurofibrillary tangles in this region.

Thorn-shaped (thorny) astrocytes show positive Gallyas and tau staining. They are seen in subpial and subependymal areas and can also be found in senile tauopathy. Glial fibrillary tangles ('tuft-shaped' or 'tufted' astrocytes) are immunoreactive against antibodies to GFAP and CD44. Tau immunoreactivity is concentrated in the cytoplasmic centre. On Gallyas staining, tufts are observed as an aggregation of conglomerated, fine or thick processes in a concentric arrangement. They are tree-shaped, branching without collaterals (see Figure 4.14). They are restricted to the grey matter and are located especially in the precentral and premotor gyri, putamen, medial thalamus, subthalamic nucleus, and tegmentum of the brainstem. Tufted astrocytes can have double nuclei. They are not specific for supranuclear palsy.

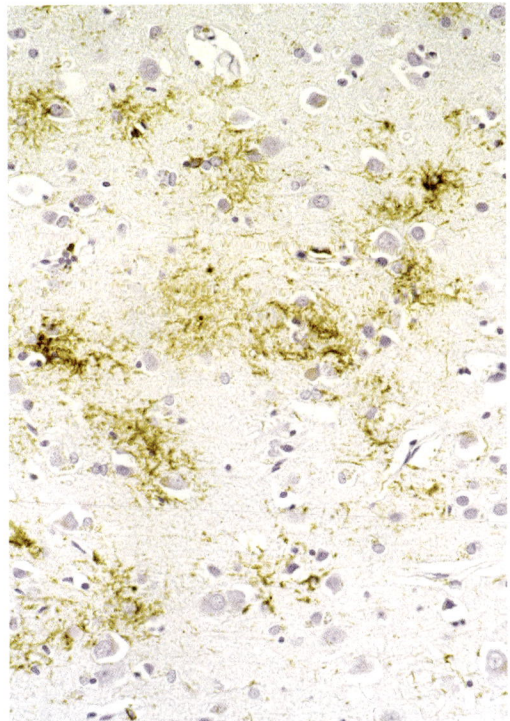

Figure 4.14
'Tufted' astrocytes in progressive supranuclear palsy (premotor cortex) (tau (AT8) staining).

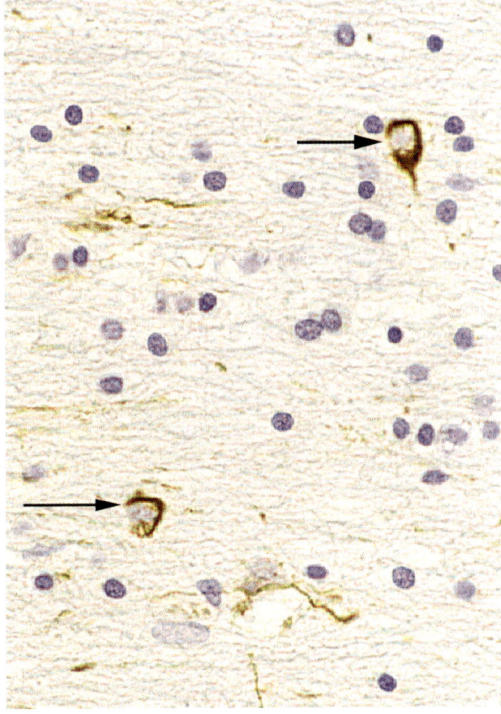

Figure 4.15
'Coiled bodies' in progressive supranuclear palsy (white matter) (tau (AT8) staining).

Coiled bodies are most consistently found in PSP. They contain enlarged nuclei with thin coil-like, thick comma-like, and spine-like structures with frequent branching (see Figure 4.15). Fine, branching coiled bodies are characteristic of PSP, while thick comma-like ones are often observed in CBD. They are limited to the precentral cortex and internal capsule, and pencil fibers to the lenticular nuclei, midbrain, and tegmentum.

Their presence in the cerebellar white matter is relatively specific to PSP. Coiled bodies are also found in CBD, PD, Pick's disease, and dementia with argyrophilic grains. Western blotting of tau from patients with PSP showed a doublet of 64 and 69 kDa consistent with 4-repeat tau forms.

Hypertrophy of the olivary nucleus, caused by lesions in the dentate nucleus, and of the central tegmental tract of the pons is occasionally seen. Furthermore, granulovacuolar degeneration can be present in the substantia nigra, red nucleus, locus ceruleus, basis pontis, and dentate nucleus. Typical 'grumose degeneration' may develop around dentate neurons, i.e. eosinophilic granular structures, some of which are stained by antibodies against phosphorylated neurofilaments. Electron microscopy reveals that they consist of clusters of axon terminals and pre-terminal axons. Ballooned (achromatic) neurons in the entorhinal/transentorhinal area/neocortex are seen less often (117).

Criteria and grading systems for PSP have been proposed (118). When a 12-tiered grading system is used based on coiled body and thread lesions in the substantia nigra, caudate and dentate nucleus, tau pathology is severest in the clinical subtype Richardson's syndrome compared to PSP-Parkinson type and the pure akinesia with gait freezing type (119). As the presence of PSP-like pathology in neurologically healthy subjects ('incidental PSP') is rare (120), the paucity

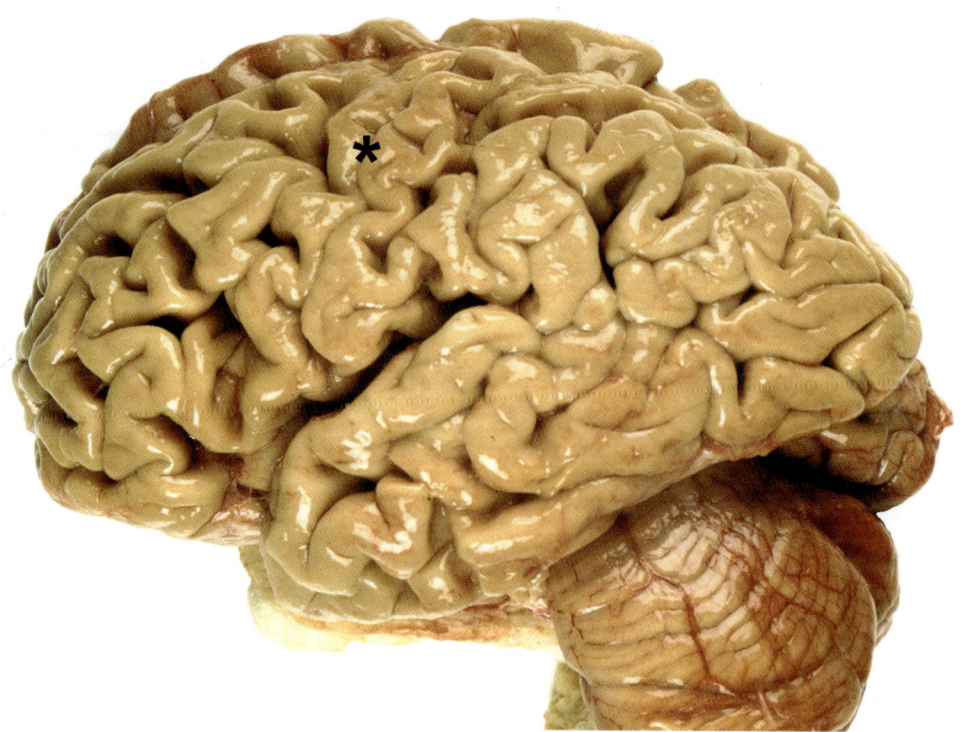

Figure 4.16
Corticobasal degeneration with severe atrophy of motor cortex. Note narrowing of gyri around central sulcus (*).

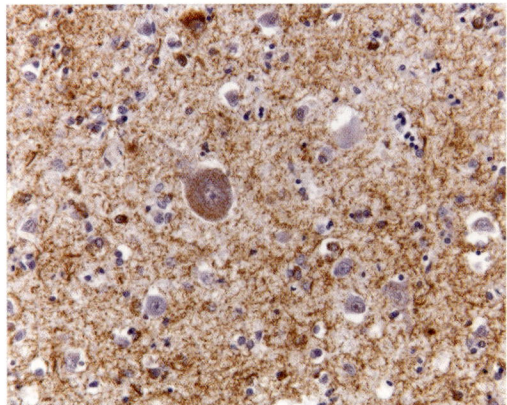

Figure 4.17
Corticobasal degeneration: AT8-immunoreactive granular staining in neurons, neuropil threads and glial cells in the motor cortex (tau (AT8) staining).

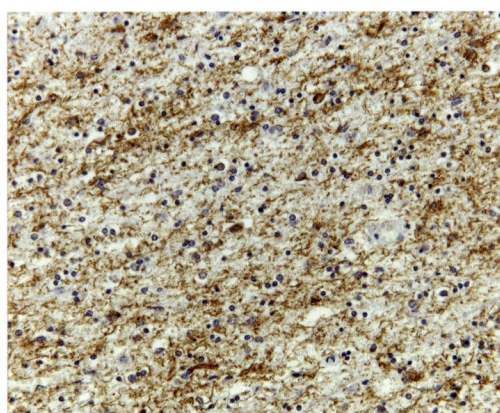

Figure 4.18
Corticobasal degeneration: white matter showing intense tau staining (tau (AT8) staining).

of such cases foreclose the collection of a large sample set necessary for the development of a staging scheme for PSP.

Corticobasal degeneration (CBD)

Macroscopically, there is a typically asymmetrical cortical atrophy of the posterior frontal, parietal and pre- and postcentral gyri contralateral to the limbs that are most severely affected in life (see Figure 4.16). The atrophy is associated with variable dilatation of the ventricular system. There is loss of pigment from the substantia nigra and locus ceruleus. The tegmentum is slightly atrophic and the aqueduct enlarged (109).

CBD is characterized by neuronal loss, astrocytosis, and microglia proliferation and is associated with four main histopathological features: swollen cortical neurons containing neurofilament protein, 4-repeat tau-containing neuropil threads, 4-repeat tau-containing astrocytes, and filamentous inclusions composed of 4-repeat tau in basal neurons and rarely in cortical neurons. A key pathological feature is the presence of swollen cortical neurons in affected areas (also termed achromatic or ballooned neurons). They are most frequent in cortical layers III, V, and VI and are apparent in H&E-stained sections as

pale large neurons, often with a surrounding artefactual area of vacuolation.

These swollen neurons are immunoreactive for phosphorylated neurofilament as well as αB-crystallin. Tau-positive (4-repeat) neuronal perinuclear fibrillary inclusions are more frequently seen in small neurons. They are less well demarcated and less round than Pick bodies and not found in the dentate gyrus, in contrast to Pick's disease. Astrocytic plaques, as collections of abnormal tau in the distal processes of astrocytes, are a characteristic finding in CBD. These plaques can be found especially in precentral and premotor gyri but also in the putamen, thalamus and subthalamicus (111).

Neuropil threads (dystrophic neurites) are numerous in CBD, being found throughout the grey matter and the white matter of affected areas of the cortex and deep grey matter (see Figure 4.17). In contrast to AD, the density of neuropil threads can be as great in the white matter as in the cortical grey matter (see Figure 4.18). Their number is larger than in PSP, but both disorders have the same tau isoforms with 4-repeat of the microtubule-binding region. Oligodendroglial 4-repeat tau inclusions, called coiled bodies and threads, are frequently found in degenerating areas like frontoparietal, deep grey and white matter, mesencephalon and pontine base (111).

The tau-positive inclusions have an annular and fibrillar appearance and are distinct both morphologically and antigenically from the round or crescent-shaped, ubiquitinated, oligodendroglial inclusions of MSA. Thick comma-like coiled bodies are often observed in CBD. In nearly all patients there is neuronal loss, pigment incontinence and gliosis of the subcortical nuclei. There is almost always cell loss and astrocytosis in the lateral portion of the substantia nigra. A characteristic feature is the presence of slightly basophilic filamentous inclusions in residual nigral neurons (originally termed corticobasal bodies), which can mimic globose tangles, characteristic of PSP (121). Mild to moderate neuronal loss, gliosis, and/or neurofibrillary tangles can be found in other subcortical and brainstem structures such as the thalamus, subthalamic nucleus, dentate nuclei, red nuclei, pons, reticular formation, and inferior olivary nuclei. The dentate nucleus shows eosinophilic degeneration as in PSP. However, in contrast with PSP, most changes are seen in the cortex and subcortical area.

Frontotemporal lobar degeneration (FTLD)

Frontotemporal lobar degeneration (FTLD) encompasses a spectrum of disorders with a variety of clinical manifestations including behavioural and executive impairment, language problems and motor dysfunction (122). Recent advances in our understanding of the neuropathological and molecular genetic basis have shown that FTLD can be classified into three main subtypes based on the most prominent immunohistochemical profile: i) FTLD-TAU, which includes Pick's disease, PSP, CBD, FTLD-17T and argyrophilic grain disease; ii) FTLD-TDP, which is subdivided further into types A-D; and iii) FTLD-FUS, which includes TDP-43 negative FTLD-U, neuronal intermediate filament inclusion disease (NIFID) and basophilic inclusions body disease (BIBD) (2,19,123,124). Ubiquitin and P62 is always positive in all

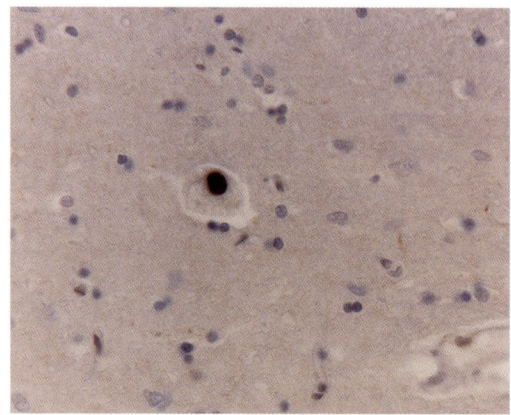

Figure 4.19
FUS inclusion in putamen using FUS antibodies in frontotemporal lobe degeneration (FUS staining).

these protein aggregations. Revised criteria for the neuropathological diagnoses of FTLD take into account existing classification methods of tauopathies and recently discovered pathologies like TDP-43 and FUS proteinopathies, intermediate filament inclusions and a subtype with cellular inclusions composed of an unidentified ubiquitinated protein (2,19,122). Using antibodies against phosphorylated TDP-43, four types can be recognized based on numbers and shape of neuronal cytoplasmic inclusions and of TDP threads and the presence of neuronal intranuclear lentiform inclusions. A small proportion

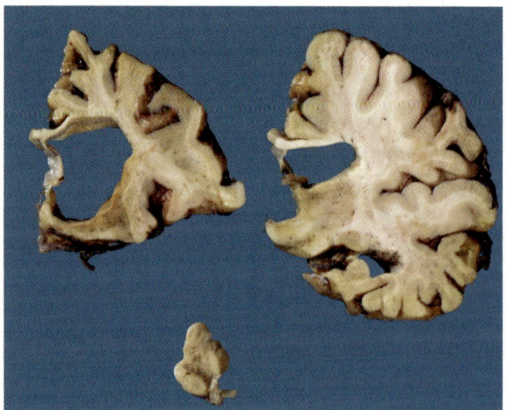

Figure 4.20
Severe atrophy of the caudate nucleus in a young patient with frontotemporal lobe degeneration, FUS subtype.

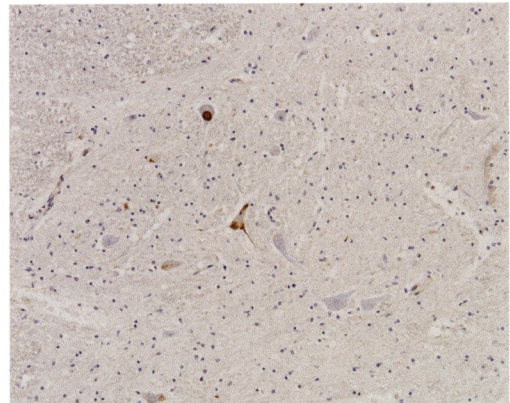

Figure 4.21
FUS immunoreactive inclusion in the spinal cord in amyloid lateral sclerosis (FUS staining).

of FTLD is caused by neuronal cytoplasmic accumulation of the FUS protein that occurs especially in young sporadic FTLD patients (see Figure 4.19). Extensive atrophy of the caudate and large lateral ventricles are seen in them (see Figure 4.20). Furthermore, the inclusions in the spinal cord in some patients with amyloid lateral sclerosis (ALS) are FUS-immunoreactive (see Figure 4.21).

Improvement of immunohistochemical techniques and novel antibodies have made FTLD 'without distinctive histological features' very rare (125). Prion mutations must be excluded in these cases and can even cause FTLD with 17 years' duration (126). Different unknown mutations in families with FTLD have to be elucidated.

FTLD-TAU

Pick's disease: sporadic FTLD with classical Pick bodies

Macroscopically, lobar or circumscribed cerebral atrophy affecting the frontal and/or anterior temporal lobes is seen, which may extend to the parietal lobe. The marked gyral atrophy is sometimes referred to as 'knife edge' atrophy or 'walnut brain' after a long duration of the disease. Areas spared include the posterior part of the superior temporal gyrus and the pre-and post-

central gyri (see Figure 4.22). The atrophy may be asymmetrical, with the dominant hemisphere (usually the left side) being more extensively affected. Temporal atrophy alone is rarely seen.

On sectioning, the cortical ribbon is thinner than usual, and the grey-white junction is indistinct. The white matter can be atrophied, rubbery and granular. The ventricles, especially the frontal and temporal horns of the lateral ventricles, are dilated. The severity of the atrophy results in a brain weight that is often less than 1000 grams. Atrophy of the corpus striatum (especially the head of the caudate nucleus) and amygdala can be found and is mild, contrasting with the atrophy that is seen in some cases of Huntington's disease, MSA, FTLD-FUS and some tau mutations.

In areas with severe pathology, the cytoarchitectural features of the cortex become obscured. There is a loss of large pyramidal neurons with collapse of the parenchyma, spongiosis, and astrocytic gliosis. This gliosis is often marked in the upper cortex and at the grey-white matter junction. Ballooned neurons are present in the middle and lower cortical layers. In the cortex, neurons contain round to irregularly shaped inclusions (Pick bodies) that are intensely argyrophilic with

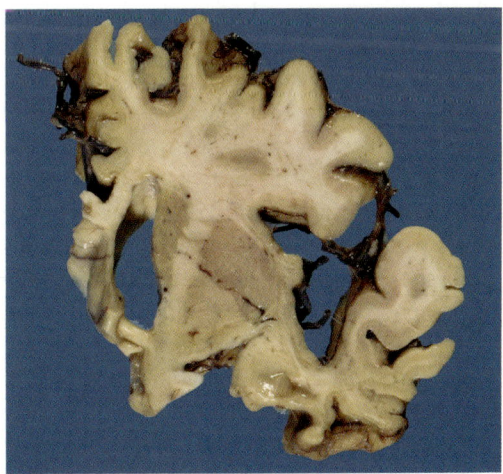

Figure 4.22
Pick's disease: note sparing of the posterior part of the first temporal gyrus.

silver impregnation methods. The position of the nucleus is remarkably eccentric. Anti-tau (3-repeat tau) and anti-neurofilament immunostains strongly label Pick bodies and Pick neurites. Characteristically, Pick bodies contain 3-repeat tau isoforms and are negative for 4-repeat tau antibodies. They are most numerous in the cingulate, insular, inferior parietal, inferior temporal, fusiform, and lingular gyri. Cell loss is greater in the frontal and temporal lobes than in the parietal lobe (127). Although Pick bodies are widespread and can be seen in different subcortical and brainstem nuclei, the hippocampal formation and amygdala are usually severely affected, with many Pick bodies in the CA1, subiculum and dentate fascia (128). They can be found in the olfactory nucleus as well. In regions where the atrophy is greatest, the subjacent white matter displays a loss of myelinated fibers, accompanied by gliosis and axonal degeneration.

Western blotting shows a pattern of two major bands (55 and 66 kDa) (129) consistent with 3-repeat tau. These isoforms also contain exon 3. Ubiquitin has been identified as another constituent of Pick bodies, but frequently the staining is weak, and it is not found in all Pick bodies. They are negative for α-synuclein, which differentiates Pick bodies from Lewy bodies. Ultrastructurally, they are composed of randomly arranged, straight filaments, ranging from 14 to 16 nm in diameter and admixed with a variable number of twisted filaments with a diameter ranging from 22 to 24 nm and with a half period of 120-160 nm. This contrasts with the twisted paired helical filaments of AD, which are 22 nm wide and have a half period of 60-80 nm. Ballooned neurons are best demonstrated with antibodies that recognize phosphorylated neurofilament epitopes. They also contain stress proteins (αB-crystallin positive). Ultrastructurally, they are composed of granulofilamentous material.

Tau-positive astrocytes have been described in the cerebral cortex and in the white matter (111,127). Most of them are 3-repeat tau-positive, and a small amount stain for 4-repeat tau. In the cerebral cortex, ramified tau-positive astrocytes are present, with a few thick processes and eccentric nuclei. In the white matter, they show dense tau-positivity and have a sharp margin. The distribution of the ramified astrocytes is limited to the affected cortex, such as the frontal, temporal and insular cortices, and to the hippocampus. Coiled bodies are far less numerous than in PSP and CBD and are limited to the affected areas (111). Neuropil threads in Pick's disease can be visualised better using 3-repeat tau antibodies and are rare with Gallyas silver staining, which especially visualises 4-repeat tau forms (130).

Hereditary FTLD with MAPT mutations (FTLD-17T)

Macroscopically, the degree of atrophy depends on the type of tau mutation and duration of the disease, but it can be severe. Atrophy of the hemispheres can be mild in intermediate stages. Frontal and temporal atrophy, especially in the anterior part of the temporal lobes, is prominently seen in later stages. On the cut surface, the substantia nigra and locus ceruleus are pale. The caudate nucleus, putamen, globus pallidus, amygdala, hippocampus, and ventral hypothalamus are variably involved. A loss of frontotemporal white matter is seen with enlargement of the ventricles. Parietal and occipital lobes are less frequently affected. The midbrain, pons and cerebellar cortex can be atrophic.

The microcopic findings vary substantially depending on the type of mutation (131-133). In general, tau can accumulate in neurons and glial cells in the cortex, basal nuclei, and brainstem nuclei and in glial cells in the white matter (see Figure 4.23). The deposits can be found in the perikaryon or in the extensions. The neuronal inclusions may resemble AD tangles (as in the P310L mutation), globose tangles or Pick-like inclusions. Glial tau inclusions resemble coiled bodies, tufted astrocytes or astrocytic plaques. The mutations in exon 10 can lead to more 4-repeat tau in neurons and glial cells. A deletion of exon 10, as seen in the deltaK 280 mutation,

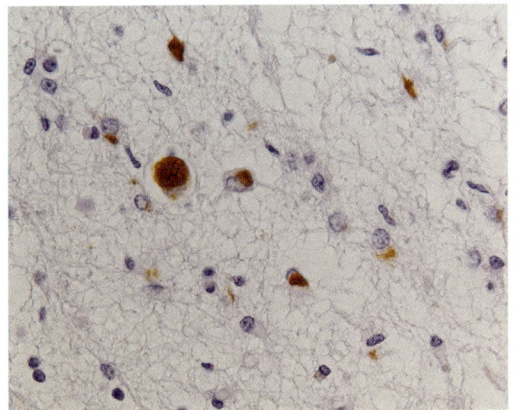

Figure 4.23
Pick like inclusions in a patient with FTLD-TAU, MAPT 315 mutation, in atrophic frontal cortex (tau (AT8) staining).

shows many Pick-like inclusions of 3-repeat tau (134). Some mutations in exons 9, 11, 12 and 13 also lead to Pick-like inclusions; they can be found in the frontotemporal cortex, caudate nucleus, pallidum, hippocampus (CA1, subiculum, facia dentata) and substantia nigra. Along with Pick-like inclusions and tangles, neuronal tau staining can be diffuse, ring-like, granular, rounded, oval and dot-like. Ballooned neurons can be visualised with αB-crystallin.

In areas with severe neuronal loss and gliosis, the architecture cannot be recognised, and spongiosis is present. The pattern in Western blotting for tau varies from Pick-like doublets to AD-like triplets and PSP-like doublets depending on the type of mutation (amount of 3-repeat tau and 4-repeat tau).

FTLD-TDP (Tardopathies)

Macroscopically, the brain is lighter than normal, and weights of less than 1000 grams are not uncommon. Cerebral atrophy is seen, principally involving the frontal, anterior parietal, and temporal lobes. The atrophy can be asymmetric. In some cases, the atrophy is confined to the frontal part, especially in type B which is associated with motor neuron disease. Others can show more temporal involvement. In general, the motor cor-

tex, sensorimotor cortex, and posterior cerebral hemispheres are largely unaffected, and the cerebellum and brainstem appear externally normal. Upon coronal section, the atrophy is obvious within the frontal, anterior temporal, anterior parietal, anterior cingulate and anterior insular regions. The amygdala is frequently atrophied, as is the caudate nucleus. The mesial temporal lobe and hippocampus can be atrophic as well. The lateral ventricles are always enlarged. In some instances, the substantia nigra is pale, but the locus ceruleus is pigmented. The ventral roots in the spinal cord can be atrophic in FTLD with motor neuron disease. The most important abnormalities on routine staining consist of microvacuolar changes in layer II and neuronal loss within the outer cortical laminae, mainly in layer II and upper layer III (see Figure 4.24). Occasionally, swollen chromatolytic neurons are seen, especially in layers V and VI (immunoreactive for αB-crystallin). Any astroglial reaction is slight, and the loss of myelin and axons is often inconspicuous. Distinctive inclusion bodies are absent in routine staining, and this distinguishes frontal lobe-type histology from Pick-type histology, where the pyramidal cell loss is accompanied by astrocytosis with intraneuronal inclusions, and the microvacuolation is not limited to the superficial layers.

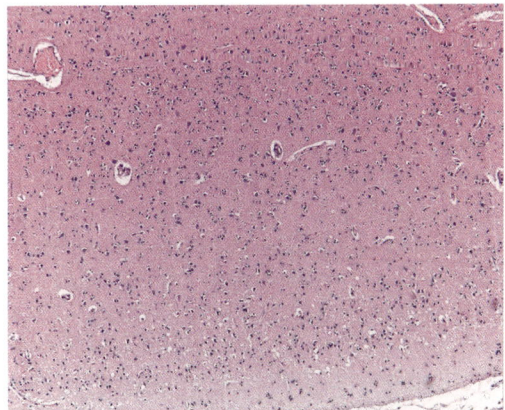

Figure 4.24
Microvacuolar changes and mild gliosis in layer II of the parietal cortex in FTLD-TDP type B (haematoxyline & eosin staining).

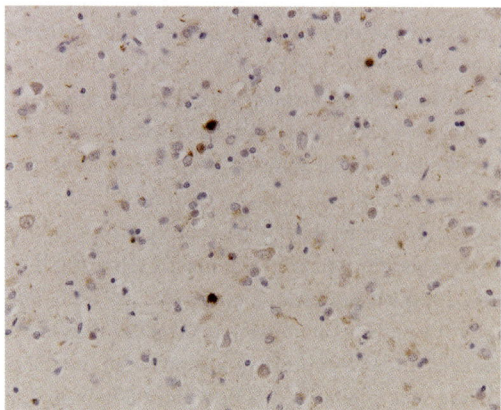

Figure 4.25
Cytoplasmic neuronal inclusions and few threads in frontal cortex of patient with FTLD-TDP type B (pTDP-43 staining).

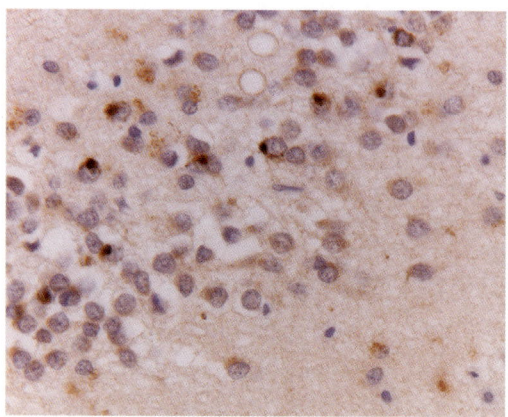

Figure 4.26
Cytoplasmic neuronal inclusions in the granular layer of the hippocampus in FTLD-TDP type B (pTDP-43 staining).

Four disease types can be recognised using antibodies against pTDP. However, using P62, even more inclusions and threads can be visualised. In the most frequent type, type A, often based on hereditary progranulin mutations, many small threads and crescentic and oval-shaped, neuronal, cytoplasmic inclusions are seen along with a few lentiform, intranuclear, neuronal inclusions. Layer II of the cerebral frontotemporal cortex is particularly affected. Sporadic mutations in progranulin also occur. A proportion of this type A is caused by hexanucleotide insertions on chromosome 9p (C9orf72), which usually causes type B.

In type B, star-shaped and rounded, neuronal, cytoplasmic inclusions are seen dispersed in all cortical layers, and small numbers of neuropil threads but rarely intranuclear inclusions can be observed. Interestingly, the number of these hexanucleotide insertions can increase with age. This type is often related to familial ALS, and patients in one family can have FTLD or ALS or both (135,136). Parkinsonism and ataxia have also been described. It is important to note that the cerebellum of these C9orf72 cases shows very small dots of P62 (but not TDP-43) immunoreactivity in the granular layer, which is pathognomonic for these C9orf72 cases and can be used for the neuropathological diagnosis. The number of these small inclusions can vary considerably from rare to numerous. Type B has characteristics of both frontotemporal dementia and motor neuron disease. In the affected frontal, temporal, and parietal cortices, there are microvacuolar changes in layer II (see Figure 4.24) and intraneuronal inclusions, which are ubiquitin and TDP-43-immunoreactive (see Figure 4.25), in all layers. Similar inclusions are present in the granule cells of the dentate gyrus of the hippocampus (see Figure 4.26). Inclusions may be seen in the cingulate cortex, basal ganglia and motor cortex as well. The substantia nigra is nearly always damaged. As in classic motor neuron disease, the characteristic skein-like or rounded, ubiquitin inclusions can be seen within the motor neurons of the anterior horns of the spinal cord and brainstem cranial nerve nuclei, accompanied by cell loss.

Type C of the TDP proteinopathies is rare and shows prominent, large, TDP-positive neuropil threads in the cortex, especially layer II, but far fewer neuronal cytoplasmic inclusions and no intranuclear inclusions. The caudate and putamen do show more cytoplasmic inclusions and fewer threads (see Figure 4.27). Type D is quite rare as well and related to mutations in the gene encoding valosine-containing protein and

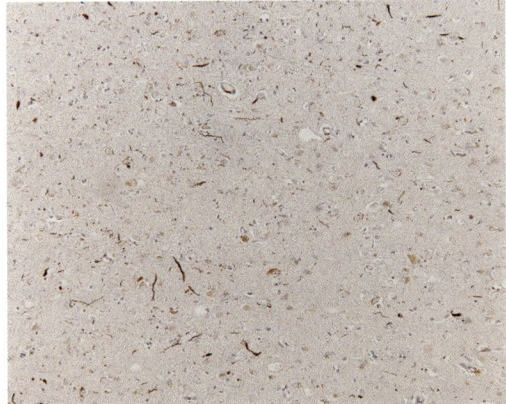

Figure 4.27
Cytoplasmic inclusions and neuropil threads in the putamen and caudate nucleus in FTLD-TDP type C (pTDP-43 staining).

has prominent neuronal intranuclear inclusions but few threads and cytoplasmic inclusions dispersed in all layers (123). As well as FTD, these patients have Paget disease of the bone and inclusion body myopathy. TDP-43 proteinopathies show glial inclusions in addition to the spectrum of neuronal inclusions (cytoplasmic, intranuclear and dystrophic neurites), which are predominantly oligodendroglial. Tau- and TDP-43-negative forms of FTLD with ubiquitin inclusions are rare disorders, like basophilic inclusion body disease charged multivesicular body protein 2B (CHMP2B) mutation and neu-

ronal intermediate filament inclusion disease, but their relation to FUS is still unclear.

Polyglutamine disorders (CAG repeat diseases)

The CAG-repeat (polyQ) disorders are hereditary neurodegenerative disorders caused by an expansion of CAG repeats and include at least Huntington's disease, spinocerebellar ataxias (SCA) type 1, 2, 3, 6, 7 and 17, dentatorubral pallidoluysian atrophy (DRPLA) and X-linked spinobulbar muscular atrophy of Kennedy (138). Specific disease-associated mutant proteins include huntingtin for Huntington's disease, atrophin-1 for DRPLA, the androgen receptor for spinobulbar muscular atrophy and ataxins 1, 2, 3 and 7 for SCA type 1, type 2, type 3, and type 7, respectively. The CAG expansion of SCA type 6 has been identified in the gene for the human alpha 1A, voltage-dependent, calcium-channel protein. Repeats in SCA 17 are in a TATA-box-binding protein. Increasing size of the CAG repeat expansion correlates with increased pathology in several of these disorders.

Huntington's disease

Macroscopically, a variable amount of atrophy can be seen with a reduced brain weight down to 30% of the normal weight. On the cut surface, the

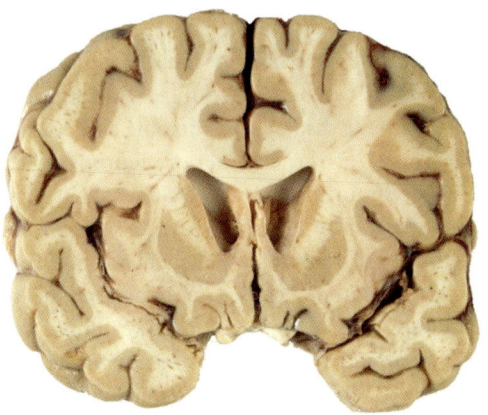
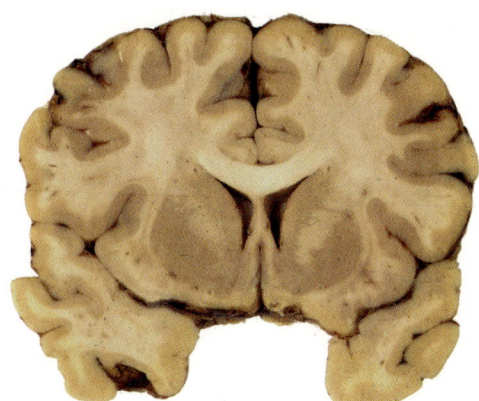

Figure 4.28
Atrophy of corpus striatum in Huntington's disease (right: control).

caudate nucleus, putamen and globus pallidus are atrophic, resulting in dilatation of the lateral ventricle, especially the frontal part (see Figure 4.28) (139). Initially, the caudate nucleus is affected. A grading system (encompassing 5 grades: 0-4) is used that combines macroscopic and microscopic features and correlates them with clinical signs (140,141). In grade 0-1 there is substantial evidence for a clinical diagnosis of Huntington's disease, but no macroscopic alterations and mild to moderate fibrillary astrocytosis and neuronal loss in the caudate nucleus (only in stage 1).

Grade 2 applies when atrophy of the head of the caudate nucleus is evident macroscopically, but the convex outline is retained. In grades 3 and 4 more microscopic changes are found – diffuse, severe nerve cell depletion and fibrillary astrocytosis in the CN and putamen – and the surface is much less convex or even concave (grade 4). Microscopically, neuronal loss is seen also outside the striatum, i.e. in the neocortex, allocortex (deep entorhinal layer), hypothalamus, thalamus, subthalamic nucleus and substantia nigra pars reticularis (142-144). In addition, Purkinje cells in the cerebellum and cortical regions may be affected (145). The presence of neuronal inclusions and abnormal neurites in the striatum and neocortex (layers III, V and VI) are important diagnostic features. They can be visualised using antibod-

ies against huntingtin and against polyglutamine (mab1C2) (see Figure 4.29) (146), but also antibodies against chaperone proteins like ubiquitin and P62. In the allocortex, these inclusions and neurites are seen in the entorhinal region, subiculum and pyramidal cells of the amygdala (147).

Spinocerebellar ataxias (SCAs)

The spinocerebellar ataxias (SCAs) represent a heterogeneous group of neurodegenerative disorders with progressive ataxia and cerebellar degeneration. The SCAs are distinguishable by their specific morphological appearance of the cerebellar, extrapyramidal and/or oculomotor systems and classified based on the underlying genetic defects and typical disease courses (148). To date, 31 SCA types have been genetically defined which result from cerebellar damage and interconnected brain nuclei (149). The SCA1, SCA2, SCA3, SCA6 and SCA7 are genetically defined, autosomal dominant, progressive cerebellar ataxias.

SCA1

Macroscopically, mild to moderate widening of the sulci, atrophy of pons, cerebellum, inferior olive and spinal cord is visible in SCA1 patients. Pallor of the substantia nigra can occur as well. Microscopically, the loss of Purkinje cells in the cerebellum is severe, and the few remaining cells exhibit pathological alterations (i.e. axonal torpedoes or altered dendritic trees). Pontine nuclei and inferior olivary nuclei also show neuronal loss, resulting in atrophy of the superior, medial and inferior cerebellar peduncle. Furthermore, SCA1 patients display considerable and consistent damage of the cholinergic neurons in the basal forebrain in contrast to SCA2, SCA3 and SCA7 (150). The thalamus reveals selective degeneration of motor, somatosensory and visual nuclei. The red nucleus and cranial nerve nuclei (including the oculomotor and vestibular nuclei) are affected as well. Apparent neuronal loss is visible in the spinal cord, in particular spinal motor neurons and neurons in the dorsal nuclei of Clarke. In the posterior columns, the nucleus

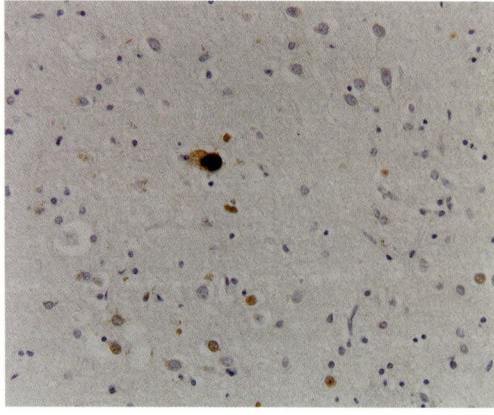

Figure 4.29
Cytoplasmic and nuclear inclusions in caudate nucleus in Huntington's disease (1C2 staining).

gracilis is variably involved. Immunohistochemically, intranuclear inclusions mimicking nucleoli can be found in broad areas of the brain, specifically in the pontine nuclei. These inclusions can be visualised using antibodies against ubiquitin, ataxin-1 and expanded polyglutamine stretches (IC2). Purkinje cells, although heavily affected in SCA1 patients, do not show prominent intranuclear inclusions (138, 150,151).

SCA2

The brain damage observed in SCA2 patients is quite similar to that in SCA1. The brain weight is largely reduced, and atrophic changes are seen in the pons, cerebellum, medulla oblongata and cranial nerves III-XII, as well as pallor of the substantia nigra. Microscopically, loss of Purkinje cells and granule cells in the cerebellum, of neurons in the pontine nuclei, thalamus, substantia nigra, nucleus ruber, and colliculi, of olivary nuclei in the dorsal columns of the spinal cord, and of dorsal nuclei of Clarke is apparent. Neuronal loss combined with astrogliosis has been described in trigeminal, facial and hypoglossal nuclei. The ambiguus nucleus and the solitary and reticular nuclei can be damaged as well (152,153). The presence of neuronal intranuclear inclusions is not prominent in SCA2, in contrast to other polyQ disorders. In the largely affected Purkinje cells, many cytoplasmic granules can be made visible with an antibody against ataxin-2, but not ubiquitin (138).

SCA3

SCA 3, also called Machado-Joseph's disease, is the most frequent but also the most heterogeneous form of the SCAs. It accounts for about 30-35% of the SCA patients. Again, neurodegeneration is largely similar to both SCA1 and SCA2. The brain weight is reduced, and macroscopic

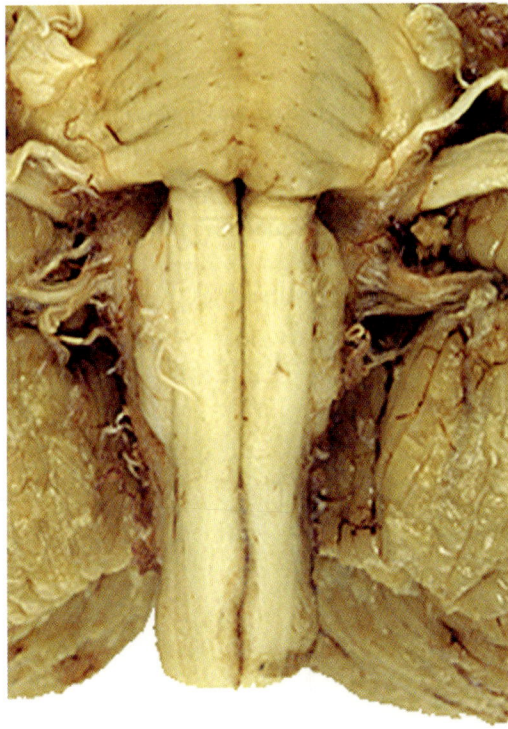
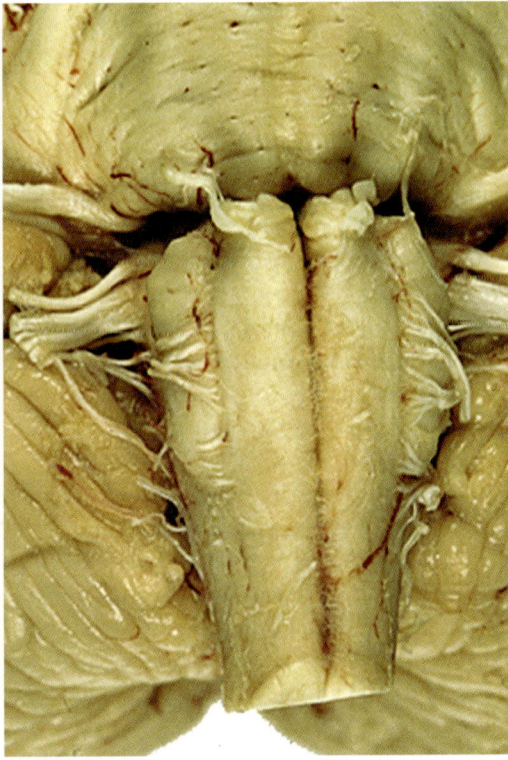

Figure 4.30
Atrophy of pons and outgoing nerves in spinocerebellar ataxia, type 3 (right: control).

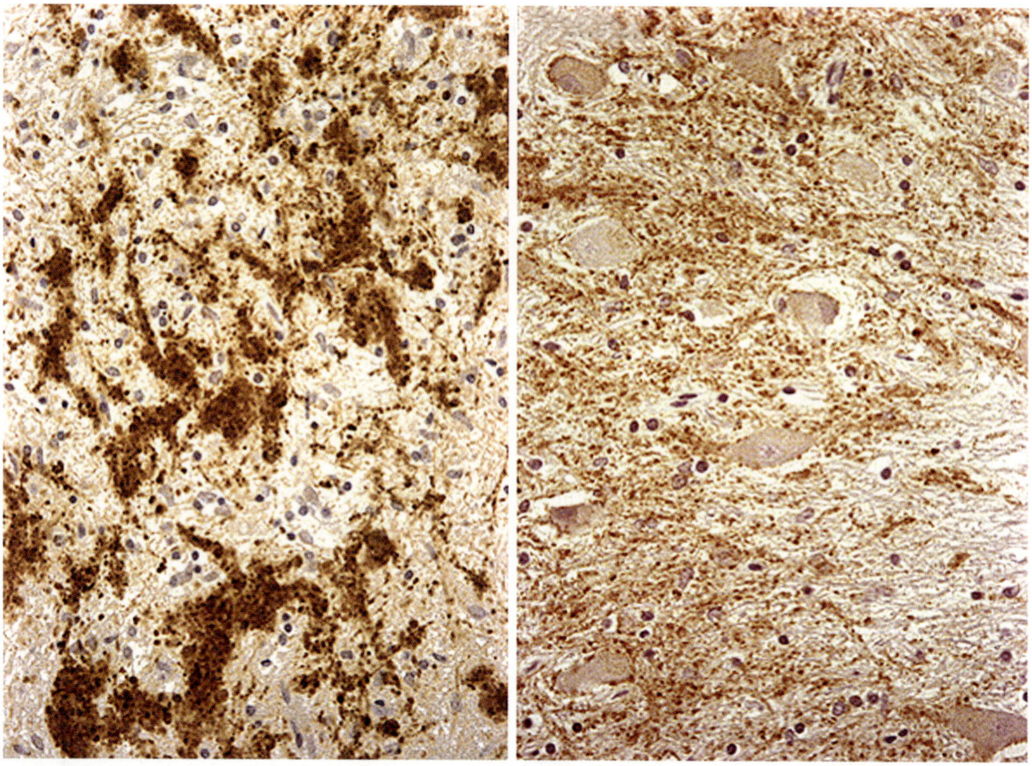

Figure 4.31
'Grumose' degeneration in cerebellum in spinocerebellar ataxia, type 3 (dentate nucleus, synaptophysin staining; right: control).

features include depigmentation of the substantia nigra and considerable atrophy of the pons, cerebellum, medulla oblongata, spinal cord and variable atrophy of the outgoing cranial nerves III-XII (see Figure 4.30). The major microscopical abnormalities are found in the spinocerebellar system (including severe neuronal loss and degeneration of Clarke's column) and anterior horn of the spinal cord, dentate nuclei ('eosinophilic grumose' degeneration that can be visualised nicely using synaptophysin staining) (see Figure 4.31), cerebellar Purkinje cells and the pontine nuclei. Changes in the extrapyramidal system include abnormalities in the globus pallidus (especially the medial internal part), thalamus, subthalamic nucleus, substantia nigra and nucleus ruber.

In the neocortex, most of the terminal SCA3 patients show a severe depletion of giant Betz py-

ramidal cells in the primary motor cortex. In the lower brainstem, in addition to the nuclei of the vestibular system, degenerative changes in the ingestion-related nuclei such as trigeminal, facial,

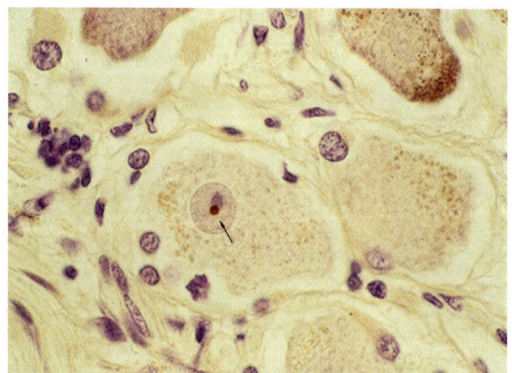

Figure 4.32
Intranuclear inclusion in dorsal ganglion in spinocerebellar ataxia, type 3 (ataxin-3 staining).

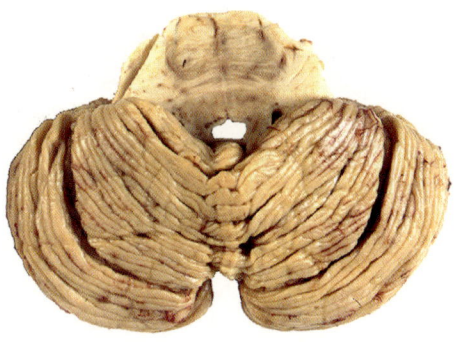
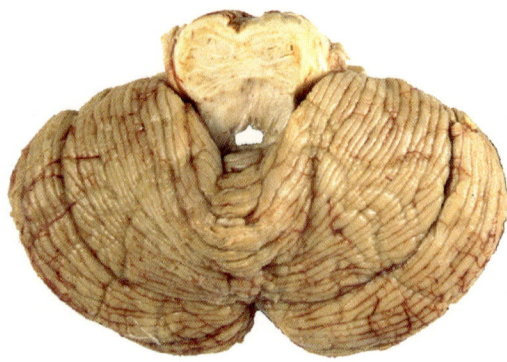

Figure 4.33
Atrophy of cerebellum in spinocerebellar ataxia, type 6 (right: control).

hypoglossal ambiguus, dmX, solitary and reticular nuclei have been described (154). Neuronal loss is associated with a marked astrogliosis.
Outside the brain, neurons in the dorsal ganglia are affected as well (see Figure 4.32). The intranuclear inclusions can be found in affected brain regions and visualised using antibodies against ataxin-3, expanded polyglutamine stretches and transcription factors. No inclusions have been observed in Purkinje cells.

SCA6

Trinucleotide CAG repeat in this type of ataxia is found in the gene coding for the α-subunit of a calcium channel (CACNA-1A) on chromosome 19. This protein is expressed strongly in Purkinje cells. Therefore, atrophy in the cerebellum is most obvious (see Figure 4.33) (155).
The severe atrophy of the cerebellum is most pronounced in the vermis and can optimally be visualized in sagittal sections (see Figure 4.34). The pons is frequently normal. Microscopic changes

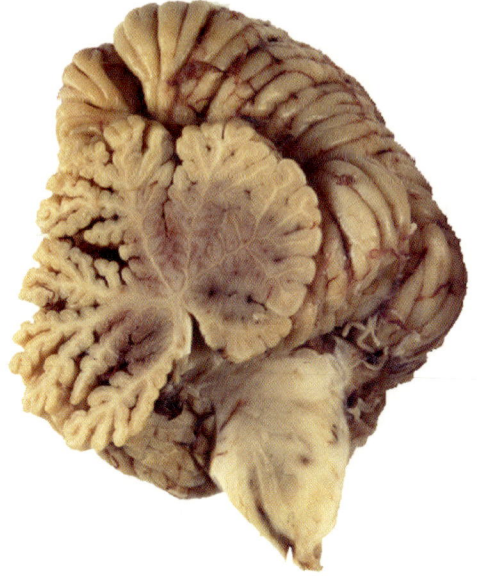
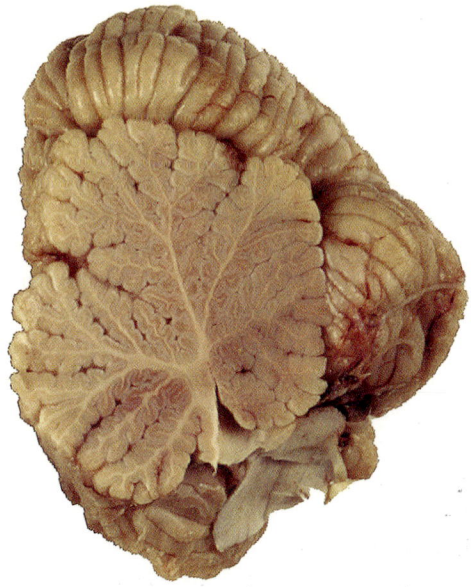

Figure 4.34
Sagittal slice of spinocerebellar ataxia, type 6, through vermis showing atrophy particularly of the anterior part (right: control).

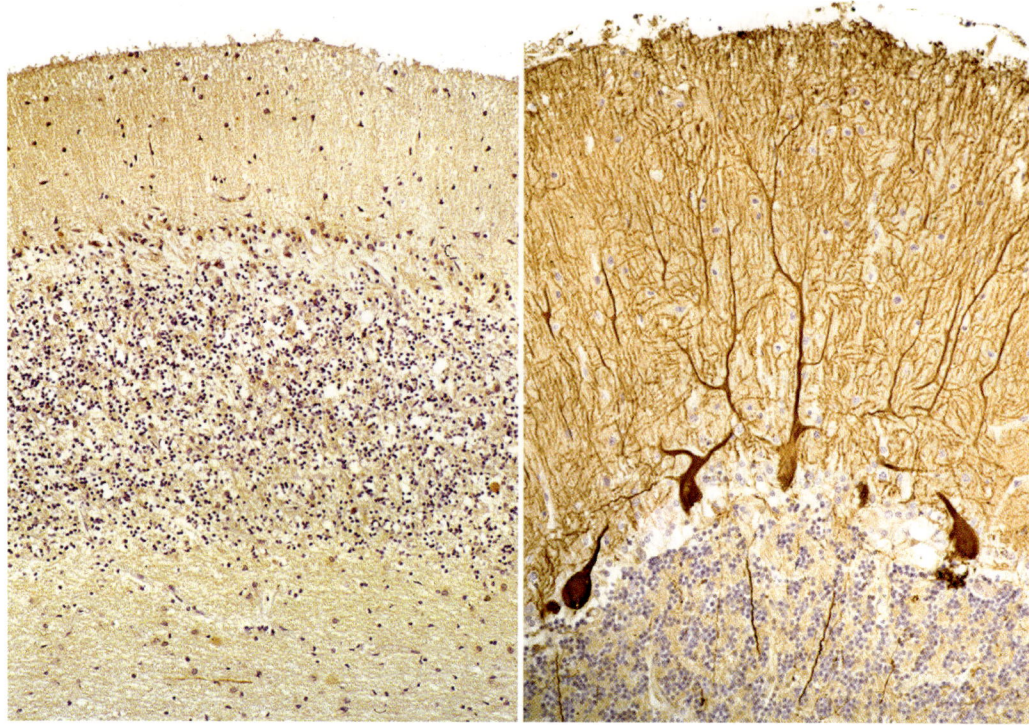

Figure 4.35
Loss of Purkinje cells in atrophic cerebellum in spinocerebellar ataxia, type 6 (vermis, calbindin staining, right: control).

in SCA6 are less severe and less widespread compared to SCA1, SCA2, SCA3, SCA4 and SCA7. Neuronal loss is visible in the Purkinje cells (see Figure 4.35), deep cerebellar nuclei and Betz pyramidal cells in the primary motor cortex. The marked loss of Purkinje cells can be demonstrated microscopically using antibodies against calbindin, a calcium-binding protein. The dendritic arborisation is almost completely lost. Changes in the vermis are most severe in the superior part. The dentate nucleus is usually normal. The inferior olives show a variable loss of neurons and gliosis, probably because of trans-synaptic degeneration. Degenerative changes have been described in some brainstem nuclei such as trigeminal nucleus, facial nucleus, solitary nucleus and reticular nucleus (154). Microglia activation can be visualized using microglia markers (CD68 of HLA-DR). Intranuclear inclusions have not been

observed. The mutated protein is found in the cytoplasm of Purkinje cells (156).

SCA7

A reduced brain weight is often noted. Atrophy of the cerebellar molecular and granular layers, loss of Purkinje cells (see Figure 4.36A and B), nerve cell loss and eosinophilic granular degeneration of the cerebellar dentate nucleus, neuronal loss in the substantia nigra, red nucleus, internal and external segments of the pallidum, thalamus and cerebral cortex have been found as well as degenerative changes in the spinal cord, motorneurons and destruction of the Clarke column (148,157). Widespread degeneration of the brainstem nuclei involved has also been seen. Immunocytochemical analysis (anti-ataxin-7) showed the presence of neuronal inclusions in degenerated brain and retinal regions as well as

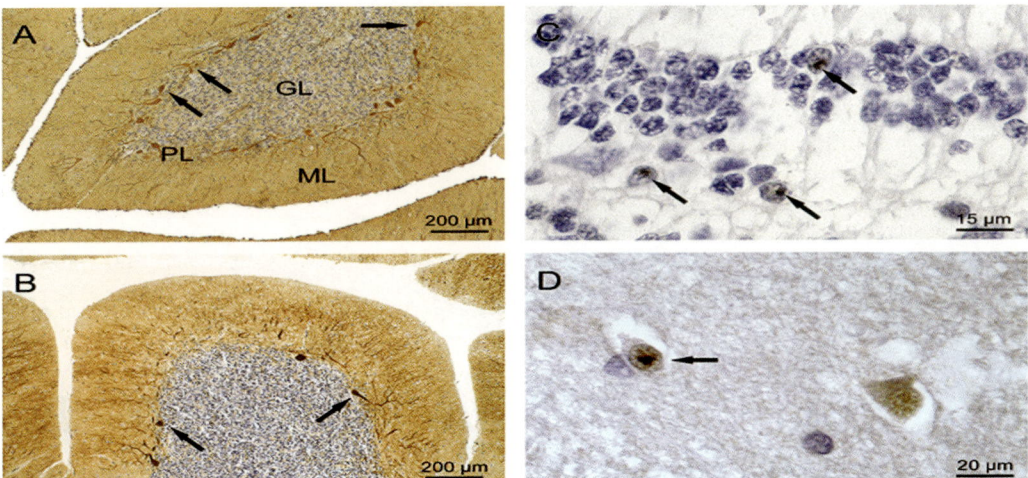

Figure 4.36
Spinocerebellar ataxia, type 7: A and B: cerebellum with few Purkinje cells and loss of dendritic network (calbindin staining). C: neuronal inclusions in retina (ataxin-7 staining). D: neuronal inclusion in facial nucleus (ataxin-7 staining).

in well-preserved brain and retina regions (see Figure 4.36C and D). In contrast to the other polyQ disorders like Huntington, SCA1, SCA2 and SCA3, their distribution is not restricted to areas of severe neuronal loss (157,158).

Prion diseases

Human prion diseases, also known as transmissible spongiform encephalopathies (TSEs), are rare, rapidly progressive, fatal, neurodegenerative disorders that exhibit a wide variety of clinical and histopathological phenotypes. The current classification allows for six major subtypes with distinctive pathological features based on the combination of the prion protein PrP^{Sc} typing (type 1 or 2) and the codon 129 polymorphism (MM, MV or VV) (159,160).
Prion diseases affect the central nervous system through alterations in the conformation of the cellular PrP, sometimes in combination with depositions of tau, α-synuclein and Aβ.

Creutzfeldt-Jakob disease
The gross appearance of the brain in Creutzfeldt-Jakob disease (CJD) and other prion disorders is remarkably variable. In most CJD patients, no recognizable abnormalities are seen, while cases with a long duration show varying degrees of cerebral, striatal, and/or cerebellar atrophy. The brain can weigh as little as 850 grams in panencephalopathic forms (walnut brains). Rare hereditary forms with atypical parkinsonian or PSP-like features can show complete loss of pigmentation in the substantia nigra.
The microscopic hallmarks of CJD and other prion disorders are spongiform degeneration of neurons and their processes, neuronal loss, reactive astrogliosis, and prion amyloid plaque formation after longer duration. These changes vary considerably from case to case and are also related to the type of prion molecule, depending on polymorphisms (especially on codon 129), glycosylation and the length of the PrP molecule (160,161). This variation in glycosylation and length leads to different electrophoretic mobility in Western blotting (type 1 band at 21 kD or type 2 band at 19 kDa). Type 2b is characteristic for variant CJD. Confirmation of the diagnosis can be done immunohistochemically with prion antibodies (mab 3F4), which can be performed after protein K pretreatment to eliminate normal prion molecules.

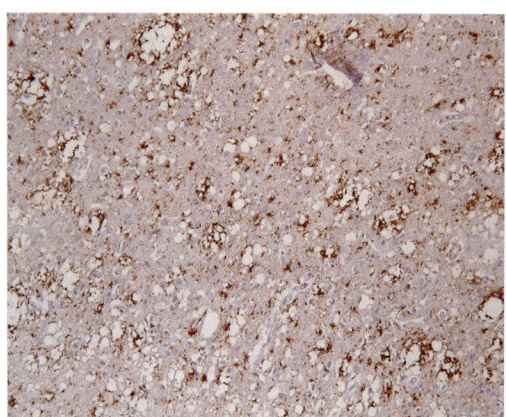

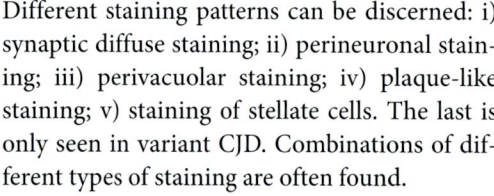

Figure 4.37
Perivacuolar and synaptic prion staining in the cerebral cortex of Creutzfeldt-Jakob disease (MV2K+C type) (3F4 staining).

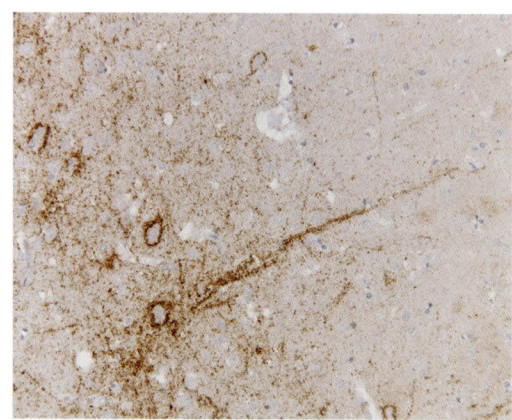

Figure 4.38
Perineuronal and synaptic prion staining in deep cortical layer in Creutzfeldt-Jakob disease (type VV2) (3F4 staining).

Different staining patterns can be discerned: i) synaptic diffuse staining; ii) perineuronal staining; iii) perivacuolar staining; iv) plaque-like staining; v) staining of stellate cells. The last is only seen in variant CJD. Combinations of different types of staining are often found.

In CJD with short duration as seen in MM1 or MV1 types, often the only histological abnormality is delicate vacuolation of the grey matter in all layers with minimal neuronal loss or astrogliosis. Immunohistochemistry with 3F4 antibodies shows synaptic and dot-like PrP staining. Spongiform degeneration can be found in the cerebral neocortex, putamen, caudate nucleus, thalamus, subiculum and cerebellar molecular layer. It is usually minimal in the brainstem and spinal cord. Vacuolation is mostly confined to nerve cell processes. Generally, the lesions in the white matter are secondary to neuronal loss and can be extensive in the panencephalopathic form, showing numerous macrophages. Occasionally, no or very weak staining can be seen in the frontal regions, and different blocks must be examined to confirm the diagnosis. Severe spongiosis in the entorhinal and temporal cortex in DLB patients can mimic CJD, but prion staining will be negative in these cases. Other main forms of CJD are MV2K with Kuru-type plaques, especially in the cerebellum,

VV2 with a band of peri-neuronal staining of the deep layers (see Figure 4.38), MM2C and MV2C with grapelike, confluating vacuoles and perivacuolar PrP staining, MM2T with prominent thalamic involvement, and the rare VV1 type with larger vacuoles sparing the occipital lobe and cerebellum. Combinations also often occur (see Figure 4.37) such as MV2K +C or MM/MV1 +2C, and atypical forms exist. Recently, several protease-sensitive (partly) prion disorders have been described, often VV2 types, that can be missed in blotting after protein K pretreatment.

Systematic examination of genetic CJD associated with the E200K mutation revealed α-synuclein pathology in ~15%, phospho-tau-immunoreactive neuritic profiles in ~92% and neurofibrillary degeneration in 38% of the CJD cases (162). Prion amyloid plaques are found in only 5-23% of sporadic and genetic CJD cases. In the bovine spongiform, encephalitis-related variant CJD, characteristic 'florid amyloid plaques' are found with a corona of vacuoles. In addition, clusters of small amyloid plaques are present. The PrP staining shows pathognomonic staining of stellate cells along with these prion plaques.

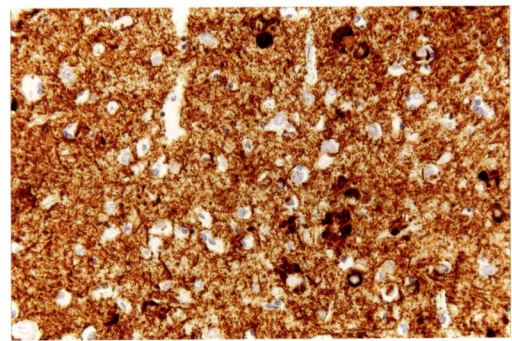

Figure 4.39
Tauopathy secondary to prion plaques in young patient with Gerstmann Sträussler Scheinker's disease, 227 mutation in prion gene (tau staining).

Gerstmann Sträussler Scheinker's (GSS) disease

In the hereditary Gerstmann Sträussler Scheinker's (GSS) disease, caused by mutations in the prion gene on chromosome 20, the prion amyloid plaques are often multicentric and especially present in the cerebellar cortex. The extend of tandem repeats in the octapeptide repeat insertion, mutated prion molecule strongly influences the formation of prion amyloid plaques in GSS. In the rare Q227X mutation with clinically atypical parkinsonian features, the histological picture can be similar to AD with numerous amyloid plaques (prion) and severe tauopathy with tangles, neuropil treads and dystrophic neurites in the cerebral cortex (126) (see Figure 4.39).

Summary

Neurodegenerative disorders, including movement disorders, are classified according to the growing number of .pathognomic protein abnormalities. α-Synuclein and tau are the important proteins that accumulate in neurons, abnormal neurites as well as glial cells in synucleinopathies (PD, DLB and MSA) and tauopathies (PSP, CBD, FTLD, TSE, Guam Parkinson-Dementia complex), respectively. Another protein, TDP-43, has been discovered that accumulates in cytoplasmic inclusions in parkin-

sonian and other neurodegenerative disorders. A uniform feature of all parkinsonian disorders is the nigrostriatal dopaminergic loss and accompanying α-synuclein pathology. However, co-morbidity with tau-immunoreactive pathology, Aβ plaques and vascular abnormalities is common in parkinsonian disorders, and these pathologies influence disease progression and clinical phenotypes.

α-Synuclein is the major substrate for LBs, LNs and the less frequently observed astrocytic inclusions in PD, DLB and α-synuclein-positive neurites and glial inclusions in MSA. Tau is the major substrate of tangles and inclusions in glial cells in PSP, CBD and FTLD-17T. To date, 17 'PARK' loci and multiple genetic associations have been associated with familial forms of PD, most of which reveal neuropathological hallmarks typical for PD, but varying histopathological features or lack of LB pathology has also been reported in these cases upon postmortem examination.

FTLD form a heterogeneous group of neurodegenerative disorders with intranuclear, intracytoplasmatic or neuritic neuronal inclusions that can be neuropathologically distinguished with tau, TDP-43 and FUS antibodies. Trinucleotide CAG repeat disorders are caused by the expansion of polyQ domains in specific disease-associated proteins, including huntingtin, atrophin and ataxins, leading to neuronal inclusions. CJD is the most common fatal prion disease in which the pathological protease resistance form PrP is often accompanied by α-synuclein, tau and Aβ pathology.

Harmonisation of the criteria and quantification of the abnormal protein deposits in a minimum set of regions is becoming more and more important for clinical correlations and monitoring of new biomarker candidates as is done in the consensus criteria for AD (22). Multiple pathologies are quite common and must be recognised and scored. In the future, new proteinopathies will be discovered in still unclassifiable disorders. In addition, shared genetic risk factors involved in various parkinsonian disorders and subtypes remain to be determined and may play an important role in developing novel therapeutic strategies aimed at preventing or stopping disease progression in these devastating disorders. Discovery of new mutations and proteins involved in the pathogenesis will lead to more biomarkers in neuropathology and will improve the further classification of neurodegenerative disorders.

Acknowledgements

This work was supported by the Stichting Internationaal Parkinson Fonds (IPF) and Neuroscience Campus Amsterdam (NCA), VU University Medical Center (VUmc) Amsterdam, the Netherlands.

We thank dr. Wouter Kamphorst, Michiel Kooreman and all other staff members of the Netherlands Brain Bank for their support. We are grateful to all patients and controls that donated their brains. In addition, we would like to thank the valuable input of dr. Rob A.I. de Vos and C. Jansen, Pathologie laboratorium Oost, Nederland, Hengelo.

References

1 Buee L, Bussiere T, Buee-Scherrer V, Delacourte A, Hof PR. Tau protein isoforms, phosphorylation and role in neurodegenerative disorders. Brain Res Brain Res Rev 2000;33:95-130.

2 Cairns NJ, Bigio EH, Mackenzie IR, et al. Neuropathologic diagnostic and nosologic criteria for frontotemporal lobar degeneration: consensus of the Consortium for Frontotemporal Lobar Degeneration. Acta Neuropathol (Berl) 2007;114:5-22.

3 Dickson DW. Tau and synuclein and their role in neuropathology. Brain Pathol 1999;9:657-61.

4 Polymeropoulos MH, Lavedan C, Leroy E, et al. Mutation in the alpha-synuclein gene identified in families with Parkinson's disease. Science 1997;276:2045-2047.

5 Spillantini MG, Schmidt ML, Lee VM, Trojanowski JQ, Jakes R, Goedert M. Alpha-synuclein in Lewy bodies. Nature 1997;388:839-840.

6 Clayton DF, George JM. The synucleins: a family of proteins involved in synaptic function, plasticity, neurodegeneration and disease. Trends Neurosci 1998;21:249-254.

7 Dickson DW, Braak H, Duda JE, et al. Neuropathological assessment of Parkinson's disease: refining the diagnostic criteria. Lancet Neurol 2009;8:1150-1157.

8 Halliday GM, Holton JL, Revesz T, Dickson DW. Neuropathology underlying clinical variability in patients with synucleinopathies. Acta Neuropathol 2011;122:187-204.

9 Farrer M, Chan P, Chen R, et al. Lewy bodies and parkinsonism in families with parkin mutations. Ann Neurol 2001;50:293-300.

10 Takahashi H, Ohama E, Suzuki S, et al. Familial juvenile parkinsonism: clinical and pathologic study in a family. Neurology 1994;44:437-441.

11 Forman MS, Schmidt ML, Kasturi S, Perl DP, Lee VM, Trojanowski JQ. Tau and alpha-synuclein pathology in amygdala of Parkinsonism-dementia complex patients of Guam. Am J Pathol 2002;160:1725-1731.

12 McKee AC, Cantu RC, Nowinski CJ, et al. Chronic traumatic encephalopathy in athletes: progressive tauopathy after repetitive head injury. J Neuropathol Exp Neurol 2009;68:709-735.

13 Irwin DJ, Cohen TJ, Grossman M, et al. Acetylated tau neuropathology in sporadic and hereditary tauopathies. Am J Pathol 2013;183:344-351.

14 Goedert M, Spillantini MG, Jakes R, Rutherford D, Crowther RA. Multiple isoforms of human microtubule-associated protein tau: sequences and localization in neurofibrillary tangles of Alzheimer's disease. Neuron 1989;3:519-526.

15 Mandelkow EM, Schweers O, Drewes G, et al. Structure, microtubule interactions, and phosphorylation of tau protein. Ann N Y Acad Sci 1996;777:96-106.

16 Iqbal K, Gong CX, Liu F. Hyperphosphorylation-induced tau oligomers. Front Neurol 2013;4:112.

17 Hutton M, Lendon CL, Rizzu P, et al. Association of missense and 5'-splice-site mutations in tau with the inherited dementia FTDP-17. Nature 1998;393:702-705.

18 Goedert M. Tau gene mutations and their effects. Mov Disord 2005;20S12:45-52.

19 Mackenzie IR, Neumann M, Bigio EH, et al. Nomenclature and nosology for neuropathologic subtypes of frontotemporal lobar degeneration: an update. Acta Neuropathol 2010;119:1-4.

20 Robitaille Y, Lopes-Cendes I, Becher M, Rouleau G, Clark AW. The neuropathology of CAG repeat diseases: review and update of genetic and molecular features. Brain Pathol 1997;7:901-926.

21 Vital A, Fernagut PO, Canron MH, et al. The nigrostriatal pathway in Creutzfeldt-Jakob disease. J Neuropathol Exp Neurol 2009;68:809-815.

22 Alafuzoff I, Ince PG, Arzberger T, et al. Staging/typing of Lewy body related alpha-synuclein pathology: a study of the BrainNet Europe Consortium. Acta Neuropathol 2009;117:635-652.

23 McKeith IG, Dickson DW, Lowe J, et al. Diagnosis and management of dementia with Lewy bodies: third report of the DLB Consortium. Neurology 2005;65:1863-1872.

24 Hyman BT, Phelps CH, Beach TG, et al. National Institute on Aging-Alzheimer's Association guidelines for the neuropathologic assessment of Alzheimer's disease. Alzheimers Dement 2012;8:1-13.

25 Schwartz AL, Ciechanover A. The ubiquitin-proteasome pathway and pathogenesis of human diseases. Annu Rev Med 1999;50:57-74.

26 Braak H, Braak E. Neuropathological stageing of Alzheimer-related changes. Acta Neuropathol (Berl) 1991;82:239-259.

27 Thal DR, Rub U, Orantes M, Braak H. Phases of A beta-deposition in the human brain and its relevance for the development of AD. Neurology 2002;58:1791-1800.

28 Braak H, Alafuzoff I, Arzberger T, Kretzschmar H, Del Tredici K. Staging of Alzheimer disease-associated neurofibrillary pathology using paraffin sections and immunocytochemistry. Acta Neuropathol (Berl) 2006;112:389-404.

29 Alafuzoff I, Gelpi E, Al-Sarraj S, et al. The need to unify neuropathological assessments of vascular alterations in the ageing brain: multicentre survey by the BrainNet Europe consortium. Exp Gerontol 2012;47:825-833.

30 Alafuzoff I, Pikkarainen M, Al-Sarraj S, et al. Interlaboratory comparison of assessments of Alzheimer disease-related lesions: a study of the BrainNet Europe Consortium. J Neuropathol Exp Neurol 2006;65:740-757.

31 Gelb DJ, Oliver E, Gilman S. Diagnostic criteria for Parkinson disease. Arch Neurol 1999;56:33-39.

32 Daniel SE, Lees AJ. Parkinson's Disease Society Brain Bank, London: overview and research. J Neural Transm Suppl 1993;39:165-172.

33 Braak H, de Vos RA, Jansen EN, Bratzke H, Braak E. Neuropathological hallmarks of Alzheimer's and Parkinson's diseases. Prog Brain Res 1998;117:267-285.

34 Marras C, Lang A. Invited article: changing concepts in Parkinson disease: moving beyond the decade of the brain. Neurology 2008;70:1996-2003.

35 Spillantini MG, Crowther RA, Jakes R, Hasegawa M, Goedert M. alpha-Synuclein in filamentous inclusions of Lewy bodies from Parkinson's disease and dementia with lewy bodies. Proc Natl Acad Sci U S A 1998;95:6469-6473.

36 Tashiro M, Kojima M, Kihara H, et al. Characterization of fibrillation process of alpha-synuclein at the initial stage. Biochem Biophys Res Commun 2008;369:910-914.

37 Anderson JP, Walker DE, Goldstein JM, et al. Phosphorylation of Ser-129 is the dominant pathological modification of alpha-synuclein in familial and sporadic Lewy body disease. J Biol Chem 2006;281:29739-29752.

38 Marques O, Outeiro TF. Alpha-synuclein: from secretion to dysfunction and death. Cell Death Dis 2012;3:e350.

39 Kanazawa T, Adachi E, Orimo S, Nakamura A, Mizusawa H, Uchihara T. Pale neurites, premature alpha-synuclein aggregates with centripetal extension from axon collaterals. Brain Pathol 2012;22:67-78.

40 Goedert M, Spillantini MG, Del TK, Braak H. 100 years of Lewy pathology. Nat Rev Neurol 2013;9:13-24.

41 Braak H, Del Tredici K, Rub U, de Vos RA, Jansen Steur EN, Braak E. Staging of brain pathology related to sporadic Parkinson's disease. Neurobiol Aging 2003;24:197-211.

42 Braak H, Bohl JR, Muller CM, Rub U, de Vos RA, Del Tredici K. Stanley Fahn Lecture 2005: The staging procedure for the inclusion body pathology associated with sporadic Parkinson's disease reconsidered. Mov Disord 2006;21:2042-2051.

43 Jellinger KA. Lewy body-related alpha-synucleinopathy in the aged human brain. J Neural Transm 2004;111:1219-1235.

44 Muller CM, de Vos RA, Maurage CA, Thal DR, Tolnay M, Braak H. Staging of sporadic Parkinson disease-related alpha-synuclein pathology: inter- and intra-rater reliability. J Neuropathol Exp Neurol 2005;64:623-638.

45 Jellinger KA. Alpha-synuclein lesions in normal aging, Parkinson disease, and Alzheimer disease: evidence from the Baltimore Longitudinal Study of Aging (BLSA). J Neuropathol Exp Neurol 2005;64:554.

46 Klos KJ, Ahlskog JE, Josephs KA, et al. Alpha-synuclein pathology in the spinal cords of neurologically asymptomatic aged individuals. Neurology 2006;66:1100-1102.

47 DelleDonne A, Klos KJ, Fujishiro H, et al. Incidental Lewy body disease and preclinical Parkinson disease. Arch Neurol 2008;65:1074-1080.

48 Buchman AS, Shulman JM, Nag S, et al. Nigral pathology and parkinsonian signs in elders without Parkinson disease. Ann Neurol 2012;71:258-266.

49 Harding AJ, Stimson E, Henderson JM, Halliday GM. Clinical correlates of selective pathology in the amygdala of patients with Parkinson's disease. Brain 2002;125:2431-2445.

50 Halliday GM. Thalamic changes in Parkinson's disease. Parkinsonism Relat Disord 2009;15S3:152-155.

51 Braak H, Sastre M, Bohl JR, de Vos RA, Del Tredici K. Parkinson's disease: lesions in dorsal horn layer I, involvement of parasympathetic and sympathetic pre- and postganglionic neurons. Acta Neuropathol (Berl) 2007;113:421-429.

52 Braak H, de Vos RA, Bohl J, Del Tredici K. Gastric alpha-synuclein immunoreactive inclusions in Meissner's and Auerbach's plexuses in cases staged for Parkinson's disease-related brain pathology. Neurosci Lett 2006;396:67-72.

53 Iwanaga K, Wakabayashi K, Yoshimoto M, et al. Lewy body-type degeneration in cardiac plexus in Parkinson's and incidental Lewy body diseases. Neurology 1999;52:1269-1271.

54 Braak H, Sastre M, Del Tredici K. Development of alpha-synuclein immunoreactive astrocytes in the forebrain parallels stages of intraneuronal pathology in sporadic Parkinson's disease. Acta Neuropathol (Berl) 2007;114:231-241.

55 Compta Y, Parkkinen L, O'Sullivan SS, et al. Lewy- and Alzheimer-type pathologies in Parkinson's disease dementia: which is more important? Brain 2011;134:1493-1505.

56 Horvath J, Herrmann FR, Burkhard PR, Bouras C, Kovari E. Neuropathology of dementia in a large cohort of patients with Parkinson's disease. Parkinsonism Relat Disord 2013;19:864-868.

57 Selikhova M, Williams DR, Kempster PA, Holton JL, Revesz T, Lees AJ. A clinico-pathological study of subtypes in Parkinson's disease. Brain 2009;132:2947-2957.

58 Selikhova M, Williams DR, Kempster PA, Holton JL, Revesz T, Lees AJ. A clinico-pathological study of subtypes in Parkinson's disease. Brain 2009;132:2947-2957.

59 van de Berg WD, Hepp DH, Dijkstra AA, Rozemuller JA, Berendse HW, Foncke E. Patterns of alpha-synuclein pathology in incidental cases and clinical subtypes of Parkinson's disease. Parkinsonism Relat Disord 2012;18S1:28-30.

60 Selikhova M, Williams DR, Kempster PA, Holton JL, Revesz T, Lees AJ. A clinico-pathological study of subtypes in Parkinson's disease. Brain 2009;132:2947-2957.

61 Houlden H, Singleton AB. The genetics and neuropathology of Parkinson's disease. Acta Neuropathol 2012;124:325-338.

62 Trinh J, Farrer M. Advances in the genetics of Parkinson disease. Nat Rev Neurol 2013;9:445-454.

63 Doherty KM, Silveira-Moriyama L, Parkkinen L, et al. Parkin disease: a clinicopathologic entity? JAMA Neurol 2013;70:571-579.

64 Zimprich A, Biskup S, Leitner P, et al. Mutations in LRRK2 cause autosomal-dominant parkinsonism

with pleomorphic pathology. Neuron 2004;44:601-607.

65 Hasegawa K, Stoessl AJ, Yokoyama T, Kowa H, Wszolek ZK, Yagishita S. Familial parkinsonism: study of original Sagamihara PARK8 (I2020T) kindred with variable clinicopathologic outcomes. Parkinsonism Relat Disord 2009;15:300-306.

66 Samaranch L, Lorenzo-Betancor O, Arbelo JM, et al. PINK1-linked parkinsonism is associated with Lewy body pathology. Brain 2010;133:1128-1142.

67 Kruer MC, Hiken M, Gregory A, et al. Novel histopathologic findings in molecularly-confirmed pantothenate kinase-associated neurodegeneration. Brain 2011;134:947-958.

68 Sidransky E, Lopez G. The link between the GBA gene and parkinsonism. Lancet Neurol 2012;11:986-998.

69 Duda JE, Giasson BI, Mabon ME, et al. Concurrence of alpha-synuclein and tau brain pathology in the Contursi kindred. Acta Neuropathol 2002;104:7-11.

70 Golbe LI, Di IG, Bonavita V, Miller DC, Duvoisin RC. A large kindred with autosomal dominant Parkinson's disease. Ann Neurol 1990;27:276-282.

71 Spira PJ, Sharpe DM, Halliday G, Cavanagh J, Nicholson GA. Clinical and pathological features of a Parkinsonian syndrome in a family with an Ala53Thr alpha-synuclein mutation. Ann Neurol 2001;49:313-319.

72 Zarranz JJ, Alegre J, Gomez-Esteban JC, et al. The new mutation, E46K, of alpha-synuclein causes Parkinson and Lewy body dementia. Ann Neurol 2004;55:164-173.

73 Obi T, Nishioka K, Ross OA, et al. Clinicopathologic study of a SNCA gene duplication patient with Parkinson disease and dementia. Neurology 2008;70:238-241.

74 Gouider-Khouja N, Larnaout A, Amouri R, et al. Autosomal recessive parkinsonism linked to parkin gene in a Tunisian family. Clinical, genetic and pathological study. Parkinsonism Relat Disord 2003;9:247-251.

75 Hayashi S, Wakabayashi K, Ishikawa A, et al. An autopsy case of autosomal-recessive juvenile par-

kinsonism with a homozygous exon 4 deletion in the parkin gene. Mov Disord 2000;15:884-888.

76 Mori H, Kondo T, Yokochi M, et al. Pathologic and biochemical studies of juvenile parkinsonism linked to chromosome 6q. Neurology 1998;51:890-89.

77 van de Warrenburg BP, Lammens M, Lucking CB, et al. Clinical and pathologic abnormalities in a family with parkinsonism and parkin gene mutations. Neurology 2001;56:555-557.

78 Sasaki S, Shirata A, Yamane K, Iwata M. Parkin-positive autosomal recessive juvenile Parkinsonism with alpha-synuclein-positive inclusions. Neurology 2004;63:678-682.

79 Pramstaller PP, Schlossmacher MG, Jacques TS, et al. Lewy body Parkinson's disease in a large pedigree with 77 Parkin mutation carriers. Ann Neurol 2005;58:411-422.

80 Gaig C, Marti MJ, Ezquerra M, Rey MJ, Cardozo A, Tolosa E. G2019S LRRK2 mutation causing Parkinson's disease without Lewy bodies. J Neurol Neurosurg Psychiatry 2007;78:626-628.

81 Khan NL, Jain S, Lynch JM, et al. Mutations in the gene LRRK2 encoding dardarin PARK8) cause familial Parkinson's disease: clinical, pathological, olfactory and functional imaging and genetic data. Brain 2005;128:2786-2796.

82 Ross OA, Toft M, Whittle AJ, et al. Lrrk2 and Lewy body disease. Ann Neurol 2006;59:388-393.

83 Marti-Masso JF, Ruiz-Martinez J, Bolano MJ, et al. Neuropathology of Parkinson's disease with the R1441G mutation in LRRK2. Mov Disord 2009;24:1998-2001.

84 Paisan-Ruiz C, Guevara R, Federoff M, E, et al. Early-onset L-dopa-responsive parkinsonism with pyramidal signs due to ATP13A2, PLA2G6, FBXO7 and spatacsin mutations. Mov Disord 2010;25:1791-1800.

85 Aarsland D, Ballard CG, Halliday G. Are Parkinson's disease with dementia and dementia with Lewy bodies the same entity? J Geriatr Psychiatry Neurol 2004;17:137-145.

86 Jellinger KA. Significance of brain lesions in Parkinson disease dementia and Lewy body dementia. Front Neurol Neurosci 2009;24:114-125.

87 Halliday GM, Song YJ, Harding AJ. Striatal beta-amyloid in dementia with Lewy bodies but not Parkinson's disease. J Neural Transm 2011;118:713-719.

88 Jellinger KA, Attems J. Does striatal pathology distinguish Parkinson disease with dementia and dementia with Lewy bodies? Acta Neuropathol 2006;112:253-260.

89 Mirra SS, Heyman A, McKeel D, et al. The Consortium to Establish a Registry for Alzheimer's Disease (CERAD). Part II. Standardization of the neuropathologic assessment of Alzheimer's disease. Neurology 1991;41:479-486.

90 Fujishiro H, Ferman TJ, Boeve BF, et al. Validation of the neuropathologic criteria of the third consortium for dementia with Lewy bodies for prospectively diagnosed cases. J Neuropathol Exp Neurol 2008;67:649-656.

91 Ballard C, Ziabreva I, Perry R, et al. Differences in neuropathologic characteristics across the Lewy body dementia spectrum. Neurology 2006;67:1931-1934.

92 Sherzai A, Edland SD, Masliah E, et al. Spongiform change in dementia with Lewy bodies and Alzheimer disease. Alzheimer Dis Assoc Disord 2013;27:157-161.

93 McKeith IG, Perry EK, Perry RH. Report of the second dementia with Lewy body international workshop: diagnosis and treatment. Consortium on Dementia with Lewy Bodies. Neurology 1999;53:902-905.

94 Wenning GK, Stefanova N, Jellinger KA, Poewe W, Schlossmacher MG. Multiple system atrophy: a primary oligodendrogliopathy. Ann Neurol 2008;64:239-246.

95 Gilman S, Wenning GK, Low PA, et al. Second consensus statement on the diagnosis of multiple system atrophy. Neurology 2008;71:670-676.

96 Papp MI, Kahn JE, Lantos PL. Glial cytoplasmic inclusions in the CNS of patients with multiple system atrophy (striatonigral degeneration, olivopontocerebellar atrophy and Shy-Drager syndrome). J Neurol Sci 1989;94:79-100.

97 Jellinger KA, Lantos PL. Papp-Lantos inclusions and the pathogenesis of multiple system atrophy: an update. Acta Neuropathol 2010;119:657-667.

98 Arima K, Murayama S, Mukoyama M, Inose T. Immunocytochemical and ultrastructural studies of neuronal and oligodendroglial cytoplasmic inclusions in multiple system atrophy. 1. Neuronal cytoplasmic inclusions. Acta Neuropathol 1992;83:453-460.

99 Gilman S, Low PA, Quinn N, et al. Consensus statement on the diagnosis of multiple system atrophy. J Auton Nerv Syst 1998;74:189-192.

100 Papp MI, Lantos PL. The distribution of oligodendroglial inclusions in multiple system atrophy and its relevance to clinical symptomatology. Brain 1994;117:235-243.

101 Sone M, Yoshida M, Hashizume Y, Hishikawa N, Sobue G. alpha-Synuclein-immunoreactive structure formation is enhanced in sympathetic ganglia of patients with multiple system atrophy. Acta Neuropathol 2005;110:19-26.

102 Nishie M, Mori F, Yoshimoto M, Takahashi H, Wakabayashi K. A quantitative investigation of neuronal cytoplasmic and intranuclear inclusions in the pontine and inferior olivary nuclei in multiple system atrophy. Neuropathol Appl Neurobiol 2004;30:546-554.

103 Kanda T, Tsukagoshi H, Oda M, Miyamoto K, Tanabe H. Changes of unmyelinated nerve fibers in sural nerve in amyotrophic lateral sclerosis, Parkinson's disease and multiple system atrophy. Acta Neuropathol (Berl) 1996;91:145-154.

104 Pramstaller PP, Wenning GK, Smith SJ, Beck RO, Quinn NP, Fowler CJ. Nerve conduction studies, skeletal muscle EMG, and sphincter EMG in multiple system atrophy. J Neurol Neurosurg Psychiatry 1995;58:618-621.

105 Matsuo A, Akiguchi I, Lee GC, McGeer EG, McGeer PL, Kimura J. Myelin degeneration in multiple system atrophy detected by unique antibodies. Am J Pathol 1998;153:735-744.

106 Jellinger KA, Seppi K, Wenning GK. Grading of neuropathology in multiple system atrophy: proposal for a novel scale. Mov Disord 2005;2 S12:29-36.

107 Fujishiro H, Ahn TB, Frigerio R, et al. Glial cytoplasmic inclusions in neurologically normal elderly: prodromal multiple system atrophy? Acta Neuropathol 2008;116:269-275.

108 Lantos PL. The neuropathology of progressive supranuclear palsy. J Neural Transm1994;42S:137-152.

109 Dickson DW. Neuropathologic differentiation of progressive supranuclear palsy and corticobasal degeneration. J Neurol 1999;246S2:6-15.

110 Ikeda K, Akiyama H, Kondo H, et al. Thorn-shaped astrocytes: possibly secondarily induced tau-positive glial fibrillary tangles. Acta Neuropathol (Berl) 1995;90:620-625.

111 Komori T. Tau-positive glial inclusions in progressive supranuclear palsy, corticobasal degeneration and Pick's disease. Brain Pathol 1999;9:663-679.

112 Yamada T, Calne DB, Akiyama H, McGeer EG, McGeer PL. Further observations on Tau-positive glia in the brains with progressive supranuclear palsy. Acta Neuropathol (Berl) 1993;85:308-315.

113 Dickson DW, Rademakers R, Hutton ML. Progressive supranuclear palsy: pathology and genetics. Brain Pathol 2007;17:74-82.

114 de Silva R, Lashley T, Gibb G, et al. Pathological inclusion bodies in tauopathies contain distinct complements of tau with three or four microtubule-binding repeat domains as demonstrated by new specific monoclonal antibodies. Neuropathol Appl Neurobiol 2003;29:288-302.

115 Verny M, Duyckaerts C, Delaere P, He Y, Hauw JJ. Cortical tangles in progressive supranuclear palsy. J Neural Transm Suppl 1994;42:179-188.

116 Feany MB, Mattlace LA, Dickson DW Neuropathologic overlap of progressive supranuclear palsy, Pick's disease and corticobasal degeneration. J Neuropathol Exp Neurol 1996;55:53-67.

117 Mackenzie IR, Hudson LP. Achromatic neurons in the cortex of progressive supranuclear palsy. Acta Neuropathol (Berl) 1995;90:615-619.

118 Litvan I, Hauw JJ, Bartko JJ, et al. Validity and reliability of the preliminary NINDS neuropathologic criteria for progressive supranuclear palsy and related disorders. J Neuropathol Exp Neurol 1996;55:97-105.

119 Williams DR, Holton JL, Strand C, et al. Pathological tau burden and distribution distinguishes progressive supranuclear palsy-parkinsonism from Richardson's syndrome. Brain 2007;130:1566-1576.

120 Evidente VG, Adler CH, Sabbagh MN, et al. Neuropathological findings of PSP in the elderly without clinical PSP: possible incidental PSP? Parkinsonism Relat Disord 2011;17:365-371.

121 Gibb WR, Luthert PJ, Marsden CD. Corticobasal degeneration. Brain 1989;112:1171-1192.

122 Josephs KA, Hodges JR, Snowden JS, et al. Neuropathological background of phenotypical variability in frontotemporal dementia. Acta Neuropathol 2011;122:137-153.

123 Mackenzie IR, Munoz DG, Kusaka H, et al. Distinct pathological subtypes of FTLD-FUS. Acta Neuropathol 2011;121:207-218.

124 Sieben A, Van LT, Engelborghs S, et al. The genetics and neuropathology of frontotemporal lobar degeneration. Acta Neuropathol 2012;124:353-372.

125 Mackenzie IR, Shi J, Shaw CL, et al. Dementia lacking distinctive histology (DLDH) revisited. Acta Neuropathol (Berl) 2006;112:551-559.

126 Jansen C, Parchi P, Capellari S, et al. Human prion diseases in the Netherlands (1998-2009): clinical, genetic and molecular aspects. PLoS One 2012;7:e36333.

127 Braak H, Braak E. Pick's disease: cytoskeletal changes in the hypothalamic lateral tuberal nucleus. Brain Res 1998;802:119-124.

128 Kovacs GG, Rozemuller AJ, van Swieten JC, et al. Neuropathology of the hippocampus in FTLD-Tau with Pick bodies: A study of the BrainNet Europe Consortium. Neuropathol Appl Neurobiol 2012; doi: 10.1111/j.1365-2990.

129 Delacourte A, Sergeant N, Wattez A, et al. Vulnerable neuronal subsets in Alzheimer's and Pick's disease are distinguished by their tau isoform distribution and phosphorylation. Ann Neurol 1998;43:193-204.

130 Uchihara T. Silver diagnosis in neuropathology: principles, practice and revised interpretation. Acta Neuropathol (Berl) 2007;113:483-99.

131 Bird TD, Nochlin D, Poorkaj P, et al. A clinical pathological comparison of three families with frontotemporal dementia and identical mutations in the tau gene (P301L). Brain 1999;122:741-756.

132 Dickson D.W. Neurodegeneration: the molecular pathology of dementia and movement disorders.

ISN Neuropath Press, Basel ed. ISN Neuropath Press, Base; 2003;414.

133 Yen SH, Hutton M, DeTure M, et al. Fibrillogenesis of tau: insights from tau missense mutations in FTDP-17. Brain Pathol 1999;9:695-705.

134 van Swieten JC, Bronner IF, Azmani A, et al. The DeltaK280 mutation in MAP tau favors exon 10 skipping in vivo. J Neuropathol Exp Neurol 2007;66:17-25.

135 van der ZJ, Gijselinck I, Dillen L, et al. A pan-European study of the C9orf72 repeat associated with FTLD: geographic prevalence, genomic instability, and intermediate repeats. Hum Mutat 2013;34:363-373.

136 jesus-Hernandez M, Mackenzie IR, Boeve BF, et al. Expanded GGGGCC hexanucleotide repeat in noncoding region of C9ORF72 causes chromosome 9p-linked FTD and ALS. Neuron 2011;72:245-256.

137 Ash PE, Bieniek KF, Gendron TF, et al. Unconventional translation of C9ORF72 GGGGCC expansion generates insoluble polypeptides specific to c9FTD/ALS. Neuron 2013;77:639-646.

138 Yamada M, Sato T, Tsuji S, et al. CAG repeat disorder models and human neuropathology: similarities and differences. Acta Neuropathol (Berl) 2007.

139 Lowe J, Lennox G, Leigh P. Disorders of movement and system degeneration. In: Greenfield's neuropathology. 6th ed ed. 2007;305-309.

140 Vonsattel JP, Myers RH, Stevens TJ, et al. Neuropathological classification of Huntington's disease. J Neuropathol Exp Neurol 1985;44:559-577.

141 Vonsattel JP, DiFiglia M. Huntington disease. J Neuropathol Exp Neurol 1998;57:369-384.

142 Braak H, Braak F. Allocortical involvement in Huntington's disease. Neuropathol Appl Neurobiol 1992;18:539-47.

143 Glass M, Faull RL, Dragunow M. Loss of cannabinoid receptors in the substantia nigra in Huntington's disease. Neuroscience 1993;56:523-527.

144 Kremer HP, Roos RA, Dingjan GM, et al. The hypothalamic lateral tuberal nucleus and the characteristics of neuronal loss in Huntington's disease. Neurosci Lett 1991;132:101-104.

145 Han I, You Y, Kordower JH, et al. Differential vulnerability of neurons in Huntington's disease:

the role of cell type-specific features. J Neurochem 2010;113:1073-1091.

146 DiFiglia M, Sapp E, Chase KO, et al. Aggregation of huntingtin in neuronal intranuclear inclusions and dystrophic neurites in brain. Science 1997;277:1990-1993.

147 Maat-Schieman ML, Dorsman JC, Smoor MA, et al. Distribution of inclusions in neuronal nuclei and dystrophic neurites in Huntington disease brain. J Neuropathol Exp Neurol 1999;58:129-137.

148 Iwabuchi K, Tsuchiya K, Uchihara T, et al. Autosomal dominant spinocerebellar degenerations. Clinical, pathological, and genetic correlations. Rev Neurol (Paris) 1999;155:255-270.

149 Seidel K, Siswanto S, Brunt ER, et al. Brain pathology of spinocerebellar ataxias. Acta Neuropathol 2012;124:1-21.

150 Rub U, Burk K, Timmann D, et al. Spinocerebellar ataxia type 1 (SCA1): new pathoanatomical and clinico-pathological insights. Neuropathol Appl Neurobiol 2012;38:665-680.

151 Duyckaerts C, Durr A, Cancel G, et al. Nuclear inclusions in spinocerebellar ataxia type 1. Acta Neuropathol (Berl) 1999;97:201-207.

152 Rub U, Gierga K, Brunt ER, et al. Spinocerebellar ataxias types 2 and 3: degeneration of the pre-cerebellar nuclei isolates the three phylogenetically defined regions of the cerebellum. J Neural Transm 2005;112:1523-1545.

153 Rub U, Schols L, Paulson H, et al. Clinical features, neurogenetics and neuropathology of the polyglutamine spinocerebellar ataxias type 1, 2, 3, 6 and 7. Prog Neurobiol 2013;104:38-66.

154 Rub U, Brunt ER, Petrasch-Parwez E, et al. Degeneration of ingestion-related brainstem nuclei in spinocerebellar ataxia type 2, 3, 6 and 7. Neuropathol Appl Neurobiol 2006;32:635-649.

155 Gomez CM, Thompson RM, Gammack JT, et al. Spinocerebellar ataxia type 6: gaze-evoked and vertical nystagmus, Purkinje cell degeneration, and variable age of onset. Ann Neurol 1997;42:933-950.

156 Ishikawa K, Fujigasaki H, Saegusa H, et al. Abundant expression and cytoplasmic aggregations of [alpha]1A voltage-dependent calcium channel protein associated with neurodegeneration in

spinocerebellar ataxia type 6. Hum Mol Genet 1999;8:1185-1193.

157 Rub U, Brunt ER, Gierga K, et al. Spinocerebellar ataxia type 7 (SCA7): first report of a systematic neuropathological study of the brain of a patient with a very short expanded CAG-repeat. Brain Pathol 2005;15:287-295.

158 Holmberg M, Duyckaerts C, Durr A, et al. Spinocerebellar ataxia type 7 (SCA7): a neurodegenerative disorder with neuronal intranuclear inclusions. Hum Mol Genet 1998;7:913-918.

159 Parchi P, Strammiello R, Notari S, et al. Incidence and spectrum of sporadic Creutzfeldt-Jakob disease variants with mixed phenotype and co-occurrence of PrPSc types: an updated classification. Acta Neuropathol 2009;118:659-671.

160 Parchi P, Strammiello R, Giese A, et al. Phenotypic variability of sporadic human prion disease and its molecular basis: past, present, and future. Acta Neuropathol 2011;121:91-112.

161 Collins SR, Douglass A, Vale RD, et al. Mechanism of prion propagation: amyloid growth occurs by monomer addition. PLoS Biol 2004;2:e321.

162 Kovacs GG, Seguin J, Quadrio I, et al. Genetic Creutzfeldt-Jakob disease associated with the E200K mutation: characterization of a complex proteinopathy. Acta Neuropathol 2011;121:39-57.

PART II

Hypokinetic Motor Behavioural Disorders

5

Parkinson's Disease

Erik Ch. Wolters, Hans de Munter & Harry Steinbusch

Until the late twentieth century, Parkinson's disease (PD) was more or less considered a synonym to motor parkinsonism, the complex of mainly motor symptoms, originally described by James Parkinson and later on by Charcot as the clinical hallmark for Parkinson's disease (PD). In this disease, (motor) parkinsonism was considered the clinical expression of a dopaminergic denervation of the basal ganglia, as the result of an abiotrophic degeneration of the dopamine-producing cells in the substantia nigra (SN). As of now, PD is considered rather the expression of a diffuse degeneration, affecting the peripheral and central nervous system. Indeed, PD, as of yet, is regarded a progressive α-synucleinopathic neurodegenerative disease, manifesting characteristically with both appendicular (hypokinesia, bradykinesia, rigidity and tremor) and/or axial (gait impairment, postural changes and postural instability) motor symptoms, though accompanied and in some cases even preceded by a multitude of non-motor signs and symptoms, with substantial variability among patients suffering this disease. Non-motor symptoms comprise autonomic dysfunctions such as cardiovascular, urogenital and gastro-intestinal manifestations, sleep-wake disorders, sensory disorders such as hyposmia or pain, impaired color vision, and neuropsychiatric disorders including mood disturbances, anxiety, cognitive deficits, dementia and psychosis. Symptomatic treatment in PD initially comprises oral dopaminomimetics, later on, to suppress dopaminomimetic-induced complications, continuous dopaminergic stimulation (CDS) with intrajejunal levodopa-carbidopa gel infusion, a subcutaneous apomorphin pump, or with deep brain stimulation (DBS) in order to continuously compensate for the intracerebral dopaminergic loss. Thanks to these therapeutical strategies, quality of life can be maintained into the latest stages of this disease. As of yet, protective treatment is not available although cell-based (1) and genetic therapies are promising.

Epidemiology

PD is a widespread disease with a world-wide incidence of about 10-20 in 100,000; a more recent overall annualized age- and gender-adjusted incidence reached 13.4 in 100,000 with a significant higher rate for men as for women, and with increasing rates in blacks (9.9), Asians (11.3), whites (13.6) and Hispanics (16.6), suggesting that the incidence varies by gender, race and ethnicity (2). PD cases are reported at all ages, but are uncommon in people aged under the age of 40 years. As the average age of onset in PD is established at about 60 years, it is principally considered to be a disease of the elderly. Younger patients, as a rule, are often found to suffer genetic parkinsonism (see Chapter 16).

Pathogenesis

Thanks to Braak and colleagues (3), following the identification of α-synuclein mutations and the realization that this protein was a core component of characteristic PD-related proteina-

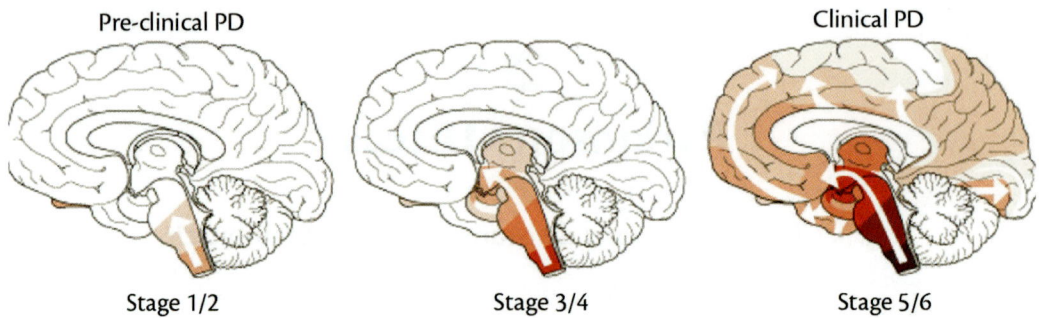

Figure 5.1
In PD, α-synucleinopathy with Lewy pathology develops in predictable stages. Starting in the olfactory bulb and dorsal motor vagus nucleus (stage 1), this pathology expands into additional brain stem nuclei (stages 2-4) and finally into the neocortex (stages 5, 6). First signs of motor parkinsonism might be expected in stages 4 and/or 5, when the loss of nigral dopaminergic cells surpasses the clinical threshold.

ceous Lewy bodies and Lewy neurites in 1997 (4), as of now, PD is hypothesized a multisystem synucleinopathic neurodegenerative process, starting (stage 1 and 2) at clearly defined sites (in the autonomic nervous system, olfactory bulb and lower brainstem) and advancing in a topographically predictable sequence (in stage 3-4 affecting the SN, ventral tegmental area, VTA, nucleus basalis of Meynert, NBM) and other nuclear grays of the basal midbrain and forebrain) into the neocortex (stage 5-6) (see Figure 5.1). It must be noted, however, that individual pathological courses may vary significantly between patients.

The same pathology is seen in incidental Lewy body disease (iLBD), which is considered an early, asymptomatic phase of PD (see also Chapter 4) and in dementia with Lewy bodies (DLB), hypothesized to be a special clinical manifestation of PD in which typical motor parkinsonism is preceded by cognitive deterioration. Although the aetiology in idiopathic PD is still essentially unknown, it is suggested that the synucleinopathy-driven neurodegeneration with Lewy bodies and neurites is the consequence of both cell-autonomous (originating within dying neurons) and non-cell-autonomous (originating from outside dying neurons) processes (5). Supposedly, cell autonomous processes comprise alter-

ations in mitochondrial bioenergetics as well as a dysregulation of calcium homeostasis (with increased mitochondrial reactive oxygen species), both leading to mitochondrial damage and a defective autophagy (by lysosomal and ubiquitin proteasome systems), resulting in accumulation of intracellular α-synuclein oligomers and aggregates. In time, the burden of mitochondrial dysfunction will reach a pathological threshold, provoking neuronal dysfunction and ultimately cell death (5,6). Non-cell-autonomous processes, on top of this, are responsible for the contingent (supposedly prion-like) (7) spreading of the synucleinic pathology over various (dopaminergic, cholinergic, serotonergic and noradrenergic) neuronal and non-neuronal (astrocytes, microglia, lymphocytes) cells across brain regions (5). As a matter of fact, the degeneration of some neurons in itself might also involve non-cell-autonomous mechanisms through their specific intraneuronal connections (such as cholinergic or noradrenergic projections to dopaminergic neurons), or through a decrease of brain-derived neurotrophic factors (8,9).

Risk factors contributing to synucleinopathic degeneration include autonomous activity, broad action potentials, low intrinsic calcium-buffering capacity, poorly myelinated axons and the use of monoamine neurotransmitters (with the formation of neuromelanin pigment)

(10). In PD, vulnerable neuronal populations comprise both peripheral (noradrenergic neurons innervating the heart and the skin, and dopaminergic neurons of the enteric nervous system) and central (dorsal motor nucleus of the vagus) autonomic neurons, olfactory neurons, and neuromelanin-containing catecholaminergic neurons in the dopaminergic SN, VTA and retro-rubral area (RRA), in the noradrenergic locus ceruleus (LC), the cholinergic, glutamatergic and GABAergic pedunculo-pontine nucleus (PPN), the serotonergic raphe nuclei (RN) and the cholinergic NBM (10).

Pathophysiology

Suggested by post-mortem cell counts of mid-brainstem dopamine-producing neuromelanin-containing cells and extrapolating the extent of dopaminergic striatal denervation as visualized by (single) photon emission tomography (SPET) or positron emission tomography (PET), using radioligands for the dopamine transporter (11), in PD, the onset of mid-brainstem dopaminergic cell loss antedates the clinical diagnosis (based on the presence of levodopa-responsive parkinsonism, which will manifest after a loss of about 50% of these cells) by several years. During this period, and probably already some years before, extra-nigral synucleinopathic pathology might have become clinically overt. According to Braak (2), as said before, synucleinopathic pathology in PD patients often starts in the peripheral autonomic nervous system, dorsal motor vagal nucleus and olfactory bulb (stage 1 and 2), before reaching the SN and the brainstem sensory relay centers (the serotoninergic raphe nuclei, the adrenergic cerulean nuclei and the cholinergic brainstem complex) in a topographically predictable sequence (stage 3 and 4). This process then will finally spread to the neocortex (stage 5-6) (see Figure 5.1). Indeed, before the first clinical manifestations of the stage 3 and 4-related degeneration of the dopamine-producing neurons in

Table 5.1
Survey of primary (premotor) *and secondary* non-motor symptoms in PD.

Autonomic dysfunction	Parasympathetic cholinergic	Dry mouth, Gastroparesis, Constipation Pollakisuria, Incontinence Erectile dysfunction Pupillomotor abnormalities
	Sympathetic cholinergic	Thermoregulatory dysfunction Hypo/hyperhidrosis (drenching sweats)
	Sympathetic noradrenergic	Cardiovascular dysfunction Baroreflex failure Orthostatic hypotension
Sleep-wake disorders	Insomnia and sleep fragmentation Fatigue, Excessive daytime sleepiness and Sleep attacks REM sleep behavioral disorder (RBD)	
Sensory disorders	Pain Hyposmia Impaired color vision	
Neuropsychiatric disorders	Apathy, Anxiety and panic attacks, Depression Mild cognitive impairment (executive domain) Dementia and Psychosis	
	Impulse control disorders	

the mid-brainstem, the so-called premotor phase, primary PD-related sensory, sleep and autonomic symptoms may bother the patients already for many years (see Table 5.1).

In 1980, Oppenheimer was the first to suggest that progressive synucleinopathic degeneration with Lewy pathology in the autonomic nervous system was associated with PD (12). In fact, his observations gave rise to the suggestion that PD's phenotype correlates with the regional localization and severity (surpassing the threshold of clinical expression) of Lewy pathology: a localization within the autonomic nervous system with autonomic failure, a midbrain-brainstem localization with motor parkinsonism and a cortical localization with dementia. Based on the same observations, Braak (13) hypothesized that – like in prion diseases- PD might originate outside the nervous system, caused by an unidentified pathogen, passing the mucosal barrier of the gastrointestinal tract to enter the central nervous system by retrograde axonal and transneuronal transport along post- and preganglionic neurons. So far, however, the exact cause of this disease has still to be unveiled.

As for the pathophysiology of motor parkinsonism, one has to understand that the loss of nigral dopaminergic neurons will result in a dopaminergic denervation of the basal ganglia. This complex keeps fully actualized motor programs available and generates impulses for the supplementary motor cortex as soon as motor action is planned in the premotor area, in order to select adequately adapted (learned) automated time- and place-coherent patterns out of this pool. In order to fully understand chapters 11, 13 and 14, dealing with the various (pharmacotherapeutic and neurosurgical) strategies of the symptomatic treatment of motor parkinsonism, it is essential to understand the functional neuro-anatomy of the basal ganglia as displayed in Figure 5.2, and as further outlined in Chapters 2 and 6. Parkinsonism, thus, characteristically manifests the striatal dopaminergic denervation-induced dysfunction of the basal ganglia, irrespective of its cause: primary (degenerative) or secondary (genetic, iatrogenic, toxic, metabolic or structural) parkinsonism (see Table 5.2).

Dopaminergic neurons in the lateral and the medial part of the pars compacta of the substantia nigra (SNc) innervate the dorsolateral (putamen) and the ventromedial (caudate) stri-

Table 5.2
Overview of primary and secondary parkinsonism.

Primary (degenerative) parkinsonism	Secondary (symptomatic) parkinsonism	
Idiopathic Parkinson's disease (PD)	iatrogenic	Benzamides, Butyrophenones, Ca-blockers, Lithium, α-Methyldopa, Phenothiazines, Reserpine, Sodium-Valproate, Tetrabenazine, Thioxanthenes
Dementia with Lewy Bodies (DLB) Genetic Parkinsonism Multiple System Atrophy (MSA)		
Progressive Supranuclear Palsy (PSP) Cortico-Basal Degeneration (CBD)	toxic	Manganese, MPTP, MG-132, CO, Methanol, Cyanide, Organophosphonates
Alzheimer's disease (AD) Fronto-Temporal Dementia with	metabolic	Wilson's disease; Hypoparathyreoidism
Parkinsonism (FTDP)	infectious	Encephalitis lethargica, HIV Prion infections (such as Creutzfeld-Jakob disease: CJD)
Neuroacanthocythosis Huntington's disease (HD) Spino-Cerebellar Atrophies (SCA)	structural	Normal-pressure hydrocephalus; Cerebrovascular infarctions, CNS traumata and/or tumors

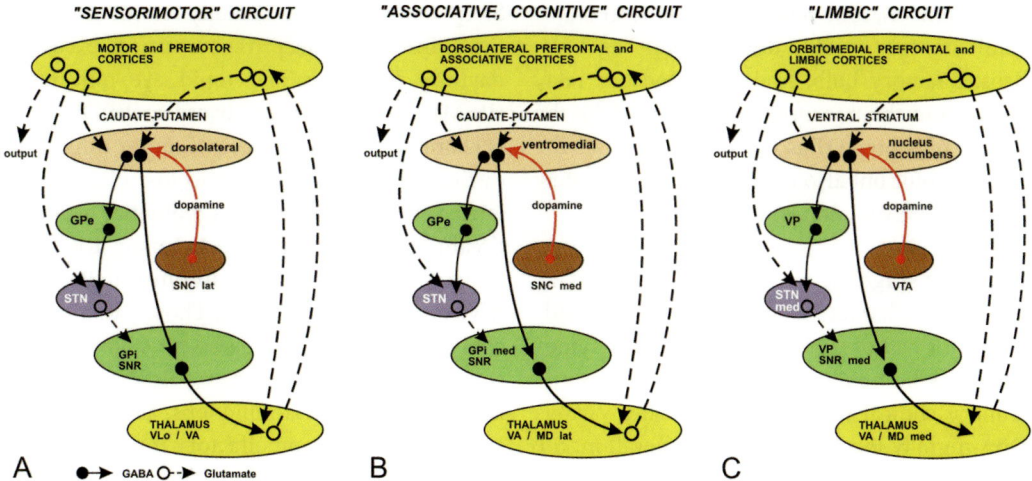

"SENSORIMOTOR" CIRCUIT — "ASSOCIATIVE, COGNITIVE" CIRCUIT — "LIMBIC" CIRCUIT

Figure 5.2

Schematic presentation of the essential neuronal connections in the basal ganglia-thalamocortical (extrapyramidal) circuit as a model for the multiple, parallel organized but functionally segregated connections within this system.

atum respectively, and in the VTA those neurons innervate the ventral striatum (nucleus accumbens), in order to modulate the neural activity respectively within the motor, cognitive and emotional basal ganglia-thalamo-cortical loops (see Figure 5.2), and to transform signals into well-organized patterns of neuronal activity with coordinated muscle contractions. The dorsolateral motor loop (including the ocular and auditory loops) is responsible for the orchestration of pure motor behaviour, while the ventromedial cognitive loop takes care of the contextual tuning, and the ventral emotional loop serves the personal flavor and limbic behaviour.

Both, spontaneous and reactive voluntary movements will be elicited by internal, autonomic or external (environmental) sensori stimuli and motivated by the limbic system. In case of a preponding putaminal denervation, mainly internally-cued, and not so much externally-generated, behaviour will be affected, resulting in bradykinesia, hypokinesia and rigidity. As these symptoms, but not tremor and postural instability, are fully levodopa-responsive, a more complicated pathophysiological mechanism might be involved in

these latter symptoms. In case of an accompanying considerable denervation of caudate and nucleus accumbens, one might also expect cognitive and emotional behavioural abnormalities with loss of mental flexibility and psychomotor retardation (loss of adaptational abilities). As the externally-cued, environmental-induced reactive behaviour as a rule is less affected, in patients suffering parkinsonism, the loss of spontaneous behaviour might be compensated by inducing externally-cued reactive behaviour. In PD, but not in other parkinsonian conditions, concomitant disease-related degeneration of serotonergic, adrenergic and cholinergic transmitter systems also play a role, and probably might down-regulate this compensatory mechanism.

Clinical presentation

As of now, PD is only diagnosed when the first signs and symptoms of motor parkinsonism become overt, and oral dopaminomimetics are found to consistently reduce these symptoms. As argued before, in PD, synucleinopathic degeneration not only involves mesencephalic dopaminergic structures (manifesting with motor parkinsonism), but also the peripheral autonomic nervous system, dorsal motor vagal nucleus, olfactory bulb, brainstem sensory relay centers and the neocortex (see Figure 5.1); the clinical phenotype thus not only comprises the typical motor but also a range of (unfortunately rather unspecific) non-motor symptoms.

Premotor stage

Pending the characteristic chronological spreading of this pathological condition, motor symptoms may be heralded or accompanied by the primary clinical manifestations of the various extra-nigrally located sites of degeneration. So, characteristically, pending the exact localization and severity, autonomic nervous system disorders, sleep-wake disorders, sensory disorders including pain and hyposmia, apathy, anxiety and mood disorders, as well as subtle cognitive (executive) dysfunction eventually may precede the first motor manifestations in PD. As a rule, more extensive cognitive dysfunction and/or dementia might accompany motor parkinsonism in the later phase, though sometimes cognitive failure with attentional deficits may precede the first signs of motor parkinsonism (this condition is called DLB: dementia with Lewy bodies).

Clinical relevant dysautonomia, variably including cardiovascular (including both cardiac sympathetic denervation with orthostatic hypotension and baroreflex failure, and cardiovascular dysregulation), gastrointestinal (dysphagia, delayed gastric emptying, constipation), urogenital (sphincter-related bladder dysfunction due to anticholinergic but not levodopa-responsive detrusor muscle hypertrophy, leading to pollakisuria and urgency; sexual disturbances with the loss of arousal, erectile dysfunction, and premature ejaculation), sudomotor, (sympathetic) thermoregulatory (drenching sweats), pupillomotor (due to synucleinopathic degeneration of the cholinergic nucleus of Westphal-Edinger), sleep and respiratory disorders, are present in the majority of PD patients, regularly already in the premotor phase (14).

Sleep-wake disorders mainly manifest as fatigue, insomnia, sleep fragmentation, excessive daytime sleepiness and rapid eye movement (REM) sleep behaviour disorder (RBD). RBD is characterized by the lack of motor inhibition during REM sleep, leading to loss of REM-related atonia and a vigorous, potential harmful, dream-enacting behaviour. In many RBD patients (without overt parkinsonism), PD may develop up to 20 years later. Those patients may concomitantly suffer progressive cognitive (executive) dysfunction with impaired verbal fluency and visuospatial functions, and may score significantly worse on olfactory threshold, odor discrimination and odor identification tests (15). Sensory disorders comprise pain, visual color discrimination problems and hyposmia with problems in both detection, discrimination and identification. Hyposmia is a well-recognized symptom in premotor PD; the prevalence in PD patients is about 80% (16). About 70% of all PD patients suffer neuropathic or nociceptive pain, in over 25% already in the premotor phase (17). Neuropsychiatric disorders including dopamine deficiency-related anhedonia, apathy and psychomotor retardation, anxiety and panic attacks, and (noradrenalin and serotonin deficiency-related) depression (with a threefold higher prevalence than in normal elderly), are also frequently bothering the patients, often already in the premotor phase. Eventually, psychosocial factors here might also play a certain role. In the initial phase of the disease, most if not all PD patients already suffer subtle cognitive loss: executive impairments including a deficit of behavioural regulation in sorting or planning tasks in combination with mild mnemonic dysfunction due to defective storage and impaired manipulation of internal representation of visuospatial stimuli. In about 80% of the patients, these mild problems may proceed to dementia. Dementia in PD (PDD) is typically characterized by a dysexecutive syndrome with attentional deficits and fluctuating cognition. PDD interferes with ADL activities and often

Table 5.3
Pathophysiology in striatal dopaminergic denervation-related parkinsonism.

Pathophysiology	Etiology	Conditions / Chemicals
Presynaptic	idiopathic	Parkinson's disease; Dementia with Lewy bodies; Segawa's disease
	genetic	Genetic parkinsonism
	toxic	6-Hydroxydopamine, MPTP, MG-132
	iatrogenic	Reserpine, Tetrabenazine
Postynaptic	iatrogenic	Benzamides, Butyrophenones, Phenothiazines, Thioxanthenes,
	toxic	Manganese, CO, Methanol, Cyanide, Organophosphonates
Pre/Postsynaptic	idiopathic	MSA, PSP, CBD
	structural	Space-occupying lesions; Traumatic lesions; Vascular parkinsonism

necessitates nursing home placement, especially when accompanied by delusions and hallucinations (18). As said before, in a small number of patients, dementia with attentional deficits and additional psychotic symptoms (DLB) might occur in the premotor phase. Clinical symptoms in PDD are comparable to those in DLB, except for the fact that DLB is a typical premotor feature, whereas PDD, as a rule, becomes only overt in the later stages of PD motor phase.

Motor stage

As of yet, clinical hallmarks in PD, enabling the diagnosis, comprise only motor parkinsonism, manifesting with typical striatal dysfunction-related appendicular and axial motor (sensorimotor, associative/cognitive and emotional) behavioural abnormalities. These abnormalities include slowing down of movements (bradykinesia), scarcity of movements (hypokinesia), tremor, rigidity, gait disturbances and postural instability. Some of these symptoms, mainly the appendicular symp-

Table 5.4
Hoehn & Yahr scale: a commonly used system for describing how the symptoms of PD progress. It was originally published in 1967 (19) and later on modified with the addition of stages 1.5 and 2.5 to help describe the intermediate course of the disease.

Stage	Hoehn and Yahr Scale	Modified Hoehn and Yahr Scale
Stage 1	Unilateral involvement only usually with minimal or no functional disability	Unilateral involvement only
Stage 1.5		Unilateral and axial involvement
Stage 2	Bilateral or midline involvement without impairment of balance	Bilateral involvement without impairment of balance
Stage 2.5		Mild bilateral disease with recovery on pull test
Stage 3	Bilateral disease: mild to moderate disability with impaired postural reflexes; physically independent	Mild to moderate bilateral disease; some postural instability; physically independent
Stage 4	Severely disabling disease; still able to walk or stand unassisted	Severe disability; still able to walk or stand unassisted
Stage 5	Confinement to bed or wheelchair unless aided	Wheelchair bound or bedridden unless aided

toms, but not all, are levodopa-responsive. This therapeutic strategy will give a lasting symptomatic relief only in case of conditions caused by a dopaminergic denervation, due to predominant presynaptic dopamine deficiency (see Table 5.3). Severity of motor parkinsonism is expressed in the (modified) Hoehn and Yahr score (19) (see Table 5.4) and the most applied clinical rating scale is the unified PD rating scale (UPDRS), adapted by the Movement Disorders Society (see also chapter 41) (20).

In the long run, after 5-10 years, due to the progressive dopaminergic denervation with the increasing loss of striatal dopamine storage, underlying a progressively more pulsatile stimulation of the postsynaptic dopaminergic receptors, the majority of patients will suffer iatrogenic purposeless motor abnormalities (see Chapter 12), namely hyper(dys)kinesia. A subset of patients, due to the treatment with dopamine agonists and irrespective of the duration of disease, might suffer from other iatrogenic treatment complications, i.e. impulse control disorders (ICD). These pathological behaviours are characterized by excessive or poorly controlled preoccupations, urges or stereotype behaviours. ICD's such as binge eating, compulsive shopping, pathological gambling and/or hypersexuality are considered the expression of a homeostatic hedonistic dysregulation, a class effect of dopamine agonists. Punding, a stereotypy normally seen in amphetamine addiction,

Table 5.5
Clinical diagnostic criteria from the UK Brain Bank Criteria (21).

PD diagnostic criteria	1	Bradykinesia (slowness of initiation of voluntary movements with progressive reduction in speed and amplitude of repetitive actions)
	2	At least one of the following: ▪ Rigidity ▪ 4-6 Hz Rest tremor ▪ Postural instability (not caused by primary visual, vestibular, cerebellar and/or proprioceptive dysfunction)
PD exclusion criteria		▪ Familiar parkinsonism ▪ Persisting strictly unilateral parkinsonism ▪ Sustained remission ▪ Levodopa-unresponsiveness ▪ Strokes with stepwise progressive parkinsonism ▪ Repeated head injuries ▪ Preceding neuroleptic treatment ▪ Supranuclear gaze palsy or oculogyric crises ▪ Early severe autonomic, cerebellar and/or pyramidal signs ▪ Early Alzheimer-type dementia ▪ Cerebral tumor, communicating hydrocephalus ▪ MPTP intoxication
PD supportive prospective positive criteria (three or more criteria required to make the diagnosis of PD definitive)		▪ Unilateral onset ▪ Progressive disorder ▪ Clinical course > 10 years ▪ Persistent asymmetry affecting side of onset ▪ Excellent levodopa-responsiveness (70-100% improvement) ▪ Persistent levodopa responsiveness (> 5 years) ▪ Levodopa-induced dyskinesias ▪ Rest tremor

is characterized by an intense fascination with the purposeless repetitive manipulation, examination, cataloguing and endless sorting of objects of common use, is seen in about 15% of the patients.

Diagnosis

As shown in Table 5.3, parkinsonism might be caused by various idiopathic neurodegenerative disorders (including PD, multiple system atrophy, MSA, progressive supranuclear palsy, PSP, corticobasal degeneration, CBD, and corticobasal syndrome, CBS; see Chapters 19-21), by genetic disorders (see Chapter 16), by cerebrovascular incidents (see Chapter 17) and by various drugs and toxins (see Chapter 18). The differentiation of PD and genetic parkinsonism (see also Chapter 10) is performed by genetic screening for the latter, whereas its differentiation from the other parkinsonistic syndromes is still mainly based on phenotypical phenomena or neuroimaging findings. As of yet, the UK Parkinson's disease Society Brain Bank (UK Brain Bank Criteria) criteria (21) (see Table 5.5), enabling the diagnosis of PD in about 80% of the cases, are still valid for clinical diagnosis.

Generally speaking, positive clinical criteria for PD-related parkinsonism (bradykinesia in combination with rigidity, resting tremor or postural instability) include the progressive character, the unilateral onset with the persistent unilateral preponderance, and a persisting levodopa responsiveness. Red flags comprise (genetic) familiar parkinsonism, (vascular) lower body half-parkinsonism and early significant postural instability, autonomic failure and cerebellar and/or pyramidal pathology. Of course, also focal cortical pathology, signs of supranuclear palsy, and

the absence of a lasting levodopa responsiveness, as well as the earlier use of neuroleptics, or the presence of hydrocephalus or brain tumors also make the diagnosis less probable.

To further improve diagnostic accuracy, various imaging techniques as well as biochemical and morphological investigation of body fluids may help (see also Chapters 10 and 45). As a rule, in presynaptic levodopa-responsive parkinsonism (see Table 5.3), functional imaging with presynaptic dopamine-transporter (DaT) single-photon emission computed tomography (SPECT) (such as [123I] FP-CIT or [123I] β-CIT SPECT) and/or positron emission tomography (PET) (such as [18F] Fluorodopa PET) will show a loss of presynaptic integrity of the dopaminergic system, whereas postsynaptic [123I] iodobenzamide (IBZM)-SPECT and/or [11C] raclopride PET evidences a normal expression of dopaminergic receptors (see Figures 5.3 and 5.4).

As of yet, (a combination of) premotor non-motor manifestations in PD, although their presence might be highly suggestive, have not yielded a reliable marker for PD. Nevertheless, the

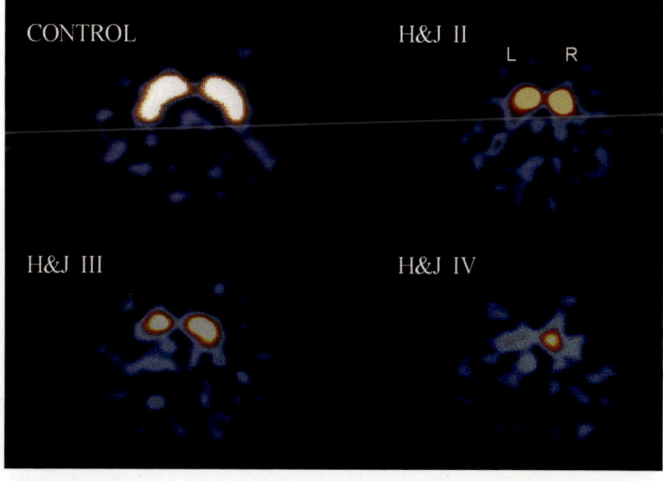

Figure 5.3
[123I] β-CIT -SPECT in a healthy control (upper left) with a normal uptake of the radio-active ligand, and in a PD patient suffering right>left body-half parkinsonism in different consecutive Hoehn & Yahr stages: H&Y 2 (upper right), H&Y 3 (lower left) and H&Y 4 with progressively reduced uptake of the radio-active ligand (lower right).

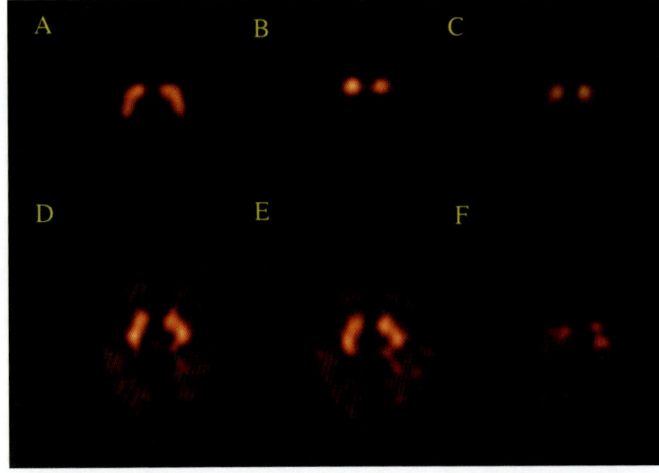

Figure 5.4
Presynaptic [^{123}I]-FP-CIT-SPECT (above) and postsynaptic [^{123}I]benzamide IB-ZM-SPECT (under) images in a healthy person (A, D) in a PD or DLB patient, showing reduced dopamine transporter binding (indicating a loss of presynaptic integrity of the nigrostriatal dopaminergic system) with a normal dopamine receptor binding (indicating a normal postsynaptic integrity of this system) (B, E) and in a MSA or PSP patient, showing a loss of integrity of both the presynaptic and the postsynaptic elements of the nigrostriatal dopaminergic system (C, F). Patients suffering iatrogenic parkinsonism will show a normal presynaptic element with a decreased integrity of the postsynaptic element (A, F), patients suffering manganism, essential tremor, Alzheimer disease and/or psychogenic parkinsonism show normal pre- and postsynaptic elements (A, D).

cerebral glucose patterns or loss of the postsynaptical cardial sympathetic neurons (see Figure 5.7), and might thus be highly suggestive for this disease (22) (see also Chapter 10).

Differential Diagnosis

The differentiation of pure presynaptic dopamine deficiency-related parkinsonian conditions (idiopathic PD, genetic parkinsonism, Segawa's disease) is based on levodopa-responsiveness, phenotypical differences and genetic screening. Other parkinsonian conditions (MSA, PSP, iatrogenic, structural and/or toxic parkinsonism) caused by dysfunctional dopaminergic receptors or other abnormalities resulting in a functional dysbalance of the basal ganglia output structures (see Table 5.2), are not, or only partly and temporarily levodopa-responsive. Therefore, in order not to frustrate patients with inadequate drugs inducing unwanted side-effects but lacking any efficacy, it is essential to reach a specific diagnosis. Patients suffering from MSA or PSP, or drug-in-

combination of these symptoms with transcranial sonography and/or functional imaging may already indicate a mild, still subclinical, progressive loss of the integrity of the dopaminergic system (see Figures 5.5 and 5.6), abnormal

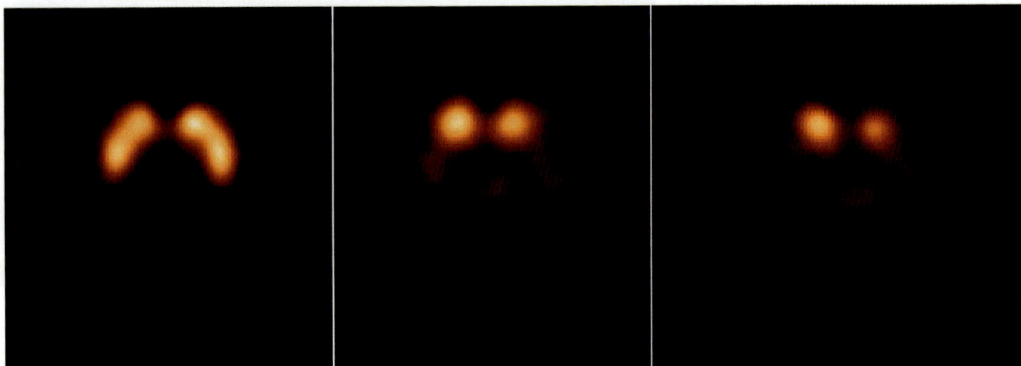

Figure 5.5
DAT-SPECT scan in a healthy control (left), and in an hyposmic man, without motor parkinsonism (middle) and three years later, suffering left>right body-half motor parkinsonism (right).

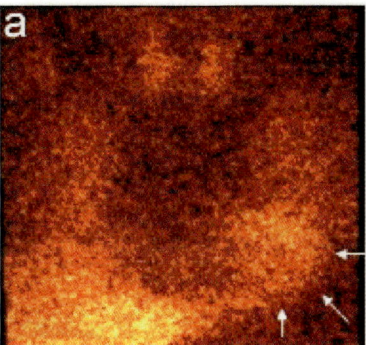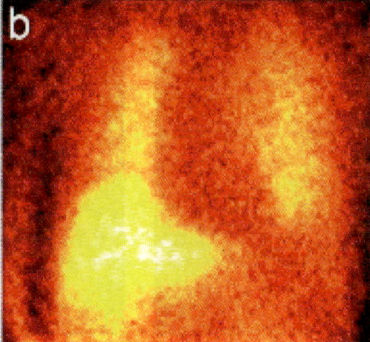

Figure 5.6
Cardiac sympathetic denervation demonstrated by ^{123}I-MBIG (metaiodobenzylgua-nidine), showing a normal myocardial uptake (arrows) of radioactivity in a MSA patient (a) and sympathetic denervation in a PD patient (courtesy H. Reichmann, Dresden).

minomimetics loses its effectiveness, as (non) motor complications such as (un)predictable motor fluctuations and dyskinesias progressively develop. Therefore, as PD progresses, adequate control of motor symptoms depends increasingly on continuous drug delivery (24) (see Chapter 14). Based on scientific evidence, guidelines and expert opinions, paramedical rehabilitation programs, including physical therapy, occupational therapy, and speech therapy, are also thought to improve mobility, activities of daily living, communication and quality of life in the different stages of this disease, and do contribute significantly to the rehabilitation of PD patients. Unmet needs still comprise neuroprotection and/or restoration. Progress has been hampered by the lack of animal models that reflect the widespread brain pathology presumed to cause both motor and non-motor symptoms of PD in humans (23). As of yet, no drugs unequivocally did establish that property, though recent preclinical (25) as well as clinical (26) studies with forced physical activity and cell-based therapies (1) did suggest that the natural worsening of symptoms associated with PD could be effectively counteracted, probably by increasing cerebral GDNF and BDNF levels. In the next future, the further development of drugs and/or cell-based and gene-therapies promoting the expression of these neurotrophic factors, therefore, seems challenging (1,27).

duced parkinsonism, might be differentiated from PD by postsynaptic raclopride-PET and/or IBZM-SPECT dopamine receptor imaging (see Figure 5.4), showing reduced uptake of the radio-ligands. Otherwise, structural, metabolic or toxin-induced postsynaptic parkinsonism, such as Wilson's disease, might be recognized by typical clinical symptoms and or abnormalities on imaging modalities such as MRI (see Figure 5.7)

Treatment

Parkinson's disease is a common, progressive, debilitating disease with substantial physical, psychological and social implications. Therefore, patients require a holistic, multidisciplinary approach to maximise quality of life for patients and their carers (23) (see also Chapter 11). Indeed, to optimal meet the patient's needs, best results seem to be reached with multidisciplinary teams, under the leadership of a clinical neurologist and/or specialized PD-nurse, combining medical (neurology, psychiatry, gerontology, rehabilitation) and paramedical care with psychological and welfare expertise.

As for motor parkinsonism, pharmacological management is complex, and should be individualised according to the needs of the patient. In time, conservative oral medication with dopa-

Prognosis

Recent developments in the understanding and the treatment of PD not only increased quality of life, but also longevity in patients suffer-

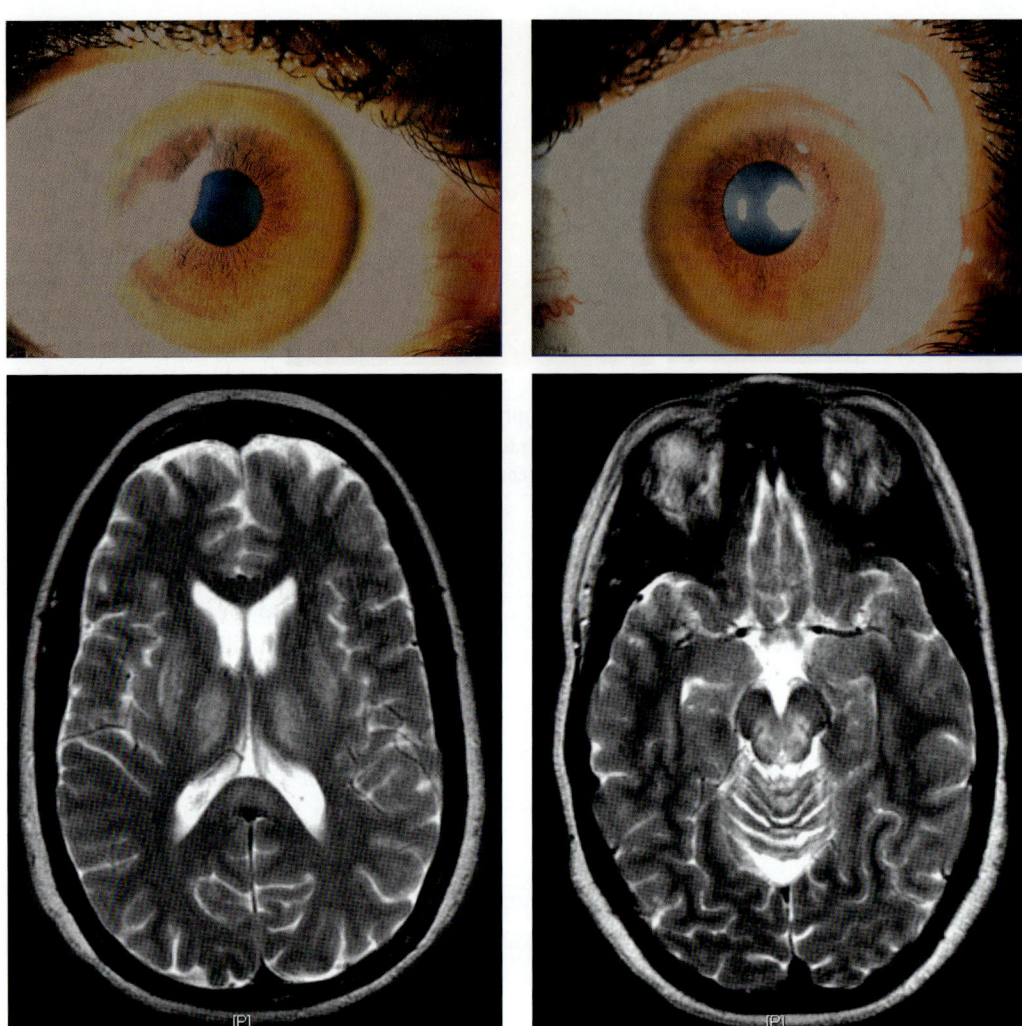

Figure 5.7
MR brain images in a patient suffering Wilson's disease with typical corneal kayer Fleischer rings (above), showing characteristic signal intensity changes in the caudate, putamen and thalamus (lower left) as well as the typical so-called face-of-a-giant-panda sign, caused by accentuation of the normal low intensity of the nucleus ruber and substantia nigra by the surrounding abnormal high intensity signal in the midbrain tegmentum (lower right).

ing this debilitating disease. PD is not any longer considered a fatal disease by itself, though life expectancy is still somewhat below normal expectations, due to complications induced by swallowing problems (choking, pneumonia), falls and psychotic manifestations. As of yet, there is only symptomatic therapy, and disease-modifying therapeutical strategies have not surfaced today. Cell-based and/or gene-thera-pies promoting the expression of cerebral neurotrophic factors, in the next future, wishfully will fulfil the unmet need for disease-modifying strategies in Parkinson's disease.

Conclusion

PD is the complex of signs and symptoms caused by an idiopathic synucleinopathic degeneration of the central and peripheral nervous system. Diagnosis is enabled when the first symptoms of levodopa-responsive motor parkinsonism become overt, as preceding non-motor signs are aspecific and biomarkers unequivocally. Improved symptomatic treatment of motor parkinsonism did increase quality of life and longevity, though disease-modifying strategies are still an unmet need.

Video fragments

Fragment 5.1
Parkinsonism (Segments 1-10)
The clinical hallmarks of (motor) parkinsonism are shown in this video fragment.
Segments 1-3 display bradykinesia, segment 4 hypokinesia, segment 5 the typical parkinsonian rest tremor, and segment 6 rigidity with the cogwheel phenomenon in various patients suffering from motor parkinsonism. Segment 7 shows the loss of postural reflexes with instability, the phenomena of propulsion (segment 8) and retropulsion (segment 9), and stooped posture (segment 10) in motor parkinsonism.

Fragment 5.2
Parkinson's disease (Segments 1-5)
This fragment shows a 60-year-old woman suffering from right > left-sided Parkinson's disease, with hypokinesia (masked face: segment 1), reduced arm swing (segment 2), tremor (segment 3), and bradykinesia in the right body-half (segments 4 and 5).

References

1 Munter H de, Wolters ECh. Cell-based therapies in parkinsonism. Transl Neurodegen 2013;2(1):13 doi 10.1186/2047-9158-2-13.

2 Van den Eeden S, Tanner C, Bernstein A., et al. Incidence of Parkinson's disease: variation by age, gender and race/ethnicity. Am J Epidemiol 2003;157:1015-1022.

3 Braak H Del Tredici K, Rub U et al. Staging of brain pathology related to sporadic Parkinson's disease. Neurobiol Aging 2003;24:197-211.

4 Polymeropoulos MH, Lavedan C, Leroy E et al. Mutation in the α-synuclein gene identified in families with Parkinson's disease. Science 1997;276:2045-2047.

5 Hirsch EC, Jenner P, Prrzedborski S. Pathogenesis of Parkinson's disease. Mov Dis 201;28(S1):24-30.

6 Olanow CW, McKnaught K. Parkinson's disease, proteins, and prions: milestones. Mov Disord 2011;26:1056-1071.

7 Prusiner SB. Cell biology. A unifying role for prions in neurodegenerative diseases. Science 2012;336:1511-1513

8 MogiM, Togari AKondo T et al. Brain-deriveed groth factor and nerve growth factor concentrations are decreased in the substantia nigra in Parkinson's disease.Neurosci lett 1999;270:45-48

9 MogiM, Togari AKondo T et al. Gial cell line-derived neurotrophic factor in the substantia nigra from control and parkinsonian brains. Neurosci lett 2001;300:179-181.

10 Sulzer D, Surmeier DJ. Neural vulnerability, pathogenesis, and Parkinson's disease. Mov Dis 2013;28(S1):41-50.

11 Booij J, Tissingh G, Winogrodzka A, van Royen EA. Imaging of the dopaminergic neurotransmission system using single-photon emission tomography in patients with parkinsonism. J Nucl Med 1999;26:171-182.

12 Oppenheimer DR. Lateral horn cells in progressive autonomic failure. J Neurol Sci 1980:46:393-404.

13 Braak H, Rub U, Gai WP, Del Tredici K. Idiopathic Parkinson's disease: possible routes by which vulnerable neuronal types may be subject to neuroin-

vasion by an unknown pathogen. J Neural transm 2003;110: 517-537.

14 Magerkuth C, Schnitzer R, Braune S. Synptoms of autonomic failure in Parkinson"s disease: prevalence and impact on daily life. Clin Auton Res 2005;15:76-82.

15 Stiassny-Kolster K, Doerr Y, Moller JC, et al. Combination of idiopathic REM sleep behavior disorder and olfactory dysfunction as possible indicator for α-synucleinopathy demonstrated by dopamine transporter FP-CIT-SPECT. Brain 2005;128:126-137.

16 Ponsen MM, Stoffers D, Booij J, van Eck-Smit BLF, Wolters ECh, Berendse HW. Idopathic hyposmia as a preclinical sign of Parkinson"s disease. Ann Neurol 2004;56:173-181.

17 Giuffrida R, Vingerhoets FJG, Bogousslavsky J, Ghika J. Pain in Parkinson"s disease. Rev Neurol (Paris) 2005;161:407-418.

18 Bosboom JLW, Stoffers D, Wolters ECh. Cognitive function in Parkinson's disease. J Neural transm 2004;111:1303-1315.

19 Hoehn M, Yahr M. Parkinsonism: onset, progression and mortality. Neurology 1967;244:2-8.

20 Goetz CG, Tilley BC, Shaftman SR, et al. Movement Disorder Society-sponsored revision of the Unified Parkinson's Disease Rating Scale (MDS-UPDRS): scale presentation and clinimetric testing results. Mov Disord. 2008;23:2129-2170.

21 Hughes AJ, Daniel SE, Kilford L, Lees AJ. The accuracy of the clinical diagnosis of Parkinson's disease. J Neurol Neurosurg Psychiatry 1992;55:181-184.

22 Truong DD, Wolters ECh. Recognition and management of Parkinson's disease during the premotor (prodromal) phase. Exp Ther Neurol 2009;9:847-857.

23 Worth PF. How to treat Parkinson's disease in 2013. Clin Med. 2013;13:93-96.

24 Zigmond MJ, Cameron JL, Leak RK et al. Triggering endogenous neuroprotective processes through exercise in models of dopamine deficiency. Parkinsonism Rel Disord 2009;15(S3):42-45.

25 Frazitta G, Bertotti G, Riboldazi G et al. Effectiviness of Intense Inpatient Rehabilitation Treatment on Disease Progression in Parkinsonian Paients: a Randomized Controlled Trial with 1-Year Follow-up. Neurorehabil Neural Repair 2012;26:144-150.

26 Zhang R, Wang Z, Howson PA et al. Smilagenin attenuates beta amyloid (25-35)-induced degeneration of neuronal cells via stimulating the gene expression of brain-derived neurotrophic factor. Neuroscience. 2012;210:275-285.

6

Synchronized Neural Oscillations and the Parkinsonian State

Ashwini Oswal, Vladimir Litvak & Peter Brown

Synchronized neural oscillations are ubiquitous within the central nervous system. Mounting evidence suggests that these rhythms may be involved in mediating normal function and in the pathogenesis of neurological disease states. In this chapter we consider how abnormalities in oscillatory activity within cortico-basal ganglia loops may play an important role in the generation of Parkinsonian phenotypes in patients. While the main emphasis will be on exploring the oscillatory correlates of motor phenotypes, we will also review evidence pointing to the role of oscillations in cognitive features of the disease.

Oscillations in motor control: early descriptions

The first description of cortical oscillatory modulations associated with movement demonstrated 20 Hz oscillations close to the central sulcus that desynchronized upon active and passive movements (1). It has subsequently been shown that physiological, cortical, oscillatory changes in multiple frequency bands, which reflect the degree and extent of synchronization of activity in a local population of neurons, are modulated by the anticipation, execution and termination of voluntary movements (2–6).
Both beta (15-30 Hz) and lower frequency alpha rhythms (8-13 Hz) demonstrate event-related desynchronisation (ERD) prior to movement, with sustained suppression during movement execution (4,6). Furthermore, beta-band activity also displays event-related synchronisation (ERS) following the termination of movement (3). Activity at higher frequencies in the gamma band (40-90 Hz) displays ERS prior to movement execution in contrast to low frequencies (7).

This pattern of reactivity is repeated in the basal ganglia in patients with Parkinson's disease, raising two important questions. First, to what extent are the oscillations detected in Parkinson's disease physiological or pathological? Second, what is the relationship of such activity between the cortical motor sites and the basal ganglia? In considering the second question, we will first briefly review the anatomy of the cortico-basal ganglia circuitry and its proposed role in the control of movement.

Cortico-basal ganglia circuit

The basal ganglia consist of several nuclei, which receive inputs from wide areas within the cerebral cortex and return outputs back to the cerebral cortex via the thalamus, hence forming a cortico-basal ganglia loop, and simultaneously outputs to the brainstem, particularly through the substantia nigra pars reticulata (SNr) (see Figure 6.1). Cortical motor projections converge on the striatum from which striatal projection neurons innervate the globus pallidum externa (GPe) and interna (GPi), forming the classical indirect and direct pathways, respectively (8,9). The subthalamic nucleus (STN), the sole excitatory (glutaminergic) nucleus of the basal gan-

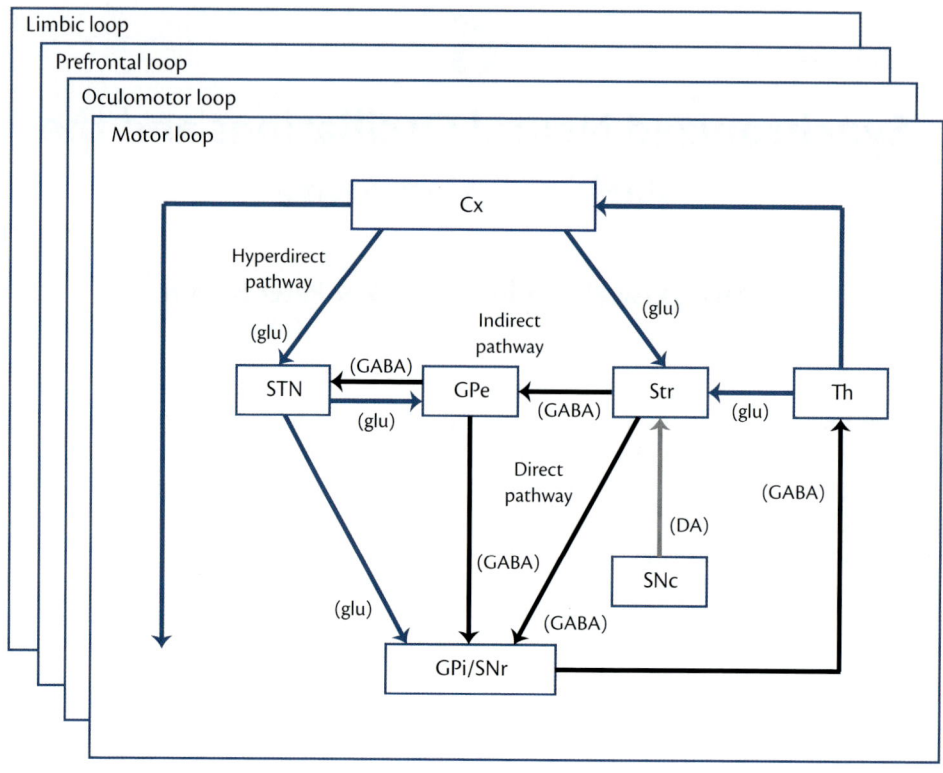

Figure 6.1

Figure 6.1: Anatomy of the cortico-basal ganglia motor loop and its neurotransmitter modulations. A hyperdirect pathway exists between Cx-STN-GPi/SNr. The direct (Cx-Str-GPi/SNr) and indirect pathways (Cx-Str-GPe-STNGPi/SNr) are also shown. Blue arrows represent excitatory glutaminergic projections whilst black arrows represent inhibitory GAB-Aergic projections. The grey arrow represents dopaminergic inputs. Cx – cortex; GPe – external segment of the globus pallidus; GPi – internal segment of the globus pallidus; SNc – substantia nigra pars compacta; SNr – substantia nigra pars reticulata; STN – subthalamic nucleus; Str – striatum; Th – thalamus. Adapted with permission from (9).

glia network, also receives direct cortical afferents through a cortico-subthalamic projection, which forms the hyperdirect pathway (10).

Broadly speaking, the direct pathway leads to the disinhibition of thalamic neurons and hence cortical excitation, which has a prokinetic effect, favouring movement. The effects of the indirect and hyperdirect pathways lead in contrast to the inhibition of cortical neurons and antikinetic effects, biasing against movement. It has been proposed that the reciprocal balance of the direct and hyperdirect/indirect pathways plays a key role in selecting specific desired motor programs and inhibiting undesired ones (9). In terms of linking this model to the pathophysiol-

ogy of the Parkinsonian state, there is evidence that dopamine depletion resulting from the degeneration of nigrostriatal neurons – and thus a reduction of dopaminergic innervation to the basal ganglia – favours the activity of the indirect pathway (11,12). This imbalance is effectively ameliorated by administration of the dopamine precursor levodopa.

Insights from the basal ganglia and cortical recordings

Most of our understanding about oscillatory activity in the basal ganglia in humans comes from patients undergoing functional neurosurgery for the insertion of electrodes for deep brain stimulation (DBS) in target nuclei, although there is increasing complementary evidence from animal models of Parkinson's disease. The most common neurosurgical targets for Parkinson's disease are the STN and GPi (13), although others like the thalamus and the pedunculopontine nucleus (PPN) are also targeted for specific indications (14). Here we will focus largely on insights provided by STN recordings. The long-term efficacy of DBS of this site in reducing motor parkinsonian symptoms has been extensively documented (15-20) . The typical improvement in motor scores assessed using the UPDRS III is around 50% (21). Postoperative doses of levodopa are reduced by around 50% (22), and there is a reduction in levodopa-induced dyskinesias of around 60% (21). Furthermore, several reports have demonstrated an improvement in quality of life following DBS surgery (19,23).

Recordings from DBS patients offer a unique insight into the functional properties of subcortical activity. Recordings in patients can be made intraoperatively from the microelectrodes used to aid functional localisation of surgical targets. Microelectrodes afford the recording of single neuronal units, the background firing of multiple units, and the local field potential (LFP). Alternatively, LFP recordings can be made postoperatively, with fewer time constraints, directly from the DBS electrode.

Local beta oscillations: a pathophysiological hallmark of Parkinson's disease?

Clinical studies have demonstrated that a hallmark of dopamine depletion in the Parkinsonian state is elevated beta-band (13-35 Hz) synchronisation in motor areas of the basal ganglia (24) (Figure 6.2). Prominent beta-band activity has been recorded from LFPs of the STN, GPi and striatum in parkinsonian patients (25–28). Approximately 95% of STN recordings from DBS electrodes demonstrate a peak in the beta-band (29). These oscillations tend to be maximal in

the dorsolateral motor territories of the STN (30-32). Although it is not entirely clear how LFP activity relates to neural spike firing, the locking of neurons to LFP activity over a wide range of frequencies provides support for its use as a measure of the pattern of the underlying neuronal synchronization (33). LFPs themselves probably result from a complex interaction of cellular and synaptic mechanisms (34), with the major influence being slow, subthreshold, post-synaptic potentials (35).

Beta-band activity has often been subdivided into upper (20-35 Hz) and lower (13-20 Hz) bands (36). LFP power tends to dominate in the lower band and is more markedly suppressed by dopaminergic agents such as apomorphine and the dopamine prodrug levodopa (37-40) (see Figure 6.2). This has fuelled the idea that beta activity is pathologically exaggerated in Parkinson's disease by the dopaminergic deficiency that is central to this condition. This hypothesis is supported by studies of patients with dystonia who have been treated with tetrabenazine, which induces a dopaminergic deficit and parkinsonism (41). These patients also exhibit prominent beta activity in their basal ganglia. Finally, studies in the 6OH-dopamine midbrain-lesioned rodent model of Parkinsonism clearly confirm that exaggerated beta synchronization develops in both the basal ganglia and cerebral cortex following lesioning (42-44).

So if beta activity is pathologically exaggerated in Parkinson's disease, what is the evidence that it relates to certain phenotypic features? MEG recordings have shown that local beta activity over the motor areas is increased at rest in patients with moderately advanced PD (45), and its suppression by movement is attenuated or even reversed in mild PD (46). Crucially, both of these features correlate with motor impairment, assessed through UPDRS motor scores. Interestingly, in the former study, although correlations between local beta synchronization and brady-kinesia subscores were significant, correlations with tremor subscores did not achieve signifi-

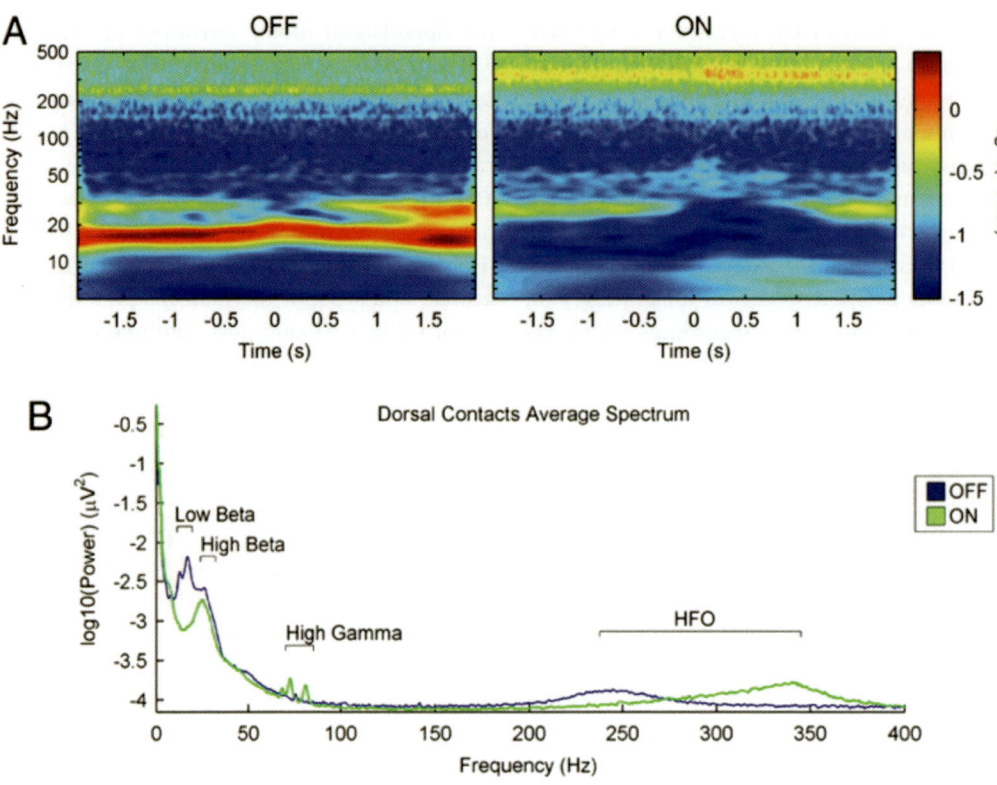

Figure 6.2
STN power spectra observed ON and OFF dopaminergic medication in a cohort of patients with Parkinson's disease.
A) Time-frequency plots showing spectra evolving over time centred at the onset of self-initiated wrist movements
(t = 0). Beta activity desynchronises prior to and during movement, particularly ON medication. This is accompanied
by a concurrent increase in gamma band and high-frequency (200-350 Hz) activity. B) The resting spectrum shows
a reduction in low-frequency, but not high-frequency beta power ON medication. There are also peaks in the theta/
alpha, gamma and high-frequency bands. Adapted with permission from (38).

cance. At the level of the STN, spontaneous fluctuations in beta activity have also been shown to correlate with the clinical state (29,47). In these studies spontaneous fluctuations in beta activity have been measured using the coefficient of variation or measures of complexity. Fluctuations could arise through variation in the strength, density and spatial extent of phase synchronisation. The latter can be inferred from the phase consistency of beta across DBS electrode contacts (48), which also correlates with the clinical state.

Evidence that beta-band oscillations contribute to motor impairment in PD also comes from several reports of levodopa-induced suppression

in LFP beta power and of the incidence of neurons oscillating over this frequency range correlating with treatment-induced improvements in bradykinesia and rigidity (49–51). Interestingly, treatment-related suppressions of beta activity have not been shown to correlate with tremor scores. Similarly, MEG studies exploring the dopaminergic modulation of cortical beta activity have revealed a correlation between improvements in motor scores and dopamine-related changes in cortical beta activity (52). Of note, however, is the observation that dopamine-related reductions in beta activity were only seen in those patients with the greatest improvements in motor scores.

The possibility of a mechanistic role for elevated beta activity in parkinsonsism would be strengthened by evidence that beta suppression occurs during DBS as well as following treatment with levodopa. Traditionally, it had been thought that DBS mimics the effect of lesioning and exerts a suppressive effect on STN output in keeping with the classic pathophysiological model of the disease (53). This idea has been challenged by two observations; firstly, an increase in SNr activity and, secondly, an increase in GPi activity during high-frequency stimulation, both of which would not be predicted by the classical model of the disease (9,54,55).

The major barrier to understanding how beta-band oscillations in the STN are modulated by DBS has been the presence of stimulation-induced electrical artifacts which are several orders of magnitude larger than spontaneous LFP fluctuations (56). Initially, an indirect approach to this problem was employed by recording either from projection sites of the STN (57,58) or by recording following the cessation of DBS effects (50,59,60). These studies revealed that suppression of the coherence between different cortical areas in the beta-band induced by STN DBS correlated with an improvement in bradykinesia and rigidity scores but not tremor scores. Furthermore, the degree of suppression of beta activity in the STN following DBS has been shown to correlate with the degree of residual motor improvement. More direct evidence of a link between STN DBS and suppression of beta-band activity has been facilitated through technical advances, specifically the development of amplifiers that allow simultaneous recordings from the STN during stimulation of this site (56). Using this approach, it has been possible to demonstrate directly that DBS suppresses beta-band activity (61).

The story outlined thus far highlights the importance of exaggerated beta oscillatory synchrony locally in the basal ganglia and cortex in the clinical phenotype of Parkinson's disease, particularly with respect to two of the three cardinal features of the condition: bradykinesia and rigidity.

Beta oscillations are synchronized across levels in Parkinson's disease

There is also evidence to suggest that excessive synchronization of beta-band activity is an important pathological process in PD not only locally, but between cortical areas and the basal ganglia (27,37,62-64). Typically, synchronization in these studies has been measured by computing coherence, a linear measure of the similarity of two signals at a particular frequency. Recently, the importance of non-linear interactions has also been emphasized, and we will discuss examples of them later in the chapter (65). Measurements of synchronization between STN and cortical sites in PD patients with DBS electrodes have involved the simultaneous recording of STN LFPs and cortical recordings with either EEG or MEG (magnetoencephalography). MEG is a functional imaging technique developed in the 1960s which measures the magnetic fields produced by electrical currents in the brain (66,67). It has a number of advantages over EEG measurements, including enhanced spatial resolution and the fact that magnetic fields, unlike electric fields, are not distorted by the presence of burr holes (37,68). Furthermore, the use of spatial filtering techniques such as beam-forming (69) has made it possible to extract physiologically meaningful data in the presence of high-amplitude artifacts caused by the presence of stainless steel wires connecting the depth electrode to the external amplifier in patients who have just undergone implantation. Resting recordings with MEG have repeatedly confirmed the existence of two spatially and spectrally distinct cortico-STN networks. A beta-band network exists between the STN and motor/premotor cortical areas whilst a diffuse alpha-band network, the potential roles of which will be discussed later, exists between the STN and temporoparietal as well as brainstem areas (37,62). A gamma-band network between the STN and motor/premotor cortical areas develops or intensifies around the time of movement (see Figure 6.3).

Using Granger causality-based estimates of the directionality of coupling between sites, it has been possible to demonstrate that although beta-band coupling is bidirectional, it is asymmetric, suggesting that cortical beta oscillations are the most likely driver of the increased beta-band activity in the Parkinsonian basal ganglia (37). Hence a pathophysiological picture emerges whereby cortical beta activity drives subcortical beta-band activity, leading to increased synchronization between and within these sites. This rather simplistic view is complicated by the observation that cortical driving at rest is primarily seen in the upper beta-band (37,62), whereas it is the lower beta-band in the STN that is most exaggerated and best suppressed following the administration of levodopa in PD (37-40). Furthermore, levodopa has not been shown to reduce cortico-STN coherence in the upper beta-frequency band. One possible explanation for these paradoxes stems from the existence of non-linear interactions between STN activities in the upper and lower beta-frequency bands, which are severely attenuated by dopamine (39). Thus, high cortical beta activity may be transformed into lower frequency activity during its transmission to subcortical structures in the dopamine-depleted state. Direct experimental evidence for this assertion is lacking as yet, however.

Task-related reactivity of beta activity in Parkinson's disease

Thus far, we have provided a picture whereby tonic levels of beta activity are elevated in PD

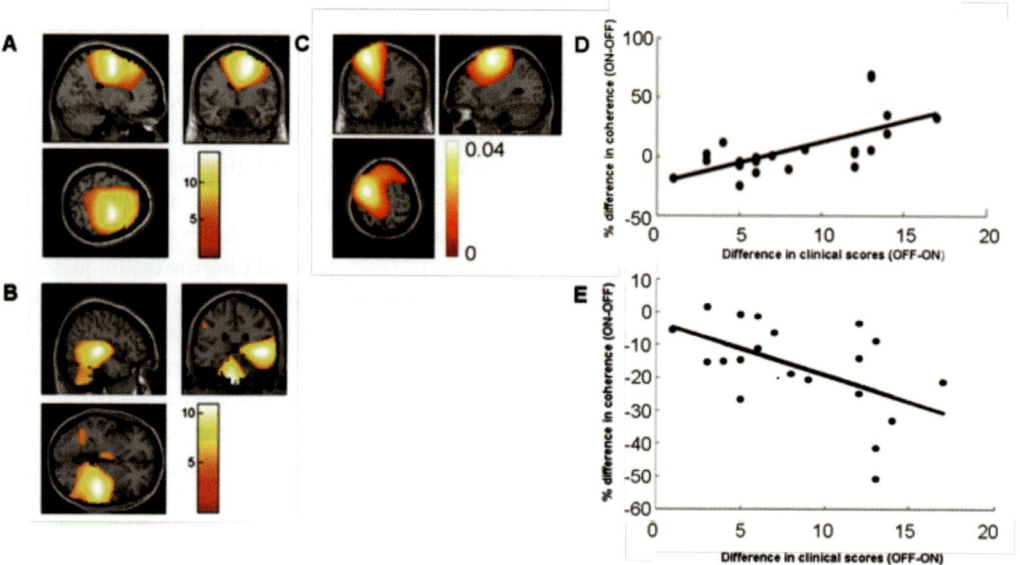

Figure 6.3
Left panel: images A and B show the topography of coherence between STN and cortical areas, at rest, averaged across PD patients. Significant coherence was seen in the alpha (B; STN-temporo-parietal-brainstem areas) and beta bands (A; STN-motor/premotor areas). The colour bars represent t-statistic values. Between half a second prior to and post movement, increased gamma band coherence between STN and M1 is also observed (C). Here the colour bar represents thresholded absolute coherence values. Right panel: during movement dopamine increases coupling between STN and M1 in the gamma band (D) and decreases coupling between STN and temporo-parietal areas in the alpha band (E). Both of these features correlate across subjects with drug induced improvements in clinical scores. Note therefore that the correlation between improvements in UPDRS motor scores and coherence changes is positive for the gamma band, but negative for the alpha band. A and B adapted with permission from ref (37); C and D adapted with permission from ref (98); E adapted with permission from ref (109).

in the basal ganglia, and possibly in the cortex, and relate to bradykinesia and rigidity. What we have not yet considered is task- or event-related reactivity in beta synchrony in the Parkinsonian state. A defining feature of beta oscillations at both the cortical and subcortical sites is their reactivity upon voluntary movement (Figure 2). Movement preparation is associated with a beta ERD, which is further exaggerated by the initiation of movement. Following the termination of movement, beta power rebounds (ERS) before normalising. Such changes in beta activity are often bilateral, although they tend to be more pronounced on the contralateral side to the movement (6).

The functional significance of task-related changes in beta activity in patients with Parkinson's disease may depend on when they occur with respect to movement and, in particular, whether they are perimovement or anticipatory. Recent work suggests that these two processes may subserve distinct functional roles and are independent at least in part (70). The timing of perimovement beta desynchronisation correlates with reaction times within and across patients (28,71). In contrast, phasic increases in beta activity are observed during successful inhibition of pre-potent responses that are seen, for example, in successful stop trials in Go/NoGo tasks (28). This has led to speculation that beta activity may dynamically antagonise motor processing (72,73), in line with views regarding the function of tonically elevated beta. Thus, beta is phasically reduced when movement is necessary, and increased when prepotent responses have to be suppressed. Changes in the coupling between motor cortex and STN are likely to have similar functional relevance. Beta-band coherence is reduced at the time of self-paced movements, with dopamine enhancing this reduction (74).

However, beta activity in the STN may show reactivity even when it is temporally divorced from motor processing. Beta is suppressed following cues indicating the likelihood of the need for a forthcoming movement, even before the nature of the required movement becomes known (70,75). This has raised the possibility that anticipatory reductions in beta activity signal the likelihood that a forthcoming action, be it cognitive or motor, will need to be performed (70,76). In fact, it has been proposed that such impaired reactivity may contribute to both the motor and cognitive slowing which are observed in PD. Crucially, both perimovement and anticipatory beta modulations are dependent upon dopamine.

Is beta an epiphenomenon or causally important in Parkinsonism?

The evidence mentioned thus far implicating beta oscillations in the pathophysiology of the parkinsonian state is largely correlative. Although it is possible that beta oscillations could be an epiphenomenon of other neural processes underscoring movement, there are a few lines of evidence from studies of both healthy subjects and parkinsonian patients that would support a causal rather than an epiphenomenal role. Firstly, it has been demonstrated that cortical stimulation at beta frequencies slows voluntary movements and force generation in healthy subjects (77,78). Secondly, DBS experiments in which chronically implanted patients are stimulated at low frequencies rather than at high frequencies reveal that stimulation at frequencies between 5-25 Hz exacerbates bradykinesia (79-82). The scale of these effects has been rather disappointing in humans, but in optogenetic rodent models it has been demonstrated that low-frequency, 20Hz stimulation of STN afferent projections markedly worsens Parkinsonian symptoms (63). Still, the quantitative importance of beta synchrony in terms of its contributions to bradykinesia and rigidity in patients is unclear, and given that this has been most intensively studied in patients undergoing functional neurosurgery, its role early on in the disease process also remains to be firmly established.

Insights into the generation and propagation of beta rhythms in PD

Recent computational modeling studies have shed light on the potential mechanisms through which dopamine depletion may lead to exaggerated beta-band synchrony in the cortico-basal ganglia circuit. Studies adopting an approach of examining model-based interactions of causal influences in the cortico-basal ganglia circuit have illuminated a number of important features of the dopamine-deficient state (83,84).

Modeling work using data from PD patients with multisite recordings has revealed that dopamine depletion results in increased connectivity between the cortex and STN, GPe and STN, and STN and GPi. Strengthening connections in any one of these pathways, as well as the pathway from STN to GPe, strongly promotes beta activity. These findings are in line with a model whereby cortical activity is required to maintain the STN-GPe circuit in a resonant state, which in turn promotes the generation and propagation of beta oscillations in the cortico-basal ganglia circuit. This is in keeping with numerous other studies highlighting strong interactions between GPe and STN as an important factor in promoting the emergence of beta-band oscillatory activity (11,85–88). Moreover, inactivation of these structures with muscimol, a potent GABA agonist, has also been shown to suppress beta oscillations in 1-methyl-4-phenyl-1,2,3,6-tetrahydropyridine-treated parkinsonian monkeys (89).

The gamma-frequency band: a prokinetic signal?

Several studies have demonstrated gamma oscillations in the spectra of LFPs recorded in the GPi, STN and thalamus of subjects at rest (6,27,38,64,74,90-95). The activity has been termed finely tuned gamma (FTG) as it is sharply tuned to a narrow frequency band within the 60-90 Hz range. It is not limited to patients with Parkinson's disease, nor a consistent feature in such patients (96). It is contralaterally enhanced during voluntary movement, so that the direction of change is opposite to that of activity in the beta-band. Akin to the beta-rhythm, however, subcortical FTG is coherent with motor/frontal cortical activity. FTG is enhanced by therapy with the dopamine prodrug levodopa (25,27,74,97,98).

FTG oscillations have been linked to arousal through demonstrations that they are increased following startling stimuli and during REM sleep, which is associated with cortical arousal (93). In contrast, FTG is absent during states of reduced arousal and during non-REM sleep (25,93). Based on these findings and on the above studies highlighting the motoric role of the FTG, it has been suggested that the role of oscillations in this frequency band may be to contribute to the vigor or effort of a motor response, which partly relates to the level of phasic arousal. Impairment of motor vigor may be an important feature of the dopamine-depleted Parkinsonian state (96).

Patients with Parkinson's disease also demonstrate broadband gamma synchronization perimovement, even in the absence of FTG in the resting spectrum (6,98). It is therefore likely that although FTG can contribute to this broadband reactivity, this is not the only factor. Whether broadband gamma reactivity also helps to encode motor effort or vigor, rather than biomechanical movement parameters like force, remains unclear. Studies that demonstrate a correlation between both drug-related increases in STN gamma activity and STN-cortical gamma-band coherence and motor improvement do not really address this point (98). Similarly, studies that show gamma-amplitude around movement correlating with the speed and scale of voluntary movements cannot disambiguate vigor from force (99–101). Indeed, whether gamma activity actually encodes anything and is causally relevant is uncertain. Cortical stimulation at gamma frequencies in healthy subjects does increase the rate of development of grip force but only by less than 10% (77).

Finally, there is also a much higher frequency ERS upon movement, extending up to 600 Hz in the STN (98). It is still unclear whether this activity is the product of multiple, dynamic, phase-coupled neuronal clusters spanning this broad frequency range or reflects the brief and asynchronous burst of activity hypothesized to be an LFP correlate of population firing (102-104).

Interestingly, the observation of impaired, but reciprocal, oscillatory activities in the beta and gamma frequency bands in PD raises the question of whether patterns of alterations in the beta and gamma frequency bands occur simultaneously in the disease process or in a staged manner. To this extent, recent work demonstrates that increases in gamma-band activity may compensate for higher levels of tonic beta activity (105). However, any suggestion that increased levels of tonic beta may precede reductions in gamma activity is at best speculative, and we await the results of studies formally relating the evolution of oscillatory features of the disease to clinical progression.

Low-frequency (theta/alpha) rhythms and PD

A peak in the alpha-band is often noted in LFP spectra from the STN in PD, but it does not appear to be substantially modulated by dopamine. Theta/alpha power in the STN is increased during cued movements (99,106,107), although its response in self-paced movements is less consistent (108,109). In addition, in PD, increased levels of theta and alpha STN power correlate with improved motor performance; specifically, power in these frequency bands correlates with force measures during the onset, maintenance and release of maximal grip, and with the latency to onset of grip and its release (99,100). These associations raise the possibility that STN activity in the theta/alpha-band might subserve a non-specific function related to movement, such as attention.

This is also in keeping with views about coherent activity at similar frequencies between the STN, parieto-temporal cortex and the brainstem of patients with PD (37,62). While formal confirmation of a putative role for the STN-cortico-brainstem alpha-band network in orienting attention is awaited, it is interesting to note that movement-related reductions in coherence in this network on and off levodopa correlate with clinical motor improvement. Hence this network may form a neural substrate for explaining how attentional deficits in PD relate to motor impairments (109). This suggestion is supported by previous correlations of attentional deficits in PD with motor impairment such as gait freezing and falls (110,111).

It is also of note that both local STN theta/alpha activity and STN-cortical coherence in this frequency band have been associated with dopamine-related side-effects, namely dyskinesias and impulse control disorders (112,113). The cortical topographies of the coherent activities relating to dyskinesias and impulse control disorders are different, however (113), indicating different anatomical territories in the aetiology of dopamine-related side-effects.

Oscillations and cognitive features of Parkinson's disease

It has become increasingly evident that cognitive impairments in patients with PD may also be associated with changes in oscillatory activity in the cortex and in non-motor regions of the STN. A general phenomenon in PD is the slowing of background oscillatory activity in cortical EEG and MEG, manifesting as a diffuse increase in theta- and alpha-band power (114,115). However, in PD dementia, this slowing becomes even more marked, so there is an increase in the power of delta rhythms at the expense of a relative reduction in alpha power (116). Reversal of oscillatory slowing in PD dementia by acetylcholine esterase inhibitors highlights that the spectral changes may be the result of cholinergic neuron loss (117). While the functional consequences or associations of such oscillatory changes remain to be elucidated, their demonstration in other, primarily cognitive disease states such as Alzheimer's disease suggests an important relationship with cognitive processing.

At the level of the basal ganglia, theta activity in the STN has been shown to be sensitive to conflicts in decision-making (118,119) and has accordingly been reported to be particularly elevated in PD patients with impulse control disorders (113). Similarly, STN activity in the alpha-band is suppressed by emotional stimuli, with the degree of suppression correlating to individual valence ratings and the affective state of the patient. It has therefore been suggested that STN alpha-band reactivity to emotional stimuli may be an important marker of depressive symptoms in PD (120-122). As already mentioned, impaired beta reactivity has also been cited as a possible correlate of cognitive slowness, or bradyphrenia (70,123).

Finally, gamma activity in the STN has also been implicated in cognitive processing. It is increased during the performance of paced random number generation and verbal fluency tests. These gamma changes correlate with a measure of randomness which indexes success in switching from automatic counting to a more controlled random generation of numbers (124) and with the ability to switch between subcategories in verbal fluency tasks (125). Together, these studies provide support for STN gamma activity in executive processes such as suppression of habitual or pre-potent responses and switching from automatic to controlled processing in cognitive tasks. Therefore, it is plausible that dopamine-dependent impairments of gamma-band activity and reactivity in PD may be partly responsible for some cognitive features, such as cognitive inflexibility.

Oscillations and tremor in Parkinson's disease

Tremor is the only one of the three cardinal features of PD that has a directly measurable oscillatory nature. Tremor-dominant types of PD have traditionally been considered distinct to brady-kinesia/rigidity-dominant subtypes (126,127), and it is hardly surprising therefore that dopamine depletion in the striatum and beta-band activity have not been shown to correlate with the severity of PD tremor (128). A key difficulty in understanding the neural basis of tremor has been the fact that tremor often displays marked variability both over time and across the body, such that the tremor activity of different limbs in a PD patient is almost never coherent (128,129). These observations suggest that multiple oscillators may drive peripheral tremor, rather than a single oscillator.

MEG studies have allowed characterization of the brain regions coherent with Parkinsonian resting tremor, revealing functional tremor networks. These studies demonstrate the presence of strong EMG coupling with the contralateral primary motor cortex (M1) and also coupling between M1 and other premotor, supplementary motor and somatosensory areas as well diencephalic and cerebellar sites (130).

The investigation of tremor frequency activity at subcortical sites has become possible with much greater spatial resolution than that afforded by MEG through intraoperative, microelectrode recordings in PD patients. Such work has revealed oscillatory peaks at tremor frequency and tremor harmonics within the STN, GPi and thalamus (25,131-134) in addition to coherence between these sites and EMG activity (135,136). Recent work has shown that both in the STN and VIM, distinct, spatially segregated tremor clusters may relate to tremor activity in specific muscle groups, pointing to multiple tremor-related subloops within subcortical structures (135,136).

In keeping with the finding of prominent, thalamic tremor-related oscillations in the ventral intermediate nucleus (VIM), there is the finding that DBS of this site is successful in the treatment of both Parkinsonian and essential tremor (137-140). Furthermore, in accord with electrophysiological studies of VIM connectivity, tractography has demonstrated that regions of the VIM adjacent to the most effective contacts for DBS have extensive connectivity with motor cortical and subcortical areas including the cerebellum and brainstem (141). Taken together, the above evidence highlights the possible existence of tremor oscillator(s) within basal ganglia-thalamo-cortical circuits. This assertion has gained theoretical support from computational models showing that both dopamine depletion and altered connectivity between nodes of the basal ganglia-thalamo-cortical circuit may lead to tremor-like spiking activity (142).

Cross-frequency interactions

We have largely focused on local synchronization and linear measures of synchronization (coherence) of activity across the cortico-basal ganglia circuit. Several lines of evidence point to the fact that activity in a particular frequency band may either influence activity in other frequency bands or interact with other frequency bands to influence behaviour. Such interactions may be either linear or non-linear (143).

Studies adopting a multivariate approach to correlating activities in multiple frequency bands with behavioural performance during maximal grip demonstrate that effects in the alpha- and gamma-bands best predict behavioural performance when other features are held constant. Thus, the relationship hitherto reported between beta activity and bradykinesia-rigidity might be tightly locked with or even secondary to effects at both lower and higher frequencies (99,100).

Another striking feature demonstrated in a variety of physiological studies is the ability of the phase of a low-frequency signal, typically in the delta, theta or alpha range, to correlate with the amplitude of a higher frequency oscillation, typically in the gamma range (144,145). Although the directionality of such phase-amplitude coupling has yet to be explored, it is often assumed that the phase of the lower frequency

signal drives the amplitude of the higher frequency one. Phase-amplitude coupling has been demonstrated in a number of brain areas including the neocortex, hippocampus and basal ganglia and has been shown to be involved in a number of cognitive processes such as learning, memory and attention (146-148), leading to the suggestion that it may play an important role in both local computation and long-range communication in large-scale brain networks (145).

Phase-amplitude coupling has recently been proposed as a mechanism for motor impairment in PD. STN LFP recordings in PD patients have demonstrated coupling between the phase of beta-band oscillations and the amplitude of high-frequency oscillations in the off-medicated state. This coupling is reduced by dopamine and by movement with movement-related modulations, correlating negatively with bradykinesia and rigidity scores (38). Furthermore, recent electrocortigraphy (ECOG) studies have demonstrated a coupling of the beta phase in the STN and in the motor cortex with broadband gamma amplitude over the motor cortex in PD. Such exaggerated coupling appears specific to PD, as it is not observed in patients undergoing neurosurgery for other conditions such as dystonia or epilepsy. It is also suppressed by DBS of the STN. Moreover, in accordance with previous studies demonstrating the cortical driving of STN beta oscillations, there is the finding that the peak modulation of gamma-band amplitude over the motor cortex precedes the peak modulation of the beta phase in the STN (149).

There is also evidence that cross-frequency interactions are not solely limited to local power but may also be observed in long-range coherence spectra. Levodopa treatment causes a frequency-selective change in the reactivity of cortico-subthalamic coherence during movement. The degree of reactivity correlates across the alpha- and gamma-bands with treatment-related improvement in motor performance (98,109). However, the analysis suggests that changes in coupling in the two frequency bands explain the same portion of the variance in the clinical response to treatment (109). Interestingly, this is the case despite frequency-dependent differences in the cortical topography of the coherences. The implication is that the dopamine-dependent disengagement of the STN from its locking to the temporal cortex at alpha-band frequencies, and the engagement of STN locking to the motor cortex in the gamma-band are two sides of the same coin (Figure 6.3).

Concluding remarks

Growing evidence suggests that synchronized neural oscillations at discrete frequencies play a key role in neural communication and information processing, both locally and within long-range brain networks. Furthermore, direct evidence of oscillatory activity being causal to behaviour rather than simply being an epiphenomenon of neural processing is being provided by experiments studying the behavioural consequences of directly manipulating oscillatory activity.

In PD, oscillatory activity has been considered as either antikinetic (beta-band) or prokinetic (gamma-band), with the balance between them contributing to the motor symptoms of bradykinesia and rigidity. However, this simplistic distinction neither captures the full functional roles of activity within these frequency bands and their cross-frequency relations, nor explains non-motor parkinsonian phenotypes. Here we have attempted to illustrate that the tonic and phasic reactivity of oscillations across multiple frequency bands and their cross-frequency interactions within spatially segregated loops of the basal ganglia-thalamo-cortical system may relate to distinct components of clinical impairment, both motor and non-motor. The hope is that an improved understanding of the role of oscillatory activity in contributing to the symptoms of parkinsonism may translate into the development of novel therapeutic interventions. This is beginning to be realised, as evinced by proof-of-principle studies demonstrating that by specifically focusing on oscillatory activity, closed-loop DBS and phase-cancelling cortical stimulation may control symptoms in PD (150,151).

References

1 Jasper H, Andrews H. Electroencephalography. III Normal differentiation of occipital and precentral regions in man. Archive Neurology Psychiatry 1938;39:96-115.

2 Pfurtscheller G, Neuper C, Kalcher J. 40-Hz oscillations during motor behavior in man. Neurosci Let 1993;164:179-182.

3 Neuper C, Pfurtscheller G. Post-movement synchronization of beta rhythms in the EEG over the cortical foot area in man. Neurosci Lett 1996;216:17-20.

4 Pfurtscheller G, Lopes da Silva FH. Event-related EEG/MEG synchronization and desynchronization: basic principles. Clin Neurophysiol 1999;110:1842-1857.

5 Foffani G, Bianchi A, Baselli G, Priori A. Movement-related frequency modulation of beta oscillatory activity in the human subthalamic nucleus. J Physiol 2005;568:699-711.

6 Alegre M, Alonso-Frech F, Rodríguez-Oroz MC, et al. Movement-related changes in oscillatory activity in the human subthalamic nucleus: ipsilateral vs. contralateral movements. Europ J Neurosci 2005;22:2315-2324.

7 Salenius S, Salmelin R, Neuper C, Pfurtscheller G, Hari R. Human cortical 40 Hz rhythm is closely related to EMG rhythmicity. Neurosci Lett 1996;213:75-78.

8 Kaneda K, Nambu A, Tokuno H, Takada M. Differential processing patterns of motor information via striatopallidal and striatonigral projections. J Neurophysiol 2002;88:1420-1432.

9 Nambu A. Seven problems on the basal ganglia. Curr Opin Neurobiol 2008;18:595-604.

10 Mathai A, Smith Y. The corticostriatal and corticosubthalamic pathways: two entries, one target. So what? Frontiers in Systems Neuroscience 2011;5:64.

11 Albin RL, Young AB, Penney JB. The functional anatomy of basal ganglia disorders. Trends in Neurosciences 1989;12:366-375.

12 DeLong MR. Primate models of movement disorders of basal ganglia origin. Trends in Neurosciences 1990;13:281-285.

13 Ponce FA, Lozano AM. Deep brain stimulation state of the art and novel stimulation targets. Progress in Brain Research 2010;184:311-324.

14 Fasano A, Daniele A, Albanese A. Treatment of motor and non-motor features of Parkinson's disease with deep brain stimulation. Lancet Neurology 2012;11:429-442.

15 Rodriguez-Oroz MC, Obeso JA, Lang AE, et al. Bilateral deep brain stimulation in Parkinson's disease: a multicentre study with 4 years follow-up. Brain 2005;128:2240-2249.

16 Deuschl G, Schade-Brittinger C, Krack P, et al. A randomized trial of deep-brain stimulation for Parkinson's disease. N Engl J Med. 2006;31;355:896-908.

17 Follett KA, Weaver FM, Stern M, et al. Pallidal versus subthalamic deep-brain stimulation for Parkinson's disease. N Engl J Med 2010;362:2077-2091.

18 Fasano A, Romito LM, Daniele A, et al. Motor and cognitive outcome in patients with Parkinson's disease 8 years after subthalamic implants. Brain 2010;133:2664-2676.

19 Weaver FM, Follett K, Stern M, et al. Bilateral deep brain stimulation vs best medical therapy for patients with advanced Parkinson disease: a randomized controlled trial. JAMA 2009;301:63-73.

20 Witjas T, Kaphan E, Régis J, et al. Effects of chronic subthalamic stimulation on nonmotor fluctuations in Parkinson's disease. Mov Disord 2007;22:1729-1234.

21 Krack P, Batir A, Van Blercom N, et al. Five-year follow-up of bilateral stimulation of the subthalamic nucleus in advanced Parkinson's disease. N Engl J Med 2003;349:1925-1934.

22 Benabid AL, Chabardes S, Mitrofanis J, Pollak P. Deep brain stimulation of the subthalamic nucleus for the treatment of Parkinson's disease. Lancet Neurology 2009;8:67-81.

23 Williams A, Gill S, Varma T, et al. Deep brain stimulation plus best medical therapy versus best medical therapy alone for advanced Parkinson's disease (PD SURG trial): a randomised, open-label trial. Lancet Neurology 2010;9:581-591.

24 Hammond C, Bergman H, Brown P. Pathological synchronization in Parkinson's disease: networks, models and treatments. Trends in Neurosciences. 2007;30:357-364.

25 Brown P, Oliviero A, Mazzone P, Insola A, Tonali P, Di Lazzaro V. Dopamine dependency of oscillations between subthalamic nucleus and pallidum in Parkinson's disease. J Neurosci 2001;21:1033-1038.

26 Sochurkova D, Rektor I. Event-related desynchronization/synchronization in the putamen. An SEEG case study. Exp Brain Res 2003;149:401-404.

27 Williams D, Tijssen M, Van Bruggen G, et al. Dopamine-dependent changes in the functional connectivity between basal ganglia and cerebral cortex in humans. Brain 2002;125:1558-1569.

28 Kühn AA, Williams D, Kupsch A, et al. Event-related beta desynchronization in human subthalamic nucleus correlates with motor performance. Brain 2004;127:735-746.

29 Little S, Pogosyan A, Kuhn AA, Brown P. β band stability over time correlates with Parkinsonian rigidity and bradykinesia. Exp Neurol 2012;236:383-388.

30 Levy R, Hutchinson W, Lozano A, Dostrovsky JO. Synchronised neuronal discharge in the basal ganglia of parkinsonia patients is limited to oscillatory activity. J Neurosci 2002;22:2855-2861.

31 Levy R, Ashby P, Hutchison WD, Lang AE, Lozano AM, Dostrovsky JO. Dependence of subthalamic nucleus oscillations on movement and dopamine in Parkinson's disease. Brain 2002;125:1196-1209.

32 Zaidel A, Spivak A, Grieb B, Bergman H, Israel Z. Subthalamic span of beta oscillations predicts deep brain stimulation efficacy for patients with Parkinson's disease. Brain 2010;133:2007-2021.

33 Moran A, Bergman H, Israel Z, Bar-Gad I. Subthalamic nucleus functional organization revealed by parkinsonian neuronal oscillations and synchrony. Brain 2008;131:3395-3409.

34 Logothetis NK, Pauls J, Augath M, Trinath T, Oeltermann A. Neurophysiological investigation of the basis of the fMRI signal. Nature 2001;412:150-157.

35 Eccles J. Interpretation of action potentials evoked in the cerebral cortex. Electroencephal Clin Neurophysiol 1951;3:449-464.

36 De Solages C, Hill BC, Koop MM, Henderson JM, Bronte-Stewart H. Bilateral symmetry and coherence of subthalamic nuclei beta band activity in Parkinson's disease. Expl Neurol 2010;221:260-266.

37 Litvak V, Jha A, Eusebio A, et al. Resting oscillatory cortico-subthalamic connectivity in patients with Parkinson's disease. Brain 2011;134:359-374.

38 López-Azcárate J, Tainta M, Rodríguez-Oroz MC, et al. Coupling between beta and high-frequency activity in the human subthalamic nucleus may be a pathophysiological mechanism in Parkinson's disease. J Neurosci 2010;30:6667-6677.

39 Marceglia S, Foffani G, Bianchi AM, et al. Dopamine-dependent non-linear correlation between subthalamic rhythms in Parkinson's disease. J Physiol 2006;571:579-591.

40 Priori A, Foffani G, Pesenti A, et al. Rhythm-specific pharmacological modulation of subthalamic activity in Parkinson's disease. Exp Neurol 2004;189:369-379.

41 Kühn AA, Brücke C, Schneider G-H, et al. Increased beta activity in dystonia patients after drug-induced dopamine deficiency. Exp Neurol 2008;214:140-143.

42 Sharott A, Magill PJ, Harnack D, Kupsch A, Meissner W, Brown P. Dopamine depletion increases the power and coherence of beta-oscillations in the cerebral cortex and subthalamic nucleus of the awake rat. Europ J Neurosci 2005;21:1413-1422.

43 Mallet N, Pogosyan A, Sharott A, et al. Disrupted dopamine transmission and the emergence of exaggerated beta oscillations in subthalamic nucleus and cerebral cortex. J Neurosci 2008;28:4795-4806.

44 Magill PJ, Bolam JP, Bevan MD. Dopamine regulates the impact of the cerebral cortex on the subthalamic nucleus-globus pallidus network. Neurosci 2001;106:313-330.

45 Stoffers D, Bosboom JLW, Deijen JB, Wolters EC, Stam CJ, Berendse HW. Increased cortico-cortical functional connectivity in early-stage Parkinson's disease: an MEG study. NeuroImage 2008;41:212-222.

46 Pollok B, Krause V, Martsch W, Wach C, Schnitzler A, Südmeyer M. Motor-cortical oscillations in early stages of Parkinson's disease. J Physiol 2012;590:3203-3212.

47 Chen CC, Hsu YT, Chan HL, et al. Complexity of subthalamic 13-35 Hz oscillatory activity directly correlates with clinical impairment in patients with Parkinson's disease. Exp Neurol 2010;224:234-240.

48 Pogosyan A, Yoshida F, Chen CC, et al. Parkinsonian impairment correlates with spatially extensive subthalamic oscillatory synchronization. Neurosci 2010;171:245-257.

49 Kühn AA, Kupsch A, Schneider G-H, Brown P. Reduction in subthalamic 8-35 Hz oscillatory activity correlates with clinical improvement in Parkinson's disease. Europ J Neurosci 2006;23:1956-1960.

50 Kühn AA, Tsui A, Aziz T, et al. Pathological synchronisation in the subthalamic nucleus of patients with Parkinson's disease relates to both bradykinesia and rigidity. Exp Neurol 2009;215:380-387.

51 Ray NJ, Jenkinson N, Wang S, et al. Local field potential beta activity in the subthalamic nucleus of patients with Parkinson's disease is associated with improvements in bradykinesia after dopamine and deep brain stimulation. Exp Neurol 2008;213:108-113.

52 Stoffers D, Bosboom JLW, Wolters EC, Stam CJ, Berendse HW. Dopaminergic modulation of cortico-cortical functional connectivity in Parkinson's disease: an MEG study. Exp Neurol 2008;213:191-195.

53 Bergman H, Wichmann T, DeLong MR. Reversal of experimental parkinsonism by lesions of the subthalamic nucleus. Science 1990;249:1436-1438.

54 Maurice N, Thierry A-M, Glowinski J, Deniau J M. Spontaneous and evoked activity of substantia nigra pars reticulata neurons during high-frequency stimulation of the subthalamic nucleus. J Neurosci 2003;23:9929-9936.

55 Hashimoto T, Elder CM, Okun MS, Patrick SK, Vitek JL. Stimulation of the subthalamic nucleus changes the firing pattern of pallidal neurons. J Neurosci 2003;23:1916-1923.

56 Rossi L, Foffani G, Marceglia S, Bracchi F, Barbieri S, Priori A. An electronic device for artefact sup-

pression in human local field potential recordings during deep brain stimulation. Journal of Neural Engineering 2007;4:96-106.

57 Silberstein P, Pogosyan A, Kühn AA, et al. Cortico-cortical coupling in Parkinson's disease and its modulation by therapy. Brain 2005;128:1277-1291.

58 Brown P, Mazzone P, Oliviero A, et al. Effects of stimulation of the subthalamic area on oscillatory pallidal activity in Parkinson's disease. Exp Neurol 2004;188:480-490.

59 Wingeier B, Tcheng T, Koop MM, Hill BC, Heit G, Bronte-Stewart HM. Intra-operative STN DBS attenuates the prominent beta rhythm in the STN in Parkinson's disease. Exp Neurol 2006;197:244-251.

60 Bronte-Stewart H, Barberini C, Koop MM, Hill BC, Henderson JM, Wingeier B. The STN beta-band profile in Parkinson's disease is stationary and shows prolonged attenuation after deep brain stimulation. Exp Neurol 2009;215:20-28.

61 Eusebio A, Thevathasan W, Doyle Gaynor L, et al. Deep brain stimulation can suppress pathological synchronisation in parkinsonian patients. J Neurol Neurosurg Psychiatry 2011;82:569-573.

62 Hirschmann J, Özkurt TE, Butz M, et al. Distinct oscillatory STN-cortical loops revealed by simultaneous MEG and local field potential recordings in patients with Parkinson's disease. NeuroImage 2011;55:1159-1168.

63 Gradinaru V, Mogri M, Thompson KR, Henderson JM, Deisseroth K. Optical deconstruction of parkinsonian neural circuitry. Science 2009;324:354-359.

64 Fogelson N, Williams D, Tijssen M, Van Bruggen G, Speelman H, Brown P. Different functional loops between cerebral cortex and the subthalmic area in Parkinson's disease. Cerebral Cortex 2006;16:64-75.

65 Wei C-S, Tsai C-H, Chiou S-M, et al. Nonlinear analysis of movement-related changes in human subthalamic local field potentials. Conference proceedings : IEEE Engineering Med Biol Soc 2010;2010:4132-4135.

66 Cohen D. Magnetoencephalography: evidence of magnetic fields produced by alpha-rhythm currents. Science 1968;161:784-786.

67 Cohen D. Magnetoencephalography: detection of the brain's electrical activity with a superconducting magnetometer. Science 1972;175:664-666.

68 Litvak V, Eusebio A, Jha A, et al. Optimized beamforming for simultaneous MEG and intracranial local field potential recordings in deep brain stimulation patients. NeuroImage 2010;50:1578-1588.

69 Van Veen BD, Van Drongelen W, Yuchtman M, Suzuki A. Localization of brain electrical activity via linearly constrained minimum variance spatial filtering. IEEE transactions on bio-medical engineering 1997;44:867-880.

70 Oswal A, Litvak V, Sauleau P, Brown P. Beta reactivity, prospective facilitation of executive processing, and its dependence on dopaminergic therapy in Parkinson's disease. J Neurosci 2012;32:9909-9916.

71 Williams D, Kühn A, Kupsch A, et al. The relationship between oscillatory activity and motor reaction time in the parkinsonian subthalamic nucleus. Europ J Neurosc. 2005;21:249-258.

72 Engel AK, Fries P. Beta-band oscillations – ignalling the status quo? Current Opin Neurobiol 2010;20:156-165.

73 Gilbertson T, Lalo E, Doyle L, Di Lazzaro V, Cioni B, Brown P. Existing motor state is favored at the expense of new movement during 13-35 Hz oscillatory synchrony in the human corticospinal system. J Neurosci 2005;25:7771.

74 Cassidy M, Mazzone P, Oliviero A, et al. Movement-related changes in synchronization in the human basal ganglia. Brain 2002;125:1235-1246.

75 Jenkinson N, Brown P. New insights into the relationship between dopamine, beta oscillations and motor function. Trends in Neurosciences 2011;34:611-618.

76 Tzagarakis C, Ince NF, Leuthold AC, Pellizzer G. Beta-band activity during motor planning reflects response uncertainty. J Neurosci 2010;30:11270-11277.

77 Joundi RA, Jenkinson N, Brittain J-S, Aziz TZ, Brown P. Driving oscillatory activity in the human cortex enhances motor performance. Curr Biol 2012;22:403-407.

78 Pogosyan A, Gaynor LD, Eusebio A, Brown P. Boosting cortical activity at Beta-band fre-

quencies slows movement in humans. Curr Biol 2009;19:1637-1641.

79 Timmermann L, Wojtecki L, Gross J, et al. Ten-Hertz stimulation of subthalamic nucleus deteriorates motor symptoms in Parkinson's disease. Mov Disord 2004;19:1328-1333.

80 Fogelson N, Kühn AA, Silberstein P, et al. Frequency dependent effects of subthalamic nucleus stimulation in Parkinson's disease. Neurosci Lett 2005;382:5-9.

81 Chen CC, Litvak V, Gilbertson T, et al. Excessive synchronization of basal ganglia neurons at 20 Hz slows movement in Parkinson's disease. Exp Neurol 2007;205:214-221.

82 Eusebio A, Chen CC, Lu CS, et al. Effects of low-frequency stimulation of the subthalamic nucleus on movement in Parkinson's disease. Exp Neurol 2008;209:125-130.

83 Moran RJ, Mallet N, Litvak V, et al. Alterations in Brain Connectivity Underlying Beta Oscillations in Parkinsonism. PLoS Computational Biology 2011;7:e1002124.

84 Marreiros AC, Cagnan H, Moran RJ, Friston KJ, Brown P. Basal ganglia-cortical interactions in Parkinsonian patients. NeuroImage 2012;66C:301-310.

85 Cruz A V, Mallet N, Magill PJ, Brown P, Averbeck BB. Effects of dopamine depletion on information flow between the subthalamic nucleus and external globus pallidus. J Neurophysiol 2011;106:2012-2023.

86 Fan KY, Baufreton J, Surmeier DJ, Chan CS, Bevan MD. Proliferation of external globus pallidus-subthalamic nucleus synapses following degeneration of midbrain dopamine neurons. J Neurosci 2012;32:13718-13728.

87 Kumar A, Cardanobile S, Rotter S, Aertsen A. The role of inhibition in generating and controlling Parkinson's disease oscillations in the Basal Ganglia. Frontiers in Systems Neuroscience 2011;5:86.

88 Holgado AJN, Terry JR, Bogacz R. Conditions for the generation of beta oscillations in the subthalamic nucleus-globus pallidus network. J Neurosci 2010;30:12340-12352.

89 Tachibana Y, Iwamuro H, Kita H, Takada M, Nambu A. Subthalamo-pallidal interactions underlying parkinsonian neuronal oscillations in the primate basal ganglia. Europ J Neurosci 2011;34:1470-1484.

90 Alonso-Frech F, Zamarbide I, Alegre M, et al. Slow oscillatory activity and levodopa-induced dyskinesias in Parkinson's disease. Brain 2006;129:1748-1757.

91 Androulidakis AG, Doyle LMF, Yarrow K, Litvak V, Gilbertson TP, Brown P. Anticipatory changes in beta synchrony in the human corticospinal system and associated improvements in task performance. Europ J Neurosci 2007;25:3758-3765.

92 Devos D, Szurhaj W, Reyns N, et al. Predominance of the contralateral movement-related activity in the subthalamo-cortical loop. Clin Neurophysiol 2006;117:2315-2327.

93 Kempf F, Brücke C, Salih F, et al. Gamma activity and reactivity in human thalamic local field potentials. Europ J Neurosci 2009;29:943-953.

94 Trottenberg T, Fogelson N, Kühn AA, et al. Subthalamic gamma activity in patients with Parkinson's disease. Exp Neurol 2006;200:56-65.

95 Pogosyan A, Kühn AA, Trottenberg T, Schneider G-H, Kupsch A, Brown P. Elevations in local gamma activity are accompanied by changes in the firing rate and information coding capacity of neurons in the region of the subthalamic nucleus in Parkinson's disease. Exp Neurol 2006;202:271-279.

96 Jenkinson N, Kühn AA, Brown P. Gamma oscillations in the human basal ganglia. Exp Neurol 2013;245:72-76.

97 Lalo E, Thobois S, Sharott A, et al. Patterns of bidirectional communication between cortex and basal ganglia during movement in patients with Parkinson disease. J Neurosci 2008;28:3008-3016.

98 Litvak V, Eusebio A, Jha A, et al. Movement-Related Changes in Local and Long-Range Synchronization in Parkinson's Disease Revealed by Simultaneous Magnetoencephalography and Intracranial Recordings. J Neurosci 2012;32:10541-10553.

99 Anzak A, Tan H, Pogosyan A, et al. Subthalamic nucleus activity optimizes maximal effort motor responses in Parkinson's disease. Brain 2012;135:2766-2778.

100 Tan H, Pogosyan A, Anzak A, et al. Frequency specific activity in subthalamic nucleus correlates with

hand bradykinesia in Parkinson's disease. Exp Neurol 2013;240:122-129.

101 Brücke C, Huebl J, Schönecker T, et al. Scaling of movement is related to pallidal γ oscillations in patients with dystonia. J Neurosci 2012;32:1008-1019.

102 Manning JR, Jacobs J, Fried I, Kahana MJ. Broadband shifts in local field potential power spectra are correlated with single-neuron spiking in humans. J Neurosci 2009;29:13613-13620.

103 Miller KJ, Sorensen LB, Ojemann JG, Den Nijs M. Power-law scaling in the brain surface electric potential. PLoS computational biology 2009;5:e1000609.

104 Ray S, Maunsell JHR. Differences in gamma frequencies across visual cortex restrict their possible use in computation. Neuron 2010;67:885-896.

105 Florin E, Erasmi R, Reck C, et al. Does increased gamma activity in patients suffering from Parkinson's disease counteract the movement inhibiting beta activity? Neuroscience 2013;237:42-50.

106 Klostermann F, Nikulin V V, Kühn AA, et al. Task-related differential dynamics of EEG alpha- and beta-band synchronization in cortico-basal motor structures. Europ J Neurosci 2007;25:1604-1615.

107 Alegre M, Lopez-Azcarate J, Obeso I, et al. The subthalamic nucleus is involved in successful inhibition in the stop-signal task: a local field potential study in Parkinson's disease. Exp Neurol 2013;239:1-12.

108 Singh A, Levin J, Mehrkens JH, Bötzel K. Alpha frequency modulation in the human basal ganglia is dependent on motor task. Europ J Neurosci 2011;33:960-967.

109 Oswal A, Brown P, Litvak V. Movement related dynamics of subthalmo-cortical alpha connectivity in Parkinson's disease. NeuroImage 2013;70:132-142.

110 Yarnall A, Rochester L, Burn DJ. The interplay of cholinergic function, attention, and falls in Parkinson's disease. Mov Disord 2011;26:2496-2503.

111 Tessitore A, Amboni M, Esposito F, et al. Resting-state brain connectivity in patients with Parkinson's disease and freezing of gait. Parkinsonism Relat Disord 2012;18:781-787.

112 Silberstein P, Kühn AA, Kupsch A, et al. Patterning of globus pallidus local field potentials differs between Parkinson's disease and dystonia. Brain 2003;126:2597-2608.

113 Rodriguez-Oroz MC, López-Azcárate J, Garcia-Garcia D, et al. Involvement of the subthalamic nucleus in impulse control disorders associated with Parkinson's disease. Brain 2011;134:36-49.

114 Stam CJ. Use of magnetoencephalography (MEG) to study functional brain networks in neurodegenerative disorders. J Neurol Sci 2010;289:128-134.

115 Stoffers D, Bosboom JLW, Deijen JB, Wolters EC, Berendse HW, Stam CJ. Slowing of oscillatory brain activity is a stable characteristic of Parkinson's disease without dementia. Brain 2007;130:1847-1860.

116 Bosboom JLW, Stoffers D, Stam CJ, et al. Resting state oscillatory brain dynamics in Parkinson's disease: an MEG study. Clin Neurophysiol 2006;117:2521-2531.

117 Bosboom JLW, Stoffers D, Stam CJ, Berendse HW, Wolters EC. Cholinergic modulation of MEG resting-state oscillatory activity in Parkinson's disease related dementia. Clin Neurophysiol 2009;120:910-915.

118 Cavanagh JF, Wiecki T V, Cohen MX, et al. Subthalamic nucleus stimulation reverses mediofrontal influence over decision threshold. Nature Neuroscience 2011;14:1462-1467.

119 Fumagalli M, Giannicola G, Rosa M, et al. Conflict-dependent dynamic of subthalamic nucleus oscillations during moral decisions. Social neuroscience 2011;6:243-256.

120 Huebl J, Schoenecker T, Siegert S, et al. Modulation of subthalamic alpha activity to emotional stimuli correlates with depressive symptoms in Parkinson's disease. Mov Disord 2011;26:477-483.

121 Brücke C, Kupsch A, Schneider G-H, et al. The subthalamic region is activated during valence-related emotional processing in patients with Parkinson's disease. Europ JNeurosci 2007;26:767-774.

122 Kühn AA, Hariz MI, Silberstein P, et al. Activation of the subthalamic region during emotional processing in Parkinson disease. Neurology 2005;65:707-713.

123 Rogers D, Lees AJ, Smith E, Trimble M, Stern GM. Bradyphrenia in Parkinson's disease and psychomotor retardation in depressive illness. An experimental study. Brain 1987;110:761-76.

124 Anzak A, Gaynor L, Beigi M, et al. Subthalamic nucleus gamma oscillations mediate a switch from automatic to controlled processing: a study of random number generation in Parkinson's disease. NeuroImage 2013;64:284-289.

125 Anzak A, Gaynor L, Beigi M, et al. A gamma band specific role of the subthalamic nucleus in switching during verbal fluency tasks in Parkinson's disease. Experimental Neurology 2011;232:136-142.

126 Rivlin-Etzion M, Marmor O, Heimer G, Raz A, Nini A, Bergman H. Basal ganglia oscillations and pathophysiology of movement disorders. Curr Opin Neurobiol 2006;16:629-637.

127 Jankovic J, McDermott M, Carter J, et al. Variable expression of Parkinson's disease: a base-line analysis of the DATATOP cohort. The Parkinson Study Group. Neurology 1990;40:1529-1534.

128 Raethjen J, Lindemann M, Schmaljohann H, Wenzelburger R, Pfister G, Deuschl G. Multiple oscillators are causing parkinsonian and essential tremor. Mov Disord 2000;15:84-94.

129 Ben-Pazi H, Bergman H, Goldberg JA, et al. Synchrony of rest tremor in multiple limbs in parkinson's disease: evidence for multiple oscillators. J Neural Transm 2001;108:287-296.

130 Timmermann L, Gross J, Dirks M, Volkmann J, Freund H-J, Schnitzler A. The cerebral oscillatory network of parkinsonian resting tremor. Brain 2003;126:199-212.

131 Levy R, Dostrovsky JO, Lang AE, Sime E, Hutchison WD, Lozano AM. Effects of apomorphine on subthalamic nucleus and globus pallidus internus neurons in patients with Parkinson's disease. J Neurophysiol 2001;86:249-260.

132 Bergman H, Wichmann T, Karmon B, DeLong MR. The primate subthalamic nucleus. II. Neuronal activity in the MPTP model of parkinsonism. J Neurophysiol 1994;72:507-520.

133 Lenz FA, Tasker RR, Kwan HC, et al. Single unit analysis of the human ventral thalamic nuclear group: correlation of thalamic "tremor cells" with the 3-6 Hz component of parkinsonian tremor. J Neurosci 1988;8:754-764.

134 Marsden JF, Ashby P, Limousin-Dowsey P, Rothwell JC, Brown P. Coherence between cerebellar thalamus, cortex and muscle in man: cerebellar thalamus interactions. Brain 2000;123:1459-1470.

135 Reck C, Florin E, Wojtecki L, et al. Characterisation of tremor-associated local field potentials in the subthalamic nucleus in Parkinson's disease. Europ JNeurosci 2009;29:599-612.

136 Pedrosa DJ, Reck C, Florin E, et al. Essential tremor and tremor in Parkinson's disease are associated with distinct "tremor clusters" in the ventral thalamus. Exp Neurol 201;237:435-443.

137 Lyons KE, Pahwa R. Deep brain stimulation and essential tremor. J Clin Neurophysiol 2004;21:2-5.

138 Barbe MT, Liebhart L, Runge M, et al. Deep brain stimulation in the nucleus ventralis intermedius in patients with essential tremor: habituation of tremor suppression. J Neurol 2011;258:434-439.

139 Koller WC, Pahwa PR, Lyons KE, Wilkinson SB. Deep brain stimulation of the Vim nucleus of the thalamus for the treatment of tremor. Neurology 2000;55S6):29-33.

140 Rehncrona S, Johnels B, Widner H, Törnqvist A-L, Hariz M, Sydow O. Long-term efficacy of thalamic deep brain stimulation for tremor: double-blind assessments. Mov Disord 2003;18:163-170.

141 Klein JC, Barbe MT, Seifried C, et al. The tremor network targeted by successful VIM deep brain stimulation in humans. Neurology 2012;78:787-795.

142 Dovzhenok A, Rubchinsky LL. On the origin of tremor in Parkinson's disease. PloS one 2012;7:e41598.

143 Chen C-C, Kilner JM, Friston KJ, Kiebel SJ, Jolly RK, Ward NS. Nonlinear coupling in the human motor system J Neurosci 2010;30:8393-8399.

144 Canolty RT, Edwards E, Dalal SS, et al. High gamma power is phase-locked to theta oscillations in human neocortex. Science 2006;313:1626-1628.

145 Canolty RT, Knight RT. The functional role of cross-frequency coupling. Trends in Cognitive Sciences 2010;14:506-515.

146 Tort ABL, Komorowski RW, Manns JR, Kopell NJ, Eichenbaum H. Theta-gamma coupling increases during the learning of item-context associations. PNAS 20098;106:20942-20947.

147 Mormann F, Fell J, Axmacher N, et al. Phase/amplitude reset and theta-gamma interaction in the

human medial temporal lobe during a continuous word recognition memory task. Hippocampus 2005;15:890-900.

148 Demiralp T, Bayraktaroglu Z, Lenz D, et al. Gamma amplitudes are coupled to theta phase in human EEG during visual perception. Int J Psychophysiol 2007;64:24-30.

149 De Hemptinne C, Ryapolova-Webb ES, Air EL, et al. Exaggerated phase-amplitude coupling in the primary motor cortex in Parkinson disease. PNAS 2013;110:4780-4785.

150 Rosin B, Slovik M, Mitelman R, et al. Closed-loop deep brain stimulation is superior in ameliorating parkinsonism. Neuron 2011;72:370-384.

151 Brittain J-S, Probert-Smith P, Aziz TZ, Brown P. Tremor Suppression by Rhythmic Transcranial Current Stimulation. Current Biology 2013;23:436-440.

7

Autonomic Manifestations in Parkinson's Disease

Elisaveta Sokolov & K. Ray Chaudhuri

Clinically, Parkinson's disease (PD) is regarded as a predominantly motor disorder characterised by rigidity, tremor and bradykinesia. However, emerging views suggest that this concept is now outdated, and a range of non-motor symptoms (NMS), including autonomic dysfunction (ADf), is integral to the diagnosis, prognosis and symptom complex of PD.

Autonomic dysfunction in Parkinson's disease

The autonomic nervous system (ANS) is a generic term and has multiple components consisting of sympathetic noradrenergic, sympathetic cholinergic, parasympathetic cholinergic, enteric, and adrenomedullary components, and these subsystems are not uniformly involved in this disease (1). There is now considerable evidence of the differential involvement of these components in PD. Clinically, ADf-related or 'associated' NMS in PD can present before the 'motor symptoms' start, and NMS as a whole are regarded as the key determinants of a patient's quality of life (QoL) (2). In addition, disorders of the autonomic nervous system can be seen as a primary, selective disease involving only the ANS or more commonly secondary to drugs and/or diseases of the peripheral nervous system (PNS) and central nervous system (CNS). Other parkinsonian syndromes such as multiple system atrophy (MSA) and dementia with Lewy bodies (DLB) can present with features of ADf,

which can complicate motor parkinsonism in these diseases from the onset of motor symptoms to the very late stage (3).

ADf is one of the key components of the burden of NMS in PD, and the extent of ANS dysfunction is often understated and under-reported, despite it having a major impact on the diagnosis, prognosis and management (4). Functionally, the ANS maintains homeostasis with afferent autonomic signals arriving from the periphery and processed within the central autonomic centres located across the brainstem and supratentorial areas, and a subsequent efferent response sent to the relevant end organ. It is relevant that the craniosacral output, implicated in the early pathology of PD and related to Braak stages 1 and 2, is involved in the control of the urinary tract and the lower digestive tract as well as a range of end organs including the heart, lacrimal and salivary glands (5). This involvement of central autonomic centres may explain the features of late-onset hyposmia, rapid eye movement (REM) sleep behaviour disorder (RBD) and constipation that are associated with cardiac sympathetic denervation as possible 'pre-motor' markers of PD. As described by Langston, the motor aspect of PD is only the tip of the iceberg, while the body of the iceberg involves many brainstem areas subserving autonomic functions and leading to peripheral and central ADf (see Figure 7.1) (6).

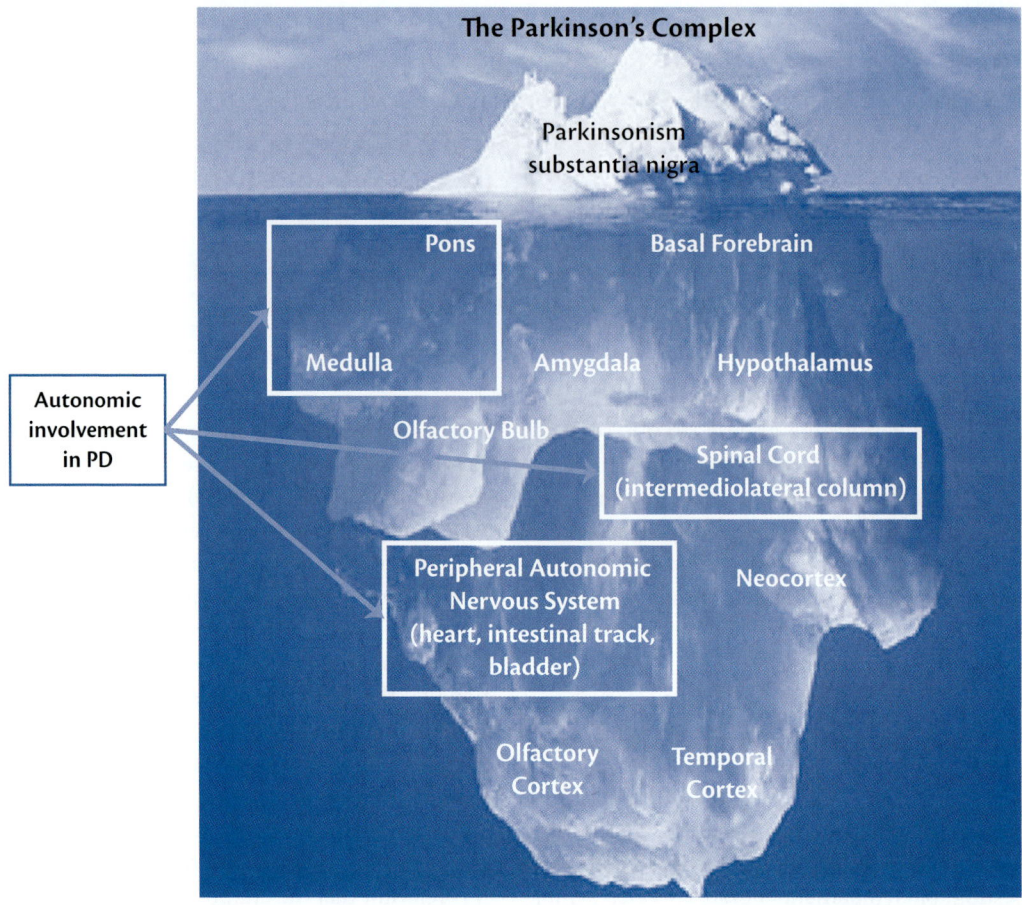

Figure 7.1
The unseen face of Parkinson's disease includes dominant autonomic areas in the central and peripheral systems.
Adapted from (6).

Epidemiology

It is important to address the prevalence and occurrence of ADf in PD in a holistic and unified manner. Clinically, the overall prevalence of dysautonomia can range from 14% to 80% in those diagnosed with PD, depending on the method used for assessing ADf as well as the type of ADf studied and the precision of the clinical diagnosis (7). Symptoms of dysautonomia are subjectively experienced by more than 50% of PD patients, while a recent population-based study of 207 newly diagnosed PD cases versus 175 healthy controls (the PARKWEST study) demonstrated that autonomic and sensory symptoms were experienced significantly more in untreated early PD patients than in healthy elders (p < 0.001) (8), although the effect on activities of daily living was minimal. In another important study, Bonuccelli et al. evaluated 60 patients with newly diagnosed, untreated, idiopathic PD. They performed autonomic function tests at study entry and followed the patients for at least 7 years to ensure diagnostic validity. Orthostatic hypotension (suggestive of sympathetic failure) was found in 14% of patients with de novo PD (decrease in systolic blood pressure of 20 mmHg), and on follow-up, 60% of these patients were subsequently reclassified as MSA. Furthermore, PD patients also had impaired sinus arrhythmia compared with controls, suggesting sympathetic and parasympathetic failure in patients with untreated PD. In another community-based study, Hobson et al. reported that PD patients had a two-fold greater risk of bladder problems and four-fold risk of autonomic problems compared with the controls (9). Erectile dysfunction was nearly twice as frequent in patients compared to controls, while depressive symptoms in the PD group were predictive of bladder problems and autonomic impairment and also poorer social functioning and dependency in activities of daily living.

Using validated tools including the non-motor symptoms questionnaire (NMSQuest) and NMS scale (NMSS), Martinez-Martin et al. and Chaudhuri et al. published the percentage rates of self-declared and interview-based frequency of occurrence of several autonomic symptoms as part of a NMS survey across Europe, USA, Asia, South America and Japan (10-12). Nocturia was one of the most common autonomic features (see Figure 7.2). These results have been replicated in a UK-based survey of over 8000 PD patients, in which urinary and cardiovascular dysfunctions

were rated as the most common and troublesome difficulties by patients (23). In a large national study conducted in Germany of 3414 patients, the difference in prevalence of autonomic symptoms was classified by gender, with orthostatic hypotension reported in 10% of women and 11% of men; urinary incontinence in 22% of women and 21% of men; sexual dysfunction in 8% of women and 30% of men; and sleep disturbance in 43% of women and 35% of men (13). A more recent study by Martinez-Martin et al. involving 951 patients reported that some Adf-related NMS, such as dribbling of saliva and sexual difficulties, were significantly more prevalent in men (14).

Sexual dysfunction is common in PD, and in a study by Bronner et al., the premorbid and current sexual functioning of 75 people with PD (32 women) was investigated (15). Women reported difficulties with arousal (87.5%), problems achieving orgasm (75.0%), low sexual desire (46.9%) and sexual dissatisfaction (37.5%), while men reported erectile dysfunction (68.4%), sexual dissatisfaction (65.1%), premature ejaculation (40.6%), and difficulties achieving orgasm (39.5%).

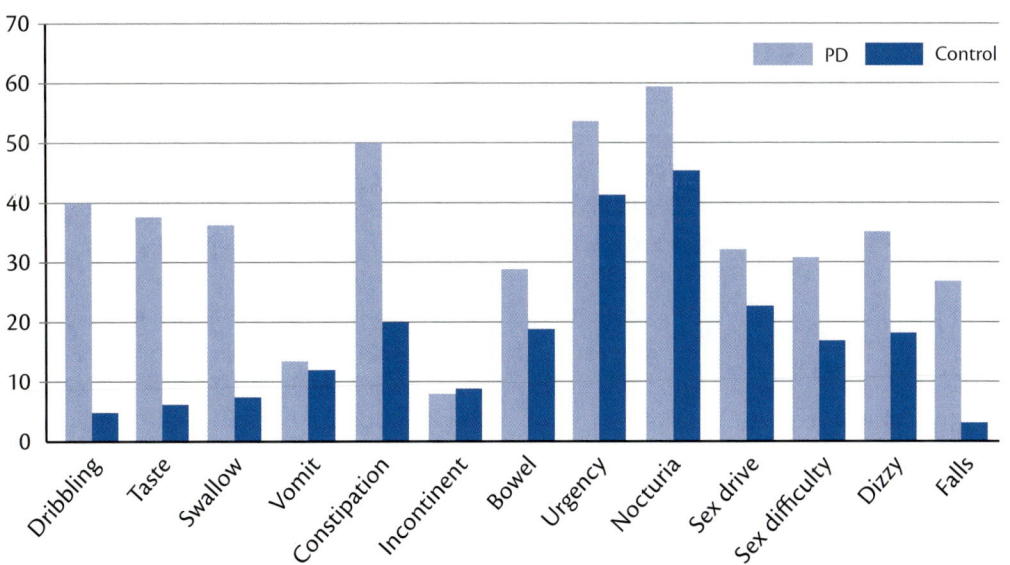

Figure 7.2
NMS Quest study reporting autonomic symptoms in PD versus control. Adapted from (10,11).

Table 7.1
Key autonomic symptoms in Parkinson's disease (PD).

	The range of non-motor Symptoms in PD related to autonomic dysfunction
Cardiac sympathetic denervation	▪ Orthostatic intolerance ▪ Orthostatic hypotension ▪ Postural orthostatic tachycardia (rare) ▪ Post prandial hypotension
Gastrointestinal	▪ Dribbling of saliva ▪ Dysphagia ▪ Ageusia ▪ Constipation ▪ Fecal incontinence (rare)
Genito-urinary	▪ Bladder urgency ▪ Bladder frequency ▪ Nocturia
Sexual dysfunction	▪ Loss of libido ▪ Erectile dysfunction ▪ Premature ejaculation ▪ Vaginal dryness ▪ Secondary dyspareunia ▪ Failure of orgasm
Thermoregulatory	▪ Hyperhidrosis ▪ Seborrhoea
Drug induced	As part of: ▪ Dopamine dysregulation syndrome ▪ Diphasic dyskinesias ▪ Parkinson hyperpyrexia syndrome ▪ Non motor fluctuations 　• Tachycardia 　• Hyperhidrosis 　• Hyperpyrexia ▪ Hypersalivation
Other possible symptoms	▪ Related to vision ▪ Pupillomotor abnormalities ▪ Sleep ▪ Fatigue

Pathophysiology

ADf-related NMS may start already in the pre-motor phase of Parkinson's disease, with neuropathological correlates implicated in Braak stages 1 and 2 involving the lower medullary nuclei elegantly reviewed by Wolters and Braak (16).

PD-related autonomic dysfunction

In PD, the possible anatomical and clinical correlates of non-motor dysfunctions are listed in Table 7.2 and mostly relate to Braak stages 1 and 2 (pre-motor by definition), but also stage 3 when there is involvement of the substantia nigra, followed by emergence of the classical motor features of PD (17). The role of the ANS in the pathogenesis of PD has also been speculated upon by Hawkes et al., who have proposed a possible 'dual-hit' hypothesis as a potential mechanism for the development of PD (18). They suggest that a neurotropic pathogen could gain entry to the brain via a nasal route, resulting in anterograde progression into the temporal lobe, while a gastric entry resulting from swallowing of nasal secretions may enter the axons of the Meissner's plexus, and transsynaptic transmission would then transfer these pathogens to the preganglionic parasympathetic motor neurons of the vagus nerve (12). There would be subsequent retrograde transport into the medulla pons and the midbrain, areas implicated in Braak stages 1-3.

The pathological involvement of the gastrointestinal system in the 'pre-motor' diagnosis of PD has been explored, and alpha-synuclein-containing inclusion bodies in neurons of the submucosal Meissner's plexus of pathologically proven PD autopsies have been reported by Braak et al. (19). Lebouvier et al. performed colonic biopsies in PD patients and reported that the number of Lewy neurites in the enteric nervous system correlated inversely with the neuronal count and positively with the levodopa-unresponsive features of ADf

Table 7.2

Pathological involvement of the central nervous system in Parkinson's disease (PD), correlation to Braak stage and clinical symptoms. (OH = orthostatic hypotension; AD = autonomic dysfunction).

Pathological Involvement within CNS	Braak Stage	Clinical Symptoms
Dorsal motor glossopharyngeal nucleus	Stage 1	Dysphagia Dribbling of saliva
Dorsal motor vagal nucleus	Stage 1	Constipation
Postganglionic parasympathetic neurons Preganglionic and postganglionic SN	Stages1/2	Bladder dysfunction Sexual dysfunction OH
Central subnucleus of the amygdala	Stage 3	Other AD
Cardiac sympathetic denervation	Stage 1 (?)	Possibly OH

and, in particular, constipation (20). Shannon et al. perfomed sigmoidoscopy-based biopsies in 10 untreated PD patients, and all were positive for alpha-synuclein and 3-nitrotyrosine, a marker for mitochondrial stress (21). In a further study by Shannon et al., alpha-synuclein-positive immunohistochemistry was found in 3 colonic biopsies, 2-5 years before the onset of motor PD, suggesting that this procedure could emerge as a biomarker for PD based on ADf (22).

Further evidence of ADf preceding the motor onset of PD comes from clinical studies reported by Abbott et al. as part of the Honolulu-Asia Aging study. The frequency of bowel movements in 6790 Japanese-American men was studied between 1971 and 1994 for incident PD for 24 years, and 96 PD cases were reported with an average time to onset of 12 years (23). The rates were 18.9 per 10,000 person-years in men with less than one bowel movement per day. This suggested that constipation could be an early marker of PD and/or susceptibility to the environmental factors that may cause PD. Goldstein et al. outlined the importance of cardiac neuroimaging with evidence of cardiac sympathetic denervation occurring several years before the motor onset of PD. They report cases where 6-[^{18}F]-fluorodopamine cardiac scans showed progressive denervation of cardiac sympathetic nerves as PD progresses and also suggest that the phenomenon of cardiac sympathetic denervation and orthostatic

hypotension (OH) (resulting from sympathetic failure) in PD may be independent of the degree of striatal dopaminergic denervation (24). OH has rarely been investigated in early or untreated PD and has been considered a typical sign, for instance, in multiple systems atrophy (MSA). However, analysis of historical data from 35 patients with PD and OH in a study from the National Institutes of Health in the USA showed that 60% had developed OH as an early feature in PD and not MSA (25). These findings have also been replicated in untreated PD by an Italian study by Bonuccelli and others (26). Erectile dysfunction (ED) has also been investigated as a pre-motor feature in PD, and Xiang et al. reported data from 32,616 men free of PD at baseline in 1986 who completed a retrospective questionnaire in 2000 on erectile dysfunction at different time periods. Of those who reported erectile function before 1986, 200 were diagnosed with PD during 1986-2002, and men with erectile dysfunction before 1986 were 3.8 times more likely to develop PD during the follow-up than those without (relative risk = 3.8, 95% confidence interval: 2.4, 6.0; P< 0.0001) (27).

Dopaminomimetics-related autonomic dysfunctions

Symptoms of ADf may arise in several drug-related complications in PD (see Table 7.1). These include non-motor fluctuations when Adf-related NMS such as hyperhidrosis, dysphagia and urinary urgency may be manifested as purely 'off'-related symptoms or worsen during off-periods (28). Respiratory difficulties can occur also as 'off'-symptoms as well as at nighttime during sleep. In Parkinson hyperpyrexia syndrome or dopamine agonist withdrawal syndrome, often precipitated by either sudden withdrawal of dopamine replacement therapies and/or concurrent infections, autonomic symptoms such as hyperhidrosis, tachycardia, urinary urgency and OH may occur (7) (see Chapter 38). OH can be a side-effect of potent dopamine agonist therapy, particularly in the elderly.

Clinical expression

ADf is a generic term for an array of symptoms ranging from OH to bladder dysfunction and symptoms, and thus can be diverse and specific to aspects of the CNS or PNS that may be specifically involved (29). Key symptoms are listed in Table 7.1. They may occur in isolation or in combination and can be present from an early untreated stage to an advanced stage. Clinically, OH, bladder dysfunction, particularly nocturia and dribbling of saliva, are often rated by patients as the most bothersome symptom (30). Another aspect of AD often overlooked is post-prandial hypotension, which could result in significant morbidity and 'afternoon off' periods in PD (31).

Little data is available in relation to the progression of ADf in PD, particularly in a holistic manner. Evidence suggests that dysautonomia is mild in the early stages of PD, and becomes a dominant, robust feature in the later stages. In a recently published follow-up study to a holistic NMS prevalence study in Italy, Antonini et al. followed up 707 patients for 24 months and reported that at 24 months, while some Adf-related NMS such as gastrointestinal and thermoregulatory problems become more prevalent, others such as cardiovascular ADf may become less prominent and prevalent (32). The Sydney multicentre study of PD demonstrated that drug-induced dyski-

nesia and end-dose failure were experienced by most patients, although the patients were most concerned by non-levodopa-responsive features of PD, many of which were related to ADf (33). Falls occurred in 87% of cases within this patient group, with 48% being symptomatic of postural hypotension. Some 71% of the patients unresponsive to levodopa experienced urinary incontinence. The prognosis of a PD patient worsens once the features of dysautonomia set in, with a poorer quality of life.

Diagnosis

The Movement Disorders Society task force recently published an article recommending and suggesting validated tools that may be used for screening and assessing aspects of ADf in PD. Several scales were evaluated, and the NMSQuest as well as the scale for outcomes in PD autonomic dysfunctions (SCOPA-AUT) were recommended as satisfactory screening tools for global dysautonomia as well as sialorrhoea, dysphagia and constipation (34). No scales met the criteria set by the MDS task force for satisfactory assessment of constipation, and the development of new tools in this area is encouraged.

Biomarkers and investigations

A whole range of cardiovascular and biochemical autonomic function tests are available and can be used to clinically assess the integrity and function of the sympathetic and parasympathetic nervous systems, but none are specific to PD. PD patients have been shown to have a loss of cardiac sympathetic innervation with the use of radiolabelled catecholamines such as $6\text{-}^{18}\text{F}$-flurodopamine (35,36). These catecholamines are substrates for cell membranes and vesicular norepinephrine transporters, as well as monoamine oxidase and catechol-O-methyltransferase, and can be used in conjunction with positron emission tomography to provide a good spatial and temporal resolution (32). ^{123}I-meta-iodobenzylguanidine (^{123}I-MIBG) can be used in conjunction with single-photon emission computed tomography (SPECT) scanning to mark and image storage vesicles within cardiac sympathetic neurons. Aberrant MIBG uptake is marked in PD patients with autonomic failure from even early stages (32,33). It is possible that cardiac sympathetic imaging may show abnormalities before the motor syndrome of PD becomes apparent (37). No or poor visualisation of the heart with intact cardiac circulation as shown in MIBG scans could be considered reasonable evidence to support a clinical diagnosis of PD (see Figure 7.3). Work by Shannon et al. and others also suggest that rectal or colonoscopy-based biopsies of rectal or colonic mucosa may emerge as an important diagnostic or pre-motor diagnosis tool in PD (15,16). These findings need to be replicated in large-scale studies.

Treatment

It is not possible to cover detailed treatment strategies for all Adf-related NMS in this review, and furthermore, two recent reviews by the American Academy of Neurology and the Movement Disorder Society (MDS) concluded that in most cases there is no level 1 evidence to support any specific treatment strategies for these symptoms in PD. Probable treatment strategies supported by levels 2-4 evidence are listed in Table 7.3.

Conclusions

In PD, ADf consists of a wide array of multi-system dysfunctions in PD prevalent from the pre-motor stage corresponding to Braak stages 1 and 2 to advanced PD. Clinically, ADf leads to the expression of a wide range of NMS with a significant impact on QoL as well as morbidity and mortality, as shown in the 15-year Sydney follow-up study. The clinical importance of ADf in PD is underpinned by the fact that aspects of NMS subserved by ADf may emerge as potential biomarkers or pre-motor markers in populations who may be at risk of developing PD.

Prognosis

The underlying pathophysiology in PD-related, non-motor symptoms involves a range of

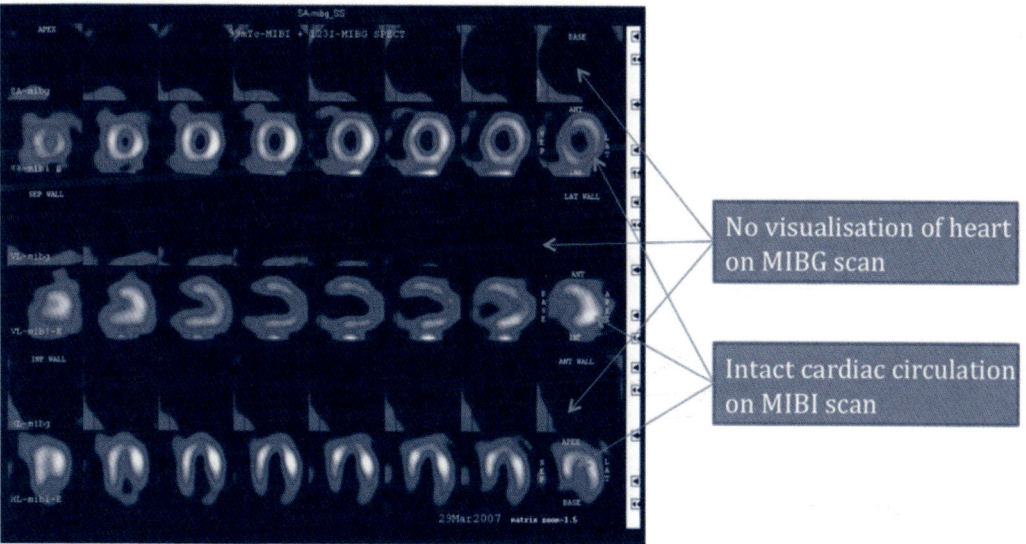

No visualisation of heart on MIBG scan

Intact cardiac circulation on MIBI scan

Figure 7.3
Data from a combined MIBI (Methoxy-Isobutyl-Isonitrile) and MIBG (meta-Iodobenzyl-Guanidine) scan of a patient with no visualisation of the heart in MIBG scan suggestive of idiopathic Parkinson's disease.

Table 7.3
Pharmacological, lifestyle and non-pharmacological strategies to address some non-motor symptoms (NMS) related to autonomic dysfunction in Parkinson's disease. Many strategies are based on weak evidence base.

NMS	Suggested strategies
Constipation	• Practical measures such as try to pass the faeces when 'on' / Soluble levodopa or apomorphine before starting defecation. • Diet rich in insoluble fibre & good hydration. • Psyllium: increases stool frequency (no effect on colonic transit time). • 5-HT4 receptor agonists (investigational). • Botulinum toxin to puborectalis muscle and/or in the external anal sphincter or in painful anismus-type dystonia. • Isosmotic macrogol (polyethylene glycol) (Recommended) • Apomorphine and intrajejunal levodopa infusion.
Sialorrhea and dribbling of saliva	• Swallow timers and head positioning. • Oral atropine drops. • Parotid and submandibular botulinum toxin injections.
Erectile dysfunction	• Psychological assessment • Sildenafil citrate
Bladder dysfunction	Assess type: Nocturia can be helped by • Avoiding night-time diuretics. • Use of D1 long acting dopamine agonists (rotigotine patch, apomorphine infusion). • Nocturnal intranasal administration of DDAVP. • Oxybutinin and related agents. • Botulinum toxin to bladder wall (can cause retention).
Orthostatic hypotension	Remove aggravating factors: • Volume depletion. • Prolonged bed rest/deconditioning. • Alcohol, Diuretics, Antihypertensives (alpha-blockers). Medical non-pharmacological treatment: • Liberalize salt intake, salt supplements. • High water intake. • Head-up tilt during the night. • Waist-high support stockings. • Exercise as tolerated, preferable in-water exercises. Pharmacological treatment: • - Sodium chloride supplementation of meal. • Fludrocortisone. • Short-acting pressor agents: Midodrine, Yohimbine. • Nocturnal intranasal administration of DDAVP. • L-threo-dops (Droxidopa). • Recombinant erythropoietin, (increases upright blood pressure and ameliorates symptoms of orthostatic hypotension in anaemic PD with OH).
Post prandial hypotension	• Frequent, small meals with a low carbohydrate. • Minimise alcohol intake. • Caffeine tablets with meals. • Timed Octreotide subcutaneous injections. • Acarbose (alpha-glucosidase inhibitor) with meal.

non-dopaminergic neuropeptides, and as such dopaminergic treatment is often ineffective, and specific treatment strategies have a poor evidence base thus far. Therefore, much work needs to be done to improve our understanding and treatment of ADf in PD, which must be regarded as a key unmet need.

Acknowledgement

We thank Ms Sandeep Bassi, coordinator at the National Parkinson Foundation Centre of Excellence for editorial and administrative assistance with this work.

References

1 Jost WH: Autonomic dysfunctions in idiopathic Parkinson's disease. J Neurol 2003;250:28–30.

2 Martinez-Martin P, Rodriguez-Blazquez C, Kurtis MM, Chaudhuri KR, on behalf of the NMSS Validation Group. The Impact of Non Motor Symptoms on Health-Related Quality of Life of patients with Parkinson's disease. Mov Disord 2011;26:399-406.

3 Müller B, Larsen JP, Wentzel-Larsen T, Skeie GO, Tysnes OB; Parkwest Study Group. Autonomic and sensory symptoms and signs in incident, untreated Parkinson's disease: frequent but mild. Mov Disord 2011;26:65-72.

4 Chaudhuri KR, Prieto-Jurcynska C, Naidu Y, Mitra T, Frades-Payo B, Tluk S et al.. The nondeclaration of nonmotor symptoms of Parkinson's disease to health care professionals: An international study using the nonmotor symptoms questionnaire. Mov Disord 2010;25:704–709.

5 Braak H, Del Tredici K, Rüb U, de Vos RA, Jansen Steur EN, Braak E. Staging of brain pathology related to sporadic Parkinson's disease. Neurobiol Aging 2003;24:197-211.

6 Langston JW. The Parkinson's complex: parkinsonism is just the tip of the iceberg. Ann Neurol 2006;59:591-596.

7 Barone P, Antonini A, Colosimo C, et al. The PRIAMO study: A multicenter assessment of nonmotor symptoms and their impact on quality of life in Parkinson's disease. Mov Disord 2009;24:1641-1649.

8 Breen KC, Drutyte G. Non-motor symptoms of Parkinson's disease: the patient's perspective. Journal Neural Transmisson 2013;120:531-535.

9 Hobson P, Meara J. Risk and incidence of dementia in a cohort of older subjects with Parkinson's disease in the United Kingdom. Mov Disord 2004;19:1043-1049.

10 Martinez-Martin P, Schapira AHV, Stocchi P et al. Prevalence of non motor symptoms in PD disease in an international setting; study using non-motor symptoms questionnaire in 545 patients. Mov Disord 2007;22:1623-1629.

11 Chaudhuri KR, Martinez-Martin P, Brown RG, Sethi K, Stocchi F, Schapira AH. The Metric Properties of a Novel Non-Motor Symptoms Scale for Parkinson's Disease: Results from an International Pilot Study. Mov Disord 2007;15:1901-1911.

12 Martinez-Martin P, Rodriguez-Blazquez C, Abe K, Bhattacharyya KB, Bloem BR, Carod-Artal FJ MD, Chaudhuri KR et al. International study on the psychometric attributes of the Non-Motor Symptoms Scale in Parkinson disease. Neurology 2009;73:1584-1591.

13 Wüllner U, Schmitz-Hübsch T, Antony G, Fimmers R, Spottke A, Oertel WH. Autonomic dysfunction in 3414 Parkinson's disease patients enrolled in the German Network on Parkinson's disease. The effect of ageing. Eur J Neurol 2007;14:1405-1408.

14 Martinez-Martin P, Pecurariu CF, Odin P, van Hilten J, Antonini A, Rojoabuin J, Chaudhuri KR. Gender-related differences in the burden of non-motor symptoms in Parkinson's disease. J Neurol 2012;259:1639-1647.

15 Bronner G, Royter V, Korczyn AD. Sexual dysfunction in Parkinson's disease. J Sex MaritTherapy 2004;30:95-105.

16 Wolters ECh, Braak H. Parkinson's disease: premotor clinico-pathological correlations. Parkinsonism Relat Disord 2006;70:309-319.

17 Del Tredici K, Rub U, De Vos RA, Bohl JR, Braak H. Where does Parkinson disease pathology begin in the brain? J Neuropathol Exp Neurol 2002;61:413-426.

18 Hawkes CH, Del Tredici K, Braak H. Parkinson's disease: a dual-hit hypothesis. Neuropathol Appl Neurobiol 2007;33:599-614.

19 Braak H, de Vos RA, Bohl J, Del Tredici K . Gastric alpha-synuclein immunoreactive inclusions in Meissner's and Auerbach's plexuses in cases staged for Parkinson's disease-related brain pathology. Neuroscience Lett 2006;396:67-72 .

20 Lebouvier T, Neunlist M, Bruley des Varannes S, Coron E, Drouard A, et al. Colonic Biopsies to Assess the Neuropathology of Parkinson's Disease and Its Relationship with Symptoms. PLoS One 2010;5:e12728.

21 Shannon K, Keshavarzian A, Mutlu E, Dodiya HB, Daian D, Jaglin JA and Kordower JH. Alpha-synuclein in colonic submucosa in early untreated Parkinson's disease. Mov Disord 201;27:709–715.

22 Shannon K, Keshavarzian A, Dodiya HB, Jakate S and Kordower JH. Is alpha-synuclein in the colon a biomarker for premotor Parkinson's Disease? Evidence from 3 cases. Mov Disord 2012;27:716–719.

23 Abbott RD, Petrovitch H, White LR, Masaki KH, Tanner CM, Curb JD, Grandinetti A, Blanchette PL, Popper JS, Ross GW. Frequency of bowel movements and the future risk of Parkinson's disease. Neurology 2001;57:456-462.

24 Goldstein DS. Cardiac denervation in patients with Parkinson disease. Cleve Clin J Med 2007;74:91-94.

25 Goldstein DS. Orthostatic hypotension as an early finding in Parkinson disease. Clin Autonom Res 2006;16:46–64.

26 Bonuccelli U, Lucetti C, Del Dotto P, Ceravolo R, Gambaccini G, Bernardini S, Rossi G, Piaggesi A. Orthostatic hypotension in de novo Parkinson disease. Arch Neurol 2003;60:1400-1404.

27 Xiang G, Chen H, Schwarzschild M, Ascherio A. A Prospective Study of Bowel Movement Frequency and Risk of Parkinson's Disease. Am J Epidem 2007;166:1446-1450.

28 Storch A, Schneider C, Wolz M, Stürwald Y, Nebe A, Odin P et al. Nonmotor fluctuations in Parkinson's disease: Severity and correlation with motor complications. Neurology 2013;80:800–809.

29 Chaudhuri KR, Healy D, Schapira AHV. The non-motor symptoms of PD disease. Diagnosis and management. Lancet Neurol 2006;5:235-245.

30 Politis M, Wu K, Molloys S, Bain PG, Ray Chaudhuri K, Piccini P. Parkinson's disease symptoms: the patient's perspectives. Mov Disord 2010;25:1646-1651.

31 Chaudhuri KR, Ellis C, Love-Jones S, Thomaides T, Clift S, Mathias CJ et al. Postprandial hypotension and parkinsian state in Parkinson's disease. Mov Disord 1997;12:877-884.

32 Antonini A, Barone P, Marconi R, Morgante L, Zappulla S, Pontieri FE et al. The progress of non-motor symptoms in Parkinsons disease and their contribution to motor disability and quality of life. J Neurol 2012;259:2621-2631.

33 Hely MA, Morris JGL, Reid WGJ, Trafficante R Sydney multicenter study of Parkinson's disease: non-L-dopa-responsive problems dominate at 15 years. Mov Disord 2005;20:190-199.

34 Evatt M, Chaudhuri, KR, Chou KL, Cubo E, Hinson V,, Kompoliti K et al. Dysautonomia Rating Scales in Parkinson's Disease: Sialorrhea, Dysphagia, and Constipation – Critique and Recommendations by Movement Disorders Task Force on Rating Scales for Parkinson's Disease, Mov Disord 2009;24:635–646.

35 Goldstein D, Holmes C, Cannon R, Eisenhofer G, Kopin I. Sympathetic cardioneuropathy in dysautonomias. N Engl J Med 1997;336:696-702.

36 Spiegel J, Hellwig D, Farmakis G, Jost WH, Samnick S, Fassbender K, Kirsch CM, Dillmann U. Myocardial sympathetic degeneration correlates with clinical phenotype of Parkinson's disease. Mov Disord 2007;22:1004-1008.

37 Goldstein DS, Sharabi Y, Karp BI, Bentho O, Saleem A, Pacak K, Eisenhofer G. Cardiac sympathetic denervation preceding motor signs in Parkinson's disease. Cleve Clin J Med 2009;76:158–172.

8

Neuropsychiatric Manifestations of Parkinson's Disease

Daniel Weintraub, Lama Chahine & Matthew B. Stern

Parkinson's disease is a neurodegenerative disorder characterized by the classic motor features of tremor, rigidity, and bradykinesia. It is often associated with several neuropsychiatric manifestations that lead to as much, if not more, morbidity like motor manifestations and have a significant negative impact on the quality of life. Affective disorders, cognitive decline, and psychosis have long been recognized as a part of PD presentation. Other common, but less well studied psychiatric disorders include impulse control disorders, anxiety symptoms, disorders of sleep and wakefulness, and apathy. Because of the increasing recognition of the prominence of non-motor features in PD, significant emphasis has been placed on this area by the research community in recent years. This has resulted in a dramatic evolution in our understanding of the wide array of neuropsychiatric manifestations in PD, though much remains to be learned. This review summarizes key issues pertaining to neuropsychiatric manifestations of PD, with an emphasis on state-of-the-art advancements in recent years.

Cognitive impairment and dementia

Epidemiology

A significant percentage of newly diagnosed PD patients have cognitive deficits (1) and experience cognitive decline over a period lasting several years (2). Approximately 25-30% of non-demented PD patients have mild cognitive impairment (MCI), and 80% of individuals with

PD eventually go on to develop dementia (PDD; see Table 8.1) (3). In PD, cognitive decline is a significant contributor to poor function and is associated with a reduced quality of life and increased caregiver burden.

A range of possible risk factors for the development of PDD have been reported, including advanced age, early executive and memory deficits, male sex, lower level of education, increased severity and longer duration of PD, atypical parkinsonism (i.e., prominent akinesia-rigidity or extensive vascular disease), and psychiatric co-morbidity (psychosis, apathy, depression) as well as rapid eye movement (REM) sleep behaviour disorder (RBD) (3).

Etiology and Pathophysiology

Our understanding of the neural changes underpinning cognitive decline in PD has grown recently. It is likely that the neuropathology of PDD is heterogeneous. While diffuse subcortical and cortical Lewy body disease pathology appears to be the major contributing pathology (27), a substantial portion of PD patients have AD-related neuropathological changes at autopsy (27). As in AD, the ∈4 allele of apolipoprotein E is associated with dementia in PD (27), and lower cerebrospinal fluid (CSF) β-amyloid$_{1-42}$ (Aβ42) levels predict cognitive decline on follow-up (28). The first serum biomarker identified to predict the occurrence of dementia in PD is epidermal growth factor (EGF) (29); non-demented PD patients with EGF levels in the low-

Table 8.1
Epidemiology of neuropsychiatric disorders in Parkinson's disease.

Neuropsychiatric Disorder		Prevalence	Comment
Depressive disorders	Major depression	17% (4)	Variable based on population studied: 2-11% in community samples (4,5), 20% in tertiary neurology clinics (5), 54% in the inpatient setting (4). Also variable based on diagnostic strategy:19% using semi-structured interview to establish DSM criteria, 7% without structured interview (4).
	Minor depression	22% (4)	Ranges from 10-30% depending on population studied
	Dysthymia	13% (4)	
	Clinically significant depressive symptomatology	35% (4)	Variable based on diagnostic strategy: 33% using semi-structured interview, 27% using Diagnostic Statistical Manual (DSM) criteria, 42% using a specific cut-off on a depression rating scale (4) In PD with dementia, clinically relevant depressive symptomatology was present in 22% (6)
Anxiety disorders	Generalized anxiety disorder	3-11% (7)	
	Panic disorder	13-30% (7,8)	Associated with earlier age of PD onset and motor fluctuations(8,9)
	Anxiety disorder not other-wise stated (NOS)	30% (8)	Anxiety disorder NOS is diagnosed in the setting of prominent anxiety when criteria for any specific anxiety disorder is not met (8).
	Anxiety in absence of for-mal diagnosis of anxiety disorder	40% (7), even in early PD (10)	
	Social phobia	8-15% (7,8)	
Apathy	Apathetic symptoms	40-45% (5)	In a sample of non-demented PD patients drawn from 2 tertiary care centers, prevalence of apathy was 17.2% (11) whereas in a mixed (demented and non-demented) sample from a movement disorders clinic, prevalence was 32% (12). A population based study found a prevalence of 38% (13)
	Apathy as the primary psy-chiatric problem (without comorbid depression)	11-39% (5,11,12,14)	Highly variable based on instrument used and population studied

Psychotic symptoms	Complex visual hallucinations	22-38% in PD samples not selected based on cognitive status (15); 13% in PD patients without dementia (16)	25% lifetime prevalence in a community based sample, 50% in clinic-based samples (17) In a 12-year population based study of psychosis in PD, 60% developed visual hallucinations or delusions (18); annual incidence was 80 per 1000 person-years
Cognitive Dysfunction	Mild cognitive impairment (MCI)	26.7% (range 18.9-38.2%) of non-demented PD patients (19)	11.3% non-amnestic single-domain, 8.9% amnestic single-domain(20)
	Dementia	30-40% in clinic based surveys (3)	8-year cumulative prevalence of dementia in PD is 78% (3)(3) 3-4% of dementia cases in general population are due to Parkinson's disease dementia (3)

est quartile for the group studied had 8 times the odds of developing dementia compared to those with levels in the highest quartile (29).

Various neurochemical changes are seen in PDD. While PDD is considered one of the non-dopaminergic manifestations of PD, some studies have shown that striatal dopamine function correlates with executive function (3). Degeneration of cholinergic neurons is present early in PD as is loss of noradrenergic locus ceruleus cells, and deficits in both neurotransmitter symptoms have been associated with PDD (3).

With regard to the genetic factors that contribute to PDD, dementia is not likely to be more common in monogenic PD than in idiopathic PD. There is accumulating evidence of increased risk of dementia in PD in the setting of apolipoprotein E ε4 genotype (30) and heterozygote pathogenetic mutations in the glucosidase beta acid *(GBA)* gene (31) (homozygote mutations of which cause Gaucher's disease). A specific polymorphism in the catechol-O-methyl-transferase (COMT) gene, val[158]met, is associated with attention and executive deficits in PD (32). In one study, the COMT val[158]met polymorphism did not predict development of PDD, while the microtubule-associated protein tau (MAPT) H1/H1 genotype did (33).

Structural imaging findings of dementia in PD have varied (3). A validated AD-spatial pattern of brain atrophy was shown to be associated with worse global cognitive performance even in non-demented PD patients, and the extent of AD-type atrophy predicted cognitive decline in non-demented PD patients, even in those with normal cognition at baseline (34).

With regard to metabolic abnormalities, deficits in metabolism, identified typically by using 18F-fluorodeoxyglucose positron emission tomography (FDG-PET) imaging, are reported in the inferior parietal and occipital cortices in PDD compared to non-demented PD patients (3). Global reductions in cerebral glucose metabolism have been reported in PDD compared to AD (3).

Clinical presentation

The concept of MCI in PD is relatively new, and its definition is evolving. MCI may be present at the time of PD diagnosis and prior to initiation of dopaminergic medications (19). The frequency of MCI in PD increases with age and PD disease duration. Mild cognitive impairment may be further subdivided into single domain or multi-domain (19). Longitudinal studies suggest that about 60% of PD patients with MCI will progress to PDD over a 4-year period, compared to 20% of PD patients with normal cognition (19).

Cognitive dysfunction in PD is marked by impairments in a range of cognitive domains, including executive (i.e., impaired planning and working memory), visuospatial, attentional, and language (3) (Table 8.2). Cognitively impaired PD patients can conform to either an Alzheimer's disease (AD) 'cortical' or PDD ('subcortical') cognitive profile (24). Compared to early AD, language deficits are less pronounced and executive impairment more pronounced in PDD (3). In dementia with Lewy bodies (DLB), probably a distinct clinical syndrome, the occurrence of preceding or coinciding dementia within 1 year of the development of motor symptoms is the key feature distinguishing this entity from PDD (3).

Diagnosis

Traditionally, PD patients were diagnosed with dementia according to the DSM-IV-TR criteria on the basis of 'dementia due to other general medical conditions'; this has been revised in the DSM-V to make PD dementia and DLB subtypes of major neurocognitive disorders (25). The Movement Disorder Society (MDS) task force proposed clinical criteria for the diagnosis of PDD (3) (see Table 8.2) and published an algorithm for diagnosing it (26). Two levels of testing were recommended: level I testing is of utility for the clinician, whereas level II testing is suggested when there is a need to specify the pattern and severity for clinical monitoring or research (21).

Table 8.2a
Clinical features and diagnostic criteria of dementia and mild cognitive impairment seen in Parkinson's disease.

Neuropsychiatric Disorder	Clinical features	Diagnostic Criteria	Comments
Dementia	Impairment in more than one cognitive domain, presenting a decline from a premorbid level, with deficits severe enough to impair daily live. The impairment in daily life is independent of the any impairment ascribable to motor or autonomic symptoms (3)	Probable Parkinson's disease dementia (3). A Core features: both of the following must be present (1) a diagnosis of PD based on Queen Square brain bank criteria (2) slow onset and progression of a dementia syndrome developing within the context of established PD and diagnosed by history, clinical, and mental examination (see definition under clinical features) B Associated clinical features: ▪ Typical profile of cognitive deficits including impairment in at least 2 of the 4 core cognitive domains (attention (impairments of which may fluctuate), executive functions, visuo-spatial functions, and free recall memory (which may improve with cueing)) ▪ Presence of at least one behavioral symptom (apathy, depressed or anxious mood, hallucinations, delusions, excessive daytime sleepiness) is supportive of diagnosis but not necessary C and D. Absence of a co-existent abnormality which by itself would cause and explain the dementia (such as metabolic encephalopathy, drug intoxication, major depression, or vascular dementia)	Diagnostic criteria for possible PDD have also been proposed in which atypical cognitive features may be present as may co-morbidities that could potentially contribute to the cognitive dysfunction (3)
Mild Cognitive Impairment	Cognitive decline that is not normal for age but without affectation of functional activities (19)	Mild cognitive impairment (21). A Level I (abbreviated assessment) ▪ Impairment on a scale of global cognitive abilities validated for use in PD or impairment on at least two tests, when a limited battery of neuropsychological tests is performed B Level II (comprehensive assessment) ▪ Neuropsychological testing that includes two tests within each of the five cognitive domains (i.e, attention and working memory, executive, language, memory, and visuospatial) ▪ Impairment on at least two neuropsychological tests, represented by either two impaired tests in one cognitive domain or one impaired test in two different cognitive domains ▪ Impairment on neuropsychological tests may be demonstrated by either performance approximately 1-2 standard deviations below appropriate norms or significant decline demonstrated on serial cognitive testing or demonstration of a significant decline from estimated premorbid levels	Among PD patients with single-domain impairment, non-amnestic MCI is more common than amnestic MCI

Table 8.2b
Clinical features and diagnostic criteria of depression seen in Parkinson's disease.

Neuropsychiatric Disorder	Clinical features	Diagnostic criteria	Comments

Major Depression	Persistent or pervasive sadness, anhedonia (inability to experience pleasure or enjoyment), diminished interests, hopelessness, helplessness	Major depressive episode (5)
		A Persistence and general pervasiveness of ≥5 of the following symptoms during the same 2-week period that represent a change from previous functioning; at least one of the symptoms is either (1) depressed mood or (2) loss of interest or pleasure that is present most of the day, nearly every day, as indicated by either subjective report or observation made by others.
		  1 Depressed mood
		  2 Markedly diminished interest or pleasure in all, or almost all, activities
		  3 Loss or gain in weight or appetite
		  4 Insomnia or hypersomnia
		  5 Psychomotor agitation or retardation
		  6 Fatigue or loss of energy
		  7 Feelings of worthlessness or excessive or inappropriate guilt
		  8 Diminished ability to think or concentrate, or indecisiveness
		  9 Recurrent thoughts of death, recurrent suicidal ideation without a specific plan, or a suicide attempt or a specific plan for committing suicide
		B Symptoms do not meet criteria for a DSM mixed episode (presence of phenomena of both a manic and a depressed episode).
		C Symptoms cause clinically significant distress or functional impairment.
		D Symptoms are not better accounted for by bereavement.
			Diagnostic criteria are based on modifications of the Diagnostic and statistical manual version 4 (DSM-IV) (22). These criteria are proposed but not yet validated

Minor Depression	See clinical features of major depression	Minor depressive episode (5) See criteria for major depression, but requires only 2 of the 9 symptoms listed. One of the symptoms must be depression/sadness or lost of interest/pleasure	

Dysthymia	See clinical features of major depression	Dysthymic disorder (22)
		A Depressed mood for most of the day, for more days than not, as indicated either by subjective account or observation by others, for at least 2 years
		B Presence, while depressed, of ≥2 of the following:
		  1 poor appetite or overeating
		  2 Insomnia or Hypersomnia
		  3 low energy or fatigue
		  4 low self-esteem
		  5 poor concentration or difficulty making decisions
		  6 feelings of hopelessness
		C During the 2-year period of the disturbance, the person has never been without the symptoms in Criteria A and B for more than 2 months at a time.
		D No major depressive episode has been present during the first 2 years of the disturbance
		E There has never been a Manic Episode, a Mixed Episode, or a Hypomanic Episode, and criteria have never been met for Cyclothymic Disorder
		F The disturbance does not occur exclusively during the course of a chronic Psychotic Disorder, such as Schizophrenia or Delusional Disorder
		G The symptoms are not due to the direct physiological effects of a substance (e.g., a drug of abuse, a medication) or a general medical condition (e.g., hypothyroidism).
		H The symptoms cause clinically significant distress or impairment in social, occupational, or other important areas of functioning
			Note that major depressive episodes may be superimposed on dysthymia (so-called 'double depression') (4)

Subsyndromal (subthreshold) Depression	See clinical features of major depression	Depressive symptoms are present and clinically relevant but do not meet criteria for other depressive disorders. As compared to major depression, symptoms are of short duration (eg not present all day or every day) (5)	It has been suggested that depressive symptoms occurring strictly in the "off" state may be classified as subsyndromal depression (5).

Table 8.2c
Clinical features and diagnostic criteria of psychosis seen in Parkinson's disease.

Neuropsychiatric disorder	Clinical features	Diagnostic criteria	Comment

Psychosis	Hallucinations (visual, auditory, tactile, gustatory, or cenesthetic (involving viscera)), illusions, and paranoid delusions	PD-associated psychosis (17)
		A Characteristic symptoms
		  Presence of at least one of the following symptoms (specify which of the symptoms fulfill the criteria): illusions, false sense of presence, hallucinations, delusions
		B Primary diagnosis
		  UK brain bank criteria for PD
		C Chronology of the onset of symptoms of psychosis: the symptoms in Criterion A occur after the onset of PD
		D Duration: the symptom(s) in Criterion A are recurrent or continuous for 1 month
		E Exclusion of other causes: The symptoms in Criterion A are not better accounted for by another cause of Parkinsonism such as dementia with Lewy bodies, psychiatric disorders such as schizophrenia, schizoaffective disorder, delusional disorder, or mood disorder with psychotic features, or a general medical condition including delirium
		F Associated features: with or without insight, dementia, or PD treatment
			These criteria are proposed but not yet validated

Table 8.2d
Clinical features and diagnostic criteria of anxiety and panick attacks seen in Parkinson's disease.

Neuropsychiatric disorder	Clinical features	Diagnostic features	Comment

Generalized Anxiety	Worry, apprehension	Generalized anxiety disorder (22)
		A Excessive anxiety and worry (apprehensive expectation), occurring more days than not and for at least 6 months, about a number of events or activities
		B The person finds it difficult to control the worry
		C The anxiety and worry are associated with ≥3 of the following 6 symptoms (with at least some symptoms present for more days than not for the past 6 months).
		  1 restlessness or feeling keyed up or on edge
		  2 being easily fatigued
		  3 difficulty concentrating or mind going blank
		  4 irritability
		  5 muscle tension
		  6 sleep disturbance (difficulty falling or staying asleep, or restless unsatisfying sleep)
		D The focus of the anxiety and worry is not confined to features of an Axis I disorder
		E The anxiety, worry, or physical symptoms cause clinically significant distress or impairment in social, occupational, or other important areas of functioning
		F The disturbance is not due to the direct physiological effects of a substance or general medical condition and does not occur exclusively during a mood disorder, a psychotic disorder or a pervasive developmental disorder
			Note that presence of PD would not negate the diagnosis (eg in regard to criterion F)

Panic Attack	Abrupt and brief episode of fear or discomfort associated with various somatic symptoms	Panic attack (22) A A discrete period of intense fear or discomfort, in which ≥4 of the following symptoms developed abruptly and reached a peak within 10 min 1 Palpitations, pounding heart, or accelerated heart rate 2 Sweating 3 Trembling or shaking 4 Sensations of shortness of breath or smothering 5 Feeling of choking 6 Chest pain or discomfort 7 Nausea or abdominal distress 8 Feeling dizzy, unsteady, lightheaded, or faint 9 Derealization (feelings of unreality) or depersonalization (being detached from oneself) 10 Fear of losing control or going crazy 11 Fear of dying 12 Paresthesias (numbness or tingling sensations) 13 Chills or hot flushes	
Panic Disorder	Recurrent panic attacks associated with significant worry about attacks with or without agoraphobia (anxiety in situations where environment is perceived as being difficult to escape or get help)	Panic disorder (22) A Both (1) and (2) 1 Recurrent unexpected panic attacks (as defined above) 2 At least one of the attacks has been followed by ≥1 month of ≥1 of the following: a Persistent concern about having additional attacks b Worry about the implications of the attack or its consequences c A significant change in behavior related to the attacks B The presence (or absence) of agoraphobia C The panic attacks are not due to the direct physiological effects of a substance or a general medical condition D The panic attacks are not better accounted for by another mental disorder	Note that presence of PD would not negate the diagnosis (eg in regard to criterion F)

Table 8.2e
Clinical features and diagnostic criteria of apathy seen in Parkinson's disease.

Neuropsychiatric disorder	Clinical features	Diagnostic criteria	Comment
Apathy	Lack of motivation, manifested by reduced goal-directed behavior and cognition, with decreased social and emotional engagement	Apathy (23) For a diagnosis of apathy the patient should fulfill the criteria A, B, C and D: A Loss of or diminished motivation in comparison to the patient's previous level of functioning and which is not consistent with his age or culture (reported by patient or observed by others) B Presence of ≥1 symptom in ≥2 of the three following domains for a period of at least 4 weeks and present most of the time Domain B1: Loss of, or diminished, goal-directed behaviour as evidenced by at least one of the following: (i) Loss of self-initiated behaviour (for example: starting conversation, doing basic tasks of day-to-day living, seeking social activities, communicating choices) (ii) Loss of environment-stimulated behavior (for example: responding to conversation, participating in social activities) Domain B2: Loss of, or diminished, goal-directed cognitive activity as evidenced by at least one of the following: (i) Loss of spontaneous ideas and curiosity for routine and new events (i.e., challenging tasks, recent news, social opportunities, personal/family and social affairs) (ii) Loss of environment-stimulated ideas and curiosity for routine and new events (i.e., in the persons residence, neighbourhood or community) Domain B3: Loss of, or diminished, emotion as evidenced by at least one of the following: (i) Loss of spontaneous emotion, observed or self-reported (for example, subjective feeling of weak or absent emotions, or observation by others of a blunted affect) (ii) Loss of emotional responsiveness to positive or negative stimuli or events (for example, observer-reports of unchanging affect, or of little emotional reaction to exciting events, personal loss, serious illness, emotional-laden news) C These symptoms (A, B) cause clinically significant impairment in personal, social, occupational, or other important areas of functioning D The symptoms (A, B) are not exclusively explained or due to physical disabilities (e.g. blindness and loss of hearing), to motor disabilities, to diminished level of consciousness or to the direct physiological effects of a substance (e.g. drug of abuse, a medication)	These criteria have been validated in PD (11) Another similar set of diagnostic criteria for apathy in PD have also been validated (12)

Treatment

As with many other neuropsychiatric manifestations of PD, there is little evidence to guide pharmacologic therapy of cognitive dysfunction and dementia in PD. Discontinuation of any potential aggravators of cognitive dysfunction such as anti-cholinergic agents is essential (35). The acetylcholinesterase inhibitor rivastigmine is the one pharmacologic intervention for dementia in PD that has a high level of evidence supporting its use and is FDA-approved for this indication (see Table 8.3). The NMDA antagonist memantine has been studied in several randomized controlled trials but with conflicting results; thus, high-quality evidence to support its use for the treatment of dementia in PD is lacking (36). There is also preliminary evidence that cognitive training or rehabilitation can improve executive abilities in non-demented patients (39), but it remains unknown if there are any acute or long-term cognitive benefits to treating PD-MCI. A 12-week, exploratory, randomized, placebo-controlled trial examined the effects of the monoamine oxidase-B (MAO-B) inhibitor rasagiline on cognition in PD patients with cognitive impairment but without dementia (40). In this trial, improvements in attention and executive functions were established.

Depression

Epidemiology

Results of epidemiological studies on the frequency of depression in PD have been highly variable (see Table 8.1), likely resulting from variations in definition, assessment methods, and the patient population studies. The prevalence of major depression in PD is lowest in community samples (2-10%) and highest in samples drawn for tertiary care neurology clinics (20%) (5).

Many correlates or risk factors for depression in PD have been reported, including female sex, a personal or family history of depression, early-onset PD, and psychiatric co-morbidity (cognitive dysfunction, anxiety, apathy, and insomnia). Co-morbid anxiety may account for at least a portion of subsyndromal depressive symptomatology (5) and thus should also be sought in a patient with such symptoms.

The consequences of depression in PD are dramatic, including functional disability, higher rates of caregiver stress, decreased quality of life, and poorer outcomes (5).

Etiology and Pathophysiology

In some PD patients, depressed mood can occur as a reaction to the diagnosis, and later in the disease due to limitations and disability. Depression in PD cannot be explained solely as a psychological process; it is more likely the result of an endogenous disorder resulting from a complex interaction of psychological and neurobiological factors (e.g., underlying neurochemical and neuropathological changes occurring as a result of the disease itself). Several lines of evidence support this. PD patients have a higher lifetime prevalence of depressive disorders than non-PD controls (44), and non-PD patients with depression are at higher risk of subsequently developing PD than non-depressed controls (45). These findings implicate depression as a potential risk factor or prodromal symptom of PD.

The neuroanatomic basis of depression in PD relates to dysfunction in the subcortical nuclei and the prefrontal cortex (PFC), striatal-thalamic-PFC circuits and the basotemporal limbic circuit; and brainstem monoamine and indolamine systems. Depressed PD patients have lower brainstem monoamine transporters compared to non-depressed PD patients (46).

Clinical presentation

The clinical manifestations of depression in PD occur along a spectrum ranging from occasional depressed mood to severe major depression. Common categorizations in the literature include, in increasing order of severity, subsyndromal or subthreshold depression, minor depression, dysthymia, and major depression (see Table 8.2). The

Table 8.3
Evidence-based Treatment of the Neuropsychiatric Manifestations of Parkinson's disease.

Neuropsychiatric Disorder	Drugs With Evidence of Efficacy	Quality of evidence for Efficacy	Comment
Dementia	Rivastigmine	Evidence supported by data from at least 1 high quality RCT without conflicting level-I data (36)	Data to support the use of other acetyl-choline esterase inhibitors including donepezil and galantamine are lacking (36)
Depression	Pramipexole(36)	Evidence supported by data from at least 1 high quality RCT without conflicting level-I data (36)	
	Notriptyline (36)	Evidence supported by data from at least 1 high quality RCT without conflicting level-I data (36)	
	Desipramine (36)(37)	Evidence supported by data from at least 1 high quality RCT without conflicting level-I data (36)	
	Paroxetine (38)	Evidence based on high quality randomized, controlled clinical trial (38)	Other SSRIs (citalopram, sertraline, paroxetine, and fluoxetine) have been widely used for the treatment of depression in PD but data supporting their use is insufficient (36).
	Venlafaxine extended release(38)	Evidence based on high quality randomized, controlled clinical trial (38)	
Psychosis	Clozapine (36)	Evidence supported by data from at least 1 high quality RCT without conflicting level-I data (36)	Regarding other atypical antipsychotics, there is insufficient evidence for use of quetiapine (36). Olanzapine is considered unlikely to be efficacious and not useful in treatment of psychosis in PD (36).

diagnosis of depression in PD can be challenging, as many of the features used to diagnose depression in the general population may be influenced by motor manifestations in PD. For example, psychomotor retardation in a PD patient could be the result of bradykinesia and bradyphrenia, or could be due to depression.

Diagnosis

Expert consensus prefers an all-inclusive approach, at least in the research setting, in order to maximize the sensitivity and reliability of diagnostic criteria of PD (5), such that an attempt to distinguish the cause of depressive symptomatology as being psychiatric versus motor is not made. In the clinical setting, this distinction could have management implications (such as whether or not to focus on dopaminergic versus anti-depressant therapy). Depression in PD is under-recognized and under-treated even in specialty care settings. Depression rating scales in PD are shown in Table 8.4.

Treatment

In recent years, several randomized, controlled trials for depression in PD have been published (see Table 8.3). Recent research shows efficacy for selective serotonin reuptake inhibitors (SSRIs), serotonin-norepinephrine reuptake inhibitors (SNRIs), tricycle anti-depressants, and cognitive behavioural therapy. SSRIs and bupropion are prescribed most commonly. Bupropion is commonly used to treat depression in PD and has the advantage of minimal adverse sexual side effects; evidence for its efficacy is lacking. An early meta-analysis suggested that the benefit of SSRI treatment is less in PD than in non-PD depression (47). In a recent controlled study, atomoxetine treatment was not efficacious for the treatment of clinically significant depressive symptoms, but was associated with improvement in global cognitive performance and daytime sleepiness (36). Non-pharmacologic treatments, including cognitive behavioural therapy, may be as efficacious and preferred by

patients (48). Other non-pharmacologic interventions for depression for which sufficient data is lacking but which are a promising avenue of active investigation include transcranial magnetic stimulation (36).

Psychosis

Epidemiology

While psychosis in PD is not common in untreated PD patients, the long-term cumulative prevalence of PD-associated psychosis was 60% in a recent prospective study (18) (see Table 8.1). Psychosis in PD is associated with older age and is typically a late feature of PD. Onset of hallucinations within 1 year of onset of parkinsonism may suggest an alternate diagnosis such as DLB (17). Common co-morbidities in PD patients with psychosis include cognitive impairment, axial impairment, sleep disturbances (including sleep fragmentation, vivid dreams, RBD), daytime somnolence, and visual disturbances, anxiety, and possibly depression (15,17,18). Psychotic symptoms are most often seen in PD patients with underlying dementia (16), with a five-fold increased prevalence in demented as compared to non-demented PD patients (18). It is important to note, however, that cognitive function does not predict a risk of future psychosis; visual hallucinations often predate dementia in PD and may in fact be a harbinger of future dementia (18). A recent study demonstrated that psychotic symptoms are also common in PD patients without dementia and are similarly co-morbid in this patient population with various non-motor features including affective disorders and a disorder of sleep-wakefulness (16). Psychosis in PD causes significant caregiver burden and increases the probability of nursing home admission (15,17).

Etiology and Pathophysiology

Higher amounts of dopaminergic medications have been associated with psychosis in PD, with a 26% increased risk of incident psychosis over a 12-year period for every 100 mg increase in

Table 8.4
Scales for assessment of neuropsychiatric symptoms in Parkinson's disease.

Neuropsychiatric Disorder	Recommended or suggested screening scales	Severity scales	Other scales/Comments
Depression	Hamilton depression scale (HAM-D), Beck depression inventory (BDI), hospital anxiety and depression scale (HADS), Montgomery-Asberg depression rating scale (MADRS), geriatric depression scale (GDS) (41)	HAM-D, BDI, MADRS, Zung self-rating depression scale (SDS) (41)	▪ The HAM-D, MADRS, BDI, and SDS are sensitive to longitudinal change of depression in PD (41)
Anxiety	Beck anxiety inventory (BAI) (to screen for panic attacks), Zung self-rated anxiety scale (SAS), Spielberger state trait anxiety inventory (STAI), Hamilton anxiety rating scale (HARS), hospital anxiety and depression scale (HADS), and anxiety subscale of neuropsychiatric inventory (NPI) (7)	Spielberger state trait anxiety inventory (STAI), anxiety subscale of neuropsychiatric inventory (NPI) ('as an estimate') (7)	▪ BAI may be used to monitor response to treatment (7) ▪ While many of the recommended or suggested scales have been used in PD, only the BAI has been validated
Apathy	Apathy scale (AS), motivation/initiative item of unified Parkinson's disease rating scale (UPDRS), apathy evaluation scale (AES), Lille apathy rating scale (LARS), apathy item of NPI (42)	AS, AES, LARS (42)	▪ Apathy should be rated in the PD 'on' state ▪ Snaith-Hamilton pleasure scale (SHAPS) can be used to assess for anhedonia (42) ▪ SHAPS and motivation/initiative item of UPDRS may be useful as longitudinal measures though have not been formally assessed for sensitivity to change (42) ▪ Other scales that have been used to assess apathy and anhedonia in PD but require additional validation: apathy inventory (AI), Chapman scales for physical and social anhedonia (42)
Psychosis	Parkinson psychosis rating scale, Parkinson psychosis questionnaire, Neuropsychiatric inventory (NPI), behavioral pathology in Alzheimer's rating scale (BPARS), brief psychiatric rating scale (BPRS), Positive and negative syndrome scale (PANSS), schedule of assessment of positive symptoms (SAPS), clinical global impression scale (43)	NPI (particularly in the cognitively impaired population), BPARS, BPRS (particularly in cognitively intact), SAPS (in non-demented) (43)	▪ BPRS and SAPS appear sensitive to change (43) ▪ For clinical trials on PD psychosis assessing new treatments, NPI (in cognitive impaired or when caregiver required), SAPS, PANSS, and BPRS (for cognitively intact) (43)

baseline levodopa-equivalent dose (18). However, extricating drug-induced psychosis from primary psychosis in PD is challenging, and the two may be inter-related, such that disease-related factors interact with medications in the genesis of psychotic symptoms in PD (15,17).

Psychosis in PD likely results from a complex interaction of medication exposure, PD pathology, aberrant REM-related phenomena, and co-morbid vulnerabilities, particularly cognitive impairment and visual disturbances. In addition to dopaminergic pathways, cholinergic and serotonergic systems may be involved as well. Greater frontal lobe atrophy has been reported in PD patients with hallucinations (49), and they also demonstrate long-term, widespread, limbic, paralimbic and neocortical gray matter loss (50).

Clinical presentation

Visual hallucinations are the most common feature of psychosis in PD, occurring in 90% of patients who experience psychosis (17), but hallucinations involving other senses as well as illusions, delusions, and paranoia are other features (see Table 8.2). In contrast to schizophrenia, auditory hallucinations are less common in PD, but co-occur with visual hallucinations in 8-13% of PD patients (17). Mild hallucinations with retained insight may be seen (17). In some PD patients however, complex psychotic symptoms occur, typically hallucinations and persecutory delusions in the context of significant cognitive impairment. These patients typically do not have insight into their psychosis, may display behavioural changes (including 'sundowning'), and typically require treatment.

Diagnosis

Various scales are available for the assessment of psychosis in PD (see Table 8.4), but none examine the full spectrum of PD psychosis (43).

Treatment

The treatment of psychosis in PD is challenging, since optimizing the management of mo-tor symptoms with antiparkinsonian therapy typically worsens the psychosis, while treating psychosis with an antipsychotic (AP) can worsen the parkinsonism. A thorough medical evaluation for delirium should be performed, any non-essential non-PD medications that might contribute to mental impairment should be discontinued, and the risk-benefit ratio of each antiparkinsonian medication should be reviewed. Based on expert recommendations (35), medications are usually discontinued in the following order: anticholinergics, MAO-B inhibitors, amantadine, dopamine agonists, catechol-O-methyltransferase (COMT) inhibitors, and finally, a reduction in levodopa dosage. This initial management strategy can be sufficient for a significant percentage of patients (51). Antipsychotic treatment (see Table 8.3) is initiated for persistent and problematic psychosis. There are significant safety concerns regarding use of these medications in PD patients; high potency APs such as haloperidol should be avoided as they can exacerbate parkinsonism. Increased morbidity and mortality has been observed with the use of both typical and atypical antipsychotics in individuals with dementia; in PD, increased 30-day mortality was reported in patients newly prescribed an AP (52).

Impulse control disorders and related behaviours

Epidemiology

Over the past decade, it has been recognised that impulse control disorders (ICDs) (see Chapter 41) occur in PD, including compulsive gambling, buying, sexual behaviour, and eating, as well as impulse control-related disorders, including the dopamine dysregulation syndrome and punding (53). In a recent multi-site observational study (DOMINION) of 3,090 PD patients, an ICD was identified in 13.6% of patients (gambling =5.0%, sexual behaviour =3.5%, buying =5.7%, and binge-eating disorder =4.3%), and 3.9% had ≥2 ICDs (54).

Etiology

A case-control study (55) demonstrated that PD itself does not confer an increased risk of ICDs; rather, ICDs in PD are the result of dopaminergic therapy, particularly dopamine agonists. In the DOMINION study (54), ICDs were more common in patients on a dopamine agonist (17.1% versus 6.9%), with similar frequencies for pramipexole and ropinirole (17.7% vs. 15.5%). Regarding other PD medication, both levodopa (particularly in higher dosages) and amantadine (54) use were associated with ICDs in this study, although to a lesser extent compared with dopamine agonist treatment. Additional variables associated with ICDs in PD are a personal or familial history of alcoholism or gambling, premorbid impulsive or novelty-seeking character traits, young age, male sex, early PD onset, being unmarried, and current cigarette smoking (53). Other rather levodopa-induced behavioural disorders include the dopamine dysregulation syndrome (DDS or compulsive PD medication use) and punding (repetitive non-goal-directed activity).

Decision-making deficits have been reported in PD patients with ICDs, with increased impulsive choice and working memory deficits when exposed to a DA compared with PD controls. Furthermore, PD patients with an ICD demonstrate intact stimulus-reinforcement learning, but have a strong preference for immediate over future rewards compared with non-ICD patients (57). PD patients with pathological gambling also demonstrate impairment in bedside tests of executive abilities (57).

One study has reported a genetic association for ICDs in PD, specifically the AA genotype of DRD3 p.S9G (a D3 receptor subtype) and the CC genotype of GRIN2B c.366C>g (a NMDA receptor subtype) (57).

Pathophysiology

PD patients with and without dopamine dysregulation syndrome underwent PET scanning with the D2/D3 receptor ligand ^{11}C-raclopride before and after levodopa oral challenge. Dopamine dysregulation syndrome patients exhibited a greater decrease in D2/D3 binding potential (i.e., enhanced levodopa-induced ventral striatal dopamine release) (57). In another ^{11}C-raclopride study, patients with pathological gambling demonstrated decreased D2/D3 binding potential at baseline and a relatively greater decrease in binding potential during performance of a gambling task compared with non-ICD PD patients (57). A recent SPECT study in PD patients with pathological gambling showed increased brain perfusion in multiple regions linked with impulse control, including the orbitofrontal cortex, hippocampus, amygdala, insula, and ventral pallidum (57). In a fMRI study using a probabilistic gain and loss learning task, ICD patients responded to dopamine agonist exposure with an increased rate of learning for gain outcomes and an increased striatal reward prediction error (RPE) activity compared with PD controls (57). Using both perfusion and blood oxygenation level-dependent (BOLD) fMRI to measure neural responses to risk-taking, ICD patients demonstrated diminished resting perfusion and BOLD activity during risk-taking in the ventral striatum compared with PD controls (58). Another fMRI study in PD patients with pathological gambling reported increased activation, compared with PD controls, on exposure to gambling-related visual cues in diffuse brain regions, including the cingulate cortex and the ventral striatum (57). Finally, PD patients with pathological gambling had diminished dopamine transporter availability in the ventral striatum compared with PD controls (57).

Clinical presentation

Each of the ICDs (including pathological gambling, hypersexuality, compulsive shopping, and compulsive eating), punding, and DDS has its own set of proposed diagnostic criteria (53). ICDs in PD may lead to significant impairments in psychosocial functioning, interpersonal relationships, physical health, and quality of life.

209

Patients may omit to report such behaviours to a treating physician, perhaps due to embarrassment, not suspecting an association with PD treatment, or ambivalence regarding stopping the behaviour. Hence, ICDs are under-recognized in clinical practice.

Diagnosis

A screening instrument, the Questionnaire for Impulsive-Compulsive Disorders in Parkinson's Disease (QUIP), was developed and validated to assess ICDs, other compulsive behaviours, and DDS in PD (56) (see Chapter 41).

Treatment

ICD behaviours often resolve after reducing the dopamine agonist dose, switching to a different dopamine agonist, or discontinuing dopamine agonist treatment entirely (57). In such cases, patients typically introduce or increase their levodopa dosage to compensate (59). However, many patients do not want or cannot tolerate dopamine agonist discontinuation, and a dopamine agonist withdrawal syndrome (DAWS) was described recently, characterized by anxiety, dysphoria, autonomic changes, and medication craving (60).

The relationship between DBS and ICDs is complex (60). On the one hand, subthalamic nucleus (STN) DBS was associated with improvement in ICD symptoms in a case series, likely due to significant reductions in the dopamine replacement therapy that occurred post-surgery (61). However, there is also anecdotal evidence that ICDs may begin or worsen transiently after STN DBS.

A range of psychiatric treatments, most commonly SSRIs, have been used to treat ICDs in PD (see also Chapter 41), but there is no empirical evidence to support their use in PD patients. There are case reports of the successful treatment of pathological gambling in PD with atypical antipsychotics (57). A recent placebo-controlled study reported a benefit with amantadine as a treatment for pathological gambling in PD

(36), although its use was associated with ICDs in a large epidemiological study (54). A small study (62) randomizing PD patients with ICDs to cognitive behavioural therapy plus standard medical care versus standard medical care alone suggested that cognitive behavioural therapy reduces the severity of impulse control behaviours in PD; further large-scale studies are needed.

Anxiety disorders

Epidemiology

Compared with depression, anxiety disorders have received little attention in PD. As with depression, the epidemiology of anxiety in PD varies according to the study population and assessments (see Table 8.1).

In a community-based sample of PD patients, 43% had an anxiety disorder, with 17% having 2 or more (8). Anxiety disorders are often co-morbid with depression in PD and present together in over two-thirds of cases (8).

Etiology and Pathophysiology

Reduced noradrenaline due to locus ceruleus dysfunction has been implicated in anxiety, and the common occurrence of anxiety disorders in PD is consistent with involvement of this nucleus by PD pathology (8).

Clinical expression

Up to 40% of PD patients experience anxiety symptoms or disorders, as defined in Table 8.2, including generalized anxiety disorder, panic attacks, obsessive compulsive disorder (OCD), and social phobia, although OCD is not clearly more common in PD than in the general population. Anxiety disorders may precede the diagnosis of PD by up to 20 years (44).

Diagnosis

A recent MDS task force did not find that any current anxiety rating scales met the criteria for 'recommended' use, highlighting the need for additional research in this area (see Table 8.4).

Treatment

There have been no controlled anxiety treatment studies in PD (63). Antidepressant treatment studies have reported a secondary benefit for anxiety symptoms. For patients who experience anxiety as part of an 'off' state, PD medication adjustments can be made in an attempt to decrease the duration and severity of these episodes. Anecdotally, clomipramine and newer antidepressants are also used for anxiety symptoms. However, many patients require treatment with benzodiazepines (most commonly low-dose lorazepam, alprazolam, and clonazepam), although this medication class must be used cautiously in PD patients due to their propensity to increase sedation, gait imbalance, and cognitive impairment.

Apathy

Epidemiology

Apathy occurs in approximately 40% of PD patients (see Table 8.1). Although there is an overlap between apathy and depression, delirium, and dementia, apathy also occurs independently of these syndromes.

Etiology and Pathophysiology

The neurochemical mechanism of apathy has not been well studied, but may involve both dopaminergic and non-dopaminergic pathways (64). A recent MRI study (65) utilizing voxel-based morphometry to determine the structural correlates of apathy found that higher apathy scores correlated with lower gray matter density in various brain regions including bilateral precentral gyri, inferior parietal gyri, inferior frontal gyri, right posterior cingulated gyrus, and right precuneus (65). It is noteworthy that apathy has been associated with reduced volume in the cingulate gyrus and inferior frontal gyrus in other populations including AD and patients with depression (65).

Clinical expression

Apathy is characterized predominantly by a reduction in motivation (see Table 8.2) and leads to significant functional impairment, particularly in relation to social activities. Apathy is usually accompanied by diminished self-awareness, so changes are typically noticed and brought to the attention of clinicians by caregivers. A common assumption is that the patient is depressed, though the lack of endorsement of sad mood and the typical cognitive changes seen in depression suggest a diagnosis of apathy instead. Apathy in PD is often co-morbid with depression and/or dementia, but may occur in isolation. Anhedonia, or inability to experience pleasure, is a symptom often seen in apathy but may also be seen in isolation or in depression (42).

Diagnosis

Diagnostic criteria for apathy in PD have been put forth and validated (11,12, 23), which will hopefully enhance research in this area. For the assessment of apathy, the apathy scale (AS) was 'recommended' for use by a MDS task force (see Table 8.4).

Treatment

Few studies have investigated the treatment of apathy in PD. As a rule, treatable co-morbid psychiatric conditions (such as depression) should be addressed initially. Data regarding the effects of levodopa and deep brain stimulation on apathy in PD are mixed (64). Anecdotally, psychostimulants (e.g., methylphenidate, dextroamphetamine) and stimulant-related compounds (e.g., modafinil) are used in clinical practice, but their efficacy is not known. The selective D2/D3 agonist piribedil was investigated and showed promise, and was well tolerated, in a small, placebo-controlled, randomized study of Parkinson's patients with apathy following withdrawal of dopamine agonist medication post-DBS (66).

Neuropsychiatric effects of deep brain stimulation surgery

The impact of DBS, primarily STN DBS, on non-motor symptoms appears to be complex. Immediately postoperatively, patients have experienced transient abnormalities such as confusional states. A meta-analysis identified significant declines in executive functions and verbal learning and memory post-DBS (67). In a controlled trial comparing DBS to the best medical therapy for advanced PD, DBS patients were more likely to experience worsening of working memory, processing speed, verbal fluency and delayed recall at 6-month follow-up (68). In additional analyses from this study, patients who received STN versus globus pallidus interna (GPi) DBS were more likely to experience worsening in processing speed (69). Psychiatric findings post-DBS have included both overall improvement and occasionally worsening of depression, anxiety, psychosis, mania, apathy, and emotional lability. In a randomized trial comparing DBS with the best medical treatment (68), there were no between-group differences in either mood or on part I of the UPDRS at 6 months after study treatment initiation. However, patients who received STN versus GPi DBS were more likely to experience a worsening in severity of depressive symptoms (69). Increased risk of suicide among the PD patients who underwent DBS was not found in that study (70).

Non-motor fluctuations

Many of the neuropsychiatric manifestations discussed above, such as depression, anxiety, irritability, and hallucinations can be strictly or nearly almost interpreted as a manifestation of the PD 'off' state (5,71). On the other hand, euphoric symptoms, hypomania, and hypersexuality may occur in the 'on' state (e.g., when dopaminergic medications are in effect). Mood fluctuations accompany motor fluctuations in over 75% of PD patients (5). Although affective fluctuations are common in patients who fluc-

tuate between 'on' and 'off' states, there is not always a correlation between affect and motor state.

Future directions

While an increase in research focus on the neuropsychiatric manifestations of PD has occurred, much remains to be elucidated. Regarding the epidemiology of neuropsychatric manifestations of PD, longitudinal epidemiological research focussing on the predictors, development, course, and impact of cognitive decline and psychiatric disorders in PD is needed, with utilization of sophisticated statistical techniques to account for the significant co-morbidity, heterogeneity, and variability in symptoms that occur. Recent efforts to establish diagnostic criteria for the various neuropsychiatric disorders in PD are a key step, but these criteria require validation and refinement. Finally, there is a significant need to improve our understanding of the neural substrate of cognitive and psychiatric complications through examination of the neuropathology, disease-specific biomarkers, neurotransmitters, brain structure, and neural circuitry. Ultimately, reducing the impact of PD on the patients and families will require improved recognition and the development of better therapies for its cognitive and psychiatric complications.

References

1 Aarsland D, Bronnick K, Alves G, et al. The spectrum of neuropsychiatric symptoms in patients with early untreated Parkinson's disease. J Neurol Neurosurg Psychiatry 2009;80:928-930.

2 Kandiah N, Narasimhalu K, Lau PN, Seah SH, Au WL, Tan LC. Cognitive decline in early Parkinson's disease. Mov Disord 2009;24:605-608.

3 Emre M, Aarsland D, Brown R, et al. Clinical diagnostic criteria for dementia associated with Parkinson's disease. Mov Disord 2007;22:1689-1707; quiz 1837.

4 Reijnders JS, Ehrt U, Weber WE, Aarsland D, Leentjens AF. A systematic review of prevalence studies

of depression in Parkinson's disease. Mov Disord 200823:183-189; quiz 313.

5 Marsh L, McDonald WM, Cummings J, Ravina B, NINDS/NIMH Work Group on Depression and Parkinson's Disease. Provisional diagnostic criteria for depression in Parkinson's disease: report of an NINDS/NIMH Work Group. Mov Disord 2006;21148-158.

6 Ehrt U, Bronnick K, De Deyn PP, et al. Subthreshold depression in patients with Parkinson's disease and dementia--clinical and demographic correlates. Int J Geriatr Psychiatry 2007;22:980-985.

7 Leentjens AF, Dujardin K, Marsh L, et al. Anxiety rating scales in Parkinson's disease: critique and recommendations. Mov Disord 2008;23:2015-2025.

8 Pontone GM, Williams JR, Anderson KE, et al. Prevalence of anxiety disorders and anxiety subtypes in patients with Parkinson's disease. Mov Disord 2009;24:1333-1338.

9 Dissanayaka NN, Sellbach A, Matheson S, et al. Anxiety disorders in Parkinson's disease: prevalence and risk factors. Mov Disord 2010;25:838-845.

10 Khoo TK, Yarnall AJ, Duncan GW, et al. The spectrum of nonmotor symptoms in early Parkinson disease. Neurology 2013;80:276-281.

11 Drijgers RL, Dujardin K, Reijnders JS, Defebvre L, Leentjens AF. Validation of diagnostic criteria for apathy in Parkinson's disease. Parkinsonism Relat Disord 2010;16:656-660.

12 Starkstein SE, Merello M, Jorge R, Brockman S, Bruce D, Power B. The syndromal validity and nosological position of apathy in Parkinson's disease. Mov Disord 2009;24:1211-1216.

13 Pedersen KF, Larsen JP, Alves G, Aarsland D. Prevalence and clinical correlates of apathy in Parkinson's disease: a community-based study. Parkinsonism Relat Disord 2009;15:295-299.

14 Kirsch-Darrow L, Fernandez HH, Marsiske M, Okun MS, Bowers D. Dissociating apathy and depression in Parkinson disease. Neurology 2006;67:33-38.

15 Fenelon G, Alves G. Epidemiology of psychosis in Parkinson's disease. J Neurol Sci 2010;15;289:12-17.

16 Lee AH, Weintraub D. Psychosis in Parkinson's disease without dementia: common and comorbid with other non-motor symptoms. Mov Disord 2012;27:858-863.

17 Ravina B, Marder K, Fernandez HH, et al. Diagnostic criteria for psychosis in Parkinson's disease: report of an NINDS, NIMH work group. Mov Disord 2007;22:1061-1068.

18 Forsaa EB, Larsen JP, Wentzel-Larsen T, et al. A 12-year population-based study of psychosis in Parkinson disease. Arch Neurol 2010;67:996-1001.

19 Litvan I, Aarsland D, Adler CH, et al. MDS Task Force on mild cognitive impairment in Parkinson's disease: critical review of PD-MCI. Mov Disord 2011;26:1814-1824.

20 Aarsland D, Bronnick K, Williams-Gray C, et al. Mild cognitive impairment in Parkinson disease: a multicenter pooled analysis. Neurology 2010;75:1062-1069.

21 Litvan I, Goldman JG, Troster AI, et al. Diagnostic criteria for mild cognitive impairment in Parkinson's disease: Movement Disorder Society Task Force guidelines. Mov Disord 2012;27:349-356.

22 Diagnostic and statistical manual of mental disorders:. DSM-IV-TR. 4th ed., text revision. ed. Washington, DC: American Psychiatric Association 2000.

23 Robert P, Onyike CU, Leentjens AF, et al. Proposed diagnostic criteria for apathy in Alzheimer's disease and other neuropsychiatric disorders. Eur Psychiatry 2009;24:98-104.

24 Weintraub D, Moberg PJ, Culbertson WC, Duda JE, Stern MB. Evidence for impaired encoding and retrieval memory profiles in Parkinson disease. Cogn Behav Neurol 2004;17:195-200.

25 American Psychiatric Association. Diagnostic and Statistical Manual of Mental Disorders. 5th ed. Arlington, VA: American Psychiatric Publishing 2013.

26 Dubois B, Burn D, Goetz C, et al. Diagnostic procedures for Parkinson's disease dementia: recommendations from the movement disorder society task force. Mov Disord 2007;22:2314-2324.

27 Irwin DJ, White MT, Toledo JB, et al. Neuropathologic substrates of Parkinson disease dementia. Ann Neurol 2012;72:587-598.

28 Siderowf A, Xie SX, Hurtig H, et al. CSF amyloid {beta} 1-42 predicts cognitive decline in Parkinson disease. Neurology 2010;75:1055-1061.

29 Chen-Plotkin AS, Hu WT, Siderowf A, et al. Plasma epidermal growth factor levels predict cognitive decline in Parkinson disease. Ann Neurol 2011;69:655-663.

30 Tsuang D, Leverenz JB, Lopez OL, et al. APOE epsilon4 increases risk for dementia in pure synucleinopathies. JAMA Neurol 2013;70:223-228.

31 Tsuang D, Leverenz JB, Lopez OL, et al. GBA mutations increase risk for Lewy body disease with and without Alzheimer's disease pathology. Neurology 2012;79:1944-1950.

32 Williams-Gray CH, Hampshire A, Barker RA, Owen AM. Attentional control in Parkinson's disease is dependent on COMT val 158 met genotype. Brain 2008;131:397-408.

33 Williams-Gray CH, Evans JR, Goris A, et al. The distinct cognitive syndromes of Parkinson's disease: 5 year follow-up of the CamPaIGN cohort. Brain 2009;132:2958-2969.

34 Weintraub D, Dietz N, Duda JE, et al. Alzheimer's disease pattern of brain atrophy predicts cognitive decline in Parkinson's disease. Brain 2012;135:170-180.

35 Horstink M, Tolosa E, Bonuccelli U, et al. Review of the therapeutic management of Parkinson's disease. Report of a joint task force of the European Federation of Neurological Societies EFNS and the Movement Disorder Society-European Section MDS-ES. Part II: late complicated Parkinson's disease. Eur J Neurol 2006;13:1186-1202.

36 Seppi K, Weintraub D, Coelho M, et al. The Movement Disorder Society Evidence-Based Medicine Review Update: Treatments for the non-motor symptoms of Parkinson's disease. Mov Disord 2011;26S3:42-80.

37 Devos D, Dujardin K, Poirot I, et al. Comparison of desipramine and citalopram treatments for depression in Parkinson's disease: a double-blind, randomized, placebo-controlled study. Mov Disord 2008;23:850-857.

38 Richard IH, McDermott MP, Kurlan R, et al. A randomized, double-blind, placebo-controlled trial of antidepressants in Parkinson disease. Neurology 2012;78:1229-1236.

39 Sammer G, Reuter I, Hullmann K, Kaps M, Vaitl D. Training of executive functions in Parkinson's disease. J Neurol Sci 2006;248:115-119.

40 Hanagasi HA, Gurvit H, Unsalan P, et al. The effects of rasagiline on cognitive deficits in Parkinson's disease patients without dementia: a randomized, double-blind, placebo-controlled, multicenter study. Mov Disord 2011;26:1851-1858.

41 Schrag A, Barone P, Brown RG, et al. Depression rating scales in Parkinson's disease: critique and recommendations. Mov Disord 2007;22:1077-1092.

42 Leentjens AF, Dujardin K, Marsh L, et al. Apathy and anhedonia rating scales in Parkinson's disease: critique and recommendations. Mov Disord 2008;23:2004-2014.

43 Fernandez HH, Aarsland D, Fenelon G, et al. Scales to assess psychosis in Parkinson's disease: Critique and recommendations. Mov Disord 2008;23:484-500.

44 Shiba M, Bower JH, Maraganore DM, et al. Anxiety disorders and depressive disorders preceding Parkinson's disease: a case-control study. Mov Disord 2000;15:669-677.

45 Fang F, Xu Q, Park Y, et al. Depression and the subsequent risk of Parkinson's disease in the NIH-AARP Diet and Health Study. Mov Disord 2010;25:1157-1162.

46 Hesse S, Meyer PM, Strecker K, et al. Monoamine transporter availability in Parkinson's disease patients with or without depression. Eur J Nucl Med Mol Imaging 2009;36:428-435.

47 Weintraub D, Morales KH, Moberg PJ, et al. Antidepressant studies in Parkinson's disease: a review and meta-analysis. Mov Disord 2005;20:1161-1169.

48 Dobkin RD, Menza M, Allen LA, et al. Cognitive-behavioral therapy for depression in Parkinson's disease: a randomized, controlled trial. Am J Psychiatry 2011;168:1066-1074.

49 Sanchez-Castaneda C, Rene R, Ramirez-Ruiz B, et al. Frontal and associative visual areas related to visual hallucinations in dementia with Lewy bodies and Parkinson's disease with dementia. Mov Disord 2010;25:615-622.

50 Ibarretxe-Bilbao N, Ramirez-Ruiz B, Junque C, et al. Differential progression of brain atrophy in Parkin-

son's disease with and without visual hallucinations. J Neurol Neurosurg Psychiatry 2010;81:650-657.

51 Thomsen TR, Panisset M, Suchowersky O, Goodridge A, Mendis T, Lang AE. Impact of standard of care for psychosis in Parkinson disease. J Neurol Neurosurg Psychiatry 2008;79:1413-1415.

52 Marras C, Gruneir A, Wang X, et al. Antipsychotics and mortality in Parkinsonism. Am J Geriatr Psychiatry 2012;20:149-158.

53 Voon V, Fox SH. Medication-related impulse control and repetitive behaviors in Parkinson disease. Arch Neurol 2007;64:1089-1096.

54 Weintraub D, Koester J, Potenza MN, et al. Impulse control disorders in Parkinson disease: a cross-sectional study of 3090 patients. Arch Neurol 2010;67:589-595.

55 Weintraub D, Papay K, Siderowf A, Parkinson's Progression Markers Initiative. Screening for impulse control symptoms in patients with de novo Parkinson disease: a case-control study. Neurology 2013;80:176-180.

56 Weintraub D, Hoops S, Shea JA, et al. Validation of the questionnaire for impulsive-compulsive disorders in Parkinson's disease. Mov Disord 2009;24:1461-1467.

57 Weintraub D, Nirenberg MJ. Impulse control and related disorders in Parkinson's disease. Neurodegener Dis 2013;11:63-71.

58 Rao H, Mamikonyan E, Detre JA, et al. Decreased ventral striatal activity with impulse control disorders in Parkinson's disease. Mov Disord 2010;25:1660-1669.

59 Mamikonyan E, Siderowf AD, Duda JE, et al. Long-term follow-up of impulse control disorders in Parkinson's disease. Mov Disord 2008;23:75-80.

60 Rabinak CA, Nirenberg MJ. Dopamine agonist withdrawal syndrome in Parkinson disease. Arch Neurol 2010;67:58-63.

61 Ardouin C, Voon V, Worbe Y, et al. Pathological gambling in Parkinson's disease improves on chronic subthalamic nucleus stimulation. Mov Disord 2006;21:1941-1946.

62 Okai D, Askey-Jones S, Samuel M, et al. Trial of CBT for impulse control behaviors affecting Par-

kinson patients and their caregivers. Neurology 2013;80:792-799.

63 Zesiewicz TA, Sullivan KL, Arnulf I, et al. Practice Parameter: treatment of nonmotor symptoms of Parkinson disease: report of the Quality Standards Subcommittee of the American Academy of Neurology. Neurology 2010;74:924-931.

64 Starkstein SE. Apathy in Parkinson's disease: diagnostic and etiological dilemmas. Mov Disord 2012;27:174-178.

65 Reijnders JS, Scholtissen B, Weber WE, Aalten P, Verhey FR, Leentjens AF. Neuroanatomical correlates of apathy in Parkinson's disease: A magnetic resonance imaging study using voxel-based morphometry. Mov Disord 2010;25:2318-2325.

66 Thobois S, Lhommee E, Klinger H, et al. Parkinsonian apathy responds to dopaminergic stimulation of D2/D3 receptors with piribedil. Brain 2013;136:1568-1577.

67 Parsons TD, Rogers SA, Braaten AJ, Woods SP, Troster AI. Cognitive sequelae of subthalamic nucleus deep brain stimulation in Parkinson's disease: a meta-analysis. Lancet Neurol 2006;5:578-588.

68 Weaver FM, Follett K, Stern M, et al. Bilateral deep brain stimulation vs best medical therapy for patients with advanced Parkinson disease: a randomized controlled trial. JAMA 2009;301:63-73.

69 Follett KA, Weaver FM, Stern M, et al. Pallidal versus subthalamic deep-brain stimulation for Parkinson's disease. N Engl J Med 2010;362:2077-2091.

70 Weintraub D, Duda JE, Carlson K, et al. Suicide ideation and behaviours after STN and GPi DBS surgery for Parkinson's disease: results from a randomised, controlled trial. J Neurol Neurosurg Psychiatry 2013;84:1113-1118.

71 Storch A, Schneider CB, Wolz M, et al. Nonmotor fluctuations in Parkinson disease: Severity and correlation with motor complications. Neurology 2013; 80:800-809.

9

Sleep-wake Disorders in Parkinson's Disease

Christian R. Baumann

Sleep-wake disturbances belong to the most frequent non-motor symptoms in Parkinson's disease (PD). They negatively interact with motor symptoms and quality of life and must therefore be carefully evaluated in every PD patient. Table 9.1 gives an overview of important sleep-wake disturbances in PD which are discussed in more detail in this chapter.

Table 9.1
Sleep-wake disturbances in Parkinson's disease.

- Insomnia
- Excessive daytime sleepiness
- Fatigue
- Rapid eye movement (REM) sleep behaviour disorder
- Non-REM (NREM) parasomnias
- Restless legs syndrome and periodic limb movement disorder
- Sleep apnea syndromes
- Circadian sleep-wake disorders

Insomnia

Epidemiology

Insomnia, a difficulty to fall asleep or to maintain sleep, is very common in PD patients. Up to 80-90% of PD patients suffer from insomnia symptoms during the course of their disease (1).

Etiology

Motor impairment during the night plays an important role: 65% of PD patients have difficulty turning around in bed (1). Furthermore, some patients suffer from pain when off dopaminer-

gic medication at night. In addition, many patients suffer from neuropsychiatric symptoms such as anxiety, depression and hallucinations, whether or not off-related, and they often negatively impact their quality of sleep. Co-morbid sleep-wake disturbances such as restless legs syndrome or sleep apnea may impair the quality of sleep, and nocturia is also associated with sleep fragmentation. Finally, PD patients are often treated with a multitude of drugs which impact sleep and wakefulness. For instance, selegiline and amantadine both may exert alerting effects and therefore should not be used in the afternoon or evening if insomnia complaints are present.

Diagnosis

Insomnia symptoms should be assessed by detailed history-taking of both patients and their relatives or caregivers. Screening questions should assess sleep latency, the number of awakenings at night, and early awakening. The Parkinson's disease sleep scale (PDSS) helps assess insomnia and its daytime consequences (see Figure 9.1) (2).

Polysomnography is usually not helpful in the diagnosis of insomnia, and in most countries, costs for polysomnography are not reimbursed unless co-morbid sleep disorders such as REM sleep behaviour disorder, restless legs syndrome or sleep apnea are suspected. On the other hand, actigraphy over 2-3 weeks may help quantifying insomnia symptoms, and differentiate them from circadian sleep-wake disorders.

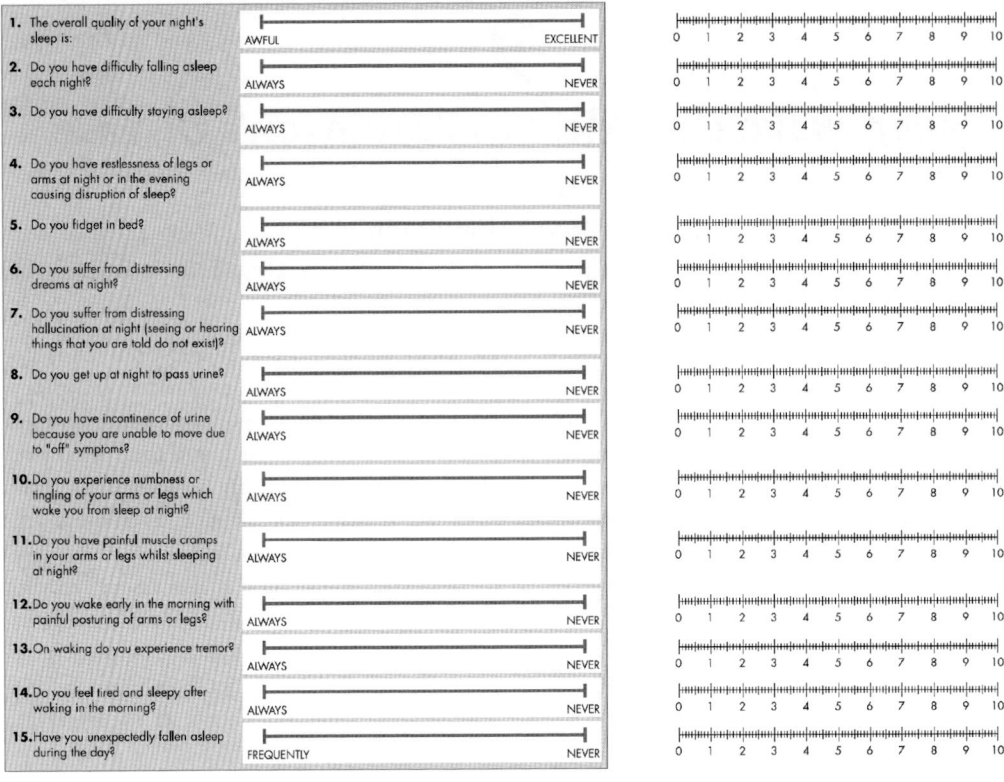

Figure 9.1
The Parkinson's disease sleep scale (PDSS) (2). Left panel: the actual scale as presented to patients, who are asked to mark their responses according to severity by placing a cross or line mark on the 10 cm line. The mm scale (right panel) which is printed on a transparency is then applied on the 10 cm lines to measure the responses in decimal figures; 10 represents excellent/never responses; 0 represents the worst score. Reproduced (2) with permission from the BMJ Publishing Group Ltd.

Treatment

Although very frequent, insomnia in PD patients is poorly studied, and treatment studies are sparse. Above all, underlying conditions should be managed. Continuous dopaminergic stimulation (CDS) (see also Chapter 14) is a good strategy to improve nocturnal motor symptoms. For instance, a multinational, double-blind, placebo-controlled trial of 287 PD subjects showed that 24-hour transdermal application of rotigotine improves both motor function and nocturnal sleep disturbances (3). Similarly, subthalamic deep brain stimulation has been shown to improve nocturnal sleep, as assessed with the PDSS (4).

Co-morbid sleep-wake disorders, if present (see below), should be treated accordingly. Sleep-inducing or sedative drugs can be tried, if necessary. Many patients who are treated with clonazepam because of co-existing REM sleep behaviour disorder (RBD) report a beneficial effect on sleep quality. High doses of melatonin (50mg) revealed a mild, objective increase of total sleep time as measured by actigraphy, but subjectively, this improvement was significant (5). In the same line, an open-label polysomnographic study showed that nocturnal sodium oxybate in split doses improved the quality of sleep (6). Sedating antidepressants such as amitriptyline or mirtazapine may also have a beneficial effect on sleep, but they may worsen or cause restless legs symptoms. Last not least, evening doses of neuroleptics including clopazine and quetiapine, which are used to treat psychotic symptoms, improve nocturnal sleep in PD patients (7).

Excessive daytime sleepiness

Epidemiology

Excessive daytime sleepiness (EDS) is characterized by an increased propensity to fall asleep in various circumstances during daytime and is a frequent condition in PD, affecting around 50% of patients (8,9). EDS may precede the onset of motor symptoms in PD (10) and is associated with severer cognitive deficits and a higher risk of falls (11).

Etiology and Pathophysiology

In most PD patients, multiple factors contribute to the expression of EDS. Most importantly, treatment with dopaminergic drugs, particularly dopamine agonists, is linked to EDS. In fact, the use of dopamine agonists increases the risk of sleep attacks by 2-3 times (12, 13). A double-blind, placebo-controlled study confirmed that pramipexole, a D2/D3 receptor agonist, objectively increases EDS in PD patients, whereas levodopa was not different from placebo (14). Still, non-dopaminergic compounds such as neuroleptics or sedative antidepressants may also contribute. In addition, co-morbidities in PD potentially aggravate EDS. First of all, sleep abnormalities including insomnia, sleep apnea, and periodic limb movements during sleep might be linked to EDS, although a clear correlation has not been shown so far. Second, neuropsychiatric disturbances including nocturnal anxiety and depression may negatively interact with daytime vigilance.

There is growing evidence that the neurodegenerative process itself also contributes to sleepiness. From a clinical perspective, it has been shown that EDS increases with disease duration and severity (15,16). This finding is mirrored by early reports of pathological changes in the brainstem of PD patients, particularly in the serotoninergic raphe nucleus and the noradrenergic locus coeruleus (17). These nuclei are critical components of the central arousal system. More recently, two groups described a partial loss of wake-promoting hypocretin (orexin) neurons in the posterior hypothalamus, and this loss was severer in PD patients with higher Hoehn and Yahr staging of the disease (18,19). Altogether, these studies suggest that non-nigrostriatal neurodegeneration in important wakefulness-mediating nuclei contributes to the expression of EDS in PD.

Diagnosis

To subjectively diagnose EDS, validated scales and questionnaires can be used. One of the most widely used tools is the Epworth sleepiness scale (ESS), which has been validated in multiple languages and in PD patients (see Figure 9.2). To objectively diagnose EDS, multiple sleep latency tests preceded by nocturnal polysomnography can be performed. In a controlled study, in comparison to controls (mean sleep latency 11.5 minutes) and PD patients in an early disease stage (12.1 minutes), advanced PD patients were much sleepier (6.0 minutes) (20).

Treatment

After identifying potential causes of EDS in PD patients, they should be primarily treated. The use and dose of any sedative drugs should be re-evaluated. Targeting of identified sleep disorders can also be beneficial, as well as sleep hygiene counseling. If these strategies fail to improve vigilance, stimulants can be tried. Modafinil has been suggested, but clinical experience and recent studies suggest that its alerting effect may be limited (21). In any PD patient with EDS, her or his ability to drive a motor vehicle must be questioned.

How likely are you to doze off or fall asleep in the following situations, in contrast to feeling just tired? This refers to your usual way of life in recent times. Even if you have not done some of these things recently, try to work out how they would have affected you. Use the following scale to choose the most appropriate number for each situation:

Situation	Chance of dosing
Sitting and reading	
Watching TV	
Sitting inactive in a public place (e.g a theater or a meeting)	
As a passenger in a car for an hour without a break	
Lying down to rest in the afternoon when circumstances permit	
Sitting and talking to someone	
Sitting quietly after a lunch without alcohol	
In a car, while stopped for a few minutes in traffic	

0 no chance of dozing; **1** slight chance of dozing; **2** moderate chance of dozing; **3** high chance of dozing

Figure 9.2
Epworth sleepiness scale to assess excessive daytime sleepiness. A score of 10 and more points suggests EDS. Along (57).

Fatigue

Fatigue is a frequent complaint in PD patients, it may affect more than 50% (8). Its definition is somewhat vague and reflects multiple – physical and mental – dimensions of this syndrome: fatigue is defined as a subjective experience and includes such symptoms as rapid inanition, persisting lack of energy, exhaustion, physical and mental tiredness, and apathy (22). There is a significant overlap with symptoms of EDS, apathy, and depression. In fact, there is evidence that depression plays an important role in PD-related fatigue (23). The observation that dopaminergic drugs are related to fatigue relief indicates that fatigue and apathy share some common dopamine-related pathways (24). Fatigue can be measured by validated scales such as the modified fatigue impact scale (MFIS) or the fatigue severity scale (FSS) (see Figure 9.3) (25,26).

There are only a few and mainly small treatment studies on fatigue in PD. Simulants are probably ineffective, but dopaminergic drugs such as rasagiline or pramipexole may work (24,28).

Rapid eye movement (REM) sleep behaviour disorder

Epidemiology

REM sleep behaviour disorder (RBD) is a parasomnia which occurs during REM sleep only and is characterized by loss of physiological REM sleep atonia and by dream-enacting behaviours. It may be observed in 30-90% of patients with synucleinopathies, while it occurs much more rarely in other proteinopathies (29). Among synucleinopathies, it is most tightly linked to multiple system atrophy (present in 90-100%) and dementia with Lewy bodies (80-100%) (30,31). In PD patients, it is observed in about 25-50% (32). Still, due to the fact that (a) the diagnostic criteria may be too narrow and (b) questionnaire-based studies may have failed to identify all cases, the true prevalence of RBD in PD patients could be markedly higher than these previously reported figures.

Most importantly, RBD may herald motor symptoms in many PD patients (33): in their seminal study, Iranzo and colleagues showed that idio-

Fatigue Severity Scale (FSS)*							
	strongly disagree					strongly agree	
	1	2	3	4	5	6	7
1 My motivation is lower when I am fatigued.	☐	☐	☐	☐	☐	☐	☐
2 Exercise brings on my fatigue.	☐	☐	☐	☐	☐	☐	☐
3 I am easily fatigued.	☐	☐	☐	☐	☐	☐	☐
4 Fatigue interferes with my physical functioning.	☐	☐	☐	☐	☐	☐	☐
5 Fatigue causes frequent problems for me.	☐	☐	☐	☐	☐	☐	☐
6 My fatigue prevents sustained physical functioning.	☐	☐	☐	☐	☐	☐	☐
7 Fatigue interferes with carrying out certain duties and responsibilities.	☐	☐	☐	☐	☐	☐	☐
8 Fatigue is among my three most disabling symptoms.	☐	☐	☐	☐	☐	☐	☐
9 Fatigue interferes with my work, family, or social life.	☐	☐	☐	☐	☐	☐	☐

*Patients are instructed to choose a number from 1 to 7 that indicates their degree of agreement with each statement where 1 indicates strongly disagree and 7, strongly agree.

Figure 9.3
The fatigue severity scale (FSS) (26), adapted from (27). A score of ≥ 4.0 indicates fatigue.

pathic RBD often antedates the development of neurodegenerative disease. Seven years later, in a follow-up study of the 44 participants from the original cohort, 82% had developed a synucleinopathy (34). The rates of neurological disease-free survival from the time of RBD diagnosis were 65% at 5 years, 27% at 10 years, and only 8% at 14 years (34). Functional brain imaging revealed pathologically decreased dopamine transporter uptake in all of the remaining disease-free subjects, suggesting that all are likely to develop clinical parkinsonism as well.

Etiology and pathophysiology

Overall, the neuronal dysfunctions underlying the loss of atonia in RBD patients still remain elusive. In 3 patients who died before antemortem diagnoses of a neurodegenerative disease, the authors found widespread neuronal loss and α-synuclein-containing Lewy bodies and Lewy neuritis, particularly in the brainstem nuclei that regulate REM sleep atonia (34). Thus, dysfunctional signaling of these particular brainstem nuclei (including the pedunculopontine nucleus (PPN) and the locus coeruleus) appears to play an important role in RBD. More specifically, motor neurons are tonically hyperpolarized and phasically excited during REM sleep (35). REM sleep atonia is probably induced by premotoneurons in the raphe magnus and the ventral medullary reticular formation. During REM sleep, these neurons are directly activated by neurons in the pontine sublaterodorsal tegmental nucleus (35). Pierre Luppi and colleagues derived from these data that RBD might be caused by degeneration of descending REM-on neurons localized in the sublaterodorsal nucleus or of the REM-on premotoneurons in the ventral medullary reticular formation, and that RBD-associated movements might be directed by descending projections of cortical motor neurons (35).

Clinical presentation

Classically, vigorous enactment of dreams is the clinical hallmark of RBD, and the dream content is often though not always (see Videofragment 9.1), frightening (see Video fragment 9.2). Thus, RBD patients often shout, kick, punch and lash out during their dreams when they are chased or attacked. It has been shown, however, that RBD is associated with a wide range of non-violent stereotype behaviours including masturbating-like behaviour and coitus-like pelvic thrusting, mimicking eating and drinking, urinating and defecating, laughing, singing, dancing, whistling, smoking a fictive cigarette, clapping and gesturing 'thumbs up', greetings, flying, building a stair, dealing textiles, inspecting the army, searching a treasure, and giving lessons (36) (see Chapter 38). Despite being off medication, PD patients' movements appear normal, and despite depressive moods during the daytime, they may exhibit high spirits at night (37). Sleepwalking-like behaviours like walking and appropriate use of objects, however, are rare in RBD patients (38).

Diagnosis

The diagnosis of RBD is primarily clinical. History-taking in spouses or close relatives is crucial, for most patients do not remember their nocturnal behaviour. Some patients remember bruises or damage to objects in the proximity of the bed. Several questionnaires have been developed for the diagnosis of RBD. Reviewing all these questionnaires would be beyond the scope of this chapter. However, a Canadian group found one single question to be a useful tool to screen for RBD comparable to earlier published longer questionnaires (39): 'Have you ever been told, or suspected yourself, that you seem to 'act out your dreams' while asleep (for example, punching, flailing your arms in the air, making running movements, etc.)?'

The gold standard to prove RBD or REM sleep without atonia, e.g. in patients with suspected RBD but without a typical history, remains nocturnal video-polysomnography. This examina-tion allows for the recording of submental electromyography (EMG) tone, limb twitching, and abnormal behaviour during REM sleep. Montplaisir and colleagues have extensively discussed the polysomnographic diagnosis of RBD: critical findings for the diagnosis of RBD are tonic ($\geq$30%) and phasic ($\geq$15%) increases of EMG activity as well as $\geq$24 leg movements per hour of REM sleep (40).

Treatment

Clonazepam and high-dose melatonin are the mainstays of RBD treatment, and these strategies are often successful. Isabelle Arnulf provided an excellent overview on RBD treatment studies (see Table 9.2).

Prognosis

There is increasing evidence that the presence of RBD may not only herald neurodegeneration per se but is also linked to an impaired prognosis in PD patients. Gagnon and colleagues found that RBD is associated with an increased risk of mild cognitive impairment, both in patients with idiopathic RBD and in PD patients (42). In our own cohort, we found that PD patients with polysomnographically confirmed RBD or REM sleep without atonia had markedly faster motor progression than patients with normal REM sleep (unpublished results).

Non-REM (NREM) parasomnias

The literature on NREM parasomnias in PD is sparse. A questionnaire-based assessment of sleepwalking revealed a prevalence of 9%, but these data must be interpreted with caution until confirmed by polysomnography (43).

Sleep-disordered breathing (Sleep apnea syndrome)

The prevalence and clinical significance of sleep-disordered breathing in PD remain the subject of controversy. Thus, the range of published

Table 9.2
Treatment of REM sleep behavior disorder (RBD). Level of evidence and study outcomes (41).

Drug (dose)	Level of evidence		Benefit
Melatonin (3-15 mg)	2	One double-blind placebo-controlled study, small groups (n < 50)	82% of positive responders. Reduction of phasic and tonic muscle activity in PSG
Clonazepam (0.5-2 mg)	4	Open studies, large groups (n > 300)	73% with complete control of RBD, 17% with partial control, 10% of non-responders
Zopiclone (3.75-7 mg)	4	Open study, large groups (n = 11)	73% of responders when used alone (n = 9) or in combination (n = 2)
Rivastigmine (4.5-6 mg)	4	Open studies in patients with DLB, small group (n = 10)	100% of responders (little data)
Donepezil (10-15 mg)	4	Open studies in patients with DLB, small group (n = 6)	66% of responders (little data)
Pramipexole (0.5-1.5 mg)	2	One double-blind placebo-controlled study (n = 11)	Open series: 45% of responders
	4	Open studies (n = 29)	Double-blind study in PD: no benefit

prevalences in the literature is wide (27-69%) (44,45). In addition, the overall clinical significance of sleep apnea in PD patients has been questioned: in one study, the authors concluded that sleepiness, nocturia and cognitive impairment are mostly caused by other, non-apneic mechanisms (46). In a retrospective analysis of our own patients (unpublished results), the prevalence and severity of EDS were similar in PD patients with and without sleep apnea. Thus, EDS might not be a good predictor for sleep-disordered breathing in PD. Instead, history-taking should focus on nocturnal apneic events, i.e. pauses in breathing or instances of shallow or infrequent breathing during sleep. Last not least, there is no evidence on whether sleep apnea in PD increases vascular morbidity or mortality. These factors may explain why there is a complete absence of trials with continuous positive airway pressure (CPAP).

Restless legs syndrome

Both restless legs syndrome (RLS) and PD benefit from dopaminergic treatment, which would suggest that these two disorders share some common final pathway. Still, the pathophysiological basis of RLS is poorly understood, and besides dopaminergic signaling, iron metabolism is likely to play an important role. An elegant study on the expression of iron management proteins in the epithelial cells of the choroid plexus and the brain microvasculature in postmortem tissues found a decrease of iron regulatory protein activity, which might underlie the problems of brain iron acquisition in RLS (47). It remains unclear, however, whether RLS is more frequent in PD than in non-PD subjects (48,49). Like in PD-related sleep apnea, the clinical significance remains unclear: a recent study found that RLS does not affect the quality of life or daytime vigilance in PD (50).

Diagnosis
If patients complain of (1) an urge to move the limbs with or without sensations, (2) improvement with activity, (3) worsening at rest, and (4) worsening in the evening or night (constituting the typical clinical tetrad of RLS symptoms), they may be considered as suffering from RLS, and treatment could be considered.

Treatment

The first choice for treatment still remains long-acting dopaminergic compounds and iron supplements, particularly in cases with low serum ferritin (below 50-80 µg/L). For instance, in PD patients treated with L-dopa, low doses of additional transdermal rotigotine (1.0-3.0mg per day) or of pramipexole (0.125-1.0mg) may alleviate RLS symptoms. Second-line treatment includes anticonvulsants such as gabapentin, pregabaline or carbamazepine, benzodiazepines, or opioids such as methadone or oxycodone.

Circadian disorders

Despite the recurrent clinical observation of circadian shifts, circadian rhythmicity in L-dopa pharmacokinetics, and circadian fluctuations of motor, autonomic and behavioural symptoms in PD patients, there are only a few small, systematical studies on circadian rhythms in PD. Actigraphy is a non-invasive method of monitoring human rest-activity cycles: subjects wear an actimeter on the non-dominant wrist to measure motor activity and light exposure.

Diagnosis

In PD patients, compared to controls, actigraphy studies revealed a decrease of peak activity levels and lower amplitudes of the rest-activity cycle (51,52). The neurohormone melatonin signaling regulates the circadian sleep–wake cycle and can be measured in the cerebrospinal fluid, saliva and plasma. An observational study found a slight but insignificant phase advance and amplitude decrease of circadian plasma melatonin secretion related to both the evolution and treatment of PD (53). On the other hand, the measurement of 24-hour core body temperature rhythms was similar in PD patients and controls (54). Altogether, larger systematic studies are needed to gain better insights into circadian function in PD.

Treatment

From a therapeutic point of view, it has been discussed whether bright light exposure might be beneficial for PD patients. Light synchronizes the human circadian system, suppresses melatonin secretion, and is often applied in circadian sleep-wake and mood disorders. Two exploratory studies exposed PD patients to bright light. One randomized, placebo-controlled, double-blind study in 36 PD patients found a significant improvement of tremor and depression after bright light exposure in the morning (55). Another study applied bright light 1 hour prior to the usual time of sleep onset and found elevated mood, improved sleep, decreased seborrhea, reduced impotence, and increased appetite in treated PD patients (56). Again, larger studies are warranted to elucidate the potential therapeutic role of bright light therapy in PD.

Video fragments

PLAY

Fragment 9.1
REM sleep behavior disorder (1)
Nocturnal video-polysomnography of a 78-year-old male patient with idiopathic Parkinson's disease and REM sleep behaviour disorder (RBD). In this patient with severe comorbid depression, RBD manifests with expression of joy and laughter.

Fragment 9.2
REM sleep behavior disorder (2)
Nocturnal video-polysomnography of a 71-year-old female patient with idiopathic Parkinson's disease. On the left side, sleep electro-encephalogram (bottom), electro-oculogram (top) and electro-myogram are visible. The patient is in rapid eye movement (REM) sleep. REM sleep behaviour in this patient manifests primarily with expression of fear and screaming, but not with motor activity.

References

1 Lees AJ, Blackburn NA, Campbell VL. The night-time problems of Parkinson's disease. Clin Neuropharmacol 1988;11:512-519.

2 Chaudhuri KR, Pal S, DiMarco A, et al. The Parkinson's disease sleep scale: a new instrument for assessing sleep and nocturnal disability in Parkinson's disease. J Neurol Neurosurg Psychiatry 2002;73:629-635

3 Trenkwalder C, Kies B, Rudzinska M, et al. Rotigotine effects on early morning motor function and sleep in Parkinson's disease: a double-blind, randomized, placebo-controlled study (RECOVER). Mov Disord 2011;26:90-99.

4 Hjort N, Østergaard K, Dupont E. Improvement of sleep quality in patients with advanced Parkinson's disease treated with deep brain stimulation of the subthalamic nucleus. Mov Disord 2004;19:196-199.

5 Dowling GA, Mastick J, Colling E, et al. Melatonin for sleep disturbances in Parkinson's disease. Sleep Med 2005;6:459-466.

6 Ondo WG, Perkins T, Swick T, et al. Sodium oxybate for excessive daytime sleepiness in Parkinson disease: an open-label polysomnographic study. Arch Neurol 2008; 65: 1337-40.

7 Linazasoro G, Martí Massó JF, Suárez JA. Nocturnal akathisia in Parkinson's disease: treatment with clozapine. Mov Disord 1993;8:171-174.

8 Valko PO, Waldvogel D, Weller M, Bassetti CL, Held U, Baumann CR. Fatigue and excessive daytime sleepiness in idiopathic Parkinson's disease differently correlate with motor symptoms, depression and dopaminergic treatment. Eur J Neurol 2010;17:1428-1436.

9 De Cock VC, Vidailhet M, Arnulf I. Sleep disturbances in patients with parkinsonism. Nat Clin Pract Neurol 2008;4:254-266.

10 Abbott RD, Ross GW, White LR, et al. Excessive daytime sleepiness and subsequent development of Parkinson disease. Neurology 2005; 65:1442-1446.

11 Spindler M, Gooneratne NS, Siderowf A, Duda JE, Cantor C, Dahodwala N. Daytime Sleepiness is Associated with Falls in Parkinson's Disease. Parkinsons Dis 2013;3:387-391.

12 Hobson DE, Lang AE, Martin WR, Razmy A, Rivest J, Fleming J. Excessive daytime sleepiness and sudden-onset sleep in Parkinson disease. A survey by the Canadian Movement Disorder Group. JAMA 2002;287:455-463.

13 Ondo WG, Dat Vuong K, Khan H, Atassi F, Kwak C, Jankovic J. Daytime sleepiness and other sleep disorders in Parkinson's disease. Neurology 2001;57:1392–1396.

14 Micallef J, Rey M, Eusebio A, et al. Antiparkinsonian drug-induced sleepiness: a double-blind placebo-controlled study of L-dopa, bromocriptine and pramipexole in healthy subjects. Br J Clin Pharmacol 2009;67:333-340.

15 Valko PO, Waldvogel D, Weller M, Bassetti CL, Held U, Baumann CR. Fatigue and excessive daytime sleepiness in idiopathic Parkinson's disease differently correlate with motor symptoms, depression and dopaminergic treatment. Eur J Neurol 2010;17:1428-1436.

16 Zoccolella S, Savarese M, Lamberti P, Manni R, Pacchetti C, Logroscino G. Sleep disorders and the natural history of Parkinson's disease: the contribution of epidemiological studies. Sleep Med Rev 2011;15:41-50.

17 Jellinger KA. Pathology of Parkinson's disease. Changes other than the nigrostriatal pathway. Mol Chem Neuropathol 1991;14:153-197.

18 Fronczek R, Overeem S, Lee SY, et al. Hypocretin (orexin) loss in Parkinson's disease. Brain 2007;130:1577-1585.

19 Thannickal TC, Lai YY, Siegel JM. Hypocretin (orexin) cell loss in Parkinson's disease. Brain 2007;130:1586-1595.

20 Wienecke M, Werth E, Poryazova R, et al. Progressive dopamine and hypocretin deficiencies in Parkinson's disease: is there an impact on sleep and wakefulness? J Sleep Res 2012;21:710-717.

21 Lohr JB, Liu L, Caligiuri MP, et al. Modafinil improves antipsychotic-induced parkinsonism but not excessive daytime sleepiness, psychiatric symptoms or cognition in schizophrenia and schizoaffective disorder: A randomized, double-blind, placebo-controlled study. Schizophr Res 2013;150:289-296.

22 Chaudhuri A, Behan PO. Fatigue in neurological disorders. Lancet 2004; 363: 978-88.

23 van Dijk JP, Havlikova E, Rosenberger J, et al. Influence of Disease Severity on Fatigue in Patients with Parkinson's Disease Is Mainly Mediated by Symptoms of Depression. Eur Neurol 2013;70:201-209.

24 Stocchi F; The ADAGIO investigators. Benefits of treatment with rasagiline for fatigue symptoms in patients with early Parkinson's disease. Eur J Neurol 2013;doi:10.1111/ene.12205.

25 Schiehser DM, Ayers CR, Liu L, Lessig S, Song DS, Filoteo JV. Validation of the Modified Fatigue Impact Scale in Parkinson's disease. Parkinsonism Relat Disord 2013;19:335-338.

26 Krupp LB, LaRocca NG, Muir-Nash J, Steinberg AD. The fatigue severity scale. Application to patients with multiple sclerosis and systemic lupus erythematosus. Arch Neurol 1989;46:1121-1123.

27 Valko PO, Bassetti CL, Bloch KE, Held U, Baumann CR. Validation of the fatigue severity scale in a Swiss cohort. Sleep 2008;31:1601-1607.

28 Morita A, Okuma Y, Kamei S, et al. Pramipexole reduces the prevalence of fatigue in patients with Parkinson's disease. Intern Med 2011;50:2163-2168.

29 Boeve BF, Silber MH, Ferman TJ, Lucas JA, Parisi JE. Association of REM sleep behavior disorder and neurodegenerative disease may reflect an underlying synucleinopathy. Mov Disord 2001;16:622-630.

30 Ferini-Strambi L, Marelli S. Sleep dysfunction in multiple system atrophy. Curr Treat Options Neurol 2012;14:464-473.

31 Pao WC, Boeve BF, Ferman TJ, et al. Polysomnographic findings in dementia with Lewy bodies. Neurologist 2013;19:1-6.

32 Comella CL, Nardine TM, Diederich NJ, Stebbins GT. Sleep-related violence, injury, and REM sleep behavior disorder in Parkinson's disease. Neurology 1998;51:526-529.

33 Iranzo A, Molinuevo JL, Santamaría J, et al. Rapid-eye-movement sleep behaviour disorder as an early marker for a neurodegenerative disorder: a descriptive study. Lancet Neurol 2006;5:572-577.

34 Iranzo A, Tolosa E, Gelpi E, et al. Neurodegenerative disease status and post-mortem pathology in idiopathic rapid-eye-movement sleep behaviour disorder: an observational cohort study. Lancet Neurol 2013;12:443-453.

35 Luppi PH, Clément O, Valencia Garcia S, Brischoux F, Fort P. New aspects in the pathophysiology of rapid eye movement sleep behavior disorder: the potential role of glutamate, gamma-aminobutyric acid, and glycine. Sleep Med 2013;14 714-718.

36 Oudiette D, De Cock VC, Lavault S, Leu S, Vidailhet M, Arnulf I. Nonviolent elaborate behaviors may also occur in REM sleep behavior disorder. Neurology 2009;72 551-557.

37 Siclari F, Wienecke M, Poryazova R, Bassetti CL, Baumann CR. Laughing as a manifestation of rapid eye movement sleep behavior disorder. Parkinsonism Relat Disord 2011;17:382-385.

38 Scaglione C, Vignatelli L, Plazzi G, et al. REM sleep behaviour disorder in Parkinson's disease: a questionnaire-based study. Neurol Sci 2005;25:316-321.

39 Postuma RB, Arnulf I, Hogl B, et al. A single-question screen for rapid eye movement sleep behavior disorder: a multicenter validation study. Mov Disord 2012;27:913-916.

40 Montplaisir J, Gagnon JF, Fantini ML, et al. Polysomnographic diagnosis of idiopathic REM sleep behavior disorder. Mov Disord 2010;25:2044-2051.

41 Arnulf I. REM sleep behavior disorder: motor manifestations and pathophysiology. Mov Disord 2012;27:677-689.

42 Gagnon JF, Vendette M, Postuma RB, et al. Mild cognitive impairment in rapid eye movement sleep behavior disorder and Parkinson's disease. Ann Neurol 2009; 66: 39-47.

43 Oberholzer M, Poryazova R, Bassetti CL. Sleepwalking in Parkinson's disease: a questionnaire-based survey. J Neurol 2011;258:1261-1267.

44 Yong MH, Fook-Chong S, Pavanni R, Lim LL, Tan EK. Case control polysomnographic studies of sleep disorders in Parkinson's disease. PLoS ONE 2011;6:e22511.

45 Trotti LM, Bliwise DL. No increased risk of obstructive sleep apnea in Parkinson's disease. Mov Disord 2010;25:2246-2249.

46 Cochen de Cock V, Abouda M, Leu S, et al. Is obstructive sleep apnea a problem in Parkinson's disease? Sleep Med 2010;11:247-252.

47 Connor JR, Ponnuru P, Wang XS, Patton SM, Allen RP, Earley CJ. Profile of altered brain iron acquisition in restless legs syndrome. Brain 2011;134:959-968.

48 Ondo WG, Vuong KD, Jankovic J. Exploring the relationship between Parkinson disease and restless legs syndrome. Arch Neurol 2002;59:421–424.

49 Tan EK, Lum SY, Wong MC. Restless legs syndrome in Parkinson's disease. J Neurol Sci 2002;196:33–36.

50 Gómez-Esteban JC, Zarranz JJ, Tijero B, et al. Restless legs syndrome in Parkinson's disease. Mov Disord 2007;22:1912-1916.

51 Whitehead DL, Davies AD, Playfer JR, Turnbull CJ. Circadian rest-activity rhythm is altered in Parkinson's disease patients with hallucinations. Mov Disord 2008;23:1137-1145.

52 van Hilten B, Hoff JI, Middelkoop HA, et al. Sleep disruption in Parkinson's disease. Assessment by continuous activity monitoring. Arch Neurol 1994;51:922-928.

53 Bordet R, Devos D, Brique S, et al. Study of circadian melatonin secretion pattern at different stages of Parkinson's disease. Clin Neuropharmacol 2003;26:65-72.

54 Pierangeli G, Provini F, Maltoni P, et al. Nocturnal body core temperature falls in Parkinson's disease but not in Multiple-System Atrophy. Mov Disord 2001;16:226-232.

55 Paus S, Schmitz-Hübsch T, Wüllner U, Vogel A, Klockgether T, Abele M. Bright light therapy in Parkinson's disease: a pilot study. Mov Disord 2007;22:1495-1498.

56 Willis GL, Turner EJ. Primary and secondary features of Parkinson's disease improve with strategic exposure to bright light: a case series study. Chronobiol Int 2007;24:521-537.

57 Johns NW. A new method for measuring daytime sleepiness: the Epworth sleepiness scale. Sleep 1991;14:540-554.

10

Diagnosis of Parkinson's Disease

Kathrin Brockmann & Daniela Berg

Parkinson´s disease (PD) is the second most frequent neurodegenerative disorder after Alzheimer's disease and affects about 1-2% of individuals above the age of 65. Clinically, most patients present with the cardinal symptoms of motor parkinsonism: bradykinesia, resting tremor, rigidity, and postural instability.

Underlying these clinical features is a progressive degeneration of dopaminergic neurons in the substantia nigra pars compacta (SNc), accompanied by an accumulation of eosinophilic intracytoplasmic protein inclusions known as Lewy bodies and Lewy neurites, both of which are the pathological hallmarks. Since twin studies in the 1980s failed to confirm evidence of familial accumulation, genetic factors were thought to play a minor role in the pathogenesis of PD and the assumption that ageing and environmental toxins cause PD was further propagated.

Does this description represent our current understanding of PD or is it time to integrate new research findings and accommodate our definition and diagnostic criteria of PD? In the following chapter we will outline the currently used diagnostic criteria/guidelines based on the UK Parkinson's disease society brain bank clinical diagnostic criteria (UK Brain Bank Criteria) (see Table 10.1) and will then discuss recent research findings that challenge these criteria and might provide future prospects for new diagnostic criteria for PD.

Motor symptoms

The clinical diagnosis of Parkinson's disease is based on the UK Brain Bank Criteria which focuses on the cardinal motor features, asymmetry of symptoms and a robust response to levodopa treatment (see Table 10.1).

Findings from clinicopathological studies reported a 90% specificity of these criteria at death (1), and the diagnosis by experienced clinicians was even better than the application of these clinical criteria in some cases. However, although a reasonable specificity can indeed be achieved by the application of these criteria, some aspects need to be reconsidered.

Postural instability, which is still in general included in the cardinal motor features, occurs only late(r) in the disease process, and an early occurrence suggests other diagnoses like atypical parkinsonian syndromes. To avoid confusion, this item should be omitted from the list of cardinal motor symptoms. Similarly, asymmetry of symptoms and response to L-dopa therapy in other movement disorders challenge these aspects of the current criteria.

We face major unforeseen challenges such as the characterization/definition of mild parkinsonian signs, especially for the early disease stages that were not recognised or considered at the time of establishing the UK Brain Bank Criteria. Several large-scale studies reported mild parkinsonian syndromes in 25-50% of elderly individuals without clinical features of PD (2-5) or α-synuclein deposition (3,6). In accordance with this unspec-

Table 10.1

UK Parkinson's Disease Society Brain Bank clinical diagnostic criteria (UK Brain Bank Criteria) according to Goetz.

Step 1 Diagnosis of parkinsonian syndrome
- Bradykinesia (slowness of initiation of voluntary movement with progressive reduction in speed and amplitude of repetitive actions) *and at least one of the following*:
- Muscular rigidity
- 4–6 Hz resting tremor
- Postural instability not caused by primary visual, vestibular, cerebellar or proprioceptive dysfunction

Step 2 Exclusion criteria for Parkinson's disease
- History of repeated strokes with stepwise progression of parkinsonian features
- History of repeated head injury
- History of definite encephalitis
- Oculogyric crises
- Neuroleptic treatment at onset of symptoms
- More than one affected relative
- Sustained remission
- Strictly unilateral features after 3 years
- Supranuclear gaze palsy
- Cerebellar signs
- Early severe autonomic involvement
- Early severe dementia with disturbances of memory, language, and praxis
- Babinski sign
- Presence of cerebral tumour or communicating hydrocephalus on CT scan
- Negative response to large doses of levodopa (if malabsorption excluded)
- Exposure to 1-methyl-4-phenyl-1,2,3,6-tetrahydropyridine

Step 3 Supportive prospective positive criteria for Parkinson's disease
(Three or more required for definite diagnosis of Parkinson's disease)
- Unilateral onset
- Rest tremor present
- Progressive disorder
- Persistent asymmetry affecting side of onset most
- Excellent response (70–100%) to levodopa
- Severe levodopa-induced chorea
- Levodopa response for 5 years or more
- Clinical course of 10 years or more

ificity of symptoms, no differences in quantitative motor assessments were obtained 1 year before death between 61 control individuals and 15 age- and sex-matched clinically healthy individuals with post-mortem identification of incidental Lewy body disease (histopathological detection of Lewy bodies in clinically healthy individuals) (7). Similarly, in the Honolulu-Asia Aging Study, the total unified Parkinson's disease rating scale (UPDRS) scores obtained about 2.9 years before death were similar for 29 participants with incidental Lewy body disease and for 50 control individuals without Lewy bodies at autopsy (8).

On the other hand, single mild motor signs such as tremor, rigidity, bradykinesia, and gait abnormalities might represent early markers of neurodegeneration (2,9) since the degree of motor impairment meets the clinical diagnostic criteria for PD when cell loss in the substantia nigra (SN) pars compacta reaches about 40-50%, with striatal dopamine depletion of about 60-70% (10). The late occurrence of manifest cardinal motor signs can be explained by compensatory mechanisms which substantially hide changes in the nigrostriatal system for many years (11). Here thorough clinical investigation and quantitative assessments are demanded: in a cohort of patients with rapid eye movement (REM) sleep behaviour disorder (RBD), abnormal (UPDRS) scores could be measured 4.5 years before diagnosis in those who developed clinical PD. Using quantitative motor assessments, abnormalities could be detected even 6-9 years before diagnosis (12). Also, the variability of gait trunk acceleration and smoothness of sway under challenging tasks measured by accelerometers positioned in the lower back are greater in non-manifesting *LRRK2* Gly-2019Ser mutation carriers than in healthy individuals without this mutation (13,14). To assess motor abnormalities earlier in the course of PD, it will be essential to identify the kind of mild motor impairment which is suggestive for early forms of PD. This will most likely necessitate the application of clearly defined specific tasks and quantitative assessments.

Moreover, regarding the general concept of the UK Brain Bank Criteria, the focus on motor features deserves reconsideration. It has been well established that PD is associated with several non-motor symptoms that vary largely in prevalence, order of appearance, rate of progression, and severity and affect many patients at some disease stages at least as much as motor symptoms do. This multisystemic character implicated by the large variety of non-motor symptoms points towards a broader approach in future criteria.

Non-motor symptoms

So far, non-motor symptoms are not part of the diagnostic criteria for PD but are listed for optional assessment.

Apart from motor impairment, PD is associated with a large variety of non-motor symptoms (NMS). They include neuropsychiatric disturbances (e.g. dementia, depression), autonomic and sensory dysfunction, and sleep-wake problems (see Figure 10.1A) (15).

NMS independently determine the course of the disease, mortality and quality of life in PD patients and do often not respond to levodopa. For diagnostic criteria, knowledge about prevalence, progression and additional modulating factors of diagnostic criteria is of major importance to obtain a more complete picture of the clinical phenotype and to finally evaluate the effect of therapeutic strategies.

So far, early severe autonomic involvement and early severe dementia with disturbances of

A Overview on non-motor symptoms in PD (known prevalences are given in %)

Neuropsychiatric	Sleep	Autonom	Gastrointestinal	Sensory
• Depression 45% • Dementia 80% • Hallucination • Obsessional behaviour	• REM-Sleep 30% behaviour disorder • Vivid dreaming • Insomnia • Exessive daytime sleepiness	• Urinary 40% dysfunction • Sexual dysfunction • Orthostatic dysfunction • Sweating	• Constipa- 80% tion • Dysphagia • Hypersalivation	• Hyposmia 80% • Pain • Paraesthesia • Color/constrast discrimination

B Overview on non-motor symptoms according to the model of a prodromal phase in PD

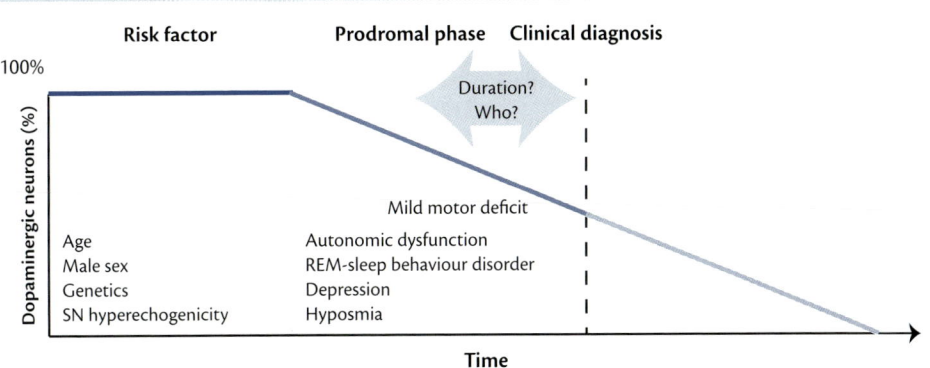

Figure 10.1A and 10.1B
Overview of non-motor symptoms (NMS) in Parkinson's disease (PD; A) and on NMS in association with the prodromal phase (B).

memory, language, and praxis have been listed as exclusion criteria for PD. With the latest knowledge about prevalence of these symptoms not only in the early stages but even before motor symptoms occur, a clearer definition of 'severe' or an alternate staging system of non-motor symptoms is necessary.

As some of these NMS such as hyposmia (16), constipation (17), depression (18), and RBD (19) precede the onset of the classic motor features at least in a subgroup of patients, they are referred to as prodromal markers indicating an already ongoing neurodegenerative process which has not reached a level sufficient enough to lead to the typical motor symptoms used in the clinical diagnostic criteria of PD (see Figure 10.1B). Although a number of studies describe the magnitude by which the risk for a later development of PD increases when a single marker is present, little is known about the effect on the risk of developing PD when a combination of markers occurs. Recent reports suggest that such a combination of various markers may be far more predictive of the risk of developing PD than one single marker alone (20-22). However, the sensitivity and specificity of these markers have not yet been sufficiently established for a reliable, cost-effective screening paradigm.

Genetics

The existence of more than one affected relative serves as an exclusion criterion for the diagnosis of PD, according to the currently used UK Brain Bank Criteria.

Since twin studies in the 1980s failed to find evidence of familial accumulation, genetic factors were thought to play a minor role in the pathogenesis of PD. It was only during the last 15 years that genes causative of monogenic forms of the disease were identified. To date, we know of 18 genes/loci (PARK1-18) causing either autosomal dominant or autosomal recessive forms of PD. Point mutations in the gene α-synuclein

(SNCA) as well as duplications and triplications of the wild-type gene are responsible for a dominant form of PD. The SNCA protein is known to be the major component of Lewy bodies and Lewy neuritis, the pathological hallmarks of PD (23). It therefore appears to play a central role in the pathogenesis of familial and sporadic PD as well as in other α-synucleinopathies. Mutations in the gene encoding leucine-rich repeat kinase 2 (LRRK2) seem to be the most frequent genetic cause of autosomal dominant PD, showing a prevalence of about 10% in familial cases, about 2% in the sporadic condition, and up to 40% in several ethnic populations, e.g. Ashkenazi Jews and North African Arabs (24). The clinical phenotype and imaging findings (TCS, MRI, SPECT, PET) mostly resemble those from sporadic PD patients without mutation, although there are some hints of a more benign, non-motor progression of cognitive and olfactory impairment in LRRK2-associated PD (25,26). Most patients show typical α-synuclein pathology at post-mortem. However, there are reports of patients with LRRK2 mutations who had nigral degeneration without Lewy pathology or with tau pathology at autopsy (27). It is still unclear whether these few patients with LRRK2 mutation exhibiting an akinetic-rigid disorder during life and showing tau-pathology at post-mortem should be classified as PD patients or rather as a different disease entity carrying a non-penetrant LRRK2 mutation accompanied by a coincidental sporadic tauopathy.

Several mutations in genes such as Parkin (PRKN), DJ-1, and PINK1 are known to cause early onset parkinsonism following an autosomal recessive pattern of inheritance. Because the phenotype of recessive PD is mostly that of dominant motor parkinsonian syndrome with less olfactory and autonomic impairment as well as rare dementia even after a long disease duration, the disease process underlying these recessive cases might differ from that of autosomal dominant cases (28,29). Most autopsy results in cases with Parkin mutations support this assumption, showing pure nigral degeneration without Lewy pathology (30). Although some cases have had Lewy bodies, these patients were mostly older than cases without Lewy bodies and could represent examples of incidental Lewy body disease (31). Conversely, the only case with a *PINK1* mutation reported at autopsy so far showed abundant Lewy pathology (32). Yet, there is evidence from cell and animal models that Parkin and *PINK1* act in the same molecular pathway in which *PINK1* deficiency can even be rescued by Parkin overexpression, suggesting loss-of-function mechanisms and neuroprotective effects of the wild-type products (33).

Moreover, there is increasing evidence that genetic variations are not only causative of monogenic forms of PD, they may also increase susceptibility to sporadic PD, which leads to the classification of genetic risk factors (34,35). Besides variations in the *SNCA* and *MAPT* genes, sequence alterations in the glucocerebrosidase (*GBA*) gene represent the most common genetic risk factor associated with sporadic PD so far (prevalence of 3% among sporadic PD patients) (36,37). Currently, great effort is being put into the evaluation of whether some of these variants also act as disease modifiers, possibly explaining the variety of the clinical phenotype with regard to disease progression and the characteristics of different NMS. Recent studies in sporadic PD patients report an association of non-coding variants in the *SNCA* gene with an earlier age at onset and a faster motor progression (38,39).

Since both monogenic and sporadic forms of PD share genetic influences, the 'more than one affected relative' item of the currently used UK Brain Bank Criteria seems outdated. Moreover, these genetic findings imply common pathogenic mechanisms and help to clarify the underlying pathophysiology since monogenetic and idiopathic forms tend to share many overlapping features that include, most importantly, parkinsonism with nigrostriatal dopaminergic degeneration. But how do mutations in closely related genes within the same signaling pathway

such as *Parkin* and *PINK1* then lead to different pathological characteristics? And should one be called Parkinson's disease but not the other? Owing to the complexity of genetics, grouping causative genes might be important: *SNCA* mutations might primarily result in misfolded protein aggregates; *Parkin*, *DJ1*, and *PINK1* mutations might be related to dysregulation of mitochondrial homeostasis (40). *GBA* is a lysosomal protein suggesting that lysosomal protein degradation is another important component (see Figure 10.2) (see also Chapter 16).

Imaging

Functional and structural imaging are not directly implemented in the clinical diagnostic criteria for PD but are listed as optional assessments to evaluate characteristics that point to an atypical or symptomatic form of parkinsonism as well as other differential diagnoses (see Table 10. 2).

The detection of nigrostriatal dysfunction with PET and SPECT has become an important supportive aid in the clinical diagnosis of PD (41,42). In contrast to findings obtained by clinical assessments, functional neuroimaging data might be more specific regarding the evaluation of a presynaptic dopaminergic dysfunction and might also be less influenced by compensatory mechanisms and could possibly enable an earlier diagnosis. This notion is supported by findings showing bilaterally reduced striatal dopaminergic activity in PD patients with purely unilateral clinical features (Hoehn and Yahr stage 1) and also by the report that mutation carriers of monogenetic forms of PD who do not show any motor symptoms have a reduced tracer uptake (43).

Additionally, evolving neuroimaging techniques visualizing structural changes of the nigrostriatal system might prove helpful to improve the diagnostic accuracy. Findings from these techniques include changes in diffusivity and frac-

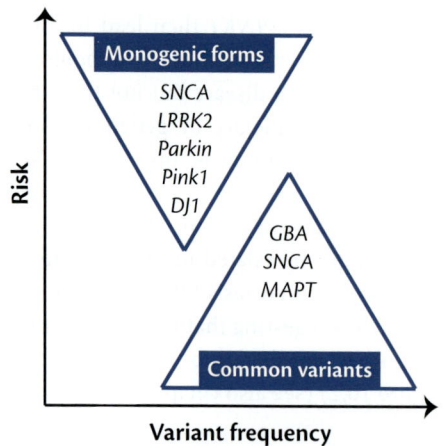

Gene	Comments
GBA	▪ Homozygousm utations cause Gaucher's disease ▪ Heterozygousm = risk factor for sporadic PD, OR 5.5 ▪ Heterozygousm utations = risk factor for DLB, OR 8
SNCA	▪ Point mutations/gene multiplication cause autosomal dominant PD ▪ Risk factor for sporadic PD, OR 1.5-2 ▪ Risk factor for MSA, OR 1.5
MAPT	▪ Mutations cause familial FTD ▪ Risk factor for sporadic PD ▪ Risk factor for PSP

	Gene	Locus	Inheritance	Onset	Clinical features
PARK1*	SNCA	4q21	AD	EO	▪ Similar to sporadic PD ▪ Cognitive/psychiatric impairment
PARK 2	PRKN	6q25	AR	EO	▪ Frequent dystonia at beginning ▪ Early dopa-induced fluctuations ▪ Slow progression
PARK 3	?	2p13	AD	LO	▪ Similar to idiopathic PD
PARK 4*	SNCA	4q21	AD	EO	▪ More severe disease progression, dementia, dysautonomia in triplications
PARK 5	UCHLI	4p14	AD	LO	▪ Similar to idiopathic PD
PARK 6	PINK1	1p35	AR	EO	▪ Slow disease progression
PARK 7	DJ-1	1p36	AR	EO	▪ Slow disease progression
PARK 8	LRRK2	12q12	AD	LO	▪ Similar to idiopathic PD
PARK 9	ATP13AZ	1p36	AR	EO	▪ Parkinsonism ▪ Pyramidal degeneration ▪ Supranuclear gaze palsy ▪ Cognitive dysfunction
PARK 10	?	1p32	AD	LO	▪ Similar to idiopathic PD
PARK 11	GIGYF2 ?	2q36	AD	LO	▪ Similar to idiopathic PD
PARK 12	?	Xq	?	LO	
PARK 13	OMI/HTRA2	2p13	AD	LO	▪ Similar to idiopathic PD
PARK 14	PLA2G6	22q13.1	AR	EO	▪ Dystonia ▪ Parkinsonism ▪ Pyramidal signs ▪ Cognitive impairment
PARK 15	FBXO7	22q12	AR	EO	▪ Parkinsonian-pyramidal syndrome (PPS)
PARK 16	?	1q32	Risk factor		
PARK 17	VPS35		AD	LO	▪ Similar to idiopathic PD
PARK 18	EIF4G1		AD	LO	▪ Similar to idiopathic PD

tional anisotropy of the SN and the striatum on diffusion-tensor imaging (DTI) MRI as well as changes in SN morphology on high-field MRI (see also Chapter 45) (42,44,45).

Substantia nigra hyperechogenicity assessed by transcranial sonography might be useful as a trait marker because it has been found in over 90% of patients with early PD and in asymptomatic carriers of mutations in *LRRK2*, *Parkin*, and *PINK1* as well as in individuals at risk for sporadic PD (46-48). Moreover, a possible contribution to an early, even premotor diagnosis of PD has been demonstrated lately by a large, multicenter, prospective trial (see also Chapter 45) (47,49).

Still, limitations are associated with each of these technical approaches: none of the functional or structural abnormalities defined so far are fully specific for PD, and we still do not know at what time point they occur in the early disease process. Moreover, none of these methods assay the basic cellular/biological changes such as α-synuclein pathology.

Pathology

> Progressive degeneration of dopaminergic neurons in the SNc accompanied by an accumulation of eosinophilic intracytoplasmic protein inclusions which mainly consist of α-synuclein and are known as Lewy bodies and Lewy neurites represent the pathological hallmarks of sporadic as well as familial PD. This histological finding is the current gold standard for PD diagnosis.

However, the notion that PD is a synucleinopathy with Lewy pathology predominantly affect-

ing the nigrostriatal system has been challenged by the following findings. First, Lewy pathology is not restricted to the dopaminergic nigrostriatal system. Rather, it is widespread with aggregates in cholinergic neurons of the nucleus basalis of Meynert, norepinephrine neurons of the locus ceruleus, serotonin neurons of the raphe nucleus, the olfactory system, the cerebral hemispheres, the upper and lower brainstem, the spinal cord, and the peripheral nervous system (see Chapter 15) (50). Braak and colleagues hypothesized that neurons are affected in a sequential and ascending manner, with dopamine cells becoming involved in the mid-stages of the disease (51). Although this hypothesis does not hold true for all cases of PD (e.g. some individuals in the prodromal non-motor phase develop cognitive decline before clinical parkinsonism, and others with pronounced Lewy pathology in the SNc do not have evidence of lower brainstem involvement), there is growing clinical and pathological evidence for the involvement of caudal brainstem structures prior to the involvement of the SN in a large proportion of cases (50).

Second, Lewy pathology also occurs in healthy individuals. At least 17% of 744 deceased individuals in a recent study (mean age at death 88.5 years) who had had global parkinsonism but did not fulfill the UK Brain Bank Criteria had Lewy pathology (i.e. incidental Lewy body disease, ILB) (52). Using a linear regression model including nigral neuronal loss and Lewy pathology as variables, only neuronal loss was significantly associated with mild parkinsonian signs, but not Lewy pathology. The authors concluded that neuronal loss mediates the association of Lewy bodies with global parkinsonism and, indirectly, that Lewy pathology alone is not suf-

Figure 10.2
Overview of monogenic forms of Parkinson's disease and risk factors associated with sporadic Parkinson's disease.
* Initially, PARK1 and PARK4 were assigned to different regions on chromosome 4 but were later assigned to the same locus. AD = autosomal dominant; AR = autsomal recessive; EO = early onset; LO = late onset. DLB = Lewy body dementia; FTD = frontotemporal dementia; *GBA* = glucocerebrosidase; *LRRK2* = leucine-rich repeat kinase 2; *MAPT* = microtubule-associated protein tau; MSA = multisystem atrophy; *PINK1* = PTEN-induced putative kinase 1; PSP = progressive supranuclear palsy; SNCA = α-synuclein.

Table 10.2
Overview of clinical and imaging characteristics in differential diagnosis of Parkinson's disease (PD).

Parkinsonian subtypes	Clinical characteristics next to parkinsonism	Funtional imaging characteristics			Morphological imaging characteristics	
		Presynaptic e.g. DATScan	Postsynaptic e.g. IBZM SPECT	PET e.g. Glucose	MRI	TCS
Sporadic PD	▪ Unilateral beginning ▪ Good dopa response	▪ Asymmetric presynaptic dopamine transporter deficit	▪ Mainly normal ▪ In early stages up-regulation, ▪ In later stages down-regulation possible	▪ Asymmetric hypometabolism of the putamen	▪ Normal	▪ Hyperechogenic SN
Atypical						
DLB	▪ Dementia within first year or even preceding parkinsonism ▪ Prominent hallucinations ▪ Fluctuations of alertness	▪ Presynaptic dopamine transporter deficit	▪ Mainly normal	▪ Parieto-occipital hypometabolism	▪ No clear findings ▪ Unspecific atrophy in later stages	▪ Hyperechogenic SN with no or hardly any side-predominance ▪ Enlarged ventricles in later stages
MSA	▪ Antecollis ▪ Severe autonomic impairment in early stages ▪ Pyramidal and cerebellar symptoms ▪ Little dopa response	▪ Some presynaptic dopamine transporter deficit	▪ Predominant Postsynaptic receptor deficit	▪ Hypometabolism of putamen, brain stem, cerebellum	▪ T2: Hot-cross-bun sign of pons ▪ T2: Hyperintense band between putamen and intern capsula	▪ Hyperechogenic basal ganglia, usually normal SN
PSP	▪ Often symmetric akinesia ▪ Early postural instability and dementia ▪ Supranuclear gaze palsy ▪ Little dopa response	▪ Some presynaptic dopamine transporter deficit	▪ Predominant postsynaptic receptor deficit	▪ Hypometabolism of putamen and caudate nucleus	▪ Mickey Mouse sign ▪ Hummingbird sign	▪ Hyperechogenic basal ganglia ▪ Enlarged 3th ventricle ▪ Sometimes SN hyperechogenicity
FTD	▪ Behavioural changes ▪ Affect lability ▪ No dopa response	▪ No data available	▪ No data available	▪ Marked fronto-temporal Hypometabolism	▪ Fronto-temporal atrophy	▪ Enlarged ventricles

CBD	▪ Unilateral impairment ▪ Pyramidal symptoms ▪ Myoclonus ▪ Alien limb phenomenon ▪ Apraxia ▪ Poor dopa response	▪ Some asymmetric presynaptic dopamine transporter deficit	▪ Asymmetric postsynaptic receptor deficit	▪ Asymmetric fronto-parietal hypometabolism (contralateral to the clinical impairment)	▪ Asymmetric fronto-parietal atrophy (contralateral to the clinical impairment)	▪ Marked hyperechogenic SN with clear side-predominance. ▪ In later stages enlarged ventricular system
Symptomatic						
Vascular	▪ Lower body parkinsonism	▪ Normal	▪ Normal		▪ Vascular lesions	▪ Normal SN echogenicity
Medication Encephalitis Tumor	▪ Symptoms according to location	▪ Normal	▪ Normal		▪ No generalizable findings	▪ Normal SN echogenicity
Other differential diagnosis						
Wilson's disease	▪ Psychiatric impairment ▪ Dystonia ▪ Kayser-Fleischer corneal ring ▪ Classic copper associated biochemistry	▪ Normal	▪ Postsynaptic receptor deficit	▪ Hypometabolism of the basal ganglia	▪ T2: hyperintense signal of the basal ganglia (gliosis) next to hypointense signal (copper)	▪ Hyperechogenic lentiform nucleus
Fahr's disease	▪ Parkinsonism ▪ Possible ataxia ▪ Possible dystonia ▪ Wide spectrum of symptoms possible	▪ Depending on involvement of basal ganglia	▪ Depending on involvement of basal ganglia	▪ Hypometabolism of the basal ganglia	▪ Calcification of basal ganglia and dentate nucleus	▪ Hyperechogenic basal ganglia
SCA2/3	▪ Parkinsonism ▪ Ataxia and other cerebellar dysfunctions	▪ Presynaptic dopamine transporter deficit	▪ Normal	▪ Cerebellar and brainstem hypometabolism	▪ Cerebellar and brainstem atrophy	▪ Hyperechogenic basal ganglia ▪ Enlarged 4th ventricle
Normal pressure hydrocephalus	▪ Gait impairment ▪ Dementia ▪ Incontinence	▪ Normal	▪ Normal	▪ Normal	▪ Enlarged ventricles	▪ Enlarged ventricles

CBD = corticobasal degeneration; DLB = Lewy Body dementia; FTD = frontotemporal dementia; MSA = multisystem atrophy; PD = Parkinson's disease; PSP = progressive supranuclear palsy; SCA = spinocerebellar ataxia; S N = substantia nigra.

ficient to induce these clinical signs (52). Incidental Lewy body disease might have evolved into clinical PD if the individuals had lived long enough. However, if short lifespan is the primary reason for not developing a PD phenotype in cases of incidental Lewy body disease, the incidence of PD in those over 85 years old should be substantially higher than in young elderly people (60–85 years), which is not the case (53). Thus, these findings challenge the notion that Lewy pathology is necessary and sufficient for PD pathogenesis.

Third, the specific effects of Lewy pathology remain uncertain (see also Chapter 15). Some researchers argue that Lewy bodies and Lewy neurites are the consequence of a protective mechanism to deal with misfolded proteins (54). In fact, there is evidence from recent studies of patients assessed post-mortem that substantial neurodegeneration and cellular dysfunction precede the occurrence of Lewy bodies and Lewy neurites in the SN (55). Moreover, presynaptic accumulation of α-synuclein leads to retraction of postsynaptic dendritic spines and neuronal dysfunction in both patients with PD and those with dementia with Lewy bodies (DLB), which might be correlated with, and thus explain, the clinical symptoms of PD better than Lewy pathology (56,57). In addition, Lewy pathology is not always present in patients diagnosed with PD. Some patients with specific genetic forms of PD do not show Lewy pathology, such as most carriers of *Parkin* mutations and some with *LRRK2* mutations (58,59) (see above). However, despite uncertainty about the role of Lewy pathology, it can be found in most patients with PD. Furthermore, there is much to learn from the finding that α-synuclein pathology can develop in previously healthy embryonic dopaminergic neurons transplanted into the brain of patients with PD and that, at least in an animal model, α-synuclein pathology can be transmitted to anatomically interconnected regions (60,61).

Biomaterial

In contrast to Alzheimer's disease, there are no biochemical markers available in PD so far.

Biomarkers which specifically mark the onset of the neurodegenerative process and also measure disease progression are desperately needed in order to improve the early detection/diagnosis and to predict disease progression. Such markers should also reflect the major pathological features underlying PD, be easily applicable, and allow for a serial examination in an individual. The identification and validation of biochemical markers that can identify molecular pathological abnormalities will contribute tremendously to a better understanding of the pathogenesis, which is the basis for disease-modulating therapy or even neuroprotection.

Summary

Recent advances in research are expanding our understanding of PD and suggest that new criteria for the diagnosis are needed. However, the redefinition of PD and consequently the development of new diagnostic criteria are hampered by:

(i) the complexity and heterogeneity in genetics, phenotypes, and underlying molecular mechanisms
(ii) the absence of biochemical markers or the ability to visualize PD-specific histopathological changes with imaging modalities
(iii) the long prodromal period during which non-motor manifestations might precede classic motor manifestations
(iv) the uncertainty about the status of disorders diagnosed clinically as PD without post-mortem Lewy pathology.

Diagnostic criteria should include new findings. Although the great value of the UK Brain Bank Criteria must be acknowledged, it also needs to serious reconsider aspects such as more than

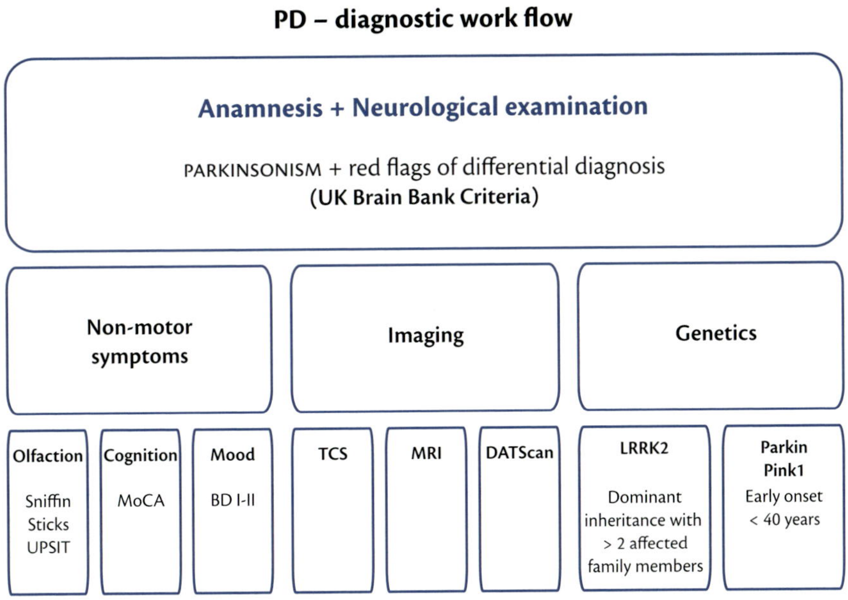

PD – diagnostic work flow

Figure 10.3
Suggestion for a PD-related diagnostic work flow.
BDI-II = Beck Depression Inventory II; MoCA = Montreal Cognitive Assessment; UPSIT = University of Pennsylvania Smell Identification Test.

one affected family member or NMS like autonomic dysfunction and dementia as exclusion criteria (see Figure 10.3). The Movement Disorders Society commissioned a task force to consider a redefinition of PD which might form the basis for creating new diagnostic criteria for PD.

References

1 Hughes AJ, Daniel SE, Lees AJ. Improved accuracy of clinical diagnosis of Lewy body Parkinson's disease. Neurology 2001;57:1497-1499.

2 Louis ED, Bennett DA. Mild Parkinsonian signs: An overview of an emerging concept. Mov Disord 2007;22:1681-1688.

3 Buchman AS, Shulman JM, Nag S, et al. Nigral pathology and parkinsonian signs in elders without Parkinson disease. Ann Neurol 2012;71:258-266.

4 Uemura Y, Wada-Isoe K, Nakashita S, Nakashima K. Mild parkinsonian signs in a community-dwelling elderly population sample in Japan. J Neurol Sci 2011;304:61-66.

5 Lost D, Tang MX, Schupf N, Mayeux R. Functional correlates and prevalence of mild parkinsonian signs in a community population of older people. ArchNeurol 2005;62:297-302.

6 Buchman AS, Nag S, Shulman JM, et al. Locus coeruleus neuron density and parkinsonism in older adults without Parkinson's disease. Mov Disord 2012; 27:1625-31.

7 Adler CH, Connor DJ, Hentz JG, et al. Incidental Lewy body disease: clinical comparison to a control cohort. Mov Disord 2010;25:642-646.

8 Ross GW, Petrovitch H, Abbott RD, et al. Parkinsonian signs and substantia nigra neuron density in decendents elders without PD. Annals of Neurology 2004;56:532-539.

9 Bennett DA, Beckett LA, Murray AM, et al. Prevalence of parkinsonian signs and associated mortality in a community population of older people. The New England journal of medicine 1996;334:71-76.

10 Fearnley JM, Lees AJ. Ageing and Parkinson's disease: substantia nigra regional selectivity. Brain 1991;114:2283-2301.

11 Bezard E, Gross CE, Brotchie JM. Presymptomatic compensation in Parkinson's disease is not dopamine-mediated. Trends Neurosci 2003;26:215-221.

12 Postuma RB, Lang AE, Gagnon JF, Pelletier A, Montplaisir JY. How does parkinsonism start? Prodromal parkinsonism motor changes in idiopathic REM sleep behaviour disorder. Brain 2012;135:1860-1870.

13 Mirelman A, Gurevich T, Giladi N, Bar-Shira A, Orr-Urtreger A, Hausdorff JM. Gait alterations in healthy carriers of the LRRK2 G2019S mutation. Annals of Neurology 2011;69:193-197.

14 Maetzler W, Mancini M, Liepelt-Scarfone I, et al. Impaired trunk stability in individuals at high risk for Parkinson's disease. PLoS One 2012 ;7:e32240.

15 Chaudhuri KR, Schapira AH. Non-motor symptoms of Parkinson's disease: dopaminergic pathophysiology and treatment. Lancet Neurol 2009;8:464-474.

16 Ross GW, Petrovitch H, Abbott RD, et al. Association of olfactory dysfunction with risk for future Parkinson's disease. Annals of neurology 2008;63:167-173.

17 Tolosa E, Compta Y, Gaig C. The premotor phase of Parkinson's disease. Parkinsonism Relat Disord 2007;13S:S2-7.

18 Leentjens AF, Van den Akker M, Metsemakers JF, Lousberg R, Verhey FR. Higher incidence of depression preceding the onset of Parkinson's disease: a register study. Mov Disord 2003;18:414-418.

19 Iranzo A, Molinuevo JL, Santamaria J, et al. Rapid-eye-movement sleep behaviour disorder as an early marker for a neurodegenerative disorder: a descriptive study. Lancet Neurol 2006;5:572-577.

20 Liepelt I, Behnke S, Schweitzer K, et al. Pre-motor signs of PD are related to SN hyperechogenicity assessed by TCS in an elderly population. Neurobiol Aging 2011;32:1599-1606.

21 Berg D, Poewe W. Can we define 'pre-motor' Parkinson's disease? Mov Disord 2012;27:595-596.

22 Postuma RB, Gagnon JF. Symmetry of Parkinson's disease and REM sleep: one piece of the puzzle. Annals of Neurology 2011;69:905; author reply 906.

23 Spillantini MG, Schmidt ML, Lee VM, Trojanowski JQ, Jakes R, Goedert M. Alpha-synuclein in Lewy bodies. Nature 1997;388:839-840.

24 Lesage S, Brice A. Parkinson's disease: from monogenic forms to genetic susceptibility factors. Human molecular genetics 2009;18(R1):R48-59.

25 Healy DG, Falchi M, O'Sullivan SS, et al. Phenotype, genotype, and worldwide genetic penetrance of LRRK2-associated Parkinson's disease: a case-control study. Lancet Neurol 2008;7:583-590.

26 Brockmann K, Groger A, Di Santo A, et al. Clinical and brain imaging characteristics in leucine-rich repeat kinase 2-associated PD and asymptomatic mutation carriers. Mov Disord 2011;26:2335-2342.

27 Hasegawa K, Stoessl AJ, Yokoyama T, Kowa H, Wszolek ZK, Yagishita S. Familial parkinsonism: study of original Sagamihara PARK8 (I2020T) kindred with variable clinicopathologic outcomes. Parkinsonism Relat Disord 2009;15:300-306.

28 Lucking CB, Durr A, Bonifati V, et al. Association between early-onset Parkinson's disease and mutations in the parkin gene. The New England journal of medicine 2000;342:1560-1567.

29 Valente EM, Bentivoglio AR, Dixon PH, et al. Localization of a novel locus for autosomal recessive early-onset parkinsonism, PARK6, on human chromosome 1p35-p36. Am J Hum Genet 2001;6:895-900.

30 van de Warrenburg BP, Lammens M, Lucking CB, et al. Clinical and pathologic abnormalities in a family with parkinsonism and parkin gene mutations. Neurology 2001;56:555-557.

31 Farrer M, Chan P, Chen R, et al. Lewy bodies and parkinsonism in families with parkin mutations. Annals of Neurology 2001;50:293-300.

32 Samaranch L, Lorenzo-Betancor O, Arbelo JM, et al. PINK1-linked parkinsonism is associated with Lewy body pathology. Brain 2010;133:1128-1142.

33 Park J, Lee SB, Lee S, et al. Mitochondrial dysfunction in Drosophila PINK1 mutants is complemented by parkin. Nature 2006;441:1157-1161.

34 Nalls MA, Plagnol V, Hernandez DG, et al. Imputation of sequence variants for identification of genetic risks for Parkinson's disease: a meta-analysis of genome-wide association studies. Lancet 2011;377:641-649.

35 Sharma M, Ioannidis JP, Aasly JO, et al. Large-scale replication and heterogeneity in Parkinson disease genetic loci. Neurology 2012;79:659-667.

36 Simon-Sanchez J, Schulte C, Bras JM, et al. Ge-
    nome-wide association study reveals genetic risk
    underlying Parkinson's disease. Nature genetics
    2009;41:1308-1312.

37 Sidransky E, Nalls MA, Aasly JO, et al. Multicenter
    analysis of glucocerebrosidase mutations in Parkin-
    son's disease. The New England journal of medicine
    2009;361:1651-1661.

38 Brockmann K, Schulte C, Hauser AK, et al. SNCA:
    Major genetic modifier of age at onset of Parkinson's
    disease. Mov Disord 2013;28:1217-1221.

39 Ritz B, Rhodes SL, Bordelon Y, Bronstein J. al-
    pha-Synuclein genetic variants predict faster motor
    symptom progression in idiopathic Parkinson dis-
    ease. PLoS One 2012;7:e36199.

40 Hardy J. Genetic analysis of pathways to Parkinson
    disease. Neuron 2010;68:201-206.

41 Stoessl AJ. Neuroimaging in Parkinson's disease.
    Neurotherapeutics 2011;8:72-81.

42 Stoessl AJ, Martin WW, McKeown MJ, Sossi V.
    Advances in imaging in Parkinson's disease. Lancet
    Neurol 2011;10:987-1001.

43 Piccini P, Burn DJ, Ceravolo R, Maraganore D,
    Brooks DJ. The role of inheritance in sporadic
    Parkinson's disease: evidence from a longitudinal
    study of dopaminergic function in twins. Annals of
    Neurology 1999;45:577-582.

44 Cho ZH, Oh SH, Kim JM, et al. Direct visualization
    of Parkinson's disease by in vivo human brain im-
    aging using 7.0T magnetic resonance imaging. Mov
    Disord 2011;26:713-718.

45 Kwon DH, Kim JM, Oh SH, et al. Seven-Tes-
    la magnetic resonance images of the substantia
    nigra in Parkinson disease. Annals of Neurology
    2012;71:267-277.

46 Berg D, Godau J, Walter U. Transcranial sonography
    in movement disorders. Lancet Neurol 2008;7:1044-
    1055.

47 Berg D, Seppi K, Behnke S, et al. Enlarged substan-
    tia nigra hyperechogenicity and risk for Parkinson
    disease: a 37-month 3-center study of 1847 older
    persons. Archives of Neurology 2011;68:932-937.

48 Brockmann K, Hagenah J. TCS in monogenic
    forms of Parkinson's disease. Int Rev Neurobiol
    2010;90:157-164.

49 Berg D, Behnke S, Seppi K, et al. Enlarged hyper-
    echogenic substantia nigra as a risk marker for
    Parkinson's disease. Mov Disord 2013;28:216-219.

50 Goedert M, Spillantini MG, Del Tredici K, Braak
    H. 100 years of Lewy pathology. Nat Rev Neurol
    2013;9:13-24.

51 Braak H, Del Tredici K, Rub U, de Vos RA, Jansen
    Steur EN, Braak E. Staging of brain pathology relat-
    ed to sporadic Parkinson's disease. Neurobiol Aging
    2003;24:197-211.

52 Buchman AS, Shulman JM, Nag S, et al. Ni-
    gral pathology and parkinsonian signs in elders
    without Parkinson disease. Annals of Neurology
    2012;71:258-266.

53 Perez F, Helmer C, Dartigues JF, Auriacombe S,
    Tison F. A 15-year population-based cohort study of
    the incidence of Parkinson's disease and dementia
    with Lewy bodies in an elderly French cohort. J
    Neurol Neurosurg Psychiatry 2010;81:742-746.

54 Olanow CW, Perl DP, DeMartino GN, McNaught
    KS. Lewy-body formation is an aggresome-related
    process: a hypothesis. Lancet Neurol 2004;3:496-
    503.

55 Milber JM, Noorigian JV, Morley JF, et al. Lewy
    pathology is not the first sign of degeneration in
    vulnerable neurons in Parkinson disease. Neurology
    2012;79:2307-2314.

56 Kramer ML, Schulz-Schaeffer WJ. Presynaptic
    alpha-synuclein aggregates, not Lewy bodies, cause
    neurodegeneration in dementia with Lewy bodies. J
    Neurosci 2007;27:1405-1410.

57 Schulz-Schaeffer WJ. The synaptic pathology of
    alpha-synuclein aggregation in dementia with Lewy
    bodies, Parkinson's disease and Parkinson's disease
    dementia. Acta Neuropathol 2010;120:131-143.

58 Hattori N, Shimura H, Kubo S, et al. Autosomal re-
    cessive juvenile parkinsonism: a key to understand-
    ing nigral degeneration in sporadic Parkinson's
    disease. Neuropathology 2000;20S:S85-90.

59 Marti-Masso JF, Ruiz-Martinez J, Bolano MJ, et
    al. Neuropathology of Parkinson's disease with
    the R1441G mutation in LRRK2. Mov Disord
    2009;24:1998-2001.

60 Kordower JH, Chu Y, Hauser RA, Freeman TB,
    Olanow CW. Lewy body-like pathology in long-

term embryonic nigral transplants in Parkinson's disease. Nature medicine 2008;14:504-506.

61 Luk KC, Kehm V, Carroll J, et al. Pathological al-pha-synuclein transmission initiates Parkinson-like neurodegeneration in nontransgenic mice. Science 2012;338:949-953.

11

Conventional Treatment in Parkinson's Disease

Jay A. van Gerpen

The symptoms of Parkinson's disease (PD) can be improved by different treatment strategies. Seminal observations have indicated that PD is associated with dopamine deficiency in the striatum secondary to the loss of dopaminergic input from the substantia nigra (1,2). Therefore, early targeted treatment involves oral dopamine replenishment in the form of levodopa plus a dopa-decarboxylase inhibitor (3,4). This therapy has enabled PD patients to have impressive, sustained improvement in bradykinesia, tremor, rigidity and quality of life for over 40 years (5,6). Furthermore, the recognition that PD is not merely a disorder affecting dopaminergic neurons and motor function (7) has widened the focus of PD treatment to include autonomic dysfunction, sleep-wake disorders, mood and perceptual disturbances, and cognitive impairment (8-11). Yet, despite this progress, neuroprotective or even curative therapies remain an elusive goal (12). However, accumulating evidence indicates that physical and cognitive exercise can directly affect the progression of PD and other neurodegenerative disorders (13-17).

This chapter will include information regarding currently available pharmacological treatments for PD, as well as a brief overview of agents under investigation. In addition, other modes of therapy will be described. The first section will cover dopaminergic and ancillary pharmacological treatment options for PD. The second section will describe complementary, alternative strat-egies for PD management including physical and cognitive exercise and repetitive transcranial magnetic stimulation (rTMS). Treatment for PD-related autonomic, neuropsychiatric and sleep disorders as well as deep brain stimulation (DBS) and continuous dopamine receptor stimulation (CDS) will be covered in chapters 7, 8, 9, 13 and 14, respectively.

Levodopa

Levodopa is the precursor to the neurotransmitters dopamine, norepinephrine (noradrenaline), and epinephrine (adrenaline) and is still the most effective pharmacological treatment overall for motor impairment of PD (5,6,18,19). Common non-motor symptoms in PD are listed in Figure 11.1. Although their treatment will be discussed in chapters 7 and 8, it is important to note that many of them are 'off' phenomena (e.g., pain and anxiety) and readily respond to dopaminergic therapy (20,22).

After oral intake and gastric passage, levodopa is absorbed from the duodenum. Unlike dopamine, levodopa crosses the blood-brain barrier and utilizes large, neutral amino acid transporters. It is then transported to the nigrostriatal nerve terminals where it is converted to dopamine (Figure 11.2) (20). To prevent the conversion of levodopa to dopamine in the periphery, it is combined with a decarboxylase inhibitor. Carbidopa and benzerazide are both decarbo-

Nonmotor Features of PD

Sensory
- Pain-may be radicular, musculoskeletal, central, or dystonia related
- Paresthesias
- Akathisia
- Restless Leg Syndrom

Cognitive-psychiatric
- Dementia
- Psychosis-hallucinations, delusions
- Anxiety/panic
- Depression
- Hypomania/mania
- Moaning/screaming
- Hypersexuality

Sleep
- Insomnia
- Excessive daytime somnolence

Autonomic
- Cardiovascular-tachycardia, hypotension
- Gastrointestinal-constipation, bloating, belching, dysphagia, sialorrhea
- Genitourinary-urinary frequency, urgency, incontinence, erectile dysfunction
- Dermatological-pallor, sweating, skin temperature changes

Respiratory
- Dyspnea

Figure 11.1
Non-motor features of PD.

xylase inhibitors, applied worldwide except that benserazide is not available in the USA (21).

The use of the decarboxylase inhibitors greatly increases the amount of levodopa that crosses the blood-brain barrier (BBB). By reducing serum dopamine levels, this minimizes the nausea that is produced by dopaminergic stimulation of the area postrema in the medulla, which lacks a BBB (20). A robust, sustained response to levo-dopa is highly indicative of a diagnosis of PD, and the converse is also true (18-20).

Formulations

Levodopa is available in a number of formulations, including immediate-release and extended-release versions. Although 10 mg of carbidopa combined with 100 mg levodopa (10/100) is available in the US, many clinicians utilize the 25/100 formulation to decrease nausea. Additionally, because of the erratic absorption of the extended-release carbidopa/levodopa (C/L), many physicians opt for immediate-release 25/100 C/L. A commonly utilized titration schedule is detailed in Figure 11.3 (22).

Extended-release C/L may be a useful bedtime adjunct when a longer efficacy during the night is desired, and can be helpful in advanced PD patients with diminished dopaminergic storage capacity, i.e. when the duration of the beneficial effect of levodopa diminishes (20). Combined use of C/L with a dopamine agonist (DA) or with monoamine oxidase type-B (MAO-B) inhibitor or catechol-O-methyltransferase (COMT) inhibitor (which further inhibits the peripheral metabolism of levodopa) (see Figure 11.2) may also be helpful in advanced PD patients with 'wearing-off' (20). Continuous intra-duodenal infusion of levodopa/carbidopa intestinal gel (LCIG) is a valuable escalation therapy for PD patients with levodopa-dependent motor fluctuations significantly lacking CNS dopamine storage capacity, to arrange for more stable levodopa serum and CNS levels (see Chapter 14) (20).

Initiation

When to initiate symptomatic, pharmacological therapy in PD patients and which agent to use have been controversial topics for many years. Given that no currently available medication conclusively provides neuroprotection in PD (i.e., retards the progression of neurodegeneration) (12) and that levodopa is demonstrably not neurotoxic (23), a reasonable approach

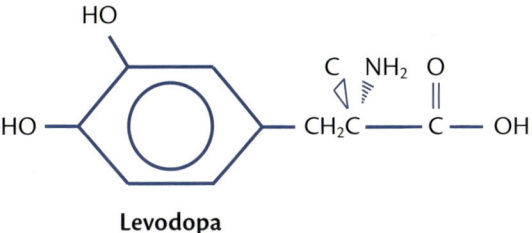

Levodopa

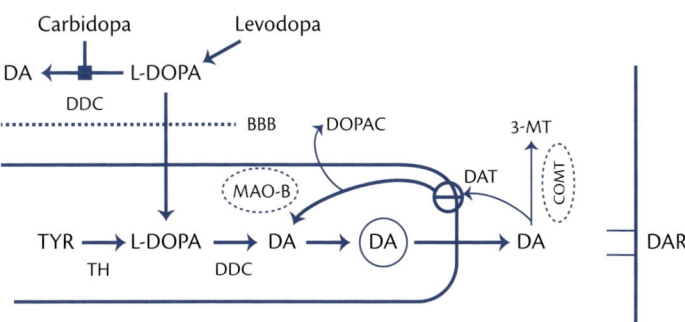

Figure 11.2

Schematic diagram of DA biosynthesis in a nigrostriatal nerve terminal. The rate-limiting enzyme, tyrosine hydroxylase (TH), converts the dietary amino acid tyrosine (TYR) into levodopa (L-DOPA). L-DOPA is then converted into dopamine (DA) by dopa-decarboxylase (DDC). DA is stored in vesicle for release into the synaptic cleft where it can be activated postsynaptic dopamine receptors (DARs). DA may be brought back into the presynaptic nerve terminal via the dopamine transporter (DaT) or may be metabolized by mitochondria monoamine oxidase type B (MAO-B) or catechol-O-methyltransferase (COMT) into 3,4-dihydroxyphenylacetic acid (DOPAC) or 3-methoxytyramine (3-MT), respectively. Peripheral DDC-mediated catabolism of levodopa is blocked by co-administration of carbidopa, thus allowing appreciable amounts of levodopa to pass across the blood brain barrier and enter the presynaptic nerve terminal where it may be enzymatically converted into DA.

significant consideration in medication choice (24).

Complications

Chronic levodopa use may elevate homocysteine levels. Theoretically, this could render patients more susceptible to vascular disease, cognitive impairment, and peripheral neuropathy (20). Therefore, periodically testing a C/L-treated patient's serum for abnormalities in homocysteine, vitamins B12 and B6, and methylmalonic acid levels should be considered. If any of these are abnormally altered, treatment with oral folate, vitamin B6 and B12 would be appropriate.

Common non-motor complications of PD are listed in Figure 11.1. Although their treatment will be discussed elsewhere in this book, it is important to note that many of them are 'off' phenomena (e.g., pain and anxiety) and readily respond to dopaminergic therapy (20,22).

is to discuss with the patient whether their PD symptoms (motor or otherwise) are sufficiently troublesome to adversely affect their daily living, and if so, to recommend medication. Other than levodopa, arguably the main choice is a DA (19). These alternative agents will be discussed below. Primary considerations include weighing the risk of levodopa-induced dyskinesias (LIDs), which are the subject of Chapter 12, against the lower efficacy and higher likelihood of various side effects with dopamine agonist treatment. Given that clinically significant LIDs are common in patients under the age of 40 and far less so in those over 60, the patient's age can be a

Dopamine Agonists

Dopamine agonists (DA) may or may not be ergot-derived. Ergot-derived DAs include bromocriptine, pergolide, cabergoline, and lisuride. Given that numerous studies have demonstrated that these agents may induce life-threatening inflammatory-fibrotic reactions of tissues with serosal membranes, including heart valves and lung pleura (25, 26), their use is discouraged; hence, they will not be discussed further in this chapter.

Dose Escalation, Carbidopa/Levodopa (25/100 immediate-release tablets)

Start with the low dose, below, and increase weekly, guided by your response. If a dose markedly improves your parkinsonian symtomps (walking difficulties, tremor, slowness, stiffness, etc.), you can continue taking that dose. Otherwise continue to escalate, up to 2½ to 3 tablets each dose. Ultimately, if several doses are equally beneficial, choose to continue taking the lowest of those equally effective doses.

Proteins in your diet may prevent absorption of levodopa; thus, the best response occurs if carbidopa/levodopa is taken on an empty stomach. Conventionally, this is done ty taking each of the 3 doses **1 or more hours before each meal**. Obviously, if you skip a meal, you can take that dose when convenient

Week 1 Start with one 25/100 carbidopa/levodopa tablet 3 times per day.

Week 2 Increase to 1½ tablets 3 times per day.

Week 3 If necessary, increase again to 2 tablets 3 times per day. For most, this dose is at the point of diminishing returns.

Option, Week 5 If there is not substantial improvement on the above dosage, you can try 1 more increment to 3 tablets 3 times per day.

Again, if several dose produce the same degree of benefit, settle on the lowest of these.

For patient with no improvement with any of the doses: You can reverse this process, decreasing your dosage every few days down to zero, or whatever dose seems to be providing benefit.

Figure 11.3
Example of a patient handout, outlining carbidopa/levodopa initiation and escalation.

Dopamine receptors

Dopamine receptors are divided into five types: D1-D5. D1 and D5 stimulate the adenylate cyclase pathway, whereas D2, D3, and D4 inhibit it (27). D1 and D2 receptors are heavily concentrated in the striatum, while D3 receptors are primarily located in mesolimbic structures, such as the nucleus accumbens (27). The major motor effects of dopamine agonists are thought to arise from D2 stimulation; however, D1 stimulation works in concert with D2 stimulation to mediate motor activity (27). DAs primarily stimulate D2 and D3 receptors and have much longer half-lives than levodopa (27). These characteristics likely contribute to the common effects of DAs. They are less likely to induce dyskinesias than levodopa, possibly because of less pulsatile dopamine receptor stimulation (28). On the other hand, these compounds are less potent at alleviating the motor impairment of PD (18-20). In addition, as discussed in chapter 12, DAs are more commonly associated with troublesome neuropsychiatric side effects including hallucinations, psychosis, and impulse control disorders than levodopa. The latter include pathological gambling, binge eating, compulsive shopping and hypersexuality, and related behaviours including punding and dopamine dysregulation syndrome (Chapter 41) (29-31). Furthermore, DA may also induce excessive daytime sleepiness including 'sleep attacks' (32), orthostatic hypotension, and pedal edema (20).

Types

Currently, the most widely distributed DAs include pramipexole and ropinirole, which are available in both immediate release and prolonged release oral formulations. Additionally, rotigotine is available as a transdermal patch, and apomorphine is available as a subcutaneous injection (Figure 11.4). As noted above, a DA may be used as the initial symptomatic therapy in PD, particularly in younger and otherwise healthy patients (24).

Characteristics of Clinically Available Non-Ergot Derived

	Metabolism	Half-Life	Therapeutic Dose (mg/Day)	High Dose (mg)	Titration (weekly)
Pramipexole	Renal	8-12 h	1.5-4.5	6	0.125 mg t.i.d. then 0.25 mg t.i.d. then 0.5 mg t.i.d.
Ropinirole	Hepatic	6 h	3-24	18-34	0.25 mg t.i.d. until 3 mg then 0.5 mg t.i.d.
Apomorphine	Hepatic	35 min	98	>100	–
Rotigotine	Renal	5-7 h (transdermal)	4-6	24	2mg/24 h

Figure 11.4
Characteristics of clinically available non-ergot derived DAs.

Use of DAs as adjunctive therapy to levodopa may be considered when the patients begin suffer from wearing-off symptoms (20). Injectable apomorphine may be used to relieve severe motor symptoms in advanced PD patients with severe, protracted wearing-off episodes. Apomorphine has strong D1, D2 and D3 agonism, which may account for its particular utility in this situation (33). Rotigotine also has slight D1 agonism; however, it remains unclear whether this mechanism will provide additional benefit over the oral DAs (34). A recent study indicates that rotigotine may ameliorate PD non-motor symptoms, including fatigue, night-time problems and depression (35). A beneficial effect on depression has also been found for pramipexole.

Non-Dopaminergic Agents

Amantadine and other N-methyl-D-aspartate-type glutamate receptor (NMDAR) agents

Amantadine and levodopa were introduced as treatments for PD around the same time (20,36). Initially developed to treat influenza, it was found serendipitously to improve the motor symptoms of PD, albeit modestly. More recently, its primary role in the treatment of PD has been to alleviate LIDs. The pharmacology of amantadine is complex, given its multiple putative actions; however, its anti-dyskinetic effects may stem from inhibition of glutamate receptors of the N-methyl-D-aspartate (NMDA) subtype (36). This is especially pertinent because excessive glutamatergic activity appears to be pivotal in the induction of LIDs (37). The dose of amantadine is typically 100 mg twice daily and may be titrated up to 300-400 mg two to three times per day. Unfortunately, the beneficial effect of amantadine may fade within weeks to months.

Recent and ongoing studies are investigating whether negative allosteric modulators (NAM) of metabotropic glutamate (mGlu) receptors, particularly the mGlu5 subtype, may also be useful in reducing LIDs (37). Early work on safinamide (a unique molecule with a novel dual mechanism of action based on potent reversible inhibition of MAO-B and inhibition of excessive release of glutamate) indicates that it may also be helpful in reducing LIDs and may prolong the action of levodopa. This medication selectively and reversibly inhibits monoamine oxidase-type B (MAO-B). It also induces use- and frequency-dependent blockade of voltage-gated sodium channels, and inhibits calcium channels. Finally, it reduces induced presynaptic glutamate release (38). It may also work synergistically with amantadine and levodopa (38). A randomized, double-blind, placebo-controlled trial of safinamide as add-on therapy in early PD patients did not demonstrate a significant improvement of motor symptoms at a dose of 200 mg/day (56). However, post-hoc analyses on an extension study indicate that safinamide 100 mg/day may be effective as add-on treatment to DA in PD (57).

Intriguingly, it has been hypothesized that *stimulation* of the glycine modulatory site of NMDARs may improve motor function and non-motor symptoms, e.g., apathy, in advanced PD (39).

Monoamine oxidase-type B (MAO-B) inhibitors

MAO-B degrades dopamine (see Figure 11.2). Currently available, irreversible MAO-B inhibitors include selegiline and rasagiline. Though there was some initial excitement that each was neuroprotective in PD (40,41), this optimism has not been validated (12). As noted above, some clinicians utilize them to prolong the effects of dopaminergic agents (20). When used as monotherapy, these compounds are strikingly less effective than levodopa and even dopamine agonists.

Catechol-O-methyl transferase inhibitors

Most of levodopa is peripherally metabolized by catechol-O-methyl transferase (COMT). Thus, even when combined with decarboxylase inhibitors, only a low percentage of orally administered levodopa gets into the brain. To improve this situation, COMT inhibitors have been introduced. The two available compounds, entacapone and tolcapone, increase the half-life of levodopa by up to 50%, and pharmakokinetically, they decrease the low trough levels seen with regular levodopa (58). Clinically, these compounds increase 'on' times by up to 25% over placebo (58).

Tolcapone acts both peripherally and centrally and is therefore probably more effective, but due to its side-effect of potentially fatal hepatic toxicity, it is mostly used as a second-line COMT inhibitor. Entacapone acts only peripherally. Its most common side-effects include diarrhea and urine and other bodily fluid decolorization. In many countries, entacapone is available in combination pills with both levodopa and carbidopa.

Other non-dopaminergic agents

In a recent review, Kalia et al. reviewed recent and ongoing trials of agents acting on cholinergic (e.g., nicotine), histaminergic (e.g., famotidine), noradrenergic (e.g., methylphenidate), GABAergic, serotonergic (e.g., pardoprunox), adenosinergic (e.g. istradefylline), and glutamatergic systems in the treatment of PD (37). Figure 11.5, borrowed from that article with permission, indicates the rationale behind the utilization of these various, non-dopaminergic neurotransmitter systems (37). It is conceivable that one or more of these agents will become a useful component of the pharmacological armamentarium to combat PD symptoms.

Physical and Cognitive Exercise

Though extant knowledge indicates that no currently available oral medication unquestionably stems the progression of neurodengeneration in PD (12), accumulating evidence suggests that vigorous physical exercise, which is defined as activity that is sufficient to increase the heart rate and oxygen demand (15), reduces the risk of developing PD and cognitive decline (15,16,42-44). However, the putative, neuroprotective effects of exercise have not been demonstrated in multiple, randomized, prospective clinical trials of PD patients (15). Such trials would be difficult to conduct for numerous reasons, including the current lack of reliable biomarkers for PD progression (15). Nonetheless, substantial indirect evidence, both from animal and human studies, indicates plausible mechanisms for such an effect.

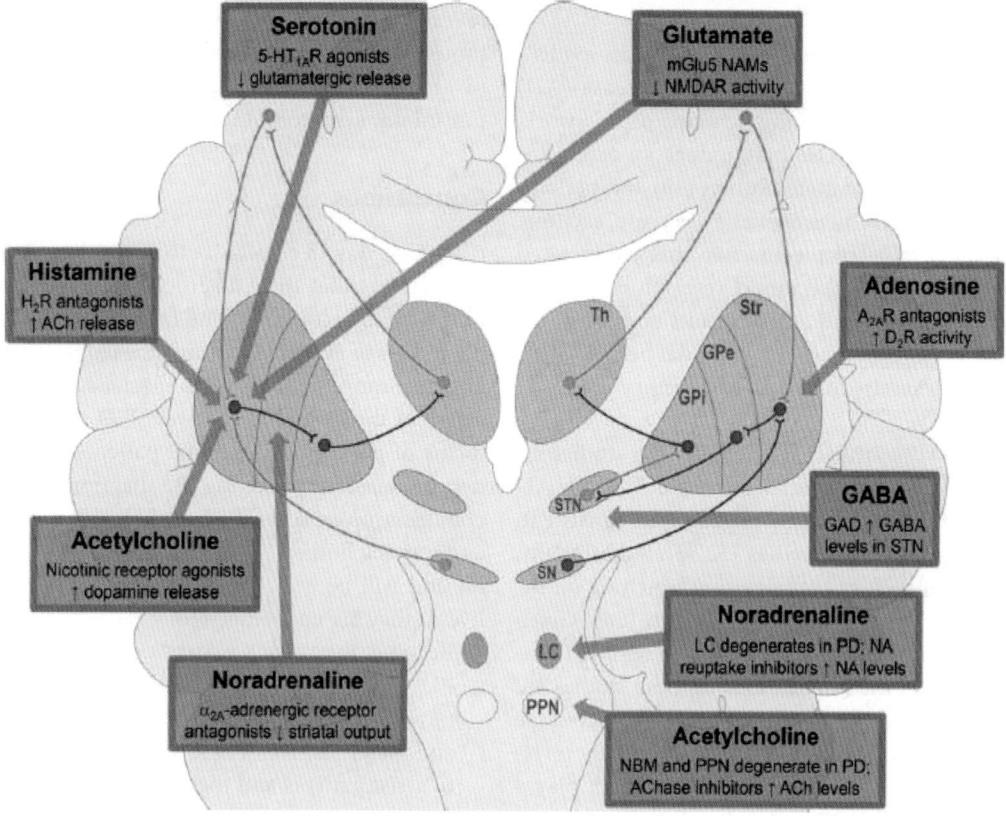

Figure 11.5
Nondopaminergic neurotransmitter systems involved in the motor features of PD. Non-dopaminergic nuclei affected in PD include the PPN and nucleus basalis of Meynert (NBM; not shown), which produce Ach, as well as the locus ceruleus (LC), which produces noradrenaline (NA). These nuclei project to the basal as well as other brain regions to supply their respective neurotransmitters. Within the basal ganglia, current drugs that target the Ach, glutamate, histamine, NA, or serotonin systems appear to modulate the direct pathway (left), whereas those that target the adenosine and GABA systems may influence the indirect pathway (right) (37). AChase = acetylcholinesterase; GPe = globus pallidus externa; GPi = globus pallidus interna; Str = striatum; Th = thalamus.

Physical exercise

Multiple rat/mouse studies have shown that exercise using running wheels or treadmills reduces the effects of the dopaminergic neurotoxins 6-hydroxydopamine (6-OH-DA) and 1-methyl,4-phenyl,1,2,3,6-tetrahydropyridine (MPTP) (45, 46). This may be the result of the exercise-induced expression of brain neurotrophic factor expression, including brain-derived neurotrophic factor (BDNF) and glial-derived neurotrophic factor (GDNF) (15). Additionally, exercise appears to enhance neuroplasticity, perhaps by increasing concentrations of synaptic proteins, e.g., synapsin I and synaptophysin. Exercise also may enhance the long-term potentiation, a measure of synaptic efficiency and increased dendritic length, complexity, and spine density (15,47). Furthermore, given that physical exercise during mid-life appears to provide at least as much protection from developing PD as tobacco and caffeine use, it may still have salutary effects on patients who have developed PD (15).

Cognitive exercise

Additionally, the benefits of exercise are evident in numerous, recent Alzheimer's disease (AD) studies (48-50). The implications of this work, namely that exercise may induce an actual increase in gray matter volumes (49) and perhaps even stimulate neurogenesis (51), are exciting. Perhaps some of the mechanisms enumerated above in PD animal model research may be involved. At any rate, these results engender further optimism about the potential beneficial effects of exercise on the natural history of PD.

The AD literature is also replete with studies indicating the substantial cognitive benefits AD patients may accrue by engaging in consistent, mind-enriching activities (52,53). Additionally, the baleful effects of television watching on intellectual function are well known (54). Given that dementia eventually occurs in many PD patients (15), the implications of these studies are clear: PD clinicians should strongly encourage their patients to not only engage in daily physical exercise, but also to regularly read, play a musical instrument, work crossword and jigsaw puzzles, participate in home repairs, or learn new skills, such as using e-mail (54).

Repetitive Transcranial Magnetic Stimulation (rTMS)

Repetitive transcranial magnetic stimulation (rTMS) allows non-invasive stimulation of the cerebral cortex by a pulsed magnetic field which stimulates electrical activity in the brain. An early placebo-controlled study in 18 PD patients applied 25 Hz rTMS and found that rTMS sessions appear to have a cumulative benefit on improving gait, as well as reducing upper-limb bradykinesia in PD patients (59). On the other hand, intermittent theta-burst TMS of the motor and prefrontal cortices improves mood, but failed to improve gait, upper-extremity bradykinesia or other motor symptoms in PD (60). A larger, randomized, controlled study in 106 PD patients revealed that 1 Hz TMS over the supplementary motor area appears to produce long-lasting (up to 11 weeks) improvement of motor but not of non-motor symptoms (61).

Conclusions

Clinicians should emphasize to newly diagnosed PD patients that their disorder, while not currently curable, could respond favorably to multiple modes of available treatment. Many patients and non-movement disorder specialists are unaware of the distinction between PD and other forms of parkinsonism. Some patients become despondent after receiving the diagnosis, often conjuring up images of wheelchairs, dementia, and nursing homes. This is not necessarily their lot and will be even less likely to darken their lives if they are encouraged to:

- Become 'the world's expert' on their case of PD to collaborate best with their treating physician. There are myriad excellent books and materials from PD foundations available to assist patients and their families including (55).
- Begin an exercise program if they are currently sedentary, including aerobic, strength training, and stretching components. They should preferably do this with their spouse or significant other to foster compliance.
- Maintain an active mind.

Video fragment

Fragment 11.1
Allied health strategies in
PD (Segments 1-2)
Patients suffering Parkinson's disease with progressive instability and/or freezings, limiting their activities of daily living, might be helped by external cues. Two examples are given: the first segment shows an elderly man, passing sliding doors without and later with acoustic cues (rhythmic ticks with his cane). The second segment shows the impact of visual cues on a late-stage PD patient with severe walking problems in the home situation (with lines on the floor).

References

1 Carlsson A.The occurrence, distribution, and physiological role of catecholamines in the nervous system Pharmacol Rev 1959;11:490-493.

2 Ehringer H, Hornykiewicz O. Verteilung von Noradrenalin und Dopamine (3-hydroxytyramin) in Gehirn des Menschen und ihr Verhalten bei Erkrankungen des extrapyramidalen Systems. Klin Wochenschr 1960;38:1236-1239.

3 Birkmayer W, Hornykiewicz O. Der L-dioxyphen-aylalanin (L-dopa) Effekt bei der Parkinson-Akine-sia. Wien Klin Wochenschr 1961;73:787-788.

4 Cotzias GC, Van Woert MH, Schiffer LM. Aromatic amino acids and modification of parkinsonism. N Engl J Med 1967;276:374-379.

5 Hoehn MM. Parkinsonism treated with levodopa: progression and mortality. J Neural Transm 1983;19(Suppl 1):253-264.

6 Uitti RJ, Ahlskog JE, Maraganore DM, et al. Levodopa therapy and survival in idiopathic Parkinson's disease: Olmsted County Project. Neurology 1993;43:1918-1926.

7 Braak H, Del Tredici K, Rüb U, de Vos RA, Jansen Steur EN, Braak E. Staging of brain pathology related to sporadic Parkinson's disease. Neurobiol Aging 2003;24:197-211.

8 Low PA, Gilden JL, Freeman R, Sheng KN, McElligott MA. Efficacy of midodrine vs placebo in neurogenic orthostatic hypotension. A randomized, double-blind multicenter study.Midodrine Study Group. JAMA 1997;277:1046-1051.

9 Boeve BF, Silber MH, Ferman TJ, Lucas JA, Parisi JE. Association of REM sleep behavior disorder and neurodegenerative disease may reflect an underlying synucleinopathy. Mov Disord 2001;16:622-630.

10 Cummings JL. Depression and Parkinson's disease: a review. Am J Psychiatry 1992;149:443-454.

11 Miyasaki JM, Shannon K, Voon V, et al. Practice parameter: evaluation and treatment of depression, psychosis, and dementia in Parkinson disease (an evidence-based review): report of the Quality Standards Subcommittee of the American Academy of Neurology. Neurology 2006;66:996-1002.

12 Suchowersky O, Gronseth G, Perlmutter J, Reich S, Zesiewicz T, Weiner WJ. Practice parameter: neuroprotective strategies and alternative therapies Parkinson disease (an evidence-based review): report of the Quality Standards Subcommittee of the American Academy of Neurology. Neurology 2006;66:976-982.

13 Dibble LE, Hale TF, Marcus RL, Droge J, Gerber JP, LaStayo PC. High-intensity resistance training amplifies muscle hypertrophy and functional gains in persons with Parkinson's disease. Mov Disord 2006;21:1444-1452.

14 Falvo MJ, Schilling BK, Earhart GM. Parkinson's disease and resistive exercises: rationale, review, and recommendations. Mov Disord 2008;23:1-11.

15 Ahlskog JE. Does vigorous exercise have a neuroprotective effect in Parkinson disease? Neurology 2011;77:288-294.

16 Ahlskog JE, Geda YE, Graff-Radford NR, Petersen RC. Physical Exercise as a preventive or disease-modifying treatment of dementia and brain aging. Mayo Clin Proc 2011;86:876-884.

17 Chou CH, Hwang CL, Wu YT. Effect of exercise on physical function, daily living activities, and quality of life in the frail older adults: a meta-analysis. Arch Phys Med Rehabil 2012;93:237-244.

18 Agid Y, Ahlskog E, Albanese A, et al Levodopa in the treatment of Parkinson's disease: a consensus meeting. Mov Disord 1999;14:911-913.

19 Miyasaki JM, Martin W, Suchowersky O, Weiner WJ, Lang AE. Practice parameter: initiation of treatment for Parkinson's disease: an evidence-based review: report of the Quality Standards Subcommittee of the American Academy of Neurology. Neurology 2002;58:11-17.

20 Goudreau JL, Ahlskog JE. Symptomatic treatment of Parkinson's disease: levodopa, in: Pfeiffer RF, Wszolek ZK, Ebadi M, eds. Parkinson's Disease, Second Edition, 2013, CRC Press, Boca Raton: 847-859.

21 Pinder RM, Brogden RN, Sawyer PR, Speight TM, Avery GS. Levodopa and decarboxylase inhibitors: a review of their clinical pharmacology and use in the treatment of parkinsonism. Drugs 1976;11:329-377.

22 Ahlskog JE. Cheaper; simpler; and better: tips for treating seniors with Parkinson disease. Mayo Clin Proc 2011;86:1211-1216.

23 Parkinson-Study Group. Does levodopa slow or hasten the rate of progression of Parkinson disease? The results of the Elldopa trial Neurology 2003;60(S1):A80.

24 Van Gerpen JA, Kumar N, Bower JH, Weigand S, Ahlskog JE. Levodopa-associated dyskinesia risk among Parkinson disease patients in Olmsted County, Minnesota, 1976-1990. Arch Neurol 2006;63:205-209.

25 Zanettini R, Antonini A, Gatto G, Gentile R, Tesei S, Pezzoli G.Valvular heart disease and the use of dopamine agonists for Parkinson's disease. N Engl J Med 2007;356:39-46.

26 Yamamoto M, Uesugi T, Nakayama T. Dopamine agonists and cardiac valvulopathy in Parkinson disease: a case-control study. Neurology 2006;67:1225-1229.

27 Gerlach M, Double K, Arzberger T, Leblhuber F, Tatschner T, Riederer P. Dopamine receptor agonists in current clinical use: comparative dopamine receptor binding profiles defined in the human striatum. J Neural Transm 2003;110:1119-1127.

28 Jenner P. Avoidance of dyskinesia: preclinical evidence for continuous dopaminergic stimulation. Neurology 2004;62(S1):S57-S55.

29 Gallagher DA, O'Sullivan SS, Evans AH, Lees AJ, Schrag A. Pathological gambling in Parkinson's disease: risk factors and differences from dopamine dysregulation. An analysis of published case series. Mov Disord 2007;22:157-1763.

30 Klos KJ, Bower JH, Josephs KA, Matsumoto JY, Ahlskog JE. Pathological hypersexuality predominantly linked to adjuvant dopamine agonist therapy in Parkinson's disease and multiple system atrophy. Parkinsonism Relat Disord 2005;11:381-386.

31 Santangelo G, Barone P, Trojano L, Vitale C. Pathological gambling in Parkinson's disease: a comprehensive review. Parkinsonism Relat Disord 2013;19:645-653.

32 Frucht S, Rogers JD, Greene PE, Gordon MF, Fahn S. Falling asleep at the wheel: motor vehicle mishaps in persons taking pramipexole and ropinirole. Neurology 1999;52:1908-1910.

33 Kolls BJ, Stacy M. Apomorphine: a rapid rescue agent for the management of motor fluctuations in advanced Parkinson disease. Clin Neuropharmacol 2006;29:292-301.

34 Watts RL, Jankovic J, Waters C, Rajput A, Boroojerdi B, Rao J. Randomized, blind, controlled trial of transdermal rotigotine in early Parkinson disease. Neurology 2007;68:272-276.

35 Chaudhuri KR, Martinez-Martin P, Antonini A, et al. Rotigotine and specific non-motor symptoms of Parkinon's disease: post hoc analysis of RECOVER. Parkinsonism Relat Disord 2013;19:660-665.

36 Rajput AH, Rajput A, Lang AE, Kumar R, Uitti RJ, Galvez-Jimenez N. New use for an old drug: amantadine benefits levodopa-induced dyskinesia. Mov Disord 1998;13:851.

37 Kalia LV, Brotchie JM, Fox SH. Novel nondopaminergic targets for motor features of Parkinson's disease: review of recent trials. Mov Disord 2013;28:131-144.

38 Gregoire L, Jourdain VA, Townsend M, Roach A, Di Paolo T. Safinamide reduces dyskinesias and prolongs L-DOPA antiparkinsonian effect in parkinsonian monkeys. Parkinsonism Relat Disord 2013;19:508-514.

39 Heresco-Levy U, Shoham S, and Javitt DC. Glycine site agonists of the N-methyl-D-aspartate receptor

and Parkinson's disease: a hypothesis. Mov Disord 2013;28:419-424.

40 Parkinson-Study-Group. Effect of deprenyl on the progression of disability in early Parkinson's disease. N Engl J Med 1989;321:1364-1371.

41 Parkinson-Study-Group. A controlled trial of rasagiline in early Parkinson disease: the TEMPO Study. Arch Neurol 2002;59:1937-1943.

42 Xu Q, Park Y, Huang X, et al. Physical activities and future risk of Parkinson disease. Neurology 2010;75:341-348.

43 Hamer M, Chida Y. Physical activity and risk of neurodegenerative disease: a systematic review of prospective evidence. Psychol Med 2009;39:3-11.

44 Baker LD, Frank LL, Foster-Schubert K, et al. Effects of aerobic exercise on mild cognitive impairment: a controlled trial. Arch Neurol 2010;67:71-79.

45 Tillerson JL, Caudle WM, Reveron ME, Miller GW. Exercise induces behavioral recovery and attenuates neurochemical deficits in rodent models of Parkinson's disease. Neuroscience 2003;119:899-911.

46 Taijiri N, Yasuhara T, Shingo T, et al. Exercise exerts neuroprotective effects on Parkinson's disease model of rats. Brain Res 2010;1310:200-207.

47 Voss MW, Prakash RS, Erickson KI, et al. Plasticity of brain networks in a randomized intervention trial of exercise training in older adults. Front Aging Neurosci 2010;2:doi:10.3389/fnagi.2010.00032.

48 Burns JM, Cronk BB, Anderson HS, et al. Cardiorespiratory fitness and brain atrophy in early Alzheimer disease. Neurology 2008;71:210-216.

49 Colcombe SJ, Erickson KI, Scalf PE, et al. Aerobic exercise training increases brain volume in aging humans. J Gerontol A Bio Sci Med Sci 2006;61:1166-1170.

50 Erickson KI, Voss MW, Prakash RS, et al. Exercise training increases size of hippocampus and improves memory. Proc Natl Acad Sci USA 2011;108:3017-3022.

51 Pereira AC, Huddleston DE, Brickman AM, et al. An in vivo correlate of exercise-induced neurogenesis in the adult dentate gyrus. Proc Natl Acad Sci USA 2007;104:5638-5643.

52 Salotti P, De Sanctis B, Clementi A, et al. Evaluation of the efficacy of a cognitive rehabilitation treatment on a group of Alzheimer's patients with moderate cognitive impairment: a pilot study. Aging Clin Exp Res 2013;108:3017-3022.

53 Toba K, Nakamura TK, Endo H, et al. Intensive rehabilitation for dementia improved cognitive function and reduced behavioral disturbance in geriatric health service facilities in Japan. Geriatr Gerontol Int 2013;doi:10.1111/ggi.12080.

54 Lindstrom HA, Fritsch T, Petot G, et al. The relationship between television viewing in midlife and the development of Alzheimer's disease in a case-control study. Brain Cogn 2005;58:157-165.

55 Ahlskog JE. The Parkinson's Disease Treatment Book, Oxford University Press, 2005.

56 Stocchi F, Borgohain R, Onofrj M, et al. A randomized, double-blind, placebo-controlled trial of safinamide as add-on therapy in early Parkinson's disease patients. Mov Disord 2012;27:106-112.

57 Schapira AH, Stocchi F, Borgohain R, et al. Long-term efficacy and safety of safinamide as add-on therapy in early Parkinson's disease. Eur J Neurol 2013;20:271-280.

58 Entacapone improves motor fluctuations in levodopa-treated Parkinson's disease patients. Parkinson Study Group. Ann Neurol. 1997;42:747–755.

59 Lomarev MP, Kanchana S, Bara-Jimenez W, Iyer M, Wassermann EM, Hallett M. Placebo-controlled study of rTMS for the treatment of Parkinson's disease. Mov Disord 2006;21:325-331.

60 Benninger DH, Berman BD, Houdayer E, et al. Intermittent theta-burst transcranial magnetic stimulation for treatment of Parkinson disease. Neurology. 2011;76:601-609.

61 Shirota Y, Ohtsu H, Hamada M, Enomoto H, Ugawa Y. Treatment of Parkinson's Disease. Supplementary motor area stimulation for Parkinson disease: a randomized controlled study. Neurology 2013;80:1400-1405.

12

Conventional Treatment-related Motor Complications: Their Prevention and Treatment

Fabrizio Stocchi

Chronic levodopa treatment for Parkinson's disease (PD) patients is frequently associated with the development of motor complications such as end-of-dose wearing-off and dyskinesias. In this chapter we provide an overview of the strategies available for dealing with these problems. Medical management in PD includes manipulation of levodopa and/or dopamine agonist dosing to establish the optimum treatment schedule. This includes improving levodopa absorption, whether or not by adding catechol-O-methyl-transferase (COMT) and/or monoamine oxidase (MAO) B inhibitors, titrating oral levodopa and dopaminergic agonists including combining these drugs, adding amantadine, and eventually changing conventional oral treatment for deep brain stimulation (DBS) (see Chapter 13) or continuous dopamine receptor stimulation (CDS) (see Chapter 14) with continuous dermal, subcutaneous or intrajejunal application of dopaminomimetics. In this chapter, the importance of initiating therapy with a strategy that reduces the risk of developing motor complications will be discussed explicitly.

Motor complications

After 40 years of clinical use, levodopa therapy remains the most effective symptomatic treatment for PD, and all PD patients eventually require levodopa therapy (1-5). However, chronic levodopa (and to a lesser extent also chronic dopamine agonist) treatment is associated with the development of motor complications in the majority of patients.

These motor complications comprise predictable and unpredictable 'on-off' motor fluctuations and dyskinesia. Predictable motor complications include 'wearing-off', nocturnal and early morning akinesia as well as delayed 'on' / no-'on' phenomena; unpredictable motor fluctuations manifest as random 'on-off' fluctuations. Dyskinesia are chorea-like and/or dystonic movements (mostly painful) which occur in a time-relationship with the dosing of levodopa: at maximum plasma levodopa levels (peak dose), during clinical efficacy of a single dose (inter-dose), related to the critical clinical threshold plasma levodopa level at the beginning or the end of the clinical efficacy (diphasic), and during low sub-clinical threshold levodopa plasma levels ('off'-period). Indeed, the ELLDOPA study indicates that in patients treated with levodopa 200 mg tid (three times a day), 16% developed dyskinesia and 20% had motor fluctuations after just 9 months of therapy (6). In a recent study in 617 parkinsonian patients (the DEEP study), predictable motor fluctuations were present in 41.8% of the subjects after less than 2.5 years' disease duration (5). Recently, the STRIDE-PD study population (6) was examined to determine the effect of levodopa dose and other risk factors on the development of dyskinesia and wearing-off. The STRIDE-PD study compared initiation of levodopa therapy with levodopa/carbidopa (LC) or levodopa/carbidopa/entaca-

Table 12.1
Overview of possible strategies that can be tried in the case of emerging motor fluctuations. COMT: catechol-O-methyltransferase; MAO: monoamine oxidase; DBS: deep brain stimulation; CDS: continuous dopaminergic stimulation, e.g. by intrajejunal or subcutaneous administration of dopaminomimetics.

Type of motor fluctuation	Definition	Possible strategies
Wearing-off and/or end-of-dose akinesia	Fading off of treatment effect a few hours after drug intake, including akinesia at night and in the morning hours.	Add dopamine agonists with prolonged efficacy, shorten intervals between levodopa adminstrations, change to prolonged-release levodopa (may not be helpful at all), or add enzyme (COMT/MAO-B) inhibitors, evaluate DBS or CDS.
Freezing in 'off' condition	Sudden freezing when walking, particularly when passing through doors or narrow passages.	Same as with wearing-off. Consider physiotherapy for gait training and/or laser sticks.
On-dyskinesia	Dyskinesia in 'on' condition, not painful and due to their non-repetitive and non-random character not to be confused with chorea.	Reduce dopaminergic total dose, consider shorter treatment intervals with lower dosages, adding adamantine, or DBS/CDS.
Off-dystonia	Dystonia, often painful, in 'off' condition, including early morning dystonia.	Same as with wearing-off. Consider rescue strategies such as soluble, fast-acting levodopa or apomorphine injections.
Diphasic (or biphasic) dyskinesia	Dyskinesia at the beginning and/or end of 'on' conditions, e.g. when levodopa plasma levels are increasing or decreasing. Dyskinesias are often uncomfortable or painful, and may exhibit dystonia-like features.	Aim at median-to-high dose dopaminergic treatment, as continuous as possible (short intervals between single doses). May be complicated by severe dyskinesias. Evaluate DBS or CDS.

pone (LCE) in patients with early PD. A total of 745 subjects participated in this 134-208 week, prospective, double-blind trial. The risk of dyskinesia in the total population was increased in a levodopa dose-dependent manner. Analysis using levodopa-equivalent doses showed comparable results. Factors predictive of dyskinesia in rank order were: young age at onset, higher levodopa dose, low body weight, North American geographic region, LCE treatment group, female gender, and severer Unified Parkinson's Disease Rating Scale (UPDRS) Part II. Risk of wearing-off also increased in a levodopa dose-dependent manner. Multivariate analyses showed similar predictors to dyskinesia, but included baseline UPDRS III and excluded weight and treatment allocation (7). In the extreme, patients can cycle between 'on' periods complicated by severe dyskinesia and 'off' periods when they are severely parkinsonian. Motor complications can be disabling, and treatment can be difficult and frustrating for patients and physicians. The difficulty of controlling motor complications in many patients illustrates the importance of employing early treatment strategies that minimize or prevent their development in the first place. It is noteworthy that none of the available medical or surgical therapies for PD has been demonstrated to provide efficacy that is superior to what can be achieved with levodopa.

Medical management of levodopa-induced motor complications

Table 12.1 provides a brief overview of strategies that can be tried by the treating neurologist, depending on the kind of motor complication.

Motor fluctuations

Manipulating levodopa dose

Levodopa is the most effective treatment for PD, but also the primary cause of motor complications. To design the optimal dosing schedule requires an appreciation of the changing response to levodopa over time. During long-term treatment there is no change in the levodopa peripheral pharmacokinetics (8); rather, changes in central pharmacokinetics and in the pharmacodynamic response are believed to underlie the development of levodopa-related motor fluctuations (9-11). The motor effects of levodopa theoretically depend on presynaptic mechanisms, such as the synthesis and storage of dopamine in the remaining nigral neurons, as well as postsynaptic events resulting from the activation of post-synaptic dopamine receptors on striatal neurons with consequent cell signalling and neurophysiologic events. The rate of motor deterioration following withdrawal from a steady-state, optimal-dose levodopa infusion is significantly faster in patients with advanced PD who exhibit motor complications compared with those in the early stages who have a stable, long-term response to the drug (9). A similar response is also observed after discontinuation of a steady-state infusion of the dopamine agonist apomorphine, which only acts postsynaptically, indicating that changes in postsynaptic mechanisms play an important role in the shortened duration of action of levodopa (11). Furthermore, in patients with asymmetric PD, the duration of motor benefit following single injections of apomorphine is shorter on the more affected side (12), suggesting that disease severity influences the postsynaptic response to dopaminergic stimulation.

When levodopa therapy is first introduced, the magnitude of its therapeutic benefit tends to reflect the dose employed. However, as fluctuations and dyskinesias emerge, this pharmacodynamic response switches from a linear dose-response to a sigmoid curve, resulting in narrowing of the 'therapeutic window' and the emergence of a 'critical levodopa threshold' for a clinical response (10). Only levodopa doses at, or above, this threshold are able to turn the patient fully 'on'. Equally, the dose that produces dyskinesias appears to decrease progressively until it becomes almost equivalent to that required to turn the patient 'on' (13). Unfortunately, this means that a reduction in levodopa dosage to relieve dyskinesias causes 'off' periods, and increased doses that turn the patient 'on' induce dyskinesias (14). When patients present with motor fluctuations, increased doses of levodopa may increase 'on' time for a while, but they eventually lead to the development, or worsening, of dyskinesia. Alternatively, more frequent administration of smaller doses may reduce dyskinesia but may increase 'off' time. Single-dose studies can be used to try to establish the critical dose required for adequate mobility, the duration of effect, and the pattern of dyskinesias. Although it might seem logical to administer this dose at repeated, overlapping intervals (as determined by the duration of its effect), it may be better to give an adequate dose of levodopa less, rather than more, frequently. This may help to avoid the build-up of dyskinesias during the course of the day, particularly in the afternoon and evening. Another strategy is to take a 'mini drug holiday' (missing the dose of levodopa at lunchtime). This can reduce late afternoon and evening dyskinesias and establish a reliable response to afternoon and evening doses (15).

With disease progression, peripheral levodopa availability becomes an increasingly important factor in determining striatal dopamine concentrations. As levodopa is primarily absorbed in the proximal small intestine, factors that delay gastric emptying may lead to a delayed clinical response or a complete dose failure (16). PD is associated with slowed gastric motility which delays gastric emptying (17). Stimulation of dopamine receptors in the stomach may further depress gastric motility (18). Excess gastric acidity can also delay gastric emptying, and excessive neutralization of stomach acid can lead to incomplete dissolution of levodopa tablets with incomplete absorption (19). Treatments directed at improving gastric emptying, such as withdrawal of anticholinergic drugs and relief of constipation, may provide a more predictable response to levodopa (20). High-protein meals may also reduce levodopa absorption, as large, neutral amino acids can compete with levodopa for transfer across the intestinal mucosa (21) and the blood-brain barrier (22). Patients wishing to be active in the afternoon may prefer to take their main meal in the evening, while those wishing to be active in the evening should do the reverse. Some have advocated taking the day's portion of protein in a single meal, but taking levodopa 1 hour before or after meals is probably sufficient. Recent studies also suggest that motor fluctuations can be associated with *Helicobacter pylori* and can be improved by antibiotic treatment (23).

Controlled-release preparations

Controlled-release (CR) preparations of levodopa, such as Madopar CR™ and Sinemet CR™, tend to cause a build-up of levodopa at the end of the day. These formulations lack the 'kick start' of conventional levodopa, so patients may take another dose, only to find that the combined effect of the two causes intolerable dyskinesias. One strategy is to combine conventional Madopar or Sinemet with the controlled-release preparations in the morning, but to take only conventional preparations in the afternoon. Treatment with CR formulations in complex patients is confounded by their relatively erratic absorption and their tendency to be associated

with low plasma levels (lower bioavailability) and the development of diphasic dyskinesias (see below), and is generally not a good means of controlling motor complications.

Water-soluble preparations

Water-soluble preparations of levodopa, such as Madopar™ dispersible, parcopa, levodopa methyl ester or levodopa ethyl ester, are absorbed more rapidly than standard levodopa. Levodopa methyl ester is a highly soluble prodrug produced by esterification of the carboxylic moiety of the levodopa molecule. It is rapidly absorbed, producing an earlier plasma peak and a more predictable clinical effect than standard levodopa preparations (24). Switching to water-soluble forms of levodopa, or dissolving standard levodopa formulations in an ascorbic acid solution or fizzy drink, may help increase uptake from the gut and reduce 'off' periods. In a double-blind, double-dummy, controlled study CHF1512 (melevodopa), a preparation of levodopa methyl ester plus carbidopa in a fizzy tablet proved to be significantly faster than standard levodopa/carbidopa preparations in turning patients 'on' in the morning and after lunch (25). Interestingly, there are naturally occurring formulations of levodopa such as those derived from the *Mucuna* plants that have long been used in traditional Ayurvedic Indian medicine for diseases including parkinsonism. In a double-blind clinical trial, it was demonstrated to have a rapid onset of action and to provide longer 'on' time without a concomitant increase in dyskinesias (26). These findings suggest that it might have advantages over traditional levodopa, and comparative studies are warranted.

In advanced cases with both motor fluctuations and dyskinesia, it often becomes increasingly difficult to find a levodopa dose that improves 'on' time and does not induce dyskinesia. Thus, levodopa dose manipulation per se, while potentially helpful in dealing with mild motor complications, is rarely a good long-term solution.

COMT Inhibition

The addition of a catechol-O-methyl transferase (COMT) inhibitor to the levodopa regimen (both standard and controlled-release) has been shown to increase 'on' time, reduce 'off' time, and improve motor scores in fluctuating PD patients (27-29). In the presence of a decarboxylase inhibitor, the main route for levodopa metabolism involves COMT. Inhibition of this metabolic pathway by a COMT inhibitor increases the elimination half-life of levodopa and provides more continuous availability of levodopa after each dose (30). Two selective inhibitors of COMT have been approved for the treatment of PD: tolcapone (Tasmar™) and entacapone (Comtess™/Comtan™). Both COMT inhibitors induce a dose-dependent increase in levodopa plasma half-life without a change in C_{max} and T_{max}. The addition of either entacapone or tolcapone to levodopa in fluctuating PD patients increases 'on' time by 1.3-1.8 hours per day with a corresponding reduction in 'off' time (27-28). Cochrane reviews indicate that benefits associated with tolcapone are greater than those seen with entacapone, consistent with this drug inducing greater COMT inhibition and also acting centrally (29). While COMT inhibitors can be helpful in controlling 'off' episodes in mild fluctuators, they can be associated with increased dyskinesia, particularly if it was pre-existent. This can sometimes be controlled by a reduction in levodopa dose, but can be a problem in more advanced cases. There has been some concern about hepatotoxicity in tolcapone-treated patients. Abnormalities in liver function tests were encountered in subjects participating in tolcapone clinical trials, and post-marketing surveillance revealed 3 cases of hepatocellular liver damage with death that were linked to the drug (31,32). It has also been associated with rare cases of neuroleptic malignant syndrome (33). As a result, its use has been restricted and regular liver function monitoring is required, although regulatory standards have recently been relaxed (34). Entacapone has not been associated with hepatotoxicity, and liver monitoring is not required. It is typically administered at a dose of 200 mg with each levodopa dose while tolcapone is administered at 100-200 mg tid. A formulation containing 200 mg of entacapone plus levodopa and carbidopa (Stalevo®) is available in a single tablet containing different levodopa doses. Another advantage of this combined formulation is its availability in many levodopa dosages (50, 75, 100, 125, 150, 175 and 200 mg).

MAO-B Inhibition

Monoamine oxidase-B (MAO-B) inhibitors block the enzymatic metabolism of dopamine in the brain, thus increasing the dopamine concentration. In fluctuating PD patients, MAO-B inhibitors can be used as an adjunct to levodopa to reduce 'off' time. Two MAO-B inhibitors are available on the market: selegeline (Eldepryl[R], Jumex[R]) and rasagiline (Azilect[R]). Selegiline in a dose of 5 mg twice a day (bid) has primarily been employed as monotherapy in early PD but was initially approved based on studies showing reduced 'off' time in fluctuating patients when used as an adjunct to levodopa (35). Rasagiline has been more extensively studied in levodopa-treated PD patients with motor fluctuations. In the PRESTO study, 472 patients were randomized to receive rasagiline 0.5 or 1 mg/day vs placebo (36), while in the LARGO study 687 patients were randomized to rasagiline 1 mg/day, entacapone 200 mg with each levodopa dose, or placebo (37). In each study, rasagiline-treated patients experienced a significant decrease in daily off time and an increase in ON time in comparison to placebo (approximately 0.5-1.2 hours; P≤.0001). The results with rasagiline were comparable to what was attained with entacapone. Indeed, in an ancillary study of LARGO on early morning, practically defined off, rasagiline but not entacapone induced a significative improvement of off severity (40). Selegiline orally disintegrating tablets (Zilopar ODT) incorporate Zydis® technology to provide a fast-dissolving, oral mucosal drug delivery system which bypasses first-pass metabolism in the liver (38). The ODT formulation provides a high bioavailability of selegiline, with five times greater area-under-the-curve values compared with an equivalent oral dose and reduced levels of selegiline metabolites. Clinical trials in fluctuating patients note a reduction in daily 'off' time of about 1.6 hours compared with placebo (P = .001) (39).

As with COMT inhibitors, the introduction of a MAO-B inhibitor can cause dopaminergic side-effects and an increase in dyskinesia. In milder cases they can be managed by a reduction in levodopa dose, but this may not be possible in more advanced patients. Non-selective MAO inhibitors can block tyramine metabolism in the gut, leading to a potentially dangerous hypertensive crisis known as the 'cheese effect'. This has not been a problem with selegiline or rasagiline, which are relatively selective inhibitors of MAO-B.

Dopamine agonists

Since the introduction of bromocriptine in the early 1980s, several dopamine agonists have become available for the treatment of PD. Dopamine agonists are frequently employed in the management of early PD as they have a relatively low potential to induce dyskinesia (41), but were initially developed as an adjunct to levodopa for more advanced patients. The addition of a dopamine agonist such as pergolide, ropinirole, pramipexole, rotigotine or cabergoline to levodopa in patients with motor complications can reduce 'off' time by about 1.1-1.8 hours per day (42-45). These benefits can be obtained in conjunction with a reduction in dyskinesia, probably by permitting a 30% reduction in the levodopa dose. However, the benefits are often not sustained. Also, many patients are already on dopamine agonists when motor complications develop, as dopamine agonists do not prevent the development of motor complications once levodopa is introduced (46). Continuous delivery of dopamine agonists is now available with

24-hour, prolonged-release formulations and a transdermal formulation of rotigotine. Double-blind, placebo-controlled trials in PD patients with motor complications have demonstrated significantly decreased 'off' time with each of these agents (47,48). In a head-to-head study, a long-acting preparation of ropinirole was more efficacious than immediate-release ropinirole in reducing 'off' time in fluctuating PD patients (49). Long-acting agents do have the potential to improve nocturnal symptoms and early morning 'off' episodes as shown by a study with a rotigotine patch (50).

Only a few studies have directly compared the efficacy of the various dopamine agonists (51-53). For the most part they are considered to be comparable, and the decision of which dopamine agonist to use generally rests on the familiarity of the physician with the drug. Dopamine agonists can cause acute side-effects such as nausea, vomiting and orthostatic hypotension. They can be minimized by slow titration and the use of peripheral dopamine antagonists such as domperidone, if available. Dopamine agonists may also be associated with cognitive impairment, psychosis, and leg swelling. Recent reports have also linked dopamine agonists with sleep disturbances and impulsive behaviours, such as pathologic gambling, compulsive eating, and hypersexuality (54-57). A more serious concern is the risk of cardiac valvulopathy that has been observed with ergot dopamine agonists. This has been reported with pergolide and cabergoline, and is thought to relate to their 5HT-2B agonist activities (58-59).

Apomorphine is a D1 and D2 receptor dopamine agonist that is extremely effective, but its short half-life and side-effects associated with oral administration preclude its routine use in PD. However, subcutaneous injections can be used to provide acute and reliable anti-parkinsonian benefits for patients with severe and/or unpredictable 'offs' (60,61). Apomorphine injections can be used: (a) to provide mobility at night either to allow the patient to return to sleep or to get up for micturition; (b) to rapidly relieve the distressing 'off' periods during the daytime; (c) to overcome end-of-dose diphasic dyskinesias; or (d) to provide a window of mobility at crucial times. In a double-blind, placebo-controlled trial, 95% of apomorphine injections reversed 'off' periods with a mean injection dose of 5.4 mg. The dose of apomorphine required to turn the patient 'on' must be individualized (usually 2-5 mg), and the drug should be initiated with EKG and blood pressure monitoring because of the associated risks of hypotension and cardiac events (63). Side-effects include dyskinesias, yawning, and injection site reactions which can be minimized by rotating the injection site. Continuous infusion of dopamine agonists such as apomorphine or lisuride can be used to control motor fluctuations that cannot be controlled with other medical therapies (64) (see discussion of infusion below). There has been recent interest in the potential of *adenosine A2A antagonists* to provide benefit for patients with motor complications based on their capacity to decrease overactive firing in striatal neurons that bear dopamine D2 receptors and comprise the indirect pathway. In 1-methyl-4-phenyl-1,2,3,6-tetrahydropyridine (MPTP) monkeys, a primate model of PD, istradefylline reduced dyskinesias associated with the introduction of levodopa (66). However, clinical trials in PD patients with established dyskinesia failed to show any benefit, but did show improvement in 'off' time. The drug is now being studied as an add-on to levodopa that reduces 'off' time.

When changing between dopaminomimetic drugs, different levodopa-equivalent efficacies must be taken into account. Table 12.2 provides an overview of the levodopa-equivalent efficacy of dopaminomimetic compounds.

Dyskinesias

Dyskinesias can be disabling. When they are mild and not troublesome to the patient, no specific treatment may be required. One should

Table 12.2
Levodopa-equivalent doses for levodopa (LD) preparations, COMT inhibitors, and dopamine agonists. For all compounds, the equivalent dose to 100 mg levodopa-carbidopa or levodopa-benserazide is given. Adapted from (116).

Controlled-release levodopa	133 mg
Duodopa	90 mg
Entacapone	LD x 0.33
Tolcapone	LD x 0.5
Pramipexole	1 mg
Ropinirole	5 mg
Rotigotine	3.3 mg
Piribedil	100 mg
Lisuride	1 mg
Bromocriptine	10 mg
Pergolide	1 mg
Cabergoline	1.5 mg

realise, though, that levodopa may be underutilized in these patients for fear of inducing worse dyskinesias. Still, as discussed in Chapter 13, DBS can already be considered at this stage.

Manipulation of levodopa dosage
Manipulation of the levodopa dosages may occasionally be helpful; in some patients, lower doses administered more frequently may reduce dyskinesia without worsening control of the parkinsonism. However, reductions in levodopa dose sufficient to decrease dyskinesia meaningfully do frequently result in impaired parkinsonian control. For patients with end-of-dose or diphasic dyskinesias, increasing plasma concentrations by using higher doses of levodopa or susbstituting regular for controlled-release formulations may be helpful.

Addition of dopamine agonists
The addition of a dopamine agonist, if the patient is not already receiving this class of drug, may permit a reduction in levodopa dose without worsening of parkinsonism. Patients may ex-

perience an additional worsening of dyskinesia with the addition of the agonist, but overall improvement can often be obtained by a subsequent downtitration in the levodopa dose. However, patients who experience severe dyskinesia are rarely controlled with this regimen, and even patients who experience initial benefit can rarely be satisfactorily controlled in the long term. Substituting high doses of a dopamine agonist for levodopa has been reported to reduce dyskinesia (68-70), but this approach is not tolerated by the majority of patients because of psychiatric side-effects.

Addition of amantadine

High doses of amantadine block NMDA receptors and have been shown to reduce the severity of dyskinesia in some PD patients without worsening parkinsonian symptoms. Double-blind, placebo-controlled studies demonstrate reductions in dyskinesia rating scales of 45-60% without adversely affecting the antiparkinsonian effect of L-dopa (71-73). Benefits are typically observed within 3 weeks, but may be transient and are often lost within 1 year. In addition, many PD patients cannot tolerate high doses of amantadine because of cognitive or neuropsychiatric side-effects.

Addition of atypical antipsychotic drugs

Low doses of the atypical antipsychotic drugs such as *clozapine* may be effective in the treatment of Ldopa-induced dyskinesia in patients with severe PD. The mechanism of the antidyskinetic action of clozapine is not known, but may result from a combination of dopamine D_1, D_2, D_4 and serotonin $5HT_2$ receptor antagonism and $5HT_{1A}$ receptor agonist properties. In a small, open-label study, clozapine significantly reduced dyskinesia scores, and this beneficial effect was maintained throughout the 4-month study period (74). In a larger, double-blind, placebo-controlled, 10-week study, clozapine reduced daily 'on' time with dyskinesia from 5.68 ± 0.66 hours to 3.98 ± 0.57 hours (75). However, clozapine has a sedative effect and requires

regular blood monitoring because of the risk of agranulocytosis. Similar results have been observed with low doses of other atypical antipsychotics including *risperidone* (103), *olanzapine* (104) and *quetiapine* (105). However, even low doses of antipsychotic medications could lead to worsening of the parkinsonism, and it is not clear that any anti-dyskinesia benefits attained are better than what could have been accomplished simply by reducing the dose of levodopa.

Addition of other agents

There are a number of other agents that are currently being explored as possible therapies for dyskinesias that target a variety of non-dopaminergic pathways. Among them, the most promising was *sarizotan*, a $5HT_{1A}$ receptor agonist and D_3 and D_4 receptor antagonist. In open-label studies, sarizotan in daily doses of 2-10 mg bid reduced dyskinesia in levodopa-treated patients by approximately 40% (79,80). However, higher doses were associated with a clear worsening in the parkinsonism. In a double-blind, placebo-controlled, fixed-dose study, sarizotan did not provide any anti-dyskinesia benefit compared to placebo, and 'off' time was significantly increased with higher doses (81). It remains to be determined if levodopa titration in combination with doses which block dyskinesia will provide additional benefits.

The antiepileptic drug *levetiracetam* has also been studied as a treatment for the dyskinesia associated with L-dopa therapy in PD. In MPTP-lesioned primates, levetiracetam significantly reduces L-dopa-induced choreic dyskinesia and potentiates the antidyskinetic effects of amantadine (82,83). In an open-label study in dyskinetic PD patients, levetiracetam increased 'on' time without dyskinesia from 43% to 61% and reduced 'on' time with troublesome dyskinesia from 23% to 11% (84). Levetiracetam treatment is associated with a high drop-out rate (50%) because of somnolence, however.

There has been considerable interest in a variety of glutamate antagonists based on a body of scientific research implicating glutamate-mediated plastic changes in the pathogenesis of dyskinesia. N-methyl-D-aspartate (NMDA) receptor antagonists such as amantadine have been shown to provide anti-dyskinetic effects in PD, but the treatment is limited because of the cognitive side-effects. *Talampanel,* a non-competitive, selective antagonist of the α-amino-3-hydroxy-5-methylisoxazole-4-propionate (AMPA) glutamate receptor, has been reported to reduce L-dopa-induced dyskinesia significantly in parkinsonian monkeys (85). When given in combination with L-dopa, talampanel enhanced its antiparkinsonian action by up to 86% but reduced dyskinesias by up to 40%. These results suggest that talampanel might be a valuable adjunct to L-dopa in the treatment of PD. However, preliminary results from the first double-blind clinical trial in PD found no benefit on parkinsonism or dyskinesia (Olanow, personal communication). Possibly more promising studies target drugs which are antagonists of NMDA receptor subunits. NMDA receptors are widely distributed, and their antagonists which have anti-dyskinetic effects, such as amantadine, are limited by psychiatric side-effects. It can be hypothesized that antagonists of NMDA receptor subunits localized to the nigrostriatal dopamine system might provide anti-dyskinetic effects without cognitive side-effects. The most interest has focused on the NR2B subunit, which is restricted to the striatum and has been shown to translocate from synaptic to extrasynaptic membranes in association with the development of levodopa-induced dyskinesia (86). Finally, *safinamide* is a MAO-B inhibitor and a glutamate release inhibitor, which is another candidate drug against PD (see also Chapter 11).

Cannabinoid agonists and antagonists have also been studied for possible anti-dyskinesia effects in PD, as cannabinoid receptors are concentrated in the basal ganglia. *Nabilone* was shown to significantly reduce dyskinesia in a small, randomized, double-blind, placebo-controlled, crossover study in seven PD patients (87). How-ever, in a larger, randomized, double-blind, placebo-controlled trial of an oral cannabis extract, there was no evidence of any effect on Ldopa-induced dyskinesia as assessed by UPDRS Part IV, items 32-34, or any other outcome measures (88). *Sildenafil* (Viagra) has attracted attention based on the observation of almost complete resolution of dyskinesia in a PD patient who took the drug as a treatment for erectile dysfunction. In a small, open-label study, sildenafil was reported to improve dyskinesia, with some patients reporting complete dyskinesia resolution (89). Patients who reported a dyskinesia benefit experienced no worsening of PD symptoms.

Continuous dopamine receptor stimulation (CDS)

Under normal circumstances, striatal dopamine levels are relatively constant, and dopamine receptors are continuously activated (90). Intermittent doses of standard levodopa in PD do not restore basal ganglia function. Rather, intermittent or pulsatile activation of brain dopamine receptors leads to molecular and physiologic changes in the basal ganglia neurons associated with the development of motor complications (91-94). These observations have led to the hypothesis that more continuous stimulation of dopamine receptors (CDS) might be more physiologic and reduce the risk of inducing motor complications (95,96). While this concept has attracted considerable attention as a means of preventing motor complications, there is also interest that CDS-based therapies might be valuable with respect to the reversal of established motor complications. Several open-label studies in PD patients have reported that continuous infusions of a dopamine agonist can reduce 'off' time and dyskinesia (97-100). In a prospective study, patients randomized to receive a continuous subcutaneous infusion of *lisuride* or levodopa experienced significant improvement in both 'off' time and dyskinesias in comparison to patients treated with oral levodopa (101).

Continuous infusion of *apomorphine* has been widely employed in European countries, but is not yet available in the USA. The infusion can be administered by a modified insulin pump, which is programmable to deliver varying infusion rates according to the patients' individual requirements. The pump is refilled every 1-2 days, and catheters of different lengths can be used to maximize comfort. Most often, the infusion is administered during waking hours and discontinued overnight in order to avoid tolerance and psychiatric side-effects. In patients not adequately controlled by the infusion, oral levodopa plus a peripheral decarboxylase inhibitor can be added. It is also possible to administer a bolus of apomorphine as a 'rescue' therapy for unpredictable 'off' periods. Although the infusion technique is demanding, it can be managed relatively easily. Unfortunately, some patients develop distressing skin reactions at the injection site. Similar results have been seen with continuous infusion of lisuride. It should be noted that many patients with disabling motor complications can be well controlled with a continous infusion of a dopamine agonist.

There is also evidence that continuous infusion of *levodopa* can provide benefit for advanced PD patients with severe motor complications. Numerous studies have shown that continuous intestinal infusion of levodopa reduces 'off' time (102-103), and benefits have been shown to persist for prolonged periods of time (104). In a prospective study, we demonstrated that continuous intraintestinal infusion of levodopa was associated with a significant improvement in both 'off' time and dyskinesia in comparison to treatment with standard oral formulations of the drug (105). The benefits of levodopa infusion have been confirmed in a placebo-controlled, double-blind, crossover study (106). A water-soluble system for delivering continuous intrajejunal levodopa (duodopa®) is available in many countries and has proven to be effective in controlling motor fluctuations and reducing dyskinesias (107-109). Levodopa infusions are generally well tolerated, but require a surgical procedure to implant a permanent intraintestinal catheter which frequently needs to be replaced because of a tendency to kink and become obstructed.

Deep brain stimulation (DBS)

In many countries, DBS became the gold standard for the control of treatment-related motor complications. This therapeutic strategy is extensively discussed in Chapter 13.

Conclusions

Levodopa-induced dyskinesias and motor fluctuations can be major problems for PD patients. They are not only a potential source of disability, they often limit the ability of physicians to utilize levodopa fully in order to better control those features that are responsive to the medication. Medical treatments may be effective in the early stages, particularly for patients with wearing-off who do not experience dyskinesia. Manipulations of levodopa or the addition of a dopamine agonist, COMT inhibitor, or MAO-B inhibitor might provide some benefit in those cases. No medical agent reliably treats established dyskinesia, with perhaps the exception of amantadine, but there are serious potential side-effects, and the benefits may be transient. Most patients with motor complications end up with polypharmacy, taking combinations of these medications. As of yet, no data are available to indicate which combination is most effective or in what order they should be employed. Thus, physician judgment is required, taking into account concurrent medication, side-effect profile, convenience, compliance, physician familiarity with the drug, and patient preference. Eventually, while these medications can provide some benefit in the early stages of wearing-off or dyskinesia, eventually they are not able to control motor complications satisfactorily in many patients, and alternate approaches must be considered.

Continuous infusion of a dopamine agonist (apomorphine, lisuride) or of levodopa (see Chapter 14) has been shown to be capable of reducing both 'off' time and dyskinesia (98,101,105), but this approach is cumbersome for the patient and caregiver. Still, it is can be an alternative to DBS (see Chapter 13) and appears to provide benefits that are comparable to surgical therapies.

Several new drugs which aim to treat motor complications are in the pipeline, and some are particularly interesting because they act on non-dopaminergic targets (1). However, none has as yet been shown to add significantly to our current armamentarium of drugs, and none has a specific anti-dyskinetic effect. Experimental surgical approaches for treating Parkinson's disease such as transplantation, stem cells, and gene therapy have caught the imagination of the neuroscience community and the popular press. Implanted fetal mesencephalic grafts have been shown to survive, reinnervate the striatum and provide motor benefits in dopamine-lesioned rodents and monkeys (110). Further, dopaminergic grafts have been reported to reduce dyskinesia in levodopa-treated rodents (111). However, no significant benefits over placebo were observed in two prospective, double-blind, placebo-controlled trials. Further, rather than improving dyskinesias, fetal nigral transplantation was complicated by the development of a previously undescribed, off-medication dyskinesia that persists even after the levodopa dose is reduced or stopped (112,113). Stem cell grafting (114) or gene delivery of key proteins (e.g. AADC, neurturin) might restore dopaminergic function in a more physiologic manner than standard dopaminergic medications. In the final analysis, while great strides have been made in the management of motor complications, and there are exciting opportunities for the future, all efforts should be made to prevent the development of motor complications in the first place (115).

Video fragments

PLAY

Fragment 12.1
Motor fluctuations in PD (Segments 1-4)
Earlier or later, PD patients will develop levodopa-induced and to a lesser extent dopamine agonists-induced complications, such as hyperkinesias (segment 1), off-related dystonia (segment 2), unpredictable 'on-off' fluctuations (segment 3) and/or diphasic dyskinesias (segment 4), which were induced in this patient by threshold concentrations of L-dopa, related to a discontinuous medication schedule.

Fragment 12.2
Peak-dose chorea
Videofragment showing typical levodopa-induced, peak-dose, choreatic hyperkinesia.

Fragment 12.3
Dopamine dysregulation syndrome
In this video, note the disabling clinical expression of the consequences of a disorder associated with the abuse (overuse) of levodopa in a young PD patient (dopamine dysregulation syndrome).

References

1 Olanow CW, Watts RL, Koller WC. An algorithm (decision tree) for the management of Parkinson's disease: treatment guidelines. Neurology 2001;56(S5):S1-S86.

2 Agid Y, Olanow C, Mizuno Y. Levodopa: why the controversy? Lancet 2002;36:575.

3 Rascol O, Goetz C, Koller W, Poewe W, Sampaio C. Treatment interventions for Parkinson's disease: an evidence-based assessment. Lancet 2002;359:1589-1598.

4 Fahn S, Oakes D, Shoulson I, et al. Does levodopa slow or hasten the rate of progression of Parkinson disease? The results of the Elldopa study. N Eng J Med 2004;351 2498-2508.

5 Stocchi F, Antonini A, Barone P, et al. Early detection of wearing off in Parkinson disease: the DEEP study. Parkinsonism Relat Disord 2013;19:

6 Stocchi F, Rascol O, Kieburtz K, et al. Initiating levodopa/carbidopa therapy with and without entacapone in early Parkinson disease: the STRIDE-PD study. Ann Neurol. 2010;68:18-27

7 Olanow CW, Kieburtz K, Rascol O, et al. Factors predictive of the development of Levodopa-induced dyskinesia and wearing-off in Parkinson's disease. Mov Disord 2013;28:1064-1071.

8 Fabbrini G, Juncos J, Mouradian MM, Serrati C, Chase TN. Levodopa pharmacokinetic mechanisms and motor fluctuations in Parkinson's disease. Ann Neurol 1987;21:370-376.

9 Fabbrini G, Mouradian MM, Juncos J, et al. Motor fluctuations in Parkinson's disease: central pathophysiological mechanisms, Part I. Ann Neurol 1988;24:366-371.

10 Mouradian MM, Juncos JL, Fabbrini G, Schlegel J, Bartko JJ, Chase TN. Wearing-off fluctuations in Parkinson's disease: central pathophysiology mechanisms, Part II. Ann Neurol 1988;24:372-378.

11 Bravi D, Mouradian MM, Roberts JW, Davis TL, Sohn YH, Chase TN. Wearing-off fluctuations in Parkinson's disease: contribution of postsynaptic mechanisms. Ann Neurol 1994;36:27-31.

12 Rodriguez M, Lera G, Vaamonde J, Luquin MR, Obeso JA. Motor response to apomorphine and levodopa in asymmetric Parkinson's disease. J Neurol Neurosurg Psychiatry 1994;57:562-566.

13 Mouradian MM, Juncos JL, Fabbrini G, Chase TN. Motor fluctuations in Parkinson's disease. Ann Neurol 1989;25:633-634.

14 Nutt JG. Levodopa-induced dyskinesia: review, observations and speculations. Neurology 1990;40:340-345.

15 Stocchi F, Nordera G, Marsden CD. Strategies for treating patients with advanced Parkinson's disease with disastrous fluctuations and dyskinesias. Clin Neuropharmacol 1997;20:95-115.

16 Baruzzi A, Contin M, Riva R, et al. Influence of meal ingestion time on pharmacokinetics of orally administered levodopa in parkinsonian patients. Clin Neuropharmacol 1987;10:527-537.

17 Edwards LL, Quingley EMM, Pfeiffer RF. Gastrointestinal dysfunction in Parkinson's disease: frequency and pathophysiology. Neurology 1992;42:726-732.

18 Valenzuela JE. Dopamine as a possible neurotransmitter in gastric relaxation. Gastroenterology 1976;71:1019-1022.

19 Leon AS, Speigel H: The effect of antacid administration on the absorption and metabolism of levodopa. J Clin Pharmacol 1972;12:263-267.

20 Kelly KA. Motility of the stomach and gastroduodenal junction. In: Johnson LR, ed. Physiology of the gastrointestinal tract. Raven Press, New York, USA 1981:394-410.

21 Nutt JG, Woodward WR, Hammerstad JP et al. The 'on-off' phenomenon in Parkinson's disease: relation to levodopa absorption and transport. N Engl J Med 1984:310:483-488.

22 Leenders Kl, Poewe WH, Palmer AJ, et al. Inhibition of L-(19F)-fluorodopa uptake into human brain by amino acids demonstrated by positron emission tomography. Ann Neurol 1986;20:258-262.

23 Pierantozzi M, Pietroiusti A, Brusa L et al. Helicobacter pylori eradication and l-dopa absorption in patients with PD and motor fluctuations. Neurology 2006;66:1824-1829.

24 Stocchi F, Barbato L, Bramante L, Nordera G, Vacca L, Ruggieri S. Fluctuating parkinsonism: a pilot study of single afternoon dose of levodopa methyl ester. J Neurol 1996;243:377-380.

25 Stocchi F, Fabbri L, Vecsei L et al. Clinical efficacy of a single afternoon dose of effervescent levodopa-carbidopa preparation (CHF 1512) in fluctuating Parkinson disease. Clin Neuropharmacol 2007;30:18-24.

26 Katzenschlager R, Evans A, Manson A, et al. Mucuna pruriens in Parkinson's disease: a double blind clinical and pharmacological study. J Neurol Neurosurg Psychiatry 2004;75:1672-1677.

27 Rinne UK, Larsen JP, Siden A, Worm-Petersen J. Entacapone enhances the response to levodopa in parkinsonian patients with motor fluctuations. Nomecomt Study Group. Neurology 1998;51:1309-1314.

28 The Parkinson Study Group. Entacapone improves motor fluctuations in levodopa-treated Parkinson's disease patients. Ann Neurol 1997;42:747-755.

29 Deane KH, Spieker S, Clarke CE. Catechol-O-methyltransferase inhibitors for levodopa-induced complications in Parkinson's disease. Cochrane Database Syst Rev 2004;4:CD004554

30 Nutt JG, Woodward WR, Beckner RM et al. Effect of peripheral catechol-O-methyltransferase inhibition on the pharmacokinetics and pharmacodynamics of levodopa in parkinsonian patients. Neurology 1994;44;913-919.

31 Olanow CW and the Tasmar advisory panel. Tolacapone and hepatotoxic effects. Arch Neurol 2000;57:263-267.

32 Assal F, Spahr L, Hadengue A, Rubbia-Brandt L, Burkhard PR, Rubbici-Brandt L. Tolcapone and fulminant hepatitis. Lancet 1998;352:958.

33 Blum MW, Siegel AM, Meier R, Hess K. Neuroleptic malignant-like syndrome and acute hepatitis during tolcapone and clozapine medication. Eur Neurol 2001;46:158-160.

34 Olanow CW, Watkins PB. Tolcapone 2007: An Efficacy and Safety Review. J Clin Neuropharm Clin Neuropharmacol 2007;30:287-294.

35 Golbe LI, Lieberman AN, Muenter MD et al. Deprenyl in the treatment of symptom fluctuations in advanced Parkinson's disease. Clin Neuropharmacol 1988;11:45-55.

36 Parkinson Study Group. A randomized placebo-controlled trial of rasagiline in levodopa-treated patients with Parkinson disease and motor fluctuations. The PRESTO study. Arch Neurol 2005;62:241-248.

37 Rascol O, Brooks DJ, Melamed E et al. Rasagiline as an adjunct to levodopa in patients with Parkinson's disease and motor fluctuations (LARGO, Lasting effect in Adjunct therapy with Rasagiline Given Once daily, study): a randomised, double-blind, parallel-group trial. Lancet 2005;365:947-954.

38 Clarke A, Brewer F, Johnson ES, et al. A new formulation of selegiline: improved bioavailability and selectivity for MAO-B inhibition. J Neural Transm 2003;110:1241-1255.

39 Waters CH, Sethi KD, Hauser RA, et al, and the Zydis Selegiline Study Group. Zydis selegiline reduces off time in Parkinson's disease patients with motor fluctuations: a 3-month, randomized, placebo-controlled study. Mov Disord 2004;19:426-432.

40 Stocchi F, Rabey JM; Effect of rasagiline as adjunct therapy to levodopa on severity of OFF in Parkinson's disease. Eur J Neurol 2011;18:1373-1378.

41 Rascol O, Brooks DJ, Korczyn AD, DeDeyn PP, Clarke CE, Lang AE. A five-year study of the incidence of dyskinesia in patients with early Parkinson's disease who were treated with ropinirole or levodopa. 065 Study Group. N Engl J Med 2000;342:1481-1491.

42 Olanow CW, Fahn S, Muenter M et al. A multi-center, double-blind, placebo-controlled trial of pergolide as an adjunct to Sinemet in Parkinson's disease. Mov Disord 1994;9:40-47.

43 Lieberman A, Olanow CW, Sethi K et al. A multi-center double blind placebo-controlled trial of ropinirole as an adjunct to L-dopa in the treatment of Parkinson's disease patients with motor fluctuations. Neurology 1998;51:1057-1062.

44 Pinter MM, Pogarell O, Oertel WH. Efficacy, safety, and tolerance of the non-ergoline dopamine agonist pramipexole in the treatment of advanced Parkinson's disease: a double blind, placebo controlled, randomised, multicentre study. J Neurol Neurosurg Psychiatry 1999;66:436-441.

45 Clarke CE, Deane KH. Cabergoline for levodopa-induced complications in Parkinson's disease. Cochrane Database Syst Rev 2001;1:CD001518.

46 Rascol O, Brooks DJ, Korczyn AD et al. Development of dyskinesias in a 5-year trial of ropinirole and L-dopa. Mov Disord. 2006;21:1844-1850.

47 Pahwa R, Stacy MA, Factor SA et al; EASE-PD. Ropinirole 24-hour prolonged release: randomized, controlled study in advanced Parkinson disease. Neurology 2007;68:1108-1115.

48 Jankovic J, Watts RL, Martin W, Boroojerdi B. Transdermal rotigotine: double-blind, placebo-controlled trial in Parkinson disease. Arch Neurol 2007;5:676-682.

49 Stocchi F, Giorgi L, Hunter B, Schapira AH. PREPARED: Comparison of prolonged and immediate release ropinirole in advanced Parkinson's disease. Mov Disord. 2011;26:1259-1265.

50 Trenkwalder C, Kies B, Rudzinska M; Rotigotine effects on early morning motor function and sleep in Parkinson's disease: a double-blind, randomized, placebo-controlled study (RECOVER) Mov Disord 2011;26:90-99.

51 Korczyn AD, Brooks DJ, Brunt ER, et al. Ropinirole versus bromocriptine in the treatment of early Parkinson's disease: a 6-month interim report of a 3-year study. 053 Study Group. Mov Disord 1998;13:46-51.

52 Guttman M. Double-blind comparison of pramipexole and bromocriptine treatment in the treatment of early Parkinson's disease. International Pramipexole-Bromocriptine Study Group. Neurology 1997;49:1060-1065.

53 Pezzoli G, Martignoni E, Pacchetti C et al. Pergolide compared with bromocriptine in Parkinson's disease: a multicenter, crossover, controlled study. Mov Disord 1994;9:431-436.

54 Stocchi F. Pathological gambling in Parkinson's disease. Lancet Neurol 2005;4:590-592.

55 Driver-Dunckley E, Samanta J, Stacy M. Pathological gambling associated with dopamine agonist therapy in Parkinson's disease. Neurology 2003;61:422-423.

56 Nirenberg MJ, Waters C. Compulsive eating and weight gain related to dopamine agonist use. Mov Disord 2006;21:524-529.

57 Brodsky MA, Godbold J, Roth T, Olanow CW. Sleepiness in Parkinson's disease: a controlled study. Mov Disord 2003;18: 668-672.

58 Zanettini R, Antonini A, Gatto G, et al. Valvular heart disease and the use of dopamine agonists for Parkinson's disease. N Engl J Med 2007;356:39-46.

59 Antonini A, Poewe W. Fibrotic heart-valve reactions to dopamine-agonist treatment in Parkinson's disease. Lancet Neurol 2007;6:826-829.

60 Frankel JP, Lees AJ, Kempster PA, Stern GM. Subcutaneous apomorphine in the treatment of Parkinson's disease. J Neurol Neurosurg Psychiatry 1990;53,96-101.

61 Hughes Aj, Bishop S, Kleedorfer B et al. Subcutaneous apomorphine in Parkinson's disease: response to chronic administration for up to five years. Mov Disord 1993;8:165-170.

62 Dewey RB Jr, Hutton JT, LeWitt PA, Factor SA. A randomized, double-blind, placebo-controlled trial of subcutaneously injected apomorphine for parkinsonian off-state events. Arch Neurol 2001;58:1385-1392.

63 Attanasio A, Capria C, Leggiardro G et al. Transient cardiac arrest during continuous intravenous infusion of apomorphine. Lancet 1990;336:1321.

64 Nutt JG, Obeso JA, Stocchi F. Continuous dopamine receptor stimulation in advanced Parkinson's disease. Trends Neurosci 2000;23:109-115.

65 Schwarzschild MA, Agnati L, Fuxe K et al. Targeting adenosine A2A receptors in Parkinson's disease. Trends Neurosci. 2006;29:647-654.

66 Bibbiani F, Oh JD, Petzer JP, et al. A2A antagonist prevents dopamine agonist-induced motor complications in animal models of Parkinson's disease. Exp Neurol 2003;184:285-294.

67 Hauser RA, Hubble JP, Truong DD; Istradefylline US-001 Study Group. Randomized trial of the adenosine A(2A) receptor antagonist istradefylline in advanced PD. Neurology 2003;61:297-303.

68 Facca A, Sanchez-Ramos J. High-dose pergolide monotherapy in the treatment of severe levodopa-induced dyskinesias. Mov Disord 1996;11:327-329.

69 Cristina S, Zangaglia R, Mancini F, Martignoni E, Nappi G, Pacchetti C. High-dose ropinirole in advanced Parkinson's disease with severe dyskinesias. Clin Neuropharmacol 2003;26:146-150.

70 Storch A, Trenkwalder C, Oehlwein C, et al. High-dose treatment with pergolide in Parkinson's dis-

ease patients with motor fluctuations and dyskinesias. Parkinsonism Relat Disord 2005;11:393-398.

71 Verhagen Metman L, Del Dotto P et al. Amantadine as treatment for dyskinesias and motor fluctuations in Parkinson's disease. Neurology 1998;50:1323-1326.

72 Luginger E, Wenning GK, Bosch S, Poewe W. Beneficial effects of amantadine on L-dopa-induced dyskinesias in Parkinson's disease. Mov Disord 2000;15:873-878.

73 Thomas A, Iacono D, Luciano AL, Armellino K, Di Iorio A, Onofrj M. Duration of amantadine benefit on dyskinesia of severe Parkinson's disease. J Neurol Neurosurg Psychiatry 2004;75:141-143.

74 Pierelli F, Adipietro A, Soldati G, Fattapposta F, Pozzessere G, Scoppetta C. Low dosage clozapine effects on L-dopa induced dyskinesias in parkinsonian patients. Acta Neurol Scand 1998;97:295-299.

75 Durif F, Debilly B, Galitzky M, et al. Clozapine improves dyskinesias in Parkinson disease: a double-blind, placebo-controlled study. Neurology 2004;62:381-388.

76 Meco G, Fabrizio E, Alessandri A et al. Risperidone in levodopa induced dyskinesiae. J Neurol Neurosurg Psychiatry 1998;64:135.

77 Manson AJ, Schrag A, Lees AJ. Low-dose olanzapine for levodopa induced dyskinesias. Neurology 2000;55:795-799.

78 Baron MS, Dalton WB. Quetiapine as treatment for dopaminergic-induced dyskinesias in Parkinson's disease. Mov Disord 2003;18:1208-1209.

79 Bara-Jimenez W, Bibbiani F, Morris MJ et al. Effects of serotonin 5-HT1A agonist in advanced Parkinson's disease. Mov Disord 2005;20:932-936.

80 Olanow CW, Damier P, Goetz CG et al. Multicenter, open-label, trial of sarizotan in Parkinson disease patients with levodopa-induced dyskinesias (the SPLENDID Study). Clin Neuropharmacol 2004;27:58-62.

81 Goetz CG, Damier P, Hicking C et al. Sarizotan as a treatment for dyskinesias in Parkinson's disease: a double-blind placebo-controlled trial. Mov Disord 2007;22:179-186.

82 Bezard E, Hill MP, Crossman AR et al. Levetiracetam improves choreic levodopa-induced

dyskinesia in the MPTP-treated macaque. Eur J Pharmacol 2004;485:159-164.

83 Hill MP, Ravenscroft P, Bezard E et al. Levetiracetam potentiates the antidyskinetic action of amantadine in the 1-methyl-4-phenyl-1,2,3,6-tetrahydropyridine (MPTP)-lesioned primate model of Parkinson's disease. J Pharmacol Exp Ther 2004;310:386-394.

84 Zesiewicz TA, Sullivan KL, Maldonado JL et al. Open-label pilot study of levetiracetam (Keppra) for the treatment of levodopa-induced dyskinesias in Parkinson's disease. Mov Disord 2005; 20: 1205-1209.

85 Konitsiotis S, Blanchet PJ, Verhagen L et al. AMPA receptor blockade improves levodopa-induced dyskinesia in MPTP monkeys. Neurology 2000;54:1589-1595.

86 Gardoni F, Picconi B, Ghiglieri V et al. A critical interaction between NR2B and MAGUK in L-DOPA induced dyskinesia. J Neurosci 2006;26:2914-2922.

87 Sieradzan KA, Fox SH, Hill M et al. Cannabinoids reduce levodopa-induced dyskinesia in Parkinson's disease: a pilot study. Neurology 2001;57:2108-2111.

88 Carroll CB, Bain PG, Teare L et al. Cannabis for dyskinesia in Parkinson disease: a randomized double-blind crossover study. Neurology 2004;63:1245-1250.

89 Swope DM, Loma L. Preliminary Report: Use of sildenafil to treat dyskinesias in patients with Parkinson's disease. Neurology 2000;54:A90.

90 Olanow CW, Obeso JA, Stocchi F. Continuous Dopamine Receptor Stimulation in the Treatment of Parkinson's Disease: Scientific Rationale and Clinical Implications. Lancet Neurology 2006;5:677-687.

91 Olanow CW, Obeso JA. Preventing levodopa-induced dyskinesia. Ann Neurol 2000;47:167-178.

92 Obeso JA, Rodriguez-Oroz MC, Rodriguez M, et al. Pathophysiology of the basal ganglia in PD. Trends Neurosci 2000;23:8-19.

93 Calon F, Grondin R, Morissette M et al. Molecular basis of levodopa-induced dyskinesias. Ann Neurol 1998;47:70-78.

94 Filion M, Tremblay L, Bedard PJ. Effects of dopamine agonists on the spontaneous activity of globus pallidus neurons in monkeys with MPTP-induced parkinsonism. Brain Res 1991;547:152-161.

95 Olanow CW, Schapira AHV, Rascol O. Continuous dopaminergic stimulation in the early treatment of PD. Trends Neurosci 2000;23:117-126.

96 Chase TN, Baronti F, Fabbrini G et al. Rationale for continous dopamimetic therapy of Parkinson's disease. Neurology 1989;39:7-10.

97 Stibe CM, Lees AJ, Kempster PA, Stern GM. Subcutaneous apomorphine in parkinsonian on-off oscillations. Lancet 1988;1:403-406.

98 Colzi A, Turner K, Lees AJ. Continuous subcutaneous waking day apomorphine in the long-term treatment of levodopa induced interdose dyskinesia in Parkinson's disease. J Neurol Neurosurg Psychiatry 1998;64:573-576.

99 Vaamonde J, Luquin MR, Obeso JA. Subcutaneous lisuride infusion in Parkinson's disease: Response to chronic administration in 34 patients. Brain 1991;114:601-614.

100 Katzenschlager R, Hughes A, Evans A et al. Continuous subcutaneous apomorphine therapy improves dyskinesias in Parkinson's disease: a prospective study using single-dose challenges. Mov Disord 2005;20:151-157.

101 Stocchi F, Ruggieri S, Vacca L, Olanow CW. Prospective randomized trial of lisuride infusion versus oral levodopa in patients with Parkinson's disease. Brain 2002;125:2058-2066.

102 Sage JI, Trooskin S, Sonsalla PK, Heikkila RE, Duvoisin RC. Longterm duodenal infusion of levodopa for motor fluctuations in parkinsonism. Ann Neurol 1998;24:87-89.

103 Kurlan R, Rubin AJ, Miller C, et al. Duodenal delivery of levodopa for on-off fluctuations in parkinsonism: Preliminary observations. Ann Neurol 1986;20:262-265.

104 Syed N, Murphy J, Zimmerman T, Mark MH, Sage JI. Ten years' experience with enteral levodopa infusions for motor fluctuations in Parkinson's disease. Mov Disord 1998;13:336-338.

105 Stocchi F, Vacca L, Ruggieri S, Olanow CW. Intermittent vs continuous levodopa administration in patients with advanced Parkinson disease: a clinical and pharmacokinetic study. Arch Neurol 2005;62:905-910.

106 Kurth MC, Tetrud JW, Tanner CM et al. Double-blind, placebocontrolled, crossover study of duodenal infusion of levodopa/carbidopa in Parkinson's disease patients with 'onoff' fluctuations. Neurology 1993;43:1698-1703.

107 Nilsson D, Hannsson L, Johansson K et al. Longterm intraduodenal infusion of a water based levodopacarbidopa dispersion in very advanced Parkinson's disease. Acta Neurol Scand 1998;97:175-183.

108 Nilsson D, Nyholm D, Aquilonius SM. Duodenal levodopa infusion in Parkinson's disease--long-term experience. Acta Neurol Scand 2001;104:343-348

109 Antonini A, Isaias IU, Canesi M, et al. Duodenal levodopa infusion for advanced Parkinson's disease: 12-month treatment outcome. Mov Disord 2007;22:1145-1149.

110 Olanow CW, Kordower JH, Freeman TB. Fetal nigral transplantation as a therapy for Parkinson's disease. Trends Neurosci 1996;19:102-109.

111 Lee CS, Cenci MA, Schulzer M, Bjorklund A. Embryonic ventral mesencephalic grafts improve levodopa-induced dyskinesia in a rat model of Parkinson's disease. Brain 2000;123:1365-1379.

112 Freed CR, Greene PE, Breeze RE, et al. Transplantation of embryonic dopamine neurons for severe Parkinson's disease. N Engl J Med 2001;344:710-719.

113 Olanow CW, Goetz CG, Kordower JH, et al. A double blind placebo-controlled trial of bilateral fetal nigral transplantation in Parkinson's disease. Ann Neurol 2003;54:403-414.

114 De Munter JP, Mochizuki H, Melamed F, Wolters ECh. Stemcells in Parkinson's disease: Why, How and When. Parkinsonism Relat Disord 2014, 2014;20(S1):

115 LeWitt PA, Rezai AR, Leehey MA et al. AAV2-GAD gene therapy for advanced Parkinson's disease: a double-blind, sham-surgery controlled, randomised trial. Lancet Neurol. 2011;10:309-319.

116 Tomlinson CL, Stowe R, Patel S, Rick C, Gray R, Clarke CE. Systematic review of levodopa dose equivalency reporting in Parkinson's disease. Mov Disord 2010;25:2649-2653.

13

Deep Brain Stimulation in Parkinson's Disease

Anne-Catherine M.L. Huys, Julien F. Bally & Pierre Pollak

In 1987, high-frequency, deep brain stimulation (DBS) was introduced as a validated therapy for Parkinson's disease (PD). It is now well established worldwide, and so far more than 100,000 patients have benefited from this treatment. In this review, the well-established facts and the most recent results will be discussed, covering in particular the indications and contraindications, the surgical considerations, the efficacy of the different targets, the adverse effects and finally, the future.

Patient selection

Careful patient selection is a crucial determinant of consistently favorable outcomes following DBS. This requires a careful evaluation by an expert multidisciplinary team involving at least a movement disorder neurologist, a neurosurgeon, a neuropsychologist, and a psychiatrist (1).

Indications

The ideal DBS candidate suffers from idiopathic Parkinson's disease or genetic parkinsonism with an excellent response to levodopa but with motor fluctuations and/or dyskinesias that are uncontrollable despite optimized medical therapy, or with medication-refractory tremor. In addition, the ideal candidate should have no levodopa-unresponsive features, no cognitive decline, psychiatric or behavioural issues, nor any major comorbidities. Except for patients with early-onset PD, most patients fall outside this ideal description. The medical art is to ap-preciate for each patient the extent to which alterations of these features can be accepted. Eventually, the patients make their decision based on detailed information of their individual risks and benefits. Candidates for DBS should have tried the main antiparkinsonian drugs. A trial of levodopa at the highest tolerated dose (ideally, at least 800 mg daily for 3 months) or an unambiguously positive levodopa challenge test is mandatory before surgical consideration.

Apart from DBS, there are currently two available strategies to reduce motor complications in advanced PD: continuous subcutaneous apomorphine infusion and continuous intestinal levodopa/carbidopa infusion gel (LCIG) (see Chapter 14). Despite very few comparative studies that help to select the best treatment for individual patients, the three procedures have a slightly different risk-benefit profile. DBS is best for younger patients and is considered the most effective treatment for drug-refractory tremor or intractable dyskinesias (7). Patients over the age of 75 are usually not good candidates, and DBS bears the risk of worsening levodopa-unresponsive dysarthria, freezing of gait or postural instability. As levodopa is the antiparkinsonian drug least likely to induce adverse psychiatric effects, LCIG is the preferred procedure for patients with cognitive impairment or psychosis, although device management may be a problem. In case of impulse control disorders, DBS (8) or LCIG are preferable because they allow discontinuation of dopamine agonists.

DBS can be safely and successfully performed in patients with previous ablative or DBS procedures at other sites and even after dopaminergic cell transplantation.

Age

Is there an age limit for DBS? The major concerns with age are cognitive dysfunction (2), co-morbidities, higher risk of surgical complications and a higher incidence of levodopa- and thus DBS-resistant symptoms, such as dysarthria, dysphagia, postural instability, and gait difficulties. All of these factors have a significant impact on the risk-benefit ratio.

The value of age as an independent outcome predictor for DBS remains debatable (3,4), but more studies and expert opinion support superior outcomes in younger patients (5-7). Although no specific age cutoff has been defined in many clinical DBS studies, most have excluded patients above the age of 75. At our institution, we tend to consider age above 75 years as a relative contraindication and age above 80 years as an almost absolute contraindication.

Nevertheless, age is less critical when considering nucleus ventralis intermedius of the thalamus (Vim) DBS in elderly patients mainly suffering from disabling tremor. Moreover, Vim DBS can be performed unilaterally, and patients suffering from the tremor-dominant type of PD often have a more benign disease course. Therefore, there is no age limit for this target.

Co-morbidities

Unsurprisingly, formal studies concerning serious systemic co-morbidities are lacking. However, common sense dictates the exclusion of patients with any serious disease, which either reduces life expectancy or considerably increases the surgical risks.

Preoperative MRI screening allows the identification of structural lesions that may increase the risk of surgery, such as vascular malformations, cortical atrophy, hydrocephalus or large cysts with brain distortion. More often than not these discoveries are circumventable by altering the implantation trajectory.

PD-related clinical characteristics

Disease severity and duration

There is no consensus on the level of disease severity that warrants DBS. Patients with the severest motor score may be dramatically improved, providing they fulfill the other clinical criteria for surgery.

Typical disease duration before DBS treatment has mostly been of the order of 10-15 years (9-14). There is currently a drive towards conducting DBS earlier, not because of a presumed neuroprotective effect, as none has been demonstrated so far, but because of the superiority of symptom control and quality of life compared to the best medical therapy. This holds true after mean disease durations of 7.5 years, and within three years after the development of levodopa-induced motor complications (15). In addition, the development of levodopa- and thus DBS-resistant symptoms with natural disease progression and the good long-term motor effects speak in favor of earlier interventions in order to maximize the years with good motor control and minimize detrimental effects on professional and personal aspects of life early on. In other words, early DBS leads to a longer period of motor benefits before the appearance of levodopa- and stimulation-unresponsive features. However, including patients with less than 5 years' disease duration carries the risk of operating on patients with atypical parkinsonism, for whom the benefit would be very limited in time, if at all, and therefore does not seem justified.

Levodopa responsiveness

So far, levodopa-responsiviness has been widely accepted as the best outcome predictor for response to DBS, especially to DBS of the subthalamic nucleus (STN) (1,3) and to a lesser extent to globus pallidus internus (GPi) DBS. It is thus mandatory to evaluate surgical candidates with a formal levodopa test, using supratherapeutic doses of levodopa. A 30% improvement in the UPDRS motor score has been considered the minimal percentage below which DBS should not be performed (1). Exceptions are levodopa-resistant severe tremor and failure to capture the worst-off or best-on motor states due to insufficiently long washout periods, sleep benefit, poor drug absorption or too low dosages at levodopa challenge tests.

Refractory postural and gait problems, dysarthria and dysphagia

Several studies indicate that patients with important gait difficulties and risks of falls despite otherwise good motor control before surgery are not improved by GPi or STN DBS (16). In other words, standard DBS should not be recommended to patients who remain disabled by freezing of gait or risk to fall during the pull test in their best on-state (7). Patients with severe dysarthria before surgery should generally not expect improvement from DBS, and speech may even worsen (see below). Dysphagia is typical of the very advanced stages of PD, generally after the age of DBS indication. DBS does not usually influence swallowing (17), but may sometimes lead to a worsening (18) and in any case does not prevent it in the long-term (5). Its presence therefore makes surgery rather unsuitable.

Dementia

Dementia, as defined by the DSM V, is the most common exclusion criterion for DBS surgery because it may be worsened, and patients will not have the leisure to take advantage of surgery-induced motor benefits. Almost all patients with PD exhibit some cognitive dysfunction, especially in the executive domain. The issue is to know to what extent this dysfunction can jeopardize the outcome of DBS. Treatable causes such as depression or medication, especially anticholinergics, must be excluded. There is no consensus on the type of testing and level of performance that should exclude patients from receiving DBS. Neuropsychological evaluation for cognitive dysfunction is mandatory, with a special emphasis on memory and exec-

utive function (19). The Mattis dementia rating scale (MDRS) (range 0–144), with a cutoff score of <124 usually distinguishing demented from non-demented patients, is mostly used for this purpose. In the case of borderline scores or cognitive complaints, it is useful to repeat the evaluation after 6-12 months to ascertain a stable cognitive function. A progressive worsening usually heralds dementia. Thus, it is wise to know the patient's cognitive performance for at least one year before DBS referral.

Depression and psychosis

Surgery is generally deferred in patients with unstable psychiatric conditions, especially depression or psychosis, until their symptoms have been adequately managed (7). Ongoing severe depression with suicidal ideation should be considered an absolute contraindication to surgery because of the increased risk of suicide (see below) (20,21).

Apathy, dopamine dysregulation syndrome, ICD and OCD

Preoperative apathy, despite high doses of dopaminergic medication, is likely to worsen with postoperative drug reduction and so will dopamine-induced creativity. Disease-related psychiatric symptoms must be distinguished from medication side effects, especially the dopamine dysregulation syndrome (DDS), punding and the impulse control disorders (ICD) (see Chapter 41). The latter three can be treated by medication reduction following STN DBS and therefore represent a good indication for surgery (8). Patients suffering from both PD and obsessive compulsive disorder (OCD) (see Chapter 40) can be good candidates for STN DBS, as this surgery has been shown to be beneficial in both diseases (19).

Personal, professional and social issues

Perceived disability can be very subjective, and individual variations in lifestyle, professional, interpersonal and social factors are an important part of the equation. They are difficult to account for in large studies but have a major impact on quality of life outcomes.

Patients' expectations are not always realistic. It is the responsibility of every neurologist to carefully assess the risk-benefit ratio for each individual patient, and provide a realistic explanation of the potential restorative benefits of DBS. Using the best on-state as a marker of what patients may expect (in addition to dyskinesia and tremor reduction) is useful in assisting patients to eliminate false hopes and set the right expectations.

Surgical issues

In PD, the two main targets for DBS are the STN and GPi, the efficacy of which will be discussed separately and then in comparison, after stressing the fact that this efficacy of course depends on the accuracy of the targeting. Finally, the eventual role of Vim DBS in Parkinson's disease will be dealt with.

The improvement of PD motor symptoms by DBS indeed depends on the accuracy of targeting. The neurosurgical procedure varies according to each team. It is based on the stereotactic method for targeting the chosen neuronal structure. The main step of targeting is imaging, which includes magnetic resonance imaging (MRI) and/or computed tomography (CT). Image-guided STN DBS without microelectrode recording was reported to lead to substantial improvements in motor disability and quality of life in well-selected PD patients, with very low morbidity (22). Intraoperative MRI facilities will enable improved guidance and successful implantation under general anaesthesia. However, many teams prefer to operate under local anaesthesia to physiologically identify the target with micro- or mac-

rorecording and stimulation. This would avoid misplacements related to brain shift due to electrode implantation and pneumocephalus due to dura mater opening. However, the use of microelectrodes is known to increase the risk of intracranial bleeding. Typically, and especially in STN DBS at the sites where microelectrode recordings show neuronal discharges characteristic of the STN, high-frequency stimulation induces a dramatic improvement in motor parkinsonism at low intensity and side effects at high intensity (wide therapeutic window). The amelioration of the symptoms can be accompanied by dyskinesias, which are a positive predictive factor for the outcome. The other side effects are induced by stimulating the surrounding areas of the STN. So far, no randomized studies have been performed to know whether surgery under general anaesthesia without microelectrode insertion provides a better benefit to risk ratio than surgery under local anaesthesia and extensive functional neurophysiology. Postoperative imaging is invaluable

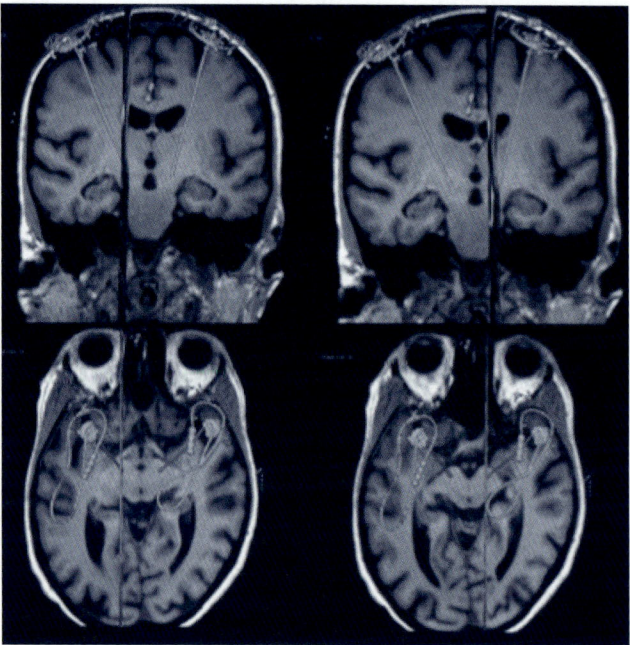

Figure 13.1
Fusion images of preoperative MRI with postoperative CT showing correct electrode placement in the STN. Courtesy of Dr M. I. Vargas, Neuroradiology Department, University Hospital of Geneva, Switzerland.

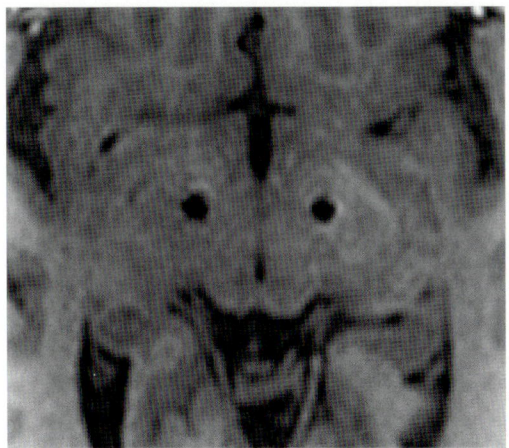

Figure 13.2
Postoperative axial T1-weighted MRI of the midbrain, showing correct electrode placement in the STN. Courtesy of Dr M. I. Vargas, Neuroradiology Department, University Hospital of Geneva, Switzerland.

for documenting the absence of complications and the location of the electrode (see Figures 13.1 and 13.2). A postoperative chest X-ray is performed to show the implanted pulse generator(s) and connecting leads, and will be useful in case of later hardware malfunction (see Figure 13.3).

Subthalamic nucleus

The STN is a small nucleus with a volume of approximately 160 mm³ (a third of the size of the GPi). The advantage is that small stimulation intensities can modulate a major part of the nucleus though the disadvantage is a higher likelihood of current spread to adjacent structures, inducing side effects. In addition, the smaller size of the STN compared to the GPi means less segregation of the limbic, associative and motor loops, making it potentially more difficult to induce selective motor effects.

Motor symptoms

After one year, bilateral STN DBS leads to an approximately 50-60% improvement in rigidity, tremor and bradykinesia in the on-stimulation/off-medication (on-stim/off-med) condition,

compared to the preoperative off-medication (off-med) state (9,10,12,17). These values have been confirmed in a large, blinded, randomised, controlled study (14). This motor improvement is maintained at around 55% improvement after 5 years (9,10,17), and at approximately 40% after 8-9 years (12,17). Analysis of the subscores of the UPDRS III at 5-10 years show approximate values of 80% improvement in tremor, 41-99% in rigidity and 8-49% in bradykinesia (9,12,17,23). Given the worsening of the baseline motor score with disease progression over time (5), these values signify that the improvement in motor function is broadly maintained over the years, especially for the cardinal motor symptoms tremor, rigidity and to a lesser degree bradykinesia. Nevertheless, part of the decline is due to the appearance of levodopa- and stimulation-resistant axial signs (dysarthria, postural instability, gait difficulties and freezing of gait). Some studies show stable off-med/off-stim UPDRS III scores at 5-10 years compared to preoperative off scores. This phenomenon is attributed to an ongoing effect of the DBS, extending for longer than the one hour that is normally allowed to elapse before testing (5, 11, 23). Currently, there are no indications that DBS of any of the known targets alters disease progression.

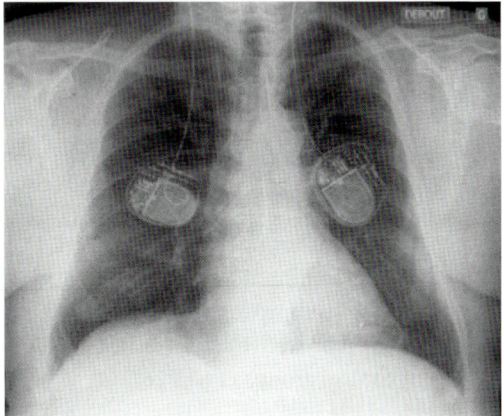

Figure 13.3
Chest X-ray showing bilateral implantable pulse generators. Courtesy of Dr M. I. Vargas, Neuroradiology Department, University Hospital of Geneva, Switzerland.

Unilateral STN-DBS has been performed in patients with very asymmetric symptoms. In this procedure, contralateral symptoms are obviously improved, but interestingly, there is also a notable benefit on the ipsilateral side of the body (24). There is a major decrease and often even complete disappearance of dyskinesias in the short and long term following bilateral STN DBS (9,11,13,14,23,25). The vast majority of authors attribute this beneficial effect on dyskinesias to the important reduction in the levodopa equivalent daily dose (LEDD) after STN-DBS. Part of the benefit could also be related to the stabilisation of the basal ganglia loop activity by continuous stimulation. The severity of off-dystonia, often particularly disabling in the early morning, is improved in about 75% of the patients, and remains so in the long term (9,11,13).

Activities of daily living and quality of life
Activities of daily living (ADL) and quality of life (QoL) are more valuable domains for the patient than pure motor aspects, even though the three obviously interact with each other.
One year after STN DBS, activities of daily living, as measured by the UPDRS part II score in the on-stim/off-med state are improved by around 60% as compared to the preoperative off-state (9-13,25). After 5 years, this improvement decreases slightly to around 45%, and by combining levodopa and stimulation, activities of daily living are improved even further (9, 10, 12). However, when comparing the postoperative on-stim/on-med scores with preoperative on-med UPDRS II scores, studies show unchanged values after 1 (12) and 5 years (12,17) and a 57-128% worsening after 8-9 years (12,17). Except for the communication item, quality of life is consistently improved following STN-DBS compared to preoperative scores or best medical treatment control groups (14,18,26).

Non-motor symptoms

Pain
Several non-motor symptoms are improved by STN-DBS. Off-period dystonia-associated pain decreases following STN DBS (9,13). In addition, pain and sensory fluctuations, other than those associated with off-period dystonias, showed a 84% improvement following STN-DBS in one study, indicating that painful conditions might in fact reinforce the indications instead of representing an exclusion criterion (27).

Sleep efficiency
Sleeptime is increased in the on-stim condition, with an increase in total sleep time of 47% (28). Several studies suggest that chronic STN-DBS may improve sleep quality through increased nocturnal mobility and reduction of sleep fragmentation. More precisely, STN stimulation greatly reduces nighttime akinesia and suppresses axial and early morning dystonia, but does not alleviate periodic leg movements or rapid eye movement (REM) sleep behaviour disorders. Daytime somnolence might be reduced by levodopa reduction.

Dysautonomia
Dysautonomic features may be improved after DBS (5,27).

Mood and cognition
Some studies support a favourable impact on mild to moderate depression and anxiety in the first postoperative year (7), but these effects are often not maintained in the long term (see below). DBS of the STN worsens verbal fluency and seems to have a mild impact on executive function in general, without worsening of global cognitive function and without a clear impact on quality of life (see below).

Dopaminomimetic co-medication
DBS of the STN allows a drastic reduction in dopamine replacement therapy. Compared to pre-

operative values, the levodopa equivalent daily doses are generally diminished by around 50% (8-14,17,18,23,25,29,30). As expected, hyperdopaminergic behaviours such as impulse control disorders and the dopamine dysregulation syndrome wane when successful STN DBS allows a significant reduction in the levodopa equivalent dose (8,17). Whether these effects are entirely due to a decrease in dopaminergic medication with desensitisation and decreased stimulation of mesolimbic dopaminergic pathways, or also due to an effect of STN DBS on pathways involved in reward and addiction, remains to be clarified (6,8). As explained below, impulse control disorders on the one hand and apathy on the other might be explained by different degrees and combinations of personal predispositions, medication and DBS.

Dopaminergic medication-induced hallucinations decrease or their appearance is delayed by medication reduction. Finally, lowering of dopaminergic drugs might unmask or worsen the presence of restless legs syndrome.

Stimulation settings

Immediately after surgery, stimulation settings are progressively increased and are mostly maintained or only mildly increased in the long term. Typical voltages are 2.8V, with a pulse width of 60 microseconds (μs) and a frequency of 130 Hertz (Hz).

Patients with severe tremor may be improved by frequencies above 130Hz. Frequencies below 130Hz may be used in the case of worsening of dysarthria or freezing of gait.

In conclusion

Taking these data together, it is clear that even though the cardinal dopaminergic features and levodopa-related motor complications remain well controlled, activities of daily living and therefore quality of life gradually deteriorate over time. Part of this can be attributed to advanced age with co-morbidities, particularly osteoarticular dysfunctions (12). The majority is probably due to natural disease progression, with unaltered deterioration of freezing of gait, postural instability, dysarthria, autonomic dysfunction and cognitive decline (1,5,9,10,12,17,23). These features are thought to be largely due to degeneration of non-dopaminergic pathways and are therefore levodopa- and stimulation-unresponsive (1,10,12,17).

Globus pallidus internus

It is important to keep in mind that there are far fewer studies of the GPi than of the STN and that very long-term studies are lacking

Motor symptoms

The UPDRS-III score performed in the off-med/on-stim compared to the baseline off-med condition shows a 35% improvement at 6 months (25) and around 40% at 3-4 years (13), with a maintenance of these effects at 5-6 years (11). Dyskinesias are dramatically improved by GPi-DBS, with a decrease by more than 70% in the on-med/on-stim condition in the short and long term (up to 5-6 years) (11,13,25). Contrary to STN DBS, this antidyskinetic effect is a direct consequence of the GPi DBS.

Off-dystonias are reported to be improved (31) or unchanged (11,13) with this therapy.

Activities of daily living and quality of life

There are few studies available, but they all show an improvement in quality of life (26,29) and activities of daily living in the short (18,25) and long term (11,13).

Non-motor symptoms

GPi DBS is generally reported not to have any influence on mood or cognition (7,13,29,32).

Dopaminometic co-medication

The levodopa equivalent daily dose (LEDD) generally remains unchanged (11,13,25,30), with a reported increase in some studies and a decrease in others (18,32).

Stimulation settings

The mean voltage is around 3.4V, with a pulse width of 90μs or more and a frequency of 130Hz or higher (25). These values remain unchanged over time (11,13). The voltage and pulse width parameters are significantly higher for the GPi-DBS than for the STN-DBS, leading to a shorter battery life in the former (18).

Subthalamic nucleus versus globus pallidus internus

In the late 1990s, a growing number of papers started to show better motor outcomes with STN-DBS than with GPi-DBS, and a substantial reduction in LEDD in the former but not in the latter. This resulted by the turn of the millennium in a tacit consensus of preferring the STN target to treat PD motor symptoms. This consensus was based on non-randomised studies until the first randomised, double-blind study of a small cohort comparing the GPi and the STN showed a similar improvement of the UPDRS-III score in the off-med/on-stim condition at 12 months compared to baseline for GPi (39% improvement) and STN (48% improvement) (30). This study started the 'rematch' opposing GPi and STN (33) and was soon followed by two large-scale, randomized, double-blind, controlled trials. Both trials concluded that STN DBS allows a greater decrease in LEDD. The North American study showed no difference in motor outcomes, as opposed to the Dutch study, which favoured STN. One item in the cognitive test was worse in the STN group in the North American study, a finding not con-

firmed in other studies (18,32). How can we deal with two well-conducted studies with opposing results concerning the motor outcome? The 25% improvement in the motor score achieved by bilateral STN DBS in the North American study is unusually low. Were the patients older than usual (23% were >70 years old), were the electrodes properly implanted (the word 'electrode' is not mentioned in the article), how were the stimulation settings adjusted? Hopefully, the Dutch study reconciles evidence-based medicine with clinical practice (34) (Figure 13.4).

Nucleus ventralis intermedius (Vim) of the thalamus

Vim was the first target used in PD DBS, and it showed an excellent effect on tremor but not on akinesia or rigidity. Not surprisingly, Vim DBS was abandoned as soon as GPi and STN DBS were proposed. However, some patients suffer mainly from severe tremor and minimal rigidity and akinesia. Thalamic surgery is generally well tolerated, whereas bilateral STN surgery

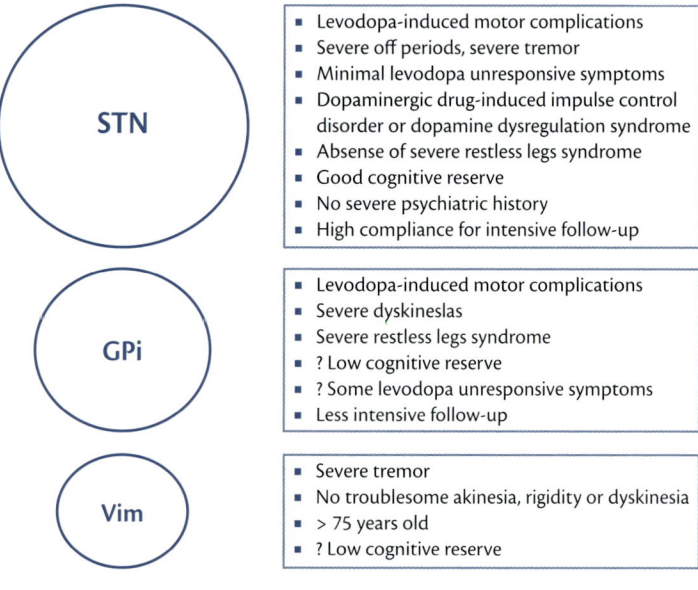

Figure 13.4
Individualised target selection for DBS.
Unclear indications are preceded by a question mark.

can worsen cognition or alter behaviour in some patients, especially in the very old. Therefore, Vim surgery can still be applied in old patients with tremor-predominant PD (see Figure 13.4). Even though Vim-DBS is well known for causing possible tolerance and rebound phenomena, the beneficial effect on tremor tends to be long-lasting (35).

Adverse effects

Two factors need to be kept in mind when evaluating the adverse effects of DBS. First, far more studies have been performed on STN than on any other target, leading to an obvious bias in overstating adverse effects associated with this location. Second, suboptimal electrode placement can certainly create a vast array of side-effects. The important question is which adverse effects are frequent or worrisome with correctly placed electrodes. Many of the earlier studies did not check the exact electrode position or did correlate it with side-effects, leading to a further potential bias.

Perioperative and hardware-associated complications

No operation is without risks. In the case of DBS, the rates of perioperative intracranial haemorrhage and stroke are generally less than 2% (1). Hardware-associated complications, which are diminishing with improvement of the hardware, include wire fractures, electrode misplacement or migration (2%), skin erosions, device malfunction (3%) and, most dreaded, infection, occurring in around 2% and then frequently requiring removal of the DBS system (1,3).

Stimulation-induced complications

Motor dysfunction

While DBS leads to a drastic improvement in overall motor function, dysarthria may worsen and certain aspects of gait difficulties persist, while controversial effects on eyelid apraxia might be seen.

Dysarthria

Even though loudness and voice tremor generally improve, this is outweighed by a general dysarthrogenic effect. About 9% of the patients develop dysarthria following STN-DBS (3,36). The mechanism is multifactorial: 90% of parkinsonian patients develop dysarthria in the course of their disease, so part of it is certainly due to natural disease progression with partial resistance to levodopa and DBS. The microlesion effect in an already fragile system probably contributes. Finally, increased dysarthria with stronger stimulation suggests a direct effect of the DBS with probable current spread to adjacent corticobulbar or cerebellothalamic pathways (36). Preliminary data suggest less dysarthria with GPi compared to STN-DBS, but more detailed studies are required (36).

Freezing of gait (FOG)

Gait is mostly improved after DBS, due to the improvement in bradykinesia, rigidity, tremor and dyskinesia (9,12,13,17,29). However, sometimes STN DBS is not as effective as levodopa for levodopa-responsive gait difficulties (7), such as freezing of gait (16), and rarely it even worsens gait, often by increasing freezing of gait (16). In the vast majority of cases, FOG is predominantly due to disease progression with levodopa- and stimulation-resistant freezing of gait and postural instability (9,10,12,17,23). A recent study suggested that freezing of gait in PD patients with STN-DBS might be improved with high doses of methylphenidate (59).

Eyelid apraxia

Apraxia of lid opening, an inability to open the eyes or to maintain the eyes open, can be induced or treated by STN-DBS (37,38). This paradoxical effect might be explained by an off-phase focal dystonia improved by STN-DBS or levodopa on the one hand, and a stimulation side-effect from current spread to corticobulbar tracts on the other (37,38). Involuntary eyelid closure might therefore be a better term than apraxia of lid opening (37).

Cognitive dysfunction

Transient postoperative confusion
Like any other brain surgery, the operation itself represents a major perturbation requiring cognitive reserves in order to be well tolerated. While postoperative transient confusion is common in DBS procedures (16%) (3), long-lasting major cognitive side effects are far less frequent.

Reduced verbal fluency
The only clearly and repeatedly demonstrated cognitive impairment with DBS is a reduction in verbal fluency. Even though some studies show an equal effect in GPi and STN-DBS (39), it is mostly reported with subthalamic stimulation; evidence shows a decline in verbal fluency compared to preoperative levels (2,8,17,20,40,41), and without worsening in the 'best medical treatment' control groups (42,43). Even though DBS is generally performed bilaterally, the left side appears to be crucial (39). Phonemic verbal fluency seems to be more affected than semantic fluency (40, 44), but some show the opposite (20) or impairment in both categories (43).

Reduced executive functions
The evidence for a negative or positive impact on other executive functions such as the Stroop, Wisconsin card sorting or trail-making tests is conflicting (2,4,8,20,41-44). Overall, even though some studies show no dysexecutive syndrome (8,44), most conclude that DBS, especially of the STN, leads to mild impairment in executive function, but without a significant impact on the quality of life (2,42,43). Other cognitive functions that have been reported to decline after STN DBS but that need further evaluation include: visuomotor processing speed (32), visuomotor coordination (39), recognition of facial emotions (45), colour naming (42) and verbal memory (42). Yet others point to an improvement in psychomotor speed and working memory in the on- versus off-state of subthalamic stimulation (41) and decreased cognitive fluctuations with mental slowness following STN DBS (27).

Global cognitive impairment
Importantly, global cognitive function as measured by the Mattis dementia rating scale generally remains unchanged in the short to medium term following STN-DBS (8-10,15,20,27,43) with only a few reports showing a worsening (29). Elderly patients, however, or those with pre-operative borderline cognitive scores might be at risk of permanent postoperative cognitive deterioration (2,9). The risk of cognitive deterioration following DBS of the GPi or Vim is thought to be even less (13,29,46).

The mechanism of verbal or other cognitive impairment following DBS remains unclear. Potential reasons are stimulation of the associative area of the STN and inhibition of cognitive loops or the reduction in dopaminergic medication, or finally the surgery itself with passage through the frontal cortex and sometimes the caudate nucleus in patients with a preexisting predisposition to subcortico-frontal dysfunction.

Mood and behavioural abnormalities

Apathy and/or impulse control disorders
Apathy can be defined as a lack of interest and motivation, with decreased emotional involvement, but without associated sadness. One in three parkinsonian patients suffers from apathy, but when cases with concomitant depression or dementia are excluded, this number falls to around 7% (47). It is commonly observed following STN-DBS (19-21,47,48). Some attribute this to high-frequency stimulation of the limbic part of the STN (49), others doubt this theory in view of a slight psychostimulant effect of STN stimulation (50,51). It is generally accepted that

lowering of dopaminergic medication favours the occurrence of apathy (21,48), and postoperative apathy tends to respond well to reaugmentation of dopamine agonists (52). However, dopamine withdrawal alone is not a sufficient cause (47). An attractive hypothesis is the notion of postoperative dopamine withdrawal unmasking an underlying hypodopaminergic state due to mesolimbic dopaminergic denervation (48). PET studies in patients developing apathy under STN-DBS show more mesocorticolimbic dopaminergic denervation than controls without apathy. The denervation is most marked in the projections to the orbitofrontal, dorsolateral prefrontal, cingulate and temporal cortices, ventral striatum and right amygdala (48). This hypothesis offers a good explanation for why apathy is not universal, but can occur both pre- and postoperatively, and given the gradual lowering of dopaminergic drugs and their long-term effect, why it tends to develop months after the intervention. Individual differences in the degree of mesolimbic dopaminergic denervation, postoperative drug management and a slight stimulating effect of STN-DBS can explain the seemingly paradoxical occurrence of postoperative apathy on the one hand or impulse control disorder on the other (48).

Depression and/or mania
The verdict on the effects of STN stimulation on depression is still out. In view of its small size of about 160mm³ and its limbic anteromedial area, it seems logical that different electrode placements in and around the STN will have different, if not opposing effects on mood. As mentioned above, the question is which impact, if any, a correctly placed dorsolateral STN electrode has. Small studies show an acute improvement in mood, independent of the motor improvement, in dorsal STN stimulation (51) and worsening of mood in more ventral locations (40). Whether such acute changes reflect long-term effects remains to be answered. Globally, most studies indicate a status quo (4,8,10, 12,17,27,49) or im-

provement (2,20,44,51) of depressive symptoms after DBS. Interestingly, most postoperative depression seems to resolve following the reintroduction of dopaminergic drugs (52). Thus, as for apathy, the higher rate of depression with STN DBS compared to GPi-DBS (13) might not be related to the stimulation, but to a more marked lowering of dopaminergic medication following STN-DBS (32). Vim DBS also seems much safer as far as mood and behavioural side-effects are concerned.

Unsurprisingly, given the frequent improvement of mood following STN-DBS, it can also induce euphoria, hypomania (4-15%), mania (<2%) (19) and mirthful laughter (53). Again, as with apathy and impulse control disorders, this apparent paradox between depression and mania might be explained by different combinations of psychostimulant effects of STN DBS, drug management and an underlying vulnerability, such as mesolimbic dopaminergic denervation.

Anxiety and stress
Anxiety, which might be linked to non-motor offs, is generally reported to decrease (7,43) or to remain unchanged (8,12,17,49) following STN-DBS. However, caution is necessary when interpreting apparent improvement in anxiety questionnaire scores as they include physical symptoms often present in PD such as tremor or an inability to relax, which are improved by DBS. Finally, one should not underestimate the psychological stress patients can experience when their well-established role suddenly changes from a dependent to an independent one with a need to re-establish their identity at home and in society. Unsurprisingly, marital difficulties are very common following DBS.

Suicide
An alarming aspect is the increased suicide rate after STN-DBS. An international study with over 5000 patients showed an attempted suicide rate of 0.9% and a completed suicide rate of 0.45% following STN-DBS (21). Since the baseline su-

icide rate in PD is the same or lower than in the general population, this indicates a substantial increase. Fifty percent of the suicides have occurred by 10 months and 75% by 17 months. The most consistent risk factor for attempted or completed suicide is postoperative depression. Other risk factors for attempted suicide are being single and a previous history of impulse control disorder or compulsive medication use (21). Of note is the high suicide rate of 3% in one study, in which all dopamine agonists were abruptly discontinued on the day of the surgery, and levodopa was reduced as much as possible within 2 weeks (8). The increased rate of suicide might be linked to an increased risk of depression, even though this in itself is still a matter of debate; it might be linked to an abrupt lowering of dopaminergic drugs; or finally it might be due to increased impulsiveness, partially linked to an executive dysfunction. The cause of suicide is certainly multifactorial, and it is of paramount importance to be vigilant to its possibility and address any contributing factors.

Weight gain

Weight gain is sometimes reported following GPi-DBS and commonly following STN-DBS (3,9,10,17,54). While part of it may be related to decreased tremor and dyskinesia, the increased mobility offsets this effect, and the weight gain generally exceeds the previous weight lost during disease evolution. The mechanism remains unclear. It might be linked to current diffusion to brain regions regulating appetite, such as the hypothalamus, as suggested by increased weight with more medially placed electrodes (55), and alterations of weight-regulating hormones, such as ghrelin, leptin, neuropeptide Y and cortisol (54).

Other complications

The immediate postoperative period can sometimes show severe but transient dyskinesia or hemiballism, resembling that seen after an acute STN stroke and therefore attributed to

the acute microlesion. Similarly, dyskinesia or even hemiballism can be caused by too strong an inhibition of the STN. Current diffusion to the corticospinal or corticobulbar tracts causes muscle contractions including eye deviation with diplopia, dysarthria or even dystonia-like postures. Current spread to the third cranial nerve in STN-DBS also causes diplopia, and diffusion to the medial lemniscus in STN-DBS or to the ventral posterior lateral thalamus in Vim DBS leads to paraesthesia. In the latter, effects on nearby cerebellar connections induce contralateral cerebellar symptoms. Effects on supranuclear connections can lead to a pseudobulbar affect, such as pseudobulbar crying. Ipsilateral mydriasis, flushing and sweating are explained by activation of sympathetic fibres in the zona incerta. Optic tract involvement in GPi DBS induces phosphenes. Other stimulation-induced side-effects include nausea and dizziness. Stimulation-related side-effects of this kind are generally easily controlled with alterations of the stimulation parameters (3).

Future developments

What does the future hold for DBS? Will it become even more common, or is it actually too expensive? At first sight, it does indeed appear to be an expensive procedure, but several studies show that the initial high investment pays off and that thanks to the medication decrease, it becomes cheaper than the best medical therapy after only a few years (57,58).

New targets: pedunculopontine nucleus

Gait difficulties such as freezing of gait and postural instability are hallmarks of the advanced stages of PD, and they become progressively more levodopa-resistant. Several basic science and clinical data point to an association of these symptoms and the dysfunction of the mesencephalic locomotion region in the pedunculopontine area. Pioneering studies showed an improvement in levodopa-unresponsive postural stability and gait with low-frequency stimulation of the mostly cholinergic pedunculopontine nucleus. However, more recent, controlled studies reported disappointing outcomes, with only a decrease in the number of falls. Some patients clearly improved, while others did not, indicating that further studies are needed to understand the factors determining the outcome (56).

New hardware: pulse generators and optogenetics

Smaller implanted pulse generators are needed. New electrodes with multiple miniature contacts or oriented electrical fields are under investigation and so are closed loop stimulation systems, allowing delivery of stimulation only when necessary. In the long term, the neuromodulation of a specific cell type or pathway will be rendered possible by techniques such as optogenetics.

References

1 Bronstein JM, Tagliati M, Alterman RL, et al. Deep brain stimulation for Parkinson disease: an expert consensus and review of key issues. Arch Neurol. 2011;68:165.

2 Saint-Cyr JA, Trepanier LL, Kumar R, Lozano AM, Lang AE. Neuropsychological consequences of chronic bilateral stimulation of the subthalamic nucleus in Parkinson's disease. Brain. 2000;123:2091-2108.

3 Kleiner-Fisman G, Herzog J, Fisman DN, et al. Subthalamic nucleus deep brain stimulation: summary and meta-analysis of outcomes. Mov Disord. 2006;21S14:S290-304.

4 Weaver FM, Follett K, Stern M, et al. Bilateral deep brain stimulation vs best medical therapy for patients with advanced Parkinson disease: a randomized controlled trial. JAMA. 2009;301:63-73.

5 Merola A, Zibetti M, Angrisano S, et al. Parkinson's disease progression at 30 years: a study of subthalamic deep brain-stimulated patients. Brain. 2011;134:2074-2084.

6 Fasano A, Daniele A, Albanese A. Treatment of motor and non-motor features of Parkinson's dis-

ease with deep brain stimulation. Lancet Neurol. 2012;11:429-442.

7 Volkmann J, Albanese A, Antonini A, et al. Selecting deep brain stimulation or infusion therapies in advanced Parkinson's disease: an evidence-based review. J Neurol. 2013

8 Lhommee E, Klinger H, Thobois S, et al. Subthalamic stimulation in Parkinson's disease: restoring the balance of motivated behaviours. Brain. 2012;135:1463-1477.

9 Krack P, Batir A, Van Blercom N, et al. Five-year follow-up of bilateral stimulation of the subthalamic nucleus in advanced Parkinson's disease. N Engl J Med. 2003;349:1925-1934.

10 Schupbach WM, Chastan N, Welter ML, et al. Stimulation of the subthalamic nucleus in Parkinson's disease: a 5 year follow up. J Neurol Neurosurg Psychiatry. 2005;76:1640-1644.

11 Moro E, Lozano AM, Pollak P, et al. Long-term results of a multicenter study on subthalamic and pallidal stimulation in Parkinson's disease. Mov Disord. 2010;25:578-586.

12 Zibetti M, Merola A, Rizzi L, et al. Beyond nine years of continuous subthalamic nucleus deep brain stimulation in Parkinson's disease. Mov Disord. 201;26:2327-2334.

13 Rodriguez-Oroz MC, Obeso JA, Lang AE, et al. Bilateral deep brain stimulation in Parkinson's disease: a multicentre study with 4 years follow-up. Brain. 2005;128:2240-2249.

14 Deuschl G, Schade-Brittinger C, Krack P, et al. A randomized trial of deep-brain stimulation for Parkinson's disease. N Engl J Med. 2006;355:896-908.

15 Schuepbach WM, Rau J, Knudsen K, et al. Neurostimulation for Parkinson's disease with early motor complications. N Engl J Med. 2013;368:610-622.

16 Ferraye MU, Debu B, Fraix V, et al. Effects of subthalamic nucleus stimulation and levodopa on freezing of gait in Parkinson disease. Neurology. 2008;70:1431-1437.

17 Fasano A, Romito LM, Daniele A, et al. Motor and cognitive outcome in patients with Parkinson's disease 8 years after subthalamic implants. Brain. 2010;133:2664-2676.

18 Odekerken VJ, van Laar T, Staal MJ, et al. Subthalamic nucleus versus globus pallidus bilateral deep brain stimulation for advanced Parkinson's disease (NSTAPS study): a randomised controlled trial. Lancet Neurol. 2013;12:37-44.

19 Voon V, Kubu C, Krack P, Houeto JL, Troster AI. Deep brain stimulation: neuropsychological and neuropsychiatric issues. Mov Disord. 2006;21S14:S305-327.

20 Funkiewiez A, Ardouin C, Caputo E, et al. Long term effects of bilateral subthalamic nucleus stimulation on cognitive function, mood, and behaviour in Parkinson's disease. J Neurol Neurosurg Psychiatry. 2004;75:834-839.

21 Voon V, Krack P, Lang AE, et al. A multicentre study on suicide outcomes following subthalamic stimulation for Parkinson's disease. Brain. 200;131:2720-2728.

22 Foltynie T, Zrinzo L, Martinez-Torres I, et al. MRI-guided STN DBS in Parkinson's disease without microelectrode recording: efficacy and safety. J Neurol Neurosurg Psychiatry. 2011;82:358-363.

23 Castrioto A, Lozano AM, Poon YY, Lang AE, Fallis M, Moro E. Ten-year outcome of subthalamic stimulation in Parkinson disease: a blinded evaluation. Arch Neurol. 201;68:1550-1556.

24 Shemisa K, Hass CJ, Foote KD, et al. Unilateral deep brain stimulation surgery in Parkinson's disease improves ipsilateral symptoms regardless of laterality. Parkinsonism Relat Disord. 201;17:745-748.

25 Group TD-BSfPsDS. Deep-brain stimulation of the subthalamic nucleus or the pars interna of the globus pallidus in Parkinson's disease. N Engl J Med. 2001;345:956-963.

26 Volkmann J, Albanese A, Kulisevsky J, et al. Long-term effects of pallidal or subthalamic deep brain stimulation on quality of life in Parkinson's disease. Mov Disord. 2009;24:1154-1161.

27 Witjas T, Kaphan E, Regis J, et al. Effects of chronic subthalamic stimulation on nonmotor fluctuations in Parkinson's disease. Mov Disord. 2007;22:1729-1734.

28 Arnulf I, Bejjani BP, Garma L, et al. Effect of low and high frequency thalamic stimulation on sleep in patients with Parkinson's disease and essential tremor. J Sleep Res. 2000;9:55-62.

29 Weaver FM, Follett KA, Stern M, et al. Randomized trial of deep brain stimulation for Parkinson disease: thirty-six-month outcomes. Neurology. 2012;79:55-65.

30 Anderson VC, Burchiel KJ, Hogarth P, Favre J, Hammerstad JP. Pallidal vs subthalamic nucleus deep brain stimulation in Parkinson disease. Arch Neurol. 2005 Apr;62(4):554-60.

31 Krack P, Pollak P, Limousin P, et al. Subthalamic nucleus or internal pallidal stimulation in young onset Parkinson's disease. Brain. 1998;121:451-457.

32 Follett KA, Weaver FM, Stern M, et al. Pallidal versus subthalamic deep-brain stimulation for Parkinson's disease. N Engl J Med. 2010;362:2077-2091.

33 Okun MS, Foote KD. Subthalamic nucleus vs globus pallidus interna deep brain stimulation, the rematch: will pallidal deep brain stimulation make a triumphant return? Arch Neurol. 2005;62:533-536.

34 Krack P, Hariz MI. Deep brain stimulation in Parkinson's disease: reconciliation of evidence-based medicine with clinical practice. Lancet Neurol. 2013;12:25-26.

35 Hariz MI, Krack P, Melvill R, et al. A quick and universal method for stereotactic visualization of the subthalamic nucleus before and after implantation of deep brain stimulation electrodes. Stereotact Funct Neurosurg. 2003;80:96-101.

36 Skodda S. Effect of deep brain stimulation on speech performance in Parkinson's disease. Parkinsons Dis. 2012;850596.

37 Weiss D, Wachter T, Breit S, et al. Involuntary eyelid closure after STN-DBS: evidence for different pathophysiological entities. J Neurol Neurosurg Psychiatry. 2010;81:1002-1007.

38 Tommasi G, Krack P, Fraix V, Pollak P. Effects of varying subthalamic nucleus stimulation on apraxia of lid opening in Parkinson's disease. J Neurol. 2012;259:1944-1950.

39 Rothlind JC, Cockshott RW, Starr PA, Marks WJ, Jr. Neuropsychological performance following staged bilateral pallidal or subthalamic nucleus deep brain stimulation for Parkinson's disease. J Int Neuropsychol Soc. 2007;13:68-79.

40 Okun MS, Fernandez HH, Wu SS, et al. Cognition and mood in Parkinson's disease in subthalamic

nucleus versus globus pallidus interna deep brain stimulation: the COMPARE trial. Ann Neurol. 2009;65:586-595.

41 Pillon B, Ardouin C, Damier P, et al. Neuropsychological changes between "off" and "on" STN or GPi stimulation in Parkinson's disease. Neurology. 2000;55:411-418.

42 Smeding HM, Speelman JD, Koning-Haanstra M, et al. Neuropsychological effects of bilateral STN stimulation in Parkinson disease: a controlled study. Neurology. 2006;66:1830-1836.

43 Witt K, Daniels C, Reiff J, et al. Neuropsychological and psychiatric changes after deep brain stimulation for Parkinson's disease: a randomised, multicentre study. Lancet Neurol. 2008;7:605-614.

44 Ardouin C, Pillon B, Peiffer E, et al. Bilateral subthalamic or pallidal stimulation for Parkinson's disease affects neither memory nor executive functions: a consecutive series of 62 patients. Ann Neurol. 1999;46:217-223.

45 Peron J, Biseul I, Leray E, et al. Subthalamic nucleus stimulation affects fear and sadness recognition in Parkinson's disease. Neuropsychology. 2010;24:1-8.

46 Hariz MI, Krack P, Alesch F, et al. Multicentre European study of thalamic stimulation for parkinsonian tremor: a 6 year follow-up. J Neurol Neurosurg Psychiatry. 2008;79:694-699.

47 Starkstein SE. Apathy in Parkinson's disease: diagnostic and etiological dilemmas. Mov Disord. 2012;27:174-178.

48 Thobois S, Ardouin C, Lhommee E, et al. Non-motor dopamine withdrawal syndrome after surgery for Parkinson's disease: predictors and underlying mesolimbic denervation. Brain. 2010;133:1111-1127.

49 Drapier D, Drapier S, Sauleau P, et al. Does subthalamic nucleus stimulation induce apathy in Parkinson's disease? J Neurol. 2006;253:1083-1091.

50 Funkiewiez A, Ardouin C, Krack P, et al. Acute psychotropic effects of bilateral subthalamic nucleus stimulation and levodopa in Parkinson's disease. Mov Disord. 2003;18:524-530.

51 Campbell MC, Black KJ, Weaver PM, et al. Mood response to deep brain stimulation of the subthalamic nucleus in Parkinson's disease. J Neuropsychiatry Clin Neurosci. 2012;24:28-36.

52 Thobois S, Lhommee E, Klinger H, et al. Parkinsonian apathy responds to dopaminergic stimulation of D2/D3 receptors with piribedil. Brain. 2013;136:1568-1577.

53 Krack P, Kumar R, Ardouin C, et al. Mirthful laughter induced by subthalamic nucleus stimulation. Mov Disord. 2001;16:867-875.

54 Markaki E, Ellul J, Kefalopoulou Z, et al. The role of ghrelin, neuropeptide Y and leptin peptides in weight gain after deep brain stimulation for Parkinson's disease. Stereotact Funct Neurosurg. 2012;90:104-112.

55 Ruzicka F, Jech R, Novakova L, Urgosik D, Vymazal J, Ruzicka E. Weight gain is associated with medial contact site of subthalamic stimulation in Parkinson's disease. PLoS One. 2012;7:e38020.

56 Ferraye MU, Debu B, Fraix V, et al. Effects of pedunculopontine nucleus area stimulation on gait disorders in Parkinson's disease. Brain. 2010;133:205-214.

57 Fraix V, Houeto JL, Lagrange C, et al. Clinical and economic results of bilateral subthalamic nucleus stimulation in Parkinson's disease. J Neurol Neurosurg Psychiatry. 2006;77:443-449.

58 Dams J, Siebert U, Bornschein B, et al. Cost-effectiveness of deep brain stimulation in patients with Parkinson's disease. Mov Disord. 2013;28:763-771.

59 Moreau C, Delval A, Defebvre L, et al. Methylphenidate for gait hypokinesia and freezing in patients with Parkinson's disease undergoing subthalamic stimulation: a multicentre, parallel, randomised, placebo-controlled trial. Lancet Neurol 2012; 11: 589-96.

14

Continuous Dopaminergic Stimulation in Parkinson's Disease

Angelo Antonini & Francesca Mancini

Continuous dopaminergic stimulation (CDS) is a therapeutic concept for the management of Parkinson's disease (PD) that proposes that continuous stimulation of striatal dopamine receptors, as opposed to discontinuous or *pulsatile* stimulation, will delay or prevent the onset of dyskinesias. Although levodopa (LD) is the most effective treatment for both motor and non-motor symptoms, its pulsatile administration likely contributes to the development of motor fluctuations and dyskinesia after a few years. All studies comparing LD versus dopamine agonists indicate that early therapy with agonists is associated with a reduced risk of motor complications, possibly because the agonists' longer half-life provides continuous dopaminergic delivery. Indeed, this therapeutic strategy may delay the onset of motor fluctuations and dyskinesia, which is essential to maintaining a satisfactory quality of life. In advanced disease, various LD-based strategies may be tried to control motor complications such as dose fragmentation (smaller, more frequent dosing) or the use of orally administered, liquid LD formulations that may reduce off-time intervals or facilitate absorption. More recently introduced, continuous LD delivery by duodenal infusion (but also apomorphine infusion) may represent a more efficacious approach to treat motor complications in advanced PD, and its effect can be perceived by improvement on both clinical scales and health-related items. Infusion therapies may reverse motor complications in patients, leading to a significant benefit on quality of life.

Etiology/pathophysiology

The hallmark of PD is loss of dopaminergic neurons of the substantia nigra pars compacta, leading to bradykinesia, rigidity and tremor. The current pharmacological treatment is therefore centred upon dopamine replacement to alleviate the symptoms. LD has been the most effective symptomatic therapy for the treatment of PD since its introduction in the late 1960s, and remains the standard against which new interventions must be compared. Most physicians initiate carbidopa/LD or benserazide/LD two or three times daily. This approach is largely based on anecdotal experience, presumably aimed at finding the lowest dose of the drug providing satisfactory clinical control, and it does not take into account what is known about the organization of the basal ganglia, nor does it attempt to replace dopamine in a physiologic manner. Indeed, there is almost no data to indicate that this is the correct or optimal way to administer LD (1). Nonetheless, progressive loss of dopamine neurons results in worsening of the motor condition and requires increasing dose and more frequent levodopa administrations. This, in turn, results in increased pulsatile dopamine release, eventually contributing to the development of motor complications. LD-induced dyskinesias were first reported by Cotzias and colleagues (2) and include dystonic and choreic movements occurring at the beginning, end, peak or even throughout the entire period of LD effect. The main treatment option to prevent dyskinesia and motor fluctuations in early PD is currently continuous dopamine agonist delivery.

Alternative methods of continuous LD delivery (including gene therapy) and new pharmacological agents that target non-dopaminergic receptor systems are currently under experimental investigation (3).

Existing and emerging pharmacological strategies for delaying dyskinesias in patients with PD involve several approaches: delaying the introduction of LD therapy, treatment with an antidyskinetic agent, use of a therapy or a delivery system that can provide CDS, or use of novel agents targeting non-dopaminergic receptors (4).

The precise mechanism responsible for why LD is so dyskinesiogenic is unknown, but increasing data suggest that it may relate to the replacement of dopamine in a non-physiological pulsatile manner (5). This hypothesis arose from studies of healthy basal ganglia demonstrating that, under normal conditions, striatal dopamine levels are maintained at a relatively constant level and the administration of LD in a discontinuous or pulsatile manner induces molecular changes in striatal neurons, and neurophysiologic changes in pallidal output neurons which lead to the development of motor complications. This concept is supported by numerous preclinical studies in MPTP-treated primates, which all showed that treatment with a long-acting dopamine agonist is associated with reduced dyskinesia compared with LD (6).

Moreover, recent findings in rats with unilateral medial forebrain bundle dopamine lesions (7) also support a role for the primary motor cortex (M1) and putative serotonin 5-HT1A receptor in LD-induced dyskinesia.

Interestingly, Lee et al. (8) examined the genetic susceptibility in the diphasic and peak-dose forms of LD-induced dyskinesias in 503 patients with PD. They showed that the presence of diphasic dyskinesia was exclusively associated with the dopamine D3 receptor (DRD3) p.S9G variant after adjusting for gender, age at PD onset, Hoehn & Yahr stage, and duration of LD treatment.

CDS in early Parkinson patients

Although most PD patients eventually require the addition of LD as the disease progresses, several current recommendations suggest initiating symptomatic treatment with a dopamine agonist in the attempt to delay motor complications (9). The exact reason why initial monotherapy with a dopamine agonist is associated with a reduced risk for dyskinesias compared to LD is not fully understood. The hypothesis claims that medications with longer half-lives provide more continuous delivery of dopaminergic medications compared to short-acting drugs such as LD. However, it should be noted that dopamine agonists provide less motor benefit than LD, at least in monotherapy, and this may also contribute to the lower incidence of dyskinesia (10). Studies using either slow-release LD or combinations of LD with the COMT-inhibitor entacapone have not found decreased incidences of motor complications over periods of up to 5 years. Moreover, the recent STRIDE-PD trial comparing initial therapy with standard LD versus combined treatment with entacapone has shown shorter latencies to the development of dyskinesias and overall increased dyskinesia rates when patients were treated with the triple combination (11). Again, this might have been due to the fact that patients with triple combination therapy had a higher central bioavailability of LD.

On the other hand, the 4- and 5-year LD-controlled monotherapy trials versus pramipexole and ropinirole both show that dyskinesia rates remain lower in the initial agonist arm, even after most patients had received adjunct LD to maintain symptomatic control (12). Six-year follow-up data for 222 of 301 patients originally randomized to the CALM PD trial continued to show reduced overall dyskinesia rates for those patients initially randomized to pramipexole (13). A similar trend was observed at a 10-year follow-up time point for the ropinirole versus LD cohort, but this was based on less than 20% of the original study cohort available for assessment (14).

How long benefits from initial agonist therapy can be maintained is being debated. The UK bromocriptine trial suggests that after 14 years of observation, the initially lower incidence of motor complications in the agonist arm was no longer present, while LD-treated patients continued to show benefits in terms of symptomatic control (15). Although the conclusions to be drawn from these data are limited by the small number of patients evaluated after 14 years, they are consistent with the eventual need for LD in almost all PD patients, which progressively diminishes differences in initial dyskinesia risk when patients are followed in the very long term. Moreover, additional factors may contribute to the development of severe disabling dyskinesias in same patients. Their rate was found to be similar at 4 years in the pramipexole versus LD trial regardless of which drug was chosen for the initial therapy, indicating possible genetic contributors, as mentioned above.

Extended release (ER) formulations of dopamine agonists (pramipexole, ropinirole) have been developed to allow a once-daily formulation and to provide more stable dopaminergic stimulation, and they may present significant advantages in terms of ensuring an improved adherence to the treatment schedule. Compared to the immediate release (IR) formulation, the substance itself is unchanged, meaning there is an identical receptor profile, identical efficacy, and identical receptor binding. The half-life is also the same, but the continuous release results in an overall prolonged plasma bioavailability. The potential advantages include maintaining more consistent dopaminergic activity with steadier plasma levels, increased tolerability, greater compliance from a simpler once-daily dosing regimen and easier dose titration (16).

Recently, a randomized, double-blind, placebo and active comparator-controlled trial of ER pramipexole in the early stage of PD was carried out by Poewe and colleagues (17). In this study, among 213 ER and 207 IR recipients, the adjusted mean 33-week UPDRS II+III change (excluding LD rescue effects) was -8.2 for ER and -8.7 for IR, a difference of -0.5 with a 95% CI of -2.3 to 1.3. Compared with placebo (n = 103), pramipexole ER and pramipexole IR were significantly superior on UPDRS II+III score amd all key secondary outcomes, and almost all other endpoints and the formulations were equally safe and well-tolerated.

In 83 patients with early PD, long-term treatment with once-daily ropinirole ER in a long-term (78 months) and open-label study (18) was not associated with any new safety concerns and was effective in maintaining the clinical status.

The introduction of the rotigotine transdermal delivery system also represents a significant development that allows a constant delivery of a non-ergot dopamine agonist using a once-daily regimen, achieving steady plasma levels. This regime has the additional advantage of bypassing the stomach, as delayed gastric emptying in PD can constitute a significant problem when administering drugs orally. Giladi and colleagues (19) investigated the rotigotine transdermal patch in 561 patients with early Parkinson's disease in a randomized, double-blind, controlled study versus placebo and ropinirole. They showed that rotigotine at doses below or equal to 8 mg/24 h were not inferior to ropinirole at doses ≤24 mg/day. In a post-hoc subgroup analysis, rotigotine ≤8 mg/24 hours had a similar efficacy to ropinirole at doses ≤12 mg/day. They reported that the most common adverse events were application-site reactions, nausea, and somnolence.

CDS in advanced Parkinson patients

Advanced PD is defined by the onset of motor response complications (MRC), characterized by 'wearing off' and dyskinesias (potentially associated with off-period dystonia), emerging in up to 80% of patients (20). Their development leads to worsening disability with a significant impact on patient and caregiver quality of life (21). Three potential mechanisms have been proposed to explain the development of motor fluctuations in levodopa-treated advanced PD patients (20,22): peripheral factors such as impaired gastric emptying and competition with dietary protein for levodopa absorption (additionally, long-chain amino acids compete with levodopa as they cross the blood-brain barrier); presynaptic factors related to nigrostriatal dopaminergic neuron loss and subsequent handling of levodopa by other neuronal and glial cells; and postsynaptic and downstream changes occurring as a result of pulsatile stimulation of dopamine receptors.

Although demonstration that a continuous supply of dopaminergic stimulation to the brain may keep PD patients from developing the potential for dyskinesias and/or motor fluctuations is still lacking, conversely, CDS with infusions can reduce both dyskinesias and motor fluctuations in PD patients who already have those problems. Based on clinical evidence, the additional potential benefits of CDS include alleviating nocturnal disturbances, avoiding priming for motor fluctuations and dyskinesia, minimizing daytime sleepiness, preventing the development of gastrointestinal dysfunction, and reducing the risk of developing psychosis or behavioural disturbances (23).

Apomorphine

Apomorphine is the oldest dopaminergic medication and was initially known for its emetic properties. It has been applied in several medical conditions such as analgesia, insomnia, alcohol dependence, schizophrenia and others. It was initially used for PD over 60 years ago but later ignored for many years following the introduction of LD. It is also the most potent dopa-

mine agonist, and its administration can provide symptom relief comparable to LD. Apomorphine exerts its antiparkinsonian effect by direct stimulation of striatal postsynaptic dopamine D1 and D2 receptors (24). The drug is rapidly absorbed after subcutaneous injection (C_{max} 20 min) and has a short half-life (almost 43 min), and this is consistent with its rapid onset of action, with effects apparent within 5–15 minutes of subcutaneous administration. Clinical studies and evidence-based reviews generally support a role for continuous subcutaneous apomorphine infusion (CSAI) (see Figure 14.1) as an effective option for patients with PD and severe fluctuations, poorly controlled by conventional oral drug treatment (25). Overall, studies report an improvement in off-time of between 50% and 80% as well as dyskinesia (26). However, these results were reported several years ago under

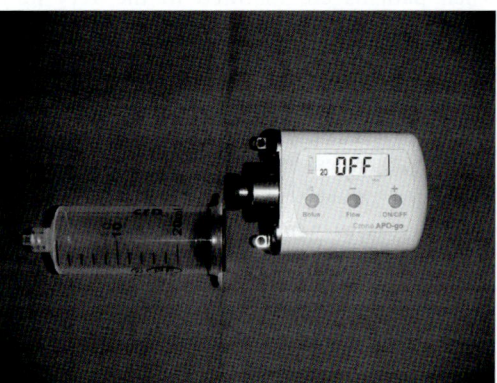

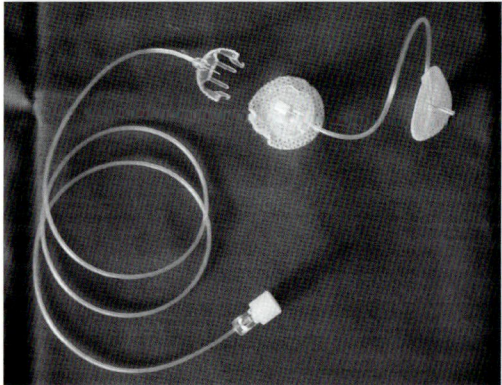

Figure 14.1
The Apo-go pump for the infusion of apomorphine.

uncontrolled conditions and mostly in individuals on LD monotherapy before the clinical application of other oral dopamine agonists had become significant. While the beneficial effect on off-time is consistent across all studies, dyskinesia improvement is somewhat controversial. The widespread use of dopamine agonists from the early disease stages usually leads to a reduction of LD doses, the main contributor to the development of involuntary movements. Dyskinesia reduction generally occurs after a few weeks or months of continuous dopaminergic stimulation as a result of a wider therapeutic window. Finally, apomorphine monotherapy can be achieved only with high doses (usually >100 mg/day) at a cost of a high risk for behavioural adverse events. The addition of LD to apomorphine causes pulsatile dopamine levels and reduces the benefits of continuous stimulation on dyskinesias.

A prospective study has compared the effects of CSAI (n = 13) with STN-DBS (n = 12) in patients with advanced PD and motor fluctuations and dyskinesias that could not be controlled with standard oral treatment (27). Patients were given the choice between the two treatments, and many chose apomorphine infusion due to the long waiting list for the DBS surgical procedure. Even if no formal randomization was possible, evaluations were performed blindly, and each cohort had a similar amount of off-time and dyskinesia at baseline. Clinical and neuropsychological outcomes were measured 12 months after the initiation of treatment. With apomorphine, patients had a 51% reduction in daily off-time and were able to reduce their levodopa dose by 29% at 12 months (27). There was no significant change in the abnormal involuntary movement scale (AIMS) scores, suggesting that apomorphine was not an effective treatment for dyskinesia. Neuropsychiatric testing revealed no significant changes in cognition or behaviour, a finding in agreement with other studies (28). Among patients who received STN-DBS for 12 months, there was a 76% reduction in off-time, a

reduction in daily levodopa dose of 62%, and an 81% reduction in AIMS scores. These improvements suggest effects on both off-time and dyskinesia. However, the neuropsychological findings were less positive for STN-DBS. There was a significant worsening of the neuropsychiatric inventory (NPI) compared with baseline, and at least 50% of patients exhibited apathy and other behavioural changes that were not apparent at baseline.

Although both apomorphine and STN-DBS produced significant clinical improvements in this study, both treatments had clear drawbacks. Apomorphine failed to treat dyskinesia, and STN-DBS was associated with behavioural problems. Experience also points to additional problems with these treatments. During more than 4 years of follow-up with 50 patients receiving apomorphine, 22 dropped out of treatment because they felt that their motor control was inadequate. In addition, patients who use long-term apomorphine (up to 16 h/day for 24 months) may develop impulse control disorders. Five patients developed such disorders, including pathological gambling, internet addiction, compulsive eating, increased libido and acute paranoia with attempted suicide. These effects are dopamine-mediated and ultimately led to treatment discontinuation (27).

Regarding the practicalities of administering CSAI, it may be helpful to pre-medicate patients with an antidopaminergic agent (such as domperidone 10 mg 3-4 times/day 3 days prior to infusion or trimethobenzamide) in order to help suppress any potential nausea and vomiting. Patients should discontinue oral dopamine agonists. The infusion should be initiated at 1 mg/hour apomorphine whilst maintaining the same dose of levodopa initially. The dose of apomorphine should be increased by 0.5/mg/hour every 2/4 hours depending on tolerance. In order to improve dyskinesias, the dose of levodopa should be reduced on a daily basis, if possible, until complete discontinuation. If adverse events occur, the infusion should be discontinued for 6-24 hours. In clinical trials, the most commonly reported adverse events associated with apomorphine infusion included nodules (70% incidence), sedation and somnolence (23%), nausea and vomiting (10%), renal impairment (6%), orthostatic hypotension (5%) and Coomb test positivity (6%). In addition, good local hygiene and changing the site of injection are important measures to help prevent panniculitis (a relatively rare event). The use of apomorphine can be limited by compliance and acute or chronic local skin reactions at the site of injection (44,45).

As with any therapy, the selection of patients suitable to receive CSAI is of fundamental importance for an optimal outcome. Appropriate candidates include patients with idiopathic PD who have responded to LD but are experiencing motor fluctuations and/or with dyskinesias that cannot be controlled with oral therapy. Patients with cognitive impairment, advanced biological age with orthostatic hypotension, severe systemic diseases (e.g., hepatic, renal or cardiac failure), or history of dopaminergic psychosis (which is a contraindication for therapy) should be excluded. Ideally, the patient should be highly motivated and have good caregiver support available. Patient (and caregiver) compliance is important to ensure optimal outcomes because drop-outs for lack of compliance usually occur during the first 1-3 months of treatment.

Continuous levodopa delivery by intestinal infusion

The principle behind constant LD infusion is to achieve CDS with an optimized dose that can be kept stable within the patient's individual therapeutic window. Gastric emptying must be bypassed to achieve this. Intravenous infusion of LD was first attempted in 1975 as 'proof of concept', and it was demonstrated that a stable constant-rate intravenous infusion of LD (and therefore stable plasma LD concentrations) ameliorated motor fluctuations in patients with PD

experiencing a fluctuating response to long-term oral LD (46,47). On the basis of these observations, it was hypothesized that the development of a sustained-release formulation of LD would lead to improved control of the response fluctuations seen with conventional LD preparations. It was found that intravenous infusion of LD cannot be maintained in an individual patient for longer than 7–10 days due to poor tolerance of venous access (LD is irritating to veins and soft tissues) and the poor water solubility of LD. The subsequent development of a stable, concentrated LD/carbidopa gel (LD/carbidopa 20/5 mg/mL in a carboxymethylcellulose mix), combined with progress in the construction and application of portable duodenal infusion systems using percutaneous endoscopic gastrostomy (see Figure 14.2), greatly facilitated the use of this treatment approach in clinical practice (48,49).

The LD/carbidopa gel is administered inside the upper intestine via a small tube inserted directly into the duodenum, allowing the potential for permanent use, and has proven to be a successful therapeutic strategy (30). It provides constant plasma LD concentrations, continuous dopamine availability and receptor stimulation which in turn result in improvement of motor complications. The reduction in motor fluctuations (through the avoidance of low plasma LD trough concentrations) translates into more continuous and predictable benefits for patients receiving LD therapy (30,31). In clinical trials, continuous LD delivery by intestinal infusion (CLDII) as monotherapy has been shown to be safe and effective with certain advantages over individually optimized combinations of conventional oral and subcutaneous medications in patients with motor fluctuations.

The pivotal trial for use of the LD/carbidopa gel is DIREQT (DUODOPA Infusion: Randomized Efficacy and Quality of life Trial) (32). This was a randomized, controlled, multicentre study involving five centres in Sweden. Patients (n = 24) with motor fluctuations and dyskinesia were studied in a crossover design to compare individualized, optimized, conventional treatment with CLDII for two periods of 3 weeks. LD infusion rates averaged about 96 mg/hour, and the average infusion time was 16.5 hours. Video scoring of motor function was assessed by blinded assessors on a global treatment response scale from −3 to 0 to +3 (severe 'off' to 'on' to 'on with severe dyskinesia'). Patients also self-assessed their own motor performance and quality of life. The primary endpoint was the percentage of ratings within the interval from −1 to +1 (functional 'on') for each treatment. Statistical analyses were performed on the intent-to-treat population. Overall, 21 patients received the LD/carbidopa gel infusion, and results from 20 patients were included for conventional treatment. The median rating for motor function from −1 to +1 was 100% with CLDII and 81.3% with conventional oral LD/carbidopa treatment (p < 0.001). Adverse effects were generally mild and similar between the two treatment regimens. Patients tended to appreciate the predictability of therapy and found the system easy to handle with the added advantage of having no fixed medication schedule. Interestingly, after completing the study, 16 patients chose to be treated with continuous daytime infusion of LD/carbidopa gel (32). A recent, multinational, observational cohort study (33) conducted in seven specialized PD clinics assessed the long-term safety and outcome of chronic treatment with CLDII in a large population of patients with advanced PD, showing improvements of motor complications and quality of life for up to 2 years. Because of between-center variations in the duration of follow-up and number of available datasets per visit, the mean 'last value reported after baseline' (LV) was calculated for each efficacy variable and compared to mean baseline using descriptive statistics and paired t-tests. The duration and severity of dyskinesias and the duration of 'off' periods assessed by the UPDRS IV items 32, 33 and 39 were all significantly reduced. The reported benefits support the long-term effectiveness of this therapeutic strategy.

As reported in another study (34), the reduction of dyskinesia severity was more pronounced compared to the decrease in the duration of dyskinesias; however, both the severity and duration of dyskinesia were consistently and significantly reduced. This is particularly remarkable since total daily doses of levodopa were higher during infusion therapy compared to baseline. Since CLDII allows stable LD plasma levels throughout the day, the significant decrease in the duration of 'off' periods observed in this and previous investigations is consistent with the primary role of LD pharmacokinetics and transport in the pathogenesis of motor fluctuations in advanced PD. While the 'on' scores of UPDRS parts II and III were significantly reduced after 6–12 months, there was no significant change of LV scores versus baseline. This is not unexpected with an approach focusing on continuous drug delivery of levodopa in patients with optimized baseline 'on' function but response fluctuations as the main clinical problem. In the present cohort, improvements in 'on' motor function might best be explained by increases in total daily administered dose with infusions in addition to better adherence and possibly to enhanced absorption of LD, while UPDRS progression over time would be expected to counterbalance such effects. The baseline LD dose on continuous infusion was 68.9 ± 31.0 mL/day (representing an average dose of 1378 mg/day), and remained a constant levodopa dose over time. No significant changes occurred over the maximal follow-up period of 2 years, arguing against the possible development of tolerance. The observed significant increase compared to previous oral therapy can be explained by the possibility of reaching higher, more constant plasma levels when LD is delivered continuously compared to oral pulsatile administration (35,36).

Olanow et al. (37) recently presented a double-blind, double-dummy trial comparing CLDII and oral administration of LD/carbidopa in IR form. For 12 weeks, PD patients selected because they had motor complications underwent active CLDII infusion and took placebo or active IR capsules and underwent placebo gel infusion. Among 66 patients who completed the study (93% of the 71 randomized subjects), decrease in 'off' time and increase in 'on' time without troublesome dyskinesia favored levodopa-carbidopa intestinal gel (LCIG) by means of -1.91 and -1.86 h/d, respectively, while 'on' time with troublesome dyskinesia showed no significant change.

Fluctuating motor performance is an important cause of impaired quality of life in advanced PD to which motor complications *per se* and psychosocial consequences of on-off fluctuations may contribute (10,47). Treatment strategies that stabilize motor performance can improve the situation. In addition to demonstrating improved short- and long-term motor outcome, CLDII may also help improve patient quality of life (38). In a 12-month study of prospective clinical and quality-of-life changes in seven patients with PD, treatment with CLDII was associated with significant improvements in four Parkinson's Disease Questionnaire (PDQ)-39 domains (mobility, activities of daily living, stigma, bodily discomfort; p < 0.05). Significant improvements in the Unified Parkinson's Disease Rating Scale (UPDRS)-II (activities of daily living) and UPDRS-IV (motor complications) in the 'on' condition (p < 0.02) were also observed (39). Significant global, functional (ADL), and quality-of-life LCIG benefits were also identified in a double-blind, double-dummy trial comparing CLDII and oral administration of LD/carbidopa in IR form (40).

Tables 14.1 and 14.2 summarize recent studies on the effect of LCIG on reduction in off time and dyskinesia.

However, adverse events can occur, and they are generally related to the device or surgical procedure. The most frequently reported complications related to the intestinal tube included dislocation, occlusion and a kink/knot in the tube. Dislocation of the distal part of the tube from the duodenum into the stomach can lead to a sudden deterioration of treatment response,

with recurring motor fluctuations. An obstruction can lead to sudden or gradual worsening of bradykinesia. Complications related to the percutaneous endoscopic gastrostomy tube included loose connectors and leakage. Adverse events related to the stoma, which may cause discomfort, include secretion from the stoma, infection, proud flesh around the stoma and pain.

Recently, several reports drew scientific attention to cases of polyneuropathy (PN) in advanced PD patients undergoing CLDII. These reports showed two general profiles of PN in CLDII patients: a less severe sensory axonal subtype that is slowly progressive, and a less common subtype that clinically resembles an acute inflammatory PN (Guillain-Barré like syndrome) and causes severe deficits (41). However, overall PN incidence can hardly be estimated from these reports, and PN also has been reported in long-term recipients of oral LD, in whom signs or symptoms develop in as many as 12% (42).

In order to assess the prevalence and features of PN in different dopaminergic treatment regimens, Mancini et al. (41) evaluated prospectively, with clinical, biochemical and neurophysiological parameters, 3 groups of consecutive PD patients, 50 on CLDII, 50 on oral levodopa (O-LD) and 50 on other dopaminergic therapy (ODT). The frequency of PN of no evident cause was 28% in CLDII, 20% in O-LD, and 6% in ODT patients. Clinically, 71% of CLDII PN patients and all O-LD and ODT PN patients displayed a subacute sensory PN. In contrast, 29% of CLDII patients presented acute motor PN. A significantly increased risk of PN for CLDII versus ODT patients was observed, and for O-LD versus ODT patients. No statistically significant difference was found for CLDII versus O-LD patients. Vitamin B12 and folate levels were significantly lower and homocysteine (hcy) levels were significantly higher in LD compared with ODT patients. No significant difference was detected when comparing CLDII with O-LD patients and SPN with APN patients. PN patients

Table 14.1
Effect of levodopa-carbidopa intestinal gel on 'off' time.

Author	Study design	Patients	Duration	Reduction in off time vs baseline
Nyholm D 2005	Randomized, controlled vs oral levodopa	24	3 + 3 weeks	Significant reduction in time in OFF (p<0.01)
Stocchi F 2005	Open	6	6 months	-78% of daily hours in OFF (p<0.001)
Eggert K 2008	Open	13	12 months	-70% of daily hours in OFF
Antonini A 2007	Open, prospective	9	12 months	-89% of mean time in OFF vs baseline (p<0.01)
Antonini A 2008	Open, prospective	22	24 months	-46% in mean OFF time duration (UPDRS IV) (p<0.05)
Santos-Garcia 2010	Open, prospective	9	6 months	-91% in OFF time (p<00.05)
Puente 2009	Open, prospective	9	18 months	Reduction of UPDRS III score, OFF from 39.7 to 29.4;(p<0.05)
Merola A. 2011	Open, retrospective vs DBS	20	15 months	Significant reduction (p<0.05) of waking day spent in OFF (item 39)

showed significantly higher hcy levels than non-PN patients LD daily dose.

A direct correlation between LD daily dose and hcy levels was observed. Cerebrospinal fluid examination, performed in 5 patients at PN onset, showed increased protein concentration with normal cell count in the 3 acute PN patients and normal values in the 2 subacute PN patients. These findings support the relationship between LD and PN and confirm that an imbalance in vitamin B12/hcy may be a key pathogenic factor. The authors suggest two different, possibly overlapping mechanisms of PN in patients on CDLII: axonal degeneration due to vitamin deficiency and inflammatory damage. Whether inflammatory damage is triggered by vitamin deficiency and/or by modifications in the intestinal micro-environment should be explored further. Proper vitamin supplementation may prevent peripheral damage in most cases.

This study confirms previous evidence (42) showing that PN is frequent in treated PD patients, particularly in the advanced phase of the disease, and supports a relationship between PN and the long-term intake of relatively high doses of LD. Furthermore, these data confirm the link between PN and vitamin B12 metabolic imbalance. LD exposure predisposes to PN with a dose-dependent effect, and intestinal infusion produces a higher LD bioavailability than oral administration. PN prevalence was not related to the route of LD administration, whereas the PN pattern differed between CLDII and O-LD patients. Indeed, all patients on O-LD and the majority of CLDII patients displayed subacute PN affecting mainly the sensory axons, whereas four CLDII patients possibly had an acute inflammatory form. Vitamin B12 deficiency and hcy increase may determine an acute imbalance between myelin toxic and trophic factors, with a subsequent increase of pro-inflammatory cytokines, toxins and free radicals and a decrease of growth factor synthesis. On the other hand, the intestinal micro-environment may be modified by local factors, such as the chronic presence of the intestinal tube and/or levodopa gel,

Table 14.2
Effect of levodopa-carbidopa intestinal gel on dyskinesia.

Author	Study design	N. Patients	Duration	Effect on invalidating dyskinesia vs baseline
Eggert K 2008	Open	13	12 months	-88% on time with disabling dyskinesia (p>0.0067)
Antonini A 2008	Open	22	24 months	-32% dyskinesia severity
Honig H 2009	Open	22	6 months	- 67% (UPDRS dyskinesia score) (p>0.0001)
Devos D 2009	Open	91	4 years	95% of patients improved dyskinesia
Santos-Garcia 2010	Open	9	6 months	-56% of patients with disabling dyskinesia (p<0.05) -67% dyskinesia duration (p<0.05)
Merola A 2011	Open vs DBS	20	15 months	Reduction of severity and duration of dyskinesia (items 32 and 33; p = NS vs baseline and DBS)

favoring a microbial overgrowth and a consequent auto-inflammatory response.

Treatment of non-motor symptoms

Published management recommendations for non-motor PD symptoms have not attempted to differentiate between symptoms intrinsic to PD and those arising as complications of PD therapy. A contributory problem may be that in clinical studies of dopaminergic options, improvement of non-motor PD symptoms, LD-related or not, has seldom been either a primary endpoint or a means for comparing treatments with potentially different abilities to produce continuous dopaminergic delivery (CDD) (43). In a double-blind, 12-week, parallel-group study of patients with early PD (44), oral LD/carbidopa/entacapone (LCE) was superior to LD/carbidopa for improving quality of life, as rated by the total score on the eight-item PDQ (PDQ-8) and by subscores for the PDQ-8 non-motor domains of depression, personal relationships, communication, and stigma. Transdermal rotigotine has recently been assessed versus placebo in a large, double-blind trial (45) in PD patients with unsatisfactory early morning motor-symptom control. On the revised Parkinson's disease sleep scale (PDSS-2) (45), a validated scale to assess sleep and its problems in PD, the mean 12-week change in total score (a co-primary outcome) was significantly improved in the rotigotine group compared with placebo from baseline to end of maintenance: the least squares (LS) mean treatment difference was -4.26 (95 % CI: -6.08 vs -2.45; p <0.0001). Difficulty in falling asleep and feeling tired and sleepy in the morning were among the ten items showing significant improvement (among the instrument's total of 15).

Improvement of non-motor PD symptoms by CLDII infusion was the primary endpoint in a prospective, open-label trial conducted in 22 patients with daily motor fluctuations and dyskinesia refractory to optimized conventional therapy with oral medications, transdermal rotigotine, or subcutaneous apomorphine infusion 47). After discontinuation of the conventional therapy (except for nighttime oral dosing with LD CR or a long-acting dopamine agonist) and its replacement by CLDII for a mean of 6.7 months, mean change in NMSS total score showed a significant improvement from baseline (-50.5, p = 0.0001). Of the nine NMSS domains, six were significantly improved: cardiovascular (-2.41, p = 0.0004), sleep/fatigue (-11.32, p = 0.0001), attention/ memory (-3.27, p = 0.002), gastrointestinal (-6.23, p = 0.0003), urinary (-6.64, p = 0.002), and miscellaneous (-7.73, p = 0.0004). The change in total NMSS score was correlated with changes in measures of motor function: UPDRS motor-complication score (-5.91, p = 0.0000), UPDRS dyskinesia subscore (-3.7, p = 0.0001), and 'off' time as a proportion of the waking day (r = 0.54, p \ 0.01). On the PDSS and PDQ-8, mean improvement in total score was also significant (-28.51; p = 0.002 and -23.4; p = 0.0003, respectively). Results on the effectiveness of LCIG on non-motor symptoms are summarized in Table 14.3.

Alternative methods of continuous LD delivery

Alternative methods to achieve continuous levodopa delivery in the central nervous system include transdermal and micro-encapsulated levodopa application, as well as cell-based therapies and gene delivery techniques.

Transdermal levodopa application
A levodopa patch has long been considered a way to provide continuous transdermal delivery of levodopa, but has proven difficult to achieve because LD is maintained in an acidic concentration (for its stability) and requires large volumes for administration (1). Alternative methods of continuous LD delivery comprise cell-based therapies and gene delivery technologies.

Micro-encapsulated levodopa application
In a recent study, LD methyl ester (LDME) and benserazide were microencapsulated into poly (lactide-co-glycolide) microspheres and then administered in a PD model in rats. The results showed that LDME/benserazide-loaded microspheres could ameliorate the expression of LD-induced dyskinesia in these rats (20).

Cell-based therapy
Cell-based therapies follow the hypothesis that implanted dopamine cells that integrate into the

host striatum might release dopamine and restore dopamine in a physiologic manner.

Gene delivery techniques
Gene delivery technology using viral vectors to deliver aromatic amino acid decarboxylase (AADC) is based on the hypothesis that enhanced expression of AADC would promote the conversion of orally administered LD to dopamine and provide a more continuous striatal dopamine level; intrastriatal infusion of glial-derived neurotrophic factor (GDNF) has been shown to protect dopamine neurons from a variety of toxins in both in vitro and in vivo models (1).

Conclusions

Current evidence indicates that the magnitude of dopamine denervation is important in the development of dyskinesia and that initiation with a dopamine agonist is effective in delaying its onset. The rationale for switching from a pulsatile to continuous dopaminergic delivery involves primarily the avoidance of peaks and troughs in plasma that may eventually widen the therapeutic window, particularly in early PD patients.

Therefore, the pharmacologic treatment of PD has been evolving, most recently, in a quest to achieve CDS or, more verifiably, continuous drug delivery. Improvements in the steadiness of the plasma concentration-versus-time profiles of various dopaminergic therapies (14) may be a sign of progress. However, improvements in the plasma profile do not necessarily translate into a more continuous stimulation of central dopamine receptors. To directly evaluate the degree of CDS that a dopaminergic drug may confer, studies assessing dopamine-receptor occupancy (as measured, e.g., by brain imaging) will be necessary. So far, clinical studies of efforts to improve PD motor symptoms using therapies expected to provide more CDS have generally been positive. However, the findings of studies comparing differing active treatments have often failed to find evidence favoring these approach-

Table 14.3
Effect of levodopa-carbidopa intestinal gel on non-motor symptoms and quality of life (QoL).

Author	Study design	N Patients	Duration	PDQ 39 – PDQ8	QoL 15D
Nyholm D 2005	Randomised, controlled vs levodopa	24	3 + 3 weeks	-28% mean change in the PDQ39 (p<0.01) Significant reduction in mean scores in 7/8 domains of the PDQ-39 (mobility, p<0.01; daily activities, p<0.03; emotional well-being, p<0.03; self-esteem, p<0.03; cognitive function, p<0.01; communication, p<0.03; pain, p<0.01)	Improvements in QoL: +7.7% in the QoL 15D (p<0.01)
Nyholm D 2008	Randomised, controlled vs APO	4	3+3 weeks	Improvement in all domains, and in particular for stigma (-25)	Improved in 3 patients (15D), unchanged in one patient
Antonini A 2007	Open	9	12 months	Significant improvement in 4/8 domains of the PDQ-39 (mobility, p<0.01; daily activities, p<0.01; self-esteem, p<0.05 and physical discomfort, p<0.05)	
Devos D 2009	Open	91	4 years		93% of patients with improvement in QoL vs baseline (48% substantial improvement)
Honig H 2009	Open	22	6 months	Significant improvement in the QoL (PDQ-8 :- 53%, p = 0.0003)	

es over an intermittent therapy. A conceivable explanation for the lack of substantial difference may be that the so-called standard- release dopamine agonists in fact have 'longish' half-lives compared with LD IR and even with LD CR. By a similar argument, continuous agonist delivery using transdermal rotigotine would lack superiority over IR ropinirole because the half-life of the oral IR agent is already fairly long. However, transdermal rotigotine is not as effective as the infusional dopaminergic therapies (apomorphine or LD), suggesting that the inherent potency of each agent is also determinative. For their part, the infusional therapies presumably

gain from accessing the bloodstream without the need for gastric transit. Currently, apomorphine is the only dopamine agonist rivaling LD in potency, and its half life is shorter. Clinical studies focusing on improving non-motor PD symptoms are becoming more common. These trials, too, have not yet clarified any potential differences across therapies with differing capacities for CDD. Nevertheless, the findings of non-motor improvement among recipients of subcutaneous apomorphine CLDII suggest that non-motor PD symptoms or complications may improve in tandem with the expected motor improvements. Future research should explore

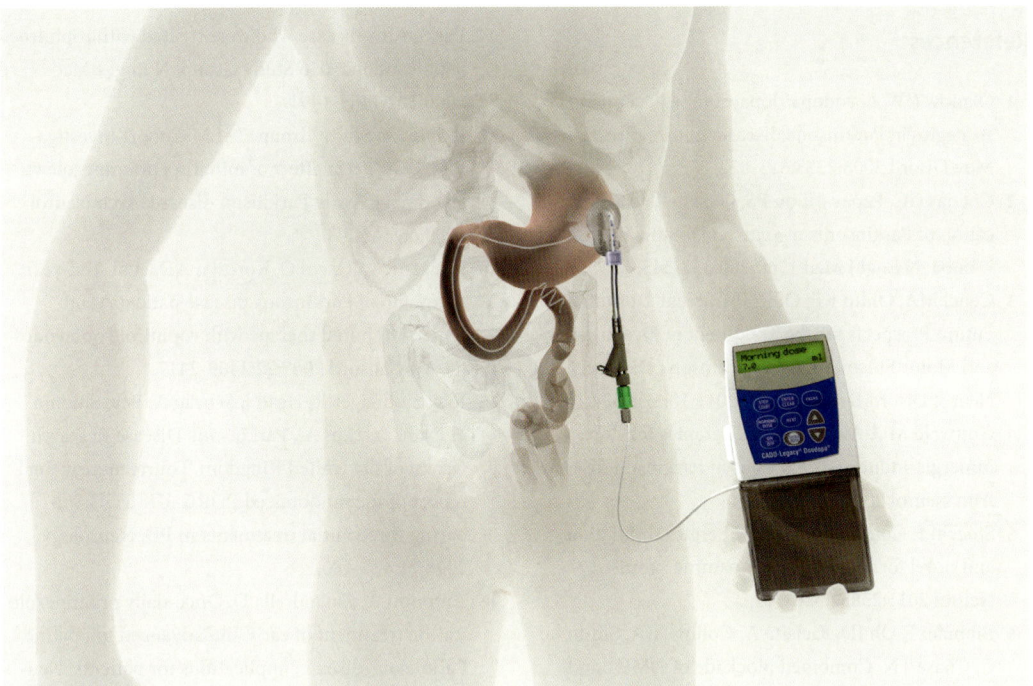

Figure 14.2
The levodopa-carbidopa intestinal gel (LCIG) infusion machinery, enabling the continuous levodopa gel infusion into the duodenum.

drug activity at dopaminergic synapses, so as to assess whether CDS is, in fact, an important determinant of clinical efficacy. Certainly, the complexities of optimal PD management, and the rationale for an underlying strategy such as CDS or CDD, have not yet been thoroughly elucidated.

Video fragments

PLAY

Fragment 14.1
CDS-LCIG (1) (segments 1-4)
This video shows a 34-year-old man, suffering since the age of 24 from right-sided, subtle motor parkinsonism, diagnosed three years later as idiopathic PD, and treated with levodopa (segment 1: off-medication). After 1.5 years of treatment, he developed motor fluctuations and dyskinesias, necessitating continuous

dopaminergic stimulation; two years later, the effects of the medication became unpredictable, with alternating, short-lived 'on' with dyskinesias (UPDRS III: 15) and akinetic 'off' (UPDRS III: 40) periods (segment 2: 'on' with dyskinesias). In segments 3 and 4 the effects of LCIG (levodopa-carbidopa intestinal gel) 700 mg/day (without bothersome dyskinesia) are evident 6 months and 3 years, respectively, after application.

Fragment 14.2
CDS-CLIG (2) (segments 1-2)
Here you see a young man suffering from idiopathic PD since the age of 11, treated with PEG-J-applied continuous CLIG (levodopa-carbidopa intestinal gel) before (segment 1) and after (segment 2) discontinuation of this application.

References

1 Olanow CW. Levodopa/dopamine replacement strategies in Parkinson's disease--future directions. Mov Disord 2008;23S3:613-622.

2 Cotzias GC, Papavasiliou PS, Gellene R. Modification of Parkinsonism – chronic treatment with L-dopa. N Engl J Med 1969;280:337-345.

3 Cenci MA, Ohlin KE, Odin P. Current Options and Future Prospects for the Treatment of Dyskinesia and Motor Fluctuations in Parkinson's Disease. CNS Neurol Disord Drug Targets. 2011;10:670-684.

4 Gottwald MD, Aminoff MJ. Therapies for dopaminergic-induced dyskinesias in Parkinson disease. Ann Neurol 2011;69:919-927.

5 Stocchi F. Continuous dopaminergic stimulation and novel formulations of dopamine agonists. J Neurol 2011;258S2:316-322.

6 Bibbiani F, Oh JD, Kielaite A, Collins MA, Smith C, Chase TN. Combined blockade of AMPA and NMDA glutamate receptors reduces levodopa-induced motor complications in animal models of PD. Exp Neurol 2005;196:422-429.

7 Ostock CY, Dupre KB, Jaunarajs KL, et al. Role of the primary motor cortex in L-DOPA-induced dyskinesia and its modulation by 5-HT1A receptor stimulation. Neuropharmacology 2011;61:753-760.

8 Lee JY, Cho J, Lee EK, Park SS, Jeon BS. Differential genetic susceptibility in diphasic and peak-dose dyskinesias in Parkinson's disease. Mov Disord 2011;26:73-79.

9 Antonini A, Tolosa E, Mizuno Y, Yamamoto M, Poewe WH. A reassessment of risks and benefits of dopamine agonists in Parkinson's disease. Lancet Neurol 2009;8:929-937.

10 Antonini A, Ursino G, Calandrella D, Bernardi L, Plebani M. Continuous dopaminergic delivery in Parkinson's disease. J Neurol 2010;257S2:305-308.

11 Stocchi F, Rascol O, Kieburtz K, et al. Initiating levodopa/carbidopa therapy with and without entacapone in early Parkinson disease: the STRIDE-PD study. Ann Neurol 2010;68:18-27.

12 Rascol O, Brooks DJ, Korczyn AD, De Deyn PP, Clarke CE, Lang AE. A five-year study of the incidence of dyskinesia in patients with early Parkinson's disease who were treated with ropinirole or levodopa. 056 Study Group. N Engl J Med 2000;342:1484-1491.

13 Parkinson Study Group CALM Cohort Investigators. Long-term effect of initiating pramipexole vs levodopa in early Parkinson disease. Arch Neurol 2009;66:563-570.

14 Hauser RA, Rascol O, Korczyn AD, et al. Ten-year follow-up of Parkinson's disease patients randomized to initial therapy with ropinirole or levodopa. Mov Disord 2007;22:2409-2417.

15 Katzenschlager R, Head J, Schrag A, Ben-Shlomo Y, Evans A, Lees AJ, Parkinson's Disease Research Group of the United Kingdom. Fourteen-year final report of the randomized PDRG-UK trial comparing three initial treatments in PD. Neurology 2008;71:474-480.

16 Antonini A, Calandrella D. Once-daily pramipexole for the treatment of early and advanced idiopathic Parkinson's disease: implications for patients. Neuropsychiatr Dis Treat 2011;7:297-302.

17 Poewe W, Rascol O, Barone P, et al. Extended-release pramipexole in early Parkinson disease: A 33-week randomized controlled trial. Neurology 2011;77:759-766.

18 Hauser RA, Reichmann H, Lew M, Asgharian A, Makumi C, Shulman KJ. Long-term,open-label study of once-daily ropinirole prolonged release in early Parkinson's disease. Int J Neurosci 2011;121:246-253.

19 Giladi N, Boroojerdi B, Korczyn AD, et al. Rotigotine transdermal patch in early Parkinson's disease: a randomized, double-blind, controlled study versus placebo and ropinirole. Mov Disord 2007;22:2398-2404.

20 Fabbrini G, Brotchie JM, Grandas F, Nomoto M, Goetz CG. Levodopa-induced dyskinesias. Mov. Disord 2007;22:1379-1389.

21 Chapuis S, Ouchchane L, Metz O, Gerbaud L, Durif F. Impact of the motor complications of Parkinson's disease on the quality of life. Mov Disord 2005;20:224-230.

22 Kurlan R, Rothfield KP, Woodward WR, et al. Erratic gastric emptying may cause 'random' fluctuations of parkinsonian mobility. Neurology 1988;38:419-421.

23 Wolters E, Lees AJ, Volkmann J, van Laar T, Hovestadt A. Managing Parkinson's disease with continuous dopaminergic stimulation. CNS Spectr 2008;13S7:1-14.

24 Tyne HL, Parsons J, Sinnott A, Fox SH, Fletcher NA, Steiger MJ. A 10 year retrospective audit of long-term apomorphine use in Parkinson's disease. J Neurol 2004; 251:1370-1374.

25 Olanow CW, Obeso JA, Stocchi F. Continuous dopamine-receptor treatment of Parkinson's disease: scientific rationale and clinical implications. Lancet Neurol 2006;5:677-687.

26 Pfeiffer RF, Gutmann L, Hull KL Jr, Bottini PB, Sherry JH; APO302 Study Investigators. Continued efficacy and safety of subcutaneous apomorphine in patients with advanced Parkinson's disease. Parkinsonism. Relat Disord 2007;13:93-100.

27 De Gaspari D, Siri C, Landi A, et al. Clinical and neuropsychological follow up at 12 months in patients with complicated Parkinson's disease treated with subcutaneous apomorphine infusion or deep brain stimulation of the subthalamic nucleus. J Neurol Neurosurg Psychiatry 2006;77:450-453.

28 Morgante L, Basile G, Epifanio A, et al. Continuous apomorphine infusion (CAI) and neuropsychiatric disorders in patients with advanced Parkinson's disease: a follow-up of two years. Arch Gerontol Geriatr 2004;S9:291-296.

29 Stocchi F, Tagliati M, Olanow CW. Treatment of levodopa-induced motor complications. Mov Disord 2008;23S3:599-5612.

30 Kurlan R, Nutt JG, Woodward WR, et al. Duodenal and gastric delivery of levodopa in Parkinsonism. Ann Neurol 1988;23:589-595.

31 Nyholm D. Enteral levodopa/carbidopa gel infusion for the treatment of motor fluctuations and dyskinesias in advanced Parkinson's disease. Expert Rev Neurother 2006;6:1403-1411.

32 Nyholm D, Nilsson Remahl AI, Dizdar N, et al. Duodenal levodopa infusion monotherapy vs oral polypharmacy in advanced Parkinson disease. Neurology 2005;64:216-223.

33 Antonini A, Odin P, Lopiano L et al. Effect and safety of duodenal levodopa infusion in advanced Parkinson's disease: a retrospective multicenter out-

come assessment in patient routine care. J Neural Transm. 2013.

34 Antonini A, Mancini F, Canesi M. Duodenal levodopa infusion improves quality of life in advanced Parkinson's disease. Neurodegener Dis 2008;5:244-246.

35 Nyholm D, Lennernas H, Gomes-Trolin C, Aquilonius SM. Levodopa pharmacokinetics and motor performance during activities of daily living in patients with Parkinson's disease on individual drug combinations. Clin Neuropharmacol 2002;25:89-96.

36 Nyholm, D, Askmark, H, Gomes-Trolin C, et al. Clinic Pharmacokinetic study comparing continuous intraduodenal levodopa infusion and oral levodopa/carbidopa in patients with advanced PD and with severe motor fluctuations. Neuropharmacol 2003;26:156-163.

37 Olanow CW, Antonini A, Kieburtz K, et al. Randomized, double- blind, double-dummy study of continuous infusion of levodopa- carbidopa intestinal gel in patients with advanced Parkinson's disease: efficacy and safety. Mov Disord 2012;27S1:411.

38 Lee MA, Walker RW, Hildreth AJ, et al. Individualized assessment of quality of life in idiopathic Parkinson's disease. Mov Disord 2006;21:1929-1934.

39 Antonini A, Isaias IU, Canesi M, et al. Duodenal levodopa infusion for advanced Parkinson's disease: 12-month treatment outcome. Mov Disord 2007;22:1145-1149.

40 Kieburtz K, Antonini A, Olanow CW, et al. Randomized, phase 3, double- blind, double-dummy study of levodopa-carbidopa intestinal gel in patients with advanced Parkinson's disease: functional and quality-of-life outcomes (abstract). Mov Disord 2012;27S1:385.

41 Mancini F, Comi C, Oggioni GD et al. Prevalence and features of peripheral neuropathy in Parkinson's disease. Parkinsonism Relat Disord. 2013;19.

42 Toth C, Breithaupt K, Ge S, et al. Levodopa, methylmalonic acid, and neuropathy in idiopathic Parkinson disease. Ann Neurol 2010;67:28-36.

43 Chaudhuri KR, Rizos A, Sethi KD. Motor and nonmotor complications in Parkinson's disease: an argument for continuous drug delivery? J Neural Transm 2013;120:1305-1320.

44 Fung VS, Herawati L, Wan Y, Movement Disorder Society of Australia Clinical Research and Trials Group, QUEST-AP Study Group. Quality of life in early Parkinson's disease treated with levodopa/carbidopa/entacapone. Mov Disord 2009;24:25-31.

45 Trenkwalder C, Kies B, Rudzinska M, Fine J, Nikl J, Honczarenko K, Recover Study Group et al. Rotigotine effects on early morning motor function and sleep in Parkinson's disease: a double-blind, randomized, placebo-controlled study (RECOVER). Mov Disord 2011;26:90-99.

46 Trenkwalder C, Kohnen R, Hogl B, et al. Parkinson disease sleep scale— validation of the revised version PDSS-2. Mov Disord 2011;26:644-652.

47 Honig H, Antonini A, Martinez-Martin P, et al. Intrajejunal levodopa infusion in Parkinson's disease: a pilot multicenter study of effects on nonmotor symptoms and quality of life. Mov Disord 2009;24:1468-1474.

15

Pathology of Parkinson's Disease

Glenda Halliday, Karen Murphy & Heidi Cartwright

Parkinson's disease (PD) is the most common, progressive, neurodegenerative movement disorder, with increasing age being the greatest risk factor for its development (1). The clinical course for idiopathic PD is long and slow, and most often there is a very lengthy disease duration. The mean age of onset of PD is around 60 years, with an average disease duration of around 15 years (1). PD patients have increased mortality, and those with coincident dementia have substantially increased mortality (2).

The disease entity is definitively diagnosed by two pathologies, the degeneration of pigmented dopamine neurons in the midbrain and α-synuclein deposited in abnormal Lewy inclusions (see Figure 15.1E) in at least some brainstem neurons (3). While historically PD was considered to be solely a disease afflicting the dopamine motor system, it is now known that PD has varied pathology affecting nearly every part of the nervous system, knowledge that has been important in better clinical definitions of the disease (see previous chapters). The aetiology of the common idiopathic form of PD remains conjecture, but numerous genes identified in familial forms of PD have provided significant clues into both genetic and environmental risks for PD. This greater understanding of the mechanisms underlying the neuronal dysfunction in PD has led to new mechanistic treatments being tried (e.g. antioxidant administration to reduce oxidative stress, trophic factor administration to promote neuronal survival, anti-inflammatory medications to counteract any inflammatory attack).

Core pathological features of Parkinson's disease

Neuronal degeneration

Macroscopic examination of post-mortem PD brains shows no significant atrophy compared to age-matched controls (see Figure 15.1A), consistent with MRI findings and the lack of neocortical volume or neuron number loss in PD brains (4). All PD patients with motor symptoms have moderate to severe loss of neuromelanin-pigmented dopaminergic neurons in the substantia nigra (see Figure 15.1C), resulting in a macroscopic pallor of this midbrain region (see Figure 15.1B). The pigmented dopamine neurons in the ventrolateral region are particularly vulnerable to degeneration (5), with cell loss beginning prior to symptom onset and progressing logarithmically over time with increasing motor dysfunction (6). On average, 80% of dopamine neurons in this region (Figure 15.1C) are lost in PD patients surviving 7-32 years after onset (7). These PD-vulnerable substantia nigra neurons project to the caudate nucleus and putamen, resulting in progressive dopaminergic denervation of the striatum (see Figure 15.2). Surprisingly, there is preservation of the dopaminergic neurons in the adjacent midbrain reticular formation (5). These extranigral dopamine cell groups innervate the thalamus, striatum, prefrontal, motor and premotor areas, and thus also affect the function of the basal ganglia and cerebral cortex.

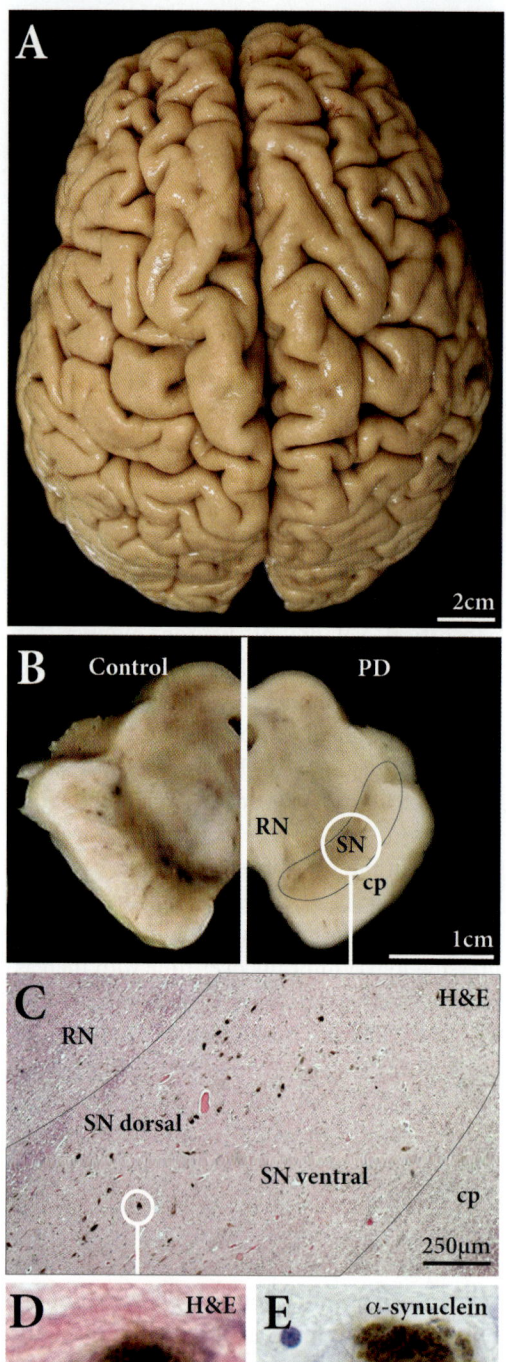

Non-dopaminergic neurons also degenerate in PD, but these regions are often affected later in the disease. Only mild cell loss is seen in the amygdala, even at end-stage disease, despite substantial α-synuclein pathology (8). The cholinergic nucleus basalis of Meynert undergoes neuron and volume loss, and hypocretin-positive hypothalamic neurons that regulate sleep and appetite degenerate at later disease stages (9). Noradrenergic locus ceruleus neurons show a disturbed phenotype without substantial loss of number, while a loss of serotonergic raphe nucleus neurons occurs at late disease stages (10). The noradrenergic dorsal vagal nucleus displays mild neuron loss despite early frequent Lewy pathology (10), in contrast to regions such as the striatal projection neurons from the caudal intralaminar nuclei of the thalamus and the corticocortical projection neurons in the pre-supplementary motor cortex (see Figure 15.2) that show significant cell loss with only limited Lewy pathology (11).

Lewy pathology

The identification of the first mutation to cause familial PD provided a new concept for its pathology. The gene was *SNCA*, which encodes the protein α-synuclein (12), a natively unfolded, soluble,

Figure 15.1
Diagnostic pathology for Parkinson's disease (PD).
A Macroscopic photo of the external superior view of a PD brain, showing no obvious atrophy.
B Macroscopic photos of transverse sections through the midbrain showing the darkly pigmented region of the substantia nigra (SN) in a control at left, and the same region depigmented in a patient with PD at right. RN = red nucleus, cp = cerebral peduncle.
C Microscopic photo of the midbrain at the same level in B of a patient with PD, stained with haematoxylin and eosin (H&E) showing the reduction in neuromelanin-pigmented neurons in the ventral part of the SN.
D Typical H&E-stained Lewy body in a surviving neuromelanin-pigmented neuron in the SN of a patient with PD. Scale equivalent to E.
E α-Synuclein immunoreactive Lewy body inclusion (arrowed) in a surviving pigmented SN neuron in a patient with PD.

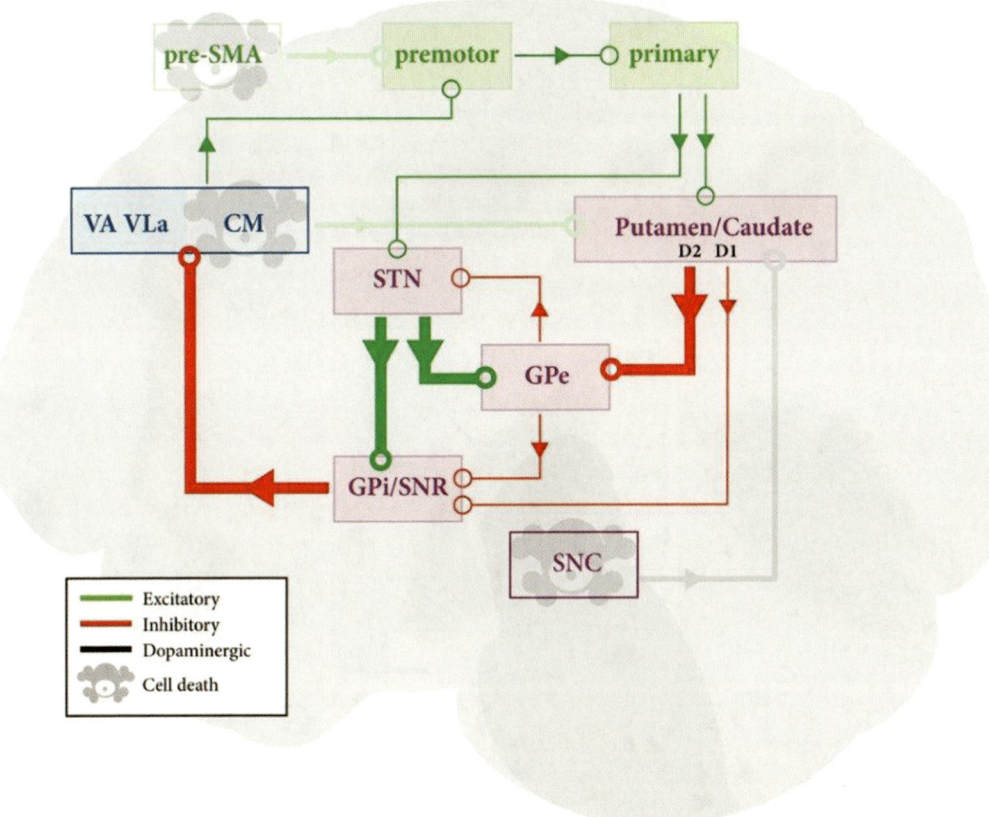

Figure 15.2 Simplified schematic diagram of circuits affected by cell loss in PD.
The loss of the pigmented dopamine cells in the substantia nigra pars compacta (SNC) disrupts the basal ganglia circuitry (in purple) by decreasing the dopaminergic input to the putamen and eventually the caudate nucleus, causing a loss of inhibition to the output nuclei, the internal globus pallidus (GPi) and substantia nigra pars reticulata (SNR), through the direct inhibitory pathway as well as by increasing the inhibition of the external globus pallidus (GPe) in the indirect pathway. The loss of inhibition to the subthalamic nucleus (STN) also increases the relative excitation to the output nuclei, which in turn inhibit the thalamic projection regions (VA, VLa) to motor cortices (premotor, primary motor) to produce the akinetic-rigid symptoms of PD. Along with this SNC cell loss, there is substantial cell loss in two non-dopaminergic cell regions, the excitatory striatal projection neurons of the thalamic caudal intralaminar nuclei (CM) and the excitatory corticocortical projection neurons in the pre-supplementary motor cortex (pre-SMA). The loss of these areas exacerbates the reduced excitatory drive caused by the dopaminergic dysregulation of the motor circuitry in PD.

140-amino acid protein expressed in high abundance in neural tissues. α-Synuclein concentrates in the presynaptic terminals of mature neurons, and interacts with synaptic vesicles and the plasma membrane through lipid rafts (13,14). It was identified as the main constituent protein accumulating in Lewy body fibrils (see Figures 15.1E and 15.3) (15), sparking many *in vitro* and *in vivo* experiments. Single- and double-knockout mice lacking α-synuclein and/or the homologous β-synuclein show that synucleins are not essential for maintaining basic synaptic functions, but are necessary for maintaining normal dopamine levels in the nigrostriatal system, and increased expression of α-synuclein in cell culture affects cell viability and enhances susceptibility to oxida-

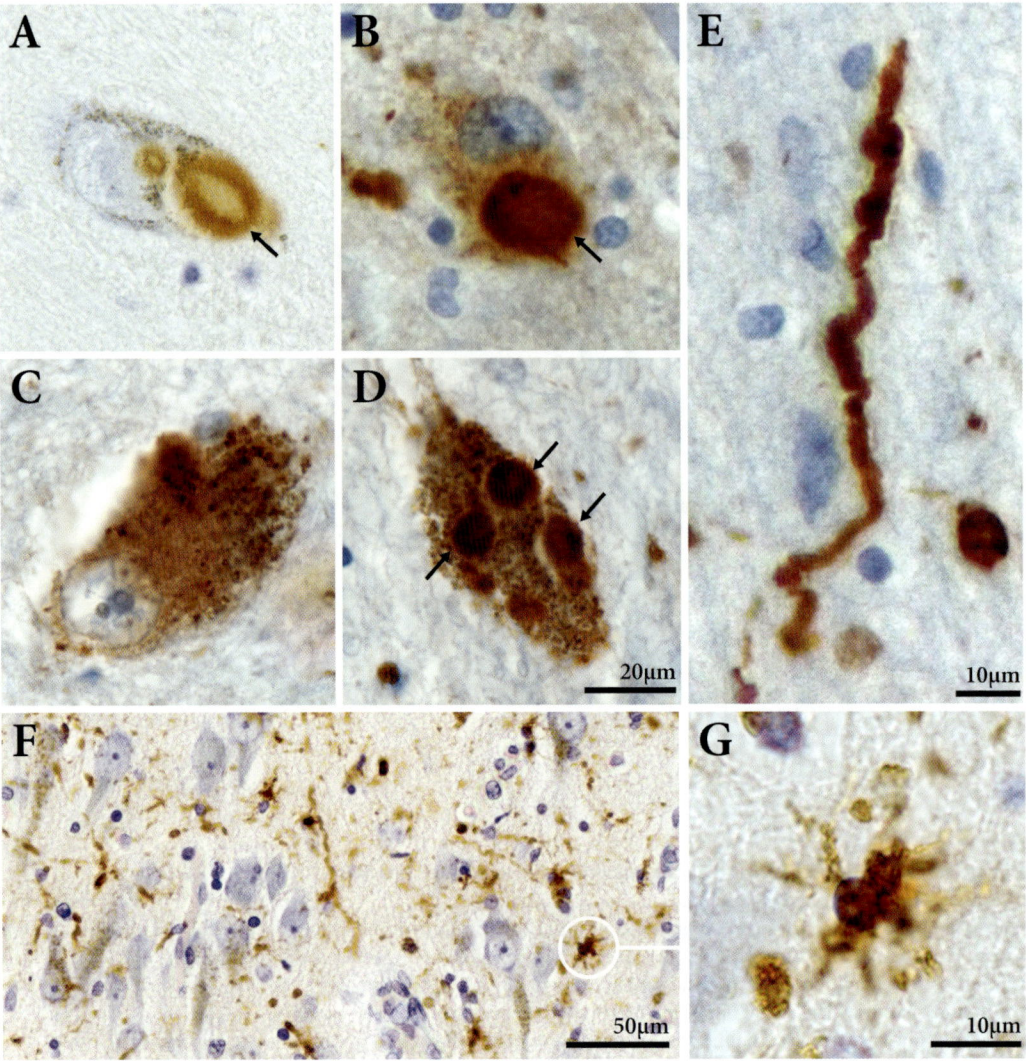

Figure 15.3 α-Synuclein-immunoreactive Lewy pathologies in PD.

A-D Intracellular neuronal deposition of α-synuclein occurs in Lewy bodies (arrows) and also as diffuse granular cytoplasmic immunostaining (B-D). Scale in D equivalent for A-D.

E High magnification of α-synuclein immunopositive Lewy neurites.

F,G Neuropil distribution of α-synuclein immunoreactive pathology in a susceptible limbic brain region, the CA2 region of the hippocampus. Both Lewy neurites and α-synuclein immunoreactive astrocytes (magnified in G) can be more prominent than Lewy bodies in such regions.

tive stress, apoptotic cell death and dopamine-induced toxicity (13). In healthy neurons, α-synuclein forms soluble monomers or oligomers, however it can undergo pathological changes to precipitate into stable fibrils that aggregate to form the insoluble Lewy body inclusions.

Lewy pathology is the collective term for the range of α-synuclein-immunoreactive inclusions found in PD that are identified using immunohistochemical staining for α-synuclein in tissue sections (see Figure 15.3). Lewy pathology is typified by the intraneuronal Lewy bodies, but incorporates inclusions in neuronal cell processes known as intraneuritic Lewy bodies, Lewy neurites, dot-like structures and axonal spheroids, as well as diffuse, granular or pleomorphic neuronal perikaryal structures (see Figure 15.3) (16). There is no consensus on how such Lewy pathology develops, or the relationship between the different types observed, but these abnormal structures may represent a continuum of abnormal α-synuclein deposition leading to Lewy body formation. In human tissue sections, α-synuclein is first evident as punctate material in cell bodies (16) and neurites (17), which then coalesce into loosely packed filaments and incorporate ubiquitin to form pale neurites and pale bodies – the structures that mature into Lewy neurites and Lewy bodies (16,17). The neuroanatomical regions that accumulate Lewy pathology in most patients with clinical PD follow a fairly consistent pattern as the disease progresses (discussed in detail below) (18), and it has been suggested that Lewy pathologies survive in degenerating neurons for 6-16 months (19). It has been noted that a common feature of cell types developing these α-synuclein inclusions is a long, thin, and poorly myelinated or unmyelinated axon (18).

In addition to α-synuclein, a wide variety of proteins are present in Lewy pathology, including structural fibril proteins (e.g. neurofilament), α-synuclein-binding proteins (e.g. synphilin-1), components of the ubiquitin-proteosome system (e.g. ubiquitin, p62/sequestome), cellular response proteins (e.g. heat shock, oxidative and cell stress proteins, Hsc70-interacting proteins), signal transduction proteins (e.g. kinases), cytoskeletal proteins (e.g. microtubule-associated proteins, tubulin), cell cycle proteins (e.g. cyclin), cytosolic proteins (e.g. tyrosine hydroxylase), lipids and mitochondrial proteins (20). Many of the proteins found in Lewy pathology show biochemical modifications, including oxidization, nitration, ubiquitylation and phosphorylation.

α-Synuclein is also observed in astroglia (see Figure 15.3J), with evidence that such pathology is not benign but may participate in the progression of PD pathology (21). *In vitro* experiments show that astrocytic α-synuclein deposition can initiate non-cell autonomous neuron death through microglial signaling (22). Astrocytes react to pathologic damage by simultaneously stimulating microglia and secreting neuroprotective agents. In PD, protoplasmic but not fibrous astrocytes become non-reactive and accumulate α-synuclein (23), with these α-synuclein-accumulating astrocytes occurring in a topographical distribution that closely parallels the distribution of Lewy pathology (24). Overall, such early α-synuclein accumulation in astrocytes is likely to cause dysfunction and potential recruitment of microglia to attack selected neurons in restricted brain regions (see below).

Biochemical changes in α-synuclein

The initiating molecular and biochemical aspects of α-synuclein accumulation and aggregation remain elusive, but show self-aggregation properties that are enhanced by the genetic α-synuclein *SNCA* mutations associated with PD (25). Furthermore, the identification of genetic *SNCA* multiplications that cause PD (26,27) suggest that toxicity may result from a simple increase in the normal monomeric form of α-synuclein, although recent studies have demonstrated no change or a progressive reduction in soluble α-synuclein in sporadic PD (28,29). In addition, there is no change in α-synuclein mRNA expression in idiopathic PD (28, 30). These studies provide compelling evidence that idiopathic PD does not result from a simple over-expression of α-synuclein protein. In contrast, there is an increase in membrane-associated α-synuclein with the formation of Lewy pathologies (29), with elevated binding of oligomeric α-synuclein to membranes suggested to be important in protein aggregation and cellular degeneration in PD (31).

Post-translational modifications assisting with this conformational change in α-synuclein protein are considered important, including phosphorylation, C-terminal truncation and ubiquitination of α-synuclein. Phosphorylation at serine 129 (S129) is the predominant modification of α-synuclein found in Lewy pathologies, with most α-synuclein in Lewy pathologies phosphorylated at this site (32,33). *In vitro* and *in vivo* models have demonstrated a role for serine 129 phosphorylation in the regulation of α-synuclein aggregation and toxicity (34), and human tissue studies have demonstrated that an increase in S129 phosphorylation of soluble α-synuclein precedes the formation of Lewy pathologies (29). These studies show that phosphorylation of α-synuclein at this site is important for the pathogenesis of Lewy pathology in PD. Truncation of α-synuclein at the C-terminus has recently been postulated to initiate α-synuclein aggregation in human tissue studies (35), supporting *in vitro* studies showing that C-terminal-truncated α-synuclein initiates its aggregation (36). C-terminal-truncated fibril transfer between neurons leads to the seeding of endogenous α-synuclein in the unaffected neuron to produce insoluble aggregates (37). These studies show that the post-translational modification of α-synuclein, rather than leading to an increase in monomeric protein, is important for its pathological toxicity.

Microglial activation (inflammation)

Glia are important in the initiation and progression of PD pathology. There is evidence for microglial activation early in PD, perhaps for clearance of extracellular α-synuclein, but the microglia transform into phagocytes that target neurons as the disease progresses (21). There are abundant reactive microglia in the PD substantia nigra found clustering around pigmented dopamine neurons and extracellular neuromelanin (38). Experimentally, dopamine neurons are particularly vulnerable to chronic microglial activation, with neuromelanin able to activate

microglia to become phagocytes. The extent of microglial activation correlates with α-synuclein deposition in PD substantia nigra, although clinical progression is not related to the severity of either pathology (39). Activated microglia are also observed in the putamen, hippocampus and cortical regions in PD, both associated with and independent of Lewy pathology. As discussed above, the upregulation of microglia in regions depositing α-synuclein may initially be a reaction to clear pathological α-synuclein. Epidemiological studies indicate that anti-inflammatory medication use in PD patients provides a slight protection, supporting the concept that microglial activation is an important component of disease progression. While the evidence supports a role for the innate activation of microglia by α-synuclein, more recent work has revealed a role for their upregulation through the adaptive immune system also, as CD8+ and CD4+ T cells have been identified in post-mortem PD brain tissue (40).

Progression of pathology in Parkinson's disease

In PD, both the regional destruction of tissue and infiltration of Lewy pathology occur in specific but divergent patterns, suggesting some separation of these degenerative processes. The pattern of neuronal loss has been discussed above, with early severe vulnerability restricted to regions involved in motor regulation. In particular, many regions concentrating early Lewy pathology have only mild neuronal loss (see above).

In contrast, the neuroanatomical regions accumulating α-synuclein pathology early in PD appear to be in the autonomic regions of the brain (18). From there, it follows a fairly consistent pattern up the brainstem to infiltrate the forebrain as the disease progresses (18), with six progressive stages of PD now identified (see Figure 15.4) (3). This system of pathological spread has become widely utilized in staging the severity of PD pathology in both diagnostic and re-

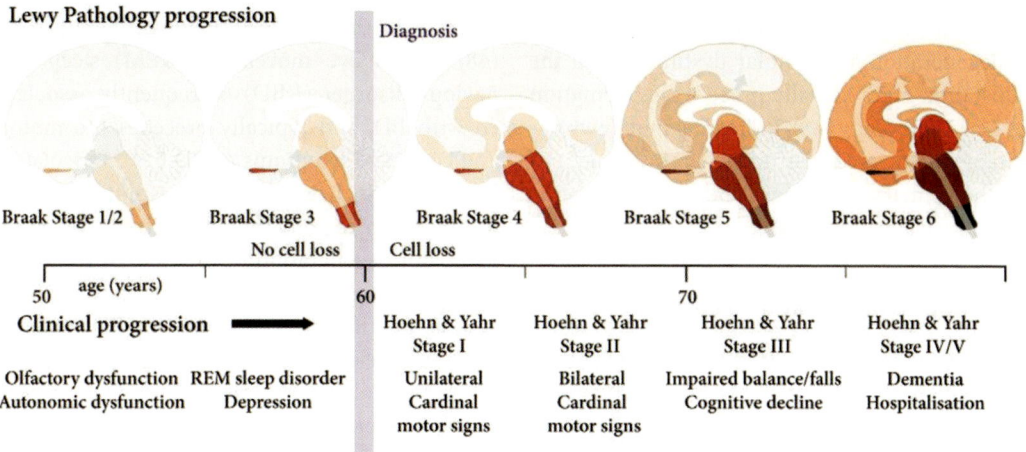

Lewy Pathology progression

Diagnosis

Braak Stage 1/2   Braak Stage 3   Braak Stage 4   Braak Stage 5   Braak Stage 6

No cell loss   Cell loss

50   age (years)   60   70

Clinical progression ➡   Hoehn & Yahr   Hoehn & Yahr   Hoehn & Yahr   Hoehn & Yahr
Stage I   Stage II   Stage III   Stage IV/V

Olfactory dysfunction REM sleep disorder   Unilateral   Bilateral   Impaired balance/falls   Dementia
Autonomic dysfunction   Depression   Cardinal   Cardinal   Cognitive decline   Hospitalisation
motor signs   motor signs

Figure 15.4 Scheme representing the progression of α-synuclein pathology in PD.
PD staging is based on both the Braak staging scheme and the Hoehn & Yahr clinical staging scheme and this illustration suggests how these two schemes are correlated. The scheme shows early α-synuclein deposition associated with non-motor symptoms affecting autonomic functions. With the spread of pathology the clinical symptoms involving motor circuits appear to affect movement, followed by those limbic brain regions as cognitive decline begins. Note that the typical clinical motor symptoms of PD only occur when there is both α-synuclein deposition and nigral cell loss.

search settings, and has particularly influenced a new clinical field of early disease indicators. The staging of PD pathology is underpinned by three premises: that α-synuclein deposition is the primary PD pathology, that the pathology occurs presymptomatically, and that the pathology spreads in a predictable manner to multiple neuronal systems. The Lewy pathology is assumed to spread progressively so that, for any grade, all the stages associated with a lower grade will show pathology (see Figure 15.4).

The assessment of different autopsy series continues to verify the validity and predictability of the Braak PD staging scheme. Only 47% of PD cases were found to fit the staging scheme in a large retrospective autopsy study by the UK PD Society Tissue Bank (41), while other studies reported no involvement of the lower brainstem in autopsy-confirmed PD cases, despite Lewy pathology in higher brainstem or cortical regions (42). An autopsy study in a population-based cohort over 65 years old revealed 37% with Lewy pathology, but only 51% conformed to the Braak staging, and surprisingly, 17% had mainly corti-

cal Lewy pathology (43). While there will probably always be outlying cases that do not conform to any staging scheme, the number with alternate distributions of Lewy pathology is greater than expected for PD. There are a number of technical reasons that may explain these differences, including the different types of pathological cohorts examined and different technical issues (amount of region sampled, staining and tissue quality issues). Another issue is that Lewy pathology is also diagnostic of other diseases, and the different distributions of Lewy pathology may indicate incidental dementia with Lewy bodies (DLB) where a different distribution of pathology would be expected based on their clinical symptoms. The longitudinal assessment of PD patients to autopsy shows that the progression of Lewy pathology is mostly consistent with the Braak PD staging scheme. In terms of the length of time between the different PD stages, at 5 years most have stage 4 disease where brainstem Lewy pathology predominates, by 13 years 50% of cases have stage 5 disease, and by 18 years all have at least this pathological stage of PD (44).

Recent work has suggested that significant neurodegeneration and cellular dysfunction in the substantia nigra actually precede the formation of Lewy pathology (45), indicating that Lewy pathology-associated neurodegeneration may not be the primary pathologic phenomenon occurring in Parkinson's disease.

Clinicopathological correlates

The presence of Lewy pathologies is required for a pathological diagnosis of PD, but the density of Lewy pathologies does not consistently relate to many clinical symptoms. Lewy pathology density in the substantia nigra does not relate to motor deficits (6), and actually remains stable over the course of PD (19). Rather, neurodegeneration of the dopamine neurons is the pathological substrate for the PD motor symptoms. The severity of pigmented dopamine cell loss in the substantia nigra relates directly to the severity of symptoms identified using the PD motor sections of the Unified PD Rating Scale (UPDRS), and specifically to bradykinesia and rigidity but not tremor (6). The degree of pigmented neuronal loss in the substantia nigra correlates with subtle changes in UPDRS scores in aged persons unaffected by PD (46). These studies indicate that cell loss occurs in a preclinical phase, with clinical symptoms sufficient for a diagnosis of PD occurring when 50-60% of the ventrolateral nigral neurons have been lost. Estimates suggest it takes approximately 5 years from the initial loss of nigral neurons to symptom onset, with rapid neuron loss during the first 5 years of symptomatic disease that tails off exponentially (6).

Early olfactory dysfunction in PD is supported by neuropathologic studies, with Lewy pathology present in the olfactory bulb, olfactory tract and anterior olfactory nucleus in preclinical Braak stages prior to significant nigral degeneration (47). Despite considerable α-synuclein deposition in the olfactory bulb in PD, there is no significant atrophy, and there is actually an increase in the number of dopaminergic cells (48). Rapid eye movement (REM) sleep behaviour disorder (RBD) is frequently associated with PD, and typically precedes the motor and cognitive symptoms of PD (49). In isolated RBD patients, Lewy pathology is not increased in brainstem regions thought to be involved in RBD, but degeneration of lower brainstem nuclei is felt to play a significant role in the pathogenesis of RBD in early premotor PD patients (49). Degeneration and dysfunction of the central and peripheral cholinergic, monoaminergic and serotonergic nuclei that mediate autonomic functions have been implicated in the development of autonomic dysfunction in the cardiovascular, gastrointestinal and urogenital systems in PD (see (50) for review). In addition, Lewy pathology is observed in the central and peripheral neurons of the cardiovascular and gastrointestinal systems that impact on autonomic functions (51). Visual hallucinations, present in more than 50% of PD patients, show strong correlations with Lewy pathology densities in temporal lobe regions, particularly the amygdala and parahippocampal cortex (8,52).

There is also a strong correlation between cortical Lewy pathology load and increasing cognitive impairment in the absence of other neurodegenerative pathologies (e.g. Alzheimer's disease, AD). Cognitive impairment in PD appears as Lewy pathology spreads from the brainstem to higher cortical areas involved in cognitive function, with evidence that subcortical pathology alone might also be sufficient to induce some cognitive decline (18,53). The risk of developing dementia increases with pathological disease progression into the cortex, and Lewy pathology density in cortical limbic areas distinguishes PD cases with dementia from those without (54). However, Lewy body load is not predictive of the onset or duration of dementia, and some PD patients develop dementia with only mild cortical Lewy pathology (54,55). A probability concept to determine the likelihood that Lewy pathology would significantly contribute to the PD-related cognitive symptoms has been developed, with a low probablility of Lewy pathology relating to cognitive impairment when only brainstem Lewy pathology is involved and the highest probability if widespread Lewy pathology is observed throughout the cortex (3). While dopamine deficiency has been implicated in cognitive impairment and dementia in PD (56), the effects of dopamine replacement therapy on cognitive symptoms is heterogeneous, suggesting that non-dopaminergic pathways are also involved. Indeed, neurodegeneration in noradrenergic, cholinergic and serotonergic nuclei have been associated with cognitive decline in PD (57, 58).

Genetics influence pathology in idiopathic PD and PD-like parkinsonisms

Data from longitudinal twin studies and nuclear families suggest heritability accounts for 35-40% of PD cases, with a strong familial genetic basis recognized in 10% of cases, although each of the genetic forms is rare overall (59). Genetic PD-like parkinsonisms often have a younger age of disease onset, and some mutations are more prevalent in certain ethnic groups. The pathogenic mechanisms of genetic mutations in parkinsonisms are not fully elucidated, but are considered to represent either a toxic gain of protein function or a loss of protein function, or contribute to the risk of developing parkinsonism. The most common mutations causing autosomal dominant parkinsonism are thought to result in a gain-of-function, while the most common mutations causing autosomal recessive parkinsonism cause a loss-of-function (see below). The risk conferred by genetic mutations that are not directly causative of PD is less well understood. The identification of causal gene mutations for common and rare forms of genetic PD, as well as risk susceptibility genes for PD, has revealed avenues for the investigation into molecular pathogenic mechanisms of the more common sporadic form of PD.

Common autosomal dominant genes have Lewy pathology

As indicated above, the first major genetic discovery in PD was the identification that mutations in the SNCA gene cause autosomal dominant PD (12). SNCA gene duplication and triplication mutations, resulting in a 50% and 100% increase in genetic load, respectively, have also been identified in families with autosomal dominant PD (26,27). As discussed above, typical Lewy pathology occurs in all PD patients with autosomal dominant SNCA gene mutations (see Table 15.1).

Mutations in the LRRK2 gene (leucine-rich repeat kinase 2 or dardarin) were also identified as a cause of autosomal dominant PD (60,61). LRRK2 mutations are the most common genetic cause of autosomal dominant, late-onset PD, and are also observed in 0.5-3.0% of 'sporadic' cases. The LRRK2 gene encodes a large cytosolic protein with multiple functional domains, including kinase and GTPase domains. While the normal function of LRRK2 protein is unknown, a role in intracellular signalling pathways is suggested by the presence of the kinase domain. In vitro studies demonstrate an increase in kinase activity with LRRK2 mutations (62), supporting a gain-of-function mechanism and suggesting increased LRRK2 enzyme activity may occur in PD. Other structural features of LRRK2 indicate possible interactions with other proteins. Typical Lewy pathology occurs in most cases with LRRK2 mutations (see Table 15.1) (63), also aligning this form of PD with common idiopathic PD. Rare cases have been described with diverse neuropathologies that include pure nigral degeneration without Lewy bodies and tau pathology similar to that seen in progressive supranuclear palsy (PSP) (61,64).

The most recently identified other autosomal dominant gene variants are in the VPS35 gene (vacuolar protein sorting 35 homologue) (65,66). The VPS35 protein is the largest subunit of the retromer complex and functions as the

Table 15.1
Neuropathological features of genetic forms of Parkinson's disease. AD, autosomal dominant; AR, autosomal recessive; S, susceptibility risk gene.

Locus	Gene symbol	Gene product	OMIM number	Mode of inheritance	Neuropathology
PARK1/4	SNCA	α-synuclein	168601	AD	Typical Lewy pathology and neuro-degeneration
PARK8	LRRK2	LRRK2	607060	AD	Typical Lewy pathology and neuro-degeneration; rare additional features
PARK2	PARK2	Parkin	600116	AR	No Lewy pathology; atypical nigro-striatal degeneration
PARK6	PINK1	PINK1	605909	AR	Rare Lewy pathology; atypical neuro-degenration
PARK7	PARK7	DJ-1	606324	AR	Unknown
PARK17	VPS35	VPS35	614203	AD	Unknown
PARK18	EIF4G1	EIF4G1	600495	AD	Typical Lewy pathology
PARK9	ATP13A2	ATP13A2	606693	AR	Unknown
PARK14/ NBIA-2	PLA2G6	PLA2G6	612953	AR	Typical Lewy pathology; additional NBIA-related and tau pathologies
NBIA-1	PANK2	PANK2	234200	AR	No Lewy pathology; some tau pathology
PARK15	FBXO7	FBXO7	260300	AR	Unknown
	C19orf12		614297	AR	Lewy pathology; additional tau pathology
	GBA1	GCase	606463	S	Typical Lewy pathology and neuro-degeneration

central platform for the assembly of VPS26 and VPS29 (67). The retromer complex is involved in retrograde transport of proteins from endosomes to the trans-Golgi, and has been implicated in a broad range of physiological, developmental and pathological processes (67). To date, the neuropathology of *VPS35*-associated PD has not been characterized (see Table 15.1).

Common autosomal recessive genes have absent or rare Lewy pathology

The first mutation identified to cause autosomal recessive, juvenile-onset PD was a homozygous deletion of exons 3-7 of the *parkin* gene, with a number of homozygous or compound heterozygous *parkin* point mutations and other small and large deletions subsequently identified that account for up to 10% of early-onset PD cases (68). The *parkin* gene encodes an ubiquitin E3 ligase in the ubiquitin-proteosome pathway, and often co-localizes with α-synuclein in Lewy pathology (69). Parkin can covalently bind oxidized dopamine *in vitro*, causing increased parkin insolubility and decreased E3 ligase activity. *Parkin* knockout mice display elevated levels of extracellular dopamine and reduced mitochondrial protein levels, supporting a loss-of-function for parkin in PD (70). Recent studies have demonstrated that parkin and PINK1 (see below) function in a common pathway to maintain mitochondrial integrity and dopaminergic neuron function through the regulation of mitochondrial fission/fusion dynamics and mito-chondrial autophagy (71,72). Autopsy studies of *parkin* mutation carriers have suggested that this disease differs significantly from idiopathic PD due to its absence of Lewy pathology (see Table 15.1) (63).

Homozygous missense and stop mutations in the *PINK1* (the phosphatase and tensin homo-logue (PTEN) induced putative kinase 1) gene also resulting in loss-of-function changes, are the second most common cause of early-onset autosomal recessive PD (73). The *PINK1* gene encodes a putative mitochondrial serine/threo-nine kinase that functions to protect cells against proteosome inhibition and apoptosis. PINK1 is ubiquitously expressed in the human brain and is found in 10% of Lewy pathology in sporadic PD (74). As described above, PINK1 and parkin interact in concert to regulate mitophagy, with *in vitro* studies demonstrating that PINK1 op-erates upstream of parkin in this pathway (75). Autopsy data on *PINK1* mutation carriers is very limited, with evidence of some Lewy pathology amid atypical neurodegeneration, suggesting *PINK1*-associated neuropathology differs from typical PD (see Table 15.1) (63).

Other rare genes often have other pathologies

Mutations in the *DJ-1* gene were also identified as a cause of autosomal recessive, early-onset PD (76), however they are rare. Putative roles for DJ-1 in neuronal oxidative stress response and protein folding and degradation have been sug-gested (59). The neuropathology of *DJ-1*-asso-ciated Parkinson's disease is currently unknown (see Table 15.1).

Homozygous and heterozygous loss-of-function mutations in the *FBXO7* gene (F-box only pro-tein 7) have been identified in rare families with autosomal recessive, early-onset PD (77). F-box proteins have been implicated in processes such as cell cycle, genome stability, development,

synapse formation, and circadian rhythms, and constitute a subunit of the F-box-contain-ing ubiquitin protein ligase complex that func-tions in phosphorylation-dependent ubiqui-tination (78). Loss of FBXO7 nuclear function is proposed as the cause of this early-onset PD syndrome with pyramidal signs (78). No neu-ropathology has been reported in patients with *FBXO7* mutations (see Table 15.1), but FP-CIT SPECT neuroimaging shows severe presynaptic nigrostriatal dopamine deficits (77).

A rare cause of autosomal dominant PD is a mu-tation in the *EIF4G1* gene (79). EIF4G1 is a large scaffolding protein that contains binding sites for other members of the multi-subunit protein complex EIF4F (80). This complex facilitates the recruitment of mRNA to the ribosome, which is a rate-limiting step during the initiation phase of protein synthesis, a process manipulated by a number of factors, including viruses and the mTOR signaling pathway (80). Typical Lewy pathologies appear present in *EIF4G1*-linked PD (Table 15.1) (79), but this needs to be con-firmed in further samples.

Homozygous mutations in the *ATP13A2* gene cause a rare form of atypical, juvenile-onset PD termed Kufor-Rakeb syndrome (81). *AT-P13A2* encodes a lysosomal member of the P5 subfamily of ATPases that function as cation transporters. ATP13A2 plays a role in cellular processes such as endoplasmic reticulum trans-location, endoplasmic reticulum-to-Golgi traf-ficking, and vesicular transport and fusion (82), with *ATP13A2* mutations causing impairment in lysosomal acidification, decreased proteo-lytic processing of lysosomal enzymes, reduced degradation of lysosomal substrates (including α-synuclein), and diminished lysosomal-medi-ated clearance of autophagosomes (83). *In vitro* studies have also suggested a role for ATP13A2 in mitochondrial maintenance. Neuropatholog-ical evaluation of *ATP13A2*-linked PD has not yet been described (see Table 15.1), but MRI studies reveal significant atrophy of the globus pallidus and the pyramids, and generalized brain atrophy in later stages (84).

Mutations in *PLA2G6* (phospholipase A2, group VI) associated with infantile neuroaxonal dystrophy or neurodegeneration with brain iron accumulation (NBIA) type 2 (85) have also been identified in rare families with early-onset parkinsonism (86). *PLA2G6* encodes a mitochondrial A2 phospholipase enzyme that catalyzes the release of fatty acids from phospholipids (85). A2 phospholipase deficiency in mice is associated with reduced fatty acid metabolism and changes in lipid-metabolizing enzyme expression and brain phospholipid fatty acid content. Patients with *PLA2G6* mutations show a widespread neuropathological phenotype with neuroaxonal dystrophy, cerebellar atrophy with or without evidence of brain iron accumulation, and significant Lewy pathology corresponding to Braak stage 6 (see Table 15.1) (86). Cortical tau-immunoreactive neurofibrillary tangles have also been documented in *PLA2G6* cases (86).

Interestingly, two other types of NBIA have been associated with rare genetic forms of autosomal recessive parkinsonism. Mutations in the *PANK2* gene (pantothenate kinase 2) cause the most common NBIA (type 1, Hallervorden-Spatz syndrome) (87). PANK2 is a kinase expressed in mitochondria and is a key regulatory enzyme in the biosynthesis of coenzyme A (CoA) (87). Patients with *PANK2* mutations do not display Lewy pathology, but neurofibrillary tangles are found in some cases (see Table 15.1) (88). Mutations in the *c19orf12* (chromosome 19 open reading frame 12) gene have been identified in patients with an unknown NBIA similar to type 1 NBIA but with later onset (89). *C19orf12* encodes a mitochondrial protein of unknown function, with this mitochondrial localization suggesting that all NBIA genes may play a role in mitochondrial lipid homeostasis

(87). A single autopsy case has detected Lewy pathology with additional tau-positive neurofibrillary tangles in *C19orf12*-associated PD (see Table 15.1) (89).

Risk genes identified in genome-wide association studies

Genome-wide association studies (GWAS) identify common genetic risk loci in an efficient yet statistically stringent manner using large disease and matched control cohorts. The first large GWAS in PD demonstrated that risk loci were present at genomic regions encoding α-synuclein and microtubule-associated protein tau (MAPT) (90,91). Subsequent GWAS and meta-analyses of multiple GWAS have validated and strengthened the association of both *SNCA* and *MAPT* with sporadic PD (92-94), particularly polymorphic associations in the promoter region of the *SNCA* gene (REP1) (95) and homozygosity for the H1 tau genotype (96).

A number of other risk loci for PD have been identified by GWAS, including loci containing genes for the human leucocyte antigen (*HLA*)-DR, cyclin G-associated kinase (*GAK*), bone marrow stromal cell antigen 1 (*BST1*), *LRRK2* and glucocerebrosidase (*GBA*) (92-94). A current meta-analysis assessment of all PD gene association studies lists *MAPT*, *SNCA*, *GBA1* and *LRRK2* as the top four genes contributing to the risk of developing PD (PDGene.org). Homozygous mutations in *GBA1* cause Gaucher disease, a lysosomal storage disorder characterized by cellular lipid accumulation due to the functional loss of the lysosomal enzyme glucocerebrosidase (GCase) (97). Clinical observations first indicated that patients with Gaucher disease, and their relatives, are affected by PD more often than expected, which ultimately led to the identification of *GBA1* mutations as a top genetic risk for PD (98). Carriers of a single *GBA1* mutant allele have a 5-fold greater risk of developing PD, with risk increased to 7-fold in Ashkenazi Jewish populations (99). The most common *GBA1* mutations are present in ~15% of Ashkenazi Jewish PD patients and ~3% of non-Ashkenazi patients, compared to ~3% and <1% in matched controls, respectively, and almost 10% of all patients with PD carry heterozygous *GBA1* mutations (100). Sporadic PD cases with heterozygous *GBA1* mutations display extensive Lewy pathology, and typical Lewy pathology is also characteristic in Gaucher disease patients who develop PD (see Table 15.1) (101). Neuropathological studies of PD cases with and without *GBA1* mutations have demonstrated no difference in Lewy pathology with no significant difference in cortical load (102). In post-mortem brain tissue from PD patients with *GBA1* mutations, GCase and α-synuclein co-localize in Lewy bodies, and aggregated forms of α-synuclein are present (103, 104). Recent human studies show reduced GCase protein levels and enzyme activity in a range of affected brain regions in all PD patients (105). Indirect CSF measures of GCase in PD show reduced activity compared with controls and AD (106). Cell and animal studies have now demonstrated that decreased wild-type GCase leads to α-synuclein accumulation, and increased α-synuclein can inhibit normal GCase function (107), highlighting the importance of this protein in PD Lewy pathology.

Conclusions

There is a distinctive pattern of pathology underlying PD that involves neuronal loss and α-synuclein deposition in the form of Lewy pathology. The distribution of these pathologies does not seem to progress in the same way, with many regions demonstrating early Lewy pathology but having only minimal neuronal loss even at end-stage disease. Genetic studies show that some genes impact more on Lewy pathology than others, lending some support to divergent pathogenic mechanisms for neuronal loss and α-synuclein accumulation. Recent studies suggest that neuronal loss may occur before the formation of Lewy pathology, at least in the vulnerable do-

pamine neurons (45), although significant cellular dysfunction due to α-synuclein accumulation must occur. Overall, these studies show that substantial early clinical deficits associate most with the complete loss of vulnerable neuronal populations, while broad and potentially milder neuronal dysfunction associates with the very slow accumulation of α-synuclein in Lewy pathology in many cell types and regions of the nervous system. Proteins influencing both types of pathologies have been identified through genetic studies. Recessive genes involved in mitochondrial function have less Lewy pathology, while genes involved in lysosomal function appear to impact most on Lewy pathology. These studies give significant support to the development of mechanistic treatments for PD.

References

1 Reider CR, Halter CA, Castelluccio PF, Oakes D, Nichols WC, Foroud T. Reliability of reported age at onset for Parkinson's disease. Mov Disord. 2003;18:275-279.

2 Willis AW, Schootman M, Kung N, Evanoff BA, Perlmutter JS, Racette BA. Predictors of survival in patients with Parkinson disease. Arch Neurol. 2012;69:601-607.

3 Dickson DW, Braak H, Duda JE, et al. Neuropathological assessment of Parkinson's disease: refining the diagnostic criteria. Lancet Neurol. 2009;8:1150-1157.

4 Pedersen KM, Marner L, Pakkenberg H, Pakkenberg B. No global loss of neocortical neurons in Parkinson's disease: a quantitative stereological study. Mov Disord. 2005;20:164-171.

5 McRitchie DA, Cartwright HR, Halliday GM. Specific A10 dopaminergic nuclei in the midbrain degenerate in Parkinson's disease. Exp Neurol. 1997;144:202-213.

6 Greffard S, Verny M, Bonnet AM, et al. Motor score of the Unified Parkinson Disease Rating Scale as a good predictor of Lewy body-associated neuronal loss in the substantia nigra. Arch Neurol. 2006;63:584-588.

7 Damier P, Hirsch EC, Agid Y, Graybiel AM. The substantia nigra of the human brain. II. Patterns of loss of dopamine-containing neurons in Parkinson's disease. Brain. 1999;122 :1437-1448.

8 Harding AJ, Stimson E, Henderson JM, Halliday GM. Clinical correlates of selective pathology in the amygdala of patients with Parkinson's disease. Brain. 2002;125:2431-2445.

9 Jellinger KA. Cell death mechanisms in Parkinson's disease. J Neural Transm. 2000;107:1-29.

10 Halliday GM, Li YW, Blumbergs PC, et al. Neuropathology of immunohistochemically identified brainstem neurons in Parkinson's disease. Ann Neurol. 1990;27:373-385.

11 Halliday GM, Macdonald V, Henderson JM. A comparison of degeneration in motor thalamus and cortex between progressive supranuclear palsy and Parkinson's disease. Brain. 2005;128:2272-2280.

12 Polymeropoulos MH, Lavedan C, Leroy E, et al. Mutation in the alpha-synuclein gene identified in families with Parkinson's disease. Science. 1997;276:2045-2047.

13 George JM. The synucleins. Genome Biol. 2002;3:REVIEWS3002.

14 Maroteaux L, Campanelli JT, Scheller RH. Synuclein: a neuron-specific protein localized to the nucleus and presynaptic nerve terminal. J Neurosci. 1988;8:2804-2815.

15 Spillantini MG, Schmidt ML, Lee VM, Trojanowski JQ, Jakes R, Goedert M. Alpha-synuclein in Lewy bodies. Nature. 1997;388:839-840.

16 Kuusisto E, Parkkinen L, Alafuzoff I. Morphogenesis of Lewy bodies: dissimilar incorporation of alpha-synuclein, ubiquitin, and p62. J Neuropathol Exp Neurol. 2003;62:1241-1253.

17 Kanazawa T, Uchihara T, Takahashi A, Nakamura A, Orimo S, Mizusawa H. Three-layered structure shared between Lewy bodies and lewy neurites-three-dimensional reconstruction of triple-labeled sections. Brain Pathol. 2008;18:415-422.

18 Braak H, Del Tredici K, Rub U, de Vos RA, Jansen Steur EN, Braak E. Staging of brain pathology related to sporadic Parkinson's disease. Neurobiol Aging. 2003;24:197-211.

19 Greffard S, Verny M, Bonnet AM, Seilhean D, Hauw JJ, Duyckaerts C. A stable proportion of Lewy body bearing neurons in the substantia nigra suggests a model in which the Lewy body causes neuronal death. Neurobiol Aging. 2010;31:99-103.

20 Wakabayashi K, Tanji K, Mori F, Takahashi H. The Lewy body in Parkinson's disease: molecules implicated in the formation and degradation of alpha-synuclein aggregates. Neuropathology. 2007;27:494-506.

21 Halliday GM, Stevens CH. Glia: initiators and progressors of pathology in Parkinson's disease. Mov Disord. 2011;26:6-17.

22 Lee HJ, Suk JE, Patrick C, et al. Direct transfer of alpha-synuclein from neuron to astroglia causes inflammatory responses in synucleinopathies. J Biol Chem. 2010;285:9262-9272.

23 Song YJ, Halliday GM, Holton JL, et al. Degeneration in different parkinsonian syndromes relates to astrocyte type and astrocyte protein expression. J Neuropathol Exp Neurol. 2009;68:1073-1083.

24 Braak H, Sastre M, Del Tredici K. Development of alpha-synuclein immunoreactive astrocytes in the forebrain parallels stages of intraneuronal pathology in sporadic Parkinson's disease. Acta Neuropathol. 2007;114:231-241.

25 Conway KA, Lee SJ, Rochet JC, Ding TT, Williamson RE, Lansbury PT, Jr. Acceleration of oligomerization, not fibrillization, is a shared property of both alpha-synuclein mutations linked to early-onset Parkinson's disease: implications for pathogenesis and therapy. Proc Natl Acad Sci USA. 2000;97:571-576.

26 Chartier-Harlin MC, Kachergus J, Roumier C, et al. Alpha-synuclein locus duplication as a cause of familial Parkinson's disease. Lancet. 2004;364:1167-1169.

27 Singleton AB, Farrer M, Johnson J, et al. alpha-Synuclein locus triplication causes Parkinson's disease. Science. 2003;302:341.

28 Quinn JG, Coulson DT, Brockbank S, et al. alpha-Synuclein mRNA and soluble alpha-synuclein protein levels in post-mortem brain from patients with Parkinson's disease, dementia with Lewy bodies, and Alzheimer's disease. Brain Res. 2012;1459:71-80.

29 Zhou J, Broe M, Huang Y, et al. Changes in the solubility and phosphorylation of alpha-synuclein over the course of Parkinson's disease. Acta Neuropathol. 2011;121:695-704.

30 Simunovic F, Yi M, Wang Y, et al. Gene expression profiling of substantia nigra dopamine neurons: further insights into Parkinson's disease pathology. Brain. 2009;132:1795-1809.

31 van Rooijen BD, Claessens MM, Subramaniam V. Membrane interactions of oligomeric alpha-synuclein: potential role in Parkinson's disease. Curr Protein Pept Sci. 2010;11:334-342.

32 Anderson JP, Walker DE, Goldstein JM, et al. Phosphorylation of Ser-129 is the dominant pathological modification of alpha-synuclein in familial and sporadic Lewy body disease. J Biol Chem. 2006;281:29739-29752.

33 Fujiwara H, Hasegawa M, Dohmae N, et al. alpha-Synuclein is phosphorylated in synucleinopathy lesions. Nat Cell Biol. 2002;4:160-164.

34 Chen L, Feany MB. Alpha-synuclein phosphorylation controls neurotoxicity and inclusion formation in a Drosophila model of Parkinson disease. Nat Neurosci. 2005;8:657-663.

35 Prasad K, Beach TG, Hedreen J, Richfield EK. Critical role of truncated alpha-synuclein and aggregates in Parkinson's disease and incidental Lewy body disease. Brain Pathol. 2012;22:811-825.

36 Ulusoy A, Febbraro F, Jensen PH, Kirik D, Romero-Ramos M. Co-expression of C-terminal truncated alpha-synuclein enhances full-length alpha-synuclein-induced pathology. Eur J Neurosci. 2010;32:409-422.

37 Luk KC, Kehm VM, Zhang B, O'Brien P, Trojanowski JQ, Lee VM. Intracerebral inoculation of pathological alpha-synuclein initiates a rapidly progressive neurodegenerative alpha-synucleinopathy in mice. J Exp Med. 2012;209:975-986.

38 McGeer PL, McGeer EG. Glial reactions in Parkinson's disease. Mov Disord. 2008;23:474-483.

39 Croisier E, Moran LB, Dexter DT, Pearce RK, Graeber MB. Microglial inflammation in the parkinsonian substantia nigra: relationship to alpha-synuclein deposition. J Neuroinflammation. 2005;2:14.

40 Brochard V, Combadiere B, Prigent A, et al. Infiltration of CD4+ lymphocytes into the brain contributes to neurodegeneration in a mouse model of Parkinson disease. J Clin Invest. 2009;119:182-192.

41 Kalaitzakis ME, Graeber MB, Gentleman SM, Pearce RK. The dorsal motor nucleus of the vagus is not an obligatory trigger site of Parkinson's disease: a critical analysis of alpha-synuclein staging. Neuropathol Appl Neurobiol. 2008;34:284-295.

42 Parkkinen L, Pirttila T, Alafuzoff I. Applicability of current staging/categorization of alpha-synuclein pathology and their clinical relevance. Acta Neuropathol. 2008;115:399-407.

43 Zaccai J, Brayne C, McKeith I, Matthews F, Ince PG. Patterns and stages of alpha-synucleinopathy: Relevance in a population-based cohort. Neurology. 2008;70:1042-1048.

44 Halliday G, Hely M, Reid W, Morris J. The progression of pathology in longitudinally followed patients with Parkinson's disease. Acta Neuropathol. 2008;115:409-415.

45 Milber JM, Noorigian JV, Morley JF, et al. Lewy pathology is not the first sign of degeneration in vulnerable neurons in Parkinson disease. Neurology. 2012;79:2307-2314.

46 Buchman AS, Shulman JM, Nag S, et al. Nigral pathology and parkinsonian signs in elders without Parkinson disease. Ann Neurol. 2012;71:258-266.

47 Del Tredici K, Rub U, De Vos RA, Bohl JR, Braak H. Where does parkinson disease pathology begin in the brain? J Neuropathol Exp Neurol. 2002;61:413-426.

48 Mundinano IC, Caballero MC, Ordonez C, et al. Increased dopaminergic cells and protein aggregates in the olfactory bulb of patients with neurodegenerative disorders. Acta Neuropathol. 2011;122:61-74.

49 Boeve BF, Silber MH, Saper CB, et al. Pathophysiology of REM sleep behaviour disorder and relevance to neurodegenerative disease. Brain. 2007;130:2770-2788.

50 Dubow JS. Autonomic dysfunction in Parkinson's disease. Dis Mon. 2007;53:265-274.

51 Wakabayashi K, Takahashi H. Neuropathology of autonomic nervous system in Parkinson's disease. Eur Neurol. 1997;38 Suppl 2:2-7.

52 Harding AJ, Broe GA, Halliday GM. Visual hallucinations in Lewy body disease relate to Lewy bodies in the temporal lobe. Brain. 2002;125:391-403.

53 Hurtig HI, Trojanowski JQ, Galvin J, et al. Alpha-synuclein cortical Lewy bodies correlate with dementia in Parkinson's disease. Neurology. 2000;54:1916-1921.

54 Braak H, Rub U, Del Tredici K. Cognitive decline correlates with neuropathological stage in Parkinson's disease. J Neurol Sci. 2006;248:255-258.

55 Colosimo C, Hughes AJ, Kilford L, Lees AJ. Lewy body cortical involvement may not always predict dementia in Parkinson's disease. J Neurol Neurosurg Psychiatry. 2003;74:852-856.

56 Rinne JO, Rummukainen J, Paljarvi L, Rinne UK. Dementia in Parkinson's disease is related to neuronal loss in the medial substantia nigra. Ann Neurol. 1989;26:47-50.

57 Bosboom JL, Stoffers D, Wolters E. Cognitive dysfunction and dementia in Parkinson's disease. J Neural Transm. 2004;111:1303-1315.

58 Del Tredici K, Braak H. Dysfunction of the locus coeruleus-norepinephrine system and related circuitry in Parkinson's disease-related dementia. J Neurol Neurosurg Psychiatry.2013;84:774-783.

59 Klein C, Westenberger A. Genetics of Parkinson's disease. Cold Spring Harb Perspect Med. 2012;2:a008888. doi: 10.1101/cshperspect.a008888

60 Funayama M, Hasegawa K, Kowa H, Saito M, Tsuji S, Obata F. A new locus for Parkinson's disease (PARK8) maps to chromosome 12p11.2-q13.1. Ann Neurol. 2002;51:296-301.

61 Zimprich A, Biskup S, Leitner P, et al. Mutations in LRRK2 cause autosomal-dominant parkinsonism with pleomorphic pathology. Neuron. 2004;44:601-607.

62 Tsika E, Moore DJ. Mechanisms of LRRK2-mediated neurodegeneration. Curr Neurol Neurosci Rep. 2012;12:251-260.

63 Poulopoulos M, Levy OA, Alcalay RN. The neuropathology of genetic Parkinson's disease. Mov Disord. 2012;27:831-842.

64 Khan NL, Jain S, Lynch JM, et al. Mutations in the gene LRRK2 encoding dardarin (PARK8) cause familial Parkinson's disease: clinical, pathological,

olfactory and functional imaging and genetic data. Brain. 2005;128:2786-2796.

65 Vilarino-Guell C, Wider C, Ross OA, et al. VPS35 mutations in Parkinson disease. Am J Hum Genet. 2011;89:162-167.

66 Zimprich A, Benet-Pages A, Struhal W, et al. A mutation in VPS35, encoding a subunit of the retromer complex, causes late-onset Parkinson disease. Am J Hum Genet. 2011;89:168-175.

67 Hierro A, Rojas AL, Rojas R, et al. Functional architecture of the retromer cargo-recognition complex. Nature. 2007;449:1063-1067.

68 Kitada T, Asakawa S, Hattori N, et al. Mutations in the parkin gene cause autosomal recessive juvenile parkinsonism. Nature. 1998;392:605-608.

69 Schlossmacher MG, Frosch MP, Gai WP, et al. Parkin localizes to the Lewy bodies of Parkinson disease and dementia with Lewy bodies. Am J Pathol. 2002;160:1655-1667.

70 Palacino JJ, Sagi D, Goldberg MS, et al. Mitochondrial dysfunction and oxidative damage in parkin-deficient mice. J Biol Chem. 2004;279:18614-18622.

71 Clark IE, Dodson MW, Jiang C, et al. Drosophila pink1 is required for mitochondrial function and interacts genetically with parkin. Nature. 2006;441:1162-1166.

72 Park J, Lee SB, Lee S, et al. Mitochondrial dysfunction in Drosophila PINK1 mutants is complemented by parkin. Nature. 2006;441:1157-1161.

73 Valente EM, Abou-Sleiman PM, Caputo V, et al. Hereditary early-onset Parkinson's disease caused by mutations in PINK1. Science. 2004;304:1158-1160.

74 Gandhi S, Muqit MM, Stanyer L, et al. PINK1 protein in normal human brain and Parkinson's disease. Brain. 2006;129:1720-1731.

75 Matsuda N, Sato S, Shiba K, et al. PINK1 stabilized by mitochondrial depolarization recruits Parkin to damaged mitochondria and activates latent Parkin for mitophagy. J Cell Biol. 2010;189:211-221.

76 Bonifati V, Rizzu P, van Baren MJ, et al. Mutations in the DJ-1 gene associated with autosomal recessive early-onset parkinsonism. Science. 2003;299:256-259.

77 Di Fonzo A, Dekker MC, Montagna P, et al. FBXO7 mutations cause autosomal recessive, early-onset parkinsonian-pyramidal syndrome. Neurology. 2009;72:240-245.

78 Ho MS, Ou C, Chan YR, Chien CT, Pi H. The utility F-box for protein destruction. Cell Mol Life Sci. 2008;65:1977-2000.

79 Chartier-Harlin MC, Dachsel JC, Vilarino-Guell C, et al. Translation initiator EIF4G1 mutations in familial Parkinson disease. Am J Hum Genet. 2011;89:398-406.

80 Walsh D. Manipulation of the host translation initiation complex eIF4F by DNA viruses. Biochem Soc Trans. 2010;38:1511-1516.

81 Ramirez A, Heimbach A, Grundemann J, et al. Hereditary parkinsonism with dementia is caused by mutations in ATP13A2, encoding a lysosomal type 5 P-type ATPase. Nat Genet. 2006;38:1184-1191.

82 Usenovic M, Knight AL, Ray A, et al. Identification of novel ATP13A2 interactors and their role in alpha-synuclein misfolding and toxicity. Hum Mol Genet. 2012;21:3785-3794.

83 Dehay B, Ramirez A, Martinez-Vicente M, et al. Loss of P-type ATPase ATP13A2/PARK9 function induces general lysosomal deficiency and leads to Parkinson disease neurodegeneration. Proc Natl Acad Sci U S A. 2012;109:9611-9616.

84 Paisan-Ruiz C, Guevara R, Federoff M, et al. Early-onset L-dopa-responsive parkinsonism with pyramidal signs due to ATP13A2, PLA2G6, FBXO7 and spatacsin mutations. Mov Disord. 2010;25:1791-1800.

85 Morgan NV, Westaway SK, Morton JE, et al. PLA2G6, encoding a phospholipase A2, is mutated in neurodegenerative disorders with high brain iron. Nat Genet. 2006;38:752-754.

86 Paisan-Ruiz C, Li A, Schneider SA, et al. Widespread Lewy body and tau accumulation in childhood and adult onset dystonia-parkinsonism cases with PLA2G6 mutations. Neurobiol Aging. 2012;33:814-823.

87 Hartig MB, Prokisch H, Meitinger T, Klopstock T. Pantothenate kinase-associated neurodegeneration. Curr Drug Targets. 2012;13:1182-1189.

88 Kruer MC, Hiken M, Gregory A, et al. Novel histopathologic findings in molecularly-confirmed pantothenate kinase-associated neurodegeneration. Brain. 2011;134:947-958.

89 Hartig MB, Iuso A, Haack T, et al. Absence of an orphan mitochondrial protein, c19orf12, causes a distinct clinical subtype of neurodegeneration with brain iron accumulation. Am J Hum Genet. 2011;89:543-550.

90 Satake W, Nakabayashi Y, Mizuta I, et al. Genome-wide association study identifies common variants at four loci as genetic risk factors for Parkinson's disease. Nat Genet. 2009;41:1303-1307.

91 Simon-Sanchez J, Schulte C, Bras JM, et al. Genome-wide association study reveals genetic risk underlying Parkinson's disease. Nat Genet. 2009;41:1308-1312.

92 Edwards TL, Scott WK, Almonte C, et al. Genome-wide association study confirms SNPs in SNCA and the MAPT region as common risk factors for Parkinson disease. Ann Hum Genet. 2010;74:97-109.

93 Consortium. A two-stage meta-analysis identifies several new loci for Parkinson's disease. PLoS Genet. 2011; 7:e1002142. doi: 10.1371/journal. pgen.1002142.

94 Pankratz N, Wilk JB, Latourelle JC, et al. Genome-wide association study for susceptibility genes contributing to familial Parkinson disease. Hum Genet. 2009;124:593-605.

95 Kruger R, Vieira-Saecker AM, Kuhn W, et al. Increased susceptibility to sporadic Parkinson's disease by a certain combined alpha-synuclein/apolipoprotein E genotype. Ann Neurol. 1999;45:611-617.

96 Farrer M, Skipper L, Berg M, et al. The tau H1 haplotype is associated with Parkinson's disease in the Norwegian population. Neurosci Lett. 2002;322:83-86.

97 Hruska KS, LaMarca ME, Scott CR, Sidransky E. Gaucher disease: mutation and polymorphism spectrum in the glucocerebrosidase gene (GBA). Hum Mutat. 2008;29:567-583.

98 Neudorfer O, Giladi N, Elstein D, et al. Occurrence of Parkinson's syndrome in type I Gaucher disease. QJM. 1996;89:691-694.

99 Aharon-Peretz J, Rosenbaum H, Gershoni-Baruch R. Mutations in the glucocerebrosidase gene and Parkinson's disease in Ashkenazi Jews. N Engl J Med. 2004;351:1972-1977.

100 Sidransky E, Nalls MA, Aasly JO, et al. Multicenter analysis of glucocerebrosidase mutations in Parkinson's disease. N Engl J Med. 2009;361:1651-1661.

101 Neumann J, Bras J, Deas E, , et al. Glucocerebrosidase mutations in clinical and pathologically proven Parkinson's disease. Brain. 2009;132:1783-1794.

102 Parkkinen L, Neumann J, O'Sullivan SS, et al. Glucocerebrosidase mutations do not cause increased Lewy body pathology in Parkinson's disease. Mol Genet Metab. 2011;103:410-412.

103 Choi JH, Stubblefield B, Cookson MR, et al. Aggregation of alpha-synuclein in brain samples from subjects with glucocerebrosidase mutations. Mol Genet Metab. 2011;104:185-188.

104 Goker-Alpan O, Stubblefield BK, Giasson BI, Sidransky E. Glucocerebrosidase is present in alpha-synuclein inclusions in Lewy body disorders. Acta Neuropathol. 2010;120:641-649.

105 Gegg ME, Burke D, Heales SJ, et al. Glucocerebrosidase deficiency in substantia nigra of parkinson disease brains. Ann Neurol. 2012;72:455-463.

106 Balducci C, Pierguidi L, Persichetti E, et al. Lysosomal hydrolases in cerebrospinal fluid from subjects with Parkinson's disease. Mov Disord. 2007;22:1481-1484.

107 Mazzulli JR, Xu YH, Sun Y, et al. Gaucher disease glucocerebrosidase and alpha-synuclein form a bidirectional pathogenic loop in synucleinopathies. Cell. 2011;146:37-52.

16

Genetic Parkinsonism

Shinsuke Fujioka & Zbigniew K. Wszolek

During the last two decades, tremendous efforts have been made to understand monogenic, Mendelian disorders with identified gene mutations. Most disorders have a monogenic cause. Despite this tremendous progress, only a small percentage of affected patients carry the known genetic defects. The identification of the associated pathogenic mutation has shed light on the underlying molecular mechanisms of the disorders. However, recent research has focused on detecting the genetic susceptibility of common disorders, including Parkinson's disease (PD), by utilizing genome-wide association studies (GWAS) and genome-wide gene-environmental studies.

We employ the term 'PD' to encompass a combination of cardinal signs that are indicative of Parkinson's disease, including bradykinesia, rigidity, resting tremor, and postural instability. These signs are usually accompanied by several additional features such as good L-dopa responsiveness and asymmetrical clinical presentation (1). Consequently, we use the term 'parkinsonism' to cover symptoms that have one or more cardinal features of PD, but do not satisfy the criteria for a diagnosis of PD (2). Patients with parkinsonism are generally less responsive to L-dopa therapy and usually manifest additional clinical features, like cognitive impairment, motor neuron disease, cerebellar ataxia, and dystonia. In some of these disorders, there is also a neurological multisystem involvement with accompanying dysfunction of the liver, lungs, and bones. Parkinsonism can be classified into three types based on clinical phenotype: akinetic-rigid type, tremor-predominant type, and mixed-type (combination of both types with the same degree of bradykinesia, rigidity, and tremor).

In this chapter, we discuss the clinical and genetic characteristics of 76 disorders with features of PD or parkinsonism. We classify them into six different groups based on a predominantly clinical phenomenology. We also discuss mitochondrial gene mutations in parkinsonian disorders, the genetic susceptibility for PD, and the issues related to diagnostic genetic tests.

Familial disorders presenting with typical features of Parkinson's disease
(Table 16.1)

PD is the second most common progressive neurodegenerative disorder after Alzheimer's disease (AD). The prevalence is estimated to be approximately 160/100,000 in the population aged 65 or older. About 10-15% of PD patients have a family history of the disease (see Chapter 5). So far, 18 genes/loci, PARK1-PARK18, have been identified. Among them, PARK1, PARK2, PARK5-PARK8, PARK17, and PARK18 have been reported to be associated with a typical PD phenotype. In this section, we discuss the clinical and genetic features related to these genetic disorders as listed in Table 16.1.

PARK1/PARK4

PARK1/PARK4 is a rare autosomal dominant form of PD, which accounts for less than 1% of familial PD. The prevalence has not been well investigated. Affected patients typically present

Table 16.1
List of familial disorders presenting with typical features of PD.

	Gene	TAAO	Clinical features	L-dopa responsiveness	Genetic tests availability
PARK1/ PARK4	SNCA	30th-60th	PD, CI, myoclonus, dysautono-mia, LP, Psy, hypoventilation, T (dystonia)	Good	I, IV, V
PARK2	PRKN	Childhood-30th	**PD, dystonia, dysautonomia, Psy,** Pyr, PN, RBD (CI)	Good	I, IV, V
PARK6	PINK1	30th-40th	**PD,** Psy, Pyr, dysautonomia (dystonia, CI, PN)	Good	I, IV, V
PARK7	DJ-1	20th-30th	**PD, dystonia, Psy,** short stature	Good	I, IV, V
PARK8	LRRK2	50th-70th	**PD, Psy,** CI, dysautonomia, sleep problems, anosmia (CBS, dystonia, P, Pyr, sleep benefit)	Good	I, II, III, IV, V
PARK17	VPS35	40th-60th	**PD,** CI, Psy, sleep benefit (dysautonomia)	Good	Not available
PARK18	EIF4G1	50th-60th	**PD, CI**	Good	Not available

CBS = corticobasal syndrome; CI = cognitive impairment; EIF4G1 = eukaryotic translation initiation factor 4 gamma, 1; LP = language problems; LRRK2 = leucine-rich repeat kinase 2; PD = Parkinson's disease; PINK1 = PTEN induced putative kinase 1; PN = peripheral neuropathy; PRKN = parkin; Pry = pyramidal signs; Psy = psychiatric symptoms; RBD = rapid eye movement sleep behaviour disorder; SNCA = α-synuclein; T = tremor; TAAO = typical age at onset; VPS35 = vacuolar protein sorting 35 homolog; I = sequence analysis of the entire coding region is available; II = sequence analysis of select exons is available; III = targeted mutation analysis is available; IV = deletion/duplication analysis is available; V = prenatal diagnosis is available; clinical features in bold are frequently seen in patients (>50% of patients); clinical features in parentheses are occasionally seen in patients (<10% of patients).

with early-onset and rapidly-progressive PD. They respond well to L-dopa therapy, especially in the initial stages of their illness. Subthalamic deep brain stimulation (STN-DBS) is also efficacious. During the course of their illness, patients may also manifest cognitive impairment, myoclonus, dysautonomia, language problems, psychiatric symptoms including depression and hallucinations, and other neurological symptoms. Cognitive impairment, dysautonomia, and psychiatric symptoms are more frequently seen in patients with α-synuclein (SNCA) multiplications than in patients with SNCA missense mutations. Routine brain magnetic resonance imaging (MRI) is usually normal. ^{18}F-fluorodopa (^{18}F-dopa) positron emission tomography (PET) and ^{11}C-raclopride

PET show reduced radiotracer uptake in the striatum, especially in the putamen.

PARK1/PARK4 is caused by mutations in the SNCA gene. α-Synuclein is a protein that is abundantly expressed in the brain, predominantly in the mitochondria in the striatum, thalamus, hippocampus, and olfactory bulb. It is associated with synaptic release and SNARE (soluble N-ethylmaleimide-sensitive-factor attachment protein receptor) complex proteins. To date, three pathogenic α-synuclein missense mutations, A30P, A53T, and E46K, as well as multiplications including duplications and triplications, have been reported to be associated with PARK1/PARK4 (3). Very recently, four additional mutations, A18T, A29T, H50Q, and G51D were identified (4-7).

PARK2

PARK2 is the most common autosomal recessive form of PD and accounts for 10-20% of early-onset, sporadic PD and about 50% of early-onset, autosomal recessive PD. Affected patients typically present with an early-onset, slowly progressive form of PD with motor fluctuations. They respond well to L-dopa therapy; however, dyskinesia and/or motor fluctuations are common. STN-DBS is efficacious. The majority of patients develop leg dystonia in the early stages of their illness. Dysautonomia and psychiatric symptoms such as depression, anxiety, and psychosis are also common. Patients sometimes manifest with hyperreflexia, peripheral neuropathy, and other neurological symptoms during the course of their illness. Routine brain MRI is usually normal. ^{18}F-dopa PET, ^{11}C-raclopride PET, and ^{11}C-2-b-carbomethoxy-3b-(4-fluorophenyl) tropane (CFT) PET shows reduced radiotracer uptake in the bilateral striatum, especially in the putamen.

PARK2 is caused by mutations in the *PRKN* gene, encoding parkinson protein 2, E3 ubiquitin protein ligase (parkin; PRKN), which is a protein that is ubiquitously expressed in the brain, including the substantia nigra. Parkin is associated with degradation of several proteins including parkin itself. To date, more than 120 pathogenic *PRKN* mutations have been reported to be associated with PARK2 (3).

PARK6

PARK6 is a rare autosomal recessive form of PD and accounts for 2-8% of familial PD. Affected patients typically present with an early-onset, slowly progressive form of PD. They respond well to L-dopa therapy; however, dyskinesia and/or motor fluctuations are common side effects. STN-DBS is efficacious. They sometimes manifest with depression, anxiety, hyperreflexia, and orthostatic hypotension during the course of their illness. Routine brain MRI is usually normal. ^{18}F-dopa PET, ^{123}I-fluoropropylcarbomethoxyiodophenylnortropane (^{18}I-FP-CIT) PET,

^{11}C-CFT PET, and ^{123}I-iodobenzamide (IBZM) single-photon emission computed tomography (SPECT) show reduced radiotracer uptake in the striatum, especially in the putamen.

PARK6 is caused by mutations in the *PINK1* gene, encoding phosphatase and tensin homolog-induced putative kinase 1 (PINK1), which is a protein that is expressed in mitochondria. PINK1 is associated with neuroprotection against mitochondrial dysfunction and proteasome-induced apoptosis. To date, more than 25 pathogenic *PINK1* mutations have been reported to be associated with PARK6 (3).

PARK7

PARK7 is an extremely rare autosomal recessive form of PD that accounts for 1-2% of familial PD. Affected patients typically present with an early-onset, slowly progressive form of PD. They respond well to L-dopa therapy. The majority of patients manifest with blepharospasm, leg dystonia, and psychiatric symptoms in the early stage of their illness. Routine brain MRI is usually normal. ^{18}I-FP-CIT PET in an affected patient showed reduced radiotracer uptake in the striatum (8).

PARK7 is caused by mutations in the *DJ-1* gene, encoding DJ-1, which is a protein that is highly expressed in both neuronal and glial cells in the brain, including basal ganglia and substantia nigra. DJ-1 is associated with the modulation of transcription, chaperone-like functions, and maintenance of mitochondrial integrity. To date, more than five pathogenic *DJ-1* mutations have been reported to be associated with PARK7.

PARK8

PARK8 is the most common form of autosomal dominant PD, and it is the most common genetic form of PD identified so far. It accounts for 1-2% of sporadic PD and 5-10% of familial PD. Affected patients typically present with a late-onset, slowly progressive form of PD. They respond well to L-dopa therapy. STN-DBS is efficacious. The majority of patients develop psychiatric symptoms such as depression, anxiety, and hallucination. They also sometimes manifest with cognitive impairment, dysautonomia, sleep problems, and anosmia during the course of their illness. Routine brain MRI is usually normal. ^{18}F-dopa PET shows reduced radiotracer uptake in the striatum, especially in the putamen.

PARK8 is caused by mutations in the *LRRK2* gene, encoding leucine-rich repeat kinase 2 (LRRK2), which is a protein that is widely expressed in human tissue, including the cerebral cortex and spinal cord (9). LRRK2 is thought to be associated with signaling cascades and cytoskeletal dyanimics. To date, seven pathogenic LRRK2 mutations, N1437H, R1441C, R1441G, R1441H, Y1699C, G2019S, and I2020T, have been reported to be associated with PARK8 (3).

PARK17

PARK17 is an extremely rare form of autosomal dominant PD. It accounts for up to 0.3 % of sporadic PD and up to 2% of familial PD. Affected patients typically present with tremor-dominant PD. They respond well to L-dopa therapy. They may also manifest with cognitive impairment and psychiatric symptoms during the course of their illness. Routine brain MRI is usually normal. ^{18}F-dopa PET in an affected patient showed asymmetrically reduced radiotracer uptake in the striatum, especially in the posterior putamen (10).

PARK17 is caused by mutations in the *VPS35* gene. *VPS35* encodes vacuolar protein sorting 35 homolog (VPS35), which is a protein that is ubiquitously expressed in the central nervous system (CNS) (9). VPS35 is associated with the transportation of proteins between the endosomes and the trans-Golgi network. To date, at least one pathogenic VPS35 mutation, D620N, has been reported (11).

PARK18

PARK18 is an extremely rare, autosomal dominant form of PD, which accounts for up to 0.2% of familial PD. Affected patients typically present with late-onset PD. They respond well to L-dopa therapy. They may also manifest with cognitive impairment during the course of their illness.

PARK18 is caused by mutations in the *EIF4G1* gene. *EIF4G1* encodes eukaryotic translation initiation factor 4 gamma, 1 (EIF4G1), a protein that is ubiquitously expressed in the CNS (9). EIF4G1 is associated with the regulation of translation of proteins involved in growth control, stress response, and bioenergetics. To date, at least one pathogenic *EIF4G1* mutation, R1205H, has been reported (12).

Familial disorders predominantly presenting with cognitive impairment accompanied by parkinsonism (Table 16.2)

Alzheimer's Disease (AD)

AD is the most common neurodegenerative disorder. Its prevalence is estimated to be approximately 1,200/100,000 in the population aged 65 or older. More than 95% of AD patients develop symptoms after the age 65 years (late-onset AD), while less than 5% develop symptoms before the age 65 years (early-onset AD; EOAD). About 25-40% of all AD patients and approximately 60% of EOAD patients have a positive family history of the disease. So far, 17 genes/loci, AD1-AD17, have been identified. Among them, AD1, AD3, and AD4 have been reported to be associated with parkinsonism. All three forms are EOAD. Affected patients with these genetic forms of EOAD typically present with an early-onset, slowly progressive form of AD, which is indistinguishable from late-onset AD. A subset of patients manifest with pyramidal signs, myoclonus, and parkinsonism during the course of their illness. Routine brain MRI usually shows gross atrophy of the brain, including the hippocampus. Low levels of beta-amyloid and elevated levels of tau in the cerebrospinal fluid (CSF) can be useful diagnostic tools. In this subsection, we discuss parkinsonism and the genetics related to these three EOAD genes.

Alzheimer Disease 1 (AD1)

AD1 is a rare EOAD, which is inherited in either an autosomal dominant or an autosomal recessive manner, and accounts for 10-15% of familial EOAD. So far, one patient in a large African-American family carrying an APP T714I mutation has developed parkinsonism during the course of his illness (13). The patient initially presented with memory problems, followed by parkinsonism, myoclonic jerking, spasticity, seizure, and behavioural problems such as aggressiveness and emotional lability. The parkinsonism that was seen in this patient included bradykinesia, rigidity, tremor, and stooped posture. L-dopa responsiveness was not reported. Another AD1 patient carrying an APP T714A mutation was described in an Iranian family. This patient evidenced a slow and wide-based gait with stooped posture and short strides during the course of the illness; however, it was not clear whether the symptom was really parkinsonism (14).

AD1 is caused by mutations in the *APP* gene, encoding the amyloid precursor protein (APP), which is a protein that is ubiquitously expressed in the CNS, especially in the cerebral cortex, thalamus, hypothalamus, and amygdala (9). APP is thought to be associated with neurite growth, axonogenesis, cell mobility, and transcription regulation. To date, more than 30 pathogenic *APP* mutations, including duplications, are associated with AD1 (15).

Alzheimer Disease 3 (AD3)

AD3 is a relatively common, autosomal dominant EOAD, and accounts for 20-70% of familial EOAD. A minority of patients develop parkinsonism during the course of their illness. The parkinsonism that is seen in AD3 patients includes rigidity and/or bradykinesia. A Japanese patient was reported to respond well to L-dopa therapy.

AD3 is caused by mutations in the *PSEN1* gene, encoding presenilin-1 (PSEN1), which is a protein that is ubiquitously expressed in the CNS,

especially in the cerebral cortex, thalamus, hypothalamus, caudate nucleus, and amygdala (9). PSEN1 is thought to be associated with intracellular signaling, gene expression, and amyloid precursor protein processing. To date, more than 180 pathogenic *PSEN1* mutations have been reported to be associated with AD3 (15).

Alzheimer Disease 4 (AD4)

AD4 is an extremely rare, autosomal dominant EOAD, and accounts for less than 5% of familial EOAD. So far, three patients in a Sardinian family have developed parkinsonism during the course of their illness (16). The parkinsonism that is seen in AD4 patients includes bradykinesia, rigidity, postural instabilities, and resting tremor. L-dopa responsiveness was not reported.

AD4 is caused by mutations in the *PSEN2* gene. *PSEN2* encodes presenilin-2 (PSEN2), which is a protein that is ubiquitously expressed in the CNS, especially in the cerebral cortex, thalamus, hypothalamus, caudate nucleus, and amygdala (9). PSEN2 is thought to be associated with intracellular signaling, gene expression, and amyloid precursor protein processing. To date, more than 10 pathogenic *PSEN2* mutations have been reported to be associated with AD4 (15).

Adult-onset Leukoencephalopathy with Axonal Spheroids and Pigmented Glia (ALSP)

ALSP is a rare, autosomal dominant, demyelinating disorder. It encompasses two distinct forms, hereditary diffuse leukoencephalopathy with spheroids (HDLS) and pigmented orthochromatic leukodystrophy (POLD). The initial symptom of affected patients is typically cognitive impairment or psychiatric symptoms. Parkinsonism, pyramidal signs, dysarthria, sleep problems, oculomotor abnormalities, urinary incontinence, etc. follow the initial symptoms. Almost all patients manifest with parkinsonism during the course of their illness, sometimes as an initial symptom. The parkinsonism that is seen in ALSP patients is characterized as the akinetic-rigid type and is rarely accompanied by

Table 16.2
Familial disorders presenting with cognitive impairment accompanied by parkinsonism.

	Gene	TAAO	Clinical features	L-dopa responsiveness	Genetic tests availability
AD1	*APP*	40th-50th	**CI**, Psy, LP, Pyr, seizure, cerebral hemorrhage, myoclonus (P)	Unknown	I, II, III, IV, V
AD3	*PSEN1*	30th-50th	**CI, myoclonus**, Psy, seizures, LP, Pyr, P (dysautonomia)	Good[†]	I, II, III, IV, V
AD4	*PSEN2*	40th-50th	**CI**, Psy, LP, seizure, myoclonus (P)	Unknown	I, V
ALSP	*CSF1R*	40th-50th	**CI, Psy, P, Pyr, dysarthria, sleep problems, OMA, UI**, dystonia, myoclonus, chorea, CA, seizure	Minimal-none	I, V
CADASIL	*NOTCH3*	40th-60th	**Recurrent stroke**, migraine, CI, Psy, Pyr, P	None	I, II, III, IV, V
FTDP-17MAPT	*MAPT*	40th-60th	**BP, PC, LP, CI**, P, Pyr, CBS, PSP, dystonia, UI, anosmia, dysphagia, sleep problems, OMA (myoclonus, PN, seizure)	Minimal-none	I, II, IV, V
FTDP-17PGRN	*PGRN*	50th-60th	**BP, LP, CI, P**, Pyr, Psy, dysphagia (MND, myoclonus, seizure)	Minimal-none	I, IV, V
FTD-3	*CHMP2B*	40th-60th	**PC, BP, CI, Psy**, LP, Pyr, P, dystonia, sleep problems, MND, OMA, myoclonus, UI,T (seizure)	Unknown	I
Kufor-Rakeb syndrome	*ATP13A2*	10th-20th	**P, CI, Pyr, OMA**, Psy, myoclonus, ptosis, T, dystonia, (CA, PN, seizure)	Good-minimal	I, IV, V
Parkinsonism/MELAS overlap syndrome	*MTCYB*	10th-20th	Migraine, hemiparesis, homonymous hemianopia, seizure, myoclonus ataxia, CI, P	Unknown	I, II, III, V
MECP2-related disorders, (classic Rett syndrome)	*MECP2*	Early childhood	**BP, DD, hand stereotypies, gait apraxia, loss of hand skills, seizure, kyphoscoliosis, bruxism, dystonia,** LP, dysautonomia, microcephaly, autistic features, P, myoclonus, T, respiratory abnormalities, CA, Psy, dysphagia	None	I, II, III, IV, V
MECP2-related disorders, (MRX)		Early childhood	**MR, Pyr, Psy, BP, T**, P, distal muscle atrophy, minor facial anomalies, LP, kyphosis, flat occiput, high-arched palate, pes cavus, CA, dysarthria, seizure	Unknown	

resting tremor. Patients respond poorly or not at all to L-dopa therapy. Routine brain MRI shows frontal lobe predominant, bilateral, and patchy white matter hyperintensities on T2-weighted image (T2WI) with deep and subcortical involvement. Atrophy and signal changes in the corpus callosum are very characteristic, but not pathognomonic.

ALSP is caused by mutations in the *CSF1R* gene, encoding colony-stimulating factor 1 recep-

Table 16.2

AD = Alzheimer's disease; ALSP = adult-onset leukoencephalopathy with axonal spheroids and pigmented glia; APP = amyloid beta precursor protein; *ATP13A2* = ATPase type 13A2; BP = behavioural problems; CA = cerebellar ataxia; CADASIL = cerebral arteriopathy with subcortical infarcts and leukoencephalopathy; CBS = corticobasal syndrome; *CHMP2B* = charged multivesicular body protein 2B; CI = cognitive impairment; *CSF1R* = colony-stimulating factor 1 receptor; DD = developmental delay; FTD-3 = frontotemporal dementia, chromosome 3-linked; FTDP-17*MAPT* = frontotemporal dementia and parkinsonism linked to chromosome 17 associated with *MAPT* mutations; FTDP-17*PGRN* = frontotemporal dementia and parkinsonism linked to chromosome 17 associated with *PGRN* mutations; LP = language problems; *MAPT* = microtubule-associated protein tau; *MECP2* = methyl-CpG-binding protein 2; MELAS = mitochondrial myopathy, encephalopathy, lactic acidosis, and stroke-like episodes; MND = motor neuron disease; MR = mental retardation; MRX = X-linked mental retardation; *MTCYB* = cytochrome b of complex III; NOTCH3 = notch homolog 3; OMA = oculomotor abnormalities; P = parkinsonism; PC = personality changes; PGRN = progranulin; PN = peripheral neuropathy; *PSEN* = presenilin; PSP = progressive supranuclear palsy; Psy = psychiatric symptoms; Pyr = pyramidal signs; T = tremor; TAAO = typical age at onset; UI = urinary incontinence; I = sequence analysis of the entire coding region is available; II = sequence analysis of select exons is available; III = targeted mutation analysis is available; IV = deletion/duplication analysis is available; V = prenatal diagnosis is available; † = only one patient has been reported; clinical features in bold are frequently seen in patients (>50% of patients); clinical features in parentheses are occasionally seen in patients (<10% of patients).

tor (CSF1R), which is a protein that is highly expressed in microglia found in the CNS (17). CSF1R is associated with the survival, proliferation, differentiation, and function of mononuclear phagocytic cells in the CNS (18). To date, 21 *CSF1R* mutations and variants have been reported to be associated with ALSP (19).

Cerebral Autosomal Dominant Arteriopathy with Subcortical Infarcts and Leukoencephalopathy (CADASIL)

CADASIL is a rare, autosomal dominant, small-vessel disease. The prevalence is estimated to be approximately 2/100,000 in the general population. Affected patients typically present with recurrent subcortical strokes and transient ischemic attacks, migraine, cognitive impairment, and psychiatric symptoms, such as depression and progressive personal neglect. Pyramidal signs and urinary incontinence are eventually seen. Parkinsonism is occasionally seen in the late stages of the illness. It is usually symmetrical and characterized as akinetic-rigid type. Patients do not respond to L-dopa therapy. Routine brain MRI shows diffuse white matter hyperintensities on T2WI, especially in the temporal lobe and external capsule.

CADASIL is caused by mutations in the *NOTCH3* gene, encoding notch homolog 3 (NOTCH 3), which is a protein that is predominantly expressed in vascular smooth muscle cells. NOTCH3 is associated with the function and survival of vascular smooth muscle cells. To date, more than 220 *NOTCH3* mutations and variants have been reported to be associated with CADASIL (19).

Frontotemporal Dementia (FTD)

FTD is a clinical umbrella term that includes disorders caused by progressive degeneration of the frontal and temporal lobes of the brain. FTD is the second most common early-onset dementia. The prevalence is estimated to be 3-15/100,000 in the population aged 45-64 years. FTD is clinically characterized by progressive personality and behavioural changes, as well as deficits in executive and language functions. Memory problems are not prominent during the early stages of the illness. Approximately 30-40% of FTD patients have a family history of the disease. So far, three genes, the microtubule-associated protein (*MAPT*), progranulin (*PGRN*), and charged multivesicular body protein 2B (*CHMP2B*), have been reported to be associated with the FTD phenotype. Parkinsonism has been described in all three genetic forms as related to these genes. These three genetic forms are discussed in more detail below.

Frontotemporal Dementia and Parkinsonism Linked to Chromosome 17 Associated with MAPT Mutations (FTDP-17MAPT)

FTDP-17MAPT is a rare, autosomal dominant, rapidly progressive, neurodegenerative disorder, which accounts for 5-14% of all FTD and 10-32% of familial FTD. Affected patients typically present with behavioural problems, which are characterized by disinhibition as an initial symptom. They also exhibit personality changes and language dysfunctions in the early stages of their illness. They usually manifest cognitive impairments, parkinsonism, and pyramidal signs in the later stages of their illness. However, cognitive impairments or parkinsonism can be a prominent, and even an initial feature in a subset of patients. The parkinsonism seen in FT-DP-17MAPT patients is characterized as akinetic-rigid type and is sometimes accompanied by resting tremor. Patients may develop asymmetrical rigidity, which is suggestive of corticobasal syndrome (CBS) (see Chapter 21), or eye movement abnormalities, which is suggestive of progressive supranuclear palsy (PSP) (see Chapter 20). Some may partially respond to L-dopa therapy, though most patients do not. Routine brain MRI usually shows frontal and/or temporal lobe atrophy. ^{18}F-dopa PET of parkinsonian patients shows asymmetrically reduced radiotracer uptake in the striatum.

FTDP-17MAPT is caused by mutations in the *MAPT* gene, encoding microtubule-associated protein (MAPT), which is ubiquitously expressed in the CNS, especially in the cerebral cortex, globus pallidus, hypothalamus, amygdala, and cerebellar peduncle (9). MAPT is associated with microtubule assembly, stabilization, neuronal morphogenesis, and axonal transport. To date, more than 40 pathogenic *MAPT* mutations have been reported to be associated with FTD (15). *MAPT* mutations have also been identified in clinically diagnosed PSP, PD, corticobasal degeneration (CBD), AD, and Pick disease cases.

Frontotemporal Dementia and Parkinsonism Linked to Chromosome 17 Associated with PGRN Mutations (FTDP-17PGRN)

FTDP-17PGRN is a rare, autosomal dominant, rapidly progressive, neurodegenerative disorder, which accounts for 5-10% of all FTD and approximately 13-25% of familial FTD. Affected patients typically present with behavioural problems that are characterized by apathy or social withdrawal as the initial and most prominent feature. They usually manifest with language problems, cognitive impairments, parkinsonism, and pyramidal signs, and psychiatric symptoms during the course of their illness. The majority of patients develop parkinsonism, which is typically characterized as the symmetrical akinetic-rigid type and is rarely accompanied by resting tremor. The parkinsonism that is seen in FTDP-17PGRN patients sometimes resembles that seen in CBD patients. Some patients may partially respond to L-dopa therapy, though most do not. Routine brain MRI shows asymmetrical frontal anterior temporal and/or parietal lobe atrophy.

FTDP-17PGRN is caused by *PGRN* mutations. *PGRN* encodes progranulin, which is a protein that is ubiquitously expressed in the CNS (9). Progranulin is associated with multiple cellular processes such as development, wound repair, and inflammation. To date, more than 60 pathogenic *PGRN* mutations and variants have been reported to be associated with FTD (15).

Frontotemporal Dementia linked to Chromosome 3 (FTD-3)

FTD-3 is an extremely rare, autosomal dominant, slowly progressive, neurodegenerative disorder. Its prevalence has not been well investigated. Affected patients typically present with personality changes, which are characterized by disinhibition and social withdrawal as the initial and most prominent feature. They usually manifest with behavioural problems, cognitive impairment including dyscalculia, depression, language problems, pyramidal signs, parkinsonism, and dystonia during the course of their illness. A minority of patients develop parkinsonism, which is characterized as the asymmetrical akinetic-rigid type and occurs a few years after symptomatic disease onset. L-dopa responsiveness has not been reported. Routine brain MRI shows general cerebral atrophy.

FTD-3 is caused by *CHMP2B* mutations. *CHMP2B* encodes charged multivesicular body protein 2B (CHMP2B), which is a protein that is predominantly expressed in the hypothalamus, amygdala, hippocampus, and spinal cord (9). CHMP2B is associated with the survival of neurons. To date, four pathogenic *CHMP2B* mutations have been reported to be associated with FTD-3 (15).

Kufor-Rakeb syndrome (KRS)

KRS, also known as PARK9, is an extremely rare, autosomal recessive, neurodegenerative disorder. Its prevalence has not been well investigated. Affected patients typically present with parkinsonism, followed by cognitive impairment and pyramidal signs in the first decade of life. They also develop supranuclear palsy, visual hallucination, myoclonus, and ptosis. The parkinsonism that is seen in KRS patients is characterized as akinetic-rigid type and is sometimes accompanied by resting tremor. Most patients respond well to L-dopa therapy. Routine brain MRI demonstrates bilaterally diffuse cerebral atrophy. ^{123}I-FP-CIT SPECT of parkinsonian patients shows reduced dopamine transporter uptake in the bilateral striatum, especially in the putamen.

KRS is caused by mutations in the *ATP13A2* gene, encoding ATPase type 13A2 (ATP13A2), which is a protein that is ubiquitously expressed in the CNS, especially in the cerebral cortex, thalamus, hypothalamus, and amygdala. ATP13A2 is thought to be associated with intracellular cation homeostasis and the maintenance of neuronal integrity. To date, five *ATP13A2* muta-

tions have been reported to be associated with KRS (19). ATP13A2 mutations have also been identified in patients with PD and parkinsonism with or without dementia.

Parkinsonism/MELAS overlap syndrome

Parkinsonism/MELAS (mitochondrial myopathy, encephalopathy, lactic acidosis and stroke-like episodes) overlap syndrome is an extremely rare mitochondrial disorder. So far, only one male patient with a 4-base pair deletion in the mitochondrial cytochrome b (MTCYB) gene has been reported (20). He presented with fine motor coordination and concentration difficulties at the age of 6 years, and gradually developed language and behavioural problems and psychiatric symptoms. Neurological examination at 14 years of age showed parkinsonism including hypomimia, resting tremor, rigidity, and reduced arm swing during walking, as well as myoclonus and pyramidal signs. At 15 years, he exhibited akinetic-rigid syndrome. He has also experienced several seizures. L-dopa responsiveness was not reported. Brain MRI of the patient showed diffuse brain atrophy and focal cerebral infarctions.

Parkinsonism/MELAS overlap syndrome is caused by mutations in the *MTCYB* gene, encoding cytochrome b, a protein that is expressed in the brain. Cytochrome b is associated with the generation of electrochemical potential coupled to ATP synthesis.

MECP2-related disorders

Since mutations in the methyl-cytosine–guanine-binding protein (*MECP2)* gene were discovered to be the cause of Rett syndrome, approximately 15 different clinical phenotypes have been reported. The prevalence has not been well investigated. Classic Rett syndrome (classic RTT) and X-linked mental retardation (MRX) have been associated with parkinsonism. Both classic RTT and MRX are caused by mutations in the *MECP2* gene, encoding methyl-CpG-binding protein 2 (MECP2), a protein that is ubiquitously expressed in the CNS, especially in the cerebral cortex and cerebellar peduncle. MECP2 is associated with chromatin remodeling and the modulation of RNA splicing. We discuss the clinical features and genetics related to classic RTT and MRX in this subsection.

Classic Rett syndrome (Classic RTT)

Classic RTT is a rare, X-linked, neurodevelopmental disorder. The incidence is estimated to be approximately 1/10,000 female births. The disorder occasionally affects males. Affected patients typically present with subtle behavioural problems as an initial symptom. They lose their motor abilities and develop language problems, and dysautonomia during the course of their illness. They eventually manifest with microcephaly, psychomotor developmental delay, hand stereotypes, mental retardation, and autistic features. More than 40% of classic RTT patients have parkinsonism in their 20's. Parkinsonism seen in classic RTT patients is characterized as akinetic-rigid type. Patients do not respond to L-dopa therapy. Brain MRI is usually normal. To date, 596 MECP mutations and variants have been reported to be associated with classic Rett syndrome (19).

X-linked mental retardation (MRX)

MRX, also known as 'primarily severe neonatal encephalopathy and manic-depressive psychosis, pyramidal signs, parkinsonism, and macroorchidism (PPM-X syndrome)', is a relatively common, X-linked, neurodevelopmental disorder. The incidence is estimated to be 1-2/600 male births. Affected females show mild intellectual impairment, while affected males present with psychomotor developmental delay in the early stages of the illness. Patients develop mental retardation, pyramidal signs, psychiatric symptoms, behavioural problems, and tremor during the course of their illness. A minority of patients manifest with parkinsonism, characterized by rigidity and resting tremor. Responsiveness to L-dopa therapy has not been noted. Routine brain MRI is usually normal. To date,

48 MECP2 mutations and variants have been reported to be associated with MRX (19).

Familial disorders presenting with motor neuron disease or muscle disease accompanied by parkinsonism
(Table 16.3)

Alexander Disease (AxD)

AxD is a rare, autosomal dominant, slowly progressive, neurodegenerative disorder that mainly affects glial cells. Its prevalence has not been well investigated. It can be classified into three different forms based on the age at symptomatic disease onset: infantile onset (50%), juvenile onset (25%), and adult onset (25%). So far, parkinsonism has been described only in adult-onset AxD (AOAxD). AOAxD patients clinically present with a variety of symptoms, including pyramidal signs, bulbar signs, cerebellar ataxia, urinary incontinence, and oculomotor abnormalities. So far, five AOAxD patients have developed parkinsonism during the course of their illness (21-24). The parkinsonism in the patients is clinically characterized by bradykinesia and/or rigidity. L-dopa responsiveness was not reported. Brain MRI usually shows a combination of extensive frontal lobe-predominant white matter changes, a periventricular rim, abnormalities of the basal ganglia, thalamus, and brain stem. There is also the presence of contrast enhancement of gray and white matter structures.

AxD is caused by mutations in the GFAP gene, encoding glial fibrillary acidic protein (GFAP), which is abundantly expressed in the CNS, especially in the cerebral cortex, olfactory bulb, thalamus, hypothalamus, caudate nucleus, amygdala, and cerebellum peduncles (9). The precise function of GFAP is not well understood. To date, 95 GFAP mutations and variants have been reported to be associated with AxD (19).

Amyotrophic Lateral Sclerosis (ALS)

ALS is a rapidly progressive neurodegenerative disorder that affects upper and lower mo-

Table 16.3
List of familial disorders presenting with motor neuron disease or muscle disease accompanied by parkinsonism.

	Gene	TAAO	Clinical features other than parkinsonism	L-dopa responsiveness	Genetic tests availability
Adult-onset Alexander disease	GFAP	30th-50th	**Pyr, dysarthria, dysphagia, CA, UI, OMA**, scoliosis, CI, dysautonomia, myoclonus, sleep problems (P, seizure)	Unknown	I, V
ALS6	FUS	40th-50th	**LMN/UMN/bulbar signs**, FTD (P)	Unknown	I, II, IV, V
ALS9	ANG	30th-60th	**LMN/UMN/bulbar signs** (FTD, P)	Unknown	I, IV, V
ALS10	TARDBP	40th-60th	**LMN/UMN/bulbar signs**, FTD, P	Good	I, II, IV, V
ALS14	VCP	20th-40th	**Myopathy, PDB**, FTD, LP, cardiomyopathy (cataracts, deafness, MND, P, PN, Pyr)	Unknown	I, V
Spastic paraplegia 10	KIF5A	Childhood-20th	**Pyr**, MR, PN, deafness, retinitis, UI, scoliosis, pes cavus	Good	I, V
Spastic paraplegia 11	KIAA0196	10th-20th	**Pyr, PN**, MR, dystonia, OMA, maculopathy (CA, MND, P)	Good-minimal	I, V
9p-linked FTD/ALS	C9orf72	50th-60th	**MND, FTD**, P, Psy, CI, CBS	Minimal-none	III, V
X-linked parkinsonism with spasticity	ATP6AP2	10th-50th	**Pyr**, seizure, CI, P	Minimal-none	I, IV, V

ALS = amyotrophic lateral sclerosis; ANG = angiogenin; ATP6AP2 = ATPase, H+ transporting, lysosomal accessory protein 2; C9orf72 = chromosome 9 open reading frame 72; CA = cerebellar ataxia; CBS = corticobasal syndrome; CI = cognitive impairment; FTD = frontotemporal dementia; FUS = fused in sarcoma; GFAP = glial fibrillary acidic protein; KIF5A = kinesin family member 5A; LMN = lower motor neuron; LP = language problems; MND = motor neuron disease; MR = mental retardation; OMA = oculomotor abnormalities; P = parkinsonism; PDB = Paget disease of bone; PN = peripheral neuropathy; Psy = psychiatric symptoms; Pyr = pyramidal signs; TAAO = typical age at onset; TARDBP = TAR DNA-binding protein; UI = urinary incontinence; UMN = upper motor neuron; VCP = valosin-containing protein; I = sequence analysis of the entire coding region is available; II = sequence analysis of select exons is available; III = targeted mutation analysis is available; IV = deletion/duplication analysis is available; V = prenatal diagnosis is available; clinical features in bold are frequently seen in patients (>50% of patients); clinical features in parentheses are occasionally seen in patients (<10% of patients).

tor neurons. Its prevalence is estimated to be up to 8/100,000 in the general population. Approximately 10% of ALS patients have a family history of the disease. ALS is clinically characterized by rapidly progressive upper motor neuron signs, lower motor neuron signs, and bulbar signs. Routine brain MRI may show frontal and/or temporal atrophy. So far, 18 genes/loci, ALS1-ALS18, have been identified. Among them, ALS6, ALS9, ALS10, ALS14, and ALS17 have been reported to be associated with parkinsonism. We discuss parkinsonism and the genetics related to these genes in this subsection.

Amyotrophic Lateral Sclerosis 6 (ALS6)

ALS6 is a rare inherited disorder, with an unclear mode of inheritance. ALS6 accounts for approximately 5% of familial ALS. So far, two patients have been reported to have developed parkinsonism during the course of their illness. One of them presented with rigidity accompanied by FTD (25). The other patient manifested with parkinsonism accompanied by dementia. However, details about parkinsonian symptomatology including L-dopa responsiveness were not reported (26). Routine brain MRI is usually normal.

ALS6 is caused by mutations in the *FUS* gene, encoding fused in sarcoma (FUS), which is a protein that is abundantly expressed in the CNS (9). FUS is associated with regulation of transcription and alternative splicing. To date, 67 *FUS* mutations and variants have been reported to be associated with ALS (65) and FTD (2) (19). *FUS* mutations have also been identified in patients with FTD.

Amyotrophic Lateral Sclerosis 9 (ALS9)

ALS9 is a rare, autosomal dominant disorder. It accounts for less than 2% of familial ALS. So far, only one ALS9 patient, carrying a K17I mutation, developed parkinsonism (27). The patient presented with akinetic-rigid type of parkinsonism as an initial symptom, followed by FTD without the ALS phenotype. L-dopa responsiveness of the patient was not described.

ALS9 is caused by mutations in the (*ANG*) gene. *ANG* encodes a protein named 'angiogenin (ANG),' which is ubiquitously expressed in the CNS (9). *ANG* is associated with angiogenesis by stimulating the growth and division of endothelial cells. Approximately 28 *ANG* mutations and variants have been reported to be associated with ALS (19). A strong association has been found between *ANG* mutations and PD (28).

Amyotrophic Lateral Sclerosis 10 (ALS10)

ALS10 is a rare, autosomal dominant disorder. It accounts for approximately 5% of familial ALS. So far, about 10 ALS10 patients have developed parkinsonism (29-32). They present with either a typical PD phenotype or a combination of parkinsonism and ALS and/or FTD. The parkinsonism that is seen in ALS10 patients is characterized as a mixed type. Patients respond well to L-dopa therapy.

ALS10 is caused by mutations in the *TARDBP* gene, encoding transactive response DNA-binding protein 43 kDa (TDP-43), which is ubiquitously expressed in the CNS (9). TDP-43 is associated with the regulation of transcription, RNA stability, and alternative splicing. To date, 56 *TARDBP* mutations and variants have been reported to be associated with ALS (50) and FTD (6) (19). *TARDBP* mutations and variants have also been identified in FTD and PD patients (N267S and A382T) (31, 32).

Inclusion body myopathy related to Paget disease of bone (IBMPDB) and/or frontotemporal dementia (IBMPFD)

IBMPFD is a rare, autosomal dominant disorder. Its prevalence has not been well investigated. Affected patients present with proximal and distal myopathy (90%), early onset PDB (50%), and FTD (30%). So far, four IBMPFD patients have developed parkinsonism (33). They presented with either mixed-type or akinetic-rigid-type parkinsonism, with a combination of myopathy, FTD, and motor neuron disease. Responsiveness to L-dopa therapy has not been reported. Elevated serum creatinine phosphokinase and alkaline phosphatase as well as elevated urine pyridinoline and deoxypyridinoline can be useful diagnostic tools. Routine brain MRI is usually normal.

IBMPFD is caused by mutations in the *VCP* genes, encoding valosin-containing protein (VCP), which is ubiquitously expressed in the CNS (9). VCP is associated with a variety of cellular pathways, such as nuclear envelope reconstruction, apoptosis, post-mitotic Golgi reassembly, and repairing damaged DNA. To date, 23 *VCP* mutations and variants have been reported to be associated with IBMPFD (19). *VCP* mutations have been also identified in patients with ALS and AD.

Hereditary Spastic Paraplegia (HSP)

HSP encompasses clinically and genetically heterogeneous neurodegenerative disorders. Its prevalence is estimated to be up to approximately 10/100,000 in the general population. It can be classified into two different forms based on clinical phenotypes: pure form and complex form. Patients with pure-form HSP show upper motor neuron signs, where patients with complex-form HSP develop additional clinical features such as seizures, cognitive impairment, psychiatric symptoms, dystonia, extrapyramidal signs, peripheral neuropathy, hearing loss, cerebellar signs, dysphagia, hydrocephalus, and dysmorphic features. So far, 48 gene/loci have been identified as associated with HSP (19). Parkinsonism has been described in patients with SPG10 and SPG11. In this subsection, we discuss the clinical features and the genetics related to these two genes.

Spastic Paraplegia 10 (SPG10)

SPG10 is a rare form of autosomal dominant HSP, and it accounts for up to approximately 9% of all HSP. Affected patients present with either pure or complex form. Spasticity, mental retardation, extrapyramidal signs, peripheral polyneuropathy, deafness, and retinitis clinically characterize the complex HSP form that is seen in SPG10 patients. So far, two SPG10 patients carrying different KIF5A mutations, Y63C and M198T, have developed parkinsonism, and it was accompanied by other features of the complex-form HSP (34). The parkinsonism that is seen in these patients included bradykinesia, rigidity, postural instability, and resting tremor. They responded well to L-dopa therapy, but developed dyskinesias shortly after initiation of the therapy. Another patient was described with limb rigidity accompanied by upper motor neuron signs; however, it is uncertain if this patient had parkinsonism (73). Routine brain MRI shows white matter changes.

SPG10 is caused by mutations in the KIF5A gene. KIF5A encodes kinesin heavy chain, which is a protein that is ubiquitously expressed in the CNS (9). Kinesin heavy chains are associated with anterograde axonal transport. To date, 21 KIF5A mutations and variants have been reported to be associated with SPG10 (19).

Spastic Paraplegia 11 (SPG11)

SPG11 is the most common form of autosomal recessive HSP. It accounts for about 20% of all HSP. Its prevalence is estimated to be 1-10/100,000. Affected patients present with either the pure form or the complex form of HSP. The complex form that is seen in SPG11 patients is clinically characterized by spasticity, peripheral neuropathy, mental retardation, dystonia, and nystagmus. So far, four patients have developed parkinsonism, which was accompanied by other features of the complex form of HSP (35-37). The parkinsonism that is seen in SPG11 patients is characterized by resting tremor, bradykinesia, rigidity, and hypomimia. Responsiveness to L-dopa therapy is variable. Wearing-off phenomenon and peak-dose dyskinesias may appear shortly after initiation of L-dopa therapy (35). Routine brain MRI shows thinning of the corpus callosum and white matter abnormalities. ^{123}I-ioflupane SPECT of one of the parkinsonian patients showed reduced ^{123}I-ioflupane uptake in the striatum bilaterally, especially in the putamen (37).

SPG11 is caused by mutations in the KIAA0196 genes. KIAA0196 encodes spatacsin, which is a protein that is ubiquitously expressed in the cytoplasm of brain neurons, including those in the basal ganglia, and spinal cord. The precise function of spatacsin is still unknown. To date, three KIAA0196 mutations have been reported to be associated with SPG11 (19).

9p-linked Frontotemporal Dementia/ Amyotrophic Lateral Sclerosis (9p-Linked FTD/ALS)

9p-linked FTD/ALS is a common, autosomal dominant, neurodegenerative disorder. It accounts for up to 21% of sporadic ALS and up to

58% of familial ALS, as well as approximately 19% of sporadic FTD and about 12-26% of familial FTD. In ALS patients, bulbar-onset type (approximately 40%) is more frequently seen. Approximately a quarter of all patients have cognitive impairment. In FTD patients, the behavioural variant is the most common phenotype (70-80%). About 35% of patients present with parkinsonism, which is characterized as akinetic-rigid type. They do not respond to L-dopa therapy. Routine brain MRI shows prominent frontal lobe atrophy. 9p-linked FTD/ALS is caused by abnormal expansions of a noncoding GGGGCC hexanucleotide repeat (700-1600 repeats: normal repeats length is up to 30) in the *C9orf72* gene, encoding chromosome 9 open reading frame 72 (C9orf72), which is a protein expressed in the neuronal cytoplasm of the presynaptic terminals in the brain. The precise function of C9orf72 is unknown. Abnormal GGGGCC expansion in the *C9orf72* gene has also been identified in patients presenting with pure AD and CBS, but not in classic PD patients.

X-linked Parkinsonism with Spasticity (XPDS)

XPDS is an extremely rare, slowly progressive, X-linked disorder. So far, only one family has been reported (38). Affected patients typically present with pyramidal signs as an initial symptom, followed by seizure, cognitive impairment, and parkinsonism. Two patients were reported to manifest only with parkinsonism. The parkinsonism seen in XPDS patients is characterized by resting tremor, bradykinesia, and hypomimia. Routine brain MRI may show diffuse cerebral atrophy. Most patients do not respond to L-dopa therapy. F-dopa PET of a parkinsonian patient showed asymmetrically reduced radiotracer uptake in the putamen (38).

XPDS is caused by mutations in the *ATP6AP2* gene, encoding ATPase, H+ transporting, lysosomal accessory protein 2 (ATP6AP2), which is abundantly expressed in the CNS, especially in the cerebral cortex, thalamus, hypothalamus, amygdala, and medulla oblongata (9). ATP6AP2 is thought to be associated with a renin-dependent cellular response. To date, only one *ATP-6AP2* mutation has been reported to be associated with XPDS (19).

Familial disorders predominantly presenting with cerebellar ataxia accompanied by parkinsonism
(Table 16.4)

Fragile X Tremor/Ataxia Syndrome (FXTAS)

FXTAS is a late-onset, X-lined disorder. ItS is the most common inherited form of mental retardation, and its prevalence is estimated to be 19-33/100,000 in the general population. Affected females may have a mild FXTAS phenotype with or without cognitive impairment. Affected males typically present with progressive intention tremor, cerebellar ataxia, or both as an initial symptom. Patients may develop parkinsonism, cognitive impairment, psychiatric problems, autonomic dysfunction, and peripheral neuropathy at least five years after symptomatic disease onset. The parkinsonism seen in FXTAS patients is usually mild and characterized by resting tremor, rigidity, bradykinesia, postural instability, and hypomimia. The majority of patients respond to L-dopa therapy. Routine brain MRI shows white matter lesions in the middle cerebellar peduncles. ^{123}I-FP-CIT SPECT in three parkinsonian patients showed symmetrically reduced radiotracer uptake in the striatum. FXTAS is caused by abnormal CGG repeat expansion (55-200: normal repeat length is 5 44) in the *FMR1* gene. *FMR1* encodes fragile X mental retardation 1 (FMR1), which is a protein that is ubiquitously expressed in the CNS, especially in the cerebral cortex and amygdala (9). FMR1 is associated with regulation of translation. To date, three mutations have been reported to be associated with FXTAS (19). Abnormal CGG repeat expansion in the *FMR1* gene has also been identified in less than 1% of patients with PD or parkinsonism.

Table 16.4
List of familial disorders presenting with cerebellar ataxia accompanied by parkinsonism.

	Gene	TAAO	Clinical features other than parkinsonism	L-dopa responsive-ness	Genetic test avail-ability
Fragile X tremor/ataxia syndrome	FMR1	50th-60th	**T, CA**, P, CI, Psy, dysautonomia, BP, PN, seizure, dysphagia, hyposmia (OMA, UI)	Good-none	I, III, IV, V
Gerstmann-Straussler disease	PRNP	40th-50th	**CA, dysarthria, CI, Pyr**, PN, Psy, P, T, myoclonus (BP, seizure, deafness, loss of taste)	Moderate-minimal	I, III, V
SCA1	ATXN1	30th-40th	**CA, dysarthria, Pyr, hyporeflexia, OMA, amyotrophy, CI, dysphagia**, PN, dystonia (chorea, P)	Unknown	III, V
SCA2	ATXN2	20th-40th	**CA, OMA, hyporeflexia**, PN, T, P, dysphagia, CI, LMN signs, UI, RBD, myoclonus, dystonia (chorea, dysautonomia, infantile MND, spasm, optic atrophy, retinitis pigmentosa)	Good	III, V
SCA3	ATXN3	20th-50th	**CA, Pyr, OMA**, PN, P, dystonia, chorea (RBD, myokimia)	Good	III, V
SCA6	CACNA1A	40th-50th	**CA, dysarthria, OMA** (CI, dysautonomia, dystonia, myoclonus, P, PN, Pyr, Psy, RLS, T)	Good-none	III, V
SCA8	ATXN8	20th-40th	**CA, dysarthria**, CI, Pyr, PN, dysphagia, Psy, T (dystonia, hyporeflexia, MND, P)	None	III, V
SCA12	PPP2R2B	40th	**T, CA, dysarthria**, hyperreflexia, CI, PN, Psy, dystonia (myokimia, P, UI)	Unknown	III, V
SCA14	PRKCG	20th-40th	**CA, dysarthria, OMA, hyperreflexia, PN**, CI, Psy, T, myoclonus (chorea, dysphagia, dystonia, MR, myokimia, P, seizure)	Unknown	I, II, IV, V
SCA17	TBP	40th-50th	**CA, dysarthria, CI, dystonia, chorea**, Psy, Pyr, P, seizures	Good	III, V
SCA23	PDYN	10th 20th	**CA, dysarthria, OMA, Pyr, T, PN, CI**, ptosis (P)	Minimum-none	I
SCA28	AFG3L2	20th-50th	**CA, dysarthria, OMA**, ptosis, Pyr, dystonia (P)	Unknown	I, V

AFG3L2 = AFG3 ATPase family member 3-like 2; BP = behavioural problems; CA = cerebellar ataxia; CACNA1A = calcium channel, voltage-dependent, P/Q type, alpha-1A subunit; CI = cognitive impairment; FMR1 = fragile X mental retardation 1; LMN = lower motor neuron; MND = motor neuron disease; OMA = oculomotor abnormalities; P = parkinsonism; PDYN = prodynorphin; PN = peripheral neuropathy; PPP2R2B = brain-specific regulatory subunit of the protein phosphatase 2; PRKCG = protein kinase C, gamma; PRNP = prion protein; Psy = psychiatric symptoms; Pyr = pyramidal signs; RBD = rapid eye movement sleep behaviour disorder; RLS = restless legs syndrome; SCA = spinocerebellar ataxia; T = tremor; TAAO = typical age at onset; TBP = TATA box binding protein; UI = urinary incontinence; I = sequence analysis of the entire coding region is available; II = sequence analysis of select exons is available; III = targeted mutation analysis is available; IV = deletion/duplication analysis is available; V = prenatal diagnosis is available; clinical features in bold are frequently seen in patients (>50% of patients); clinical features in parentheses are occasionally seen in patients (<10% of patients).

Gerstmann-Straussler Disease (GSD)

GSS is a rare, autosomal dominant, slowly progressive, transmissible neurodegenerative disease. The prevalence is estimated to be 1-10/100,000,000 in the general population. Affected patients typically present with progressive cerebellar ataxia as an initial symptom. Patients develop cognitive impairment, pyramidal signs, lower motor neuron (LMN) signs in lower limbs, psychiatric symptoms, and parkinsonism during the course of their illness. Almost half of GSD patients manifest with parkinsonism, characterized by bradykinesia, rigidity, and hypomimia. Responsiveness to L-dopa therapy is variable. Routine brain MRI may show mild to moderate generalized atrophy as well as hypointensity of the basal ganglia on T2WI.

GSD is caused by mutations in the *PRNP* gene, encoding prion protein (PRNP), which is a protein that is abundantly expressed in the CNS, especially in the cerebral cortex, globus, pallidus, thalamus, hypothalamus, amygdala, and medulla oblongata (9). PRNP is thought to be associated with neuronal development and synaptic plasticity. To date, 16 *PRNP* mutations and variants have been reported to be associated with GSD (19). A *PRNP* mutation has been identified in patients of PD.

Autosomal Dominant Cerebellar Ataxia (ADCA)

ADCA is a clinically and genetically heterogeneous group of progressive, autosomal dominant, neurodegenerative disorders (see Chapters 33, 34). The prevalence is estimated to be 1-3/100,000 in the general population. So far, 36 genes/loci, spinocerebellar ataxia (SCA)1-SCA36, have been identified. Among them, SCA1, SCA2, SCA3, SCA6, SCA8, SCA12, SCA14, SCA17, SCA23, SCA28, and SCA36 have been reported to be associated with parkinsonism. In this subsection, we discuss the clinical features and the genetics related to these eleven genes.

Spinocerebellar Ataxia Type 1 (SCA1)

SCA1 is a rare disorder that accounts for approximately 6% of all ADCA. Its prevalence is estimated to be 1-2/100,000 in the general population. Affected patients typically present with progressive cerebellar ataxia, including limb ataxia and dysarthria, and pyramidal signs. They manifest wtih proprioceptive loss, hyporeflexia, eye movement abnormalities such as nystagmus, saccadic abnormalities, and ophthalmoplegia during the course of their illness. They eventually exibit manifest cognition impairment, amyotrophy, and severe dysphagia. Only a minority of patients develop parkinsonism (39). The parkinsonism seen in these patients is characterized by rigidity and/or bradykinesia that is accompanied by cerebellar signs and also frequently by orthostatic dysregulation. Responsiveness to L-dopa therapy has not been reported. Routine brain MRI shows atrophy of cerebellum and brainstem.

SCA1 is caused by abnormal CAG repeat (39-82; normal repeat length is 6-35) in the *ATXN1* gene, encoding ataxin-1, which is a protein that is widely expressed in the CNS, especially in Purkinje cells in the cerebellum. Ataxin-1 is thought to be associated with transcriptional repression.

Spinocerebellar Ataxia Type 2 (SCA2)

SCA2 is a relatively common disorder and accounts for approximately 15% of all ADCA. Affected patients typically present with progressive cerebellar ataxia, including gait ataxia and dysarthria, eye movement abnormalities, such as slowed saccades and nystagmus, hyporeflexia, and decreased vibration sense in the lower limbs. A minority of patients have intention tremor, parkinsonism, dysphagia, and cognitive impairment. Parkinsonism can be the most prominent or unique symptom in a subset of patients. The parkinsonism that is seen in SCA2 patients is characterized by symmetrical bradykinesia, resting tremor and rigidity, and less frequently by postural instability and freezing gait. Most of patients respond well to L-dopa therapy. Routine brain MRI shows olivoponto-cerebellar atrophy (OPCA) and spinal atrophy. ^{18}F-dopa PET of parkinsonian patients shows reduced radiotracer uptake in the bilateral striatum. ^{123}I-FP-CIT SPECT in both patients with parkinsonism and patients without parkinsonism showed symmetrically reduced radiotracer uptake in the striatum.

SCA2 is caused by an abnormal CAG repeat expansion (more than 32; normal repeat length is less than 31) in the *ATXN2* gene. *ATXN2* encodes ataxin 2 (ATXN2), which is a protein that is abundantly expressed in the CNS, especially in the cerebral cortex, olfactory bulb, hypothalamus, amygdala, and cerebellar peduncle (9). The precise function of ATXN2 is still unknown. Abnormal CAG expansion in the *ATXN2* gene has also been identified in up to 2% of sporadic PD patients and about 5% of autosomal dominant parkinsonism patients.

Spinocerebellar Ataxia Type 3 (SCA3)

SCA3, also known as Machado-Joseph disease, is a common disorder and accounts for approximately 21% of all ADCA. Affected patients typically present with slowly progressive cerebellar ataxia that is accompanied by pyramidal signs, peripheral neuropathy, and parkinsonism. Patients occasionally manifest with ophthalmoplegia, dystonia, and other symptoms. Up to 23% of patients develop parkinsonism. The parkinsonism that is seen in SCA3 patients is characterized as akinetic-rigid type and is occasionally accompanied by resting tremor. A subset of patients responds well to L-dopa therapy. Routine brain MRI shows mild OPCA. 99mTc-TRODAT-1 SPECT of parkinsonian patients shows reduced radiotracer uptake in the striatum bilaterally.

SCA3 is caused by an abnormal CAG repeat expansion (more than 52; normal repeat length is 13-41) in the *ATXN3* gene, encoding ataxin 3 (ATXN3), which is a protein expressed in the cytoplasm of many types of cells outside of the CNS. ATXN3 is associated with proteasomal degradation of ubiquitinated substrates. Abnor-

mal CAG expansion in the *ATXN3* gene was not identified in PD patients or patients with autosomal dominant parkinsonism.

Spinocerebellar Ataxia Type 6 (SCA6)

SCA6 is a common disorder and accounts for up to approximately 15% of all ADCA (40). Affected patients typically present with slowly progressive pure cerebellar ataxia, including truncal and limb ataxia, and dysarthria, as well as nystagmus. They occasionally manifest with cognitive impairment, dysautonomia, dystonia, myoclonus, and parkinsonism during the course of their illness. The parkinsonism that is seen in SCA6 patients is characterized as akinetic-rigid type. Most patients do not respond to L-dopa therapy. Routine brain MRI shows severe cerebellar atrophy accompanied by mild atrophy of the middle cerebellar peduncle, pons, and red nucleus. ^{18}F-dopa PET and 99mTc-TRODAT-1 SPECT of parkinsonian patients shows reduced radiotracer uptake in the bilateral striatum, especially in the putamen.

SCA6 is caused by an abnormal CAG repeat expansion (20-33; normal repeat length is 4-18) in the *CACNA1A* gene. *CACNA1A* encodes calcium channel, voltage-dependent, P/Q type, alpha-1A subunit (CACNA1A), which is a protein expressed in the granule cells and Purkinje cells of the cerebellar cortex. CACNA1A is thought to be associated with synaptic transmission.

Spinocerebellar Ataxia Type 8 (SCA8)

SCA8 is a rare disorder and accounts for approximately 3% of all ADCA. Affected patients typically present with slowly progressive cerebellar ataxia, including dysarthria, slow speech, and gait instability, as an initial symptom. A minority of patients develops cognitive impairment, pyramidal signs, peripheral neuropathy, and dysphagia during the course of their illness. Patients occasionally manifest with a form of parkinsonism that varies from L-dopa responsive parkinsonism to CBS. However, even in the most typical presentation, L-dopa responsiveness is variable. Routine brain MRI shows cerebellar atrophy.

SCA8 is caused by an abnormal CTG repeat expansion (71-1300; normal expansion is 15-50) in the *ATXN8* gene. *ATXN8* encodes ataxin 8 (ATXN8), which is a protein expressed in the cerebral cortex and cerebellum (9). The precise function of ATXN8 is still unknown. Abnormal CTG repeat expansions in the *ATXN8* gene have also been identified in approximately 2% of sporadic PD patients.

Spinocerebellar Ataxia Type 12 (SCA12)

SCA12 is a rare disorder. So far, a German-American family, two Italian families, and a single ethnic group in India have been reported (41-43). Affected patients typically present with action tremor as an initial symptom, followed by slowly progressive cerebellar ataxia, as well as hyperreflexia and cognitive impairment. They occasionally manifest with parkinsonism in the later course of their illness. The parkinsonism that is seen in SCA12 patients is characterized by bradykinesia. L-dopa responsiveness has not been reported. Routine brain MRI shows cerebral and cerebellar atrophy.

SCA12 is caused by an abnormal CAG repeat expansion (55-78: normal expansion is 4-32) in the *PPP2R2B* gene. *PPP2R2B* encodes the brain-specific regulatory subunit of the protein phosphatase 2 (PPP2R2B), which is predominantly expressed in Purkinje cells in the cerebellum. PPP2R2B is associated with negative control of cell growth and division. Abnormal CAG repeat expansions in the *PPP2R2B* gene have not been identified in PD patients.

Spinocerebellar Ataxia Type 14 (SCA14)

SCA14 is an extremely rare disorder. So far, fewer than 30 families have been documented. Affected patients typically present with slowly progressive cerebellar ataxia, including limb and truncal ataxia, dysarthria, and eye movement abnormalities such as saccadic pursuit and nystagmus. They often manifest with hyperreflexia

and decreased vibration sense during the course of their illness. A minority of patients exhibit cognitive impairment, depression, dystonia, and postural tremor. So far, four patients have developed parkinsonism, which included rigidity (44-46) and resting tremor (47). Responsiveness to L-dopa therapy has not been noted. Routine brain MRI shows cerebellar atrophy.

SCA14 is caused by mutations in the *PRKCG* gene. PRKCG encodes protein kinase Cγ (PKCγ), which is a protein that is abundantly expressed in the neurons, especially in Purkinje cells in the cerebellum. PKCγ is thought to be associated with signal transduction, cell differentiation, and synaptic transmission. To date, 29 *PRKCG* mutations and variants have been reported to be associated with SCA14 (19).

Spinocerebellar Ataxia Type 17 (SCA17)

SCA17 is a rare disorder. Its prevalence is estimated to be less than 0.2/100,000 in the general population. Affected patients typically present with cerebellar ataxia, cognitive impairment, dystonia, chorea, psychiatric symptoms, parkinsonism, pyramidal signs, and seizures. The parkinsonism that is seen in SCA17 patients is characterized as akinetic-rigid type and is sometimes accompanied by resting tremor. Most of the patients respond to L-dopa therapy. Routine brain MRI shows atrophy of cerebellum, brainstem, and cerebrum.

SCA17 is caused by abnormal CAG repeat expansion (more than 41; normal expansion is 25-40) in the *TBP* gene. *TBP* encodes TATA box-binding protein (TBP), which is ubiquitously expressed in the CNS. TBP is associated with transcription and the regulation of activity of a wide range of genes. Abnormal CAG repeat expansion in the *TBP* gene has been identified in idiopathic PD patients, but not in patients with autosomal dominant parkinsonism.

Spinocerebellar Ataxia Type 23 (SCA23)

SCA23 is an extremely rare disorder. So far, only a single Dutch family has been documented.

SCA23 accounts for less than 0.5% of ataxia patients in Netherlands. Affected patients typically present with slowly progressive cerebellar ataxia, which includes truncal ataxia, limb ataxia, and dysarthria, as well as slowed saccades. They also have a combination of pyramidal signs, tremor, and peripheral neuropathy. So far, only one patient, carrying a PDYN L211S mutation, has developed subtle parkinsonism, which was accompanied by progressive gait and upper limb ataxia, oculomotor abnormalities, distal sensory neuropathy, and pyramidal signs of the legs (48). L-dopa responsiveness was not reported. Routine brain MRI shows cerebellar atrophy or diffuse brain atrophy.

SCA23 is caused by mutations in the *PDYN* gene, encoding prodynorphin (PDYN), which is a protein that is ubiquitously expressed in the CNS, especially in the caudate nucleus and pons (9). PDYN is associated with pain perception and responses to stress. To date, four *PDYN* mutations have been reported to be associated with SCA23 (19).

Spinocerebellar Ataxia Type 28 (SCA28)

SCA28 is an extremely rare disorder and accounts for approximately 1.5% of all European ADCA patients. So far, only 10 families have been documented. Affected patients typically present with slowly progressive cerebellar ataxia, which includes truncal ataxia, limb ataxia, and dysarthria. Patients also develop oculomotor abnormalities such as ophthalmoplegia, gaze-evoked nystagmus, and slowed saccades, as well as ptosis, pyramidal signs, and dystonia later in the course of their illness. Up to 10% of patients manifest with parkinsonism; however, this was possibly related to treatment with neuroleptics. L-dopa responsiveness was not reported. Routine brain MRI shows cerebellar atrophy.

SCA28 is caused by mutations in the *AFG3L2* gene, encoding ATPase family gene 3 (AFG3)-like 2 (AFG3L2), which is a protein that is highly expressed in Purkinje cells in the cerebellum. AFG3L2 is associated with maintenance of the mitochondorial proteome. To date, 12 *AFG3L2* mutations and variants have been reported to be associated with SCA28 (19).

Familial disorders predominantly presenting with dystonia and/or chorea accompanied by parkinsonism (Table 16.5)

Choreoacanthocytosis

Choreoacanthocytosis is a rare, autosomal recessive, neurodegenerative disorder (see Chapter 29). Its prevalence has not been well investigated. Affected patients typically present with slowly progressive cognitive impairment and psychiatric symptoms in the early stages of their illness. They develop chorea, orolingual dystonia, tongue and lip biting, tics, peripheral neuropathy, behavioural problems, and generalized or partial seizure during the course of their illness. They occasionally manifest with parkinsonism in the later stages of their illness. Parkinsonism can occasionally be the prominent feature. The parkinsonism that is seen in choreoacanthocytosis patients is characterized as the akinetic-rigid type and is sometimes accompanied by resting tremor. L-dopa responsiveness is variable. Acanthocytosis and elevated serum levels of creatine phosphokinase can be useful diagnostic tools. Routine brain MRI usually shows atrophy of the caudate nuclei and hyperintensity in the striatum on T2WI. ^{18}F-dopa PET of parkinsonian patients shows reduced radiotracer uptake in the striatum bilaterally.

Choreoacanthocytosis is caused by mutations in the *VPS13A* gene. *VPS13A* encodes chorein, which is a protein ubiquitously expressed in human tissues, especially in the brain, erythroid precursors, and skeletal muscle. Chorein is thought to be associated with maintenance of the plasma membrane. To date, more than 100 *VPS13A* mutations and variants have been reported to be associated with choreoacanthocytosis (19).

Table16.5
List of familial disorders presenting with dystonia or chorea accompanied by parkinsonism.

	Gene	TAAO	Clinical features other than parkinsonism	L-dopa responsiveness	Genetic test availability
Choreoacanthocytosis	VPS13A	20th-30th	Chorea, CI, Psy, dystonia, tongue and lip biting, PN, BP, seizure, dysarthria, dysphagia, PN, myopathy, P (dysautonomia, OMA)	Good-none	I, V
DYT3	TAF1	30th-50th	Dystonia, P, T, chorea, myoclonus, myorhythmia, chorea-ballism, hyposmia	Minimal-none	I, III, V
DYT5a	GCH1	Childhood	Dystonia, P, T, diurnal fluctuation, Pyr, Psy (MR, myoclonus, RLS)	Good	I, IV, V
DYT5b, infantile parkinsonism	TH	Infancy	DD, truncal hypotonia, dystonia, MR, Psy, P, OMA, HPA, ptosis, diurnal fluctuation, T, dysautonomia	Good-minimal	I, IV, V
DYT5b	SPR	Infancy	Dystonia, CI, DD, OMA, diurnal fluctuation, hypotonia, P, Pyr, dysarthria, dysphagia, T, CA (myoclonus)	Good-moderate	I, V
DYT10	PRRT2	Childhood-adolescence	Paroxysmal kinesigenic dystonia/choreoathetosis/ballism, seizure, hemiplegic migraine, speech delay, apraxia (P)	Good	I, IV, V
DYT12	ATP1A3	10th-20th	Dystonia, P, dysarthria, dysphagia, Psy, seizure, apraxia (T)	Minimal to none	I, IV, V
DYT16	PRKRA	Childhood-adolescence	Dystonia, P, dysarthria, DD, dysphagia, Pyr	Minimal to none	I, IV, V
Huntington disease	HTT	30th-40th	Psy, chorea, CI, dysarthria, dysphagia, dystonia, LP, P, OMA (RBD)	Unknown	III, V
Huntington disease-like 2	JPH3	20th-40th	Chorea, poor coordination, weight loss, dystonia, P, dysarthria, Pyr, CI, Psy, BP, OMA (short stature)	None	III, V
HMDPC (childhood-onset)	SLC30A10	Childhood	Dystonia, liver disease, P, dysarthria, T (BP, CI, spastic paraparesis)	Minimal-none	I, IV
HMDPC (adulthood-onset)		50th-60th	P, liver disease (PN)	None	
IBGC 3	SLC20A2	30th-50th	Dystonia, P, T, CI, Psy, headache, seizure, CA, DD, BP, dysarthria, dysphagia, sleep problems (CA, chorea, scoliosis)	Good	I, IV, V
IBGC 4	PDGFRB	Adulthood		Good	NA
Infantile parkinsonism-dystonia	SLC6A3	Early childhood	Dystonia, P, axial hypotonia, Pyr, DD, bulbar signs, OMA	None	I
NBIA1 (classic form)	PANK2	10th	Dystonia, dysarthria, Pyr, CI, pigmentary retinopathy, dysphagia, chorea, Psy, CI, DD, OMA, P (PN, seizure)	Unknown	I, IV, V

NBIA1 (atypical form)	PANK2	20th-30th	**LP, Psy, P, Pyr, dystonia, hypotonia,** chorea, DD, OMA, dysarthria, dysphagia, CI, BP (ballismus, CA, pigmentary retinopathy)	Initially good	I, IV, V
NBIA2 (PLA2G6-related dystonia-parkinsonism)	PLA2G6	Early childhood-adolescence	**Dystonia, P, CI, Psy, OMA,** myoclonus, dysarthria, dysphagia, dysautomia	Good	I, IV, V
NBIA3	FTL	30th-50th	**Dystonia, chorea, dysarthria,** P, CI, dysphagia, CA, Pyr (OMA, T)	None	I, V
NBIA4	C19orf12	Childhood	**Dystonia, Pyr, CI, Psy, dysarthria, dysphagia, optic atrophy,** P, PN, Psy, UI (seizure, MND, RBD)	Good-none	I, V
NBIA5	WDR45	Early childhood	**Psychomotor retardation, seizure, dystonia, P, CI, Psy**	Unknown	I, IV, V

ATP1A3 = ATPase, Na+/K+ transporting, alpha 3 polypeptide; BP = behavioural problems; CA = cerebellar ataxia; CI = cognitive impairment; C19orf12 = chromosome 19 open reading frame 12; DD = developmental delay; FTL = ferritin, light polypeptide; GCH1 = GTP cyclohydrolase 1; HMDPC = hypermanganesemia with dystonia, polycythemia, and cirrhosis; HPA = hyperphenylalaninemia; HTT = huntingtin; IBGC = idiopathic basal ganglia calcification; JPH3 = junctophilin 3; LP = language problems; MND = motor neuron disease; MR = mental retardation; NBIA = neurodegeneration with brain iron accumulation; OMA = oculomotor abnormalities; P = parkinsonism; PANK2 = pantothenate kinase 2; PDGFRB = platelet-derived growth factor receptor, beta polypeptide; PLA2G6 = phospholipase A2, group VI; PN = peripheral neuropathy; PRKRA = protein kinase, interferon-inducible, double-stranded RNA-dependent activator; PRRT2 = proline-rich transmembrane protein 2; Psy = psychiatric symptoms; Pyr = pyramidal signs; RBD = rapid eye movement sleep behaviour disorder; RLS = restless legs syndrome; SLC6A3 = solute carrier family 6; SLC20A2 = solute carrier family 20 (phosphate transporter), member 2; SLC30A10 = solute carrier family 30, member 10; SPR = sepiapterin reductase; T = tremor; TAAO = typical age at onset; TAF1 = TAF1 RNA polymerase II, TATA box-binding protein (TBP)-associated factor, 250kDa; TH = tyrosine hydroxylase; VPS13A = vacuolar protein sorting 13, yeast, homolog of, A; WDR45 = WD-repeated domain 45; I = sequence analysis of the entire coding region is available; II = sequence analysis of select exons is available; III = targeted mutation analysis is available; IV = deletion/duplication analysis is available; V = prenatal diagnosis is available; clinical features in bold are frequently seen in patients (>50% of patients); clinical features in parentheses are occasionally seen in patients (<10% of patients).

Dystonia

Dystonia is a syndrome that is defined as a prolonged co-contraction of the opposing agonist and antagonist muscles. Dystonia is the third most common neurodegenerative movement disorder after PD and essential tremor (see Chapters 22-24). Its prevalence is estimated to be up to approximately 50/100,000 in the general population. About 11-30% of dystonia patients have a family history of the disease. So far, 25 genes/loci, DYT1-DYT25, have been identified. Among them, DYT3, DYT5, DYT10, DYT12,

and DYT16 have been reported to be associated with parkinsonism. In this subsection, we discuss the clinical features and the genetics related to these five genes.

Dystonia 3 (DYT3)

DYT3, also known as X-linked dystonia-Parkinsonism or Lubag syndrome, is a relatively rare, X-linked disorder. It is prevalent in the Philippines, and the overall prevalence is estimated to be 5-19/100,000 in the general population. This disorder mainly affects males (99%); however, female patients have occasionally been affected. Affected males typically present with focal dystonia as an initial symptom and develop generalized dystonia within five years. They often manifest with parkinsonism after they already have dystonia; however, parkinsonism can be the initial symptom. The parkinsonism that is seen in DYT3 patients is characterized by bradykinesia and postural instability and is sometimes accompanied by rigidity and resting tremor. Patients either respond poorly to L-dopa therapy or not at all. Deep brain stimulation (DBS) of the bilateral globus pallidus interna (GPi-DBS) is efficacious for them. Some patients have action or postural tremor, chorea, and myoclonus during the course of their illness. Female patients generally show a more benign phenotype and older age of disease onset than males. Routine brain MRI may show mild, generalized cerebral atrophy. ^{18}F-dopa PET of parkinsonian patients shows normal or reduced radiotracer uptake in the striatum.

DYT3 is caused by mutations in the *TAF1* genes, encoding TAF1 RNA polymerase II, TATA box-binding protein-associated factor, 250kDa (TAF1), which is a protein that is ubiquitously expressed in the CNS (9). TAF1 is associated with transcriptional regulations. To date, only one *TAF1* mutation has been reported to be associated with DYT3 (19).

Dystonia 5 (DYT5)

DYT5, also known as 'dopa-responsive dystonia (DRD)' or 'Segawa disease' is a relatively rare disorder. It accounts for approximately 5% of all childhood-onset dystonia. The prevalence is estimated to be 0.5-1/1,000,000 in the general population. DYT5 can be classified into two major forms based on manner of inheritance: DYT5a and DYT5b. DYT5a is inherited in an autosomal dominant manner and is caused by *GCH1* mutations. DYT5b is inherited in an autosomal recessive manner and is caused by either *TH* or *SPR* mutations. All three genes are associated with dopamine biosynthesis.

DYT5a is the most common form of DYT5 and accounts for approximately 50-87% of DYT5. Affected patients typically present with foot dystonia in childhood, which eventually leads to generalized dystonia. They usually develop parkinsonism, postural tremor, and diurnal fluctuation of symptoms during the course of their illness. The parkinsonism that is seen in DYT5a patients is typically of akinetic-rigid type and is sometimes accompanied by resting tremor. Patients respond dramatically to a low dose of L-dopa therapy. Low CSF levels of neopterin and biopterin can be useful diagnostic tools. Routine brain MRI is usually normal. ^{11}C-raclopride PET shows elevated radiotracer uptake in the striatum. ^{123}I-FP-CIT SPECT of parkinsonian patients shows normal radiotracer uptake in the striatum bilaterally. Adverse motor side effects, such as dyskinesia and wearing-off, are rare for DYT5a patients despite long-term L-dopa therapy.

GCH1 encodes GTP cyclohydrolase 1 (GCH1), which is a protein that is ubiquitously expressed in the CNS (9). To date, more than 170 *GCH1* mutations and variants have been reported to be associated with DYT5 (19). A *GCH1* mutation has been identified in patients with the PD phenotype.

DYT5b with TH mutations (DYT5b-TH) is a rare form of DYT5. Affected patients can present with a wide-range of phenotypes from a mild form, including dopa-responsive dystonia or myoclonus-dystonia syndrome, to a severe form such as infantile parkinsonism (moderate) or progressive infantile encephalopathy (severe form). The severity of disease depends on the degree of residual TH enzymatic activity. Diurnal fluctuations are not typically seen. The parkinsonism seen in DYT5b-TH patients is characterized as the akinetic-rigid type. Patients respond to L-dopa therapy; however, it is not dramatically effective in patients with the severe form. The dose of L-dopa should be slowly increased to avoid side effects such as hyperkinesia and ballism. Combination of L-dopa and selegiline therapy may provide better results. Low CSF levels of homovanillic acid (HVA) and 3-methoxy-4-hydroxyphenylglycol (MHPG) can be useful diagnostic tools. Routine brain MRI is usually normal.

TH encodes tyrosine hydroxylase (TH), which is a protein expressed in the catecholaminergic neurons and adrenal medulla (49). To date, more than 40 *TH* mutations and variants have been reported to be associated with DYT5b (19). *TH* mutations have been also identified in patients with L-dopa-responsive parkinsonism.

DYT5b with SPR mutations (DYT5b-SPR) is an extremely rare form of DYT5. Affected patients present with a wide range of phenotypes, which are similar to those found in DYT5b-TH. However, diurnal fluctuations and a combination of oculogyric crises and retrocollis are more frequently seen in DYT5b-SPR patients than in DYT5b-TH patients (50). L-dopa therapy ameliorates all symptoms, except for cognitive functions. The patients may need a higher dose of L-dopa in hot weather. The dose of L-dopa should be slowly increased to avoid side effects such as dyskinesia and myoclonic movements. Low levels of CSF HVA, MHPG, and 5-hydroxyindoleacetic acid (5-HIAA) can be useful diagnostic tools. Routine brain MRI is usually normal. [123]I- IBZM SPECT and [123]I- FP-CIT SPECT of parkinsonian patients shows normal radiotracers uptake in the striatum bilaterally.

SPR encodes sepiapterin reductase (SPR), which is a protein ubiquitously expressed in the CNS (9). SPR is associated with the tetrahydrobiopterin synthetic pathway. To date, more than five *SPR* mutations and variants have been reported to be associated with DYT5b.(19)

Dystonia 10 (DYT10)

DYT10, also known as episodic kinesigenic dyskinesia 1, is a rare, autosomal dominant disorder. Its prevalence is estimated to be approximately 1/100,000 in the general population. Affected patients typically present with recurrent and brief attacks of dystonia, chorea, ballism, or a combination, triggered by a sudden voluntary movement. The attacks typically occur at least once a day and last from seconds to minutes. DYT10 shows intra- and interfamilial variability in clinical expression. Some affected patients in DYT10 families manifest with infantile convulsions or paroxysmal choreoathetosis. So far, only one patient has developed parkinsonism (51). The patient with a history of carbamazepine-responsive adventitious limb movements had L-dopa responsive parkinsonism during the course of the illness. The parkinsonism that was seen in the patient was characterized as the akinetic-rigid type. However, this patient was described before the discovery of the causative gene for DYT10. Routine brain MRI is usually normal.

DYT10 is caused by mutations in the *PRRT2* gene, encoding proline-rich transmembrane protein 2 (PRRT2), which is a protein expressed in the brain and spinal cord. To date, more than 20 *PRRT2* mutations and variants associated with DYT10 have been identified (19).

Dystonia 12 (DYT12)

DYT12, also known as rapid-onset dystonia-parkinsonism, is a rare, autosomal dominant disorder. Its prevalence has not been well investigated. Affected patients typically present with an abrupt onset of dystonic spasm with parkinsonism, dysphagia, and dysarthria that progresses over hours to days. For almost half of all patients, the initial symptoms are triggered by physical or emotional stress. Patients show rostrocaudal (face>arm>leg) gradient of involvement. The status of disease becomes stabilized over the course of a month. The patients then show minimal to no progression. A minority of patients show mild limb dystonia before the abrupt onset. The parkinsonism seen in DYT12 patients is characterized by bradykinesia and postural instability, and is sometimes accompanied by rigidity. Parkinsonism can occasionally be an initial feature and the most prominent one. Patients either respond poorly to L-dopa therapy or not at all. GPi-DBS could potentially be effective. Routine brain MRI is usually normal. ^{123}I-FP-CIT SPECT of parkinsonian patients shows normal radiotracer uptake in the striatum bilaterally.

DYT12 is caused by mutations in the *ATP1A3* gene. *ATP1A3* encodes ATPase, Na+/K+ transporting, alpha 3 polypeptide (ATP1A3), which is a protein that is ubiquitously expressed, especially in cerebral cortex, thalamus, amygdala, and medullar oblongata (9). ATP1A3 is associated with restoring the resting membrane potential in neurons. To date, seven *ATP1A3* mutations and variants have been reported to be associated with DYT12 (19).

Dystonia 16 (DYT16)

DYT16, also known as young-onset dystonia-parkinsonism, is an extremely rare, autosomal recessive, neurodegenerative disorder. So far, only two unrelated Brazilian families and one sporadic German patient have been documented (52, 53). Affected patients typically present with focal limb dystonia as an initial symptom, which gradually spreads to other parts of body. More than half of patients develop parkinsonism over 10 years after the initial symptoms. The parkinsonism seen in DYT16 patients is characterized by bradykinesia, and occasionally by rigidity and resting tremor. Patients either respond poorly to L-dopa therapy or not at all. Routine brain MRI is usually normal.

DYT16 is caused by mutations in the *PRKRA* gene. *PRKRA* encodes protein kinase, interferon-inducible, double-stranded RNA-dependent activator (PRKRA), which is a protein that is ubiquitously expressed in the CNS (9). PKR is thought to be associated with the apoptosis pathway. To date, two *PRKRA* mutations have been reported to be associated with DYT16 (19).

Huntington Disease (HD)

HD is a relatively common, autosomal dominant, neurodegenerative disorder. Its prevalence is estimated to be around 15/100,000 in the general population. Affected patients typically present with psychiatric symptoms such as apathy and depression in the early stages. They develop chorea, dystonia, and language problems during the course of their illness. These patients also eventually manifest with parkinsonism and dysphagia. The parkinsonism that is seen in HD patients is characterized as akinetic-rigid type. However, L-dopa therapy may provide benefit in patients with childhood onset Westphal variant HD. Routine brain MRI shows atrophy of the caudate nucleus and putamen. ^{11}C-raclopride PET, ^{123}I-FP-CIT SPECT, and ^{123}I-epidepride-SPECT of parkinsonian patients show reduced radiotracer uptake in the striatum.

HD is caused by abnormal CAG repeats in the *HTT* gene (more than 36; normal expansion is less than 26), encoding huntingtin, which is a protein that is ubiquitously expressed in the CNS. Huntingtin is thought to be associated with transcriptional regulation, axonal transport, and apoptosis regulation.

Huntington Disease-Like 2 (HDL2)

HDL2 is an extremely rare, autosomal dominant, neurodegenerative disorder. So far, fewer than 50 families have been documented worldwide, and most of them are of African ancestry. There are two different clinical courses for HDL2 patients. Patients of the first type predominantly present with poor coordination, weight loss, parkinsonism, dysarthria, action tremor, cognitive impairment, behavioural problems, and psychiatric symptoms, accompanied by mild chorea. Patients of the second type present with chorea, accompanied by mild dystonia, parkinsonism, tremor, hyperreflexia, dysarthria, psychiatric symptoms, and cognitive impairment. The majority of HDL2 patients develop parkinsonism, which is characterized as akinetic-rigid type, and is occasionally accompanied by resting tremor. Patients do not respond to L-dopa therapy, and indeed L-dopa therapy may exaggerate the chorea. Routine brain MRI shows atrophy of the bilateral caudate nuclei and cerebral cortex.

HDL2 is caused by abnormal CTG/CAG repeat expansions (more than 40; normal expansion is 6-28) in the *JPH3* gene. *JPH3* encodes a protein named junctophilins-3 (JPH3), which is ubiquitously expressed in the CNS (9). It is thought to be associated with the formation of junctional membrane structures.

Hypermanganesemia with Dystonia, Polycythemia, and Cirrhosis (HMDPC)

HMDPC is an extremely rare, autosomal recessive, metabolic disorder. So far, fewer than 30 patients have been documented. They can be divided into two clinical forms labelled childhood-onset and adulthood-onset. Affected childhood-onset HMDPC patients present with generalized dystonia, parkinsonism, and dysarthria. Affected adult-onset HMDPC patients mainly present with parkinsonism. The parkinsonism that is seen in HMDPC patients is characterized as akinetic-rigid type. Patients usually do not respond to L-dopa therapy. Chelation therapy with disodium calcium edetate improves the clinical features and normalizes the laboratory data. Polycythemia and elevated serum manganese levels can be useful diagnostic tools. Routine brain MRI shows symmetrical hyperintensities of the basal ganglia, midbrain, and cerebellum on T1-weighted image (T1WI), which is suggestive of manganese accumulation.

HMDPC is caused by mutations in the *SLC30A10* gene. This gene encodes solute carrier family 30, member 10 (SLC30A10), which is a protein that is expressed in the liver and brain including the basal ganglia. SLC30A10 is associated with manganese transport. To date, 10 *SLC30A10* mutations and variants have been reported to be associated with HMDPC (19).

Idiopathic Basal Ganglia Calcification (IBGC)

Familial IBGC, also known as Fahr disease, is a rare, inherited, neurological disease. Its prevalence has not been well investigated. IBGC is caused by the deposition of calcium in the brain, including the basal ganglia. It is clinically characterized by focal dystonia, parkinsonism, tremor, cognitive impairment, psychiatric symptoms, chronic headache, epilepsy, and cerebellar ataxia. Routine brain CT usually shows symmetrical calcifications in the basal ganglia, thalamus, cerebellum, cerebral cortex, and subcortical regions. So far, four genes/loci, *IBGC1-IBGC4*, have been identified. Among them, *IBGC3* and *IBGC4* have been reported to be associated with parkinsonism. We discuss parkinsonism and the genetics related to these two genes in this subsection.

Idiopathic Basal Ganglia Calcification 3 (IBGC3)

IBGC3 is a common form of IBGC, accounting for approximately 40%. The parkinsonism that is seen in IBGC3 patients is characterized as the akinetic-rigid type. Some patients respond to L-dopa therapy.

IBGC3 is caused by mutations in the *SLC20A2* gene. *SLC20A2* encodes the sodium-dependent phosphate transporter 2 (SLC20A2), which is a protein that is ubiquitously expressed in human tissue, especially in the brain, including the basal ganglia (54). SLC20A2 is associated with phosphate transport. To date, 20 SLC20A2 mutations and variants have been reported to be associated with IBGC3 (19).

Idiopathic Basal Ganglia Calcification 4 (IBGC4)

IBGC4 is an extremely rare form of IBGC. So far, only one French family has been documented (55). Parkinsonism has been reported in only one patient in the family. That patient manifested with bilateral asymmetrical parkinsonism in his 5th decade, followed by cognitive impairment. The patient responded well to L-dopa therapy and developed on-off fluctuations and dyskinesia.

IBGC4 is caused by mutations in the *PDGFRB* gene. *PDGFRB* encodes platelet-derived growth factor receptor-β (PDGFRβ), which is a protein expressed in the CNS, especially in the basal ganglia and dentate nucleus of the cerebellum. PDGFRβ is associated with cellular proliferation, differentiation, survival, and migration. To date, two *PDGFRβ* mutations have been reported to be associated with IBGC4 (19).

Infantile parkinsonism-Dystonia (PKDYS)

PKDYS is an extremely rare, autosomal recessive disorder. So far, fewer than 20 patients have been documented (56-58). Affected patients typically present with dystonia, parkinsonism, irritability, feeding difficulties, and/or axial hypotonia as the initial symptoms. They develop pyramidal signs, dyskinesia, chorea, and motor developmental delay in the early stage of their illness. They show oculomotor abnormality, bulbar dysfunctions, and other motor symptoms during the course of the illness. The parkinsonism that is seen in PKDYS patients is characterized by bradykinesia, rigidity, hypomimia, and resting tremor. Patients do not respond to L-dopa therapy. DBS can potentially be effective. An elevated ratio of CSF homovanillic acid/5-hydroxyindoleacetic acid is a useful diagnostic tool. ^{123}I-FT-CIT SPECT of parkinsonian patients shows symmetrical, severely reduced dopamine transporter uptake in the striatum bilaterally.

PKDYS is caused by mutations in the *SLC6A3* gene. *SLC6A3* encodes solute carrier family 6 (neurotransmitter transporter, dopamine), member 3 (SLC6A3), which is a protein that is ubiquitously expressed in the CNS. SLC6A3 is associated with the transportation of amine and the termination of the action of dopamine. To date, three *SLC6A3* mutations have been reported to be associated with PKDYS (19).

Neurodegeneration with Brain Iron Accumulation (NBIA)

NBIA is a rare syndrome that encompasses inherited disorders that are characterized by iron accumulation in the brain. The prevalence is estimated to be 1-3/1,000,000 in the general population. So far, nine forms of NBIA have been identified, NBIA1, NBIA2, NBIA3, NBIA4, NBIA5,

fatty acid hydroxylase-associated neurodegeneration, Kufor-Rakeb syndrome, aceruloplasminemia, and Woodhouse-Sakati syndrome. Among them, NBIA1, NBIA2, NBIA3, NBIA4, NBIA5, Kufor-Rakeb syndrome, aceruloplasminemia, and Woodhouse-Sakati syndrome have been reported to be associated with parkinsonism. We discuss the clinical features and the genetics related to NBIA1, NBIA2, NBIA3, NBIA4, and NBIA5 in this subsection. We describe Kufor-Rakeb syndrome, aceruloplasminemia, and Woodhouse-Sakati syndrome in other sections of this chapter.

Neurodegeneration with Brain Iron Accumulation 1 (NBIA1)

NBIA1, also known as pantothenate kinase-associated neurodegeneration, is an autosomal recessive disorder. NBIA1 is the most common form and accounts for approximately 50% of all NBIA. Patients can be divided into two clinical forms based on the clinical course: early-onset, rapidly progressive form (classic) and late-onset, slowly progressive form (atypical). The classic form accounts for 60-70% of all NBIA1. Patients usually present with dystonia, dysarthria, and limb rigidity, which is accompanied by cognitive impairment and retinal pigmentary degeneration. Patients with the atypical form usually present with language problems, psychiatric symptoms, parkinsonism, and pyramidal signs. Parkinsonism is more frequently seen in atypical form NBIA1 patients (70%) than in classic form NBIA1 patients (10%). The parkinsonism that is seen in NBIA1 patients is characterized as akinetic-rigid type and is sometimes accompanied by resting tremor. Freezing gait may be more prominent in the atypical form. Routine brain MRI shows the 'eye-of-the-tiger' sign, which is characterized by hypointensity of the bilateral globus pallidus with hyperintense foci on T2WI. ^{123}I-FP-CIT SPECT of parkinsonian patients shows asymmetrically reduced dopamine transporter uptake in the striatum.

NBIA1 is caused by mutations in the *PANK2* gene, encoding 'pantothenate kinase 2 (PANK2),' which is a protein that is ubiquitously expressed in the CNS, especially in the hypothalamus and amygdala (9). PANK2 is associated with the formation of coenzyme A. To date, more than 120 *PANK2* mutations and variants have been reported to be associated with NBIA1 (19).

Neurodegeneration with Brain Iron Accumulation 2 (NBIA2)

NBIA2, also known as PLA2G6-associated neurodegeneration (PLAN), is an autosomal recessive disorder and accounts for approximately 20% of all NBIA. Patients can be divided into three clinical forms based on the clinical phenotype: classic infantile neuroaxonal dystrophy (INAD), atypical INAD, and PLA2G6-related dystonia-parkinsonism. Parkinsonism is seen only in PLA2G6-related dystonia-parkinsonism patients: they prominently exhibit dystonia, parkinsonism, cognitive impairment, and psychiatric symptoms such as depression and aggression. The parkinsonism seen in these patients is characterized by resting tremor, rigidity, bradykinesia, and postural instability. Patients respond well to L-dopa therapy, but develop early dyskinesia. Routine brain MRI shows hypointensity of the globus pallidus in about half of patients on T2WI.

NBIA2 is caused by mutations in the *PLA2G6* gene. *PLA2G6* encodes a protein named 'phospholipase A2, group VI (PLA2G6),' which is ubiquitously expressed in the CNS (9). PLA2G6 is thought to be associated with cell membrane homeostasis, cell proliferation, and apoptosis. To date, 26 *PLA2G6* mutations and variants have been reported to be associated with NBIA2 (19). *PLA2G6* mutations have been also identified in patients with PD phenotype and L-dopa-responsive parkinsonism with dementia.

Neurodegeneration with Brain Iron Accumulation 3 (NBIA3)

NBIA3, also known as neuroferritinopathy, is an extremely rare, autosomal dominant disorder, accounting for less than 1% of all NBIA. Affected patients typically present with dystonia, chorea, dysarthria, parkinsonism, and other neurological symptoms. They also develop cognitive impairment and dysphagia in the later stages of the illness. Less than half of the patients manifest with parkinsonism, and this is characterized as akinetic-rigid type and is occasionally accompanied by resting tremor. Parkinsonism can sometimes be the most prominent feature. Patients do not respond to L-dopa therapy. Low serum ferritin can be a useful diagnostic tool. Routine brain MRI shows hypointensity of the basal ganglia, substantia nigra, and red nuclei on T2WI, which is suggestive of iron accumulation. The signals are eventually followed by symmetrical cystic changes in the basal ganglia. ^{18}F-dopa PET of parkinsonian patients shows normal radiotracer uptake in the striatum.

NBIA3 is caused by mutations in the *FTL1* gene, encoding ferritin light chain (FTL), which is a protein abundantly expressed in the CNS (9). FTL1 is associated with storage and homeostasis of iron. To date, seven *FTL1* mutations have been reported to be associated with NBIA3 (19).

Neurodegeneration with Brain Iron Accumulation 4 (NBIA4)

NBIA4, also known as mitochondrial protein-associated neurodegeneration (MPAN), is an extremely rare, autosomal recessive disorder, accounting for 5% of all NBIA. So far, approximately 50 cases have been reported. Affected patients typically present with dystonia, pyramidal signs, cognitive impairment, psychiatric symptoms, dysarthria, dysphagia, and optic atrophy. A minority of patients manifest with parkinsonism that is characterized by bradykinesia, rigidity, tremor, and postural instability. Response to L-dopa therapy is variable. Routine brain MRI shows hypointensity of the bilateral globus pallidus and substantia nigra on T2WI, which is suggestive of iron deposition, typically without the 'eye of the tiger sign'.

NBIA4 is caused by mutations in the *C19orf12* gene. *C19orf12* encodes chromosome 19 open reading frame 12 (C19orf12), which is a protein that is ubiquitously expressed in the CNS (9). The precise function of C19orf12 is still unknown. To date, 11 *C19orf12* mutations have been reported to be associated with NBIA4 (19). *C19orf12* mutations and variants have also been identified in a patient with the typical PD phenotype.

Neurodegeneration with Brain Iron Accumulation 5 (NBIA5)

NBIA5, also known as beta-propeller protein-associated neurodegeneration or static encephalopathy of childhood with neurodegeneration in adulthood, is an extremely rare, X-linked disorder, accounting for approximately 2% of all NBIA. All reported patients have been sporadic. Affected patients typically present with psychomotor retardation and seizures in the early stages of the illness. The symptoms remain static for a long period of time, and patients suddenly develop progressive dystonia-parkinsonism, dementia, and psychiatric problems in their twenties. The parkinsonism that is seen in NBIA5 patients is characterized as the akinetic-rigid type and is occasionally accompanied by resting tremor. Responsiveness to L-dopa therapy has not been noted. Routine brain MRI shows hyperintensity of the substantia nigra on T1WI with a central band of hypointensity, as well as hypointensity of the globus pallidus on T2WI, which is suggestive of iron deposition. Cerebral and cerebellar atrophy are also seen.

NBIA5 is caused by mutations in the *WDR45* gene. *WDR45* encodes WD-repeated domain 45 (WDR45), which is a protein that is ubiquitously expressed in the CNS. WDR45 is associated with the autophagy pathway. To date, 19 *WDR45* mutations and variants have been reported to be associated with NBIA5 (19).

Familial disorders presenting with parkinsonism accompanied by multi-system dysfunctions (Table 16.6)

Aceruloplasminemia

Aceruloplasminemia is a rare, autosomal recessive disease that affects the iron metabolism. Its prevalence is estimated to be 1/2,000,000 in non-consanguineous marriages. Approximately 20% of patients present with parkinsonism, which is characterized as akinetic-rigid type. Patients do not respond to L-dopa therapy. Low levels of serum ceruloplasmin, copper, and iron, low activity levels of plasma ceruloplasmin ferroxidase, and elevated levels of serum ferritin can be useful diagnostic tools. Routine brain MRI shows abnormal hypointensities of the striatum, thalamus, midbrain, and dentate nucleus of cerebellum on T1WI and T2WI.

Aceruloplasminemia is caused by mutations in the *CP* gene. *CP* encodes ceruloplasmin (CP), which is a protein expressed in the astrocytes in the brain. CP is associated with iron metabolism and neuronal survival in the CNS. To date, 41 *CP* mutations and variants have been reported to be associated with aceruloplasminemia (19).

Acid Sphingomyelinase Deficiency (ASD)

ASD, also known as Niemann-Pick disease, is a rare, autosomal recessive, lysosomal lipid storage disorder. Its prevalence is estimated to be approximately 1/250,000. Patients can be divided into two clinical forms based on the clinical course: infantile form (neuronopathic form ASD) and later-onset form (non-neuronopathic form ASD). So far, only one non-neuronopathic ASD patient, carrying an ASM delR608 mutation, has been reported to have developed parkinsonism (59). The patient had a short stature, unexplained cholestatic liver disease, early menopause, and hallux valgus as a child. She had resting tremor at age 51. She was treated with several anti- parkinsonian medications including L-dopa, but her symptoms progressed very rapidly. Low levels of acid sphingomyelinase activity in peripheral blood lymphocytes and li-pid-laden macrophages in the bone marrow are useful diagnostic tools.

ASD is caused by mutations in the *SMPD1* gene. *SMPD1* encodes sphingomyelinase (ASM), which is a protein expressed in the lysosome. ASM is associated with normal membrane turn-over through the hydrolysis of sphingomyelin. To date, 159 *SMPD1* mutations and variants have been reported to be associated with ASD (19).

Achalasia-Addisonianism-Alacrima Syndrome (AAA syndrome)

AAA syndrome, also known as Allgrove syndrome, is a rare, autosomal recessive disorder. Its prevalence has not been well investigated. So far, three AAA syndrome patients have developed parkinsonism, which was characterized as akinetic-rigid type (60, 61). Responsiveness to L-dopa therapy has not been noted. Routine brain MRI is usually normal.

AAA syndrome is caused by mutations in the *AAAS* gene, encoding alacrima–achalasia–adrenal insufficiency neurologic disorder (ALADIN), which is a protein that is ubiquitously expressed in human tissues, especially in the adrenal and pituitary glands, cerebellum, gastrointestinal organs, and kidney. ALADIN is thought to be associated with nucleocytoplasmic molecular transport. To date, approximately 66 *AAAS* mutations and variants have been reported to be associated with AAA syndrome (19).

Cerebrotendinous Xanthomatosis (CTX)

CTX is a rare, autosomal recessive, lipid storage disorder. Its prevalence has not been well investigated. A minority of patients present with parkinsonism during the course of their illness. The parkinsonism that is seen in CTX patients is characterized by bradykinesia, rigidity, resting tremor, hypomimia, and shuffling gait. Occasionally, it is also accompanied by resting tremor. Parkinsonism can be a prominent feature. Responsiveness to L-dopa therapy is varia-

ble, but the majority of patients respond poorly. Motor fluctuations and dyskinesias may appear shortly after the initiation of L-dopa therapy. Elevated levels of serum cholestanol and urine bile alcohols are useful diagnostic tools. Routine brain MRI shows cerebellar atrophy, cerebral atrophy, and white matter changes around the dentate nuclei of the cerebellum. ^{18}F-dopa PET and ^{99m}Tc-TRODAT-1 SPECT of parkinsonian patients show reduced radiotracer uptake in the putamen bilaterally.

CTX is caused by mutations in the *CYP27A1* gene. *CYP27A1* encodes cytochrome P450, family 27, subfamily A, polypeptide 1 (CYP27A1), which is a protein that is ubiquitously expressed in the CNS (9). CYP27A1 is associated with the metabolic pathway that converts cholesterol to biliary acids. To date, 79 *CYP27A1* mutations and variants have been reported to be associated with CTX (19).

Neuronal Ceroid-Lipofuscinoses (NCL)

NCL is a rare group of inherited lysosomal storage disorders. Its prevalence is estimated to be approximately 1-9/1,000,000 in the general population. NCL can be classified into five different forms based on clinical phenotypes: infantile NCL1 (INCL1), late-infantile NCL1 (LINCL1), juvenile NCL1 (JNCL1), adult NCL1 (ANCL1), and Northern epilepsy. INCL1 patients initially present with developmental delays, seizures, and microcephaly, which is followed by visual loss and progressive loss of motor skills. LINCL1 patients initially manifest with seizures, followed by developmental delays, cognitive impairment, cerebellar ataxia, extrapyramidal and pyramidal signs, and visual loss. JNLC1 patients initially show progressive visual loss, followed by mental retardation, seizures, extrapyramidal signs, dysarthria, deterioration of motor skills, and psychiatric symptoms. ANCL1 patients initially have progressive myoclonic seizures or behaviour problems, as well as cognitive impairment, cerebellar ataxia, and pyramidal and extrapyramidal signs. Northern epilepsy patients initially develop sei-

Table 16.6
List of familial disorders presenting with multisystem dysfunction accompanied by parkinsonism.

	Gene	TAAO	Clinical features other than parkinsonism	L-dopa responsive-ness	Genetic test availability
Aceruloplas-minemia	CP	20th-60th	Anemia, retinal degeneration, DM, CA, dystonia, T, chorea, dysarthria, CI, P, Psy	None	I, V
ASD (non-neuro-pathic form)	SMPD1	Childhood	Hepatosplenomegaly, pulmonary insuffi-ciency, DD, CA, CI, macular abnormalities, cardiovascular disease, Psy, PN (P)	None	I, III, IV, V
AAA syn-drome	AAAS	Late child-hood	Adrenal insufficiency, alacrimia, achalasia, PN, Pyr, dysautonomia, dysphagia, optic atrophy, CA, MR, CI, microcephaly, dysar-thria, seizure, MND, dermatological features, osteoporosis, short stature, glossitis fissured tongue, xerostomia, ophthalmic manifesta-tions (myoclonus, P)	Unknown	I, II, IV, V
CTX	CYP27A1	Late child-hood	Juvenile cataract, tendon xanthomas, CI, Pyr, CA, MR, seizure, diarrhea, seizure, Psy, PN, dysarthria, dysphagia, osteopenia, dystonia	Good-min-imal	I, IV, V
Ceroid-Lipo-fuscinoses 1	PPT1	Juvenile	INCL, LINCL, JNCL, ANCL (P)	None	I, II, IV, V
Ceroid-Lipo-fuscinoses 3	CLN3	Infantile-ju-venile	JNCL, P	Good-min-imal	I, II, IV, V
Chediak-Higashi syndrome	LYST	Early child-hood-early adulthood	Immunodeficiency, partial oculocuta-neuous albinism, bleeding tendency, CI, T, CA, PN, photophobia, OMA, Pyr, albinism, seizure, dystonia (P)	Good-min-imal	I, IV, V
Gaucher disease, type 1	GBA	Infantile-early child-hood	Bone disease, hepatosplenomegaly, cytope-nia, CI, pulmonary disease, OMA, Psy, can-cers, P (deafness, myoclonus, PN, seizure, T)	Good-none	I, II, III, V
Gaucher disease, type 3		Childhood	Dysarthria, dysphagia, OMA, Pyr, CI, CA, seizure, bone disease, hepatomegaly, spleno-megaly, cytopenia, pulmonary disease (P)	Good	
GM1-gan-gliosidosis, type III	GLB1	Childhood	Dysarthria, dysphagia, dystonia, Pyr, MR, bone dysplasia, scoliosis, short stature, P, CA, corneal opacity, macular spots, cataract	Mini-mal-none	I, IV, V
Hereditary hemochro-matosis	HFE	40th-50th	Hepatic disease, DM, cardiomyopathy, hypogonadism, arthritis, skin pigmentation (CA, dysautonomia, dystonia, P, RLS)	Good-none	I, II, III, IV, V
HPABH4A	PTS	Infantile	MR, hypotonia, Pyr, seizure, dysphagia, blond hair, microcephaly, eczema, short stature, hypotonia (CA, dystonia, P, ptosis)	Good*	I, IV, V

MERRF	MT-TK	Childhood	**Myoclonus, seizure, CA, muscle weakness, CI, deafness, PN, short stature**, Psy, optic atrophy, stroke-like episodes, Pyr, retinopathy, cardiomyopathy, OMA (P)	Good	I, II, III, V
PEOA1	POLG	20th-30th	**PEOA, ptosis, cataracts, myopathy, PN,** dysphagia, deafness, CA, Psy, hypogonadism, CI, T, DM, P, heart disease (deafness, migraine, seizure)	Good-moderate	I, V
PEOA3	C10orf2	20th-50th	**PEOA, ptosis, myopathy, PN,** dysphagia, deafness, CA, Psy, CI (cataract^, hypogonadism, deafness, DM, heart disease, migraine, P, seizure, T)	Good	I, IV, V
Perry syndrome	DCTN1	40th-50th	**Hypoventilation, Psy, weight loss, P, dysphagia,** CI (dysautonomia, OMA)	Good-none	I, II, IV, V
Wilson disease	ATP7B	Childhood-40th	**Liver disease, Kayser-Fleischer rings,** dysarthria, T, P, dystonia, CA, Pyr, bulbar signs, Psy, BP (chorea, choreoathetosis, myoclonus)	Minimal-none	I, II, III, IV, V
Woodhouse-Sakati Syndrome	DCAF17	Childhood	**Frontal alopecia, hypogonadism, thyroid dysfunctions, DM, CI, deafness, dystonia, chorea,** dysarthria, seizure (acanthosis nigrans, keratoconus, hypothyroidism, PN, Pyr, syndactyly, UI)	Unknown	I, V

AAA = achalasia-addisonianism-alacrima; *AAAS* = adrenocortical insufficiency, alacrima; ANCL = adult ceroid lipofuscinoses; ASD = acid sphingomyelinase deficiency; ATP7B = ATPase, Cu++ transporting, beta polypeptide; *C10orf2* = chromosome 10 open reading frame 2; CA = cerebellar ataxia; CI = cognitive impairment; *CLN3* = ceroid-lipofuscinosis, neuronal 3; *CP* = ceruloplasmin; CTX = cerebrotendinous xanthomatosis; *CYP27A1* = cytochrome P450, family 27, subfamily A, polypeptide 1; *DCAF17* = DDB1 and CUL4 associated factor 17; *DCTN1* = dynactin 1; DD = developmental delay: DM = diabetes mellitus; *GBA* = glucosidase, beta, acid; *GLB1* = galactosidase, beta 1; *HFE* = hemochromatosis; HPABH4A = hyperphenylalanimemia, BH4-deficient, A; INCL = infantile ceroid lipofuscinoses; JNCL = juvenile ceroid lipofuscinoses; LINCL = late-onset infantile ceroid lipofuscinoses; *LYST* = lysosomal trafficking regulator; MERRF = myoclonic epilepsy associated with ragged-red fibers; MND = motor neurism disease; MR = mental retardation; MT-TK = mitochondrially encoded tRNA lysine, OMA = oculomotor abnormalities; P = Parkinsonism; PEOA = progressive external ophthalmo plegia with mitochondrial DNA deletions, autosomal dominant; PN = peripheral neuropathy; *PPT1* = palmitoyl-protein thioesterase 1; *POLG* = polymerase, gamma; Psy = psychiatric symptoms; PTS = 6-pyruvoyltetrahydropterin synthase; Pyr = pyramidal signs; RLS = restless legs syndrome; *SMPD1* = sphingomyelin phosphodiesterase 1, acid lysosomal; T = tremor; TAAO = typical age at onset; UI = urinary incontinence; I = sequence analysis of the entire coding region is available; II = sequence analysis of select exons is available; III = targeted mutation analysis is available; IV = deletion/duplication analysis is available; V = prenatal diagnosis is available; *combination therapy with L-dopa and 5-hydroxytryptophan; ^cataract is less frequently seen in PEOA3; clinical features in bold are frequently seen in patients (>50% of patients); clinical features in parentheses are occasionally seen in patients (<10% of patients).

zures, intellectual impairments, and motor dysfunctions. So far, nine different genes are known to be associated with ANCL: *PPT1* (CLN1), *TPP1* (CLN2), *CLN3* (CLN3), *CLN5* (CLN5), *CLN6* (CLN6), *MFSD8* (CLN7), *CNL8* (CLN8), *CTSD* (CLN10), and *PGRN* (CLN11). Parkinsonism has been described in CLN1 and CLN3 patients. We discuss parkinsonism and the genetics related to these two genes in this subsection.

Ceroid-Lipofuscinose 1 (CLN1)

CLN1, also known as Santavuori-Haltia disease, is a rare, autosomal recessive disorder. So far, two ANCL1 patients, carrying the same PPT1 double mutations, delR151X and G108R, have developed parkinsonism during the course of their illness (62). The parkinsonism that is seen in the patients with ANCL1 includes rigidity, bradykinesia, and postural instability. One patient was treated with L-dopa without any benefit. Routine brain MRI shows cerebral atrophy. CLN1 is caused by mutations in the *PPT1* gene. *PPT1* encodes palmitoyl-protein thioesterase 1 (PPT1), which is a protein abundantly expressed in the CNS, especially in the cerebral cortex, hypothalamus, caudate nucleus, and amygdala (9). PPT1 is thought to be associated with apoptosis, endocytosis, vesicular trafficking, synaptic function, and lipid metabolism. To date, 64 *PPT1* mutations and variants have been reported to be associated with CLN1 (19).

Ceroid-Lipofuscinose 3 (CLN3)

CLN3, also known as Batten disease, is a rare, autosomal recessive disorder. A minority of CLN3 patients present with parkinsonism. The parkinsonism is characterized as akinetic-rigid type and is sometimes accompanied by resting tremor. Responsiveness to L-dopa therapy is variable. Routine brain MRI may show cerebral and cerebellar atrophy. ^{123}I-β-CIT SPECT of parkinsonian patients shows hypoperfusion in the basal ganglia, especially in the putamen.

CLN3 is caused by mutations in the *CLN3* gene. *CLN3* encodes battenin, which is a protein that is ubiquitously expressed in the CNS (9). Battenin is thought to be associated with lysosomal acidification, lysosomal arginine import, membrane fusion, vesicular transport, cytoskeletal linked function, autophagy, apoptosis, and proteolipid modification. To date, 55 *CLN3* mutations and variant have been reported to be associated with CLN3 (19).

Chediak-Higashi Syndrome (CHS)

CHS is a rare, autosomal recessive, lysosomal storage disorder. Its prevalence has not been well investigated. In patients who have symptoms during adulthood, the systemic symptoms are mild. The neurological symptoms, including parkinsonism, are more frequently seen than in those who manifest symptoms in childhood. So far, fewer than 15 patients have developed parkinsonism (63-65). The parkinsonism seen in CHS patients is characterized by bradykinesia, rigidity, resting tremor, postural instability, reduced arm swing, and hypomimia. Responsiveness to L-dopa therapy is variable. Large peroxidase-positive panleukocytic granules within leukocytes on blood smear can be a useful diagnostic tool. Routine brain MRI images vary from normal to severe atrophy of the cerebrum and cerebellum. ^{123}I-FP-CIT SPECT of parkinsonian patients shows symmetrically reduced dopamine transporter uptake in the putamen. IBZM-SPECT of parkinsonian patients shows normal dopamine transporter uptake in the striatum bilaterally.

CHS is caused by mutations in the *LYST* gene. *LYST* encodes the lysosomal trafficking regulator (LYST), which is a protein that is ubiquitously expressed in the CNS (9). LYST is thought to be associated with the regulation of intracellular protein trafficking to and from the lysosome. To date, 50 *LYST* mutations and variants have been reported to be associated with CHS (19).

Gaucher Disease (GD)

GD is a rare, autosomal recessive, lysosomal storage disorder. Its prevalence is estimated to be 1-2/100,000. Affected patients manifest with a wide spectrum of clinical phenotypes. GD is classified into three different forms based on clinical phenotypes and age at onset: non-neuropathic form (GD type 1), acute-onset neuropathic form (GD type 2), and subacute-onset neuropathic form (GD type 3). GD type 1 is the most common form (99%). A subset of GD type 1 patients and a few GD type 3 patients (66) have developed parkinsonism, primarily after other symptoms of GD (67). The parkinsonism that is seen in GD patients has a relatively early-onset (e.g., fourth or fifth decade of life), is rapidly progressive, and is characterized as akinetic-rigid type. It is sometimes accompanied by resting tremor. Responsiveness to L-dopa therapy is variable, but the majority of patients respond poorly. Gaucher cells in the bone marrow and reduced leukocyte β-glucosidase activity are useful diagnostic tools. Routine brain MRI may show mild cerebral atrophy. ^{11}C-CFT PET of parkinsonian patients shows reduced radiotracer uptake in the striatum.

GD is caused by mutations in the *GBA* gene, encoding glucosylceramidase, which is a protein that is ubiquitously expressed in the CNS (9). Glucosylceramidase is associated with catalyzation of glucosylceramide, sphingomyelin generation, and prevention of glycolipid accumulation. To date, 348 *GBA* mutations have been reported to be associated with GD (19). *GBA* mutations and variants have also been identified in patients with typical PD phenotype and PD with dementia.

Hereditary hemochromatosis (HH)

HH is a rare, autosomal recessive disorder that affects iron metabolism. Its prevalence has not been well investigated. So far, nine HH patients have developed parkinsonism during the course of their illness (68-71). The parkinsonism is either mixed-type or akinetic-rigid type. Most patients respond to L-dopa therapy. Elevated transferrin-iron saturation and serum ferritin levels can be useful diagnostic tools. Routine brain MRI may show hyperintensity of the basal ganglia.

HH is caused by mutations in the *HFE* gene. *HFE* encodes hemochromatosis (HFE), which is a protein that is ubiquitously expressed in the CNS, especially in choroid plexus epithelial cells, endothelial cells of the microvasculature, and ependymal cells. HFE is associated with the regulation of iron homeostasis and a range of cellular functions, including innate immunity.

To date, 40 *HFE* mutations have been reported to be associated with HH (19). *HFE* mutations and variants have been identified in patients with AD, ALS, PD, or ischemic stroke (72).

GM1-Gangliosidosis, Type III (GM1G-III)

GM1-Gangliosidosis is a rare, autosomal dominant, lysosomal storage disorder. GM1-Gangliosidosis can be classified into three different forms based on the clinical course of the illness: infantile form (Type I), juvenile form (Type II), and adult form (Type III). Parkinsonism is seen in approximately 50% of GM1G-III patients and includes bradykinesia, rigidity, resting tremor, postural instability, reduced arm swing, and hypomimia. Patients do not respond well to L-dopa therapy. Low leukocyte β-galactosidase activity and the presence of Gaucher-like foam cells in the bone marrow can be useful diagnostic tools. Routine brain MRI shows bilateral, symmetrical hyperintensities in the putamen on T2WI.

GM1G-III is caused by mutations in the *GLB1* gene. *GLB1* encodes β-galactosidase, which is a protein that is ubiquitously expressed in the CNS (9). β-galactosidase is associated with catalyzing the hydrolysis of β-galactosides. To date, more than 150 *GLB1* mutations and variants have been reported to be associated with GM1G-III (19).

Hyperphenylalaninemia, BH4-Deficient, A (HPBH4A)

Hyperphenylalaninemia is a rare, autosomal dominant disorder that affects amino acid metabolism. A minority of HPBH4A patients develop parkinsonism in the early stages of their illness. The parkinsonism is characterized by either rigidity or bradykinesia. Patients respond to a combination of L-dopa therapy and 5-hydroxytryptophan or monotherapy with tetrahydrobiopterin. Routine brain MRI shows prominent sulci and fissures, subcortical cyst-like lesions on T1WI, and hyperintensities of the periventricular white matter on T2WI.

HPBH4A is caused by mutations in the *PTS* gene, encoding 6-pyruvoyltetrahydropterin synthase (PTS), which is a protein that is ubiquitously expressed in the CNS, especially in the hypothalamus and amygdala (9). PTS is associated with the biosynthesis of tetrahydrobiopterin. To date, more than 40 *PTS* mutations and variants have been reported to be associated with HPBH4A (19).

Myoclonic Epilepsy associated with Ragged-Red Fibers (MERRF)

MERRF is a rare mitochondrial disorder (see Chapter 32) that is transmitted by maternal inheritance. The prevalence is estimated to be less than 2/100,000. So far, only one MERRF patient has developed parkinsonism during the course of his illness (73). The patient, carrying a MT-TK A8344G mutation, manifested with resting tremor, rigidity, and bradykinesia at the age of 58 years. On neurological examination, the patient had a typical PD phenotype, as well as bilateral hearing loss, muscle weakness, and peripheral neuropathy. He responded well to parkinsonian therapy, including L-dopa. Elevated levels of lactate and pyruvate in both serum and CSF are useful diagnostic tools. Routine brain MRI shows brain atrophy and calcification of the basal ganglia.

MERRF is caused by mutations in the *MT-TK* gene. *MT-TK* encodes mitochondrially encoded tRNA lysine (MT-TK), which is a protein that is expressed in the brain (9). The precise function of MT-TK is not well known.

Progressive External Ophthalmoplegia with Mitochondrial DNA Deletions

Progressive external ophthalmoplegia (PEO) is a condition that is caused by multiple mitochondrial DNA deletions (see also Chapter 32). Its prevalence is estimated to be approximately 1/100,000 in the adult population. PEO is inherited in either an autosomal dominant or autosomal recessive manner. Autosomal dominant PEOA can be caused by mutations in five different genes, *POLG* (PEOA1), *SLC25A4* (PEOA2), *C10orf2* (PEOA3), *POLG2* (PEOA4),

and *RRM2B* (PEOA5). *POLG* also can cause autosomal recessive PEO. Parkinsonism has been described in patients with PEOA1 and PEOA3. We discuss parkinsonism and the genetics related to these two genes in this subsection.

Progressive External Ophthalmoplegia with Mitochondrial DNA Deletions 1 (PEOA1)

A minority of PEOA1 patients present with parkinsonism. The parkinsonism is characterized as mixed-type, and usually occurs at least five years after the initial symptoms of PEO or ptosis. Patients respond well to L-dopa therapy. Routine brain MRI may show leukoencephalopathy that is accompanied by atrophy of the cerebrum, cerebellum and/or basal ganglia. ^{18}Fluorine-CFT PET of parkinsonian patients shows reduced radiotracer uptake in the striatum bilaterally (74). PEOA1 is caused by mutations in the *POLG* gene, encoding the α-subunit of polymerase γ (POLG), which is a protein that is ubiquitously expressed in the CNS (9). POLG is associated with the synthesis and repair of mitochondrial DNA in mammalian cells. To date, more than 60 *POLG* mutations and variants have been reported to be associated with PEOA1 (19). *POLG* mutations have also been identified in patients with PD.

Progressive External Ophthalmoplegia with Mitochondrial DNA Deletions 3 (PEOA3)

A minority of PEOA3 patients present with parkinsonism. The parkinsonism is characterized as mixed-type and usually occurs at least 20 years after the initial symptom of PEO or ptosis. Patients respond well to L-dopa therapy. Routine brain MRI may show leukoencephalopathy, accompanied by atrophy of the cerebrum, cerebellum, and/or basal ganglia. ^{123}I-FP-CIT SPECT of parkinsonian patients shows reduced radiotracer uptake in the putamen bilaterally.

PEOA3 is caused by mutations in the *C10orf2* gene. *C10orf2* encodes twinkle, a protein that is expressed in mitochondrial nucleoids. Twinkle is associated with mitochondrial DNA replication and stability. To date, approximately 40 C10orf2 mutations and variants have been reported to be associated with PEOA3 (19).

Perry Syndrome (PS)

PS is an extremely rare neurodegenerative disease. Its prevalence has not been well investigated. The vast majority of patients present with rapidly progressive parkinsonism, which is characterized as akinetic-rigid type and is occasionally accompanied by resting tremor. Patients usually respond to high doses of L-dopa therapy. Routine brain MRI is usually normal.

PS is caused by mutations in the DCTN1 gene. DCTN1 encodes dynactin-1, which is a protein that is abundantly expressed in the CNS (9). Dynactin-1 is associated with dynein-related retrograde movement of vesicles and organelles in the cytoplasm and along the microtubules. To date, five DCTN1 mutations have been reported to be associated with PS (19).

Wilson Disease (WD)

WD is a common, autosomal recessive disease that affects copper metabolism. The prevalence is estimated to be approximately 1-3/100,000 in the general population. The majority of patients present with parkinsonism that is characterized by bradykinesia, hypomimia, rigidity, and resting tremor. Patients may partially respond to L-dopa therapy. Chelation therapy with penicillamine improves the clinical features, including tremor and parkinsonism. Low levels of serum copper and ceruloplasmin concentrations and elevated urinary copper excretion can be useful diagnostic tools. Routine brain MRI shows hyperintensity in the caudate nucleus, globus pallidus, putamen, and thalamus on T2WI, as well as atrophy of the cerebrum and brainstem. ^{123}I-CIT PET and ^{123}I-IBZM SPECT of parkinsonian patients show reduced radiotracer uptake in the striatum.

WD is caused by mutations in the ATP7B gene. ATP7B encodes ATPase, Cu^{2+}-transporting, beta polypeptide (ATP7B), which is a protein that is ubiquitously expressed in the CNS (9). ATP7B is associated with the export of copper out of cells. To date, 647 ATP7B mutations and variants have been reported to be associated with WD (19). ATP7B mutations have been also identified in patients with early-onset PD and AD.

Woodhouse-Sakati Syndrome (WSS)

WSS, also known as hypogonadism, alopecia, diabetes mellitus, mental retardation, and extrapyramidal syndrome, is a rare, autosomal recessive, neuroendocrine and ectodermal disorder. Its prevalence has not been well investigated. So far, only one patient, carrying a DCAF17 G906A mutation, has developed parkinsonism during the course of the illness (75). The parkinsonism was characterized as mixed-type. L-dopa responsiveness was not reported. Low levels of serum insulin-like growth factor-1 and testosterone can be useful diagnostic tools. Routine brain MRI is usually normal.

WSS is caused by mutations in the DCAF17 gene, which is also called C2orf37 gene. DCAF17 encodes DDB1 and CUL4-associated factor 17 (DCAF17), which is a protein that is expressed in the CNS, liver, and skin tissues. The precise function of DCAF17 is not fully understood. To date, nine DCAF17 mutations and variants have been reported to be associated with WSS (19).

Familial parkinsonism with provisional gene mutations or without known gene mutations (Table 16.7)

Many other familial disorders that present with pure PD phenotype or parkinsonism have been reported without known causative genes. We have listed examples of these disorders in Table 16.7.

Summary

In this chapter, we provided the clinical and genetic characteristics of 76 disorders that can present with PD or parkinsonism during the

Table16.7
Example of familial disorders with provisional gene mutations or without known gene mutations with parkinsonism as one of the symptoms.

	Gene	Clinical features	L-dopa responsiveness
Corticobasal degeneration	Unknown	**P, CI, Pyr, dystonia**, LP, CA, dysautonomia	Minimal-none
CMT disease with ptosis and parkinsonism	Unknown	**Ppes cavus, PN, ptosis**, P, mild CI, dysautonomia, central hypoventilation, dystonic-choreiform movement	Good-none
Dementia/parkinsonism/with non-Alzheimer amyloid plaques	Unknown	**CI, P**, dysarthria, BP, T, LP, Psy, Pyr	None
Dementia with Lewy body disease	Unknown	**CI, Psy, P, RBD**, neuroleptic sensitivity	Minimal-none
IBGC 1	Unknown	**P**, CI, CA, Psy, Pyr, dysarthria, UI, CA, MR, DD, chorea, PN (athetosis, dyskinesia, dystonia, seizure, T, tics)	None
IBGC 2	Unknown	**CI**, Psy, dysarthria, LP, P chorea, hyperreflexia, CA, short stature (amyotrophy)	Unknown
Multiple system atrophy	Unknown	**Dysautonomia, UI, P, CA, RBD**, Pyr, OMA	Moderate-none
PARK3	Unknown	**PD** (T, CI)	Good
PARK5	Unknown	**PD**	Good
PARK10	Unknown	**PD**	Good
PARK11	GIGYF2	**PD**	Good
PARK12	Unknown	**PD**	Good
PARK13	HTRA2	**PD**	Good
PARK15	FBXO7	**PD, Pyr, Psy**, dystonia, dysarthria, dysphagia, CI, slow saccades	Good
PARK16	Unknown	**PD**	Good
Progressive supranuclear palsy	Unknown	**P, CI, PC, Pyr, OMA, dystonia, dysarthria, dysphagia, UI**, T, CA (anosmia, dysautonomia, dyskinesia, myoclonus, PN)	Minimal-none*
SCA9	Unknown	**CA**, OMA, Pyr, muscle weakness, P	Unknown
SCA20	Unknown	**CA, dysarthria, OMA, P, T**, Pyr	Unknown
SCA21	Unknown	**CA**, dysgraphia, hyporeflexia, T, P, CI	None
Waisman parkinsonism-mental retardation syndrome	Unknown	**P, MR, frontal bossing**, seizure, megalencephaly, strabismus	Unknown

course of the illness. In addition, we have also discussed the mitochondrial gene mutations associated with PD or parkinsonism phenotypes (76). Several gene mutations have been reported to be risk factors for PD. Common polymorphisms in two genes, *SNCA* and *LRRK2*, as well as variations in two other genes, *MAPT* and *GBA,* have been identified to be risk factors for PD (77). Additionally, several recent, genome-wide association studies (GWAS) (77) have nominated susceptibility genetic variants associated with PD. From these studies, we have learned that *SNCA* and *MAPT* are the most frequently replicated genes in PD cases, followed by *LRRK2, BST1, GAK, PARK16,* and others. GWAS studies require large sample sizes and can be expensive. To manage these challenges, new genetic techniques have emerged such as next-generation sequencing, which includes whole-exome or whole-genome sequencing. These new techniques allow us to sequence the entire human genome.

Detailed medical interviews and precise neurological examinations are crucial initial steps toward a correct diagnosis. A well gathered medical history provides important information on family history, clinical course, ethnic background, and other important details that are essential for making a correct diagnosis. Family history is crucial, because most patients with genetic disorders have other affected family members. This information also helps to delineate the possible mode of inheritance. However, several factors such as reduced or incomplete penetrance (78), recessive form of inheritance, de novo mutations, intrafamilial variability of clinical phenotypes, false paternity, or undisclosed adaption may mask the presence of genetic disorders. Clustering the disease in a cer-

tain population may indicate the associated genetic and environmental factors. Several environmental factors, including pesticides, industrial agents, heavy metals, farming, a history of drinking well water, a history of obesity, exposure to head trauma, or a history of emotional stress have been reported to be associated with an increased risk for PD (79). If a patient's clinical course is similar to that seen in a known genetic disorder, it may be suggestive of the presence of the same genetic factor. Ethnic background is sometimes useful to estimate potential causative genes. For examples, the LRRK2 G2019S mutation is frequently identified in populations of Ashkenazi Jewish or Northern Berber origin. *TAF1* mutations are frequently reported in populations from the Philippines. Precise neurological examination is vital. Parkinsonian features can potentially be misdiagnosed. Spasticity without muscle weakness could masquerade as bradykinesia. However, gegenhalten due to frontal lobe involvement can rarely be mistaken as muscle rigidity.

There are several limitations associated with genetic tests, such as phenocopy, digenic inheritance, and false negative/positive genetic results. Phenocopy is a condition in which a non-genetic phenotype is identical to another family member who is afflicted with a genetic disorder. Phenocopies may represent up to five percent of PD with *SNCA, LRRK2, PRKN,* and *PINK1* mutations (80). Digenic inheritance is a condition in which patients carry heterozygous mutations in two different genes (81). Finally, we have received false-negative and false-positive genetic results from commercial laboratories. We were able to catch these laboratory errors only because the same patients participated in our research studies, and the commercial results did not match the

BP = behavioural problems; CA = cerebellar ataxia; CI = cognitive impairment; CMT = Charcot-Marie-Tooth; DD = developmental delay; FBXO7 = F-box protein 7; GIGYF2 = GRB10 interacting GYF protein 2; HTRA2 = HtrA serine peptidase 2; IBGC = idiopathic ganglia calcification; LP = language problems; MR = mental retardation; OMA = oculomotor abnormalities; P = Parkinsonism; PD = Parkinson disease; PN = peripheral neuropathy; Psy = psychiatric symptoms; Pyr = pyramidal signs; RBD = rapid eye movement sleep behaviour disorder; SCA = spinocerebellar ataxia; T = tremor; UI = urinary incontinence; *a subset of cases respond to L-dopa therapy well; clinical features in bold are frequently seen in patients (>50% of patients); clinical features in parentheses are occasionally seen in patients (<10% of patients).

research results. Therefore, we advocate caution in trusting the commercially available genetic results provided to physicians. If there are any doubts, another genetic test is indicated, perhaps in a different commercial laboratory. Genetic testing is new; therefore, the possibility of false-negative or false-positive results must always be considered by the treating physician. Given that curative therapeutics are not currently available for most parkinsonian disorders, genetic counseling, education on specific disorders, symptomatic treatment, psychiatric support, comprehensive management involving the input of several specialties, and referral to support groups are critical. Several useful websites are publically available for patients (19, 82-84). Additionally, sharing the clinical and genetic information with appropriate ethical/IRB committee approval is essential to understand many of these rare genetic disorders (85). Diagnostic genetic testing is available for almost all genes discussed in this chapter (see Tables 16.1-16.6).

The genetic causes of many monogenic forms of PD and parkinsonism with a Mendelian pattern of inheritance have already been revealed, but many more still await discovery. The genetic factors do not explain the entire aetiology of these disorders. Thus, a combination of inherited and environmental factors may play a crucial role in their causation. Comprehensive research on these disorders is just getting started. We hope that a better understanding of the underlying pathogenesis of parkinsonian disorders will lead to the discovery of etiologic-based radical treatments that will be specific to the particular genetic defects.

Acknowledgements

ZKW is partially supported by the NIH/NINDS P50 NS072187, Mayo Clinic Center for Regenerative Medicine, Dystonia Medical Research Foundation, The Michael J. Fox Foundation for Parkinson's Research, and the gift from Carl Edward Bolch, Jr., and Susan Bass Bolch. We thank Kelly E. Viola for her editorial assistance.

References

1 Jankovic J. Parkinson's disease: clinical features and diagnosis. J Neurol Neurosurg Psychiatry 2008;79:368-376.

2 Gelb DJ, Oliver E, Gilman S. Diagnostic criteria for Parkinson disease. Arch Neurol 1999;56:33-39.

3 Parkinson Disease Mutation Database. [cited 2013 5/6]; Available from: www.molgen.vib-ua.be/PD-mutDB.

4 Appel-Cresswell S, Vilarino-Guell C, Encarnacion M, et al. Alpha-synuclein p.H50Q, a novel pathogenic mutation for Parkinson's disease. Mov Disord 2013; 28:811-833.

5 Proukakis C, Dudzik CG, Brier T, et al. A novel alpha-synuclein missense mutation in Parkinson disease. Neurology 2013;80:1062-1064.

6 Kiely AP, Asi YT, Kara E, et al. alpha-Synucleinopathy associated with G51D SNCA mutation: a link between Parkinson's disease and multiple system atrophy? Acta Neuropathol 2013;125:753-769.

7 Lesage S, Anheim M, Letournel F, et al. G51D alpha-synuclein mutation causes a novel parkinsonian-pyramidal syndrome. Ann Neurol 2013;doi: 10.1002/ana.23894.

8 Hering R, Strauss KM, Tao X, et al. Novel homozygous p.E64D mutation in DJ1 in early onset Parkinson disease (PARK7). Hum Mutat 2004;24:321-329.

9 Gene Cards. [cited 2013 5/7]; available from: gene4.weizmann.ac.il.

10 Wider C, Skipper L, Solida A, et al. Autosomal dominant dopa-responsive parkinsonism in a multigenerational Swiss family. parkinsonism Relat Disord 2008;14:465-470.

11 Vilarino-Guell C, Wider C, Ross OA, et al. VPS35 mutations in Parkinson disease. Am J Hum Genet 2011;89:162-167.

12 Chartier-Harlin MC, Dachsel JC, Vilarino-Guell C, et al. Translation initiator EIF4G1 mutations in familial Parkinson disease. Am J Hum Genet 2011;89:398-406.

13 Edwards-Lee T, Ringman JM, Chung J, et al. An African American family with early-onset Alzheimer disease and an APP (T714I) mutation. Neurology 2005;64:377-379.

14 Pasalar P, Najmabadi H, Noorian AR, et al. An Iranian family with Alzheimer's disease caused by a novel APP mutation (Thr714Ala). Neurology 2002;58:1574-1575.

15 Alzheimer Disease & Frontotemporal Dementia Mutation Database. [cited 2013 5/7]; Available from: www.molgen.vib-ua.be/FTDMutations.

16 Piscopo P, Marcon G, Piras MR, et al. A novel PSEN2 mutation associated with a peculiar phenotype. Neurology 2008;70:1549-1554.

17 Akiyama H, Nishimura T, Kondo H, Ikeda K, Hayashi Y, McGeer PL. Expression of the receptor for macrophage colony stimulating factor by brain microglia and its upregulation in brains of patients with Alzheimer's disease and amyotrophic lateral sclerosis. Brain Res 1994;639:171-174.

18 Stanley ER, Berg KL, Einstein DB, et al. Biology and action of colony – stimulating factor-1. Mol Reprod Dev 1997;46:4-10.

19 The Human Gene Mutation Database. [cited 2013 4/25]; available from: www.hgmd.cf.ac.uk/ac/index.php.

20 De Coo IF, Renier WO, Ruitenbeek W, et al. A 4-base pair deletion in the mitochondrial cytochrome b gene associated with parkinsonism/MELAS overlap syndrome. Ann Neurol 1999;45:130-133.

21 Howard KL, Hall DA, Moon M, Agarwal P, Newman E, Brenner M. Adult-onset Alexander disease with progressive ataxia and palatal tremor. Mov Disord 2008;23:118-122.

22 Salvi F, Aoki Y, Della Nave R, et al. Adult Alexander's disease without leukoencephalopathy. Ann Neurol 2005;58:813-814.

23 Li R, Johnson AB, Salomons G, et al. Glial fibrillary acidic protein mutations in infantile, juvenile, and adult forms of Alexander disease. Ann Neurol 2005;57:310-326.

24 Yoshida T, Sasayama H, Mizuta I, et al. Glial fibrillary acidic protein mutations in adult-onset Alexander disease: clinical features observed in 12 Japanese patients. Acta Neurol Scand 2011;124:104-108.

25 Van Langenhove T, van der Zee J, Sleegers K, et al. Genetic contribution of FUS to frontotemporal lobar degeneration. Neurology 2010;74:366-371.

26 Yan J, Deng HX, Siddique N, et al. Frameshift and novel mutations in FUS in familial amyotrophic lateral sclerosis and ALS/dementia. Neurology 2010;75:807-814.

27 van Es MA, Diekstra FP, Veldink JH, et al. A case of ALS-FTD in a large FALS pedigree with a K17I ANG mutation. Neurology 2009;72:287-288.

28 van Es MA, Schelhaas HJ, van Vught PW, et al. Angiogenin variants in Parkinson disease and amyotrophic lateral sclerosis. Ann Neurol 2011;70:964-973.

29 Borghero G, Floris G, Cannas A, et al. A patient carrying a homozygous p.A382T TARDBP missense mutation shows a syndrome including ALS, extrapyramidal symptoms, and FTD. Neurobiol Aging 2011;32:2327 e1-5.

30 Mosca L, Lunetta C, Tarlarini C, al. Wide phenotypic spectrum of the TARDBP gene: homozygosity of A382T mutation in a patient presenting with amyotrophic lateral sclerosis, Parkinson's disease, and frontotemporal lobar degeneration, and in neurologically healthy subject. Neurobiol Aging 2012;33:1846 e1-4.

31 Quadri M, Cossu G, Saddi V, et al. Broadening the phenotype of TARDBP mutations: the TARDBP Ala382Thr mutation and Parkinson's disease in Sardinia. Neurogenetics 2011;12:203-209.

32 Rayaprolu S, Fujioka S, Traynor S, et al. TARDBP mutations in Parkinson's disease. Parkinsonism Relat Disord 2013;19:312-315.

33 Spina S, Van Laar AD, Murrell JR, et al. Phenotypic variability in three families with valosin-containing protein mutation. Eur J Neurol 2013;20:251-258.

34 Goizet C, Boukhris A, Mundwiller E, et al. Complicated forms of autosomal dominant hereditary spastic paraplegia are frequent in SPG10. Hum Mutat 2009;30:376-385.

35 Guidubaldi A, Piano C, Santorelli FM, et al. Novel mutations in SPG11 cause hereditary spastic paraplegia associated with early-onset levodopa-responsive parkinsonism. Mov Disord 2011;26:553-556.

36 Everett CM, Kara E, Maresh KE, Houlden H. Clinical variability and L-Dopa responsive parkinsonism in hereditary spastic paraplegia 11. J Neurol 2012;259:2726-2728.

37 Anheim M, Lagier-Tourenne C, Stevanin G, et al. SPG11 spastic paraplegia. A new cause of juvenile parkinsonism. J Neurol 2009;256:104-108.

38 Poorkaj P, Raskind WH, Leverenz JB, et al. A novel X-linked four-repeat tauopathy with parkinsonism and spasticity. Mov Disord 2010;25:1409-1417.

39 Mori N, Adachi Y, Takeshima T, Kashiwaya Y, Okada A, Nakashima K. Branched-chain amino acid therapy for spinocerebellar degeneration: a pilot clinical crossover trial. Intern Med 1999;38:40140-6.

40 Schols L, Bauer P, Schmidt T, Schulte T, Riess O. Autosomal dominant cerebellar ataxias: clinical features, genetics, and pathogenesis. Lancet Neurol 2004;3:291-304.

41 Holmes SE, Hearn EO, Ross CA, Margolis RL. SCA12: an unusual mutation leads to an unusual spinocerebellar ataxia. Brain Res Bull 2001;56:397-403.

42 Holmes SE, O'Hearn EE, McInnis MG, et al. Expansion of a novel CAG trinucleotide repeat in the 5' region of PPP2R2B is associated with SCA12. Nat Genet 1999;23:391-392.

43 Brussino A, Graziano C, Giobbe D, et al. Spinocerebellar ataxia type 12 identified in two Italian families may mimic sporadic ataxia. Mov Disord 2010;25:1269-1273.

44 van de Warrenburg BP, Verbeek DS, Piersma SJ, et al. Identification of a novel SCA14 mutation in a Dutch autosomal dominant cerebellar ataxia family. Neurology 2003;61:1760-1765.

45 Stevanin G, Hahn V, Lohmann E, et al. Mutation in the catalytic domain of protein kinase C gamma and extension of the phenotype associated with spinocerebellar ataxia type 14. Arch Neurol 2004;61:1242-1248.

46 Klebe S, Durr A, Rentschler A, et al. New mutations in protein kinase Cgamma associated with spinocerebellar ataxia type 14. Ann Neurol 2005;58:720-729.

47 Visser JE, Bloem BR, van de Warrenburg BP. PRKCG mutation (SCA-14) causing a Ramsay Hunt phenotype. Mov Disord 2007;22:1024-1026.

48 Bakalkin G, Watanabe H, Jezierska J, et al. Prodynorphin mutations cause the neurodegenerative disorder spinocerebellar ataxia type 23. Am J Hum Genet 2010;87:593-603.

49 Cooper JR, Bloom FE. The biochemical basis of neuropharmacology. 7th ed. New York: Oxford University Press 1996.

50 Dill P, Wagner M, Somerville A, Thony B, Blau N, Weber P. Child neurology: paroxysmal stiffening, upward gaze, and hypotonia: hallmarks of sepiapterin reductase deficiency. Neurology 2012;78:29-32.

51 Lipton J, Rivkin MJ. 16p11.2-related paroxysmal kinesigenic dyskinesia and dopa-responsive parkinsonism in a child. Neurology 2009;73:479-480.

52 Camargos S, Scholz S, Simon-Sanchez J, et al. DYT16, a novel young-onset dystonia-parkinsonism disorder: identification of a segregating mutation in the stress-response protein PRKRA. Lancet Neurol 2008;7:207-215.

53 Seibler P, Djarmati A, Langpap B, et al. A heterozygous frameshift mutation in PRKRA (DYT16) associated with generalised dystonia in a German patient. Lancet Neurol 2008;7:380-381.

54 Lagrue E, Abe H, Lavanya M, et al. Regional characterization of energy metabolism in the brain of normal and MPTP-intoxicated mice using new markers of glucose and phosphate transport. J Biomed Sci 2010;17:91.

55 Nicolas G, Pottier C, Maltete D, et al. Mutation of the PDGFRB gene as a cause of idiopathic basal ganglia calcification. Neurology 2013;80:181-187.

56 Kurian MA, Li Y, Zhen J, et al. Clinical and molecular characterisation of hereditary dopamine transporter deficiency syndrome: an observational cohort and experimental study. Lancet Neurol 2011;10:54-62.

57 Kurian MA, Zhen J, Cheng SY, et al. Homozygous loss-of-function mutations in the gene encoding the dopamine transporter are associated with infantile parkinsonism-dystonia. J Clin Invest 2009;119:1595-1603.

58 Puffenberger EG, Jinks RN, Sougnez C, et al. Genetic mapping and exome sequencing identify variants associated with five novel diseases. PLoS One 2012;7:e28936.

59 Volders P, Van Hove J, Lories RJ, et al. Niemann-Pick disease type B: an unusual clinical presentation

with multiple vertebral fractures. Am J Med Genet 2002;109:42-51.

60 Grant DB, Dunger DB, Smith I, Hyland K. Familial glucocorticoid deficiency with achalasia of the cardia associated with mixed neuropathy, long-tract degeneration and mild dementia. Eur J Pediatr 1992;151:85-89.

61 Houlden H, Smith S, De Carvalho M, et al. Clinical and genetic characterization of families with triple A (Allgrove) syndrome. Brain 2002;125:2681-2690.

62 van Diggelen OP, Thobois S, Tilikete C, et al. Adult neuronal ceroid lipofuscinosis with palmi-toyl-protein thioesterase deficiency: first adult-on-set patients of a childhood disease. Ann Neurol 2001;50:269-272.

63 Silveira-Moriyama L, Moriyama TS, Gabbi TV, Ran-vaud R, Barbosa ER. Chediak-Higashi syndrome with parkinsonism. Mov Disord 2004;19:472-475.

64 Uyama E, Hirano T, Ito K, et al. Adult Chediak-Hi-gashi syndrome presenting as parkinsonism and dementia. Acta Neurol Scand 1994;89:175-183.

65 Jacobi C, Koerner C, Fruehauf S, Rottenburger C, Storch-Hagenlocher B, Grau AJ. Presynaptic dopaminergic pathology in Chediak-Higashi syn-drome with parkinsonian syndrome. Neurology 2005;64:1814-1815.

66 Goker-Alpan O, Schiffmann R, LaMarca ME, Nussbaum RL, McInerney-Leo A, Sidransky E. par-kinsonism among Gaucher disease carriers. J Med Genet 2004;41:937-940.

67 Machaczka M, Rucinska M, Skotnicki AB, Ju-rczak W. Parkinson's syndrome preceding clinical manifestation of Gaucher's disease. Am J Hematol 1999;61:216-217.

68 Costello DJ, Walsh SL, Harrington HJ, Walsh CH. Concurrent hereditary haemochromatosis and idiopathic Parkinson's disease: a case report series. J Neurol Neurosurg Psychiatry 2004;75:631-633.

69 Demarquay G, Setiey A, Morel Y, Trepo C, Chazot G, Broussolle E. Clinical report of three patients with hereditary hemochromatosis and movement disorders. Mov Disord 2000;15:1204-1209.

70 Jones HR, Jr., Hedley-Whyte ET. Idiopathic hemo-chromatosis (IHC): dementia and ataxia as present-ing signs. Neurology 1983;33:1479-1483.

71 Nielsen JE, Jensen LN, Krabbe K. Hereditary haemochromatosis: a case of iron accumulation in the basal ganglia associated with a parkinso-nian syndrome. J Neurol Neurosurg Psychiatry 1995;59:318-321.

72 Nandar W, Connor JR. HFE gene variants affect iron in the brain. J Nutr 2011;141:729-739.

73 Horvath R, Kley RA, Lochmuller H, Vorgerd M. Parkinson syndrome, neuropathy, and myopathy caused by the mutation A8344G (MERRF) in tR-NALys. Neurology 2007;68:56-58.

74 Luoma P, Melberg A, Rinne JO, et al. parkinsonism, premature menopause, and mitochondrial DNA polymerase gamma mutations: clinical and molecu-lar genetic study. Lancet 2004;364:875-882.

75 Steindl K, Alazami AM, Bhatia KP, et al. A novel C2orf37 mutation causes the first Italian cas-es of Woodhouse Sakati syndrome. Clin Genet 2010;78:594-597.

76 Finsterer J. Parkinson's syndrome and Parkinson's disease in mitochondrial disorders. Mov Disord 2011;26:784-791.

77 Pahwa R, Lyons KE. Handbook of Parkinson's Dis-ease. 5th ed. New York: Informa Healthcare 2013.

78 Sierra M, Gonzalez-Aramburu I, Sanchez-Juan P, et al. High frequency and reduced penetrance of LRRK2 G2019S mutation among Parkinson's disease patients in Cantabria (Spain). Mov Disord 2011;26:2343-2346.

79 Pfeiffer R, Wszolek ZK, Ebadi MS. Parkinson's dis-ease. 2nd ed. Boca Raton, FL: CRC Press 2013.

80 Klein C, Chuang R, Marras C, Lang AE. The cu rious case of phenocopies in families with genetic Parkinson's disease. Mov Disord 2011;26:1793-1802.

81 Funayama M, Li Y, Tsoi TH, et al. Familial parkin-sonism with digenic parkin and PINK1 mutations. Mov Disord 2008;23:1461-1465.

82 GeneTests. Available from: http://www.ncbi.nlm.nih.gov/sites/GeneTests/lab?db=GeneTests.

83 GeneReviews. Available from: http://www.ncbi.nlm.nih.gov/sites/GeneTests/review.

84 OMIM: www.omim.org.

85 Genetic Epidemiology of Parkinson's Disease. [cited 2013 5/14]; Available from: http://www.geopd.org/.

17

Vascular Parkinsonism

Barbara Pickut

Vascular parkinsonism (VP) as a clinical entity can be situated within the broader context of parkinsonism syndromes and is comprised of an array of clinical features including characteristic parkinsonism, gait disorder, corticospinal and pseudobulbar signs and symptoms. As the name suggests, etiologically VP may be defined as a syndrome occurring in relation to ischemic cerebrovascular disease (CVD) and is thus classified as secondary parkinsonism. VP is also known as vascular pseudo-parkinsonism, arteriosclerotic parkinsonism, arteriosclerotic pseudo-parkinsonism, lower-body (half) parkinsonism, and cerebrovascular gait disorder.

The first conceptualization of VP was made by Critchley in 1929. Coining the term 'arteriosclerotic parkinsonism', he described a spectrum of parkinson-like clinical presentations in the elderly and ascribed them to CVD. He identified the most common type as forming the basis for the disease entity. This consisted of rigidity, masked face, and a short-stepping gait. The addition of pseudobulbar features constituted the second type; coexisting with dementia and urinary incontinence as the third type; additional occurrence with pyramidal signs as the fourth type; and occurring together with cerebellar signs as the fifth type (1). In the ensuing years Critchley's concept was criticised. It was thought that the co-occurrence of a cerebrovascular accident and idiopathic Parkinson's disease could yield clinical presentations similar to those described by Critchley, and as such could represent merely incidental findings. There was also a lack of clinicopathological data as a basis of diagnosis to substantiate Critchley's concept (2,3). Later, Critchley refined his definition to 'arteriosclerotic *pseudo*parkinsonism', in an attempt to differentiate it from Parkinson's disease (PD) both clinically and pathologically (4).

This brief history illustrates that the mechanisms involved in the causes and development of VP may overlap in the clinical presentation. This may confound a clinical diagnosis and thus yield therapeutic challenges. Although the subsequent development of neuroimaging has provided support for the original concept, a direct correlation between vascular load or specific vascular lesions and VP in any given patient suffering from suspected VP may still be difficult to establish, if at all possible. Furthermore, post-mortem studies have yielded evidence showing that patients with vascular lesions may present with clinical syndromes similar to PD - including levodopa responsiveness (5). Nevertheless, current clinical descriptions of VP closely resemble the original work of Critchley whose findings were made without the benefit of the diagnostic technologies now available.

VP is still considered by some as a loose constellation of various clinical features (6) and a distinct clinical entity by others (7) and as such remains a controversial concept. It is widely accepted that CVD can cause elements of parkinsonism and that VP is a clinical entity necessitating a therapeutic approach differing from that in idiopathic PD. Nevertheless, the heterogeneous extent of the underlying pathologies of VP, as well as the clinical presentation and possible levodopa responsiveness, make a concise and practical, clinically useful definition of VP challenging.

Epidemiology

Prevalence figures are mostly based on brain bank autopsy data including patients with previously diagnosed idiopathic PD and other causes of parkinsonism. In the UK Parkinson disease society brain bank series and other population-based studies, VP accounted for 1.4-3% of all cases of parkinsonism, although these figures may be an underestimate (8). Jellinger reported that in three personal, consecutive, 45-year autopsy series of 759 patients with clinical parkinsonism in Vienna, Austria (1957-2002), the prevalence of neuropathologically confirmed VP was 3.4% (9). He also indicated that about 6% of 400 parkinsonism cases in an autopsy series could be classified as having disease of vascular origin, showing multi-infarct atrophy, hypertensive or Binswanger-type encephalopathy, and/or multiple vascular lesions in the basal ganglia and brain stem, with no or only mild degenerative nigral damage. In a series of 387 cases of Lewy body disease (LBD), including both idiopathic PD and dementia with Lewy bodies (DLB) patients, Jellinger found 64.5% to be free of cerebrovascular pathology except for minor to moderate amyloid angiopathy not associated with ischemic damage (10). Similar observations were made in age-matched controls, and the differences were therefore not significant (10). However, in most of these series, parkinsonism was poorly defined, and the location and extent of vascular lesions were not adequately documented. Furthermore, 9.3% of VP patients had Lewy bodies in the substantia nigra (SN), outnumbering the rate of incidental Lewy body disease (iLBD) cases. According to Sibon et al., pathological reclassification of patients diagnosed as having idiopathic PD during life revealed VP in 1-3% (11). Therefore, it seems justified to estimate the prevalence of VP in a series

of parkinsonistic patients between 1% and 6%. At present, even an estimate of incidence is not available and can only indirectly be derived from the incidence of parkinsonism. Reliable clinical diagnostic criteria may well enhance the reliability of incidence and prevalence figures (7).

Aetiology

The association of VP with transient ischemic attacks and/or stroke, as well as with cardiovascular risk factors such as arterial hypertension, coronary heart disease, atrial fibrillation, myocardial infarction, diabetes mellitus, history of smoking, or hyperlipidemia, is somewhat controversial. Of all patients who have suffered CVD, only a small proportion develops parkinsonism. This is true for patients suffering a single infarct as well as ones who suffered multiple small infarcts. Ischemic damage to the SN is quite rare, and therefore, parkinsonism is seldom caused by a mesencephalic infarct. Parkinsonism has been reported more frequently in association with infarcts affecting the basal ganglia or the anterior cerebral artery territory. Some rare cases of unilateral parkinsonism following infarcts in the territories of the lenticulostriate arteries have also been reported. Rather than a single infarct, widespread periventricular and frontal lobe white-matter lesions may underlie bilateral gait disturbances, and multiple lesions of the striatum have been associated with parkinsonism. Multiple white-matter lesions have also been incriminated, but as they are frequently found in elderly patients, these lesions are probably more of a nonspecific marker. Small-vessel CVD in the white matter and basal ganglia is often a complication of hypertension or diabetes (12).

VP might also complicate idiopathic PD. Incidental ischemic lesions have been documented in a quarter of patients with pathologically proven PD (8,13) and might have contributed to the progression of symptoms in PD (14).

In addition to corticospinal and pseudobulbar symptoms, other (strategic) ischemic lesion-induced signs and symptoms might be seen in VP, including subcortical-type dementia.

Pathophysiology

The putative pathophysiology of VP varies according to the type of lesions and symptoms observed. For example, the pathophysiology of abrupt-onset parkinsonism due to a large infarct affecting the basal ganglia may differ from that of insidious parkinsonism or 'pseudoparkinsonism' due to lacunar or chronic ischemic changes affecting the subcortical white matter. Quite typically, in VP, symptoms mainly and mostly affect the lower body half. This might be understood from the neuropathology.

Neuropathology

The neuropathology of VP is as diverse as its clinical presentation. Vascular lesions in patients with PD are quite common and may not be sufficient to cause an extrapyramidal syndrome (EPS), but they certainly contribute to clinical worsening. Jellinger described his personal experience with an autopsy series of 700 cases clinically diagnosed with parkinsonism (1957-2000) (15). PD of Lewy body type was confirmed in over 80% of these cases, with co-existing cerebrovascular lesions in about 20%, mostly subcortical white-matter changes or basal ganglia lacunes. Yamanouchi et al. described clinico-neuropathological findings in a series of 24 pathologically confirmed VP patients with normal preservation of SN pigmented neurons (16), and compared the findings with those in 30 PD patients. Compared to PD (50%), only < 5% of VP patients suffered from tremor. Some 80% of those patients, but not PD patients, displayed pyramidal tract signs, with clinical hemiparesis in half of them. Pseudobulbar palsies were found in half of VP patients. Zijlmans et al. described a series of 17 elderly patients with suspected VP (a clinical diagnosis of PD lacking neuropatho-

logical confirmation of LBD) and particularly studied white-matter changes including perivascular pallor, gliosis, arteriolar hyaline thickening, and enlargement of perivascular spaces as well as macroscopically visible infarcts (7) and compared these results with their findings in 10 age-matched control patients with hypertension but lacking parkinsonism. Less than half of the VP patients suffered from hypertension. Macroscopically visible lacunar infarcts or lacunae caused by enlarged perivascular spaces were observed in the caudate, putamen, and globus pallidus of VP but not PD patients. Four of their supposed VP patients showed a remarkably significant loss of SN dopaminergic neurons (in two cases > 50%). Also of note, half of the VP patients showed rest, postural or kinetic tremor, traditionally considered absent in VP. Thirteen of the 17 suspected VP patients presented with a gait abnormality (reduced steppage or shuffling), nine presented with postural instability, leading to falls and even fractures during the first year. At the time of death, all VP patients suffered bradykinesia, gait abnormality, and instability.

Motor parkinsonism

According to a widely accepted model of basal ganglia circuitry, the cause of VP might be an underlying ischemic lesion of the putamen and external globus pallidus rather than the internal pallidum, motor cortex and/or pyramidal tract. Such lesions might result in subthalamic and internal pallidum overactivity, inducing akinesia through overinhibition of the motor thalamus (see earlier chapters). Some authors, though, hypothesize that lesions potentially inducing VP can be situated anywhere in the cortico-subcortical basal ganglia motor loops (17).

Focal lesions of the basal ganglia rarely cause parkinsonism (18). Akyol et al. described an 80-year-old male patient with slowness of movement, rest tremor of his left hand, and tremor of the lower limbs in an upright position, which occurred suddenly and was due to a lacunar infarct

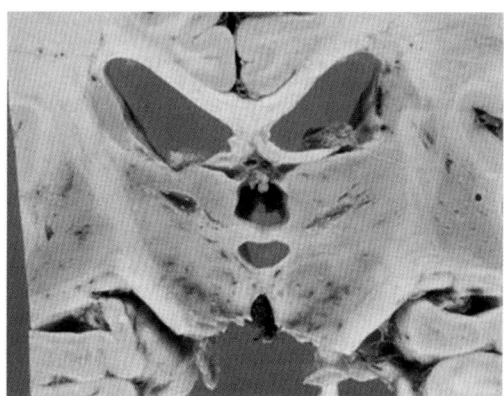

Figure 17.1
Multiple lacunes in both pallida and thalamus (cribriform state).

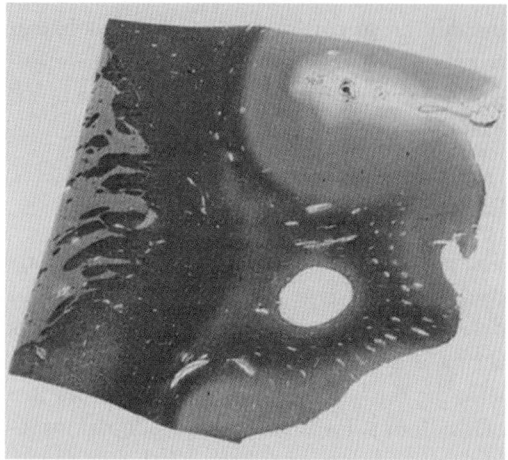

Figure 17.2
Large subcortical lacune and smaller lacunes in striatum.

in the SN and did not respond to levodopa therapy (19). Midbrain lesions, probably secondary to supratentorial pathology, are more common in VP and could also be related to other clinical features, including pseudobulbar signs (20). In exceptional cases, strategic infarcts may cause VP. More commonly, however, multiple basal ganglia or white-matter lesions are assumed to be involved. In 1843, Durand-Fardel described a lacunar state 'avant la lettre' with 'numerous canals or small round holes in the cerebral tissue' referring to this as 'état criblé', meaning 'riddled with shot or sieve-like' (21). The 'cribriform state' corresponds to dilatations of the perivascular spaces leading to a particular type of lacune (22) (see Figure 17.1).

Other types of lacunes are associated with lipohyalinosis of the arteriolar media, leading to vascular occlusion, ischemia and gliosis. These multiple lacunar infarcts in the internal capsule, centrum semiovale, and basal ganglia are characterized by white-matter rarefaction and proliferation of astrocytes and are associated with subcortical atrophy and hydrocephalus 'ex vacuo'. Parkinsonism has been associated with cribriform lesions of the striatum. Reider-Groswasser estimated the frequency of parkinsonism in patients with lacunar lesions of the basal ganglia at 38% (23), and Laitinen et al.'s MRI study of patients with idiopathic PD (IPD) showed lacunes in the posteroventral aspects of the lateral pallidal and posteroventral putaminal regions (24).

Multiple lacunes affecting the basal ganglia and the 'Binswanger type' of white-matter vasculopathy are the anatomical substrates of the white-matter MRI T2-hyperintensities, sometimes resulting in confluent leukoencephalopathy. Tohgi et al. correlated MRI abnormalities with clinical features and suggested that patients with parkinsonism and with a lacunar state in the putamen or confluent white-matter hyperintensity signals may have VP but also IPD (25). These authors suggested that an absence of 4-6 Hz tremor and cogwheel rigidity, and the reduction in the substantia nigra pars compacta width, could be indicators for differentiating VP from true IPD. However, in general, SN width is not considered a reliable parameter for the integrity of dopaminergic neurons.

Gait disturbances

If the theory that VP is caused by multiple lacunar infarctions is correct, what would be the underlying mechanism causing gait disturbances? Since the basal ganglia output is mainly to the supplementary motor area, strategic lesions

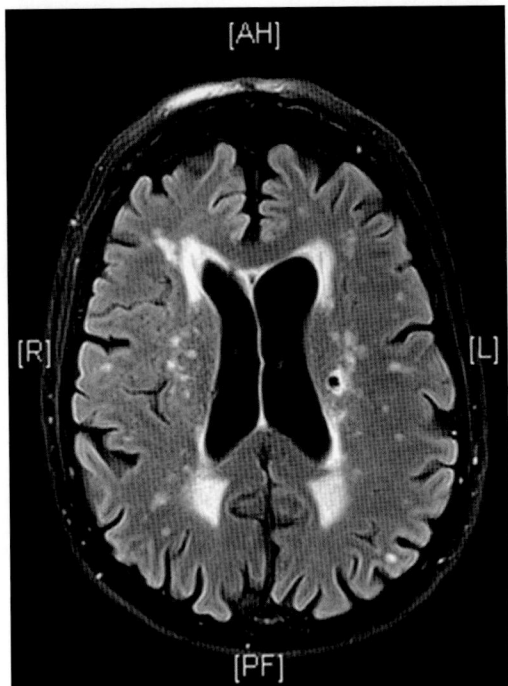

Figure 17.3
White-matter MRI T2-hyperintensities in a 84-year-old male patient suffering from a non-levodopa-responsive, lower-body (half) parkinsonism.

in these projection pathways due to these small infarctions could cause gait apraxia, with disturbed programming and sequence of gait. VP patients are able to use visual, auditory, or other cues, such as pacing or stepping over objects, to facilitate ambulation, illustrating the preservation of cognitive coping mechanisms (26).

Clinical presentation

Classically, VP presents as a bilaterally symmetrical, lower-body half parkinsonism with bradykinesia, rigidity, and a gait disorder due to reduced steppage or a broad-based shuffling, characteristically with an intact arm swing (see Video fragment 17.1). The gait disturbance may be accompanied by a variable stride length (parkinsonian-ataxic gait) in the absence of festination (27). Other authors report festination or motor blocking in the clinical presentation (26). Mobility may be further compromised by

difficulties such as start hesitation, postural instability (retropulsion), and tendency toward falls. The standing posture may be upright with a wide-based stance (12,28). Sometimes, upper body or axial signs and symptoms may also be seen in VP patients.

Bradykinesia is a clinical hallmark (5,29), although perhaps less pronounced than in PD (16,28,30). Hypertonia (spasticity) in combination with rigidity (mostly less pronounced as compared to PD) may present as paratonia or gegenhalten (13,26,28,29,31).

Tremor, if present, typically does not occur as a main feature and is rather of a postural or kinetic type (28). If rest tremor is noted, it is rarely of the pill-rolling type (28,30). Pathological reflexes including hyperreflexia and Hoffman-Tromner's and Babinski's signs can be seen in VP as an expression of corticospinal tract involvement (13,16,28,30). Pseudobulbar signs mainly present as dysphagia, dysarthria or emotional lability (13,16). Sometimes, cognitive decline and urinary incontinence may also be found at presentation (12,32). Patients are typically slightly older at presentation in comparison to PD (13,26,29,30).

In a recent systematic review on differentiating VP from PD, Kalra (6) concluded that VP patients were slightly older, had a shorter duration of symptoms at presentation, and suffered symmetrical gait difficulties. Further clinical features of VP comprised postural instability, falls, dementia, pyramidal signs, pseudobulbar palsy, and incontinence. Bradykinesia and rigidity tended to be less frequent in VP than PD, and occasional tremor in VP was of the postural type.

The typical clinical hallmarks are summarized in Table 17.1

Diagnosis

Unfortunately, no consensus diagnostic criteria for VP are currently available. Several criteria are suggested as helpful, though. Winikates and Jankovic proposed a vascular rating scale for VP

Table 17.1
Clinical hallmarks in VP.

Symptom	Remarks
Age	Slightly older
Bradykinesia	May be less pronounced than in PD
Cognition	Subcortical dementia
Disease duration	Shorter at presentation
Disease progression	Acute, subacute, progressive, stepwise, insidious
Freezing	Present or absent
Gait abnormality	Bilateral gait difficulties: wide-based shuffling, relatively preserved arm swing
Levodopa response	May be less robust if at all, may exhibit intolerance
Lower-body involvement	Typical
Pain	Non-dopa-responsive
Postural instability and falling	May present early
Pseudobulbar findings	May occur as dysphagia, dysarthria, emotional lability
Pyramidal signs	Secondary to ischemic lesions
Rigidity	Mixed-type, paratonic, gegenhalten. May be less pronounced than in PD
Sensory disturbances secondary to stroke	May occur
Symmetry	More or less symmetric
Tremor	Not a main feature. Rarely pill-rolling type
Urinary incontinence	May occur
Visual hallucinations	Uncommon

Table 17.2
Vascular rating scale for VP.

Feature	Points
Pathological or angiographic evidence of diffuse vascular disease	2
Onset of parkinsonism within one month after stroke	1
History of two or more strokes	1
History of two or more vascular risk factors for stroke	1
Neuroimaging evidence of vascular disease in two or more vascular territories	1

including pathologic, angiographic or neuroimaging evidence, onset time in relation to stroke, and vascular risk factors (see Table 17.2) (13). Zijlmans, based on his clinicopathological study, suggested that bradykinesia with gait difficulties together with either tremor and/or postural instability is characteristically more common in VP (7). However, the various authors have stated that evidence on imaging or clinical examination of CVD should be present to support the diagnosis and to correlate with the above-mentioned clinical features. The existence of a bilateral or acute onset and the presence of an early shuffling gait, falls, cognitive impairment, urinary incontinence, and corticospinal or pseudobulbar signs or symptoms are also considered indicative for VP by the authors, though not formally included in the criteria. They further emphasized the need for prospective and retrospective studies to establish the sensitivity, specificity, and predictive values of their proposed criteria (7) (see Table 17.3).

The above-mentioned criteria may serve as a basis for further research designed to formulate accepted diagnostic criteria (6). The patient's history may also provide some clues, e.g. transient ischemic attacks, stroke and cardiovascular risk factors such as arterial hypertension, coronary heart disease, atrial fibrillation, myocardial infarction, diabetes mellitus, history of smoking,

Table 17.3

Possible criteria for the clinical diagnosis of VP (adapted from (7)).

a Bradykinesia including the presence of reduced step length with at least one of the following:
   1 Tremor at rest
   2 Postural instability (visual, vestibular or proprioceptive causes excluded)

b Cerebrovascular disease with evidence from at least one of the following:
   1 Neuroimaging (CT or MRI)
   2 Focal signs or symptoms that are consistent with stroke

c A relationship between the above two disorders. In practice:
   1 An acute or delayed progressive onset with infarcts in or near areas that:
      1.1 increase the basal ganglia motor output (GPe or SNpc)
      1.2 decrease the thalamocortical drive directly (VL of the thalamus or large frontal infarct)
      1.3 consist of a parkinsonian syndrome of contralateral bradykinetic rigidity and shuffling gait within 1 year after a stroke (VPa)
   2 An insidious onset of parkinsonism with extensive subcortical white-matter lesions, bilateral symptoms at onset, and the presence of early shuffling gait or early cognitive dysfunction (VPi)
   3 Exclusion criteria for VP:
      ▪ History of repeated head injury
      ▪ Definite encephalitis
      ▪ Neuroleptic treatment at onset of symptoms
      ▪ Presence of cerebral tumor on CT/MRI
      ▪ Presence of communicating hydrocephalus on CT/MRI
      ▪ Other alternative explanation for parkinsonism

or hyperlipidemia. Co-morbidities may be noted, such as vascular subcortical cognitive deterioration or dementia, as a rule without visual hallucinations (29), with worse performance on frontal/executive tasks compared to PD (32).

The course of the disease in VP might also help with the diagnosis; it may be acute, acute progressive, stepwise or insidious, and disease duration as a rule is also shorter at presentation than in PD. Strategic infarcts in the midbrain and basal ganglia, for example, may cause an acute onset of parkinsonism, whereas a more progressive disease course is seen in small-vessel CVD.

In summary, none of the discussed clinical or imaging criteria taken alone are specific for the diagnosis. Rather, a combination of convergent clinical and imaging clues are necessary to improve the accuracy of the diagnosis. Some degree of certainty may only be achieved when underlying levodopa-responsive idiopathic PD is excluded. However, even here a subcortical ischemic burden in any given PD patient may contribute to the phenomenology, i.e. the presence of (sub)acute severe and/or disproportionate non-levodopa-responsive gait disturbance, bradykinesia, and rigidity, in a patient with otherwise levodopa-responsive parkinsonism, as well as pyramidal and/or bulbar signs and symptoms.

Differential diagnosis

The most important consideration when making a diagnosis in the context of apparent parkinsonism is to differentiate VP from both PD- and not PD related parkinsonism, also referred to as atypical parkinsonism (AP). This distinction has both prognostic and therapeutic implications. The differential diagnosis is lengthy and includes PD as well as other neurodegenerative diseases such as multiple system atrophy (MSA), progressive supranuclear palsy (PSP), corticobasal degeneration (CBD), and dementia with Lewy bodies (DLB), which are known to present clinically with motor parkinsonism (see Chapter 5). A three-pronged approach to a differential diagnosis in AP has been proposed (33).

Clinical differentiation

The salient clinical features in VP which differentiate it from PD are a symmetrical presentation with postural instability and falls, gait accompanied by a wide base stance and variable stride length rather than shuffling, preserved associated arm swing, lack of upper-limb rest tremor, frequent occurrence of pyramidal or corticospinal signs, and early subcortical dementia (27). Advanced age and lack of visual hallucinations may also be apparent (29). Response to levodopa may be less robust or not evident (5).

Neuroimaging

Structural neuroimaging, especially with MRI, may be necessary to differentiate VP from PD, but it does not establish a cause and effect relationship, given that only a limited proportion of patients with white-matter lesions do develop parkinsonism. Functional imaging, such as positron emission tomography (PET) and single photon emission computed tomography (SPECT), may show a reduction in striatal uptake ratios in PD or a lower mean asymmetry index in VP and can be used to supplement morphological imaging to investigate the integrity of the dopaminergic system. In the VADO study, ^{123}I-FP-CIT-SPECT was used to support the identification of patients with mixed PD and VP (34). This type of imaging may be abnormal in VP if there is focal basal ganglia infarction. As illustrated by Marshall and Grosset, this situation may exhibit a 'punched-out' SPECT deficit (35). By documenting dopaminergic deficits, patients could be identified who presented with IPD, VP, or an overlap between both, and those who could possibly be treated with dopaminergic agents (34). Radioisotopic measurement of myocardial innervation using iodine-123-metaiobenzylguanidine (^{123}I-MIBG) reduction has been shown in the earliest stages of PD and not in other parkinsonian syndromes (36). Diverse alternative techniques have been reported to differentiate VP from PD. Testing olfactory dysfunction using a smell identification test may help in identifying PD in order to differentiate it from VP. Moreover, this test can be accessible to the clinician in an outpatient setting (37). Given the diversity of the VP study population in general and lack of prospective or comparative studies with PD using these methods, it is difficult to reach a conclusion as to their utility in formulating a differential diagnosis at this time. However, neither clinical nor neuroimaging data alone yield a specific differential diagnosis.

Treatment

Pharmacological strategies

The current pharmacological options in VP are limited to levodopa, and a poor or non-sustained response to levodopa is another differentiating feature between VP and PD. However, patients with clinically suspected VP have been reported to experience a positive response to dopaminergic therapy (5). This may be seen in those patients with lesions in or close to the nigrostriatal pathway. It has been postulated that this response can be due to the presence of an adequate remaining complement of striatal dopaminergic nerve cell terminals within a dysfunctional nigrostriatal pathway to convert exogenous L-dopa into dopamine and thus to restore the intrinsic dopaminergic drive (38). Therefore, a trial with levodopa should be considered in the interest of the patient's functioning in the context of the activities of daily living.

Non-pharmacological strategies

Non-pharmacological therapy may also be considered in VP. Physical activity may slow the progression of white-matter changes with an impact on gait and balance (39). Cueing strategies making use of counting, a metronome, music, transverse stripes, and walkers or canes with lasers can have a positive effect on gait in both PD and VP (40). However, the subcortical cerebrovascular load has been shown to be inversely related to successful rehabilitation, as measured by changes in the unified Parkinson's disease rating scale (UPDRS) in patients with L-dopa refractory parkinsonism (41). As common sense might dictate, the primary and secondary prevention of CVD should be considered. Further, there is a need to evaluate these approaches systematically in the context of VP.

Prognosis

The prognosis in VP, pending cardiovascular co-morbidity, may include partial to (in)complete recovery consistent with a natural history of stroke. As a rule, the clinical presentation in VP is ultimately progressive.

Video fragment

Fragment 17.1
Vascular parkinsonism
Typical walking pattern of a hypertensive man, with small steps, difficulty with turning, freezing episodes, and a well preserved arm swing (lower body-half parkinsonism).

References

1 Critchley M. Arteriosclerotic parkinsonism. Brain 1929;52:23-83.

2 Schwab RS, England AC. Parkinson syndromes due to various specific causes. In PJ Vinken, GW Bruyn (Eds.), North-Holland Publishing Co, Amsterdam, 1968; 6:227-247.

3 Parkes JD, Marsden CD, Rees JE, Curzon G, Kantamaneni BD, Knill-Jones R et al. Parkinson's disease, cerebroarteriosclerosis, and senile dementia. Clinical features and response to levodopa. Q J Med. 1974;43:49-61.

4 Critchley M. Arteriosclerotic pseudoparkinsonism. In: FC Rose, R Capildeo (Eds.). Pitman, London, 1981;745-752.

5 Zijlmans JC, Katzenschlager R, Daniel SE, Lees AJ. The L-dopa response in vascular parkinsonism. J Neurol Neurosurg Psychiatry. 2004;75:545-547.

6 Kalra S, Grosset DG, Benamer HT. Differentiating vascular parkinsonism from idiopathic Parkinson's disease: a systematic review. Mov Disord. 2010;25:149-156.

7 Zijlmans JC, Daniel SE, Hughes AJ, Révész T, Lees AJ. Clinicopathological investigation of vascular parkinsonism, including clinical criteria for diagnosis. Mov Disord. 2004;19:630-640.

8 Hughes AJ, Daniel SE, Kilford L, Lees AJ. Accuracy of clinical diagnosis of idiopathic Parkinson's disease: a clinico-pathological study of 100 cases. J Neurol Neurosurg Psychiatr. 1992;55:181-184.

9 Jellinger KA. Vascular parkinsonism. Therapy. Future Medicine Ltd London, UK; 2008;5:237-255.

10 Jellinger KA. Prevalence of vascular lesions in Dementia with Lewy Bodies. A postmortem study. Journal Neural Transmission 2003;110:771-778.

11 Sibon I, Fenelon G, Quinn NP, Tison F. Vascular parkinsonism. J Neurol. 2004;251:513-524.

12 Erkinjuntti T. Subcortical vascular dementia. Cerebrovasc Dis. 2002;13S2:58-60.

13 Winikates J, Jankovic J. Clinical correlates of vascular parkinsonism. Arch Neurol. 1999;56:98-102.

14 Jellinger KA, Attems J. Prevalence and impact of vascular and Alzheimer pathologies in Lewy body disease. Acta Neuropathol. 2008;115:427-436.

15 Jellinger KA. Vascular parkinsonism-neuropathological findings. Acta Neurol Scand. 2002;105:414-415.

16 Yamanouchi H, Nagura H. Neurological signs and frontal white matter lesions in vascular parkinsonism. A clinicopathologic study. Stroke. 1997,28.965-969.

17 DeLong MR, Wichmann T. Circuits and circuit disorders of the basal ganglia. Arch Neurol. 2007;64:20-24.

18 Bhatia KP, Marsden CD. The behavioural and motor consequences of focal lesions of the basal ganglia in man. Brain. 1994;117:859-876.

19 Akyol A, Akyildiz UO, Tataroglu C. Vascular Parkinsonism: a case of lacunar infarction localized to mesencephalic substantia nigra. Parkinsonism Relat Disord. 2006;12:459-461.

20 Choi SM, Kim BC, Nam TS, Kim JT, Lee SH, Park MS, et al. Midbrain atrophy in vascular Parkinsonism. Eur Neurol. 2011;65:296-301.

21 Durand-Fardel M. Traite du ramollissement du cerveau. Bailliere, Paris. 1843.

22 Fisher CM. Lacunar infarcts: a review. Cerebrovasc Dis. 1991.

23 Reider-Groswasser I, Bornstein NM, Korczyn AD. Parkinsonism in patients with lacunar infarcts of the basal ganglia. Eur Neurol. 1995;35:46-49.

24 Laitinen LV, Chudy D, Tengvar M, Hariz MI, Bergenheim AT. Dilated perivascular spaces in the putamen and pallidum in patients with Parkinson's disease scheduled for pallidotomy: a comparison between MRI findings and clinical symptoms and signs. Mov Disord. 2000;15:1139-1144.

25 Tohgi H, Takahashi S, Abe T, Utsugisawa K. Symptomatic characteristics of parkinsonism and the width of substantia nigra pars compacta on MRI according to ischemic changes in the putamen and cerebral white matter: Implications for the diagnosis of vascular parkinsonism. Eur Neurol. 2001;46:1-10.

26 FitzGerald PM, Jankovic J. Lower body parkinsonism: evidence for vascular etiology. Mov Disord. 1989;4:249-260.

27 Gupta D, Kruruvilla A. Vascular parkinsonism: what makes it different? Postgrad Med J. 2011;87:829-836.

28 Demirkiran M, Bozdemir H, Sarica Y. Vascular parkinsonism: a distinct, heterogeneous clinical entity. Acta Neurol Scand. 2001;104:63-67.

29 Glass PG, Lees AJ, Bacellar A, Zijlmans J, Katzenschlager R, Silveira-Moriyama L. The clinical features of pathologically confirmed vascular parkinsonism. J Neurol Neurosurg Psychiatry. 2012;83:1027-1029.

30 Rampello L, Alvano A, Battaglia G, Raffaele R, Vecchio I, Malaguarnera M. Different clinical and evolutional patterns in late idiopathic and vascular parkinsonism. J Neurol. 2005;252:1045-1049.

31 Thanvi B, Lo N, Robinson T. Vascular parkinsonism-an important cause of parkinsonism in older people. Age Ageing. 2005;34:114-119.

32 Santangelo G, Vitale C, Trojano L, De Gaspari D, Bilo L, Antonini A, et al. Differential neuropsychological profiles in Parkinsonian patients with or without vascular lesions. Mov Disord. 2010;25:50-56.

33 Aerts MB, Esselink RA, Post B, van de Warrenburg BP, Bloem BR. Improving the diagnostic accuracy in parkinsonism: a three-pronged approach. Pract Neurol. 2012;12:77-87.

34 Antonini A, Vitale C, Barone P, Cilia R, Righini A, Bonucelli U, et al. The relationship between cerebral vascular disease and parkinsonism: The VADO study. Parkinsonism Relat Disord. 2012;18:775-780.

35 Marshall V, Grosset DG. Role of dopamine transporter imaging in the diagnosis of atypical tremor disorders. Mov Disord. 2003;18S7:S22-27.

36 Taki J, Nakajima K, Hwang EH, Matsunari I, Komai K, Yoshita M, et al. Peripheral sympathetic dysfunction in patients with Parkinson's disease without autonomic failure is heart selective and disease specific. Eur J Nucl Med. 2000;27:566-573.

37 Katzenschlager R, Zijlmans J, Evans A, Watt H, Lees AJ. Olfactory function distinguishes vascular parkinsonism from Parkinson's disease. J Neurol Neurosurg Psychiatry. 2004;75:1749-1752.

38 Leduc V, Montagne B, Destée A. Parkinsonism consecutive to an hemorrhagic lesion of the substantia nigra. Mov Disord 1997;12S1:2.

39 Baezner H, Blahak C, Poggesi A, Pantoni L, Inzitari D, Chabriat H, et al. Association of gait and balance disorders with age-related white matter changes: the LADIS study. Neurology. 2008;70:935-942.

40 Nieuwboer A, Kwakkel G, Rochester L, Jones D, van Wegen E, Willems AM, et al. Cueing training in the home improves gait-related mobility in Parkinson's disease: the RESCUE trial. J Neurol Neurosurg Psychiatry. 2007;78:134-140.

41 Guerini F, Frisoni GB, Bellwald C, Rossi R, Bellelli G, Trabucchi M. Subcortical vascular lesions predict functional recovery after rehabilitation in patients with L-dopa refractory parkinsonism. J Am Geriatr Soc. 2004;52:252-256.

18

Drug-induced Parkinsonism

Andrzej Friedman, Yanush Sanotsky & Erik Ch. Wolters

The pharmacological treatment of psychiatric diseases began with the French neurologist Philippe Pinel (at the end of eighteenth century), who decided to unchain psychiatric patients and treat them with psychotherapy and other methods like bloodletting and showers. In some cases he tried to use pharmacological substances, mostly opium and camphor (1). It is interesting to note that opium is known to cause effects similar to those seen in typical Parkinson's disease (PD), e.g. constipation, sexual dysfunction and sleep problems.

The treatment proposed by Pinel was effective only in a minority of patients, but for the development of new pharmacological substances that really interfered with psychotic symptoms, patients had to wait for almost 200 years. In 1950 French surgeon Henri Laborit noticed the hibernating effect of chlorpromazine in an operated patient and predicted the possible use of this product in psychiatry (2). Indeed, shortly after its introduction, its favorable effect on psychosis was acknowledged. However, it took only months to recognize that this medication caused extrapyramidal effects similar to parkinsonism (3). Soon after, the concept of drug-induced parkinsonism (DIP) appeared in the literature. Later on, not only antipsychotics, but also anti-emetics, calcium channel blockers, selective serotonin reuptake inhibitors and, occasionally, some anti-epileptics, immunosuppressants, anti-arrhythmics and statins were found to induce DIP. Some street drugs, such as MPTP and ecstasy, as well as other toxic compounds, including manganese and ephedrone, cyanide, organic solvents and cycas circinalis, have also been identified as inducing motor parkinsonism.

Clinical expression

Clinical symptoms of DIP are similar to those of Parkinson's disease (PD) and include bradykinesia, hypokinesia, rigidity, impaired postural reflexes and tremor. Gait abnormalities and dysphagia are also typical symptoms of DIP. Neuroimaging studies usually do not show any structural abnormalities related to the clinical symptoms, but magnetic resonance spectroscopy of patients with DIP has demonstrated a significant correlation between the severity of DIP and the choline concentration in the putamen (4). The significance of this finding remains to be clarified.

Autopsy studies of the brains of patients with a clinical diagnosis of DIP usually do not show significant changes, although in some cases typical Parkinson's disease-related pathology with Lewy bodies has been detected (5), suggesting that in some cases the treatment with neuroleptics unmasks incidental Lewy body disease (iLBD) or subclinical PD before the intake of antipsychotic therapy.

Differential diagnosis

DIP is characterized by motor parkinsonism, which also constitutes the clinical hallmark and backbone of the clinical diagnosis of PD. The diagnosis of Parkinson's disease is presented elsewhere (see Chapters 5 and 10). As drug-induced parkinsonism resembles PD but its treatment is different, it is essential to be aware of the differences between both conditions. The arguments favoring the diagnosis of DIP and caveats related to them are presented in Table 18.1.

Table 18.1
Arguments suggesting drug-induced parkinsonism.

- use of possibly causative drugs before the onset of motor parkinsonism
- acute or sub-acute onset of levodopa-unresponsive motor parkinsonism
- symmetric (bilateral) parkinsonian symptoms
- improvement of motor parkinsonism after discontinuation of the suspected drug
- presence of tardive dyskinesia
- normal binding of radioactive DaT in single photon emission computed tomography (SPECT) (6)
- normal fluorodopa binding in positron-emission tomography (PET)
- reduced raclopride binding in positron-emission tomography (PET)
- no hyperechogenicity of the substantia nigra in transcranial sonography

However, it should be remembered that DIP may also be asymmetric (7), and the use of medication causing DIP may unmask incidental Lewy body disease (iLBD) and/or PD (5). In the same vein, improvement of motor parkinsonism after discontinuation of the causative drug is not always observed. It should also be kept in mind that in some PD patients, normal echogenicity is seen: the diagnostic accuracy of transcranial sonography in Parkinson's disease is not adequate for routine clinical practice (8). Finally, symptoms of drug-induced parkinsonism, confirmed by a normal SPECT and/or PET scan, may persist in some patients long after withdrawal of the causative drug (9).

Risk factors

Individuals with incidental Lewy body disease, or premotor parkinsonism, are at high risk for the development of motor parkinsonism when treated with dopamine receptor-blocking and/or dopamine-depleting drugs. Other risk factors for DIP include age (10) and female gender (11). This later observation is very interesting as PD is more common in males (12). It was hypothesized that estrogens may suppress the expression of dopamine receptors (13). More recently, experimental studies suggest that estrogens promote neuroprotection (14).

Genetic predisposition may also play a role in DIP. In a study aimed at assessing the prevalence of human leucocyte antigens (HLA) in a group of 52 male subjects who developed DIP after antipsychotic treatment, a high correlation was found between HLA-B44 and the presence of DIP, with the relative risk for the carriers being 7.16 higher than for non-carriers (15).

Marketed drug-induced parkinsonism

Antipsychotic drugs

Antipsychotic drugs may cause parkinsonism either by blocking dopamine receptors or by depleting dopamine from presynaptic nerve terminals. The classic or so-called typical neuroleptics produced parkinsonian symptoms in more than 40% of patients treated, and initially it was even believed that the antipsychotic effect could be achieved only when the medication generates symptoms of DIP (16). The introduction of new atypical neuroleptics, which are able to improve the psychosis without producing parkinsonism, demonstrated that this was not the case.

In a large study evaluating the prevalence of extrapyramidal symptoms in 1559 patients treated with neuroleptics, parkinsonism was diagnosed in 302 of them (19%) (17). There are significant geographical variations concerning the prevalence of drug-induced parkinsonism ranging from 'very uncommon' in the English Midlands (18) up to 22% in central Spain (19). It is estimated that DIP is second after PD in causing motor parkinsonism; it represents up to 37% of all cases with parkinsonism (20).

Regarding their interference with the dopaminergic system, antipsychotics are either typical or atypical. Typical antipsychotics such as phenothiazine derivates (like chlorpromazine, perphenazine, fluphenazine, promethazine), butyrophenones (like haloperidol), diphenylbutylpiperidine (pimozide) and benzamide substitutes (sulpiride) frequently cause DIP. On the other hand, the atypical antipsychotics such as risperidone, olanzapine, ziprasidone and aripiprazole were found to be less inclined to induce those side-effects. The difference in inducing parkinsonism between the two types is attributed to the presumably higher affinity of atypical antipsychotics to serotonin-2A receptors than to dopamine receptors (21). This theory was disputed by the 'hit-and-run' concept of fast dissociation of atypical antipsychotics from the D2 receptors after the blockade, which should also lower the risk for DIP (22). However, more recently, the role of serotonin 1A receptors' blockade was presented as a possible cause of the difference in DIP induction (23).

Although newer atypical antipsychotics seemed to be much safer concerning induction of DIP, it turns out that most if not all of them in fact may cause this side-effect as well (24). Clozapine is very unlikely to produce DIP and, therefore, might be used safely in the treatment of psychosis in PD (25). In a PET study, it was shown that clozapine at therapeutic doses causes much lower occupancy of D2 receptors than typical neuroleptics, an occupancy far below that producing DIP (26). It should be remembered, however, that clozapine may induce agranulocytosis, although the risk of this side-effect is related to high doses of this medication (27). More recently, another new generation atypical antipsychotic, quetiapine, was established to induce DIP at a significantly lower level than the other typical and atypical antipsychotics (28).

Dopamine depleters

The first dopamine depleter used for the treatment of psychosis was reserpine (29). Nowadays, reserpine is only rarely used for the treatment of psychosis, although some authors claim that it may be effective in combination with other antipsychotics (30). Another dopamine depleter which is more commonly used is tetrabenazine, which is registered for the treatment of hyperkinetic disorders. Dopamine depleters, as might be expected, are frequently associated with the induction of motor parkinsonism (31). A meta-analysis of clinical trials with over 1100 cases, in which tetrabenazine was applied for the treatment of hyperkinetic disorders, revealed parkinsonism as an adverse effect of the treatment in 27% of patients (32).

Antiemetics

The antiemetics or gastrointestinal motility-interfering drugs comprise metoclopramide, levosulpiride, clebopride, itopride and domperidone. They have long been known to block enteric inhibitory D2 receptors (33). Metoclopramide has been shown to produce extrapyramidal side-effects, both tardive dyskinesia and parkinsonism. The first analysis of the literature data concerning the movement disorders caused by metoclopramide was published by Miller and Jankovic (34). Although tardive dyskinesia was found to be the most common extrapyramidal side-effect of metoclopramide, motor parkinsonism was second with a prevalence of about 30%. Only domperidone, as opposed to all other antiemetics, does not cross the blood-brain barrier and therefore supposedly will not cause DIP or any other extrapyramidal side effect (35). Its lack of penetration into the brain could be explained by its active removal by P-glycoprotein residing in the blood-brain barrier (36). Domperidone is therefore recommended for the prevention of nausea and vomiting related to the treatment of PD with dopaminergic drugs (37).

Calcium channel blockers

The original description of drug-induced parkinsonian symptoms induced by the calcium channel blocker flunarizine dates back to 1984 at the Brazilian World Congress of Neurology, when De Melo-Souza presented 5 elderly female patients treated with flunarizine who developed bradykinesia, rigidity and tremor. Later on, he and Ragazzo (38) presented a larger series of 28 patients with flunarizine-induced parkinsonian symptoms. It is interesting to note that most of them were female (25 of 28). The authors therefore suggested that the use of flunarizine in elderly depressed women frequently leads to the development of parkinsonism (38). Similar observations concern the use of another calcium channel blocker: cinnarizine (39).

Although the induction of parkinsonism by these compounds has been known for many years, the exact mechanism of this side-effect is still not fully understood. Animal studies did suggest a direct blockade of dopamine receptors (40), though it was also shown that both flunarazine and cinnarazine inhibit the energy-dependent vesicular dopamine uptake, thus reducing the presynaptic dopamine level (41).

Antidepressants

Selective serotonin reuptake inhibitors (SSRI), such as fluoxetine but also lithium, were linked to DIP in several case reports (42). As serotonin modulates dopamine in the basal ganglia by inhibiting its production and release, it was postulated that an increase in serotonergic transmission might cause parkinsonism, particularly in susceptible patients (43).

On the other hand, in a recently published, randomized, double-blind, placebo-controlled trial of antidepressants in PD, no worsening of motor functioning was found in patients treated with another SSRI, paroxetine (44). The impact of the selective serotonin reuptake inhibitors on motor function remains to be clarified, therefore.

Antiepileptics

Valproic acid is well known for its tremor-inducing properties (45). It seems, however, that this drug may also cause parkinsonism. Several authors described sporadic cases of DIP as the result of treatment with valproic acid, and an overview of the 21 cases described so far was recently published (46).

The mechanism by which valproic acid may cause parkinsonian symptoms remains unclear. There are studies showing a direct toxic effect of valproic acid on neurons (47).

Another possible explanation is related to mitochondrial dysfunction and impaired oxidative phosphorylation (see Chapter 32) caused by valproic acid (48). Concerning other antiepileptic drugs, there were also some case reports describing DIP after carbamazepine (49) and phenytoin (50).

In general, the risk of developing DIP using antiepileptic medication seems to be low. Most parkinsonian side-effects are noted with valproic acid, but there are insufficient data to establish its prevalence. Recent studies suggest that the risk of DIP is lower with the new generation antiepileptics, e.g. lamotrigine, topiramate, vigabatrin and gabapentin (51).

Immunosuppressants

Some case reports suggest a link between immunosuppressants and DIP. Among all immunosuppressants, only cyclosporine was reported to produce parkinsonian symptoms, although very rarely (52). Tracrolimus, another immunosuppressant, although sometimes cited as being associated with DIP (53), is only reported to induce hyperkinetic extrapyramidal symptoms extremely rarely, such as tremor and dystonia, but without any sign of motor parkinsonism (54).

Anti-arrhythmics

Some of the anti-arrhythmic drugs, particularly amiodarone (55), were also associated with motor parkinsonism. Although there are several case reports (55, 56), amiodarone-related DIP appears to be very rare. This also holds for another anti-arrhythmic drug, procaine, which may sometimes induce motor parkinsonism (56).

Statins

Lovastatin is sometimes cited as a causative factor of DIP (53). This observation is based on only one case report dating back to 1995 (57). As a matter of fact, statins may play a protective rather than a deleterious role in parkinsonism (58).

Street drug-induced parkinsonism

MPTP

Motor parkinsonism in young adults as a consequence of the use of synthetic heroin was described for the first time in 1983 (59). The byproduct of this synthesis, 1-methyl-4-phenyl-1,2,3,6-tetrahydropyridine, was quickly found to be responsible for the degeneration of the dopamine-producing cells in the substantia nigra underlying clinical motor parkinsonism (60). The mechanism of action is related to an active metabolite of MPTP, MPP+, which stimulates oxidative stress injury (61) (see also Chapter 32). Currently, MPTP is widely applied in experimental animals to create a model of non-progressive motor parkinsonism.

Ecstasy

Some animal studies showed that 3,4-methylene-dioxymethamphetamine (MDMA), better known as ecstasy, attacks not only the serotonergic but also the dopaminergic pathways. In the literature there is one case report describing a 38-year-old male patient who developed rapidly progressive, levodopa-unresponsive parkinsonism. As this patient was known to have abused ecstasy for a long time, the authors suggested that his clinical condition could represent a case of DIP (62). As the number of such case reports is extremely low, it is difficult, however, to determine the possible role of MDMA in induction of DIP.

Toxin-induced parkinsonism

Manganese

Neurologic consequences of manganese toxicity, tremors and other neurological symptoms resembling PD as well as various psychiatric behavioural disorders, have been recognized since 1837. Manganese neurotoxicity is a concern in occupational settings, especially for those working in the welding, steel-making, and mining industries. From a public health perspective, manganese has been approved for use in gasoline in many parts of the world with the potential for increased exposure to the general population. In manganese-induced parkinsonism, the problem is not caused by a degeneration of the dopaminergic system but rather by the brain's inability to release the available dopamine into the synapses (63). As a consequence, the therapeutic application of levodopa is far less effective than in PD.

A new form of presumed manganese poisoning has been reported in drug-addicted persons from Eastern Europe and the Baltic states who have intravenously injected self-prepared methcathinone hydrochloride (ephedrone, sometimes called 'cat' or 'jeff'), which is synthesized from a mixture of commercial cold remedy compounds containing phenylpropanolamine and acetic acid with potassium permanganate ($KMnO_4$) as a potent oxidant. An ephedrone-induced manganese encephalopathy underlies clinical signs of motor parkinsonism (64). The first reports describing young people who developed signs of a spastic-hypokinetic dysarthria, postural instability with falling, 'cock-gait', parkinsonian signs (hypokinesia, hypomimia, cogwheel rigidity), bradyphrenia, hypersomnia, and myoclonus after intravenous injections of ephedrone came from Russia (65). MRI of these patients showed a transient hyperintense T1 signal in the globus pallidus and putamen (see Figure 18.1A and 18.1B). The MRI changes may subsequently disappear, but the clinical symptoms remain unchanged. The related video (see Video fragment 18.1) shows typical symptoms of ephedrone encephalopathy. No treatment was found to be effective in these patients (66). This clinical syndrome is under-recognized outside Eastern Europe.

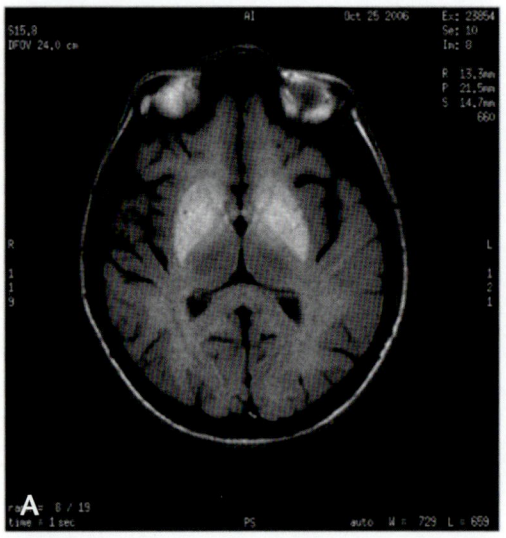 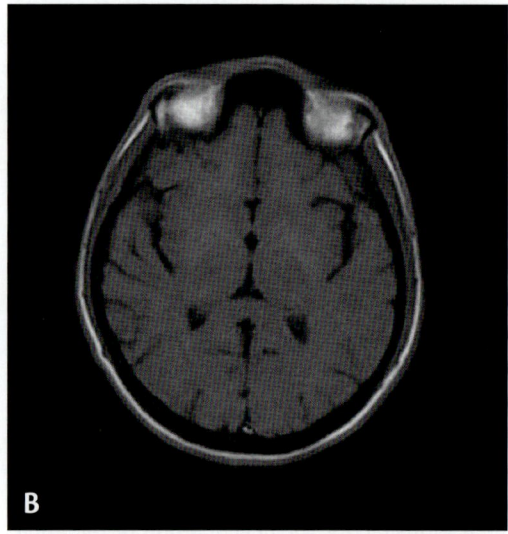

Figure 18.1

Typical hyperintensive T1 signal from the basal ganglia in a patient with ephedrone-induced manganese encephalopathy (A), fully disappearing within one year of follow-up (B), although clinical symptoms remained unchanged (unpublished material).

Pesticides

In the past, numerous population-based samples were screened for neurologic disease and occupational pesticide exposure. Based on the findings in these studies, it was concluded that elderly persons with past occupational pesticide (including paraquat, maneb, endosulfan, ziram and zineb) exposure, not only farmers working with these molecules but also people living or working close to fields sprayed with those chemicals, most probably have an increased risk of parkinsonism. This increased risk is thought to be caused by oxidative stress and subsequent neurodegeneration (67, 68). Those exposed to a combination of ziram, maneb, and paraquat were found to experience the greatest increase in PD risk (69). Clinical signs of pesticide-induced symptoms include cognitive deficits and motor parkinsonism, especially tremor and reduced dexterity.

Cyanide

Hydrogen cyanide and its solutions may be fatal following exposure via all routes. Cyanide is rapidly absorbed and distributed following in-

halation, oral or dermal exposure, and especially after inhalation and/or ingestion, the onset of signs and symptoms following exposure is rapid. It blocks oxidative respiration, causing failure of oxygen usage with tissue hypoxia leading to metabolic acidosis with a cyanide-induced apoptosis. Lactic acidosis is a key feature and correlates with the severity of cyanide intoxication. Its clinical expression mostly comprises non-specific symptoms, including headache, nausea, dizziness and dyspnea. In high concentrations, it will induce loss of consciousness, cardiac arrhythmias, coma and death. Profound neurological impairment manifests as motor parkinsonism, which may develop and persist after survival from severe intoxication (70).

Organic solvents

Solvents are widespread neurotoxic agents present in the workplace and ambient environment. They pose a considerable health risk for humans, due to the wealth of applications, copious production and consumption volumes as well as their ability to easily cross biological barriers. Case reports of parkinsonism have been asso-

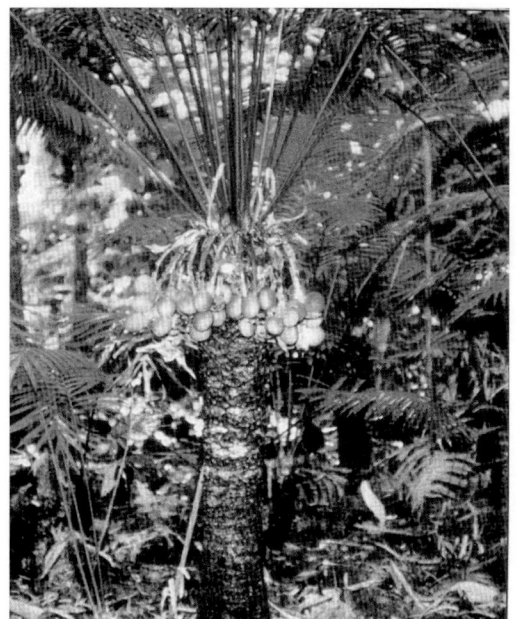

Figure 18.2
The Cycas Micronesia (cycad) with its fruits, containing cycad seeds with β-N-methylamino-l-alanine (BMAA) and cycasi.

ciated with exposure to various solvents, most notably trichloroethylene (71,72). Methanol and carbon monoxide may also induce delayed motor parkinsonism with dystonia (73) or motor parkinsonism (rigidity and bradykinesia) with intellectual impairment, respectively (74). Animal experiments did establish a solvent-related potential for inducing nigral system damage. Dopamine transporter imaging did show nigral dopaminergic cell loss, whereas magnetic resonance spectroscopy revealed transient severe white matter damage. As a rule, neurological and neuropsychological examinations also show gradual recovery from parkinsonism as well as intellectual impairment over time (74).

Cycas circinalis

A high incidence of amyotrophic lateral sclerosis (ALS) in Guam was first described in the 1940s, and by the early 1960s another co-morbid neurodegenerative disease was identified as the Guam ALS-parkinsonism-dementia complex (75).

These diseases have been linked to the ingestion of cycad seed flour tortillas, prepared after careful washing of the seeds. Epidemiologic evidence supported a causal link between the consumption of flour made from the washed seeds of *Cycas micronesica* (cycad) (see Figure 18.2) by the Chamorro population of Guam (see Figure 18.3) and the development of this complex neurodegenerative disease (76). As a matter of fact, the Chamorros already realized that unwashed seeds, which were later found to contain the neurotoxins β-N-methylamino-l-alanine (BMAA) and cycasin, were poisonous. However, they were unaware that washed cycad seeds still contained these toxins and could even produce this neurodegeneration years later (77).

Treatment

The treatment of choice in drug-induced parkinsonism, of course, is to avoid any medication with a risk of inducing it, especially in patients at risk. Therefore, the use of less risky antipsychotic drugs such as clozapine and quetiapine is always advised. When the symptoms of DIP are already present, discontinuation of the causative drug is suggested, although there might be a long time between the cessation of the drug and disappearance of DIP.

In the pharmacological treatment of pure antipsychotic-induced DIP, there is no place for levodopa and dopamine agonists as the postsynaptic dopaminergic receptors are blocked. Some improvement might be seen with anticholinergics (78), but they are contraindicated, particularly in elderly patients, as they may cause cognitive problems. Another possible treatment is amantadine, which was found to be as equally effective as anticholinergics in alleviating symptoms of DIP in schizophrenia patients at a dose of 100 mg b.i.d. (79). Electroconvulsive therapy was also described as potentially effective in the treatment of DIP (80), though a lack of randomized studies hampers the assessment of effectiveness as well as the routine application of this strategy.

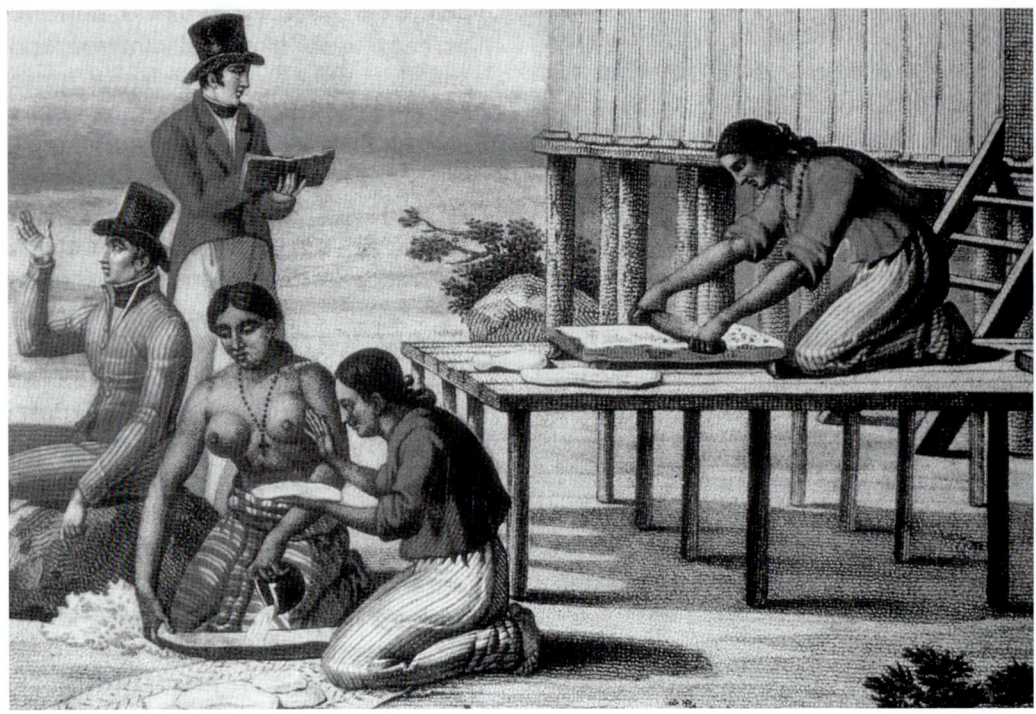

Figure 18.3
The traditional preparation of cycad tortillas in Guam.

Conclusion

Drug-induced parkinsonism is a frequent clinical condition which needs to be recognized and treated quickly. The case history is essential for a correct diagnosis, but it should be remembered that the intake of drugs known to cause DIP does not exclude other etiologies of the symptoms. An appropriate diagnosis must include neuroimaging (functional) to exclude structural brain damage as well as eventually underlying dementia with Lewy bodies (DLB) and/or PD.

Video fragment

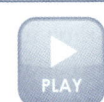

Fragment 18.1
Ephedrine-induced parkinsonism
(Segments 1-3)
This videotape displays the clinical presentation of an ephedrine-induced encephalopathy manifesting with bradykinesia and hypokinesia (segment 1), the typical cock gait (segment 2) and the specific dysarthria (segment 3).

References

1 Gerard Dl- Chiarugi and Pinel considered: soul's brain/person's mind. J Hist Behav Sci 1997;33:381-403.

2 Stip E- Happy birthday neuroleptics! 50 years later: la folie du doute. Eur Psychiatry 2002;17:115-119.

3 Delay J, Deniker P- Neuroleptic effects of chlorpromazine in therapeutics of neuropsychiatry. J Clin Exp Psychopathol 1955;16:104-112.

4 Yamasue H, Fukui T, Fukuda R, Kasai K, Iwanami A, Kato N, Kato T. Drug-induced parkinsonism in relation to choline-containing compounds measured by 1H-MR spectroscopy in putamen of chronically medicated patients with schizophrenia. Int J Neuropsychopharmacol. 2003;6:353-360.

5 Bower JH, Dickson DW, Taylor L, Maraganore DM, Rocca WA. Clinical correlates of the pathology underlying parkinsonism: a population perspective. Mov Disord 2002;17:910-916.

6 Lorberboym M, Treves TA, Melamed E, Lampl Y, Hellmann M, Djaldetti R. 123I-FP/CIT SPECT imaging for distinguishing drug-induced parkinsonism from Parkinson's disease. Mov Disord. 2006;21:510-514.

7 Caligiuri MP, Bracha HS, Lohr JB. Asymmetry of neuroleptic-induced rigidity: development of quantitative methods and clinical correlates. Psychiatry Res. 1989;30:275-284.

8 Bouwmans AE, Vlaar AM, Mess WH, Kessels A, Weber WE. Specificity and sensitivity of transcranial sonography of the substantia nigra in the diagnosis of Parkinson's disease: prospective cohort study in 196 patients. BMJ Open. 2013;3:pii:e002613. doi:10.1136.

9 Lim TT, Ahmed A, Itin I, Gostkowski M, Rudolph J, Cooper S, Fernandez HH. Is 6 months of neuroleptic withdrawal sufficient to distinguish drug-induced parkinsonism from Parkinson's disease? Int J Neurosci. 2013;123:170-174.

10 Thanvi B, Treadwell S. Drug induced parkinsonism: a common cause of parkinsonism in older people. Postgrad Med J 2009;85:322-326.

11 Stephen PJ, Williamson J. Drug-induced parkinsonism in the elderly. Lancet 1984;2:1082-1083.

12 Haaxma CA, Bloem BR, Borm GF, et al. Gender differences in Parkinson's disease. J Neurol Neurosurg Psychiatry 2007;78:819-824.

13 Bedard P, Langelier P, Villeneuve A. Oestrogens and extrapyramidal system. Lancet 1977;2:1367-1368.

14 Brann DW, Dhandapani K, Wakade C, Mahesh VB, Khan MM. Neurotrophic and neuroprotective actions of estrogen: basic mechanisms and clinical implications. Steroids 2007;72:381-405.

15 Metzer SW, Newton JEO, Steele RW, et al. HLA antigens in drug-induced parkinsonism. Mov Disord 1989;4:121-128.

16 Ayd FJ. A survey of drug-induced extrapyramidal reactions. JAMA 1961;175:1054-1060.

17 Muscettola G, Barbato G, Pampallona S, Casiello M, Bollini P. Extrapyramidal syndromes in neuroleptic-treated patients: prevalence, risk factors, and association with tardive dyskinesia. J Clin Psychopharmacol 1999;19:203-208.

18 Aronson TA. Persistent drug-induced parkinsonism. Biol Psychiatry 1985;20:795-798.

19 Benito-León J, Bermejo-Pareja F, Rodríguez J, Molina JA, Gabriel R, Morales JM. Neurological Disorders in Central Spain NEDICES Study Group. Prevalence of PD and other types of parkinsonism in three elderly populations of central Spain. Mov Disord 2003;18:267-274.

20 Barbosa MT, Caramelli P, Maia DP, Cunningham MC, Guerra HL, Lima-Costa MF, Cardoso F. Parkinsonism and Parkinson's disease in the elderly: a community-based survey in Brazil the Bambuí study. Mov Disord 2006;21:800 808.

21 Ossowska K. Neuronal basis of neuroleptic-induced extrapyramidal side-effects. Pol J Pharmacol 2002;54:299-312.

22 Kapur S, Seeman P. Does fast dissociation from dopamine D2 receptor explain the action of atypical antipsychotics?: a new hypothesis. Am J Psychiatry 2001;158:360-369.

23 Bortolozzi A, Masana M, Díaz-Mataix L, at al. Dopamine release induced by atypical antipsychotics in prefrontal cortex requires 5-HT1A receptors but not 5-HT2A receptors. Int J Neuropsychopharmacol. 2010;13:1299-1314.

24 Chan HY, Chang CJ, Chiang SC, et al. A randomised controlled study of risperidone and olanzapine for schizophrenic patients with neuroleptic-induced acute dystonia or parkinsonism. J Psychopharmacol 2010;24:91-98.

25 Friedman JH. Parkinson disease psychosis: update. Behav Neurol 2012 doi 10.3233/BEN-129016

26 Farde L, Nordström AL, Wiesel FA, Pauli S, Halldin C, Sedvall G. Positron emission tomographic analysis of central D1 and D2 dopamine receptor occupancy in patients treated with classical neuroleptics and clozapine. Relation to extrapyramidal side-effects. Arch Gen Psychiatry. 1992;49:538-440.

27 Llorca PM, Pere JJ. Leponex 10 ans après – une revue clinique. Encephale 2004;30:474-491.

28 Lieberman JA, Stroup TS, McEvoy JP, et al. Clinical Antipsychotic Trials of Intervention Effectiveness CATIE Investigators- Effectiveness of antipsychotic drugs in patients with chronic schizophrenia. N Engl J Med. 2005;353:1209-1223.

29 Ferguson RS. Reserpine and chronic psychosis: two-year outcome in a treatment group. J Ment Sci 1959;105:251-255.

30 Solon EN. Risperidone-reserpine combination in refractory psychosis. Schizophrenia Res 1996;22:265-266.

31 Frank S. Tetrabenazine as anti-chorea therapy in Huntington disease: an open-label continuation study. BMC Neurol 2009;9:62 doi:10.1186/1471-2377-9-62.

32 Guay DRP. Tetrabenazine, a monoamine-depleting drug used in the treatment of hyperkinetic movement disorders. Am J Geriatr Pharmacother 2010; 8:331-373.

33 Schuurkes JA, Van Nueten JM. Domperidone improves myogenically transmitted antroduodenal coordination by blocking dopaminergic receptor sites. Scand J Gastroenterol Suppl 1984;96:101–110.

34 Miller LG, Jankovic J. Metoclopramide-induced movement disorders. Clinical findings with a review of the literature. Arch Intern Med 1989;149:2486-2492.

35 Reddymasu SC, Soykan I, McCallum RW. Domperidone: review of pharmacology and clinical applications in gastroenterology. Am J Gastroenterol. 2007;102:2036-2045.

36 Schinkel AH,Wagenaar EL, Mol CAAM, Van Deemter L. P-Glycoprotein in the blood–brain barrier of mice influences the brain penetration and pharmacological activity of many drugs. J Clin Invest 1996;97:2517–2524.

37 Bowron A. Practical considerations in the use of apomorphine injectable. Neurology 2004; 62S4:32-36.

38 De Melo-Souza SE, Ragazzo PC. Neurologic side-effects of flunarizine. Neurology 1989;39S1:390.

39 Marti-Masso J, Poza JJ. Cinnarizine-induced parkinsonism: ten years later. Mov Disord 1998;13:453-456.

40 Kariya S, Isozaki S, Masubuchi Y, Suzuki T, Narimatsu S. Possible pharmacokinetic and pharmacodynamic factors affecting parkinsonism inducement by cinnarizine and flunarizine. Biochem Pharmacol. 1995;50:1645-1650.

41 Terland O, Flatmark T. Drug-induced parkinsonism: Cinnarizine and flunarizine are potent uncouplers of the vacuolar H+-ATPase in catecholamine storage esicles. Neuropharmacology 1999;38:879–882.

42 Christodoulou C, Papadopoulou A, Rizos E, et al. Extrapyramidal side-effects and suicidal ideation under fluoxetine treatment: a case report. Ann Gen Psychiatry. 2010;9:5. doi:10.1186/1744-859X-9-5.

43 Micheli PE, Cersosimo MG. Drug-induced parkinsonism. In: Koller WC, Melamed E eds. Handbook of Clinical Neurology 2007;84:399-416.

44 Richard IH, McDermott MP, Kurlan R, et al. SAD-PD Study Group- A randomized double-blind placebo-controlled trial of antidepressants in Parkinson's disease. Neurology 2012;78:1229-1236.

45 Onofrj M, Thomas A, Paci C. Reversible parkinsonism induced by prolonged treatment with valproate. J Neurol 1998;245:794–796.

46 Mahmoud F, Tampi RR. Valproic acid-induced parkinsonism in the elderly: a comprehensive review of the literature. Am J Geriatr Pharmacother 2011;9:405-412.

47 Lai JS, Zhao C, Warsh JJ, Li PP. Cytoprotection by lithium and valporate varies between cell types and cellular stresses. Eur J Pharmacol 2006;539:18-26.

48 Luís PB, Ruiter JP, Aires CC, et al.Valproic acid metabolites inhibit dihydrolipoyl dehydrogenase activity leading to impaired 2-oxoglutarate-driven oxidative phosphorylation. Biochim Biophys Acta. 2007;1767:1126-1133.

49 Froomes PR, Stewart MR. A reversible parkinsonian syndrome and hepatotoxicity following addition of carbamazepine to sodium valproate. Aust N Z J Med 1994;24:413–414.

50 Goni M, Jimenez M, Seijoo M. Parkinsonism induced by phenytoin. Clin Neuropharmacol 1985; 8: 383–384.

51 Zadikoff C, Munhoz RP, Asante AN, et al. Movement disorders in patients taking anticonvulsants. J Neurol Neurosurg Psychiatry. 2007;8:147-151.

52 Ling H, Bhidayasiri R. Reversible parkinsonism after chronic cyclosporine treatment in renal transplantation. Mov Disord 2009;24:1848-1849.

53 Lopez-Sendon J, Mena MA, de Yebenes JG. Drug-induced parkinsonism. Expert Opin Drug Saf 2013; doi.10.1517/14740338.2013.787065.

54 Emiroglu R, Ayvaz I, Moray G, Karakayali H, Haberal M. Tacrolimus-related neurologic and renal complications in liver transplantation: A single-center experience. Transplant Proc. 2006;38:619-621.

55 Dotti MT, Federico A. Amiodarone-induced parkinsonism: a case report and pathogenic discussion. Mov Disord 1995;10:233-234.

56 Gjerris F. Transitory procaine-induced parkinsonism. J Neurol Neurosurg Psychiatry 1971;34:20-22.

57 Muller T, Kuhn W, Pöhlau D, Przuntek H. Parkinsonism unmasked by lovastatin. Ann Neurol 1995;37:685-686.

58 Gao X, Simon KC, Schwarzschild MA, Ascherio A. Prospective study of statin use and risk of Parkinson disease. Arch Neurol 2012;69:380-384.

59 Langston JW, Ballard P, Tetrud JW, Irwin I. Chronic parkinsonism in humans due to a product of meperidine analog synthesis. Science 1983;219:979-980.

60 Bradbury AJ, Costall B, Domeney AM, et al. 1-methyl-4-phenylpyridine is neurotoxic to the nigrostriatal dopamine pathway. Nature 1986;319:56-57.

61 Przedborski S, Jackson-Lewis V, Djaldetti R, et al. The parkinsonian toxin MPTP: action and mechanism. Restor Neurol Neurosci 2000;16:135-142.

62 O'Suilleabhain P, Giller C. Rapidly progressive parkinsonism in a self-reported user of ecstasy and other drugs. Mov Disord 2003;18:1378-1381.

63 Guilarte TR. Manganese and Parkinson's Disease: A Critical Review and New Findings. Environ Health Perspect. 2010;118:1071–1080.

64 Sanotsky Y, Lesyk R, Fedoryshyn L, Komnatska I, Matviyenko Y, Fahn S. Manganic encephalopathy due to 'ephedrone' abuse. Mov Disord 2007;22:1337-1343.

65 Levin OS. 'Ephedrone' encephalopathy. Zh Nevrol Psikhiatr Im S S Korsakova 2005;105:12-20.

66 Selikhova M, Fedoryshyn L, Matviyenko Y, et al. Parkinsonism and dystonia caused by the illicit use of ephedrone--a longitudinal study. Mov Disord. 2008;23:2224-2231.

67 Steenland K, Wesseling C, Roman N, Quiros I, Juncos JL. Occupational pesticide exposure and screening tests for neurodegenerative disease among an elderly population in Costa Rica. Environmental Research 2013;120:96-101.

68 Tanner CM, Ross GW, Jewell SA, et al.. Occupation and risk of parkinsonism: a multicenter case-control study. Arch Neurol 2009;66:1106-1113.

69 Wang A, Costello S, Cockburn M, Zhang X, Bronstein J, Ritz B. Parkinson's disease risk from ambient exposure to pesticides. Eur J Epidemiol 2011;26:547-555.

70 Uitti RJ, Rajput AH, Ashenhurst EM, Rozdilsky B. Cyanide-induced parkinsonism: a clinicopathologic report. Neurology 1985;35:921-925.

71 Gralewicz S, Dyzma M. Organic solvents and the dopaminergic system. Int J Occup Med Environ Health 2005;18:103-113.

72 Lock EA, Zhang J, Checkoway H. Solvents and Parkinson disease: a systematic review of toxicological and epidemiological evidence. Toxicol Appl Pharmacol 2013;266:345-355.

73 Franquet E, Salvadó-Figueres M, Lorenzo-Bosquet C, et al. Nigrostriatal pathway dysfunction in a methanol-induced delayed dystonia-parkinsonism. Mov Disord 2012;27:1220-1221.

74 Sohn YH, Jeong Y, Kim HS, Im JH, Kim JS. The brain lesion responsible for parkinsonism after carbon monoxide poisoning. Arch Neurol 2000;57:1214-1218.

75 Hirano A, Kurland LT, Krooth RS, et al. Parkinsonism-dementia complex, an endemic disease on the island of Guam: 1. Clinical Features. Brain 1961;84:642–661.

76 Kurland LT. Amyotrophic lateral sclerosis and Parkinson's disease complex on Guam linked to an environmental neurotoxin. Trends Neurosci 1988;11:51–54.

77 Borenstein AR, Mortimer JA, Schofield E, et al. Cycad exposure and risk of dementia, MCI, and PDC in the Chamorro population of Guam. Neurology 2007;68:1764–1771.

78 Saltz BL, Woerner MG, Robinson DG, Kane JM. Side-effects of antipsychotic drugs. Avoiding and minimizing their impact in elderly patients. Postgrad Med. 2000;107:169-178.

79 Silver H, Geraisy N, Schwartz M. No difference in the effect of biperiden and amantadine on parkinsonian- and tardive dyskinesia-type involuntary movements: a double-blind crossover, placebo-controlled study in medicated chronic schizophrenic patients. J Clin Psychiatry 1995;56:167-170.

80 Sadananda SK, Holla B, Viswanath B, et al. Effectiveness of electroconvulsive therapy for drug-induced parkinsonism in the elderly. J ECT 2013;29:6-7.

19
Multiple System Atrophy

Florian Krismer & Gregor K. Wenning

Multiple system atrophy (MSA) is an adult-onset, rapidly progressive, neurodegenerative disorder characterized by an abnormal accumulation of α-synuclein (αSYN) in oligodendrocytes associated with multifocal neuronal degeneration. The disease is characterized clinically by either (more or less) levodopa-refractory parkinsonism or cerebellar ataxia accompanied by autonomic failure (1-3).

The term multiple system atrophy was first introduced in 1969 when Graham and Oppenheimer (4) provided evidence that olivopontocerebellar atrophy (OPCA) (5), striatonigral degeneration (SND) (6) and Shy-Drager Syndrome (SDS) (7) show substantial overlap in both clinical and neuropathological features, suggesting that these disorders represent a single disease. This observation was confirmed twenty years later when Papp et al. demonstrated argyrophilic glial cytoplasmic inclusions (GCIs) in MSA brains irrespective of their clinical presentation (8). Subsequently, argyrophilic GCIs became the neuropathological hallmark of the disease. Neuronal loss commonly occurs in the basal ganglia, cerebellum, pons, inferior olivary nuclei, and spinal cord and is usually accompanied by gliosis (2). Misfolded, hyperphosphorylated, fibrillar α-synuclein represents the principal component of GCIs, a finding that places MSA firmly within the spectrum of α-synucleinopathies, along with Parkinson's disease, dementia with Lewy bodies and pure autonomic failure (9).

The clinical recognition of MSA improved dramatically after the introduction of diagnostic criteria. Niall Quinn provided the first set of diagnostic criteria that distinguished two motor subtypes, parkinsonism and cerebellar ataxia (10). Nowadays, MSA consensus diagnostic criteria still largely rely on clinical diagnostic criteria, but they also include warning signs ('red flags') and neuroimaging features (1).

Epidemiology

MSA affects both sexes equally, and the mean age at onset is around 55 years. This fatal disorder progresses relentlessly until death with a median survival of nine years. However, there is a considerable variation in disease progression, with individual cases surviving up to 15 years (11-16). In the Olmsted County study, the annual incidence rate was estimated to 0.6 cases per 100,000 with no single case occurring before 50 years of age (17). Similar numbers were observed in a nationwide study in Iceland, reporting an incidence rate of 0.7 (18). In contrast, a population-based study in northern Sweden determined higher incidence rates of 2.4 per 100,000 population (19), and a Russian population-based study yielded a substantially lower incidence rate of 0.1 per 100,000 (20). Estimates of the age-adjusted prevalence range from 1.9 to 4.9 cases per 100,000 (21,22). Surprisingly, a door-to-door survey in a rural Bavarian population identified three MSA cases in 982 people who were older than 65 years, resulting in a prevalence rate of 0.31% (23).

Etiology

MSA is commonly regarded as a sporadic disorder, although in recent years, rare familial aggregations of MSA were reported (24-28). Wüllner and co-workers described a German family with an autosomal dominant inheritance of MSA. Fourteen living family members in three generations were studied with two members in two successive generations being affected (27). Post-mortem verification confirmed a diagnosis of MSA in one of the affected family members (28). The marked difference in age at disease onset in the two affected family members (anticipation) might suggest an unidentified trinucleotide repeat disorder (27). Four Japanese MSA families with multiple affected siblings have been reported (25). This study involved eight MSA patients (one patient had confirmed MSA, five patients had probable MSA, and two patients had possible MSA) with the pedigree suggesting a single-gene disorder and autosomal recessive inheritance. Mutational analysis of the coding regions of SNCA failed to identify any mutation (25). In addition, a study involving a pair of monozygotic twins discordant for the MSA phenotype showed a copy number variation in the src homology 2 domain containing transforming protein 2 (SHC2), suggesting a causal link of copy number loss in the SHC2 region to MSA (29). Recently, functionally impaired variants of the COQ2 gene (part of the coenzyme Q10 pathway) were shown to be associated with an increased risk of MSA in multiplex families and patients with sporadic disease (24).

A case control study reported an increased MSA risk resulting from occupational exposure to organic solvents, plastic monomers and additives, pesticides and metals (30). Furthermore, an Italian multi-center case-control study observed a significantly higher risk of developing MSA in subjects who worked in agriculture (31). By contrast, a French case-control study revealed that MSA was not associated with exposure to pesticides, solvents, and other occupational toxics in the assessed cohort. This study also revealed that aspirin intake, alcohol consumption, and fish and seafood consumption was more common within the control group (32).

Pathophysiology

A growing body of evidence has been collected in the past few years with regard to the pathogenesis of MSA. As mentioned earlier, the core feature of MSA pathology is the widespread appearance of GCIs containing αSYN correlating with the neuronal deterioration and disease duration (33). Abnormal accumulation of fibrillar αSYN is not restricted to oligodendrocytes, it has also been reported in the cytoplasm and the nucleus of neurons (NCIs and NNIs) as well as in neurites in MSA brains (34). Although these inclusions were not accepted as a defining neuropathological criterion of MSA (2), they are likely to be relevant for the disease process. Post-mortem studies have suggested that NNIs develop early in the disease process in the pontine nuclei and inferior olives of MSA brains (35,36). In addition, oxidative stress, mitochondrial dysfunction, excitotoxicity, inflammation, and conformational and posttranslational protein changes may be important factors in the pathogenesis of MSA (37). However, the crucial role of oligodendroglial pathology in MSA pathogenesis has been highlighted by the discovery of the early accumulation of another protein p25α in oligodendrocytes from patients with MSA (38, 39). p25α is a phosphoprotein confined to oligodendrocytes that is functionally involved in the myelination and stabilization of microtubules (40). Under physiological conditions, p25α resides in the myelin sheath, but in MSA patients it shifts to the cytoplasm. This is usually observed prior to αSYN aggregation (41). In addition, cell culture experiments have clearly shown that p25α accelerates αSYN aggregation (42). This acceleration was accompanied by caspase 3 activation and apoptotic cell death (43). Altogether, recent studies suggest that cellular interactions between myelin basic protein and p25α are disrupted early in the disease process, leading to oligodendroglial dysfunction and subsequent neurodegeneration and strengthening the hypothesis of a primary oligodendrogliopathy that precedes neuronal degeneration in MSA (44).

GCI-associated αSYN usually undergoes various posttranslational modifications, including oxidative modification, nitration, and phosphorylation at serine 129 (44-51), indicating a role for oxidative stress in MSA. Most of the αSYN in MSA was SDS-soluble, with a small amount being SDS-insoluble (SDS is a detergent used to lyse cells and to release soluble proteins). These protein alterations were also present in areas with low GCI load, suggesting that altered solubility precedes the formation of GCIs (47,52).

The origin of oligodendroglial αSYN remains elusive, as illustrated by the lack of evidence of αSYN expression in oligodendroglia of healthy and MSA brains (53-55). This gives rise to the notion that αSYN is taken up into oligodendrocytes from the extracellular space, with αSYN most likely being secreted by neurons. However, it has to be emphasized that the exact mechanisms underlying this prion-like transfer and the relative contribution of soluble and oligomeric species of αSYN as well as of other pathogenic proteins in this propagation process require further investigation (37,56-58).

Neuroinflammation may be important in the development of MSA. In the white matter, microglial activation is more prominent in areas of mild-to-moderate tissue damage compared with those areas with severe white matter degeneration (59). Misfolded αSYN directly activates microglia via a classical activation pathway (60-62) inducing the production and release of proinflammatory molecules, including interleukins, tumor necrosis factor-α (TNFα), interferon-γ (63) as well as increasing antioxidant response enzyme expression in vivo and in cultured microglia. The specific structure of misfolded αSYN is important for the induction of this proinflammatory pathway (64). Furthermore, in vitro evidence suggests that human microglia activated by αSYN mediate neurotoxic effects (61, 65).

Clinical Presentation

MSA is characterized clinically by a variable combination of parkinsonism, cerebellar dysfunction, autonomic failure and pyramidal signs. According to the clinical diagnostic criteria, two major subtypes may be distinguished by their predominant motor feature: a parkinsonian variant characterized by rapidly progressive, levodopa-refractory, akinetic-rigid parkinsonism (MSA-P) and a cerebellar variant with ataxia as the main motor presentation (MSA-C) (1). In a series of 100 cases of clinically probable MSA (15), 97% of the patients had autonomic failure, 91% had parkinsonism, 52% had cerebellar features and 61% had pyramidal features at the last evaluation.

Presenting features

Levodopa-refractory, akinetic-rigid parkinsonism is the most common presenting symptom of MSA, reported in over 60% of patients at the first visit (10,66-68). Cerebellar disorders and genitourinary dysfunction are also common presenting features of MSA (66, 68). Interestingly, MSA-C outnumbered MSA-P in a Japanese cohort (14), while in the Western hemisphere, MSA-P is the more common presentation (69).

Features of established disease

Parkinsonism
Bradykinesia, rigidity, postural tremor as well as disequilibrium and gait unsteadiness characterize parkinsonism associated with MSA. Jerky postural tremor and less commonly tremor at rest may be observed. Frequently, patients exhibit orofacial dystonia associated with a characteristic quivering, high-pitched dysarthria. Postural stability is compromised early as well, but in contrast to PSP, recurrent falls at disease onset are unusual. Although MSA patients are

commonly regarded as levodopa-unresponsive, up to 40% show beneficial treatment effects as suggested in a recent clinical series (69). Unfortunately, these effects are usually transient, lasting for less than two years (11,69,70).

Cerebellar symptoms

The cerebellar disorder comprises gait ataxia, limb kinetic ataxia and scanning dysarthria as well as cerebellar oculomotor disturbances. The most common manifestation is a wide-based ataxic gait occurring in 34-59% of patients (68, 71). Spontaneous and/or gaze-evoked nystagmus, often subtle, was detected in 23-25% of patients (15,68). The finding of a mixed dysarthria with combinations of hypokinetic, ataxic, and spastic components is consistent with the overall clinical and neuropathologic changes in MSA (72). Patients with MSA-C usually develop additional non-cerebellar symptoms and signs, but in its early stages MSA-C may be indistinguishable from other patients with idiopathic, late-onset cerebellar ataxia (73).

Autonomic dysfunction

Autonomic dysfunction involving primarily urogenital and orthostatic domains universally develops in the course of MSA (69), and a retrospective analysis of pathologically confirmed MSA cases suggests that early autonomic symptoms (within two years of disease onset) occur in more than half of the patients with MSA (11).

Urogenital dysfunction

In a clinical series, urge incontinence was the most frequent symptom, followed by incomplete bladder emptying in 73% and 48%, respectively. In one-third of patients with MSA, both symptoms were present (69). Urinary retention may be unmasked or exacerbated by benign prostatic hypertrophy or, in women, by perineal laxity secondary to complications during labour or uterine descent. In a series of patients with probable MSA, 43% of males had undergone futile prostatic or bladder neck surgery before the correct diagnosis was made, although more than half of them had neurological symptoms or signs at the time of the procedure (74). Stress incontinence occurred in 57% of the women, and half of them underwent surgery with disappointing results (74, 75).

In a series of 62 male MSA patients, impotence occurred in 96% of the men and was the first symptom in 37% (74). These results were supported by a recent prospective study observing erectile dysfunction in 84% (69). Reduced genital sensitivity with or without impaired libido has been reported in the majority of female MSA patients (76).

Orthostatic dysfunction

Applicable consensus criteria require a systolic blood pressure drop of at least 30 mmHg or a fall in diastolic blood pressure of 15 mmHg for the diagnosis of MSA-related orthostatic hypotension (1). Characteristic symptoms of orthostatic hypotension include light-headedness, visual blurring, dizziness, and presyncope. However, severe orthostatic hypotension with recurrent falls (more than three) was only reported in 15% of subjects, while postural faintness was present in up to 53% of cases (15,77). Postural hypotension is frequently associated with an inadequately low increase in heart rate. Orthostatic symptoms may be further aggravated by drugs such as dopaminergic compounds, fluid depletion, food ingestion, an increased temperature and physical deconditioning. Patients with autonomic failure are susceptible to substantial drops in blood pressure after high carbohydrate intake, and sufficient fluid intake may improve orthostatic intolerance (78-80). In severe cardiovascular autonomic failure, the loss of baroreflexes may cause recumbent arterial hypertension, which has been observed in only a few patients. Furthermore, the evolution of early autonomic failure in MSA patients (within 2.5 years after disease onset) is an independent predictive factor for rapid disease progression and reduced survival (11, 81).

Other autonomic symptoms

Anhidrosis or hypohidrosis occurs frequently in patients with MSA (82). However, the underlying site of the lesion is not well established. Although postganglionic structures may be involved, anhidrosis in patients with MSA is largely caused by preganglionic dysfunction. A recent prospective study suggested that severe and diffuse anhidrosis is predictive of MSA (83). Impaired sympathetic skin response, reduced heat tolerance and skin temperature dysregulation have also been described in MSA (82,84,85). Patients with MSA often experience cold, dusky, violaceous hands, with poor circulatory return after blanching by pressure, suggestive of a defect in the neurovascular control of distal extremities (86). This so-called 'cold hand sign' is another clinical 'red flag' that may raise the suspicion of MSA (87).

Other clinical features

Besides the poor response to levodopa and the additional presence of pyramidal or cerebellar signs, other features may suggest MSA – these early warnings signs of MSA are usually termed 'red flags' (10,87).

Rapid clinical deterioration (Hoehn and Yahr stage III within 3 years of disease onset) despite dopaminergic treatment is highly suspicious of MSA (87). Postural instability with recurrent falls causes major disability in many MSA patients. In a clinical series, postural instability was present in 93% of the MSA patients (15). However, unlike PSP patients, only a few MSA patients experienced falls in the first year (71,77). The pathophysiological basis of postural instability in MSA remains unresolved, but neuronal depletion of the pedunculopontine nucleus may contribute (88). The development of a disproportionate antecollis is another important pointer towards a diagnosis of MSA (10,89-91), hampering feeding, communication and vision. The pathophysiological basis remains uncertain. Intriguingly, levodopa treatment may worsen dystonic movements in the absence of any an-

tiparkinsonian benefit (89). Tremulous myoclonic jerks of small amplitude, usually affecting the fingers, occur in a number of patients with MSA but are otherwise rare in non-demented parkinsonian patients (10,92). In a series of postmortem-confirmed MSA patients, inspiratory stridor was documented in 9-34% and occurred at any time point in the disease process (68). Nocturnal stridor was shown to be associated with a poor prognosis (93). Speech impairment develops in virtually all MSA patients and is largely related to laryngeal dysfunction. It tends to be dominated by hypophonic monotony or a scanning quality according to clinical subtype (72). A quivering, irregular, severely hypophonic or slurring dysarthria is 'often so characteristic that the diagnosis can be suggested by listening to the patient on the telephone' (90). Severe dysarthria tends to develop earlier and is also commonly associated with dysphagia in MSA compared with PD patients (94).

Diagnosis

Since misfolded α-synuclein has been recognized as the main constituent of GCIs in MSA (9), widespread α-synuclein-positive GCI pathology with concomitant neurodegenerative changes of striatonigral or olivopontocerebellar type is currently required to achieve a diagnosis of definite MSA. Clinically probable MSA is defined as a sporadic, progressive, adult-onset (> 30 years of age) disease characterized by severe autonomic failure as defined by either urinary incontinence (with erectile dysfunction in men) or orthostatic hypotension (with blood pressure falls ≥ 30 mmHg systolic or ≥ 15 mmHg diastolic) and, additionally, a poorly levodopa-responsive parkinsonism or a cerebellar syndrome. For the diagnosis of possible MSA, parkinsonism or a cerebellar syndrome must be accompanied by at least one feature suggesting autonomic dysfunction, plus more than one additional feature suggestive of MSA. Among others, MRI evidence of putaminal, middle cerebellar peduncle, pontine or cerebellar atrophy as well putaminal, brainstem or cerebellar hypometabolism on FDG-PET are accepted as supporting features (1).

Differential Diagnosis

The main differential diagnosis of MSA is PD as they share not only parkinsonian features, but numerous non-motor symptoms as well. In a clinicopathologic study conducted by Litvan et al. (95), primary neurologists identified only 25% of MSA patients correctly at the first visit. Although formal diagnostic criteria (1) yield satisfactory specificity, their sensitivity is currently insufficient, hampering an early diagnosis of MSA (96).

Red flags may be useful to facilitate a diagnosis of MSA (87). Axial as well as orofacial dystonia and contractures of the hands and feet have been shown to occur more frequently in MSA as compared with PD and were therefore included among MSA red flags (87). Signs of thermoregulatory and respiratory autonomic failure, like cold hands or feet and inspiratory sighs or snoring, have been shown to precede overt autonomic failure in MSA (86,87,97). Moreover, although not exclusive of MSA, severe dysphonia and dysarthria as well as emotional incontinence are also indicated as supportive of a MSA diagnosis (1).

MSA patients frequently show myoclonic jerks or action tremor of the upper limbs (red flag). The classic PD pill-rolling tremor has been reported in only a minority of MSA cases (68) and was therefore included among the non-supporting features of MSA. Additionally, a disease onset above the age of 75 and a positive family history of ataxia or parkinsonism should cast doubt on a diagnosis of MSA, although MSA pedigrees and monogenic MSA cases have been reported recently (24,98). Finally, no white matter lesions suggesting multiple sclerosis must be present upon routine MRI investigation (1).

Treatment

Thus far, disease-modifying medical treatments are lacking, despite intensified efforts to develop inteventional strategies. A placebo-controlled double-blind trial of recombinant human growth hormone (r-HGH) failed to slow motor progression (99). After neuroprotective effects of minocycline were demonstrated in a transgenic mouse model of MSA (100), the clinical study was negative in all primary and key secondary outcome measures, although a strong biological effect of reduced microglial activation was observed (101). Riluzole, an antiglutamatergic agent, was assessed in a randomized-controlled double-blind trial, but also failed to prolong survival in this fatal disease (66). Low dose rasagiline treatment could not halt progression in MSA (102). Likewise, a randomized, double-blind, placebo-controlled clinical safety and efficacy study of rifampicin in 100 MSA patients was prematurely terminated because statistical criteria for futility were met in a planned interim analysis (103). Finally, a randomized controlled trial demonstrated a neuroprotective effect of mesenchymal stem cells in MSA patients (104). However, it currently appears impossible to treat MSA patients routinely with mesenchymal stem cells and it remains to be seen, whether these encouraging findings can be replicated by independent research groups. Therefore, the management of MSA patients largely concerns the alleviation of parkinsonian and autonomic symptoms. Although autonomic failure is almost universally present in MSA, only one-third of affected patients receive appropriate pharmacological treatment (69).

Autonomic dysfunction

Orthostatic hypotension
A broad range of drugs has been used in the treatment of orthostatic hypotension. However, the benefits and side-effects of many of them have not been evaluated in MSA patients in a rand-

omized, controlled fashion. Non-pharmacological options to counteract postural blood pressure drop include sufficient fluid intake, high salt diet, spreading of daily carbohydrate intake and elastic body garments (105). At night, a head-up tilt increases intravasal volume by up to 1 litre within a week, which is particular helpful to improve early morning hypotension. The beneficial effects of this approach may be enhanced by the prescription of fludrocortisone, which further supports sodium retention (79). The directly acting α-agonist midodrine is the only vasoactive agent that complies with the criteria of evidence-based medicine (105, 106). Side-effects are usually mild and rarely require withdrawal of treatment (105, 106). Additionally, the parasympathomimetic and reversible cholinesterase inhibitor pyridostigmine provides a moderate but significant improvement in orthostatic hypotension due to enhancement of sympathetic activity (107). Another promising drug appears to be the norepinephrine precursor L-threo-dihydroxy-phenylserine (L-threo-DOPS, droxidopa), which is widely used in Japan and whose efficacy has been proved by two double-blind, placebo-controlled trials (108, 109). However, neither the European (EMA) nor the American (FDA) drug administration has approved its use. Furthermore, octreotide, which is a somatostatin analogue, might alleviate postprandial hypotension without causing or increasing nocturnal hypertension (110). This effect is most likely mediated by the inhibition of the release of vasodilatory gastrointestinal peptides (111). Additionally, the vasopressin analogue desmopressin, which acts on renal tubular vasopressin-2 receptors, reduces nocturnal polyuria and improves early morning postural hypotension (112). Sympathomimetics, such as ephedrine, have both direct and indirect effects which might be useful in central autonomic dysfunction. However, with higher doses, side-effects arise, including tremulousness, loss of appetite, and urinary retention, particularly in men.

Voiding problems

In terms of neurogenic bladder dysfunction, presenting with post-void residual volumes, clean intermittent catheterization three to four times per day is a widely accepted approach to prevent secondary consequences. If mechanical obstruction in the urethra or motor symptoms of MSA prevent uncomplicated catheterization, a permanent transcutaneous suprapubic catheterization may become necessary (113). Pharmacological options including anticholinergic, procholinergic and adrenergic substances are not usually successful in altering the post-void residual volume in MSA. However, anticholinergic agents such as oxybutynin may improve the symptoms of detrusor hyperreflexia or sphincter-detrusor dyssynergia in the early course of the disease (74). The use of anticholinergic treatment is frequently limited by central nervous adverse effects. More recently, a peripherally acting anticholinergic agent, trospium chloride, has been shown to be equally effective in patients with detrusor hyperreflexia without causing central nervous adverse effects (114). Finally, α-adrenergic receptor antagonists (prazosin and moxisylyte) have been shown to improve voiding with reduction of residual volumes in MSA patients (115).

Sexual dysfunction

The requirement for a specific treatment of sexual dysfunction needs to be evaluated individually in each patient. The phosphodiesterase type 5 inhibitor sildenafil improved male erectile function in a placebo-controlled, double-blind study (116). However, sildenafil may only be prescribed after exclusion of severe postural hypotension as this compound may unmask or worsen orthostatic hypotension.

Constipation

In terms of gastrointestinal symptoms, such as constipation, non-pharmacological treatment should be considered first. This includes daily exercise, high fluid and high fiber intake, and the consumption of fruit juices. If laxative therapy becomes necessary, polycarbophil and mosapride citrate may relieve constipation symptoms as suggested by two small, open-label studies (117). Nonetheless, an increase of intraluminal fluid which may be achieved by a macrogol-water solution may alleviate such symptoms as well (118).

Parkinsonism

Parkinsonism is another major target for symptomatic treatment. Despite the lack of randomized, controlled trials, levodopa is the most frequently used antiparkinsonian agent in MSA. An analysis of a multi-site patient registry revealed that up to 40% of MSA patients benefit from levodopa treatment (69). Unfortunately, this response is often a transient effect, usually lasting for less than 3 years (70). Pre-existing orthostatic hypotension is often unmasked or exacerbated by levodopa treatment in patients with MSA. Treatment with dopamine agonists has been disappointing. Severe psychiatric side-effects occurred in a double-blind, crossover trial of 6 patients treated with lisuride, with nightmares, visual hallucinations and toxic confusional states (119). Wenning et al. reported a response to oral dopamine agonists in only 4 of 41 patients, none of 30 patients receiving bromocriptine improved, but 3 of 10 who received pergolide experienced some benefit (15). Of the levodopa responders, 22% had a good or excellent response to at least one dopamine agonist (15). A randomized, placebo-controlled study demonstrated a tendency towards the beneficial effects of amantadine treatment in MSA patients (120).

Local botulinum toxin injections are useful in the treatment of orofacial dystonia, including blepharospasm and limb dystonia (121). However, botulinum toxin injections should be avoided in the therapy of disproportionate antecollis as severe dysphagia resulting in admissions to intensive care units have been reported (122). Botulinum toxin injections into the parotid and submandibular glands were shown to be useful to alleviate siallorhea (123).

Cerebellar ataxia

Cerebellar ataxia is the clinical hallmark of MSA-C and present in nearly two-thirds of MSA patients (69). Currently, there is no effective pharmacological treatment for MSA-associated cerebellar ataxia, although several case reports suggest beneficial effects mediated by a variety of compounds including cholinergics, NMDA receptor antagonists, derivates from γ-aminobutyric acid, non-selective beta-blockers, 5-hydroxytryptophan and isoniazid. However, none of these medications proved to be effective in larger case series (124).

Prognosis

MSA is a fatal and progressive disorder associated with a reduced life expectancy. Death occurs on average within 10 years of symptom onset. Common causes of death in MSA include urinary tract infections, aspiration pneumonia, cardiopulmonary arrest with pulmonary embolism, and the wasting syndrome (125). However, sudden death frequently occurring during sleep remains another common cause of death in MSA, with loss of serotonergic neurons in the ventrolateral medulla causing dysregulation of cardiovascular and respiratory systems likely being involved (81).

References

1 Gilman S, Wenning GK, Low PA, et al. Second consensus statement on the diagnosis of multiple system atrophy. Neurology 2008;71:670-676.

2 Trojanowski JQ, Revesz T. Proposed neuropathological criteria for the post mortem diagnosis of multiple system atrophy. Neuropath Appl Neurobiology 2007;33:615-620.

3 Wenning GK, Colosimo C, Geser F, Poewe W. Multiple system atrophy. Lancet Neurol 2004;3:93-103.

4 Graham JG, Oppenheimer DR. Orthostatic hypotension and nicotine sensitivity in a case of multiple system atrophy. J Neurol Neurosurg Psychiatry. 1969;32:28-34.

5 Dejerine J, Thomas A. L'atrophie olivo-ponto-cer-ebelleuse. Nouvelle iconographie de la Salpetriere: Clinique des malacies du systeme nerveux. 1900;13:330-370.

6 Adams MR, Van Bogaert L, van der Eecken H. [Nigro-striate and cerebello-nigro-striate degeneration. (Clinical uniqueness and pathological variability of presenile degeneration of the extrapyramidal rigidity type.]. Psychiatr Neurol (Basel). 1961;142:219-259.

7 Shy GM, Drager GA. A neurological syndrome associated with orthostatic hypotension: a clinical-pathologic study. Arch Neurol 1960;2:511-527.

8 Papp MI, Kahn JE, Lantos PL. Glial cytoplasmic inclusions in the CNS of patients with multiple system atrophy (striatonigral degeneration, olivopontocerebellar atrophy and Shy-Drager syndrome). J Neurol Sci 1989;94:79-100.

9 Spillantini MG, Crowther RA, Jakes R, Cairns NJ, Lantos PL, Goedert M. Filamentous alpha-synuclein inclusions link multiple system atrophy with Parkinson's disease and dementia with Lewy bodies. Neurosci Lett 1998;251:205-208.

10 Quinn N. Multiple system atrophy--the nature of the beast. J Neurol Neurosurg Psychiatry 1989;Suppl:78-89.

11 O'Sullivan SS, Massey LA, Williams DR, et al. Clinical outcomes of progressive supranuclear palsy and multiple system atrophy. Brain 2008;131:1362-1372.

12 Schrag A, Wenning GK, Quinn N, Ben-Shlomo Y. Survival in multiple system atrophy. Mov Disord 2008;23:294-296.

13 Testa D, Filippini G, Farinotti M, Palazzini E, Caraceni T. Survival in multiple system atrophy: a study of prognostic factors in 59 cases. J Neurol 1996;243:401-404.

14 Watanabe H, Saito Y, Terao S, et al. Progression and prognosis in multiple system atrophy: an analysis of 230 Japanese patients. Brain 2002;125:1070-1083.

15 Wenning GK, Ben Shlomo Y, Magalhaes M, Daniel SE, Quinn NP. Clinical features and natural history of multiple system atrophy. An analysis of 100 cases. Brain 1994;117:835-845.

16 Wenning GK, Geser F, Krismer F, et al. The natural history of multiple system atrophy: a prospective European cohort study. Lancet Neurol 2013;12:264-274.

17 Bower JH, Maraganore DM, McDonnell SK, Rocca WA. Incidence of progressive supranuclear palsy and multiple system atrophy in Olmsted County, Minnesota, 1976 to 1990. Neurology 1997;49:1284-1288.

18 Bjornsdottir A, Gudmundsson G, Blondal H, Olafsson E. Incidence and prevalence of multiple system atrophy: a nationwide study in Iceland. J Neurol Neurosurg Psychiatry 2013;84:136-140.

19 Linder J, Stenlund H, Forsgren L. Incidence of Parkinson's disease and parkinsonism in northern Sweden: a population-based study. Mov Disord 2010;25:341-348.

20 Winter Y, Bezdolnyy Y, Katunina E, et al. Incidence of Parkinson's disease and atypical parkinsonism: Russian population-based study. Mov Disord 2010;25:349-356.

21 Schrag A, Ben-Shlomo Y, Quinn NP. Prevalence of progressive supranuclear palsy and multiple system atrophy: a cross-sectional study. Lancet 1999;354:1771-5.

22 Tison F, Yekhlef F, Chrysostome V, Sourgen C. Prevalence of multiple system atrophy. Lancet 2000;355:495-496.

23 Trenkwalder C, Schwarz J, Gebhard J, et al. Starnberg trial on epidemiology of Parkinsonism and hypertension in the elderly. Prevalence of Parkinson's disease and related disorders assessed by a door-to-door survey of inhabitants older than 65 years. Arch Neurol 1995;52:1017-1022.

24 Multiple-System Atrophy Research Collaboration. Mutations in COQ2 in Familial and Sporadic Multiple-System Atrophy. N Engl J Med 2013.

25 Hara K, Momose Y, Tokiguchi S, et al. Multiplex families with multiple system atrophy. Arch Neurol 2007;64:545-551.

26 Soma H, Yabe I, Takei A, Fujiki N, Yanagihara T, Sasaki H. Heredity in multiple system atrophy. J Neurol Sci 2006;240:107-110.

27 Wullner U, Abele M, Schmitz-Huebsch T, et al. Probable multiple system atrophy in a German family. J Neurol Neurosurg Psychiatry 2004;75:924-925.

28 Wullner U, Schmitt I, Kammal M, Kretzschmar HA, Neumann M. Definite multiple system atrophy in a German family. J Neurol Neurosurg Psychiatry 2009;80:449-450.

29 Sasaki H, Emi M, Iijima H, et al. Copy number loss of (src homology 2 domain containing)-transforming protein 2 (SHC2) gene: discordant loss in monozygotic twins and frequent loss in patients with multiple system atrophy. Mol Brain 2011;4:24.

30 Nee LE, Gomez MR, Dambrosia J, Bale S, Eldridge R, Polinsky RJ. Environmental-occupational risk factors and familial associations in multiple system atrophy: a preliminary investigation. Clin Auton Res 1991;1:9-13.

31 Vanacore N, Bonifati V, Fabbrini G, et al. Case-control study of multiple system atrophy. Mov Disord 2005;20:158-163.

32 Vidal JS, Vidailhet M, Elbaz A, Derkinderen P, Tzourio C, Alperovitch A. Risk factors of multiple system atrophy: a case-control study in French patients. Mov Disord 2008;23:797-803.

33 Ozawa T, Paviour D, Quinn NP, et al. The spectrum of pathological involvement of the striatonigral and olivopontocerebellar systems in multiple system atrophy: clinicopathological correlations. Brain 2004;127:2657-2671.

34 Yoshida M. Multiple system atrophy: alpha-synuclein and neuronal degeneration. Neuropathol 2007;27:484-493.

35 Nishie M, Mori F, Yoshimoto M, Takahashi H, Wakabayashi K. A quantitative investigation of neuronal cytoplasmic and intranuclear inclusions in the pontine and inferior olivary nuclei in multiple system atrophy. Neuropathol Appl Neurobiol ogy 2004;30:546-554.

36 Wakabayashi K, Mori F, Nishie M, et al. An autopsy case of early („minimal change") olivopontocerebellar atrophy (multiple system atrophy-cerebellar). Acta Neuropath 2005;110:185-190.

37 Jellinger K. The role of α-synuclein in neurodegeneration – An update. Transl Neurosci 2012;3:75-122.

38 Orosz F, Kovacs GG, Lehotzky A, Olah J, Vincze O, Ovadi J. TPPP/p25: from unfolded protein to misfolding disease: prediction and experiments. Biol Cell. 2004;96:701-711.

39 Kovacs GG, Laszlo L, Kovacs J, et al. Natively unfolded tubulin polymerization promoting protein TPPP/p25 is a common marker of alpha-synucleinopathies. Neurobiol Dis 2004;17:155-162.

40 Ovadi J, Orosz F. An unstructured protein with destructive potential: TPPP/p25 in neurodegeneration. Bioessays 2009;31:676-686.

41 Song YJ, Lundvig DM, Huang Y, et al. p25alpha relocalizes in oligodendroglia from myelin to cytoplasmic inclusions in multiple system atrophy. Am J Pathol 2007;171:1291-1303.

42 Lindersson E, Lundvig D, Petersen C, et al. p25alpha Stimulates alpha-synuclein aggregation and is co-localized with aggregated alpha-synuclein in alpha-synucleinopathies. J Biol Chem 2005;280:5703-5715.

43 Hasegawa T, Baba T, Kobayashi M, et al. Role of TPPP/p25 on alpha-synuclein-mediated oligodendroglial degeneration and the protective effect of SIRT2 inhibition in a cellular model of multiple system atrophy. Neurochem Int 2010;57:857-866.

44 Wenning GK, Stefanova N, Jellinger KA, Poewe W, Schlossmacher MG. Multiple system atrophy: a primary oligodendrogliopathy. Ann Neurol 2008;64:239-246.

45 Beyer K. Alpha-synuclein structure, posttranslational modification and alternative splicing as aggregation enhancers. Acta Neuropath 2006;112:237-251.

46 Beyer K, Ariza A. Protein aggregation mechanisms in synucleinopathies: commonalities and differences. J Neuropathol Exp Neurol 2007;66:965-974.

47 Duda JE, Giasson BI, Gur TL, et al. Immunohistochemical and biochemical studies demonstrate a distinct profile of alpha-synuclein permutations in multiple system atrophy. J Neuropathol Exp Neurol 2000;59:830-841.

48 Fujiwara H, Hasegawa M, Dohmae N, et al. alpha-Synuclein is phosphorylated in synucleinopathy lesions. Nat Cell Biol 2002;4:160-164.

49 Giasson BI, Duda JE, Murray IV, et al. Oxidative damage linked to neurodegeneration by selective alpha-synuclein nitration in synucleinopathy lesions. Science 2000;290:985-989.

50 Ischiropoulos H. Oxidative modifications of alpha-synuclein. Ann N Y Acad Sci 2003;991:93-100.

51 Kahle PJ, Neumann M, Ozmen L, et al. Hyperphos-phorylation and insolubility of alpha-synuclein in transgenic mouse oligodendrocytes. EMBO Reports 2002;3:583-588.

52 Duda JE, Giasson BI, Chen Q, et al. Widespread nitration of pathological inclusions in neuro-degenerative synucleinopathies. Am J Pathol 2000;157:1439-1445.

53 Jin H, Ishikawa K, Tsunemi T, Ishiguro T, Amino T, Mizusawa H. Analyses of copy number and mRNA expression level of the alpha-synuclein gene in multiple system atrophy. J Med Dent Sci 2008;55:145-153.

54 Miller DW, Johnson JM, Solano SM, Holling-sworth ZR, Standaert DG, Young AB. Absence of alpha-synuclein mRNA expression in normal and multiple system atrophy oligodendroglia. J Neural Transm 2005;112:1613-1624.

55 Ozawa T, Okuizumi K, Ikeuchi T, Wakabayashi K, Takahashi H, Tsuji S. Analysis of the expression level of alpha-synuclein mRNA using postmor-tem brain samples from pathologically confirmed cases of multiple system atrophy. Acta Neuropath 2001;102:188-190.

56 Frost B, Diamond MI. Prion-like mechanisms in neurodegenerative diseases. Nat Rev Neurosci 2010;11:155-159.

57 Lee SJ, Desplats P, Sigurdson C, Tsigelny I, Masliah E. Cell-to-cell transmission of non-prion protein aggregates. Nat Rev Neurol 2010;6:702-706.

58 Walker LC, Diamond MI, Duff KE, Hyman BT. Mechanisms of protein seeding in neurodegenera-tive diseases. JAMA Neurol 2013;70:304-310.

59 Wakabayashi K, Ikeuchi T, Ishikawa A, Takahashi H. Multiple system atrophy with severe involve-ment of the motor cortical areas and cerebral white matter. J Neurol Sci 1998;156:114-117.

60 Reynolds AD, Kadiu I, Garg SK, et al. Nitrated alpha-synuclein and microglial neuroregulatory ac-tivities. J Neuroimmune Pharmacol 2008;3:59-74.

61 Su X, Federoff HJ, Maguire-Zeiss KA. Mutant al-pha-synuclein overexpression mediates early proin-flammatory activity. Neurotox Res 2009;16:238-254.

62 Su X, Maguire-Zeiss KA, Giuliano R, Prifti L, Ven-katesh K, Federoff HJ. Synuclein activates micro-glia in a model of Parkinson's disease. Neurobiol Aging 2008;29:1690-1701.

63 Bartels AL, Willemsen AT, Doorduin J, de Vries EF, Dierckx RA, Leenders KL. [11C]-PK11195 PET: quantification of neuroinflammation and a moni-tor of anti-inflammatory treatment in Parkinson's disease? Parkinsonism Relat Disord 2010;16:57-59.

64 Beraud D, Hathaway HA, Trecki J, et al. Microglial activation and antioxidant responses induced by the Parkinson's disease protein alpha-synuclein. J Neuroimmune Pharmacol 2013;8:94-117.

65 Klegeris A, Pelech S, Giasson BI, et al. Alpha-syn-uclein activates stress signaling protein kinases in THP-1 cells and microglia. Neurobiol Aging 2008;29:739-752.

66 Bensimon G, Ludolph A, Agid Y, Vidailhet M, Payan C, Leigh PN. Riluzole treatment, survival and diagnostic criteria in Parkinson plus disorders: the NNIPPS study. Brain 2009;132:156-171.

67 Schwarz J, Tatsch K, Arnold G, et al. 123I-iodoben-zamide-SPECT predicts dopaminergic respon-siveness in patients with de novo parkinsonism. Neurology 1992;42:556-561.

68 Wenning GK, Tison F, Ben Shlomo Y, Daniel SE, Quinn NP. Multiple system atrophy: a review of 203 pathologically proven cases. Mov Disord 1997;12:133-147.

69 Kollensperger M, Geser F, Ndayisaba JP, et al. Pres-entation, diagnosis, and management of multiple system atrophy in Europe: Final analysis of the European multiple system atrophy registry. Mov Disord. 2010;25:2604-2612.

70 Geser F, Wenning GK, Seppi K, et al. Progression of multiple system atrophy (MSA): A prospective natural history study by the European MSA Study Group (EMSA SG). Mov Disord 2006;21:179-186.

71 Wenning GK, Ben Shlomo Y, Hughes A, Daniel SE, Lees A, Quinn NP. What clinical features are most useful to distinguish definite multiple system atro-phy from Parkinson's disease? J Neurol Neurosurg Psychiatry 2000;68:434-440.

72 Kluin KJ, Gilman S, Lohman M, Junck L. Char-acteristics of the dysarthria of multiple system atro-phy. Arch Neurol 1996;53:545-548.

73 Abele M, Burk K, Schols L, et al. The aetiology of sporadic adult-onset ataxia. Brain 2002;125:961-968.

74 Beck RO, Betts CD, Fowler CJ. Genitourinary dysfunction in multiple system atrophy: clinical features and treatment in 62 cases. J Urol 1994;151:1336-1341.

75 Chandiramani VA, Palace J, Fowler CJ. How to recognize patients with parkinsonism who should not have urological surgery. Brit J Urol 1997;80:100-104.

76 Oertel WH, Wachter T, Quinn NP, Ulm G, Brandstadter D. Reduced genital sensitivity in female patients with multiple system atrophy of parkinsonian type. Mov Disord 2003;18:430-432.

77 Wenning GK, Scherfler C, Granata R, et al. Time course of symptomatic orthostatic hypotension and urinary incontinence in patients with postmortem confirmed parkinsonian syndromes: a clinicopathological study. J Neurol Neurosurg Psychiatry 1999;67:620-623.

78 Deguchi K, Ikeda K, Sasaki I, et al. Effects of daily water drinking on orthostatic and postprandial hypotension in patients with multiple system atrophy. J Neurol 2007;254:735-740.

79 Freeman R. Current pharmacologic treatment for orthostatic hypotension. Clin Auton Res 2008;18 Suppl 1:14-18.

80 Lipsitz LA, Ryan SM, Parker JA, Freeman R, Wei JY, Goldberger AL. Hemodynamic and autonomic nervous system responses to mixed meal ingestion in healthy young and old subjects and dysautonomic patients with postprandial hypotension. Circulation 1993;87:391-400.

81 Tada M, Onodera O, Ozawa T, et al. Early development of autonomic dysfunction may predict poor prognosis in patients with multiple system atrophy. Arch Neurol 2007;64:256-260.

82 Cohen J, Low P, Fealey R, Sheps S, Jiang NS. Somatic and autonomic function in progressive autonomic failure and multiple system atrophy. Ann Neurol 1987;22:692-629.

83 Lipp A, Sandroni P, Ahlskog JE, et al. Prospective differentiation of multiple system atrophy from Parkinson disease, with and without autonomic failure. Arch Neurol 2009;66:742-750.

84 Kihara M, Sugenoya J, Takahashi A. The assessment of sudomotor dysfunction in multiple system atrophy. Clin Auton Res 1991;1:297-302.

85 Sandroni P, Ahlskog JE, Fealey RD, Low PA. Autonomic involvement in extrapyramidal and cerebellar disorders. Clin Auton Res 1991;1:147-155.

86 Klein C, Brown R, Wenning G, Quinn N. The „cold hands sign" in multiple system atrophy. Mov Disord 1997;12:514-518.

87 Kollensperger M, Geser F, Seppi K, et al. Red flags for multiple system atrophy. Mov Disord 2008;23:1093-1099.

88 Benarroch EE. Pedunculopontine nucleus: functional organization and clinical implications. Neurology 2013;80:1148-1155.

89 Boesch SM, Wenning GK, Ransmayr G, Poewe W. Dystonia in multiple system atrophy. J Neurol Neurosurg Psychiatry 2002;72:300-303.

90 Caplan LR. Clinical features of sporadic (Dejerine-Thomas) olivopontocerebellar atrophy. Adv Neurol 1984;41:217-224.

91 Rivest J, Quinn N, Marsden CD. Dystonia in Parkinson's disease, multiple system atrophy, and progressive supranuclear palsy. Neurology 1990;40:1571-1578.

92 Salazar G, Valls-Sole J, Marti MJ, Chang H, Tolosa ES. Postural and action myoclonus in patients with parkinsonian type multiple system atrophy. Mov Disord 2000;15:77-83.

93 Silber MH, Levine S. Stridor and death in multiple system atrophy. Mov Disord 2000;15:699-704.

94 Muller J, Wenning GK, Verny M, et al. Progression of dysarthria and dysphagia in postmortem-confirmed parkinsonian disorders. Arch Neurol 2001;58:259-264.

95 Litvan I, Goetz CG, Jankovic J, et al. What is the accuracy of the clinical diagnosis of multiple system atrophy? A clinicopathologic study. Arch Neurol 1997;54:937-944.

96 Osaki Y, Ben-Shlomo Y, Lees AJ, Wenning GK, Quinn NP. A validation exercise on the new consensus criteria for multiple system atrophy. Mov Disord 2009;24:2272-2276.

97 Ghorayeb I, Yekhlef F, Chrysostome V, Balestre E, Bioulac B, Tison F. Sleep disorders and their

determinants in multiple system atrophy. J Neurol Neurosurg Psychiatry 2002;72:798-800.

98 Ahmed Z, Asi YT, Sailer A, et al. The neuropathology, pathophysiology and genetics of multiple system atrophy. Neuropath Appl Neurobiol 2012;38:4-24.

99 Holmberg B, Johansson JO, Poewe W, et al. Safety and tolerability of growth hormone therapy in multiple system atrophy: a double-blind, placebo-controlled study. Mov Disord 2007;22:1138-1144.

100 Stefanova N, Reindl M, Neumann M, Kahle PJ, Poewe W, Wenning GK. Microglial activation mediates neurodegeneration related to oligodendroglial alpha-synucleinopathy: implications for multiple system atrophy. Mov Disord 2007;22:2196-2203.

101 Dodel R, Spottke A, Gerhard A, et al. Minocycline 1-year therapy in multiple-system-atrophy: effect on clinical symptoms and [(11)C] (R)-PK11195 PET (MEMSA-trial). Mov Disord 2010;25:97-107.

102 Poewe W, Barone P, Giladi N, et al. A randomized, placebo-controlled clinical trial to assess the effects of rasagiline in patients with multiple system atrophy of the parkinsonian subtype. Mov Disord 2012;27(S1):1182.

103 Low P, Robertson D, Gilman S, et al. Randomized treatment trial of rifampicin in MSA patients. Movement Disorders 2013;28(S1):418.

104 Lee PH, Lee JE, Kim HS, et al. A randomized trial of mesenchymal stem cells in multiple system atrophy. Ann Neurol 2012;72:32-40.

105 Low PA, Singer W. Management of neurogenic orthostatic hypotension: an update. Lancet Neurol 2008;7:451-458.

106 Jankovic J, Gilden JL, Hiner BC, et al. Neurogenic orthostatic hypotension: a double-blind, placebo-controlled study with midodrine. Am J Med 1993;95:38-48.

107 Singer W, Sandroni P, Opfer-Gehrking TL, et al. Pyridostigmine treatment trial in neurogenic orthostatic hypotension. Arch Neurol 2006;63:513-518.

108 Kaufmann H. L-dihydroxyphenylserine (Droxidopa): a new therapy for neurogenic orthostatic hypotension: the US experience. Clin Autonom Res 2008;18(S1):19-24.

109 Mathias CJ. L-dihydroxyphenylserine (Droxidopa) in the treatment of orthostatic hypotension: the European experience. Clin Autonom Res 2008;18 Suppl 1:25-29.

110 Alam M, Smith G, Bleasdale-Barr K, Pavitt DV, Mathias CJ. Effects of the peptide release inhibitor, octreotide, on daytime hypotension and on nocturnal hypertension in primary autonomic failure. J Hypertens 1995;13:1664-1669.

111 Raimbach SJ, Cortelli P, Kooner JS, Bannister R, Bloom SR, Mathias CJ. Prevention of glucose-induced hypotension by the somatostatin analogue octreotide (SMS 201-995) in chronic autonomic failure: haemodynamic and hormonal changes. Clin Sci (Lond) 1989;77:623-628.

112 Mathias CJ, Fosbraey P, da Costa DF, Thornley A, Bannister R. The effect of desmopressin on nocturnal polyuria, overnight weight loss, and morning postural hypotension in patients with autonomic failure. Br Med J 1986;293:353-354.

113 Fowler CJ, O'Malley KJ. Investigation and management of neurogenic bladder dysfunction. J Neurol Neurosurg Psychiatry 2003;74(S4):iv27-iv31.

114 Halaska M, Ralph G, Wiedemann A, et al. Controlled, double-blind, multicentre clinical trial to investigate long-term tolerability and efficacy of trospium chloride in patients with detrusor instability. World J Urol 2003;20:392-329.

115 Sakakibara R, Hattori T, Uchiyama T, et al. Are alpha-blockers involved in lower urinary tract dysfunction in multiple system atrophy? A comparison of prazosin and moxisylyte. J Anton Nerv Syst 2000;79:191-195.

116 Hussain IF, Brady CM, Swinn MJ, Mathias CJ, Fowler CJ. Treatment of erectile dysfunction with sildenafil citrate (Viagra) in parkinsonism due to Parkinson's disease or multiple system atrophy with observations on orthostatic hypotension. J Neurol Neurosurg Psychiatry 2001;71:371-374.

117 Sakakibara R, Yamaguchi T, Uchiyama T, et al. Calcium polycarbophil improves constipation in primary autonomic failure and multiple system atrophy subjects. Mov Disord 2007;22:1672-1673.

118 Eichhorn TE, Oertel WH. Macrogol 3350/electrolyte improves constipation in Parkinson's

disease and multiple system atrophy. Mov Disord 2001;16:1176-1177.

119 Lees AJ, Bannister R. The use of lisuride in the treatment of multiple system atrophy with autonomic failure (Shy-Drager syndrome). J Neurol Neurosurg Psychiatry 1981;44:347-351.

120 Wenning GK. Placebo-controlled trial of amantadine in multiple-system atrophy. Clin Neuropharmacol 2005;28:225-227.

121 Muller J, Wenning GK, Wissel J, Seppi K, Poewe W. Botulinum toxin treatment in atypical parkinsonian disorders associated with disabling focal dystonia. J Neurol 2002;249:300-304.

122 Thobois S, Broussolle E, Toureille L, Vial C. Severe dysphagia after botulinum toxin injection for

cervical dystonia in multiple system atrophy. Mov Disord 2001;16:764-765.

123 Mancini F, Zangaglia R, Cristina S, et al. Double-blind, placebo-controlled study to evaluate the efficacy and safety of botulinum toxin type A in the treatment of drooling in parkinsonism. Mov Disord 2003;18:685-688.

124 Wenning GK, Geser F, Stampfer-Kountchev M, Tison F. Multiple system atrophy: an update. Mov Disord 2003;18:S34-S42.

125 Papapetropoulos S, Tuchman A, Laufer D, Papatsoris AG, Papapetropoulos N, Mash DC. Causes of death in multiple system atrophy. J Neurol Neurosurg Psychiatry 2007;78:327-329.

20

Progressive Supranuclear Palsy

Christian R. Baumann & Andrew J. Lees

Progressive supranuclear palsy (PSP), also called Steele-Richardson-Olszewski syndrome, was identified by J.C. Richardson, J.C. Steele and J. Olszewski in 1963 (1). They described an 'unusual syndrome' characterised by axial rigidity, bradykinesia, postural instability with falls, cognitive deficits, and supranuclear vertical gaze palsy with the accumulation of brain stem neurofibrillary tangles. Several clinical subtypes have now been described and the disease is characterized by the presence of tufted astrocytes and neuropil threads as well as tangles on histological examination. Abnormal accumulation of hyperphosphorylated 4 repeat tau protein in the brain has aligned it closely with the rarer corticobasal degeneration and distinguished it from Pick's disease.

Epidemiology

The prevalence of PSP is about 5.3 per 100,000 (2,3) with no significant difference between the sexes and the incidence increases sharply with age with no convincing cases reported below the age of 45.

Aetiology

The cause is unknown and the large majority of cases have no positive family history for PSP. Several common genetic variants influencing the risk of PSP have been identified, however. Few PSP cases are autosomally dominantly inherited, and sporadic PSP patients have more first-degree relatives with parkinsonism than controls (4). In particular, a genome-wide association study in over 1,000 PSP patients and more than 3,000 controls confirmed two independent variants in microtubule-associated protein tau (MAPT) genes on chromosome 17 that influence the risk of developing PSP (5). This suggests that the genetic background of an individual plays a key role in the pathogenesis of PSP. Indeed, MAPT gene mutations, changing the way the gene's instructions are used to build the tau protein, are widely found to be causative of monogenic autosomal dominant fronto-temporal dementia-parkinsonism, and in sporadic cases the H1 MAPT haplotype has been consistently associated with PSP, while the H2 haplotype seems protective (6,7).

A study examining familial and sporadic, autopsy-proven PSP found surprisingly few clinical, pathologic, and genetic differences between the two groups (8). Familial cases resembling PSP tended to have less tau pathology, but a stronger association with H1 MAPT. Thus, H1 MAPT may not necessarily increase the severity of tau pathology (8). The H1 haplotype is also highly prevalent among healthy controls, which suggests that other predisposing conditions such as environmental or additional co-factors are important for triggering the disease. Additional genetic contributors probably exist, e.g. on chromosome 11, but environmental factors that increase the risk of PSP have not been identified (9,10).

There is increasing evidence that mitochondrial dysfunction plays a role in the pathogenesis of neurodegenerative diseases. Mitochondria are the most important cellular source for the production of reactive oxygen species. In PSP, failure in mitochondrial energy production is probably involved in both tau aggregation and neuronal cell death (11). In several post-mortem studies, increased oxidative stress was found in the brains of PSP patients (11). Indirect evidence suggests that mitochondrial dysfunction occurs as a primary phenomenon in PSP, but it remains unclear whether this is due to changes in mitochondrial DNA, to the presence of mitochondrial toxins such as lipophilic complex I inhibitors, or to tau oligomers which damage mitochondrial membranes (11). It has been found that the potency of lipophilic complex I inhibitors to decrease adenosine triphosphate (ATP) levels correlated with their potency to induce tau redistribution, which strongly suggests that cellular energy depletion plays a crucial role in tau pathology (12,13).

Pathophysiology

Microtubules are part of the cytoskeleton. They exert important cellular functions including the maintenance of the cell structure and providing platforms for intracellular transport. By forming mitotic spindles, they also play a role in cell division. Microtubules are stabilized by tau proteins, produced by alternative splicing from the MAPT gene (14). In tauopathies, the microtubule-associated tau protein is the most important component of neurofibrillary tangles (15). In PSP, there is a pathological accumulation of specific MAPT isoforms, characterized by four 31 amino acid repeats (4R) in the microtubule-binding domain (16). Normally, concentrations of 3R tau and 4R tau are similar, but in PSP, 4R tau outnumbers R3 tau. Therefore, PSP is considered a 4R tauopathy (17).

Along with neurofibrillary tangles with TAU antigen, the pathology in PSP includes astrocytic tufts, both considered characteristic for all tauopathies, including not only AD, CBD, Pick's disease and FTDP-7 but also postencephalitic parkinsonism and the parkinsonian syndromes of Guam and Guadeloupe (18-20) (see Figure 20.1).

To make the story even more complicated, PSP is clinically heterogeneous, and its clinical phenotype is mainly determined by the neuroanatomical distribution of tau pathology (20). The classical view is that the tau protein and neuropil threads accumulation appears mainly in the subthalamic nucleus, red nucleus, substantia nigra, pontine tegmentum, striatum, oculomotor nucleus, medulla, and dentate nucleus (20-22). However, there is growing evidence that cortical tau pathology is also common in PSP (18). Two post-mortem studies addressed the pathological

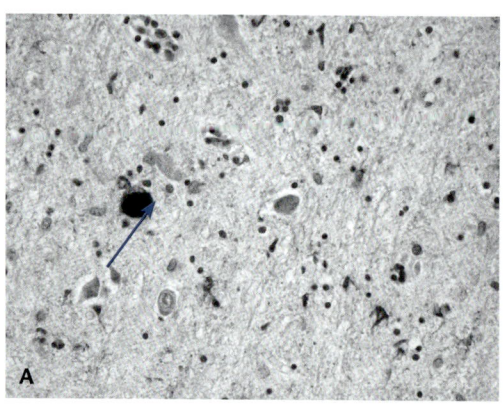
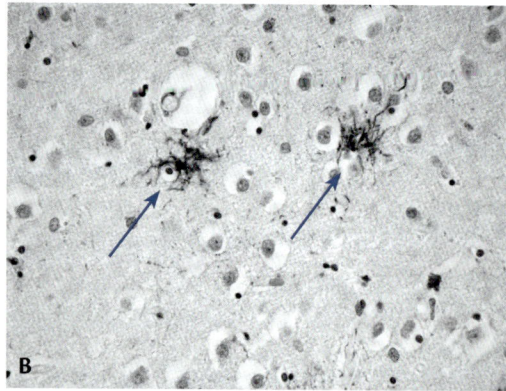

Figure 20.1

Characteristic neuropathological changes in PSP: A) globoid neurofibrillary tangle and B) tufted astrocytes. Both images visualized with antibody against tau (AT8).

Table 20.1
Clinical and functional imaging signs in different phenotypes of PSP and PD (from (20)).

	Richardson's	PSP-P	PSP-PAGF	PSP-CBS	PSP-PNFA	PD
Rigidity	Axial>limb	Axial≤limb	Axial	Yes	Sometimes	Limb>axial
Bradykinesia	Mild	Moderate	Moderate	Yes	Mild	Moderate
Tremor	No	Sometimes	No	No	No	Yes (at rest)
Early falls	Yes	No	No	Sometimes	Sometimes	No
Early postural instability	Yes	No	Yes	–	–	No
Early cognitive decline	Often	No	No	No	Yes	No
Early abnormalities of eye movement	Yes	No	No	No	Sometimes	No
Response to levodopa	No	Often	No	No	No	Usually
Hyposmia	No	No	–	–	–	Yes
Cardiac MIBG	Normal	Normal*	Normal*	–	–	Abnormal

MIGB = ^{131}I-labelled meta-iodobenzylguanidine; ·· = unknown. *Author's unpublished data. Abbreviations: see text.

heterogeneity of PSP and found major pathological differences between clinical syndromes associated with PSP-related tau pathology (23,24). Based on these findings as well as smaller clinicopathological studies, Williams and Lees and later on Dickson et al. discussed a novel clinicopathological classification of PSP syndromes (20,25). These clinical syndromes with specifically underlying neuropathology will be discussed later in this chapter.

Regarding functional dysfunction in PSP, a task-free functional MRI study has shown that patients with PSP have significant connectivity disruptions, particularly within cortico-subcortical and cortico-brainstem networks (26), associated with functional impairment.

Clinical presentation

To distinguish the different phenotypes in PSP, the Queen Square group under the direction of one of us (AJL) performed hierarchical cluster analyses without a priori assumptions in pathologically confirmed PSP cases (27,28). This sem-

inal work ultimately led to the identification of several subtypes of PSP (20,25). Table 20.1 gives an overview of the specific clinical findings in the five PSP variants distinguished, reflecting the differences in local expression of tauopathic degeneration: the classical (PSP) type, the parkinsonistic type (PSP-P), PSP with pure akinesia and freezing-of-gait (PSP-PAGF), the corticobasal type (PSP-CBS), and the variant with progressive non-fluent aphasia (PSP-PNFA).

PSP classical type

Classical PSP (also named Richardson's syndrome or Steele-Richardson-Olszewski syndrome) is characterized by a variety of clinical findings that are summarized in Table 20.2. Clinicians often look particularly for vertical gaze palsy but should keep in mind that this important diagnostic feature may be absent or appear very late in the course of the illness. Slowing of vertical saccades is a much earlier sign. Significant and multimodal functional impairment is present already early in the course of classical PSP (29), and its course is fast and leads to de-

Table 20.2
Clinical findings and neuropathological correlates in classical PSP (1,20-22,25,30-34).

Clinical findings
- Lurching gait with postural instability and early falls backwards.
- Supranuclear (initially mostly downward) (voluntary > pursuit) gaze palsy with early slowing of vertical saccades and preserved oculocephalic reflex.
- Eyelid retraction leading to a staring gaze and occasionally eyelid apraxia with involuntary eyelid closure.
- Axial > limb rigidity with dystonic posturing of the neck.
- Personality change with frontal lobe dysfunction and cognitive slowing, impaired attention, leading to subcortical dementia.
- Frequent dysarthria and dysphagia (in later phase).

Major neuropathological findings
- Tufted astrocytes in motor cortex and striatum, and predominant nuclear tau-pathology in globus pallidus, subthalamic nucleus, substantia nigra, and brainstem nuclei, but not in the cortex.

Table 20.3
Clinical findings and neuropathological correlates in PSP-P (1,20,25,35-36).

Clinical findings
- Asymmetric, modestly levodopa-responsive parkinsonism with predominant limb bradykinesia, rigidity, and tremor (jerky and postural, but also 4-6 Hz rest), followed later on by falls and cognitive impairment.
- Occasional levodopa-induced dyskinesias, autonomic dysfunction and visual hallucinations (less frequent than in PD).
- Regular extra-axial dystonia.
- Occasional vertical gaze palsy.
- In the end-stage, after 6 years or more, the clinical phenotype may become similar to classical PSP.

Major neuropathological findings
- Tau pathology is probably less severe than in classical PSP, particularly in the frontal lobes, caudate nucleus, globus pallidus interna, substantia nigra, pons, and cerebellum.

pendency within 3-4 years of diagnosis due to severe dysphagia and dysarthria, dementia, and frequent falls (32). Median survival is 5-8 years, and death is most often caused by aspiration pneumonia, pulmonary emboli, or neurogenic respiratory failure (32,33).

PSP parkinsonistic type

PSP-P is a distinct phenotype with prominent features of levodopa-responsive parkinsonism. This disorder is not always easy to distinguish from classical PSP and PD. Table 20.3 summarizes the clinical and neuropathological features of PSP-P. Compared to classical PSP, the course is a bit slower, with a survival time that is about 3 years longer (20,38).

PSP with pure akinesia and freezings-of-gait

The third phenotype is PSP-PAGF, PSP with pure akinesia and freezing-of-gait (28), although akinetic forms in PSP were already described in 1974 (37). PAGF patients reveal almost no tau pathology in cortical structures, but severe involvement of basal ganglia structures (25,38). Table 20.4 gives an overview of the clinical and neuropathological findings in PAGF patients. Their median survival time is again longer than in classical PSP, with a median survival time of about 11 years (14).

PSP corticobasal type

A fourth phenotype is PSP-CBS, which reflects some overlap with another tauopathy: corticobasal degeneration (see Table 20.5). However, the neuropathological substrate confirms corticobasal degeneration in not all patients with PSP-CBS, i.e. specimens with achromatic and balloon-shaped neurons and prominent diffuse cortical glial tau pathology (41). Those cases may involve overlap with AD or FTLD-17 (33).

Table 20.4
Clinical findings and neuropathological correlates in PSP with pure akinesia with gait freezing (PSP-PAGF) (1,20,25,38,39).

Clinical findings
- Asymmetric, non-levodopa-responsive symptoms.
- Early predominant pure akinesia with freezing-of-gait.
- Akinetic stammering speech and micrographia.
- Axial rigidity with pronounced neck stiffness, but not limb dystonia.
- Occasional tremor.
- Occasional late vertical gaze palsy and postural instability with falls.
- Mild cognitive impairment, less distinct than in classical PSP.

Major neuropathological findings
- Tau pathology (predominantly in the globus pallidus, the substantia nigra and the subthalamic nucleus, and only to a lesser extent in the striatum, pons and cerebellum) is much milder in the cortical structures and superior cerebellar peduncle compared to classical PSP.

PSP with progressive non-fluent aphasia

A last variant of PSP with predominant cortical involvement is PNFA, progressive non-flu-

Table 20.5
Clinical findings and neuropathological correlates in PSP with corticobasal syndrome (PSP-CBS) (1,20,25,40-42).

Clinical findings
- Corticobasal syndrome with very asymmetric, not levodopa-responsive parkinsonism (rigidity, bradykinesia), apraxia, cortical sensory loss, alien limb phenomenon, dystonia and/or myclonus.
- Late postural instability and falls.
- Most prominent oculomotor feature is increased latency to initiate saccadic eye movements.

Major neuropathological findings
- Pronounced tau pathology in frontal and parietal association cortices, contralateral to the clinical signs.

Table 20.6
Clinical findings and neuropathological correlates in PNFA, progressive non-fluent aphasia (1,20,25,43-45).

Clinical findings
- Non-fluent aphasia with disturbed speech production, sometimes similar to Broca's aphasia.
- Speech apraxia with errors in timing, coordination and initiation of speech, resulting in slow, segmented and groping speech.

Major neuropathological findings
- Disproportionately severe tau pathology in the frontal lobes.

ent aphasia (20). Although most PSP patients suffer from subcortical dementia, only some of them express signs of frontotemporal dementia (43,44). This syndrome shares many features with FTLD (see Table 20.6). Small case series revealed that PSP-tau pathology often underlies PNFA (45). Other pathologies included corticobasal degeneration and Pick's disease.

Altogether, PSP variants may be placed in a spectrum from predominantly subcortical basal ganglia and brainstem pathology with akinesia (PSP-PAGF and PSP-P) to predominantly cortical pathology with focal cortical symptomatology (PSP-CBS, PNFA) (25).

Diagnosis

The diagnosis of PSP and its variants is primarily based on careful clinical examination. Nevertheless, because of a significant overlap with other disorders, the diagnosis can sometimes be difficult, particularly in the early stages of the disease. In 1996, Litvan and colleagues introduced the National Institute of Neurological Disorders and Stroke and the Society for PSP (NINDS-SPSP)research criteria for the clinical diagnosis of PSP (Table 20.7) (46).

Autopsy is necessary to confirm the clinical diagnosis with certainty. A study to evaluate the NINDS-SPSP criteria clinicopathologically showed that the 'probable' criteria should be

Table 20.7
The National Institute of Neurological Disorders and Stroke and the Society for PSP (NINDS-SPSP) criteria for the clinical diagnosis of PSP.

In case of a gradually progressive disorder, starting at age ≥40 years and without signs of other disorders that might explain the symptoms

Possible PSP	▪ Vertical supranuclear palsy (upwards or downwards) **or** ▪ Slowing of vertical saccades **and** postural instability with falls within one year of disease onset
Probable PSP	▪ Vertical supranuclear palsy (upwards or downwards) **and** ▪ Postural instability with falls within one year of disease onset
Definite PSP	▪ Clinically probable or possible PSP **and** ▪ Histopathological signs of typical PSP

preferred for clinical trials, but for routine clinical care, the combined 'possible' and 'probable' criteria should be used because higher sensitivity leads to a shorter time to diagnosis and higher positive predictive values (47).

Several studies have examined whether MRI findings might serve as biomarkers for PSP. Classical findings in neuro-imaging that were linked to PSP, including the 'hummingbird' and

the 'morning-glory sign', were indeed found to be more specific though less sensitive than PSP clinical diagnostic criteria (48). This observation raised the need for more quantitative measures for the diagnosis of PSP.

In 2011, Morelli and colleagues introduced the magnetic resonance parkinsonism index (MRPI) to accurately differentiate between PSP patients and those with idiopathic PD or unclassified parkinsonism (49,50) (see Figure 20.2). They proved this index to be more accurate than the midbrain/pons ratio for the differentiation of PSP from PD patients, and superior to clinical features for differentiating PSP from clinically unclassifiable parkinsonism.

More recently, another group re-introduced the midbrain/pons ratio (51). This ratio is derived by dividing the midbrain measurements by the pons measurements (see Figure 20.3). The authors found that a midbrain measurement of <9.35mm and a ratio of ≤0.52 were 100% specific for PSP. Altogether, they concluded that this simple ratio provides both high sensitivity and specificity for the diagnosis of PSP.

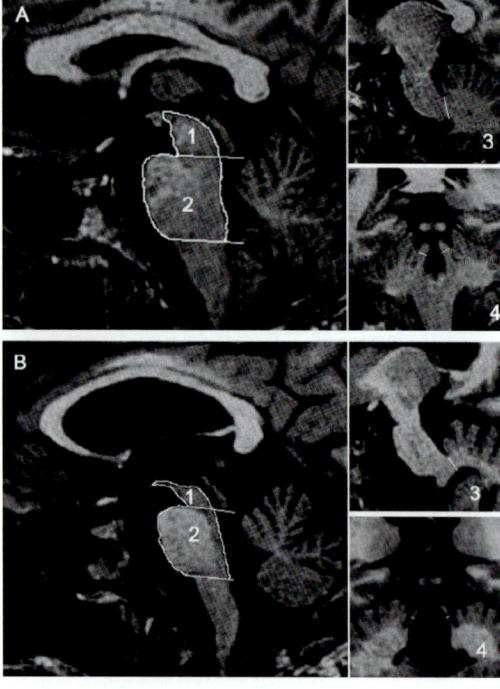

Figure 20.2
Calculation of the magnetic resonance parkinsonism index (MRPI), as introduced by (49,50). Images of a patient with clinically unclassifiable parkinsonism with normal MRPI (A) and a patient with clinically unclassifiable parkinsonism with abnormal MRPI (B). For the image assessment, the midbrain area (1) (M) and pons area (2) (P) were measured on midsagittal, T1-weighted, volumetric, spoiled gradient-echo MRI. Measurement of middle cerebellar peduncle width (3) (MCP) was performed on sagittal, T1-weighted, volumetric, spoiled gradient-echo MRI and of superior cerebellar peduncle width (4) (SCP) on the T1-weighted, volumetric, spoiled gradient-echo, high-spatial-resolution, oblique, coronal MRI. MRPI was calculated by multiplying the P/M ratio by MCP/SCP ratio: (P/M) x (MCP/SCP). MRPI values were considered abnormal if they exceeded the cutoff of 13.55. Figure reproduced with permission from (49).

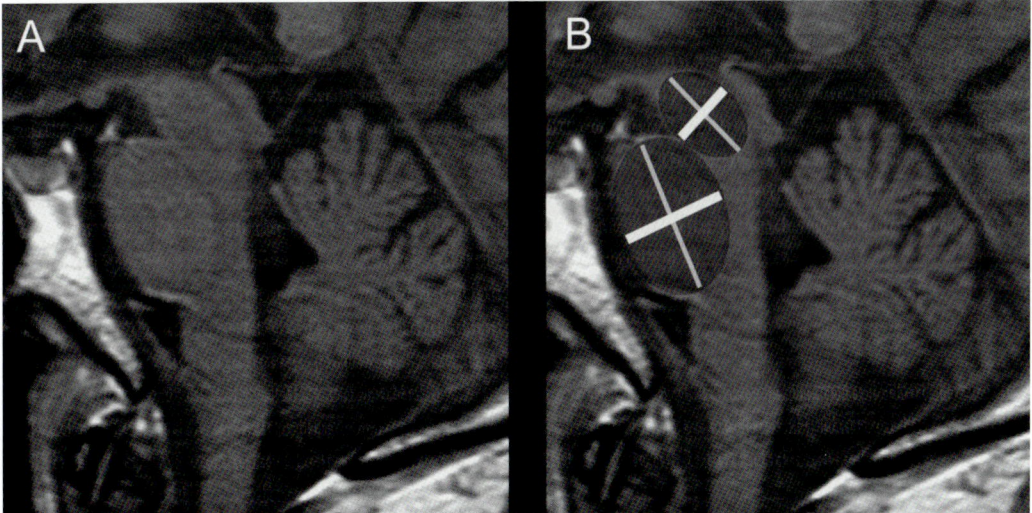

Figure 20.3
Assessment of the midbrain to pons ratio by measuring the anterior-posterior distance of the pons and midbrain, as introduced by (51). In a midsagittal T1 MRI image (A), elliptical regions of interest are placed over pons and midbrain (B). The major axes of the ellipses are introduced by two lines, and the maximal measurement (thick lines) perpendicular to the major axis (thin lines) is used for the calculations. Note that the pontine tegmentum and midbrain collicular plate are not included. Figure reproduced with permission from (51).

Differential diagnosis

PSP and its variants must certainly be differentiated from PD and other atypical Parkinson syndromes. The detailed clinical characteristics given above and in the chapters on PD (Chapters 5 and 10), multiple system atrophy (MSA) (Chapter 19), and corticobasal degeneration (CBD) (Chapter 21) might be useful for this purpose. For the distinction of psychogenic movement disorders, Chapter 37 provides further insights. There is growing evidence, however, that 'new' genetic conditions may also present with signs of PSP. Maria Stamelou and colleagues summarized these 'atypical' parkinsonistic conditions in a comprehensive review (Table 20.8) (52).

Treatment

Only about 10% of PSP patients experience some benefit from dopaminergic drugs such as levodopa and benefit is mostly partial and transient. If treatment with levodopa up to 1000 mg per day for three months fails to produce benefit then the drug should be tailed off and it is not worth trying dopamine agonists. Anticholinergic drugs are equally ineffective but on the other hand many physicians feel that amantadine may be of modest benefit in improving motor symptoms in some cases. There is some weak evidence that amitriptyline (up to 150 mg per day) might improve motor symptoms in PSP, but neuropsychiatric side effects may occur (53,54).

Keeping in mind that mitochondrial complex I appears to be dysfunctional in PSP, coenzyme Q10 (which is a physiological co-factor of this complex) might exert some beneficial effects as suggested by Stamelou and colleagues, who established some slight but significant clinical improvement in a phase II trial with coenzyme Q10 compared to placebo (55). This improvement was mirrored by increased ratios of high-energy to low-energy metabolites (ATP/ADP) in the living brain, as measured by functional imaging. Therefore, recently, a phase III trial was started (NCT00382824) in order to study a potential

Table 20.8
Important genetic PSP look-alikes with findings that may help to differentiate them in the presence of PSP features (52).

Frontotemporal lobar degeneration	
MAPT mutations	<ul><li>earlier age of onset (3rd to 5th decade)</li><li>positive family history</li><li>early episodic memory impairment and semantic dementia</li><li>symmetric frontotemporal atrophy on MRI</li><li>sequential testing for microtubule-associated protein tau</li></ul>
PGRN mutations	<ul><li>positive family history not always present</li><li>parietal signs including dyscalculia, limb apraxia or cortical sensory dysfunction</li><li>hallucinations may occur</li><li>asymmetric frontotemporal atrophy on MRI</li><li>sequential testing for progranulin</li></ul>
Perry syndrome (DCTN1)	<ul><li>earlier age of onset (30-61 years)</li><li>positive family history</li><li>central hypoventilation</li><li>extreme weight loss</li><li>athymhormia, apathy, hallucinations</li><li>genetic testing for dynactin</li></ul>
Kufor-Rakeb syndrome (ATP13A2)	<ul><li>earlier age of onset (12-29 years)</li><li>levodopa-responsive parkinsonism (with dyskinesias)</li><li>oculogyric dystonic spasms, pyramidal signs</li><li>facial-faucial finger mini-myoclonus</li><li>brain iron accumulation on T2* MRI may be observed</li><li>mutation in the ATP13A2 gene</li></ul>
Niemann-Pick C (NPC)	<ul><li>extreme clinical variability</li><li>cerebellar ataxia</li><li>splenomegaly, hepatomegaly</li><li>mutation analysis of NPC1 and more rarely NPC2</li></ul>
Gaucher's disease (GBA)	<ul><li>more prevalent in Ashkenazy Jews</li><li>slow horizontal saccades</li><li>increased horizontal saccadic latency</li><li>head thrusting, ataxia, seizures, spasticity</li><li>splenomegaly, hepatomegaly, bone crisis, anemia, thrombocytopenia</li><li>mutations in the glucocerebrosidase gene</li></ul>
Mitochondrial disorders	<ul><li>ptosis, deafness, migraine, epilepsy</li><li>infranuclear rather than supranuclear ophthalmoplegia</li><li>POLG-related parkinsonism: levodopa-responsive</li></ul>
Genetic Creuzfeldt-Jakob (PRNP)	<ul><li>rapid evolution</li><li>cerebellar signs, spasticity</li><li>stimulus-sensitive myoclonus</li><li>bilateral putaminal and caudate hyperintensities on MRI</li><li>mutations within the prion protein gene</li></ul>

disease-modifying or even neuroprotective effect of coenzyme Q10.

On the other hand, a treatment directly targeting tau dysfunction would be most elegant, for instance targeting the increased 4R/3R tau ratio (thus the modification of tau mRNA splicing), the pharmacological reduction of tau levels (at gene expression or protein clearance level), hyperphosphorylation of tau, or introducing small molecules such as tau-aggregation inhibitors (11). Several trials in this regard have been initiated. Besides pharmacological treatment and in the absence of curative or neuroprotective therapies, physiotherapy, ergotherapy, logotherapy and social counseling remain the mainstays in the treatment of PSP patients.

Video Fragments

Fragment 20.1
Progressive supranuclear palsy (1)
(segments 1-5)
Patient suffering PSP with typical, vertical, supranuclear, downward gaze paralysis (segment 1), bradykinesia (segment 2), pseudobulbar speech (segment 3), micrography (segment 4) and postural instability with falls (segment 5).

Fragment 20.2
Progressive supranuclear palsy (2)
(segments 1-5)
71-year-old patient with progressive supranuclear palsy. Segment 1 shows the patient's hypophonia, segment 2 the bilateral bradykinesia. In segment 3 and 4, the patient's postural instability and bradykinetic gait might be appreciated. Typical slow vertical saccades are shown in segment 5.

References

1 Steele JC, Richardson JC, Olszewski J. Progressive supranuclear palsy: a heterogeneous degeneration involving brain stem, basal ganglia and cerebellum with vertical gaze and pseudobulbar palsy, nuchal dystonia and dementia. Arch Neurol 1964;10:333-59.

2 Savica R, Grossardt BR, Bower JH, Ahlskog JE, Rocca WA. Incidence and Pathology of Synucleinopathies and Tauopathies Related to Parkinsonism. JAMA Neurol 2013;70:859-866.

3 Nath U, Ben-Shlomo Y, Thomson RG, et al. The prevalence of progressive supranuclear palsy (Steele-Richardson-Olszewski syndrome) in the UK. Brain 2001;124:1438-49.

4 Donker Kaat L, Boon AJ, Azmani A, et al. Familial aggregation of parkinsonism in progressive supranuclear palsy. Neurology 2009;73:98-105.

5 Höglinger GU, Melhem NM, Dickson DW, et al. Identification of common variants influencing risk of the tauopathy progressive supranuclear palsy. Nat Genet 2011;43:699-705.

6 Borroni B, Agosti C, Magnani E, Di Luca M, Padovani A. Genetic bases of Progressive Supranuclear Palsy: the MAPT tau disease. Curr Med Chem 2011;18:2655-2660.

7 Myers AJ, Pittman AM, Zhao AS, et al. The MAPT H1c risk haplotype is associated with increased expression of tau and especially of 4 repeat containing transcripts. Neurobiol Dis 2007;25:561-570.

8 Fujioka S, Algom AA, Murray ME, et al. Similarities between familial and sporadic autopsy-proven progressive supranuclear palsy. Neurology 2013;80:2076-2078

9 Vidal JS, Vidailhet M, Derkinderen P, de Gaillarbois TD, Tzourio C, Alpérovitch A. Risk factors for progressive supranuclear palsy: a case-control study in France. J Neurol Neurosurg Psychiatry 2009;80:1271-1274.

10 Melquist S, Craig DW, Huentelman MJ, et al. Identification of a novel risk locus for progressive supranuclear palsy by a pooled genomewide scan of 500,288 single-nucleotide polymorphisms. Am J Hum Genet 2007;80:769-778.

11 Stamelou M, de Silva R, Arias-Carrión O, et al. Rational therapeutic approaches to progressive supranuclear palsy. Brain 2010;133:1578-1590.

12 Escobar-Khondiker M, Höllerhage M, Muriel MP, et al. Annonacin, a natural mitochondrial complex I inhibitor, causes tau pathology in cultured neurons. J Neurosci 2007;27:7827-7837.

13 Höllerhage M, Matusch A, Champy P, et al. Natural lipophilic inhibitors of mitochondrial complex I are candidate toxins for sporadic neurodegenerative tau pathologies. Exp Neurol 2009;220:133-142.

14 Goedert M, Wischik CM, Crowther RA, Walker JE, Klug A. Cloning and sequencing of the cDNA encoding a core protein of the paired helical filament of Alzheimer disease: identification as the microtubule-associated protein tau. Proc Natl Acad Sci U.S.A. 1988;85:4051-4055.

15 Lee VM, Goedert M, Trojanowski JQ. Neurodegenerative tauopathies. Annu Rev Neurosci 2001;24:1121-1159.

16 Dickson DW, Ahmed Z, Algom AA, Tsuboi Y, Josephs KA. Neuropathology of variants of progressive supranuclear palsy. Curr Opin Neurol 2010;23:394-400.

17 Goedert M. Tau protein and neurodegeneration. Semin Cell Dev Biol 2004;15:45-49.

18 Hauw JJ, Dickson DW. Tauopathies. Neurodegeneration: the molecular pathology of dementia and movement disorders. ISN Neuropath Press, Basel;2003:82-154.

19 Yamazaki M, Makifuchi T, Chen KM, et al. Acta Neuropathol 2001;102:510-514.

20 Williams DR, Lees AJ. Progressive supranuclear palsy: clinicopathological concepts and diagnostic challenges. Lancet Neurol 2009;8:270-279.

21 Hauw JJ, Daniel SE, Dickson D, et al. Preliminary NINDS neuropathologic criteria for Steele-Richardson-Olszewski syndrome (progressive supranuclear palsy). Neurology 1994;44:2015-2019.

22 Litvan I, Hauw JJ, Bartko JJ, et al. Validity and reliability of the preliminary NINDS neuropathologic criteria for progressive supranuclear palsy and related disorders. J Neuropathol Exp Neurol 1996;55:97-105.

23 Williams DR, Holton J, Strand C , et al. Pathological tau burden and distribution distinguishes progressive supranuclear palsy-parkinsonism from Richardson's syndrome. Brain 2007;130:1566-1576.

24 Jellinger KA. Different tau pathology pattern in two clinical phenotypes of progressive supranuclear palsy. Neurodegenerative Dis 2008;5:339-346.

25 Dickson DW, Ahmed Z, Algom AA, Tsuboi Y, Josephs KA. Neuropathology of variants of progressive supranuclear palsy. Curr Opin Neurol 2010;23:394-400.

26 Gardner RC, Boxer AL, Trujillo A, et al. Intrinsic connectivity network disruption in progressive supranuclear palsy. Ann Neurol 2013;73:603-616.

27 Williams DR, de Silva R, Paviour DC, et al. Characteristics of two distinct clinical phenotypes in pathologically proven progressive supranuclear palsy: Richardson's syndrome and PSP-parkinsonism. Brain 2005;128:1247-1258.

28 Williams DR, Holton JL, Strand K, Revesz T, Lees AJ. Pure akinesia with gait freezing: A third clinical phenotype of progressive supranuclear palsy. Mov Disord 2007;22:2235-2241.

29 Duff K, Gerstenecker A, Litvan I; investigators and coordinators of the ENGENE-PSP Study Group. Functional impairment in progressive supranuclear palsy. Neurology 2013; 80: 380-384.

30 Hauw JJ, Verny M, Delaère P, Cervera P, He Y, Duyckaerts C. Constant neurofibrillary changes in the neocortex in progressive supranuclear palsy. Basic differences with Alzheimer's disease and aging. Neurosci Lett 1990;119:182-186.

31 Matsusaka H, Ikeda K, Akiyama H, Arai T, Inoue M, Yagishita S. Astrocytic pathology in progressive supranuclear palsy: significance for neuropathological diagnosis. Acta Neuropathol 1998;96:248-252.

32 Nath U, Ben-Shlomo Y, Thomson RG, Lees AJ, Burn DJ. Clinical features and natural history of progressive supranuclear palsy: a clinical cohort study. Neurology 2003;60:910-916.

33 Goetz CG, Leurgans S, Lang AE, Litvan I. Progression of gait, speech and swallowing deficits in progressive supranuclear palsy. Neurology 2003;60:917-922.

34 Golbe LI. Progressive supranuclear palsy. In: Jankovic J, Tolosa E, eds. Parkinson's disease and movement disorders. 2nd ed. Baltimore: Williams and Wilkins; 1993:145-161.

35 Williams DR, Lees AJ. What features improve the accuracy of the clinical diagnosis of progressive supranuclear palsy-parkinsonism (PSP-P)? Mov Disord 2010;25:357-362.

36 Jellinger KA. Different tau pathology pattern in two clinical phenotypes of progressive supranuclear palsy. Neurodegener Dis 2008;5:339-346.

37 Imai H, Narabayashi H. Akinesia—concerning 2 cases of pure akinesia. Adv Neurol Sci (Tokyo) 1974;18:787-794.

38 Ahmed Z, Josephs KA, Gonzalez J, DelleDonne A, Dickson DW. Clinical and neuropathologic features of progressive supranuclear palsy with severe pallido-nigro-luysial degeneration and axonal dystrophy. Brain 2008;131:460-472.

39 Mizusawa H, Mochizuki A, Ohkoshi N, Yoshizawa K, Kanazawa I, Imai H. Progressive supranuclear palsy presenting with pure akinesia. Adv Neurol 1993; 60: 618-621.

40 Rivaud-Pechoux S, Vidailhet M, Gallouedec G, Litvan I, Gaymard B, Pierrot-Deseilligny C. Longitudinal ocular motor study in corticobasal degeneration and progressive supranuclear palsy. Neurology 2000;54:1029-1032.

41 Boeve BF, Maraganore DM, Parisi JE, et al. Pathologic heterogeneity in clinically diagnosed corticobasal degeneration. Neurology 1999;53:795-800.

42 Tsuboi Y, Josephs KA, Boeve BF, et al. Increased tau burden in the cortices of progressive supranuclear palsy presenting with corticobasal syndrome. Mov Disord 2005 20:982-988.

43 Hu WT, Parisi JE, Knopman DS, et al. Clinical features and survival of 3R and 4R tauopathies presenting as behavioral variant frontotemporal dementia. Alzheimer Dis Assoc Disord 2007;21:S39-43.

44 Neary D, Snowden JS, Gustafson L, et al. Frontotemporal lobar degeneration: a consensus on clinical diagnostic criteria. Neurology 1998;51:1546-1554.

45 Josephs KA, Duffy JR, Strand EA, et al. Clinicopathological and imaging correlates of progressive aphasia and apraxia of speech. Brain 2006;129:1385-1398.

46 Litvan I, Agid Y, Jankovic J, et al. Accuracy of clinical criteria for the diagnosis of progressive supranuclear palsy (Steele-Richardson-Olszewski syndrome). Neurology 1996;46:922-930.

47 Respondek G, Roeber S, Kretzschmar H, et al. Accuracy of the National Institute for Neurological Disorders and Stroke/Society for Progressive Supranuclear Palsy and neuroprotection and natural history in Parkinson plus syndromes criteria for the diagnosis of progressive supranuclear palsy. Mov Disord 2013;28:504-509.

48 Massey LA, Micallef C, Paviour DC, et al. Conventional magnetic resonance imaging in confirmed progressive supranuclear palsy and multiple system atrophy. Mov Disord 2012;27:1754-1762.

49 Morelli M, Arabia G, Novellino F, et al. MRI measurements predict PSP in unclassifiable parkinsonisms: a cohort study. Neurology 2011;77:1042-1047.

50 Morelli M, Arabia G, Salsone M, et al. Accuracy of magnetic resonance parkinsonism index for differentiation of progressive supranuclear palsy from probable or possible Parkinson disease. Mov Disord 2011;26:527-533.

51 Massey LA, Jäger HR, Paviour DC, et al. The midbrain to pons ratio: a simple and specific MRI sign of progressive supranuclear palsy. Neurology 2013;80:1856-1861.

52 Stamelou M, Quinn NP, Bhatia KP. "Atypical" atypical parkinsonism: New genetic conditions presenting with features of progressive supranuclear palsy, corticobasal degeneration, or multiple system atrophy-A diagnostic guide. Mov Disord 2013;28:1184-1199.

53 Nieforth KA, Golbe LI. Retrospective study of drug response in 87 patients with progressive supranuclear palsy. Clin Neuropharmacol 1993;16:338-346.

54 Engel PA. Treatment of progressive supranuclear palsy with amitriptyline: therapeutic and toxic effects. J Am Geriatr Soc 1996;44:1072-1074.

55 Stamelou M, Reuss A, Pilatus U, et al. Short-term effects of coenzyme Q10 in progressive supranuclear palsy: a randomized, placebo-controlled trial. Mov Disord 2008;23:942-949.

21
Corticobasal Degeneration and Corticobasal Syndrome

Melissa J. Armstrong & Anthony E. Lang

Vocabulary is critical to the discussion of corticobasal degeneration (CBD) and corticobasal syndrome (CBS), the topics for this chapter. CBD is a pathologic entity resulting from the abnormal aggregation of hyperphosphorylated tau, particularly tau isoforms with 4 conserved repeat sequences (4R tau). The pathologic diagnosis is made by applying criteria published by the Office of Rare Diseases in 2002 (see Table 21.1) (1). CBD is typically a sporadic neurodegenerative disorder associated with various clinical phenotypes, discussed further below.

The first series of patients with 'CBD' were described by specialists in movement disorders based on their experience in tertiary movement disorders clinics. This experience encouraged the initial concept that CBD represented a very distinct clinical-pathological syndrome where the diagnosis could be made in life based on the characteristic and unique clinical picture of manifesting motor features including asymmetric parkinsonism, limb dystonia, myoclonus, and gait abnormalities, and higher cortical features including apraxia, alien limb phenomenon, and cortical sensory loss. However, subsequent experience has taught us that the clinical features once believed to be pathognomonic of CBD can also be associated with many other pathologies and that this clinical presentation is only one of several possible presentations of patients found to have CBD pathology, most notably including cognitive and behavioural disturbances.

It is only in recent years that medical publications have adopted terminology distinguishing between the classical clinical phenotype (corticobasal syndrome or CBS) and the pathologic diagnosis (CBD), so readers must be discerning when reviewing the literature dealing with these diagnoses. The distinction also raises a challenge: how do we describe research participants who we suspect have CBD but for whom an autopsy is not yet available? The term CBS alone is insufficient for this group as it is only one of several clinical presentations of the pathological entity CBD. To address this, new criteria for the clinical diagnosis of CBD were published in 2013 (2). These criteria, developed by an international consortium of behavioural neurology, neuropsychology, and movement disorders specialists, are the first ones to incorporate clinical phenotypes other than just CBS. These criteria propose additional new vocabulary for clinical syndromes that may represent pathologic CBD: clinical research criteria for probable CBD (cr-CBD), which are restrictive and therefore aim at correctly diagnosing classic CBD; and possible CBD criteria (p-CBD), which are more open but still emphasize presentations consistent with underlying tau pathology. Whether these new categories will be widely adopted is yet to be established.

Table 21.1
Pathologic criteria for the diagnosis of corticobasal degeneration.

Core features	1	Neuronal and glial lesions with tau pathology including thread-like lesions and astrocytic plaques in the gray and white matter and prominent tau immunoreactivity in cell processes
	2	Tau-immunoreactive lesions in the caudate and putamen
	3	Demonstration of moderate-marked neuronal loss in the substantia nigra
	4	Cortical neuronal loss and astrogliosis (typically most prominent in the superior frontal, superior parietal, and pre- and post-central gyri)
Supportive features	1	Gross findings including cortical gyri narrowing (often parasagittal and peri-Rolandic), cortical atrophy (particularly posterior frontal), cortical spongiosis, thinning of the corpus callosum, flattening of the caudate head, small thalamic volume, pale substantia nigra
	2	Swollen, 'achromatic', or 'ballooned' neurons
	3	Neurofibrillary lesions in brainstem monoaminergic nuclei (e.g. locus ceruleus and substantia nigra) (previously called 'corticobasal bodies')
	4	Oligodendroglial tau-positive argyrophilic inclusions, sometimes named 'coiled bodies'
	5	Sparing of hippocampus and parahippocampal gyrus
Exclusion criteria*	1	Senile plaques and Alzheimer-type neurofibrillary tangles
	2	Classic Pick bodies with sharply defined margins
	3	Lewy bodies, alpha-synuclein pathology
	4	Ubiquitin immunoreactivity
	5	Focal ischemic damage such as related to infarcts or hemorrhages

*When cases meet full criteria for both CBD and a separate diagnosis, 'mixed' pathologic diagnoses can be assigned.
Adapted from (1).

Epidemiology

Both CBS and CBD are rare, but few formal epidemiological studies exist. In a series of movement disorders patients proceeding to autopsy, four of 143 patients (2.8%) presenting with parkinsonism were diagnosed with CBD, but autopsies were only performed on a small percentage of patients, and thus this sample may not be representative of the wider population (3). A subsequent publication from the same center described that 21 (1.5%) of all autopsied cases presented with CBS and 19 (1.3%) were diagnosed pathologically with CBD (only sometimes overlapping) (4). By making various assumptions regarding diagnosis and survival, the incidence and prevalence of CBD in the United States have been estimated as 0.62-0.92/100,000 and 13,000-20,000, respectively (5). In a Moscow population-based study of incident parkinsonism, CBS had a crude incidence of 0.03 (95% CI 0.01-0.18) per 100,000 person-years and an age-adjusted incidence of 0.02 (95% CI 0.01-0.12) per 100,000 person-years (6).

Aetiology

CBD is generally considered to be a sporadic disorder, but there have been case reports of CBD pathology in patients with identified tau mutations including P301L (7) and N296N (8,9). Recently, a patient with a C9orf72 mutation evidenced CBD pathology on autopsy, though this mutation is more often associated with tau-negative processes (10). There is currently no consensus regarding whether sporadic and mutation-related CBD represent the same process. The CBS clinical phenotype, in contrast, has been associated with various etiologies ranging from identified genetic mutations to sporadic neurodegenerations to infections and mass lesions (see Table 21.2).

Pathophysiology

The pathophysiology of CBD remains poorly understood. CBD is classified as a 4R tauopathy, reflecting the pathologic accumulation of the 4R tau isoform in the brain. Tau is a microtubule-associated protein with six isoforms resulting from different splicing patterns. In particular, alternative splicing of exon 10 of tau will result in isoforms with either three (3R) or four (4R) microtubule-binding repeats. Normally, 3R-tau and 4R-tau are expressed in approximately equal amounts in the brain. Accumulation of different isoforms results in different diseases; CBD and progressive supranuclear palsy (PSP) are the primary 4R tauopathies resulting from accumulation of this isoform (11,12). The mechanism causing abnormal 4R tau levels in CBD is currently unknown.

The appearance and location of the tau accumulations in the brain distinguish CBD from PSP. CBD and PSP are now generally considered to exist on a single spectrum, but with astrocytic plaques as the pathologic hallmark of CBD and tufted astrocytes as the pathologic hallmark of PSP, in addition to other neuropathologic differences (12). Classically, CBD patients demonstrate tau accumulation in the cortex, basal ganglia, thalamus, and brainstem (1,12), while PSP patients show accumulation in the basal ganglia, thalamus, brainstem and cerebellum, with generally less cortical involvement (13) (see also chapter 20). However, lesions can involve the cortex, brainstem, basal ganglia, and other brain structures to varying degrees in both pathologies, and it is the distribution of pathology, not the histopathologic details, that drives clinical presentations. It is for this reason that clinical phenotypes are not perfectly predictive of specific neurodegenerations.

Imaging studies to date have provided little additional insight into the underlying pathophy-

Table 21.2
Reported etiologies of corticobasal syndrome.*

Neuro-degenerative diseases	▪ Corticobasal degeneration ▪ Progressive supranuclear palsy ▪ Pick's disease ▪ Parkinson's disease* ▪ Alzheimer's disease ▪ Frontotemporal lobar degeneration ▪ Motor neuron disease-inclusion dementia (FTD-U) ▪ Neurofilament inclusion body disease
Infectious	▪ Creutzfeldt-Jakob disease ▪ Progressive multifocal leukoencephalopathy
Acquired focal lesions	▪ Ischemic disease ▪ Fahr's disease* ▪ Mass lesions
Other	▪ Primary antiphospholipid syndrome ▪ Spinocerebellar ataxia type 8

*Etiologies as reported in the literature; the rigor with which corticobasal criteria were applied to the cases varies, and in some cases, patients may not have met standard criteria.

siology of CBD. Most imaging studies have been performed in CBS patients without pathological confirmation, and findings simply reflect the asymmetrical cortical and subcortical syndrome seen on examination without further exploration of the pathophysiology. Recent studies in CBS patients with known and varied pathologies suggest that subtle differences in atrophy patterns on magnetic resonance imaging (MRI) voxel-based morphometry (VBM) in patients with this phenotype may suggest different pathologic diagnoses including CBD (14,15), but the predictive value of these findings has yet to be determined, and they do not provide further insights into the underlying pathophysiology of CBD. Neurochemical imaging which might contribute to our understanding of the pathophysiology is rare in pathologically confirmed CBD cases. Dopamine D2 receptor SPECT imaging of two CBD cases produced conflicting results, with reduced striatal binding in one case and normal striatal binding in the other, though both studies showed asymmetries matching the patients' clinical presentations (16).

Clinical presentation

By definition, the clinical presentation of CBS involves both a progressive, asymmetric, akinetic-rigid syndrome and signs of higher cortical dysfunction (see Table 21.3). Not all features need be present for patients to be categorized as CBS. CBS is only one of the clinical presentations of CBD, however. In a review of the final clinical diagnosis for over 200 pathologically proven CBD cases, five phenotypes were suggested, capturing 87.1% (183/210) of reviewed cases: CBS (37.1%, 78/210), progressive supranuclear palsy (PSP) syndrome (also called Richardson syndrome) (23.3%, 49/210), frontotemporal dementia (FTD) (13.8%, 29/210), Alzheimer's disease (AD)-like dementia (8.1%), and aphasia (4.8%, 10/210), typically categorized as primary progressive aphasia (PPA) or progressive non-fluent aphasia (PNFA). An additional 5.7% (12/210) were mixed diagnoses involving these phenotypes. Parkinson's disease (PD) was diagnosed in 3.8% (8/210). In 129 patients with an *initial* presentation, CBS was the most common presenting diagnosis (27.1%,

35/129), followed by FTD and PD/atypical PD (each 15.5%, 20/129), aphasia (14.7%, 19/129), AD/dementia (9.3%, 12/129), and PSP (6.2%, 8/129) (2).

When considering the motor features of CBD, approximately three-quarters of CBD patients with parkinsonism demonstrate asymmetry in this feature. At presentation, over half of CBD patients have documented limb rigidity. Bradykinesia and postural instability are the other most common motor features, followed by falls and abnormal gait. Limb dystonia and myoclonus – classical features of CBS – are described at presentation in 20% or less of cases (2). All CBD motor features become more common as the disease progresses, with limb rigidity, bradykinesia, postural instability, and falls all described in at least 75% of CBD cases at some point. Axial rigidity also becomes more common, present in 69% of cases. Tremor, limb dystonia, and myoclonus remain the least commonly demonstrated motor features (2). Most patients who develop dystonia will do so within the first two years of symptoms, typically involving the upper extremities and often co-existing with myoclonus (17).

The frequencies of various higher cortical features are also variable in CBD. Cognitive impairment is the most common higher cortical feature at presentation, described in over half of CBD patients. Behavioural changes, limb apraxia, and aphasia are also common. Alien limb phenomena and cortical sensory loss are the least commonly described higher cortical features at presentation, found in 25% or less of cases. While the frequency of cognitive impairment, behavioural changes, and limb apraxia increases as the disease progresses, there is a minimal increase in the frequency of alien limb phenomena or cortical sensory loss (2).

The cognitive impairment of CBD typically involves prominent frontal-executive dysfunction (18,19). This includes cognitive deficits such as poor planning and impaired judgment (18,19) but also frontal behavioural features such as

Table 21.3
Clinical presentation of corticobasal syndrome.

Movement disorder features	▪ Asymmetric akinetic rigid syndrome ▪ Dystonia ▪ Myoclonus ▪ Postural instability and falls
Higher cortical dysfunction features	▪ Cognitive-behavioural changes ▪ Aphasia ▪ Apraxia (orobuccal or limb) ▪ Alien limb phenomena (more than simple levitation) ▪ Cortical sensory loss

Table 21.4
Presenting phenotypes of corticobasal degeneration.

Corticobasal Syndrome (CBS)		Frontal Behavioural Spatial Syndrome (FBS)	Non-Fluent/Agrammatic Variant of Primary Progressive Aphasia (naPPA)	Progressive supranuclear palsy syndrome (PSPS)
Probable	Possible			
At least 2 of 3: limb rigidity and/or akinesia, limb dystonia, limb myoclonus	At least 1 of 3: limb rigidity and/or akinesia, limb dystonia, limb myoclonus	At least 2 of 3: executive dysfunction, behavioural and/or personality changes, visuospatial deficits	Effortful, agrammatic speech plus at least 1 of 2: impaired grammar/sentence comprehension with relatively preserved single word comprehension, or groping, distorted speech production	At least 3 of 5: axial and/or symmetric limb rigidity or akinesia, postural instability or falls, urinary incontinence, behavioural changes, supranuclear vertical gaze palsy or decreased velocity of vertical saccades
At least 2 of 3: orobuccal or limb apraxia, cortical sensory deficit, alien limb phenomena	At least 1 of 3: orobuccal or limb apraxia, cortical sensory deficit, alien limb phenomena			
Asymmetric	Symmetric or asymmetric			

Adapted from [2].

compulsive, bizarre or antisocial behaviour, personality changes, irritability, disinhibition, excessive eating, hypersexuality, apathy, and depression (2,4,18,20-22). These features can be the most prominent signs at onset in some CBD patients, prompting inclusion of a frontal behavioural-spatial syndrome (FBS) phenotype in the new CBD criteria (Table 21.4) (2). CBD patients not meeting criteria for this phenotype are still likely to have some frontal-executive dysfunction, particularly as the disease progresses.

Language deficits are also common in CBD. While performance on neuropsychological testing of language function in CBD cohorts has been varied (18,19), likely representing some bias in the enrolled study populations, language impairments are clearly present in many CBD patients. When language dysfunction appears early and prominent, patients may meet criteria for the non-fluent/agrammatic variant of primary progressive aphasia (naPPA), and this is now one of the identified presenting phenotypes of CBD (2). Patients with this phenotype demonstrate effortful, agrammatic speech, impaired grammar/sentence comprehension with relatively preserved single word comprehension, and/or apraxia of speech (AOS) with groping, distorted speech production (see Table 21.4) (2). While frontal-executive and language domains are the most commonly affected areas of cognition in CBD, patients may also have involvement of other cognitive domains. For example, visuospatial impairments are described to varying degrees in CBD patients (18,19). Memory difficulties are a common early complaint of CBD patients, but deficits are not always found on formal testing (18). The frequency with which CBD patients are misdiagnosed clinically as having an AD or dementia, though, suggests that memory can be an issue in these patients. In a recent review of over 200 CBD cases, 11.5% were diagnosed with AD/dementia at presentation and 8.1% carried the diagnosis later in the disease (2). As with other parkinsonisms, it is possible that memory impairments seen in CBD may represent more frontally mediated impairments in encoding and retrieval rather than the classic medial temporal memory deficits of AD. Not surprisingly, the pattern of cognitive deficits seen in CBD patients varies by presenting phenotype. In a series comparing 18 CBD patients divided into clinical phenotypes of an executive-motor syndrome, PNFA, behavioural variant frontotemporal dementia (bvFTD), or posterior cortical atrophy (PCA), the CBD patients presenting with the bvFTD phenotype performed worse on most cognitive measures (15). These patients also tended to have the highest scores on the neuropsychiatric inventory (NPI), a measure of ten behavioural disturbances. NPI scores were lowest in CBD patients presenting with PNFA (15). When considering exclusively patients with a CBS phenotype, attempts to identify CBD pathology versus other pathologies based on neuropsychological presentations have had mixed results. When comparing CBS due to CBD versus AD, neuropsychological testing in one study showed similar degrees of memory and executive impairment between patients with the two pathologies (23), but another study found that CBD pathology was predicted by early frontal-behavioural symptoms, nonfluent language impairments, orobuccal apraxia and utilization behaviour while early episodic memory concerns and poor orientation and memory testing predicted AD pathology (24). CBS patients with AD pathology may perform worse on figure copying, delayed recall, and calculation tasks compared to CBS patients due to various other pathologies (15), though calculations can also be poor in CBD (15, 18). In patients with a PSPS phenotype, executive and behavioural abnormalities may be more common in those with underlying CBD than in those with PSP pathology (25).

Besides the classic motor and higher cortical findings, 60% of CBD cases have some type of abnormal eye movements documented over the course of their disease (2). This contributes to the difficulty in clinically distinguishing some cases of CBD and PSP (see also chapter 20). It has been suggested that supranuclear vertical gaze palsy within 2 years of symptom onset may exclude CBD (4), but other studies have not found any clinical features that reliably distinguish CBD

from PSP (4,25,26). The common belief that saccadic speeds and latency reliably differentiate PSP (slowed speeds and normal latency) from CBD (normal speeds and prolonged latencies) was based on studies that lacked pathological confirmation of the patients diagnosed with CBS (27). A recent study with pathologic confirmation of diagnoses showed that subjects with AD had increased saccadic latency whereas three of four CBD patients had visually guided saccades that were indistinguishable from normal controls. PSP patients had impairments in vertical saccade velocity and gains in both the vertical and horizontal directions. Antisaccade performance was abnormal in all cases (26). Thus, while eye movements may play a role in distinguishing between neurodegenerations, the description of prolonged latencies in CBS more likely reflects patients with AD pathology than CBD.

Diagnosis and differential diagnosis

The diagnosis of CBS is simply based on the presence of the motor and higher cortical signs outlined in Table 21.3. These features are formally described in many of the diagnostic criteria self-labeled as criteria for CBD (28-34) which actually reflect signs and symptoms of CBS. The 2013 clinical research criteria for the diagnosis of corticobasal degeneration (2) incorporate the CBS phenotype but also other presenting phenotypes: FBS, naPPA, and PSPS (see Table 21.4). These criteria were developed following an extensive review of all CBD case series containing five or more patients with clinical-pathological correlation. For a clinical diagnosis under this scheme, which can be probable or possible, patients must have insidious onset and gradual progression, at least one year of symptoms, and at least some features of the CBS phenotype with or without other phenotypes (see Table 21.5). Findings suggesting alternate diagnoses, such as a classic PD resting tremor, sustained levodopa responsiveness, hallucinations, dysautonomia, prominent cerebellar signs, upper or lower motor neuron findings, se-

Table 21.5
Clinical research criteria for corticobasal degeneration (CBD).

Presentation	Probable sporadic CBD (cr-CBD)	Possible CBD (possible-CBD)
	Insidious onset and gradual progression	
Minimum duration of symptoms	1 year	
Age at onset	≥50 years-old	No minimum
Family history (2 or more relatives)	Exclusion	Permitted
Permitted phenotypes (see Table 21.4 for criteria)	Probable CBS *or* FBS or NAV *plus* at least one CBS feature	Possible CBS *or* FBS or NAV *or* PSPS *plus* at least one CBS feature (other than rigidity/akinesia)
Genetic mutation affecting tau (e.g. MAPT)	Exclusion	Permitted

Adapted from (2). CBS = corticobasal syndrome; FBS = frontal behavioural spatial syndrome; NAV = non fluent/agrammatic variant of primary progressive aphasia.

mantic- or logopenic-variant primary progressive aphasia (PPA), corresponding structural lesions, select genetic mutations, or biomarker evidence of AD must be absent (2) (see Table 21.6). Of course, a true diagnosis of CBD can only be made neuropathologically.

Currently, there is no formal role for ancillary testing in making the diagnosis of CBD. Most studies of imaging, neurophysiological and laboratory tests (including CSF) in this setting have been performed in CBS patients without known pathology, and thus the diagnostic implications of these tests remain uncertain. It is prudent to obtain neuroimaging to exclude rare focal causes of the CBS phenotype (Table 21.2). As mentioned above, recent publications suggest that VBM analysis of atrophy patterns may be predictive of the underlying pathology in CBS patients (14,15), but these findings need confirmation before they can be widely applied. For patients in whom there is a reason to consider both AD and CBD, amyloid imaging and CSF Aβ42/tau ratio may be helpful to support or discourage a diagnosis of AD, though these tests have not been formally studied in CBD and thus their predictive value in this context is not certain. In select patients, genetic testing (see Chapter 16) may be reasonable; mu-

tations in the *PSEN1* and *PSEN2* or *APP* genes are associated with AD rather than CBD, and *PGRN*, *TARDBP*, *C9orf72* and *FUS* mutations are suggestive of non-tau pathologies. As stated earlier, mutations in the *MAPT* gene have been associated with both the clinical and pathological features of CBD. However, testing for tau mutations in patients suspected to have CBD is not currently recommended unless there is a strong family history. The differential diagnosis in patients presenting with CBS is broad (see Table 21.2). Patients eventually diagnosed with CBD share features with other diagnoses such as frontotemporal lobar degeneration (FTLD), AD, and PSP, as discussed above. The pathology of CBD is correctly predicted *antemortem* in only 25-56% of cases (3,4,18,20,35-37), possibly reflecting traditional reliance on criteria based only on the CBS phenotype. Whether the diagnostic accuracy will improve with the newly proposed diagnostic criteria remains to be determined.

Treatment

Treatment for CBS and CBD is symptomatic and based largely on clinical experience and limited case series. Levodopa is the treatment of choice

Table 21.6
Exclusionary criteria for clinical research criteria for corticobasal degeneration.

- Evidence suggestive of Lewy body disease (e.g. classical 4-6-Hz Parkinson's disease resting tremor, excellent and sustained levodopa response, or hallucinations)
- Evidence suggestive of multiple system atrophy (e.g. dysautonomia or prominent cerebellar signs)
- Evidence suggestive of amyotrophic lateral sclerosis (e.g. presence of both upper and lower motor neuron signs)
- Semantic- or logopenic-variant primary progressive aphasia
- Structural lesion suggestive of focal cause
- Granulin mutation or reduced plasma progranulin levels; TDP-43 mutations; FUS mutations
- Evidence supportive of Alzheimer's disease (e.g. laboratory findings strongly suggestive of AD such as low CSF A-beta42 to tau ratio or positive 11C-PIB PET; or genetic mutation suggesting AD [e.g. presenilin, amyloid precursor protein])

Adapted from [2].

for the parkinsonism in these conditions, but usually results in minimal clinical benefit (an observation reflected in the diagnostic criteria). Transient mild to moderate benefits have been described in both CBS and CBD (4,32,38,39), and dyskinesias may rarely occur even in pathologically confirmed CBD patients (4,40). Oral medications are rarely helpful for the dystonia in CBS and CBD, but targeted botulinum toxin injections may provide some relief (38,41,42). Myoclonus is typically treated with benzodiazepines, particularly clonazepam (31,38,43), or levetiracetam (44,45). CBS and CBD patients do not benefit from subthalamic or pallidal deep brain stimulation. Acetylcholinesterase inhibitors and selective serotonin uptake inhibitors are used for cognitive and behavioural features of CBS and CBD without disease-specific evidence. Physical and cognitive-behavioural therapies have been recommended, but their utility depends on the ability of patients to participate. While not technically treatments, social work, supportive services, and sometimes hospice programs are important aspects of effectively caring for CBS and CBD patients and their families.

Research on potential disease-modifying therapies targeting tauopathies such as CBD is progressing. CBS and PSPS patients were recently enrolled in a pilot study of lithium, a glycogen synthase kinase 3-beta (GSK-3ß) inhibitor which may decrease kinase activity contributing to tau hyperphosphorylation (ClinicalTrials.gov identifier NCT00703677), but the study was terminated early when 13 of 14 enrolled subjects were unable to tolerate the lithium. A different GSK-3β inhibitor, NP031112 (tideglusib), has been studied in patients with PSPS (ClinicalTrials.gov identifier NCT01049399); the results have not yet been reported. Patients with suspected tau pathology presenting with different phenotypes including CBS, PSPS, PNFA, and frontotemporal dementia with parkinsonism linked to chromosome 17 (FTDP-17) have recently participated in a study of intranasal davunetide (NAPVSIPQ), an octapeptide which interacts with microtubules and may reduce tau pathology (ClinicalTrials.gov identifier NCT01056965). In the larger PSPS group, this failed to slow the progression of disease in comparison to placebo, and further studies using davunetide have been halted. It is likely that most therapeutic trials for CBD will continue to target tauopathies in general given the difficulties in predicting underlying pathology using clinical criteria alone and the hope of modifying the presumed tau-based pathologic mechanism of the disease.

Prognosis

Until disease-modifying therapies are identified, CBD remains a relentlessly progressive neurodegeneration. In two studies where it was described, mean CBD disease duration was 6.6 years (SD 2.4, range 2.0-12.5) (18,39). CBS cases that progress rapidly to death in less than one year are more suggestive of an alternate pathology such as Creutzfeldt-Jakob disease (46,47). Not surprisingly, CBD patients develop increasingly severe symptomatology as the disease progresses. When considering pathologies grouped under the heading the 'Pick Complex,' which includes CBD, patients almost always gradually acquire features of all three of the described phenotypes of CBS, FTD, and progressive aphasia, regardless of the final pathology (48-50). This is also evident in FTD/FTLD clinicopathological studies where CBD is considered one of the tau-positive FTLD pathologies, and most subjects progress to global motor, cognitive/behavioural, and language impairments regardless of presenting symptoms (51). In a small CBD natural history study, predictors of shorter survival included first visit findings of bilateral bradykinesia, a frontal syndrome, or the presence of at least two of three extrapyramidal features (tremor, rigidity, or bradykinesia). All patients with available postmortem cause of death died of bronchopneumonia (39).

Conclusion

Our understanding of CBD has continued to evolve since its initial description over 40 years ago. Precise use of terminology is critical for a common basis of understanding in discussions of the clinical phenotype CBS, the attempted clinical diagnosis of CBD with its many presenting phenotypes, and the true pathologic diagnosis of CBD. Ongoing research needs to focus on validation of criteria for the clinical diagnosis of pathologic CBD, identification of biological markers that can reliably predict underlying pathology, and therapeutic studies targeting CBD as a member of the broader family of tauopathies in attempts to develop disease-modifying therapies for this progressive neurodegeneration.

References

1 Dickson DW, Bergeron C, Chin SS, et al. Office of Rare Diseases neuropathologic criteria for corticobasal degeneration. J of Neuropathol Exp Neurol. 2002;61:935-946.

2 Armstrong MJ, Litvan I, Lang AE, et al. Criteria for the diagnosis of corticobasal degeneration. Neurology. 2013;80:496-503.

3 Hughes AJ, Daniel SE, Ben-Shlomo Y, Lees AJ. The accuracy of diagnosis of parkinsonian syndromes in a specialist movement disorder service. Brain. 2002;125:861-870.

4 Ling H, O'Sullivan SS, Holton JL, et al. Does corticobasal degeneration exist? A clinicopathological re-evaluation. Brain. 2010;133:2045-2057.

5 Togasaki DM, Tanner CM. Epidemiologic aspects. Adv Neurol. 2000;82:53-59.

6 Winter Y, Bezdolnyy Y, Katunina E, et al. Incidence of Parkinson's disease and atypical parkinsonism: Russian population-based study. Mov Disord. 2010;25:349-356.

7 Mirra SS, Murrell JR, Gearing M, et al. Tau pathology in a family with dementia and a P301L mutation in tau. J Neuropathol Exp Neurol. 1999;58:335-345.

8 Spillantini MG, Yoshida H, Rizzini C, et al. A novel tau mutation (N296N) in familial dementia with swollen achromatic neurons and corticobasal inclusion bodies. Ann Neurol. 2000;48:939-943.

9 Brown J, Lantos PL, Roques P, Fidani L, Rossor MN. Familial dementia with swollen achromatic neurons and corticobasal inclusion bodies: A clinical and pathological study. J Neurol Sci. 1996;135:21-30.

10 Snowden JS, Rollinson S, Thompson JC, et al. Distinct clinical and pathological characteristics of frontotemporal dementia associated with C9ORF72 mutations. Brain. 2012;135:693-708.

11 Liu F, Gong CX. Tau exon 10 alternative splicing and tauopathies. Mol Neurodegener. 2008;3:8.

12 Dickson DW, Kouri N, Murray ME, Josephs KA. Neuropathology of frontotemporal lobar degeneration-tau (FTLD-tau). J Mol Neurosci. 2011;45:384-389.

13 Dickson DW, Ahmed Z, Algom AA, Tsuboi Y, Josephs KA. Neuropathology of variants of pro-

gressive supranuclear palsy. Curr Opin Neurol. 2010;23:394-400.

14 Whitwell JL, Jack CR, Jr., Boeve BF, et al. Imaging correlates of pathology in corticobasal syndrome. Neurology. 2010 Nov 23;75:1879-1887.

15 Lee SE, Rabinovici GD, Mayo MC, et al. Clinicopathological correlations in corticobasal degeneration. Ann Neurol. 2011;70:327-340.

16 Pirker S, Perju-Dumbrava L, Kovacs GG, Traub-Weidinger T, Asenbaum S, Pirker W. Dopamine D2 receptor SPECT in corticobasal syndrome and autopsy-confirmed corticobasal degeneration. Parkinsonism Relat Disord. 2013;19:222-226.

17 Stamelou M, Alonso-Canovas A, Bhatia KP. Dystonia in corticobasal degeneration: a review of the literature on 404 pathologically proven cases. Mov Disord. 2012;27:696-702.

18 Murray R, Neumann M, Forman MS, et al. Cognitive and motor assessment in autopsy-proven corticobasal degeneration. Neurology. 2007;68:1274-1283.

19 Vanvoorst WA, Greenaway MC, Boeve BF, et al. Neuropsychological findings in clinically atypical autopsy confirmed corticobasal degeneration and progressive supranuclear palsy. Parkinsonism Relat Disord. 2008;14:376-378.

20 Grimes DA, Lang AE, Bergeron CB. Dementia as the most common presentation of cortical-basal ganglionic degeneration. Neurology. 1999;53:1969-1974.

21 Forman MS, Zhukareva V, Bergeron C, et al. Signature tau neuropathology in gray and white matter of corticobasal degeneration. Am J Pathol. 2002;160:2045-2053.

22 Geda YE, Boeve BF, Negash S, et al. Neuropsychiatric features in 36 pathologically confirmed cases of corticobasal degeneration. J Neuropsychiatry Clin Neurosci. 2007;19:77-80.

23 Hu WT, Rippon GW, Boeve BF, et al. Alzheimer's disease and corticobasal degeneration presenting as corticobasal syndrome. Mov Disord. 2009;24:1375-1379.

24 Shelley BP, Hodges JR, Kipps CM, Xuereb JH, Bak TH. Is the pathology of corticobasal syndrome predictable in life? Mov Disord. 2009;24:1593-1599.

25 Kouri N, Murray ME, Hassan A, et al. Neuropathological features of corticobasal degeneration presenting as corticobasal syndrome or Richardson syndrome. Brain. 2011;134:3264-3275.

26 Boxer AL, Garbutt S, Seeley WW, et al. Saccade abnormalities in autopsy-confirmed frontotemporal lobar degeneration and Alzheimer's disease. Arch Neurol. 2012;69:509-517.

27 Rivaud-Péchoux S, Vidailhet M, Gallouedec G, Litvan I, Gaymard B, Pierrot-Deseilligny C. Longitudinal ocular motor study in corticobasal degeneration and progressive supranuclear palsy. Neurology. 2000;54:1029-1032.

28 Lang AE, Riley DE, Bergeron C. Cortical-Basal Ganglionic Degeneration. In: Calne DB, ed. Neurodegenerative Diseases. Philadelphia: W.B.Saunders; 1994:877-894.

29 Watts RL, Mirra SS, Richardson EP. Cortical-basal ganglionic degeneration. In: Marsden CD, Fahn S, ed. Movement Disorders, 3rd vol. Oxford: Butterworth Heinemann; 1994:282-299.

30 Litvan I, Cummings JL, Mega M. Neuropsychiatric features of corticobasal degeneration. J Neurol Neurosurg Psychiatry. 1998;65:717-721.

31 Riley DE, Lang AE, Lewis A, et al. Cortical-basal ganglionic degeneration. Neurology. 1990;40:1203-1212.

32 Kumar R, Bergeron C, Pollanen M, Lang AE. Cortical-basal Ganglionic Degeneration. In: Jankovic J, Tolosa E, eds. Parkinson's Disease & Movement Disorders. Baltimore, MD: Williams & Wilkins; 1998:297-316.

33 Halpern C, McMillan C, Moore P, Dennis K, Grossman M. Calculation impairment in neurodegenerative diseases. J Neurol Sci. 2003;208:31-38.

34 Bak TH, Hodges JR. Corticobasal degeneration: clinical aspects. Handb Clin Neurol. 2008;89:509-521.

35 Boeve BF, Maraganore DM, Parisi JE, et al. Pathologic heterogeneity in clinically diagnosed corticobasal degeneration. Neurology. 1999;53:795-800.

36 Boeve B. Corticobasal degeneration: the syndrome and the disease. In: Litvan I, editor. Atypical Parkinsonian Disorders: Clinial and Research Aspects. New Jersey: Humana Press; 2005:309-334.

37 Litvan I, Agid Y, Goetz C, et al. Accuracy of the clinical diagnosis of corticobasal degeneration: A clinicopathologic study. Neurology. 1997;48:119-125.

38 Kompoliti K, Goetz CG, Boeve BF, et al. Clinical presentation and pharmacological therapy in corticobasal degeneration. Arch Neurol. 1998;55:957-961.

39 Wenning GK, Litvan I, Jankovic J, et al. Natural history and survival of 14 patients with corticobasal degeneration confirmed at postmortem examination. J Neurol Neurosurg Psychiatry. 1998;64:184-189.

40 Frucht S, Fahn S, Chin S, Dhawan V, Eidelberg D. Levodopa-induced dyskinesias in autopsy-proven cortical-basal ganglionic degeneration. Mov Disord. 2000;15:340-343.

41 Vanek Z, Jankovic J. Dystonia in corticobasal degeneration. Mov Disord. 2001;16:252-257.

42 Cordivari C, Misra VP, Catania S, Lees AJ. Treatment of dystonic clenched fist with botulinum toxin. Movement Disorders. 2001;16:907-913.

43 Boeve BF, Josephs KA, Drubach DA. Current and future management of the corticobasal syndrome and corticobasal degeneration. Handb Clin Neurol. 2008;89:533-548.

44 Rossi G, Marelli C, Farina L, Laurà M, Maria Basile A, Ciano C, et al. The G389R mutation in the MAPT gene presenting as sporadic corticobasal syndrome. Mov Disord. 2008;23:892 895.

45 Kovács T, Farsang M, Vitaszil E, et al. Levetiracetam reduces myoclonus in corticobasal degeneration: report of two cases. J Neural Transm. 2009;116:1631-1634.

46 Josephs KA, Ahlskog JE, Parisi JE, et al. Rapidly progressive neurodegenerative dementias. Arch Neurol. 2009;66:201-207.

47 Lee W, Simpson M, Ling H, McLean C, Collins S, Williams DR. Characterising the uncommon corticobasal syndrome presentation of sporadic Creutzfeldt-Jakob disease. Parkinsonism Relat Disord. 2013;19:81-85.

48 Kertesz A, McMonagle P, Blair M, Davidson W, Munoz DG. The evolution and pathology of frontotemporal dementia. Brain. 2005;128:1996-2005.

49 McMonagle P, Blair M, Kertesz A. Corticobasal degeneration and progressive aphasia. Neurology. 2006;67:1444-1451.

50 Kertesz A, Martinez-Lage P, Davidson W, Munoz DG. The corticobasal degeneration syndrome overlaps progressive aphasia and frontotemporal dementia. Neurology. 2000;55:1368-1375.

51 Forman MS, Farmer J, Johnson JK, et al. Frontotemporal dementia: clinicopathological correlations. Ann Neurol. 2006;59:952-962.

PART III

Hyperkinetic Motor Behavioural Disorders

22

The Classification of Dystonia

Karen Frei & Daniel Truong

Dystonia is a neurological condition which produces sustained or intermittent muscle contractions causing abnormal, often repetitive, movements, postures, or both. Dystonia can be part of another disorder such as Parkinson's disease, or it can be a disorder of its own.

Classification of dystonia

Classification of dystonia can be based upon the aetiology, age of onset, regions affected or body parts involved. Dystonia can be considered to be primary, usually of unknown aetiology, or secondary, caused by a known entity, such as medication-induced dystonia. Genetic forms of dystonia are considered to be primary dystonia. Another classification involves using the nomenclature derived from the Human Genome Organization (HUGO).

The classification of the human genome organization (HUGO)

The HUGO classification is numbered DYT1-DYT21 (see Table 22.1) and is based on the chronologic order of gene mapping or clinical description. To date, there are 21 forms of hereditary dystonia that have been identified. The DYT classification lumps together pure dystonia, dystonia plus Parkinsonism or myoclonus and paroxysmal dyskinesias with dystonia. In most cases, hereditary dystonia is inherited in an autosomal dominant fashion with incomplete penetrance. In other words, family members may inherit the gene mutation but may not

have dystonia, or they can have varying degrees of dystonia. One family member may have cervical dystonia and another, blepharospasm or writer's cramp. Hereditary forms of dystonia usually begin in childhood and in one extremity. The autosomal dominant dystonias include DYT1, DYT5, DYT6, DYT11, rapid-onset dystonia-parkinsonism (DYT12), neuroferritinopathy, dentatorubral-pallidoluysian atrophy and Huntington's disease. The autosomal recessive dystonias include DYT2, DYT16 (1, 2), Wilson's disease, PLA2G6-associated neurodegeneration (PLAN), type 2 juvenile Parkinson disease (PARK2), and various metabolic disorders. The X-linked recessive inherited dystonia forms encompass Lubag (DYT3) (3), Lesch-Nyhan syndrome, and Mohr-Tranebjaerg syndrome (4, 5). Mitochondrial inheritance gives rise to Leigh syndrome (6) and Leber hereditary optic neuropathy (LHON) with dystonia (7).

The DYT classification, however, has various limitations such as the assignment of DYT14 as a novel form of dopa-responsive dystonia, although it is just a mutation of the GCH1 (DYT5) gene; a shared causative gene was named separately such as in the case of DYT9 and 18. Furthermore, even though they are labelled DYT disorders, DYT3 (Lubag) and DYT12 (rapid-onset dystonia-parkinsonism) are clinically dominated by parkinsonism rather than dystonia. Furthermore, there are many inherited disorders with dystonia which were described before the introduction of the DYT classification and were therefore not included. Such disorders include Wilson's disease, Lesch-Nyhan disease,

Table 22.1
DYT classification of hereditary forms of dystonia.

DYT designation	Description of disorder	Mode of inheritance	Gene identified	Type of dystonia
DYT 1	Early-onset torsion dystonia	AD	9q34.11 Tor 1 A	Pure dystonia
DYT 2	Dystonia musculorum deformans 2	AR		Pure dystonia
DYT 3	Lubag	XR	X13.1 TAF 1	Dystonia plus parkinsonism
DYT 4	Whispering dysphonia	AD		Pure dystonia
DYT 5	GCH 1; Dopa-responsive dystonia (Segawa's syndrome)	AD AR	14q22.2 GCH 1 11p15.5 TH	Dystonia plus parkinsonism
DYT 6	Adult-onset, mixed-type torsion dystonia	AD	8p11.21 Thap 1	Pure dystonia
DYT 7	Adult-onset focal dystonia	AD	18p?	Pure dystonia
DYT 8	Paroxysmal nonkinesogenic dyskinesia; Dystonic choreoathetosis	AD	2q37-35	Paroxysmal dyskinesia plus dystonia
DYT 9	Paroxysmal choreoathetosis with episodic ataxia and spasticity	AD	1p	Paroxysmal dyskinesia plus dystonia
DYT 10	Episodic/paroxysmal kinesogenic dyskinesia	AD	16p11.2	Paroxysmal dyskinesia plus dystonia
DYT 11	Myoclonus dystonia	AD	7q21.3 epsilon sarcoglycan 11p23.2 DRD2	Dystonia plus myoclonus
DYT 12	Rapid-onset dystonia-parkinsonism	AD	19q13.2 ATP1A3	Dystonia plus parkinsonism
DYT 13	Multifocal/ segmental dystonia	AD	1p36.32-36.13	Pure dystonia
DYT 15	Myoclonic dystonia	AD	18p11	Dystonia plus myoclonus
DYT 16	Young-onset dystonia-parkinsonism	AR	2q31.2 PRKRA	Dystonia plus parkinsonism
DYT 17	Autosomal recessive torsion dystonia	AR	20pq	Pure dystonia
DYT 19	Episodic kinesogenic dyskinesia-2	AD	16q	Paroxysmal dyskinesia plus dystonia
DYT 20	Paroxysmal nonkinesogenic dyskinesia-2	AD	2q	Paroxysmal dyskinesia plus dystonia
DYT21	adult-onset, generalized / multifocal dystonia	AD	2q14.3–q21.3	Pure dystonia

* AD autosomal dominant; AR autosomal recessive; XR X-linked recessive.
Modified from Online Mendelian Inheritance of Man (OMIM) (www.omim.org).

glutaric aciduria, or deafness dystonia syndrome. Genetic loci have been determined for most of the HUGO dystonia subtypes, except for DYT2, which is an autosomal recessive dystonia in the Spanish Roma population (8), and whispering dysphonia, DYT4 (9).

Primary dystonia

The following overview describes the pure dystonia forms in the DYT classification including DYT1, DYT2, DYT4, DYT6, DYT7, DYT13, DYT17 and DYT21, and dystonia plus forms.

DYT1

In 1911, Oppenheim's dystonia (DYT1) was first described in 4 young patients (10, 11). Earlier, Schwalbe had described three affected Jewish siblings from Lithuana who were presented orally by Ziehen (12). Oppenheimer coined the term 'dystonia' to describe the increase in muscle tone seen in this disorder that is different from post-stroke spasticity. DYT1 is an autosomal dominant inherited, early-onset torsion dystonia. It tends to begin in the foot or leg, with initial symptoms usually in childhood and later generalized within 3 years. Speech abnormalities are not seen. The clinical expression of DYT1 dystonia is very variable, even within families: 70% of gene carriers have no definite signs of dystonia, and among the remaining 30%, dystonia ranges from mild focal to severe generalized (13) (see Video fragment 22.1). The disorder is about five times more frequent in Ashkenazi Jews compared to non-Ashkenazim (14). It has an incomplete penetrance of about 30% and variable phenotypes. Age of onset has been reported to be from 3 up to 26 years. Despite the broad clinical spectrum, including both childhood and adult-onset and variable progression, the majority of carriers conforms to a characteristic phenotype and is similar in both Ashkenazi Jewish (AJ) and non-Jewish (NJ) populations. It frequently affects an arm or leg first, spreads to other limbs, occasionally to the neck, and rarely to cranial muscles (13). In about 65% of patients,

the disease progresses over a period of 5-10 years to a generalized or multifocal distribution; the remainder has segmental (10%) or focal (25%) involvement. A higher proportion of NJ carriers had leg rather than arm onset, and generalized disease (14). DYT1 dystonia is co-morbid with early-onset, recurrent, major depression. This association is independent of motor manifestations of dystonia and begins early in life. It occurs in both manifesting and non-manifesting carriers when compared with non-carriers. There are, however, no associations with the severity of motor signs (15). The DYT1 gene is located on chromosome 9q34.11 and encodes for a protein known as Torsin 1A. The predominant mutation is a GAG nucleotide deletion.

DYT2

DYT2 is an autosomal recessive form of generalized dystonia with clinical symptoms similar to DYT1. It usually begins in the hands or feet in infancy or early childhood and then generalizes with predominant craniocervical dystonia and prominent orofacial involvement (8,16). It was first reported in three families of consanguineous Spanish gypsies. Its gene has not been identified.

DYT3

Lubag (DYT3) is a form of dystonia inherited as an X-linked recessive, trait-linked TAF1 (TATA binding protein-associated factor 1 gene) multiple transcript system (17). It occurs in Filipino male adults with maternal roots from the Philippine island of Panay. It causes progressive dystonia, with or without parkinsonism. The phenotypic spectrum may include tremor, myoclonus, chorea and myorhythmia (18,19). Rarely, it can also occur in women and presents with mild dystonia and chorea (20,21). When presenting with parkinsonism only, it is considered a benign form (22). Neuropathologic studies show degeneration and gliosis of the putamen, striatum, and caudate, and within the neostriatum, the matrix compartment is relatively spared in a unique fashion, whereas the striosomes are severely depleted (23).

DYT4

Whispering dysphonia (DYT4) was described in an Australian family. Afflicted individuals whisper when talking and can only shout or yell when in an emotional state. They talk normally after drinking alcohol. Additional forms of dystonia including torticollis and generalized torsion dystonia were also found in this family (9).

DYT5

DYT5 is dopa-responsive dystonia (DRD), also known as Segawa syndrome. It is remarkable for the strong therapeutic effect of levodopa (24,25). DRD is caused by mutations in the DYT5 gene GTP cyclohydrolase 1 (GCH1) with a wide spectrum of phenotypes ranging from infantile cerebral palsy look-alikes to non-progressive, adult-onset parkinsonism. Patients often present with dystonic equinovarus foot posture at a young age and may generalize over the subsequent 10-15 years (25). Patients may become wheelchair-bound unless treated with levodopa. Postural, dystonic tremor rather than resting tremor may also develop. In some patients, the symptom remains subtle and may remain undiagnosed. In its classic form, the transmission is autosomal dominant, with variable penetrance. A recent study has identified DYT14 as a mutation of GCH1 (DYT5) (26).

DYT6

DYT6 differs from DYT1 in that the initial symptoms tend to affect the cranial and cervical muscles. Mutations in the THAP1 (Thanatos-associated, protein domain-containing, apoptosis-associated protein 1) gene were shown to be associated with DYT6, an autosomal dominantly inherited form of generalized dystonia with an estimated penetrance of approximately 60% (27). Initial symptoms most often begin in the arm and then generalize. In contrast to DYT1, laryngeal dystonia producing speech abnormalities is common. DYT6 was first identified in Amish/Mennonite families (28). The gene for DYT6 is located at 8p11.21. Both the gene and the gene product are known as THAP1. THAPs are thought to serve as chromatin-binding factors that regulate transcription, either directly or in complex with other proteins. It is noted that a heterogeneous collection of THAP1 sequence variants is associated with varied anatomical distributions and ages of onset of both familial and sporadic primary dystonia (29).

DYT7

Focal, adult-onset dystonia (DYT7) most commonly results in cervical dystonia. Blepharospasm and writer's cramp are also seen. It does not tend to generalize. It was identified in a German family (30). Age of onset ranged between 28 and 70 years. A locus on chromosome 18 was identified for DYT7. This location has been questioned, however (31).

DYT8-10, 19 and 20

DYT8, DYT9, DYT10, DYT19 and DYT20 are paroxysmal disorders. They are autosomal dominant. DYT8 and DYT20 are non-kinesigenic, DYT9, 10 and 19 are kinesigenic (32). DYT9 and DYT18 are identical.

DYT11

DYT11 or myoclonus dystonia (MD) is a childhood-onset movement disorder (mean onset 6 years) characterized by a combination of myoclonic jerks and dystonia. Benign essential myoclonus is a subtype of MD, where the dystonia is only subtle or absent. MD is the second most common dystonia-plus syndrome after DRD. There is a dramatic response to alcohol ingestion. In its familial form, MD has an autosomal-dominant inheritance pattern and is caused by a mutation at the epsilon-sarcoglycan gene (33,34). Myoclonus dystonia is also seen in DYT15 with a locus on chromosome 18 in a large Canadian family (35,36). It has an autosomal dominant transmission.

DYT12

DYT12 is a rapid-onset dystonia parkinsonism (RPD) characterized by dystonia and parkinsonism with abrupt onset associated with specific triggers such as physical (fever, running, childbirth, excessive alcohol ingestion) or psychological stress. RDP develops over minutes to 30 days and then stabilizes. Its dystonia has a clear rostro-caudal (face>arm>leg) gradient of involvement. Patients also suffer from dysarthria and dysphagia. L-dopa therapy is not effective (37,38). Its inheritance mode is autosomal dominant with a reduced penetrance. A mutation in the ATP1A3 is responsible for the RPD (39). DYT12 is not a neurodegenerative disorder.

DYT13

DYT13 was found in a large, non-Jewish, Italian family with mild, purely focal dystonia involving only one body part (cranial, cervical or arm). The inheritance was autosomal dominant, with affected individuals spanning three consecutive generations and male-to-male transmission. Age at onset ranged from 5 to 43 years. It begins with focal or segmental onset and occasional generalization. The DYT13 locus was mapped to chromosome 1p36 in this family. The causative gene is still missing. DYT13 tends to have a mild course (40).

DYT17

DYT 17 is an autosomal recessive disorder and usually begins in the teenage years with focal dystonia which later progresses to segmental or generalized dystonia. It was found in a large consanguineous Lebanese family with three affected individuals and was linked to chromosome 20 (41). Torticollis, dysphonia and dysarthria are features of this disorder.

DYT21

DYT21 is an autosomal dominant with adult-onset, generalized/multifocal dystonia, often starting with blepharospasm. DYT21 was mapped to 2q14.3-q21.3 (42).

Secondary dystonia

Secondary dystonia refers to dystonia that occurs as a result of another illness or insult. Table 22.2 lists some of the causes of dystonia. Secondary forms are usually accompanied by other neurological or movement disorders or additional symptoms that are more prominent than the dystonia (see Chapter 23).

Dystonia can also be part of another disorder such as a neurodegenerative disorder. Parkinson's disease (PD), corticobasal degeneration (CBD), multiple system atrophy (MSA) and progressive supranuclear palsy (PSP) are all examples of neurodegenerative disorders that may present with dystonia. Heredodegenerative disorders such as homocystinuria, Lesch-Nyhan syndrome, Wilson's disease (WD), neuroacanthocytosis, Niemann-Pick C, Leigh's disease, mitochondrial myopathy, encephalopathy, lactic acidosis and stroke-like episodes (MELAS) and Hallervorden Spatz pantothenate kinase-associated neurodegeneration (PKAN) as well as the Mohr-Tranebjearg syndrome (see Video fragment 22.2) have dystonia as part of the disorder.

Other conditions such as hypoxic brain injury, especially when involving the globus pallidus or basal ganglia, can result in dystonia, sometimes presenting many years after injury. Hypoparathyroidism and hyperthyroidism can also phenotypically include dystonia as part of the disorder. Finally, paraneoplastic disorders with underlying cervix, breast and lung malignancies have been reported to manifest with dystonia.

Classification by age of onset

Further ways to classify dystonia include age of onset. Early onset refers to symptoms initiating in childhood. Late onset usually refers to an adult age of onset of the dystonia. Generally speaking, early-onset dystonia usually begins in the leg, tends to generalize and is a hereditary form. The most commonly suggested age for separating early from adult onset is 26 years, which is utilized in formulating DYT1 testing guidelines (13). Dysto-

Table 22.2
Secondary causes of dystonia.

Heredo-degenerative disorders	▪ Wilson's disease ▪ Aceruloplasminemia ▪ Neuroacanthocytosis ▪ Lesch-Nyhan syndrome ▪ Homocystinuria ▪ Niemann-Pick C ▪ Hartnup disease ▪ GM1/GM2 gangliosidosis ▪ Ataxia-telangiectasia ▪ Cockayne's syndrome ▪ Gaucher's disease ▪ MELAS ▪ Leigh syndrome ▪ Leber's disease ▪ Kearn-Sayre syndrome
Metabolic disorders	▪ Hypoparathyroidism ▪ Hyperthyroidism
Brain lesions	▪ Anoxia ▪ Tumors ▪ Multiple sclerosis ▪ Arteriovenous malformations (AVM) ▪ Trauma
Infectious disease	▪ Encephalitis ▪ Tuberculous meningitis ▪ Cerebral malaria ▪ M. pneumoniae infection ▪ Toxoplasmosis
Toxins	▪ Methanol ▪ Cyanide ▪ Carbon monoxide ▪ Carbon disulfide ▪ Mycotoxin
Drugs	▪ Dopaminergic agents ▪ Neuroleptics ▪ Antihistamine ▪ Antidepressants ▪ Anxiolytics ▪ Antiepileptics
Autoimmune disorders	▪ Systemic lupus erythematosus ▪ Celiac disease ▪ Neuro-Behçet's disease

* Based upon (43).

nia that occurs during the first year of life is likely to be caused by an inherited metabolic disorder. Dystonia that emerges after a latent normal period such as a delayed onset dystonia or after developmental motor delay is more consistent with dystonic cerebral palsy.

Classification by involved regions

The regions affected can be another way to classify dystonia (see Table 22.3). Focal dystonia refers to a single region being affected, for example cervical dystonia affects the neck. Segmental dystonia refers to more than one contiguous region affected. Meige's syndrome involves the eyes, craniofacial muscles and neck. It can be considered a segmental dystonia. Generalized dystonia affects the entire body, limbs, trunk, neck and face.

Classification by involved body parts

Another way to classify dystonia is according to the body parts involved (see Table 22.3). When affecting the eyes, it is known as blepharospasm. Cranial dystonia affects the mouth and facial muscles. Oromandibular dystonia affects the jaw, laryngeal dystonia the larynx. Cervical dystonia or torticollis (cervical dystonia with rotation of the head) involves the neck (see Video fragment 22.3). Additional forms of cervical dystonia include laterocollis, antecollis and retrocollis. Writer's cramp is the term used to describe dystonia involving the hand and arm that becomes apparent when writing. Truncal or axial dystonia involves the trunk.

Classification by clinical expressions and aetiology

Recently, a new classification based on clinical features and aetiology (see Table 22.4) was proposed. It combines two axes to describe most cases of dystonia (44): a clinical axis and an aetiology axis.

Table 22.3
Distribution of dystonia to region and body parts involved.

Region involved	Body part involved
Focal Only one body region is affected	■ blepharospasm ■ oromandibular dystonia ■ laryngeal dystonia ■ cervical dystonia (including laterocollis, antero-collis and retrocollis) ■ writer's cramp ■ truncal dystonia ■ axial dystonia
Segmental Two or more contiguous body regions are affected	■ cranial dystonia (blepharospasm with lower facial and jaw or tongue involvement) ■ bibrachial dystonia.
Multifocal Two noncontiguous or more (contiguous or not) body regions are involved	
Generalized The trunk and at least 2 other sites are involved	■ leg involvement is annotated as additional feature
Hemidystonia More body regions restricted to one body side are involved.	

The clinical axis includes the clinical characteristics of the dystonia (the age of onset, body distribution, and temporal pattern) and associated features which specify further if the dystonia is isolated or combined, and the occurrence of other neurological or systemic manifestations. The classification by body distribution has implications for both diagnosis and therapy. Generalized dystonia treatment often involves medication and surgery, while focal dystonia is often treated with botulinum neurotoxin. The age at onset has been shown to be clinically important for diagnostic testing and prognostic value (44). The temporal pattern is an important characteristic that facilitates the diagnosis and treatment choice. The disease course can be static or progressive. The temporal pattern describes variability like persistence, action specificity, diurnal fluctuations and eventual paroxysmal occurrence. Diurnal fluctuations are used to describe the variability of the dystonia symptoms through the day. Paroxysmal dystonia means that the same trigger might or might not induce an attack, and when it does the dystonia attack only lasts for a short time after the trigger has ended. In task-specific dystonia, the same activity will characteristically always induce the dystonia, and the dystonia will typically improve after the cessation of the task. The description of the associated features in the classification of dystonia is used to differentiate the isolated dystonia from combined dystonia, in cases where the dystonia is combined with other movement disorders. Most cases previously described under 'dystonia plus' or 'heredodegenerative' would fall under this category. Unlike 'heredodegenerative', however, this description does not imply an aetiology. The description of the occurrence of other neurological or systemic manifestations is an important feature in the description of dystonia. In this classification, other non-dystonic manifestations of Wilson's disease would be described here.

Table 22.4
Proposed classification of dystonia (44).

Axis I: clinical characteristics	Axis II: aetiology
Clinical characteristics of dystonia	**Nervous system pathology**
Age at onset • Infancy (birth to 2 years) • Childhood (3–12 years) • Adolescence (13–20 years) • Early adulthood (21–40 years) • Late adulthood (>40 years)	Evidence of degeneration • Evidence of structural (often static) lesions • No evidence of degeneration or structural lesion

Body distribution
• Focal
• Segmental
• Multifocal
• Generalized (with or without leg involvement)
• Hemidystonia
	Inherited or acquired
	• Inherited
	  Autosomal dominant
	  Autosomal recessive
	  X-linked recessive
	  Mitochondrial
	• Acquired
	  Perinatal brain injury
	  Infection
	  Drug

Temporal pattern • Disease course • Static • Progressive • Variability • Persistent • Action-specific • Diurnal • Paroxysmal	Toxic Vascular Neoplastic Brain injury Psychogenic Idiopathic • Sporadic • Familial
Associated features • Isolated dystonia • Combined dystonia	
Occurrence of other neurological or systemic manifestations	

The second axis of the classification deals with the aetiology. Here, two complementary characteristics may be useful for classification: identifiable anatomical changes and pattern of inheritance (see Table 22.4). As of yet, two useful characteristics can be differentiated with the current technology: anatomical change and pattern of inheritance. It allows further classification into degenerative, static or not-degenerative or structural lesion-induced disorders. Also, the pattern of inheritance allows further subtyping. Inherited dystonias can be differentiated into autosomal dominant or recessive, X-linked re-

cessive and mitochondrial (44). The acquired dystonia is caused by a variety of specific causes. They include perinatal brain injury, infection, neoplasm, drug, intoxication and injury. Psychogenic dystonia is also included in this category (44). Furthermore, there are many conditions with unknown causes. They can be classified as sporadic or familial and eventually modified later when new dystonia genes are discovered.

Video fragments

Fragment 22.1
DYT1 dystonia
Young man with a DYT1 mutation (early-onset torsion dystonia), showing a generalized torsion dystonia.

Fragment 22.2
Secondary dystonia (Segments 1-2)
The first patient suffers from a pantothenate kinase-associated neurodegeneration (PKAN), formerly called Hallervorden-Spatz disease (segment 1). The second patient suffers from the X-linked dystonia-deafness syndrome (Mohr-Tranebjaerg syndrome) (segment 2).

Fragment 22.3
Focal/segmental dystonia (Segments1-4)
The first patient shows mainly focal blepharospasms with a slight dystonia of the perioral muscles (segment 1), the second patient suffers from a severe, segmental Meige syndrome with overflow to the trapezius muscles (segment 2), the third patient suffers from a focal torticollis spasmodica (segment 3), and the fourth patient from a focal spasmodic dysphonia. This last segment shows this patient's initially normal breathing, followed by supraglottic hyper-adduction during phonation, resulting in a typical dysphonic speech. The final part of this segment evidences the significant improvement after injection with botulinum toxin in the thyro-arythenoid muscles, producing reduced supraglottic adduction (segment 4).

References

1 Camargos S, Scholz S, Simon-Sanchez J, et al. DYT16, a novel young-onset dystonia-parkinsonism disorder: identification of a segregating mutation in the stress-response protein PRKRA. Lancet Neurol 2008;7:207-215.

2 Seibler P, Djarmati A, Langpap B, et al. A heterozygous frameshift mutation in PRKRA (DYT16) associated with generalised dystonia in a German patient. Lancet Neurol 2008;380-381.

3 Lee LV, Munoz EL, Tan KT, Reyes MT. Sex linked recessive dystonia parkinsonism of Panay, Philippines (XDP). Mol Pathol 2001;54:362-368.

4 Ha AD, Parratt KL, Rendtorff ND, et al. The phenotypic spectrum of dystonia in Mohr-Tranebjaerg syndrome. Mov Disord 2012;27:1034-1040.

5 Tranebjaerg L, Schwartz C, Eriksen H, et al. A new X linked recessive deafness syndrome with blindness, dystonia, fractures, and mental deficiency is linked to Xq22. J Med Genet 1995;32:257-263.

6 Lera G, Bhatia K, Marsden CD. Dystonia as the major manifestation of Leigh's syndrome. Mov Disord 1994;9:642-649.

7 Watanabe M, Mita S, Takita T, Goto Y, Uchino M, Imamura S. Leber's hereditary optic neuropathy with dystonia in a Japanese family. J Neurol Sci 2006;243:31-34.

8 Gimenez-Roldan S, Delgado G, Marin M, Villanueva JA, Mateo D. Hereditary torsion dystonia in gypsies. Adv Neurol 1988;50:73-81.

9 Parker N. 1985. Hereditary whispering dysphonia. J Neurol Neurosurg Psychiatry 1985;48:218-224.

10 Klein C, Fahn S. Translation of Oppenheim's 1911 paper on dystonia. Mov Disord 2013;28:851-862.

11 Oppenheim H. Uber eine eigenartige Krampfkrankheit des kindlichen und jugendlichen Alters (Dysbasia lordotica progressiva, Dystonia musculorum deformans). Neurol Centrabl 1911;30:1090–1107.

12 Truong DD, Fahn S. An early description of dystonia: translation of Schwalbe's thesis and information on his life. Adv Neurol 1988;50:651-564.

13 Bressman SB, Sabatti C, Raymond D, et al. The DYT1 phenotype and guidelines for diagnostic testing. Neurology 2000;54:1746-1752.

14 Zeman W, Dyken P. Dystonia musculorum deformans. Clinical, genetic and pathoanatomical studies. Psychiatr Neurol Neurochir 1967;70:77-121.

15 Heiman GA, Ottman R, Saunders-Pullman RJ, Ozelius LJ, Risch NJ, Bressman SB. Increased risk for recurrent major depression in DYT1 dystonia mutation carriers. Neurology 2004;63:631-637.

16 Khan NL, Wood NW, Bhatia KP. Autosomal recessive, DYT2-like primary torsion dystonia: a new family. Neurology 2003;61:1801-1803.

17 Makino S, Kaji R, Ando S, et al. Reduced neuron-specific expression of the TAF1 gene is associated with X-linked dystonia-parkinsonism. Am Jf Hum Genet 2007;80:393-406.

18 Evidente VG, Advincula J, Esteban R, et al. Phenomenology of 'Lubag' or X-linked dystonia-parkinsonism. Mov Disord 2002;17:1271-1277.

19 Lee MA, Walker RW, Hildreth TJ, Prentice WM. A survey of pain in idiopathic Parkinson's disease. J Pain Symptom Manage 2006;32:462-469.

20 Evidente VG, Nolte D, Niemann S, et al. Phenotypic and molecular analyses of X-linked dystonia-parkinsonism ('lubag') in women. Arch Neurol 2004;61:1956-1959.

21 Waters CH, Takahashi H, Wilhelmsen KC, et al. Phenotypic expression of X-linked dystonia-parkinsonism (lubag) in two women. Neurology 1993;43:1555-1558.

22 Evidente VG, Gwinn-Hardy K, Hardy J, Hernandez D, Singleton A. X-linked dystonia ('Lubag') presenting predominantly with parkinsonism: a more benign phenotype? Mov Disord 2002;17:200-202.

23 Goto S, Lee LV, Munoz EL, et al. Functional anatomy of the basal ganglia in X-linked recessive dystonia-parkinsonism. Ann Neurol 2005;58:7-17.

24 Nygaard TG, Marsden CD, Duvoisin RC. Dopa-responsive dystonia. Adv Neurol 1988;50:377-384.

25 Segawa M, Nomura Y, Nishiyama N. 2003. Autosomal dominant guanosine triphosphate cyclohydrolase I deficiency (Segawa disease). Ann Neurol 54S6:32-45.

26 Wider C, Melquist S, Hauf M, et al. Study of a Swiss dopa-responsive dystonia family with a deletion in GCH1: redefining DYT14 as DYT5. Neurology 2008;70:1377-1383.

27 Fuchs T, Gavarini S, Saunders-Pullman R, et al. Mutations in the THAP1 gene are responsible for DYT6 primary torsion dystonia. Nat Genet 2009;41:2288.

28 Almasy L, Bressman SB, Raymond D, et al. Idiopathic torsion dystonia linked to chromosome 8 in two Mennonite families. Ann Neurol 1997;42:670-673.

29 Xiao J, Zhao Y, Bastian RW, et al. Novel THAP1 sequence variants in primary dystonia. Neurology 2010;74:229-238.

30 Leube B, Rudnicki D, Ratzlaff T, Kessler KR, Benecke R, Auburger G. Idiopathic torsion dystonia: assignment of a gene to chromosome 18p in a German family with adult onset, autosomal dominant inheritance and purely focal distribution. Hum Mol Genet 1996;5:1673-1677.

31 Winter P, Kamm C, Biskup S, et al. DYT7 gene locus for cervical dystonia on chromosome 18p is questionable. Mov Disord 2012;27:1819-1821.

32 Petrucci S, Valente EM. 2013. Genetic issues in the diagnosis of dystonias. Front Neurol 2013;4:doi.10.3389/fneur.2012.00034.

33 Asmus F, Zimprich A, Tezenas Du Montcel S, et al. Myoclonus-dystonia syndrome: epsilon-sarcoglycan mutations and phenotype. Ann Neurol 2002;52:489-492.

34 Zimprich A, Grabowski M, Asmus F, et al. Mutations in the gene encoding epsilon-sarcoglycan cause myoclonus-dystonia syndrome. Nature Genetics 2001; 29:66-69.

35 Grimes DA, Han F, Lang AE, St George-Hyssop P, Racacho L, Bulman DE. A novel locus for inherited myoclonus-dystonia on 18p11. Neurology 2002;59:1183-1186.

36 Han F, Racacho L, Lang AE, Bulman DE, Grimes DA. Refinement of the DYT15 locus in myoclonus dystonia. Mov Disord 2007;22:888-892.

37 Brashear A, Dobyns WB, de Carvalho Aguiar P, et al. The phenotypic spectrum of rapid-onset dystonia-parkinsonism (RDP) and mutations in the ATP1A3 gene. Brain 2007;130:828-835.

38 Brashear A, Sweadner K, Ozelius L. Rapid-Onset Dystonia-Parkinsonism In Pagon RA, Adam MO, Bird TD, et al., eds. GeneReviews, Seattle, University of Washington, Seattle. 1993-2013 [online].

39 de Carvalho Aguiar P, Sweadner KJ, Penniston JT, et al. Mutations in the Na+/K+ -ATPase alpha3 gene ATP1A3 are associated with rapid-onset dystonia parkinsonism. Neuron 2004;43:169-175.

40 Bentivoglio AR, Ialongo T, Contarino MF, Valente EM, Albanese A. Phenotypic characterization of DYT13 primary torsion dystonia. Mov Disord 2004;19:200-206.

41 Chouery E, Kfoury J, Delague V, et al. A novel locus for autosomal recessive primary torsion dystonia (DYT17) maps to 20p11.22-q13.12. Neurogenetics 20089:287-293.

42 Norgren N, Mattson E, Forsgren L, Holmberg M. A high-penetrance form of late-onset torsion dystonia maps to a novel locus (DYT21) on chromosome 2q14.3-q21.3. Neurogenetics 2011;12:137-143.

43 Barton B, Zauber SE, Goetz CG. Movement disorders caused by medical disease. Semin Neurol 2009;29:97-110.

44 Albanese A, Bhatia K, Bressman SB, et al. Phenomenology and classification of dystonia: A consensus update. Mov Disord 2013;28:863-873.

23

Dystonia in Neurological Diseases

Franziska Hopfner & Susanne A. Schneider

Dystonia is a hyperkinetic movement disorder characterized by involuntary, sustained muscle contraction resulting in twisting and repetitive movements or abnormal postures (1).

Historically, the term 'Dystonia musculorum deformans' was coined by Oppenheim in 1911 for a syndrome that he could not assign to other known clinical phenomena (2). His patients presented with fluctuating muscular tone ranging from hypertonia to hypotonia. Similar clinical features were, however, described three years earlier by Schwalbe who reported bizarre tonic cramps in a family (3). In 1919 Mendel supported use of the term 'torsional dystonia', again emphasizing that this clinical condition is a shift between hyper- and hypotonia. The first diagnostic criteria for dystonic syndromes were established by Herz in 1944, who investigated dystonic movements using electrophysiology and cinematography (4). Using prospective observational studies, Marsden and Harrison demonstrated that there is a link between the age of onset and the clinical progression in this syndrome. Patients with a disease onset in childhood exhibited a severer disease progression with a tendency to develop generalized dystonia starting from the legs. In late-onset patients symptoms often remained restricted to one part, mostly the upper part of the body (5,6).

On the basis of these observations, three axes to classify dystonia are recognized: according to the onset age, distribution and aetiology. Thus, dystonic syndromes may first be classified by the age of the onset (young – onset: prior to age 26; late – onset: age 26 or older). Second, they may be classified by the body region affected (focal dystonia: one region of the body affected; segmental dystonia: symptoms limited to neighbouring regions of the body; multifocal dystonia: affected areas are not adjacent to each other; hemidystonia: only one side of the body affected; generalized dystonia: several neighbouring regions of the body are affected, including at least one region in the lower extremities). Depending on the localization, dystonia may be described as facial, cranial, brachial, axial, or crural dystonia, etc. Third, dystonia may be classified by aetiology. It may be the sole manifestation (as seen in primary dystonias) or occur in the context of other conditions (neurological and non-neurological). Generally, before a diagnosis of primary dystonia is made, a secondary form should be excluded. They may be caused by a wide variety of vascular, traumatic, infectious, toxic or other processes affecting the central or peripheral nervous systems. As a general rule: while the disease onset is usually slow in primary dystonia (with the exception of the genetic form of 'Rapid Onset Dystonia Parkinsonism', DYT 12), acute onset may be a pointer towards secondary dystonia.

Anatomical considerations

The concept of 'strategic lesions' derived from findings of pathological studies which promoted the understanding of topographical and functional neuroanatomy. Precise phenotype descriptions in combination with thorough brain pathology elucidated the function of the basal ganglia and its relation to movement disorders.

Thus, while motor parkinsonism is typically attributed to changes in the substantia nigra, dystonia is most commonly ascribed to dysfunction of the putamen rather than other basal ganglia nuclei. However, dystonia may also be related to lesions in the thalamus, the brainstem, the cerebellum or the frontal subcortical pathways. It has been repeatedly shown that abnormalities in these structures are more likely to cause dystonia than other forms of movement disorders.

Pathological data were confirmed by imaging studies which linked dystonia to basal ganglia lesions. Notably, abnormal basal ganglia function may be demonstrated by functional imaging techniques even when anatomical lesions are not apparent (7-9).

Depending on the localization and size of the lesion in the putaminal network, dystonia may manifest as focal (e.g. torticollis, oro-facial dystonia, lingual dystonia, cranial dystonia), hemidystonia, or generalized dystonia (10-15). As a rule of thumb, unilateral lesions typically produce contralateral signs. For example, in a large study of 240 dystonia patients with lesions in the basal ganglia, 80% of those with hemidystonia had lesions in the contralateral basal ganglia system, mainly in the putamen or thalamus (10). Thus, the presence of unilateral clinical signs should prompt an investigation for a contralateral structural lesion.

Secondary dystonia

While numerous reviews focused on primary dystonias, here we will discuss dystonia in neurological disease. There is an enormous variety of neurological disorders in which dystonia may occur, including neurodegenerative, metabolic, mitochondrial disorders and others. The most frequent diseases in which dystonia may occur are listed in Table 23.1.

In the following, we will only touch base on a few examples, namely dystonia in vascular and metabolic disease and in the context of other movement disorders.

Dystonia in cerebrovascular lesions

The most common cause of secondary dystonia is vascular in nature, mostly related to ischemic or hemorrhagic strokes, but bleeding or vascular malformations, etc. have also been reported. However, as outlined above, as well as in other chapters of this book, other types of movement disorders (like chorea, tremor, limb shaking or parkinsonism) may also occur in the context of vascular lesions (16,17). With vascular lesions, onset in the acute phase and delayed onset have to be distinguished (18). While chorea and hemiballismus typically occur in the acute stages, dystonia tends to manifest after weeks or several months or years, when patients have almost or completely recovered from the initial motor deficit (17,19). It may be transient or persistent. In contrast, dystonia is rarely observed during the acute stage of vascular events, i.e. stroke in adults. The delay between the vascular event, i.e. stroke and the onset of the movement disorder may be explained by the time required for the unbalanced but successful partial recovery of motor function and the subsequent development of pathological pathways reflecting the neuroplasticity (changes in synapse activity) (16,17,20).

In general, following ischemia the prevalence of dyskinesia in the acute stage is around 1%;

Table 23.1
(Secondary) dystonia in the context of other disease.

- Dystonia in vascular diseases
- Dystonia in metabolic diseases
- Dystonia in demyelinating diseases (such as multiple sclerosis)
- Dystonia in autoimmune diseases (such as thyroid, auto-immune encephalites)
- Dystonia in infectious disease (such as AIDS)
- Dystonia in other movement disorders
- Dystonia in mitochondrial diseases
- Dystonia as manifestation of space-occupying lesions (tumors, calcification)
- Drug- and toxin-induced dystonia (such as dopamine antagonist treatment)

and the prevalence of movement disorders with delayed onset after stroke ranges from 1.1% to 3.9% based on hospital data (18,19). An age-dependent presentation has been observed: while chorea tends to occur in elderly stroke patients, dystonia occurs more frequently in young stroke patients (16).

Posthemiplegic dystonia is the most frequent clinical feature. In most cases, dystonia after stroke manifests as hemidystonia affecting the contralateral arm and leg or as focal or segmental dystonia. Athetosis or choreatic movements may be associated features. Hemidystonia is typically due to contralateral lesions in the striatopallidal complex, thalamus, brainstem and cerebellum (21). Focal dystonia mostly involves the upper limb, with a predominantly distal distribution and a characteristic hand posture with lesions found in the parietal and thalamic area or putaminocapsular, thalamocapsular or frontal areas (18,19,20,22). Lingual, facial, oromandibular, blepharospasm and cervical dystonia have also been reported (18). The prognosis varies. In one series, 31% experienced complete recovery, while the recovery was partial in 62.5% of poststroke dystonia patients.

Several different hypotheses on the pathophysiology of dystonia have been proposed in the literature. Lesions in the striatopallidal complex may interrupt the cortico striato-pallido-thalamo-cortical loop (both the direct and indirect pathways), leading to increased thalamocortical drive and overactivity in primary and accessory motor areas (23). Dystonia induced by thalamic lesions has a different pathophysiological basis, although it induces overactivity in motor cortical areas (23). Lesions of the centromedial (CM) nucleus of the thalamus, especially lesions involving input from the pedunculopontine complex, may induce dystonia (24). The mesial thalamus (including the CM) plays an inhibitory role in the ventral lateral nucleus, which receives pallidal inputs and thus induces an increased thalamocortical drive (24). In addition, dystonia following

midbrain lesions may be induced by dopaminergic dysfunction (24). In these cases, lesions are mostly confined to the ventromesial mesencephalon and red nucleus areas, including the substantia nigra, nigrostriatal and cerebellothalamic fibers. The degree of dopaminergic denervation correlates with the severity of the dystonia (25).

Many authors suggest that dystonia is most probably associated with thalamofrontal disinhibition with disruption of basal ganglia inhibitory control, resulting in altered firing patterns, synchronized oscillations, and widened receptive fields (23). Although poststroke dystonia is usually associated with lesions of the lentiform nucleus, several case reports suggest that both the cerebello-thalamo-cortical pathway and the parietal-cortical pathway play an important role in the pathogenesis of dystonia, too (26-29). The same pathophysiological underpinnings may apply to other forms of dystonia caused by structural lesions, e.g. due to demyelination or space-occupying lesions (30). Their specific manifestations are beyond the scope of this review. Treatment of dystonia in these cases is mostly symptomatic.

Dystonia in parkinsonian disorders

Dystonia in Parkinson's disease (PD)

Parkinsonism is characterized by cardinal motor symptoms, including bradykinesia, hypokinesia, rigidity, resting tremor, and postural instability (31).

Parkinsonian syndromes can be divided into four subtypes: primary or idiopathic Parkinson's disease (PD) (Chapter 5), hereditary parkinsonism (Chapter 16), secondary or acquired parkinsonism (Chapters 17,18), and Parkinson plus syndromes (31). Parkinson plus syndromes are characterized by the presence of complicating features in addition to parkinsonism (32). They include multiple system atrophy (Chapter 19), progressive supranuclear palsy (Chapter 20) and corticobasal degeneration (Chapter 21).

Dystonic symptoms have been described in PD as well as in other parkinsonian syndromes. Notably, dystonia may precede the onset of parkinsonism in PD by many years, particularly in young-onset PD (see below); or it may occur as a complication of long-term treatment with dopaminergic agents (33). It may manifest as unilateral equinovarus foot, upper arm-forearm or forearm-hand flexion, oro-mandibular dystonia, torticollis, and different combinations of these symptoms (34,35). Some patients may develop dystonic contractures leading to fixed, painless, treatment-related deformities, mainly involving the hands and toes (33,36-38).

Young-onset PD, defined by consensus as PD first manifesting between 20 and 40 years of age, is particularly prone to exhibit limb dystonia (39-41). This may manifest as early morning or wearing-off dystonia with a predilection for painful, exercise-induced foot inversion, but may also manifest as a variety of segmental syndromes. Generally, 14–50% of young-onset PD patients have dystonia as the presenting feature. Thus, dystonic findings in a young individual should raise the suspicion of young-onset PD (and regular follow-up would be appropriate) (42,43). Rare variants in the parkin gene (accounting for the 50% of familial cases before age 45, and up to 20% of sporadic cases of young-onset parkinsonism), for example, cause dystonic features in about 40% of cases (44,45). Homozygous mutation carriers for variants in the gene DJ-1 and PINK-1 occasionally present with limb dystonia, laterocollis, or blepharospasm (46-48). Therapeutic application of levodopa and dopamine agonists may worsen rather than improve dystonia in some of these young-onset PD cases (34).

In PD, dystonia may also be a complication of long-term treatment: In general, dystonia usually occurs in PD as an off-period phenomenon (off-period dystonia) but may also present as peak-dose dystonia or diphasic dystonia mostly involving the foot (see also chapter 12) (49).

About 30% of chronically levodopa-treated PD patients develop off-dystonia with a broad range of manifestations (50). To avoid off-dystonia in the early morning, it is reasonable to prescribe a sustained-release preparation of levodopa at night or to administer a quick-acting levodopa medication in the early morning which can be taken before getting out of bed (51). Anticholinergic treatment, amantadine benzodiazepines, baclofen or botulinum toxin may also be helpful (52,53). Deep brain stimulation of the subthalamic nucleus permanently reduces off-dystonia in up to 90% of patients (54).

Dementia with Lewy bodies (DLB) is mostly considered a subtype of PD in which progressive cognitive decline with fluctuating alertness and attention (such as drowsiness, lethargy, lengthy periods of time spent staring into space), disorganized speech and recurrent visual hallucinations precede motor parkinsonism, and occasionally, segmental dystonic features may be observed. There are also several reports of Meige's syndrome (combination of blepharospasm and oromandibular dystonia) in DLB (55-59).

Dystonia in multiple system atrophy (MSA)

MSA includes two major subtypes within its phenotypic spectrum: a parkinsonian subtype (MSA-P) with a predominant nigrostriatal degeneration, and a cerebellar subtype (MSA-C) predominantly presenting with olivopontocerebellar atrophy (60). Of these, the majority of MSA patients present with parkinsonism (61). Patients additionally develop isolated autonomic failure such as loss of bladder control or abnormal blood-pressure regulation. The average remaining lifespan after the onset of symptoms in patients with MSA is 7.9 years (60) (see Chapter 19).

In MSA, dystonia may be more common than previously reported, occurring in 42% of levodopa-naive patients. In PD, although there are no prospective series, dystonia has been reported in only 16% of levodopa-naive patients in a retrospective survey. This suggests that dystonia is more common in untreated MSA compared with untreated PD. There is a broad phenotype of dystonia in MSA including antecollis and truncal dystonia (camptocormia and Pisa syndrome). In fact, antecollis is considered one of the characteristic features of this disease (62-65). It has been suggested that dystonia in the initial stages of MSA responds to levodopa treatment. This may reflect early nigrostriatal dysfunction due to a decrease of endogenous dopaminergic stimulation rather than postsynaptic striatal pathology (62,66-69).

Dystonia in progressive supranuclear palsy (PSP)

PSP, also known as Steele-Richardson-Olszewski syndrome (after those who first characterized its pathology), presents as a symmetrical rather than asymmetrical, akinetic-rigid syndrome (in contrast to PD and MSA) (see Chapter 20). There is often prominent axial involvement with early postural and gait instability leading to falls (typically backwards) and a dystonic posture with a flexed trunk but an extended neck (60, 70). Laryngeal dystonia, oromandibular dystonia and blepharospasm have been reported in PSP (33,71-75).

Dystonia in corticobasal degeneration (CBD)

CBD is typically strikingly asymmetrical in its presentation (76) Patients typically complain of a clumsy stiff limb, and apraxia is a hallmark feature of CBD (see Chapter 21). The most common presenting dystonic symptom in patients with corticobasal degeneration is unilateral arm dystonia with occurrence in 59% to more than 90% of patients (77-80). More than two-thirds of patients also develop a so-called 'alien limb': they feel the limb no longer belongs to them, it is as if it belongs to somebody else (81). The affected limb (typically an arm) may involuntarily perform apparently purposeful movements (77,82). Cortical sensory loss with simultagnosia and dysgraphaesthesia is frequent. Thus, pa-tients have problems recognizing objects in their pockets by tactile impressions, though crude light touch and pin prick sensation remain preserved.

Dystonia in metabolic disease

Metabolic disorders are multi-systemic diseases that often involve the central nervous system. In most cases the disease onset is in childhood or adolescence, and the mode of inheritance is recessive. In Table 22.2 and Table 23.2, an incomplete overview is presented of heredodegenerative metabolic syndromes that may be a cause of dystonia.

Wilson's disease

In this chapter, Wilson's disease will be discussed as an example of metabolic causes since it is treatable and apparently not as rare as previously considered.

Wilson's disease was first observed in the 19th century, and it is named after Samuel Alexander Kinnier Wilson (1878-1937), the British neurologist who first described the condition in 1912 in his dissertation entitled 'Progressive lenticular degeneration: A familial nervous disease associated with cirrhosis of the liver'. Today, the term 'hepatolenticular degeneration' has become obsolete in view of the much wider distribution of pathology (rather than affecting the nucleus lentiformis only). The main pathophysiological feature is an accumulation of copper leading to hepatic damage and neurological symptoms of variable degree. Wilson's disease is inherited in an autosomal recessive pattern. In the general population Wilson's disease is estimated to occur in between 1 in 5,000 and 1 in 30,000 people, and the frequency of heterozygous carriers is about 1%-2% (83-85). However, the estimated number of unreported cases may be much higher. Both new sequencing methods that provide cheaper and faster genotyping and DNA microarray analysis may help to detect mutations in the future more

Table 23.2
Incomplete list of heredodegenerative causes of dystonia.

Group of disorder	Condition	Gene	Pattern of inheritance	Main characteristics
Neuro-acanthocytoses	Choreoacanthocytosis	VPS13A	AR	Involuntary movements, mainly chorea and dystonia, epilepsy and acanthocytes on blood smear
Lysosomal storage disorder	Ceroid-lipofuscinosis	several genes	AR	Progressive dementia, seizures, and progressive visual failure
	Metachromatic leukodystrophy	ARSA	AR	Mental deterioration, bulbar palsies, motor symptoms, (dystonia, rigidity, spasticity), mental deterioration, and sometimes convulsions
	Niemann-Pick disease type 1/2	NPC1/2	AR	Ataxia, spasticity, dystonia, vertical supranuclear gaze palsy, seizures, dementia, and psychiatric symptoms, hepatosplenomegaly
	Tay-Sachs disease	HEXA	AR	Developmental retardation, paralysis, dementia, and blindness, usually fatal by age 2–3 years
	Fucosidosis	FUCA1	AR	Mental retardation, seizures, and neuropathy
Leukodystrophy	Pelizaeus-Merzbacher disease	PLP1	XR	Progressive pyramidal and cerebellar signs, and rolling head tremor
Disorder of purine metabolism	Lesch-Nyhan syndrome	HPRT	XR	Mental retardation, motor delay, and spasticity, choreoathetosis, and self-destructive biting; uric acid urinary stones
Deficiency of Glutaryl-CoA Dehydrogenase	Glutaric acidemia I	GCDH	AR	Infantile encephalopathy with dystonic choreoathetosis
Dystonia-parkinsonism	DYT3	TAF1	XR	Torsion dystonia, parkinsonian symptoms; in Filipino patients
Early-onset parkinsonism with deficits in mitochondrial homeostasis	PARK2	Parkin	AR	Early-onset dopa-sensitive parkinsonism, foot dystonia
	DJ-	DJ-1	AR	Early-onset dopa-sensitive parkinsonism

			Clinical features
Mitochondrial disease	Mohr-Tranebjaerg syndrome	TIMM8A	XR	Progressive deafness and dystonia leading to cortical blindness, fractures, and mental deficiency
	Leber hereditary optic neuropathy	several genes	M	Optic atrophy, tremor, and dystonia
	Leigh syndrome	several genes	XR, M, AR	Early onset, rapid progression, and clinical heterogeneity
Trinucleotide repeat disorders	Dentatorubra-pallidoluysian atrophy	ATN1	AD	Ataxia, chorea, and dementia, seizures
	Huntington's disease	IT15	AD	Chorea, personality change, and dementia. In young-onset cases: parkinsonism
	SCA3	ATXN3	AD	Ataxia, spasticity, and ocular movement abnormalities
	SCA17	TBP	AD	Ataxia, parkinsonism, chorea, dystonia, and dementia
Metal storage disorders	Wilson's disease	ATP7B	AR	Tremor, dystonia, and parkinsonian features, ataxia, psychiatric features, liver involvement
	Neuroferritinopathy	FTL	AD	Extrapyramidal features similar to those of Huntington's disease
	Pantothenate Kinase-Associated Neurodegeneration	PANK2	AR	Early-onset pyramidal extrapyramidal signs, cognitive decline, retinitis pigmentosa, neurodegeneration with brain iron accumulation type 1, usually eye of the tiger sign on MRI
Neuro-developmental disorder	Rett syndrome	MECP2	XD	Mental retardation, motor delay, stereotypies with hand washing movements, autism, and epilepsy

AR = autosomal recessive; AD = autosomal dominant; M = mitochondrial; XR = x-linked.

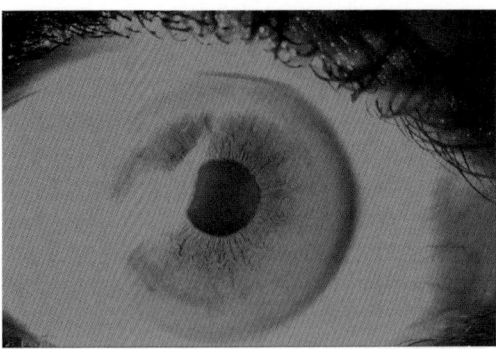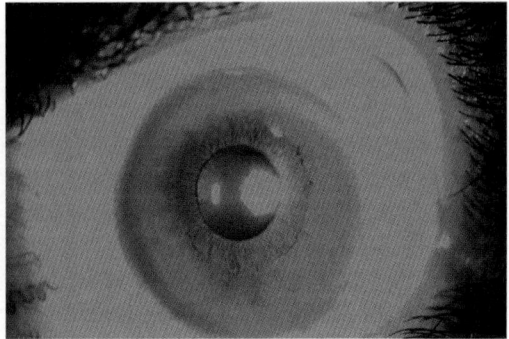

Figure 23.1
Corneal Kayser-Fleischer rings, as seen in Wilson's disease, caused by granular copper depositions in the Descement's membrane of the cornea.

easily and will allow a more precise estimation of mutation rates in different populations.

The defective gene, ATP7B, is located on chromosome 13 and encodes an ATPase, copper-transporting, beta-polypeptide, which is expressed predominantly in the liver, and plays a key role in human copper metabolism (85-87). Currently, more than 340 different, often private ATP7B mutations have been identified, of which the majority are located in the transmembrane region of the associated protein (88). Due to the variety of mutations, there is no overt genotype–phenotype correlation.

Clinical presentation

The clinical presentation of Wilson's disease is highly variable. Symptoms usually appear between the ages of 6 and 20 years, but late-onset cases have also been described (83,89). The majority of patients present with a hepatic phenotype. In patients with predominantly neuropsychiatric symptoms, there is often additional, clinically asymptomatic or symptomatic liver involvement.

The onset of hepatic Wilson's disease tends to occur earlier in life compared to the neurological type of Wilson's disease. Patients with hepatic Wilson's disease (manifestation between 8 and 18 years) exhibit features ranging from acute hepatitis, fulminant hepatic failure, or progressive chronic liver disease in the form of either chronic active hepatitis or cirrhosis of the macronodular type to mild elevations of certain liver enzymes (84,90,91). In general, the younger the age of the patient at symptom onset, the greater the degree of liver involvement (84).

The neurological form is variable, with a mean age of onset in the second to third decade, although onset has been reported as late as 72 years of age (92). The majority of patients become symptomatic before the age of 50 (91,92). Initial symptoms are often unspecific, mild, and may not be recognised. Patients commonly present with extrapyramidal (see Video fragment 23.1), cerebellar and cerebral-related symptoms, in either a subacute or chronic fashion (93). Neurological signs include asymmetric postural hand tremor, a flapping tremor, (negative) myoclonus (so-called asterixis), intention tremor, and sometimes tremor of the trunk and head, dysarthria, dysphagia and difficulties with writing.

Dystonia is found in a third of patients with Wilson's disease. Patients present with facial grimacing, tongue dyskinesia, blepharospasm and fixed, so-called 'sardonic' smiling (91). Symptoms are generalized in half of them, some have segmental, some multifocal, and some bilateral foot dystonia (94). Dystonia may be the presenting sign and may also occur later in the disease. Features of parkinsonism (i.e. rigidity and bradykinesia) commonly occur in combination (84). Initially, patients may also present with bulbar symptoms

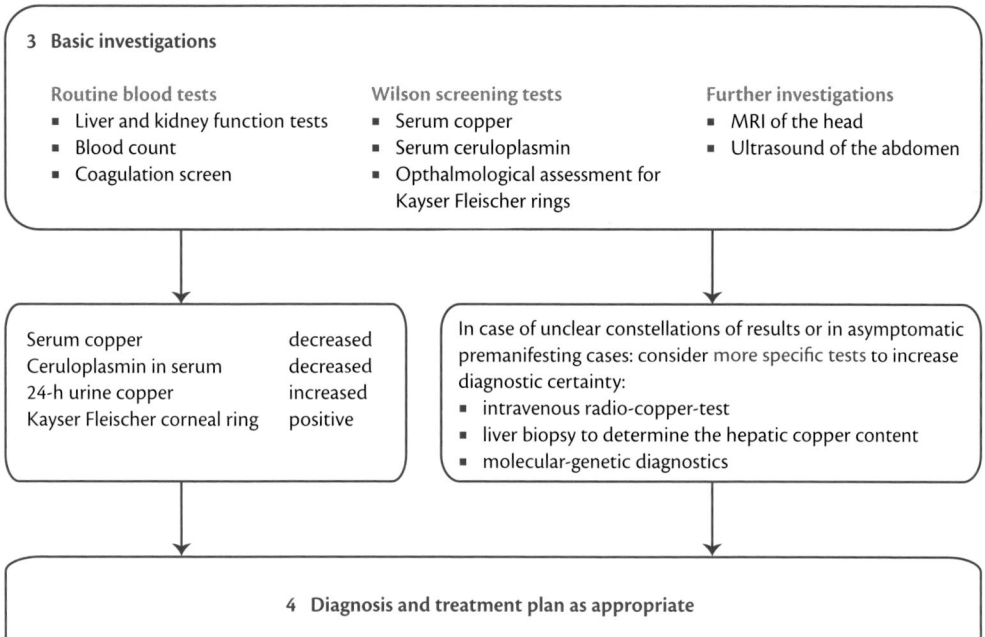

1 **Medical history**
- Disease onset age 5-45th year of life
- Unclear movement disorder or neuropsychiatric symptoms and/or
- Unclear liver dysfunction

2 **Neurological findings**
Basal ganglia and/or cerebellar symptoms
± pyramidal signs ± psychiatric involvement

3 **Basic investigations**

Routine blood tests	Wilson screening tests	Further investigations
▪ Liver and kidney function tests	▪ Serum copper	▪ MRI of the head
▪ Blood count	▪ Serum ceruloplasmin	▪ Ultrasound of the abdomen
▪ Coagulation screen	▪ Opthalmological assessment for Kayser Fleischer rings	

Serum copper	decreased
Ceruloplasmin in serum	decreased
24-h urine copper	increased
Kayser Fleischer corneal ring	positive

In case of unclear constellations of results or in asymptomatic premanifesting cases: consider more specific tests to increase diagnostic certainty:
- intravenous radio-copper-test
- liver biopsy to determine the hepatic copper content
- molecular-genetic diagnostics

4 **Diagnosis and treatment plan as appropriate**

Figure 23.2
Diagnostic algorithm for the diagnosis of Wilson's disease.

characterized by difficulties with speech, swallowing, and drooling related to dystonia of the bulbar muscles, or pseudobulbar palsy (93).

Up to one-third of patients may suffer from psychiatric symptoms, including attention deficit, attention-deficit hyperactivity disorder, impulsivity, paranoid psychosis, obsessive behaviour, depression, suicidal tendencies or bizarre behaviour (91,95). Myoclonic or tonic–clonic seizure disorders – of either the generalized or partial variety – are rarely seen (91).

Up to 95% of individuals with the neurologic form of Wilson's disease and 50-60% of cases in the absence of neurologic symptoms show a so-called Kayser–Fleischer ring that results from granular copper depositions in Descement's membrane of the cornea (see Figure 23.1) (95). The pathophysiological underpinnings of Wilson's disease is dysfunction of the copper metabolism. Investigations reveal paradoxically low serum copper (< 60 µg/dl) and coeruloplasmin levels (< 20 mg/dl) but elevated urine copper. For diagnostic purposes, urine should be col-

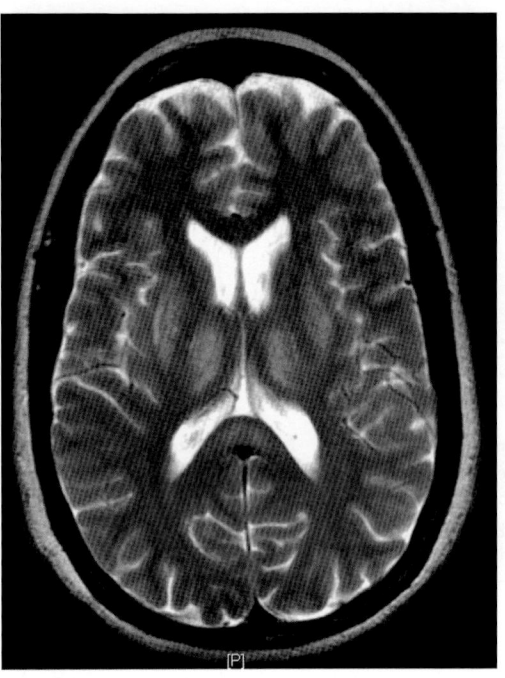 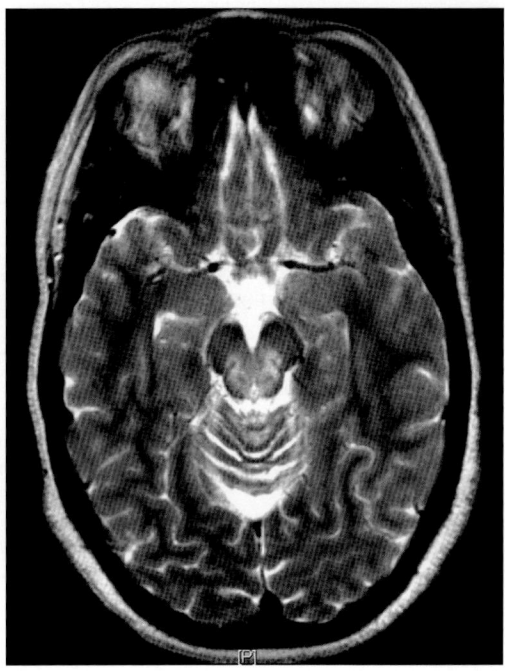

Figure 23.3
MR brain images in a patient suffering Wilson's disease, showing the characteristic signal intensity changes in the caudate, putamen and thalamus (left) as well as the typical so-called face-of-the-giant-panda sign, caused by accentuation of the normal low intensity of the red nuclei and nigral substance by the surrounding abnormal high-intensity signal in the midbrain tegmentum (right).

lected for 24 hours in a bottle with a copper-free liner. Levels above 80μg/24h are indicative of the diagnosis (83). Thus, copper studies are the clue to the diagnosis and should be performed in all young patients (before 45th year of life) presenting with a movement disorder. Furthermore, liver biopsy demonstrates elevated copper levels (> 250 μg/g dry weight) and is diagnostic of Wilson's disease (83,95). Figure 23.2 shows an algorithm for the diagnosis of Wilson's disease.

MRI studies may demonstrate the characteristic 'face of the giant panda' pattern, which is seen in T2-weighted images of the midbrain, and the 'face of the miniature panda' pattern, which can be seen in the tegmentum region of the pons in the same sequence (see Figure 23.3). Sometimes, T2-weighted images show hypointensity in the basal ganglia region as a result of deposition of iron (84). Comparing the clinical subtypes of Wilson's disease, the putamen is the main struc-

ture significantly more frequently involved in patients presenting with dystonic features than those without dystonia, suggesting a relation between abnormalities in this brain region and dystonic movements in Wilson's disease (94). In half of all patients with Wilson's disease, abnormalities in the globus pallidus, caudate, and thalami are also reported.

Treatment

The treatment of Wilson's disease aims at the removal of toxic deposits of copper to produce a negative copper balance, and the prevention of its re-accumulation. Thus, the first-line therapy consists of treatment with copper-chelating agents and restriction of dietary copper (avoiding copper-rich foods such as liver, chocolate and some forms of fish). For medical treatment the following 'anti-copper drugs' with several modes of action are currently approved and available: zinc acetate, D-penicillamine, trientine and ammonium tetrathiomolybdate (84). In patients with progressive or acute liver failure from fulminant hepatitis with or without intravenous hemolysis, orthotropic hepatic transplantation is an efficient treatment (96). The success of therapy is measured in terms of a restoration of normal levels of free serum copper and its excretion in the urine (84). It is important to mention that both psychiatric and neurologic symptoms have an organic basis and may disappear in response to adequate therapy (95).

Conclusion

Dystonia may be due to a variety of causes. Here we reviewed some of the important causes of non-primary dystonia. Large studies on secondary dystonia are lacking, and data about its prevalence remain limited. Clinical clues and characteristic investigational findings may be directive in the diagnostic process and facilitate making the correct diagnosis and thus allow the ideal treatment to be initiated. Syndromic association may give a clue and should be looked for (97).

Video fragment

PLAY

Fragment 23.1
Wilson's disease (Segments 1-6)
Mild signs of parkinsonism can be appreciated in this video fragment of a young woman suffering Wilson's disease: hypokinesia (segment 1), resting tremor (segment 2), intention tremor (segment 3), bradykinesia (segment 4), instability and loss of postural reflexes with retropulsion (segment 5) as well as the typical corneal Kayser-Fleischer rings (segment 6).

References

1 Fahn S. Concept and classification of dystonia. Adv Neurol 1988;50:1-8.

2 Oppenheim H. Über eine eigenartige Krampfkrankheit des kindlichen und jugendlichen Alters (Dysbasia lordotica progressiva, Dystonia musculorum deformans). Neurologie Centralblatt 1911;30:1090-1107.

3 Schwalbe W. Eine eigentümliche tonische Krampfform mit hysterischen symptomen. Inauguraldissertation. Universitätsdruckerei Gustav Schade, Berlin 1908.

4 Herz E. Dystonia I Historical review: Analysis of dystonic symptoms and physiologic mechanisms involved. Arch Neurol Psychiatry 1944;51:305-318.

5 Marsden CD HM, Bundey S. Natural history of idiopathic torsion dystonia. Adv Neurol 1976;14:177-187.

6 Marsden CD HM. Idiopathic Torsion Dystonia (Dystonia Musculorum Deformans) A review of forty-two patients. Brain 1974;97:793-810.

7 Marsden CD, Obeso JA, Zarranz JJ, Lang AE. The anatomical basis of symptomatic hemidystonia. Brain 1985;108:463-483.

8 Meunier S, Lehericy S, Garnero L, Vidailhet M. Dystonia: lessons from brain mapping. Neuroscientist 2003;9:76-81.

9 Eidelberg D, Moeller JR, Antonini A, et al. Functional brain networks in DYT1 dystonia. Ann Neurol 1998;44:303-312.

10 Bhatia KP, Marsden CD. The behavioural and motor consequences of focal lesions of the basal ganglia in man. Brain 1994;117:859-876.

11 Quinn NP, Lang AE, Sheehy MP, Marsden CD. Lisuride in dystonia. Neurology 1985;35:766-769.

12 Messimy R, Diebler C, Metzger J. (Torsion dystonia of the left upper limb probably due to a head injury. Calcification of the head of the right caudate nucleus discovered by tomodensitometric examination). Rev Neurol (Paris) 1977;133:199-206.

13 Jabbari B, Paul J, Scherokman B, Van Dam B. Posttraumatic segmental axial dystonia. Mov Disord 1992;7:78-81.

14 Pettigrew LC, Jankovic J. Hemidystonia: a report of 22 patients and a review of the literature. J Neurol Neurosurg Psychiatry 1985;48:650-657.

15 Grimes JD, Hassan MN, Quarrington AM, D'Alton J. Delayed-onset posthemiplegic dystonia: CT demonstration of basal ganglia pathology. Neurology 1982;32:1033-1035.

16 Bejot Y, Giroud M, Moreau T, Benatru I. Clinical spectrum of movement disorders after stroke in childhood and adulthood. Eur Neurol 2012;68:59-64.

17 Scott BL, Jankovic J. Delayed-onset progressive movement disorders after static brain lesions. Neurology 1996;46:68-74.

18 Alarcon F, Zijlmans JC, Duenas G, Cevallos N. Post-stroke movement disorders: report of 56 patients. J Neurol Neurosurg Psychiatry 2004;75:1568-1574.

19 Ghika-Schmid F, Ghika J, Regli F, Bogousslavsky J. Hyperkinetic movement disorders during and after acute stroke: the Lausanne Stroke Registry. J Neurol Sci 1997;146:109-116.

20 Kim JS. Delayed onset mixed involuntary movements after thalamic stroke: clinical, radiological and pathophysiological findings. Brain 2001;124:299-309.

21 Giroud M, Lemesle M, Madinier G, Billiar T, Dumas R. Unilateral lenticular infarcts: radiological and clinical syndromes, aetiology, and prognosis. J Neurol Neurosurg Psychiatry 1997;63:611-615.

22 Burguera JA, Bataller L, Valero C. Action hand dystonia after cortical parietal infarction. Mov Disord 2001;16:1183-1185.

23 Ceballos-Baumann AO, Passingham RE, Marsden CD, Brooks DJ. Motor reorganization in acquired hemidystonia. Ann Neurol 1995;37:746-757.

24 Krystkowiak P, Martinat P, Defebvre L, Pruvo JP, Leys D, Destee A. Dystonia after striatopallidal and thalamic stroke: clinicoradiological correlations and pathophysiological mechanisms. J Neurol Neurosurg Psychiatry 1998;65:703-708.

25 Vidailhet M, Dupel C, Lehericy S, et al. Dopaminergic dysfunction in midbrain dystonia: anatomoclinical study using 3-dimensional magnetic resonance imaging and fluorodopa F 18 positron emission tomography. Arch Neurol 1999;56:982-989.

26 Zadro I, Brinar VV, Barun B, Ozretic D, Habek M. Cervical dystonia due to cerebellar stroke. Mov Disord 2008;23:919-920.

27 Jinnah HA, Hess EJ. A new twist on the anatomy of dystonia: the basal ganglia and the cerebellum? Neurology 2006;67:1740-1741.

28 de Vries PM, Johnson KA, de Jong BM, et al. Changed patterns of cerebral activation related to clinically normal hand movement in cervical dystonia. Clin Neurol Neurosurg 2008;110:120-128.

29 Obermann M, Vollrath C, de Greiff A, et al. Sensory disinhibition on passive movement in cervical dystonia. Mov Disord 2010;25:2627-2633.

30 Shneyder N, Harris MK, Minagar A. Movement disorders in patients with multiple sclerosis. Handbook of clinical neurology 2011;100:307-314.

31 Jankovic J. Parkinson's disease: clinical features and diagnosis. J Neurol Neurosurg Psychiatry 2008;79:368-376.

32 Samii A, Nutt JG, Ransom BR. Parkinson's disease. Lancet 2004;363:1783-1793.

33 Tolosa E, Compta Y. Dystonia in Parkinson's disease. J Neurol 2006;253:VII7-13.

34 Klawans HL, Paleologos N. Dystonia-Parkinson syndrome: differential effects of levodopa and dopamine agonists. Clin Neuropharmacol 1986;9:298-302.

35 Katchen M, Duvoisin RC. Parkinsonism following dystonia in three patients. Mov Disord 1986;1:151-157.

36 Jankovic J, Tintner R. Dystonia and parkinsonism. Parkinsonism Relat Disord 2001;8:109-121.

37 Hu MT, Bland J, Clough C, Ellis CM, Chaudhuri KR. Limb contractures in levodopa-responsive parkinsonism: a clinical and investigational study of seven new cases. J Neurol 1999;246:671-676.

38 Hariz GM, Lindberg M, Bergenheim AT. Impact of thalamic deep brain stimulation on disability and health-related quality of life in patients with essential tremor. J Neurol Neurosurg Psychiatry 2002;72:47-52.

39 Golbe LI. Young-onset Parkinson's disease: a clinical review. Neurology 1991;41:168-173.

40 Schrag A, Ben-Shlomo Y, Brown R, Marsden CD, Quinn N. Young-onset Parkinson's disease revisit-

ed--clinical features, natural history, and mortality. Mov Disord 1998;13:885-894.

41 Quinn N, Critchley P, Marsden CD. Young onset Parkinson's disease. Mov Disord 1987;2:73-91.

42 Gershanik OS, Leist A. Juvenile onset Parkinson's disease. Adv Neurol 1987;45:213-216.

43 Quinn NP. Parkinsonism and dystonia, pseudo-parkinsonism and pseudodystonia. Adv Neurol 1993;60:540-543.

44 Kitada T, Asakawa S, Hattori N, et al. Mutations in the parkin gene cause autosomal recessive juvenile parkinsonism. Nature 1998;392:605-608.

45 Lucking CB, Durr A, Bonifati V, et al. Association between early-onset Parkinson's disease and mutations in the parkin gene. N Engl J Med 2000;342:1560-1567.

46 Bonifati V, Rizzu P, van Baren MJ, et al. Mutations in the DJ-1 gene associated with autosomal recessive early-onset parkinsonism. Science 2003;299:256-259.

47 Bonifati V, Rohe CF, Breedveld GJ, et al. Early-onset parkinsonism associated with PINK1 mutations: frequency, genotypes, and phenotypes. Neurology 2005;65:87-95.

48 van Duijn CM, Dekker MC, Bonifati V, et al. Park7, a novel locus for autosomal recessive early-onset parkinsonism, on chromosome 1p36. Am J Hum Genet 2001;69:629-634.

49 Melamed E. Early-morning dystonia. A late side effect of long-term levodopa therapy in Parkinson's disease. Arch Neurol 1979;36:308-310.

50 Kidron D, Melamed E. Forms of dystonia in patients with Parkinson's disease. Neurology 1987;37:1009-1011.

51 Juncos JL, Fabbrini G, Mouradian MM, Chase TN. Controlled release levodopa-carbidopa (CR-5) in the management of parkinsonian motor fluctuations. Arch Neurol 1987;44:1010-1012.

52 Poewe WH, Lees AJ, Stern GM. Dystonia in Parkinson's disease: clinical and pharmacological features. Ann Neurol 1988;23:73-78.

53 Poewe WH, Lees AJ. The pharmacology of foot dystonia in parkinsonism. Clin Neuropharmacol 1987;10:47-56.

54 Krack P, Pollak P, Limousin P, Benazzouz A, Deuschl G, Benabid AL. From off-period dystonia to peak-dose chorea. The clinical spectrum of varying subthalamic nucleus activity. Brain 1999;122:1133-1146.

55 Bonanni L, Thomas A, Onofrj M. Diagnosis and management of dementia with Lewy bodies: third report of the DLB Consortium. Neurology 2006;66:1455

56 McKeith IG, Dickson DW, Lowe J, et al. Diagnosis and management of dementia with Lewy bodies: third report of the DLB Consortium. Neurology 2005;65:1863-1872.

57 Tabet N, Sivaloganathan S. Meige's syndrome in dementia with Lewy bodies. J R Soc Med 2002;95:201-202.

58 Mark MH, Sage JI, Dickson DW, et al. Meige syndrome in the spectrum of Lewy body disease. Neurology 1994;44:1432-1436.

59 Kim HJ, Lee MC, Kim JS, Chung SJ, Kwon M, Shin HW. Lingual dystonia as a manifestation of thalamic infarction. Mov Disord 2009;24:1703-1704.

60 O'Sullivan SS, Massey LA, Williams DR, et al. Clinical outcomes of progressive supranuclear palsy and multiple system atrophy. Brain 2008;131:1362-1372.

61 Wenning GK, Colosimo C, Geser F, Poewe W. Multiple system atrophy. Lancet Neurol 2004;3:93-103.

62 Boesch SM, Wenning GK, Ransmayr G, Poewe W. Dystonia in multiple system atrophy. J Neurol Neurosurg Psychiatry 2002;72:300-303.

63 Merlo IM, Occhini A, Pacchetti C, Alfonsi E. Not paralysis, but dystonia causes stridor in multiple system atrophy. Neurology 2002;58:649-652.

64 Slawek J, Derejko M, Lass P, Dubaniewicz M. Camptocormia or Pisa syndrome in multiple system atrophy. Clin Neurol Neurosurg 2006;108:699-704.

65 Hozumi I, Piao YS, Inuzuka T, et al. Marked asymmetry of putaminal pathology in an MSA-P patient with Pisa syndrome. Mov Disord 2004;19:470-472.

66 Poewe W, Lees AJ, Steiger D, Stern GM. Foot dystonia in Parkinson's disease: clinical phenomenology and neuropharmacology. Adv Neurol 1987;45:357-360.

67 Poewe WH, Wenning GK. The natural history of Parkinson's disease. Ann Neurol 1998;44:S1-9.

68 Schober R, Langston JW, Forno LS. Idiopathic orthostatic hypotension. Biochemical and pathologic observations in 2 cases. Eur Neurol 1975;13:177-188.

69 Boudin G, Guillard A, Mikol J, Galle P. (Striato-nigral degeneration. Apropos of a clinical, therapeutic, and anatomic study of 2 cases). Rev Neurol (Paris) 1976;132:137-156.

70 Scaravilli T, Tolosa E, Ferrer I. Progressive supranuclear palsy and corticobasal degeneration: lumping versus splitting. Mov Disord 2005;20S12:21-28.

71 Panegyres PK, Hillman D, Dunne JW. Laryngeal dystonia causing upper airway obstruction in progressive supranuclear palsy. J Clin Neurosci 2007;14:380-381.

72 Lamberti P, De Mari M, Zenzola A, Aniello MS, Defazio G. Frequency of apraxia of eyelid opening in the general population and in patients with extrapyramidal disorders. Neurol Sci 2002;23S2:81-82.

73 Tan EK, Chan LL, Wong MC. Levodopa-induced oromandibular dystonia in progressive supranuclear palsy. Clin Neurol Neurosurg 2003;105:132-134.

74 Oide T, Ohara S, Yazawa M, et al. Progressive supranuclear palsy with asymmetric tau pathology presenting with unilateral limb dystonia. Acta Neuropathol 2002;104:209-214.

75 Barclay CL, Lang AE. Dystonia in progressive supranuclear palsy. J Neurol Neurosurg Psychiatry 1997;62:352-356.

76 Murray R, Neumann M, Forman MS, et al. Cognitive and motor assessment in autopsy-proven corticobasal degeneration. Neurology 2007;68:1274-1283.

77 Wadia PM, Lang AE. The many faces of corticobasal degeneration. Parkinsonism Relat Disord 2007;13 Suppl 3:336-340.

78 Belfor N, Amici S, Boxer AL, et al. Clinical and neuropsychological features of corticobasal degeneration. Mech Ageing Dev 2006;127:203-207.

79 Vanek Z, Jankovic J. Dystonia in corticobasal degeneration. Mov Disord 2001;16:252-257.

80 Stamelou M, Alonso-Canovas A, Bhatia KP. Dystonia in corticobasal degeneration: a review of the literature on 404 pathologically proven cases. Mov Disord 2012;27:696-702.

81 Soliveri P, Piacentini S, Girotti F. Limb apraxia in corticobasal degeneration and progressive supranuclear palsy. Neurology 2005;64:448-453.

82 Fitzgerald DB, Drago V, Jeong Y, Chang YL, White KD, Heilman KM. Asymmetrical alien hands in corticobasal degeneration. Mov Disord 2007;22:581-584.

83 Ala A, Walker AP, Ashkan K, Dooley JS, Schilsky ML. Wilson's disease. Lancet 2007;369:397-408.

84 Das SK, Ray K. Wilson's disease: an update. Nat Clin Pract Neurol 2006;2:482-493.

85 Figus A, Angius A, Loudianos G, et al. Molecular pathology and haplotype analysis of Wilson disease in Mediterranean populations. Am J Hum Genet 1995;57:1318-1324.

86 Frydman M, Bonne-Tamir B, Farrer LA, et al. Assignment of the gene for Wilson disease to chromosome 13: linkage to the esterase D locus. Proc Natl Acad Sci U S A 1985;82:1819-1821.

87 Yamaguchi Y, Heiny ME, Gitlin JD. Isolation and characterization of a human liver cDNA as a candidate gene for Wilson disease. Biochem Biophys Res Commun 1993;197:271-277.

88 Wilson Disease Mutation Database, Department of Medical Genetics, University of Alberta. (http://wwwuofa-medical-geneticsorg/wilson/indexphp) 2006).

89 Ferenci P, Czlonkowska A, Merle U, et al. Late-onset Wilson's disease. Gastroenterology 2007;132:1294-1298.

90 Roberts EA, Schilsky ML. Diagnosis and treatment of Wilson disease: an update. Hepatology 2008;47:2089-2111.

91 Lorincz MT. Neurologic Wilson's disease. Ann N Y Acad Sci 2010;1184:173-187.

92 Ala A, Borjigin J, Rochwarger A, Schilsky M. Wilson disease in septuagenarian siblings: Raising the bar for diagnosis. Hepatology 2005;41:668-670.

93 Starosta-Rubinstein S, Young AB, Kluin K, et al. Clinical assessment of 31 patients with Wilson's disease. Correlations with structural changes on magnetic resonance imaging. Arch Neurol 1987;44:365-370.

94 Svetel M, Kozic D, Stefanova E, Semnic R, Dragasevic N, Kostic VS. Dystonia in Wilson's disease. Mov
Disord 2001;16:719-723.

95 Ferenci P. Pathophysiology and clinical features of
Wilson disease. Metab Brain Dis 2004;19:229-239.

96 Schilsky ML, Scheinberg IH, Sternlieb I. Liver
transplantation for Wilson's disease: indications and
outcome. Hepatology 1994;19:583-587.

97 Schneider SA, Bhatia KP. Secondary dystonia – clinical clues and syndromic associations. Eur J Neurol.
2010;17S1:52-7.

24

Treatment of Dystonia

Dirk Dressler

Dystonias may be classified according to their aetiology as idiopathic and symptomatic (see Chapters 22 and 23). Only a minor proportion are symptomatic. As their aetiology is known, they offer the opportunity for causal or near-causal treatment. The cause of idiopathic dystonias has not been identified yet. In this group of dystonias, by far the largest, the treatment is only symptomatic. As this is only partly effective, the best results might be achieved with multimodal treatment options, taking advantage of allied health strategies. This chapter gives an overview of currently available treatment options with botulinum toxin and common oral drug therapies, as well as more specialized pharmacotherapeutical and surgical interventions and allied health strategies (see Figure 24.1). It will also hint at emerging treatment strategies and future developments. It will not cover practical aspects or details of their specific applications. Its aim is to provide a strategic view and to emphasize and encourage a multimodal therapeutic approach.

Botulinum toxin therapy

History

The therapeutic use of botulinum toxin (BT) was pioneered by Alan B. Scott, who first published this entirely new therapeutic principle in 1973 (1). It was soon adopted in neurology, with blepharospasm and cervical dystonia being the first indications.

Mode of action

BT therapy is based on the fully reversible, easily controllable and strictly local paralysing effect of BT. With this, the dystonic muscle hyperactivity can be directly reduced, and muscular pain will respond subsequently. Additional central nervous system effects on dystonia as well as intrinsic analgesic effects have been discussed. BT's effect starts within a few days after application and will gradually fade away after 8-12 weeks, necessitating reapplication. Long-term follow-up over more than 25 years demonstrates that this procedure can be repeated without loss of efficacy or additive adverse effects.

Adverse effects

Reduction of the dystonic muscle activity also reduces the target muscle's voluntary muscle activity. This inherent adverse effect can be reduced by dose adjustment and the use of agonistic muscles to overtake the target muscle's function. Other possible adverse effects are local paresis (usually mild) and hypotonia, caused by BT spread into adjacent muscles. As of yet, no systemic adverse effects whatsoever have been reported, not even when higher BT doses were applied.

Dosing

The therapeutic BT doses used vary enormously, depending on the target muscle size, the degree of their dystonic involvement, and the number of target muscles identified. Target muscle selection is highly individual. It depends on skilful analyses of the dystonic postures or movements. Palpation as well as active and pas-

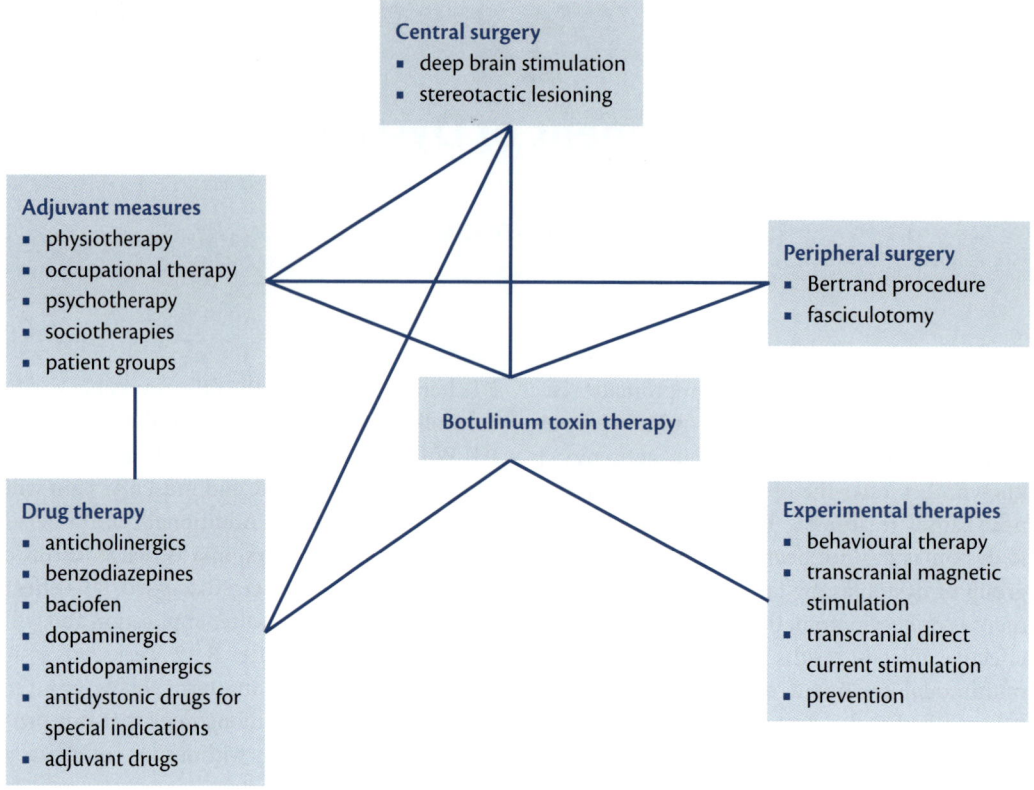

Figure 24.1
Overview of treatment modalities for dystonia. Lines indicate which treatment modalities can be combined.

sive manoeuvres can help to identify the target muscle and exclude antagonistic muscle activities and preventive postures. Occasionally, electromyography can help to improve the target muscle selection. Once the injection scheme has been developed, the actual BT application is performed using palpation and anatomical landmarks. For muscles of the forearm and deep muscles in the lower extremity, ultrasound guidance can be helpful. In those cases, similar results can be produced by recording electromyographic signals from the target muscle through a special injection needle. Additional electrostimulation through this special injection needle can further improve the precision of BT placement.

Marketed botulinum toxin drugs

BT drugs registered in major industrialised countries include onabotulinumtoxinA (Botox®, Allergan, Irvine, CA, USA), abobotulinumtoxinA (Dysport®, Ipsen Ltd, Slough, Berks, UK) and incobotulinumtoxinA (Xeomin®, Merz Pharmaceuticals, Frankfurt/M, Germany). All of these drugs are based upon BT type A. They have similar properties, except for Xeomin® which lacks complexing proteins and contains neurotoxin with an improved purity. RimabotulinumtoxinB (Myobloc®, US World Drugs, Louisville, KY, USA; NeuroBloc®, Eisai, Hatfield, Herts, UK) is the only BT type B drug available. Its market share is marginal because of substantial, systemic, anticholinergic adverse effects and because of high antigenicity.

Indications

Focal / segmental / multifocal dystonia

BT therapy is used to treat cervical dystonia. Overall, about 80% of patients report a good or very good therapeutic effect. It works best on tonic torticollis. Local adverse effects include dysphagia and reduced neck stability. Adjacent muscles in the shoulder are often included in the injection scheme. Another well established indication for BT therapy is blepharospasm. The outcome is similar to cervical dystonia. Mandibular muscles can also be approached by BT therapy.

In spasmodic dysphonia, perioral or transcutaneous BT injections into the opening or closing muscles of the vocal cord can produce extremely satisfying effects for the patient. Reproducibility of the therapy effects, however, can sometimes be problematic.

Writer's cramps are difficult to treat due to the complexity of the muscular system in the forearm and the narrowness of the therapeutic window of the forearm muscles. Paretic adverse effects and insufficient therapeutic effects are notoriously difficult to separate by dose adjustments. About half of the patients are satisfied with the therapeutic effect of BT therapy, the other half quits treatment. Ultrasound and electromyography guidance are crucial to produce satisfactory results. Musicians' dystonias, affecting forearm muscles as well as facial muscles, produce even less favourable results since the functional requirements for performing musicians are extremely high.

Generalized dystonia

Apart from focal dystonias, more widespread dystonias such as hemidystonia and generalized dystonia can also be treated effectively with BT therapy. The concept of high-dose therapy was recently introduced for this purpose (2). This concept is based on a lack of systemic toxicity and immunologic acceptance of high doses of Xeomin® (400 to 1200MU), thus allowing more target muscles to be treated than previously be-lieved. Even in generalised dystonia, BT therapy can be helpful when functional or pain foci can be identified. In widespread, painful and severe dystonias, especially in young patients, deep brain stimulation is the therapy of choice.

Failure of botulinum toxin therapy

Failure of BT therapy is relatively rare when it is performed by experienced staff. Less favourable results are obtained in special subforms of dystonias such as antecollis, tremulous forms and alternating activation patterns in cervical dystonia or additional apraxia of eyelid opening in blepharospasm, especially when it occurs with progressive supranuclear palsy. Pretarsal injections and a lid suspension operation can then be helpful. In writer's cramp, the predominant involvement of finger muscles as opposed to the involvement of wrist muscles generally leads to reduced therapy effects. In spasmodic dysphonia, abductor forms may have less favourable outcomes than adductor forms. Psychiatric co-morbidity and unsolved social benefit issues may also interfere with the therapy outcome.

In general, most cases of reduced therapy outcome are caused by inadequate injection schemes applying insufficient BT doses to too few target muscles or using inappropriate target muscles. In some patients the formation of antibodies against botulinum neurotoxin may partially or completely block the biological action of BT, thus reducing the therapeutic effect. Risk factors include the total BT dose, interinjection intervals, application of booster injections and the immunological quality of the BT drug applied.

Common oral drug therapy

Indications

Drug treatment is disappointing in general, evaluating the efficacy of the various challenges and establishing the best treatment options are time consuming, and the adverse effects are substantial. Oral drugs have been used for many years to treat dystonia. No single drug produces a really striking result. Oral drugs may be used in monotherapy for mild dystonias and in combination with BT therapy or deep brain stimulation when residual symptoms are still present, or at the end of the BT treatment cycle. Usually, they are introduced sequentially in a special order, always starting with anticholinergics and then followed by benzodiazepines, baclofen, and dopaminergic and antidopaminergic drugs such as tetrabenazine and clozapine. The order after anticholinergics has been challenged repeatedly. There are no robust comparative studies between different antidystonic drugs available.

In severely affected children and in exacerbated generalised dystonia (dystonic storm), a cocktail introduced by Marsden that includes anticholinergics, benzodiazepines and tetrabenazine may be tried (3). For some special and rare conditions (see below), rather effective antidystonic drugs and/or surgical procedures are available.

Anticholinergics

Anticholinergics are the drugs with the best antidystonic effect. They may be considered the antidystonic drugs of choice. The best studied compound is trihexyphenidyl (Artane'). It comes in tablets of 2.0-5.0 mg. To reduce the adverse effects, it should be initiated at extremely low doses, and the dose increased very slowly until adequate effects are obtained or the adverse effects become intolerable. Typical anticholinergic adverse effects include dryness of mouth, blurred vision when reading, memory impairment, nervousness, drowsiness, urinary retention and constipation. Effectivity usually starts at doses of around 8-10 mg/day. Adverse effects, which are all fully reversible, may start at the same doses. If anticholinergics are tolerated in doses of up to 14 or 16 mg per day, there is a chance of adequate therapeutic benefit for the patient. Interestingly, children tolerate much higher doses and, therefore, have a better chance for a therapeutic benefit. Other anticholinergic substances include benztropine, biperidene, ethopropazine and diphenhydramine. There is no reason to assume they have very different therapeutic efficacies or adverse effect profiles.

Benzodiazepines

GABA-A agonists including clonazepam and diazepam have direct antidystonic properties. They are dosed individually. Anxiolytic effects and mental relaxation may induce uncontrolled dose expansion which needs to be avoided by controlled prescriptions. Withdrawal of benzodiazepines may reveal physical dependency. Immediate adverse effects include reduced reaction times, leading to driving restrictions, memory impairment, apathy and drowsiness. In patients with strong stress induction of the dystonic symptoms, punctual interventions with rapid-onset and short-acting benzodiazepines may be helpful.

Baclofen

Baclofen (Lioresal'), a GABA-B agonist, has antispastic and less powerful antidystonic effects. It may also have some analgesic effects. Its dose is slowly titrated upwards until satisfactory effects or intolerable adverse effects occur. The upper dose limit is around 120 mg per day. Adverse effects include drowsiness and nausea. Withdrawal may provoke seizures. In some patients, continuous intrathecal baclofen was given through an implanted radio-controlled pump, but this procedure did not produce robust results.

Dopaminergics

Occasionally, levodopa can have mild antidystonic effects. This effect has to be distinguished from the often dramatic effect levodopa can have on true dopa-responsive dystonia. Adverse effects are mild, including self-limiting, mostly short-lived hypotension and nausea.

Antidopaminergics

D2 receptor-blocking agents may have antidystonic effects. Interestingly, at the same time, these drugs may also induce tardive dystonias. Given this reason, they should not be used in idiopathic dystonia except under extraordinary circumstances. They are contraindicated in tardive dystonias. Clozapine is an atypical dopamine receptor blocker that does not produce tardive dystonia. Its antidystonic potency is only moderate. It can produce drowsiness. Dopamine levels within the central nervous system can also be reduced by dopamine-depleting agents blocking the re-uptake of dopamine into the presynaptic nerve terminals. Tetrabenazine and reserpine are the best described dopamine depletors. Their antidystonic effects are mild and somewhat unpredictable. Both frequently produce motor parkinsonism-like symptoms and, to a lesser extent, depression. With reserpine, hypotension is another adverse effect. Tardive dystonia has not yet been reported as an adverse effect of these dopamine depletors.

Specialized antidystonic strategies

Pharmacotherapeutic strategies
In dopa-responsive dystonia (Segawa disease), dystonia and parkinsonism with typical diurnal fluctuations are caused by a lack of dopamine due to various enzyme defects. Levodopa produces dramatic, long-term symptom relief. Most patients respond to levodopa at a dose of 5 mg/kg body weight/day. Lack of efficacy to levodopa doses of more than 600 mg per day makes dopa-responsive dystonia unlikely. Dyskinesias may occur, but are mild, while fluctuations do not as there is a normally intact dopamine storage capacity. The use of dopamine agonists has not been sufficiently studied.

Paroxysmal kinesigenic and to some extent also non-kinesigenic dyskinesia responds well to anticonvulsants such as carbamazepine. For these dyskinesias, benzodiazepam might be tried instead. The precipitating factors of emotional stress, fatigue, alcohol or caffeine should be avoided. Paroxysmal exercise-induced dyskinesia may respond only partially to carbamazepine and benzodiazepines. Physical exercise, a precipitating factor in those dyskinesias, should be avoided.

In myoclonic dystonias, anticonvulsants may occasionally be helpful. If dystonic tremor does not respond sufficiently to the common oral antidystonic drugs, beta-blockers may sometimes work. In more severe dystonias, pain may be the leading symptom. If antidystonic treatment is not sufficient, analgesics may be added at least temporarily. If there is a strong stress induction of the dystonic symptoms, rapid-onset benzodiazepines may help.

Surgical strategies
Surgery has long been used to treat dystonias. The initial strategies focussed on peripheral interventions, later on central interventions were developed.

Peripheral surgery
Since the 19th century, myotomy (muscle dissection) and myectomy (muscle resection) have been performed, and as soon as electric stimulation became available, denervation techniques of dystonic muscles were developed. The results were problematic since the therapeutic effects are difficult to control, and inadequate therapeutic effects or paretic adverse effects could easily occur. For blepharospasm, denervation and myectomy alone or in combination could be performed, though often with long-lasting pain syndromes after denervation. Denervation surgery was also applied in spasmodic dysphonia. These surgical procedures are now largely abandoned, and replaced by chemical denervation using BT. However, in young patients with dystonia in isolated muscles, myectomy or denervation might still be preferred to a prolonged BT therapy, as is also the case in spastic-dystonic conditions of the lower limb which might be treated with selective fasciculotomy. In cervical dystonia, a combination of myectomy, peripheral denervation and anterior ramizectomy, as developed by Claude Bertrand of Montreal in the 1980s (4,5), may also give the same results as BT therapy. Therefore, this regime is still considered in case of antibody-induced failure of BT

therapy, when patients are hesitant to undergo brain surgery. Adverse effects often include substantial muscle atrophy.

Brain surgery

Brain surgery for movement disorders was developed in the 1950s (6). It is based upon stereotaxy, i.e a local intervention in the depth of the brain controlled by a 3-dimensional geometric coordinate system referring to morphological reference points. Because of mixed results, it was reserved for severe cases of dystonia. With the advent of advanced imaging techniques, stereotaxy was revived in the 1980s. Originally, stereotactic procedures were applied for ablative strategies with thermocoagulation, cryocoagulation (to a lesser extent) and chemocoagulation. From the early 1990s, thermocoagulation was replaced more and more by high-frequency stimulation techniques (deep brain stimulation, DBS) blocking central nervous system nuclei in the same way as ablative techniques. In time, the adjustment of the electrodes to the exact target became possible without moving the stimulation electrode after implantation. Currently, improved imaging techniques and additional neurophysiological recordings of the firing patterns of different neuron populations allow even more precise targeting precision.

DBS for dystonia was introduced in 1996 (7). It is usually performed bilaterally, thus improving the therapeutic outcome. The target point with the best antidystonic effect is the globus pallidus internus (GPi-DBS). Thalamic stimulation (VIM-DBS) produces much less robust effects Therapeutic effects on phasic components of dystonia tend to start within several days. Therapeutic effects on tonic components can take weeks to months to develop fully.

GPi-DBS can produce substantial improvement of idiopathic generalised dystonia, and the extent of this improvement is far superior to that obtained by BT therapy. Whether patients with a DYT1 gene defect show better results than patients with other gene defects remains open. In

segmental dystonia and in symptomatic, structural lesion-induced dystonia, the DBS-induced improvement seems less. BT therapy in those conditions may provide a similar level of improvement, especially when high-dose therapy is applied. In focal dystonias, the antidystonic efficacy of DBS and BT therapy are similar.

Suboptimal results and adverse effects can be caused by suboptimal electrode positions, intraoperative or postoperative infections, intraoperative haemorrhage, electrode displacements and electrode disconnections. The disadvantages of DBS include high costs, need for a highly specialised neurosurgical team, time-consuming postoperative programming, and stimulator replacement after battery discharge (usually after 3-5 years).

DBS can and usually will be combined with BT therapy, oral drugs and allied health strategies.

Allied health strategies

In most cases BT therapy will have to be accompanied by physiotherapy to enhance its effect by readjustment of the body image, training of antagonistic muscles and stretching of the target muscles. Occupational therapy may also be helpful to transfer the BT effect into functional improvement. Antidystonic drugs and analgesics may be used at the end of the BT effect before BT injections are repeated. Physiotherapy can help to activate antidystonic muscles, readjust impaired body posture and stretch target muscles of BT therapy, thus preventing contractures. BT therapy should only be performed when it is combined with physiotherapy. The scientific evidence for the efficacy of physiotherapy in dystonia is scarce, however. Occupational therapy can improve impaired functioning. Adequate communication with the patient and family members helps to clarify the nature and prognosis of dystonia and its treatment options. Psychotherapy can improve coping with a chronic disease with all its private and professional consequences. In severe cases, the psychotherapy should include the caregivers. Sociotherapy helps the patient to claim his various social benefits. Introduction to a dystonia patient group is welcome by many, but not all patients.

Experimental strategies

Behavioural therapies including constraint use, re-training and feedback elements may produce mild and temporary effects best studied in writer's cramps and in some musicians' cramps (8-10). Transcranial magnetic brain stimulation also may produce mild and temporary effects (11,12), while transcranial direct current stimulation does not seem to be effective (13,14). Preventive strategies may be helpful in musicians' dystonias.

Treatment Algorithm

Given the enormous variability of dystonia with respect to localisation and severity, there is no straightforward treatment algorithm. Treatment has to be individualised and should consider all possible options. The best results will be obtained when multiple treatment options can be combined. The individual treatment scheme is based upon the dystonia's localisation and severity, the presence of pain, the patient's age, compliance, his personal preferences and logistical considerations. In mild forms of dystonia when there is no functional impairment, no pain and no stigmatisation, treatment might best be postponed. Counselling of the patient and his family about the nature of dystonia and its prognosis should be performed. As soon as treatment is required, the first choice is BT, not only for focal but also for more widespread forms.

When the dystonia is severe, BT is still the first treatment to try. As a rule, in focal dystonia, BT will usually produce satisfactory results. The therapeutic outcome is less effective though in writer's cramp, tremulous dystonias, severe antagonistic forms, antecollis and apraxia of eyelid opening. In those patients, additional oral anti-dystonic drugs may be tried. If pain is a leading symptom, analgesics should be added, in tremulous dystonia, beta blockers and in myoclonic dystonia, anticonvulsants. If there is a strong stress induction of symptoms, lorazepam (Tavor 1.0 Expidet⁰) should be used preventively before stressful situations arise. Additional physiotherapy and occupational therapy should be offered. Psychotherapy for coping and the training of self-relaxation techniques may be helpful. Counselling of the patient and his/her relatives and sociotherapy can add to the patient's well-being. If all this does not produce satisfactory results, DBS should be offered. In most cases, additional measures will need to be continued. In functionally impairing and/or stigmatizing segmental and generalised dystonias, therapy could start with BT followed by additional drug therapy and allied health strategies. Most of these patients will ultimately choose DBS procedures.

Outlook

In symptomatic dystonia, the challenge will be to develop more and improved causal treatments. For optimal preventive, restorative and/or disease-modifying therapies in idiopathic dystonia, the underlying causes must be better understood. Most probably, therefore, symptomatic treatment will remain the mainstay of treatment for many years to come, and the best results will be obtained by multidisciplinary approaches.

References

1 Scott AB, Rosenbaum A, Collins CC. Pharmacologic weakening of extraocular muscles. Invest Ophthalmol 1973;12:924-927.

2 Dressler D, Adib Saberi F. First high dose use of complex free botulinum toxin type A. Mov Disord 2006;21(S15):S640.

3 Marsden CD, Marion MH, Quinn N. The treatment of severe dystonia in children and adults. J Neurol Neurosurg Psychiatry 1984;47:1166-1173.

4   Bertrand C, Molina Negro P, Martinez SN. Technical aspects of selective peripheral denervation for spasmodic torticollis. Appl Neurophysiol 1982;45:326-330.

5   Bertrand CM. Selective peripheral denervation for spasmodic torticollis: surgical technique, results, and observations in 260 cases. Surg Neurol 1993;40:96-103.

6   Cooper IS. An investigation of neurosurgical alleviation of parkinsonism, chorea, athetosis and dystonia. Ann Intern Med 1956;45:381-392.

7   Iacono RP, Kuniyoshi SM, Lonser RR, Maeda G, Inae AM, Ashwal S. Simultaneous bilateral pallidoansotomy for idiopathic dystonia musculorum deformans. Pediatr Neurol 1996;14:145-148.

8   Berque P, Gray H, Harkness C, McFadyen A. A combination of constraint-induced therapy and motor control retraining in the treatment of focal hand dystonia in musicians. Med Probl Perform Art 2010;25:149-161.

9   Zeuner KE, Molloy FM. Abnormal reorganization in focal hand dystonia--sensory and motor training programs to retrain cortical function. NeuroRehabilitation 2008;23:43-53.

10 O'Neill MA, Gwinn KA, Adler CH. Biofeedback for writer's cramp. Am J Occup Ther 1997;51:605-607.

11 Kieslinger K, Höller Y, Bergmann J, Golaszewski S, Staffen W. Successful treatment of musician's dystonia using repetitive transcranial magnetic stimulation. Clin Neurol Neurosurg 2013;115:1871-1872.

12 Borich M, Arora S, Kimberley TJ. Lasting effects of repeated rTMS application in focal hand dystonia. Restor Neurol Neurosci 2009;27:55-65.

13 Benninger DH, Lomarev M, Lopez G, Pal N, Luckenbaugh DA, Hallett M.Transcranial direct current stimulation for the treatment of focal hand dystonia. Mov Disord. 2011;26:1698-1702.

14 Buttkus F, Baur V, Jabusch HC, et al. Single-session tDCS-supported retraining does not improve fine motor control in musician's dystonia. Restor Neurol Neurosci 2011;29:85-90.

25

The Pathophysiology of Tremor

Rick C. Helmich

Tremor is characterized by involuntary, rhythmic and sinusoidal, alternating movements of one or more body parts. The movement does not necessarily involve a limb, as tremor can affect almost any body part, including the head, chin and soft palate. In this chapter the pathophysiology of tremor will be discussed. The clinical characteristics, diagnosis and treatment of tremor are covered in another chapter. After summarizing the functional anatomy of the basal ganglia and cerebellum (relevant for understanding tremor), the pathophysiology of the two most common tremors, essential tremor (ET) and Parkinson's disease (PD) tremor, will be considered. Finally, the pathophysiology of less prevalent tremors will be discussed, including Holmes' tremor, orthostatic tremor, dystonic tremor and palatal tremor.

Central and peripheral mechanisms

The tremors discussed in this chapter are mainly caused by central mechanisms. Evidence for this view comes from work showing that peripheral deafferentation, peripheral anesthesia of tremulous muscles, and mechanical perturbations have little effect on, for example, Parkinson's tremor. An example of a mechanical perturbation is that loading of the tremulous limb alters the peak frequency of the EMG in the case of a peripheral cause (for example, demyelinating neuropathy or metabolic causes), but not in the case of a central cause (for example, PD tremor or ET). Nevertheless, central and peripheral mechanisms may interact, for example periph-

eral reflexes (muscle stretch) and central oscillations. It seems both factors play a role in most tremor types.

The anatomy of tremor

As might be appreciated in Figure 25.1, tremor is associated with dysfunction of the basal ganglia (open boxes), the cerebellar circuit (gray), and several neurotransmitter systems projecting to both these circuits (shown in dark gray). The basal ganglia and cerebellum project to separate thalamic nuclei: the globus pallidus, internal part (GPi) sends gamma-aminobutyric acid (GABA)-ergic, inhibitory projections to the anterior ventrolateral (VLa) and ventral anterior (VA) nuclei of the thalamus, and the cerebellar nuclei send glutamatergic, excitatory projections to the posterior ventrolateral nucleus of the thalamus (VLp). Therefore, activity of the cerebellar output nuclei reinforces or facilitates motor cortical activity, while activity of the GPi inhibits motor cortical activity. The cerebellum is reciprocally connected with the contralateral inferior olive: the cerebellar nuclei send GABA-ergic, inhibitory projections to the inferior olive, which sends excitatory projections to the Purkinje cells in the cerebellar cortex (climbing fibers) and cerebellar nuclei. The basal ganglia and cerebellar circuits are anatomically connected (dashed lines). This makes the subthalamic nucleus (STN) an important connectional hub in the tremor circuit, linking the basal ganglia and the cerebellar circuits. For anatomical details, see (1).

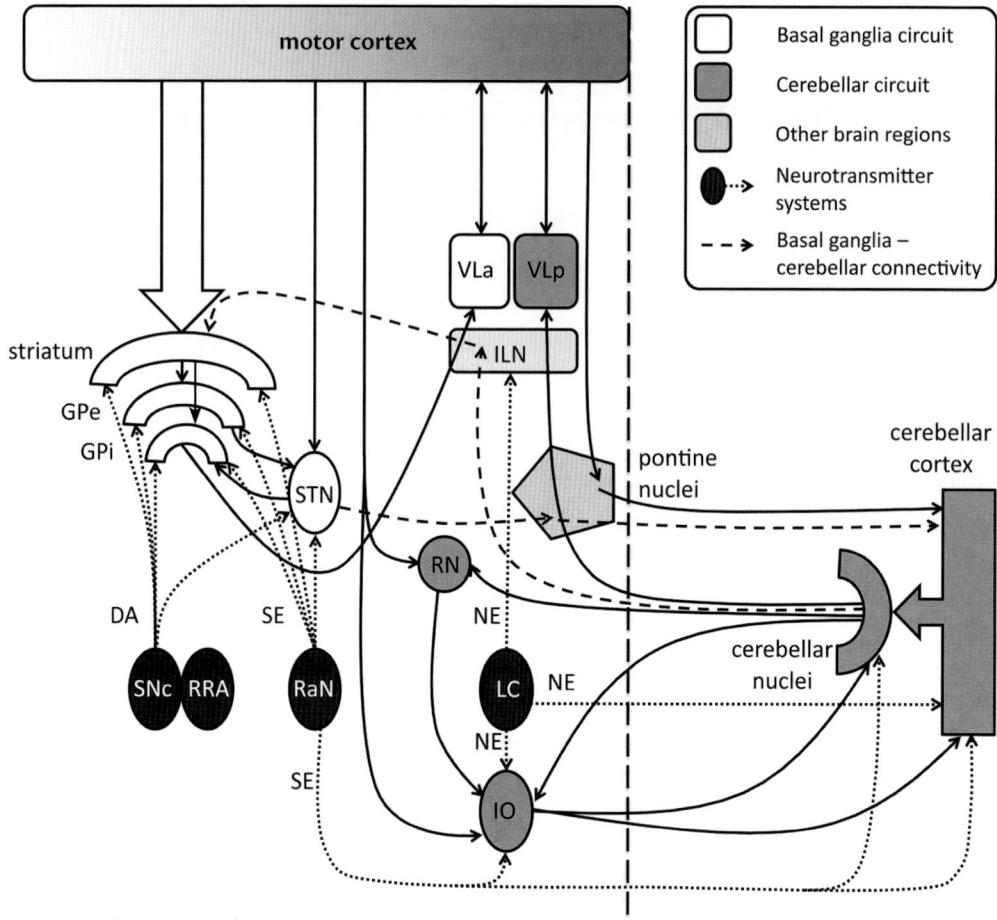

Figure 25.1 The anatomy of tremor.
The basal ganglia are shown as open boxes, the cerebellar system as gray boxes. Modulatory neurotransmitters projections are shown in dark gray. Anatomical connections between basal ganglia and cerebellum are shown in dashed lines. DA, dopamine; GPi, globus pallidus, internal part; GPe, globus pallidus, externa part; ILN, thalamic interlaminar nuclei; IO, inferior olive; LC, locus ceruleus; NE, norepinephrine; RaN, raphe nuclei; RN, red nucleus; RRA, retrorubral area; SNc, substantia nigra, pars compacta; STN, subthalamic nucleus; VLa, ventrolateral thalamus, anterior part; VLp, ventrolateral thalamus, posterior part.

Essential tremor (ET)

Classical ET is characterized by action tremor, which affects the upper limbs in at least 95% of patients. It is defined according to the Movement Disorders Society consensus statement (see chapter 26). ET is characterized by marked clinical heterogeneity, which is reflected in heterogeneous pathophysiological findings. We discuss below the pathophysiology of ET, focusing on findings from animal models and from neuropathological, neurochemical, and neuroimaging studies in human patients. These four approaches give rise to four mutually non-exclusive hypotheses about the pathophysiology of ET: the olivary pacemaker hypothesis, the neurodegeneration hypothesis, the GABA hypothesis, and the oscillating network hypothesis (see Figure 25.2).

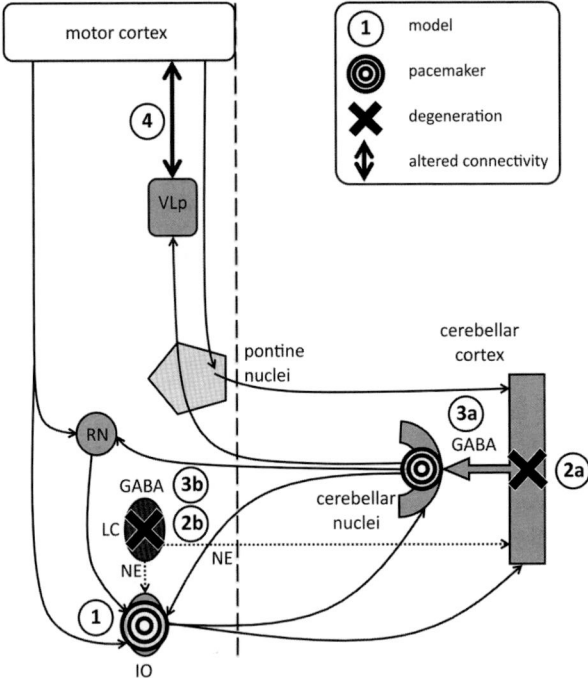

Figure 25.2 The pathophysiology of essential tremor.
This figure shows 4 mutually non-exclusive theories about the pathophysiology of ET. (1) The olivary pacemaker hypothesis, based on animal models of ET (harmaline tremor); (2) The neurode-generation hypothesis, based on post-mortem studies showing neuropathological abnormalities in the cerebellum (2a) and locus ceruleus (2b) of ET patients; (3) the GABA hypothesis, based on post-mortem and imaging studies showing altered GABA concentrations in the vermis (3a) and locus ceruleus (3b) of ET patients; (4) the oscillating network hypothesis, based on neuroimaging studies showing synchronization within a large cerebello-thalamo-cortical circuit, with differences between pathological and physiological tremors mainly in the thalamo-cortical axis. For abbreviations, see Figure 25.1.

Essential tremor is a heterogeneous disorder

There is marked heterogeneity in the published neuroimaging and pathological findings, which is partly explained by the selection of patients studied. Most importantly, there is a risk of misdiagnosis. ET is a clinical diagnosis that relies heavily on the exclusion of alternative causes of action tremor. There is no post-mortem gold standard, such as the presence of Lewy bodies in the substantia nigra pars compacta (SNc) of PD patients. In one study, 37% of 71 patients with a previous

diagnosis of ET (79% by a neurologist) received a different diagnosis from a tertiary referral centre (Columbia University, New York). The most commonly missed diagnoses were PD and dystonia (2). Although the group of ET patients visiting a tertiary referral centre is a selected sample, this study illustrates that it may be difficult to select a group of 'pure ET'. Even within the group of ET patients, there is marked clinical heterogeneity in the site of the tremor, the occurrence of non-tremulous symptoms (such as ataxia or cognitive disturbances), and the response of tremor to different drugs. Therefore, there may be different ET subtypes, leading to the concept of a 'family of essential tremors' (3). Others have divided ET into hereditary ET, sporadic ET, and senile ET (4). The presence of different ET subtypes within a study cohort may lead to heterogeneous findings, especially with small samples.

Animal models of essential tremor

The most common animal model used for investigating ET and physiological tremor is the harmaline model (5). This model is based on the property of harmaline to induce an 8-12 Hz rest and postural tremor in several species, including mice and primates. Harmine, a β-carboline related to harmaline, induces severe tremor in humans that shares some features with ET. β-carboline is found in brewed coffee, cigarettes, and the blood of patients with ET. In animals, harmaline induces synchronized rhythmic activity of neurons in the olivary nucleus, and this activity is transferred to the cerebello-thalamo-cortical circuit (Figure 25.2). The synchronized olivary activity is explained by increased electronic coupling of olivary neurons, which is mediated through GABA-receptor-controlled gap junctions. Harmaline is thought to block these inhibitory receptors, thereby increasing the natural tendency of olivary neurons towards rhythmic oscillations. A recent animal study suggested that low-threshold, voltage-dependent Ca^{2+} channels (T-type) in the inferior olive mediate these rhythmic oscillations: mice lacking the CaV3.1 gene did not show rhythmic olivary activity, and elective knockdown of CaV3.1 gene in the inferior olive suppressed the harmaline-induced tremor (6). Harmaline tremor certainly shares some features with ET, but it is far from clear that similar cerebral mechanisms play a role in ET. For instance, post-mortem studies have failed to find olivary abnormalities in human patients with ET (7) (see below).

The neuropathology of essential tremor

There continues to be a vivid discussion about whether or not ET is a neurodegenerative disease. Prominent advocates of this hypothesis are Louis and colleagues (8). The arguments they put forward are the fact that ET begins insidiously, follows a progressive course, and is associated with age. Furthermore, in some studies ET is associated with an increased risk of PD and Alzheimer's disease (AD), two recognized neurodegenerative diseases. Prominent opponents of this hypothesis are Rajput and colleagues, who argue that many pathological abnormalities fall within the normal range and do not correlate with the duration of ET (9).

There are few pathological studies in ET, and most studies included low numbers of patients. These studies have focused on three brain regions: the cerebellum, inferior olive, and locus ceruleus. The most evidence has been gathered for cerebellar pathology. The largest post-mortem study to date was performed in 33 ET patients and 21 healthy controls (10). In that study, eight ET cases (24%) had Lewy bodies in the locus ceruleus, and the average amount of cerebellar Purkinje cells was 25% lower in ET than in controls. This suggests that there may be two ET subtypes, one associated with brain stem pathology and the other with cerebellar pathology (Figure 25.2). Later studies

by the same group confirmed Purkinje cell loss, and they showed increased Purkinje cell axonal swellings ('torpedoes') in the neo-cerebellum and vermis of ET patients (8). Another study in 24 different ET cases and 21 healthy controls reported cerebellar pathology in seven ET cases (Purkinje cell loss, cerebellar cortical sclerosis, and proliferation of Bergmann glia), but there was no evidence for increased Lewy body pathology in the locus ceruleus (11). Rajput and colleagues reported similar cerebellar Purkinje cell counts in ET patients and controls, and no ET patients with Lewy bodies (9). Finally, only one study specifically focused on the inferior olive, and reported normal neuronal density and morphology in 14 ET cases vs. 15 controls (7). Neuroimaging findings also give an incongruent picture of cerebellar pathology in ET (reviewed in (12)). For example, diffusion tensor imaging (DTI) studies in ET showed normal cerebellar fractional anisotropy (FA; fractional anisotropy in diffusion tensor imaging: a marker of white matter integrity), reduced FA in the inferior cerebellar peduncle, and reduced FA in the dentate nucleus and superior cerebellar peduncle. Voxel-based morphometry (VBM) studies in ET showed widespread cerebellar atrophy, cerebral and cerebellar atrophy, and no gray matter reductions. Finally, magnetic resonance spectroscopy studies showed reduced N-acetyl-l-aspartate (NAA) levels in the cerebellum of ET patients, suggesting cerebellar neurodegeneration (13).

Taken together, there is evidence for neurodegeneration of the cerebellum in ET, although more independent samples are necessary to confirm this. There is some evidence for neurodegeneration of the LC, but there is no evidence for inferior olive pathology.

The neurochemistry of essential tremor

Several lines of evidence support the idea that ET is associated with abnormal functioning of the inhibitory neurotransmitter GABA.

First, drugs that increase GABA-ergic transmission, such as primidone, topiramate, gabapentin and ethanol, are effective in treating ET.

Second, reduced GABA has been found in the cerebrospinal fluid of ET patients (14).

Third, experimental interference with GABA-ergic transmission in animals can evoke an ET-like postural tremor. For example, harmaline has been suggested to evoke tremor by inhibiting GABA-A receptors, resulting in enhanced electrical coupling of cerebellar afferents in the inferior olive (5).

Fourth, nuclear imaging studies found altered binding to GABA receptors in ET. Using positron emission tomography (PET) in eight ET patients and healthy controls, Boecker and colleagues reported increased ^{11}C-flumazenil binding to GABA-A receptors in the ventrolateral thalamus, the dentate nucleus of the cerebellum, and the premotor cortex (15).

Fifth, a post-mortem study by Paris-Robidas and colleagues compared 10 ET patients with 10 PD patients and 16 controls, showing a decrease in GABA-A (35% reduction) and GABA-B (22–31% reduction) receptors in the dentate nucleus of the cerebellum in ET, compared with controls or PD patients (16). These effects seemed to be specific for GABA: the authors did not find evidence for a general neurodegenerative process in the dentate nucleus. The authors also dismiss the possibility that the decrease in GABA-A and GABA-B receptors is a post-synaptic consequence of increased GABA input from Purkinje cells, since there was no significant overall increase in cerebellar GABA. Instead, they suggest that the reduction of dentate GABA receptors may be a primary deficit in ET, restricting the post-synaptic action of GABA released from Purkinje cell axons, and thereby disinhibiting deep cerebellar nuclei neurons. The ensuing overactivity of deep cerebellar nuclei neurons may spread up through the cerebello-thalamo-cortical circuit, possibly resulting in tremor (see Figure 25.2).

This finding of reduced GABA-A receptors in the dentate nucleus of ET appears to contradict the increased binding of flumazenil to GABA-A receptors in ET reported by Boecker and colleagues. One possibility is that ET tremor patients have both a reduction in dentate GABA receptors and a functional receptor abnormality that changes the affinity of these receptors to flumazenil. In a similar vein, a post-mortem study by Shill and colleagues reported that parvalbumin, a marker of GABA-ergic neurons, was significantly reduced in the locus ceruleus and pons of ET cases. In contrast, cerebellar parvalbumin and markers of dopaminergic and noradrenergic innervation were normal in ET (17). A subgroup analysis showed that this finding was most pronounced in patients with late-onset ET, and not present in patients with early-onset and long-standing ET. This fits with the hypothesis that late-onset ET, or so-called senile tremor, has neuropathological underpinnings that might differ from classic ET, which typically begins at a much earlier age. The GABA-ergic abnormalities in ET do not have a known genetic basis: several studies have failed to find a relationship between GABA receptor and transporter polymorphisms and ET. Taken together, there is firm evidence for a reduction of GABA-ergic tone in ET, which, interestingly, is localized in the same areas (cerebellum and locus ceruleus) where neurodegenerative changes have been found.

The electrophysiological basis of essential tremor

Several studies have used electrophysiological recordings such as electroencephalography (EEG), magnetoencephalography (MEG), and deep brain electrodes to test for cerebral activity that is coherent with peripheral tremor. Using MEG, Schnitzler and colleagues have shown that ET (as measured with electromyography; EMG) is coherent with oscillatory activity in the contralateral primary motor cortex, premotor cortex, thalamus, brainstem, and the ipsilateral

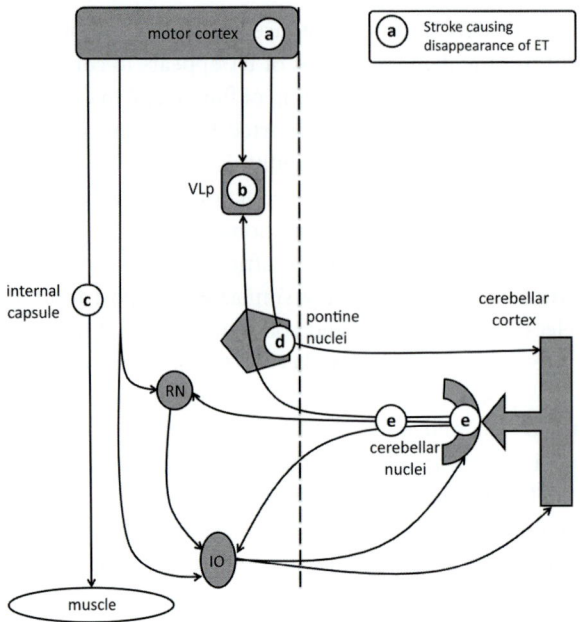

Figure 25.3 The disappearance of essential tremor after stroke. This figure is based on (22), which summarizes the case reports reporting disappearance of ET after stroke in the motor cortex or its subcortical connections (a), the ventrolateral thalamus (b), the posterior limb of the internal capsule (c), the pons (d), or the cerebellum (e). For abbreviations, see Figure 25.1.

pathological tremors (ET, PD tremor). This study showed that all tremors arise from the same cerebello-thalamo-cortical circuit, but that only the pathological tremors show bidirectional thalamo-cortical interactions (see Figure 25.2) (21). Taken together, these studies show that ET arises from a cerebello-thalamo-cortical network; the exact spatial topography of that network may dynamically change, and network properties such as thalamo-cortical connectivity may explain differences in voluntary tremor.

Several case reports have shown that stroke in ET patients can abolish tremor, indicating a causal relationship between the affected brain regions and tremor. A recent study summarized these different case reports, showing that lesions at several locations within the cerebello-thalamo-cortical circuit can abolish ET (22) (see Figure 25.3). Conversely, there are no studies reporting that lesions in the inferior olive abolish tremor. This is possibly because the inferior olive lies between the anteromedial and lateral medullar arterial territories, and there have been few strokes that selectively affect that region. These findings emphasize that the whole cerebello-thalamo-cortical circuit is required for the production of tremor, arguing against a single oscillator.

cerebellum (18). The limited spatial resolution of MEG does not allow a further localization of the brainstem activity to, for example, the inferior olive. Using EEG, Raethjen and colleagues have shown that ET is coherent with cerebral activity in the contralateral primary motor cortex. Interestingly, they found that cortico-muscular coherence in ET was lost intermittently without observable changes in peripheral tremor activity (19). This finding suggests a shifting mode of cooperation between all the constituents of the tremor network, such that the exact network composition is continuously changing. This idea is further supported by studies using thalamic deep brain stimulation (DBS) electrodes in patients with ET, showing that multiple, spatially separated tremor clusters within the posterior ventrolateral nucleus of the thalamus (VLp) are capable of driving the tremor (20). Finally, an MEG study compared voluntary tremor with

The genetics of essential tremor
For a recent review, see (23). Linkage studies have identified three loci in a low number of families with apparently autosomal dominant ET: (ETM)-1 (chromosome 3q13), ETM2 (chromosome 2p) and ETM3 (chromosome 6p23). However, these links could not be replicated in other ET families, the responsible genes have not been identified, and they only explain a small percentage of ET heritability. Two genome-wide

association studies (GWAS) found an association between two single-nucleotide polymorphism (SNPs) in the Leucine-rich repeat and Ig domain containing Nogo receptor interacting protein-1 gene (LINGO1), and an intronic variant in the solute carrier family 1- glial affinity glutamate transporter, member 2 (SLC1A2) gene with ET. These results have been replicated by some but not other studies (23). Clinical differences between ET patients and diagnostic uncertainty may partly explain these differences. LINGO1 is a transmembrane protein expressed in neural cells and oligodendrocytes, which inhibits the differentiation of oligodendrocyte precursors into mature oligodendrocytes and interferes with myelination and remyelination neuronal processes. The LINGO1 gene shares structural properties with Leucine-Rich Repeat Kinase 2 gene (LRRK2) linked to familial PD. The SLC1A2 gene encodes the predominant glutamate reuptake transporter (excitatory amino acid transporter 2), which removes glutamate from the synaptic cleft. Interestingly, SLC1A2 is strongly expressed in the inferior olive but not in other structures of the brainstem. In summary, there are data suggesting an association between LINGO1 and SLC1A2 variants and ET, but further studies are necessary to replicate these findings before establishing a role of these genes in the pathophysiology of ET.

Parkinson's resting tremor

Three out of four PD patients develop tremor during the course of their disease. The typical PD tremor occurs at rest, i.e. in a body part that is not voluntarily activated and is completely supported against gravity. The frequency of resting tremor in PD is relatively slow, typically within a bandwidth of 4-6 Hz.

The neuropathology of Parkinson's resting tremor

Tremor-dominant PD patients have milder cell loss in the substantia nigra pars compacta (par-ticularly in the lateral portion) and in the locus ceruleus than non-tremor PD patients (24). This suggests that tremor-dominant PD patients have less dopaminergic (and possibly also less noradrenergic) dysfunction than non-tremor patients. This could explain some of the clinical advantages that are associated with tremor. On the other hand, tremor-dominant PD patients have considerably more cell loss in the retrorubral area of the midbrain, as assessed in a post-mortem study comparing six tremulous PD patients to five non-tremor PD patients (25). The small sample size in this study warrants caution, although confirmatory evidence came from animal work. In non-human primates, the RRA contains about 10% of the mesencephalic dopaminergic neurons, as compared to 76% in the substantia nigra pars compacta and 14% in the ventral tegmental area. Injection of 1-methyl-4-phenyl-1,2,3,6-tetrahydropyridine (MPTP) destroys these dopaminergic neurons, but with marked differences between species. Clinically, rhesus (Macaca mulatta) monkeys develop infrequent and brief episodes of high-frequency tremor, whereas vervet (African green) monkeys frequently have prolonged episodes of low-frequency resting tremor (26). Both species develop akinesia, rigidity, and severe postural instability. Thus, vervet monkeys resemble the tremulous PD subtype, while rhesus monkeys resemble the non-tremor PD subtype. There are no studies directly comparing the spatial topography of MPTP-induced neural damage between these species, but in vervet monkeys the retrorubral area (A8) is preferentially damaged (27), while in rhesus monkeys the substantia nigra pars compacta (A9) is more affected (28). Although circumstantial, these observations lend further support to the idea that tremor is related to – and possibly caused by – dopaminergic cell loss in the retrorubral area. The retrorubral area could produce tremor via its dopaminergic projections to, among other regions, the subthalamic region and the pallidum (29). Accordingly, a study in parkinsonian vervet monkeys found that tremor severity correlated exclusively with dopaminergic fibers in the external globus pallidus (GPe) (30). Similarly, a post-mortem study in PD patients showed that clinical tremor severity was correlated exclusively with concentrations of the dopamine metabolite homovanillic acid in the pallidum (31). Taken together, these data suggest that tremor might result from pallidal dysfunction, triggered by a specific loss of dopaminergic projections from the retrorubral area. Note that not all findings consistently point in this direction: a recent post-mortem study showed *higher* dopamine levels in the ventral internal globus pallidus (GPi) of tremor-dominant than of non-tremor PD patients (32). However, only few data points were measured (a single hemisphere of two tremor-dominant patients), which limits the interpretation of these results.

The neurochemical basis of Parkinson's resting tremor

The core pathological process in PD involves dopaminergic cell loss in the substantia nigra pars compacta, particularly the lateral ventral tier. This leads to dopamine depletion in the striatum, particularly in the dorsolateral putamen. These changes are strongly linked to bradykinesia, but not to tremor (33,34). Several ^{123}I-FP-CIT SPECT studies described differences in striatal dopamine binding between tremor-dominant and non-tremor PD patients. Most of these studies showed that tremor-dominant PD patients had less striatal dopamine depletion than non-tremor PD patients (33,35). These findings fit with the milder nigral pathology of tremor-dominant patients noted earlier (24). Two SPECT studies compared pallidal dopamine levels between tremor-dominant and non-tremor PD patients. One study found reduced pallidal dopamine in the most-affected hemisphere of tremor-dominant patients, and a correlation between pallidal dopamine depletion and tremor severity (35) (see Figure 25.4C). However, the other study did not confirm pallidal dopamine depletion in tremor-dominant versus non-tremor PD (36). As out-

lined above, the reduced pallidal dopamine levels may be explained by more extensive neuronal cell loss in the retrorubral area in tremor-dominant PD (25), which projects to the pallidum (29). Finally, there is evidence for the involvement of other neurotransmitters in PD resting tremor. Two imaging studies indicate a role for serotonin: one study found an association between reduced midbrain raphe 5-HT1A binding and increased tremor severity (37), and another study found that tremor-dominant PD patients had lower levels of thalamic serotonin transporters than non-tremor patients (38). This opens the possibility that abnormalities in the serotonergic system are involved in generating resting tremor in PD, although this hypothesis remains to be tested in e.g. post-mortem studies.

Several studies have identified cells firing at tremor frequency in both the basal ganglia (subthalamic nucleus, STN, and pallidum) (39,40) and the VLp (41) (see Figure 25.4). Within the basal ganglia-cortical circuit, tremor activity is organized in parallel and partly segregated subloops: intraoperative recording of local field potentials in the STN of tremor-dominant PD patients revealed clusters of tremor-associated coupling between STN and tremor EMG that were spatially distinct for different muscles (42). Similar findings were shown for the cerebello-thalamo-cortical circuit, i.e. the VLp (20). Importantly, the synchronicity of basal ganglia and thalamic activity with tremor varies between regions. Pallidal neurons are only transiently and inconsistently coherent with tremor (43) (see Figure 25.4B), while VLp neurons are highly synchronous with tremor (41) (see Figure 25.4A). These findings suggest that the basal ganglia (or at least, the GPi) cannot be the driving force behind resting tremor. Magnetoencephalography work supports this view, showing that a cerebello-thalamo-cortical circuit fires in synchrony with ongoing resting tremor in PD rather than the basal ganglia (21,44).

A *Peri-operative VLp recordings in a tremor-dominant PD patient*

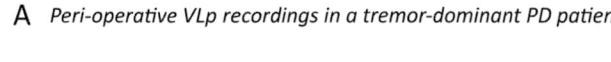

digitized spike train

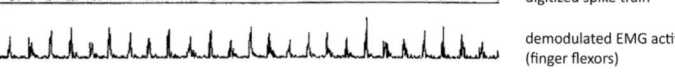

demodulated EMG activity
(finger flexors)

B *Peri-operative GPi recordings in a tremor-dominant PD patient*

GPi-EMG synchronization   No GPi-EMG synchronization

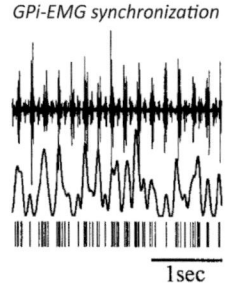

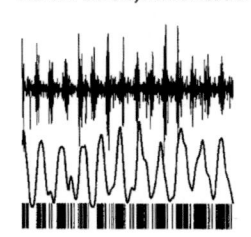

triceps EMG

spike density
function

spike train

1 sec

Figure 25.4 Electrophysiological correlates of Parkinson's resting tremor.
(A) Simultaneous recording of thalamic VLp single-unit activity and peripheral EMG during tremor in a parkinsonian patient. These data show continuous synchronization between GPi activity and peripheral EMG. Reprinted from (63), with permission from the Society for Neuroscience.
(B) Simultaneous recording of GPi multi-unit activity and peripheral EMG during tremor in a PD patient. The two plots illustrate the raw signals of two epochs of data sampled 5 min apart. Note that in the left trace the peaks in the spike density function coincide with the EMG bursts, whereas in the right trace the oscillations in the spike density function occur at a lower frequency than the EMG. These data show that synchronization between neuronal activity in GPi and peripheral EMG is transient in nature. Reprinted from (43). Copyright (2013) National Academy of Sciences, USA.

Metabolic imaging in Parkinson's resting tremor

PET studies investigated how cerebral activity changed after VLp-DBS, which reduces tremor amplitude. This revealed that VLp stimulation was associated with reduced activity in the cerebellum, motor cortex, and medial frontal cortex (45). Other PET studies compared baseline cerebral perfusion between tremor-dominant and non-tremor PD patients. They found that tremor-dominant patients had relatively increased perfusion of the thalamus, pons, and premotor cortex, compared to non-tremor patients (46). Compared to healthy controls, both PD groups had increased pallido–thalamic and pontine activity, and reduced activity in premotor cortex,

supplementary motor area and parietal cortex (46). Another PET study combined these approaches, describing a tremor-related network consisting of the sensorimotor cortex, cerebellum (lobules IV/V and dentate), cingulate cortex and, to a lesser extent, putamen (47). Activity in this network was correlated with clinical tremor scores, it was higher in tremor-dominant than non-tremor PD patients, it increased with disease progression, and it was suppressed by both VLp and STN DBS. Importantly, the metabolic effects of VLp and STN DBS overlapped in a single region: the motor cortex. This suggests that the basal ganglia and cerebellar tremor circuits converge in the motor cortex (see also Figure 25.1).

One study used functional magnetic resonance imaging (fMRI), combined with EMG recordings during scanning, to test for cerebral activity associated with fluctuations in tremor amplitude (35). PD tremor has spontaneous and abrupt changes in amplitude, which allows testing for cerebral activity that is specifically increased at the onset of tremor episodes. This study showed that tremor-dominant PD patients have transiently increased activity in the basal ganglia (pallidum and putamen) at the onset of tremor episodes, while activity in the cerebello-thalamo-cortical circuit is correlated with ongoing fluctuations in tremor amplitude. Furthermore, fMRI allows testing for inter-regional connectivity, and the same study showed that tremor-dominant PD patients have

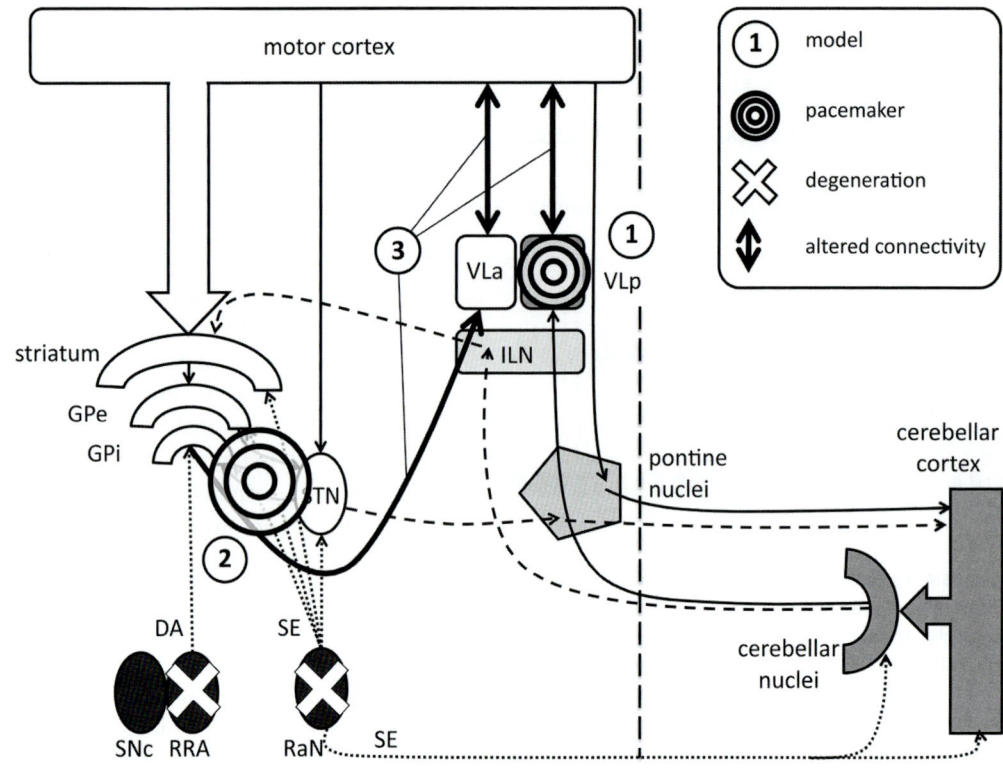

Figure 25.5 The pathophysiology of Parkinson's resting tremor.
This figure summarizes three different accounts on the pathophysiology of PD resting tremor.
(1) The thalamic pacemaker hypothesis; (2) The basal ganglia pacemaker hypothesis; (3) The dimmer-switch hypothesis, which emphasizes the increased coupling between basal ganglia and cerebello-thalamo-cortical circuits in tremor-dominant PD. According to this hypothesis, the basal ganglia trigger the onset of tremor, while the cerebello-thalamo-cortical circuit actually produce the tremor. Neurodegeneration of either the dopaminergic retrorubral area (RRA) and/or the serotonergic raphe nuclei in tremor-dominant PD may lead to neurochemical differences in the basal ganglia of tremor-dominant patients. For abbreviations, see Figure 25.1.

increased connectivity between the basal ganglia and the cerebello-thalamo-cortical circuit than non-tremor PD patients or healthy controls (35). These data suggest that Parkinson's tremor is associated with abnormal activity in both the basal ganglia and the cerebello-thalamo-cortical circuit, and by abnormal coupling between both circuits.

The effect of deep brain stimulation on Parkinson's tremor

The findings reviewed above provide evidence for the involvement of both the cerebello-thalamo-cortical circuit *and* the basal ganglia in PD

resting tremor. The arrest of tremor by focused interventions in either of these circuits further confirms that both are causally related to tremor, see review (48). That is, DBS targeted towards either the basal ganglia (pallidum or STN) or the cerebellar loop (VLp) reduces tremor severity in PD. The efficacy of VLp and STN DBS on PD tremor appears to be comparable: unified Parkinson's disease rating scale (UPDRS) tremor scores (items 20 and 21, off-medication) decreased by 75-84% with STN-DBS, and by 77-88% with VLp-DBS. Earlier studies found that 58–88% of PD patients had a total suppression of tremor 3-6 months after VLp-DBS.

Traditionally, PD tremor has been explained by localizing a central pacemaker either in the thalamus or in the basal ganglia. More recent studies have emphasized the importance of network parameters, such as interregional connectivity. Below three hypotheses explaining PD tremor will be discussed: the thalamic pacemaker hypothesis, the basal ganglia pacemaker hypothesis, and the dimmer-switch hypothesis (see Figure 25.5).

The thalamic pacemaker hypothesis

The key assumption of this model is that thalamic neurons (single), not the basal ganglia circuitry, form the tremor pacemaker. This hypothesis is based on in vitro preparations of guinea pig thalamic neurons, where it was found that the intrinsic biophysical properties of thalamic neurons allow them to serve as relay systems and as single cell oscillators at two distinct frequencies, 9-10 and 5-6 Hz. Specifically, slightly depolarized thalamic cells tend to oscillate at 10 Hz, while hyperpolarized cells oscillate at 6 Hz. These two frequencies coincide with the frequency of physiological tremor and PD tremor, respectively. However, *in vivo* measurements in the thalamus of PD patients have questioned the presence of these thalamic pacemaker cells. While the 6 Hz oscillatory mode in the animal model is associated with low-threshold calcium spike bursts (LTS), this pattern was not observed (with rare exceptions) in the thalamus of PD patients with tremor. Another question is which mechanisms drive thalamic cells into an oscillatory mode in PD. In theory, any mechanism that engenders membrane hyperpolarization, whether through reduction of excitatory drive (dysfacilitation) or excess inhibition, will trigger low-frequency rhythmicity of thalamic neurons. Several different mechanisms have been suggested. First, according to the classical model of PD, the GPi sends increased (inhibitory) output to the thalamus, which may hyperpolarize the thalamic neurons and thus trigger oscillations at 5-6 Hz. However, this mechanism would predict a predominant role for the pallidal thalamus, VLa, in tremor genesis. This does not fit with findings from deep brain surgery, which show that interference with the cerebellar thalamus, VLp, is superior for treating tremor, or with the finding that there are more tremor cells in the VLp than VLa. Other possible brain regions that may hyperpolarize thalamic neurons are the zona incerta (ZI), which is connected to the basal ganglia and sends GABA-ergic projections to the VLp, or the cerebellar nuclei, which receive input from the STN through the pons and cerebellar cortex (although the cerebellar nuclei send excitatory projections to the thalamus, raising the question of how this may hyperpolarize thalamic neurons). An appealing feature of the thalamic pacemaker hypothesis is that it explains the causal role of the cerebellar thalamus (VLp) in PD tremor. A disadvantage is that it remains to be tested how the cerebello-thalamic circuit becomes entrained in tremor, and it does not explain why DBS of the basal ganglia can also suppress tremor.

The basal ganglia pacemaker hypothesis

Several authors have argued that the tremor pacemaker resides in the basal ganglia. The key feature of these models is that the basal ganglia circuitry, not the thalamus, forms the tremor pacemaker. There are several variants. First, Bergman and colleagues have put forward the loss of segregation hypothesis (49). This hypothesis is based on the finding that – in normal primates – the activity of neighbouring pallidal neurons is completely uncorrelated, while parkinsonian primates develop markedly increased correlations between remotely situated pallidal neurons. This could lead to excessive synchronization in the basal ganglia, resulting in tremor. Second, the STN-GPe pacemaker hypothesis was based on in vitro data. This hypothesis proposes that the STN and GPe constitute a central pacemaker that is modulated by striatal inhibition of GPe neurons (50). However, these oscillations occurred at frequencies between 0.4 and 1.8 Hz, and it is unclear whether they have any relationship with parkinsonian tremor, given the lack of in vivo measurements. Third, a recent computational model built on the idea that the basal-ganglia-thalamo-cortical circuit, and in particular the STN and GPe, is prone to tremor-like burst firing. They found that the firing was dependent on feedback to the STN and GPe, which they modelled as a single unit. Dopamine depletion makes the elements of the basal ganglia circuitry more functionally connected, thereby increasing feedback and thus enhancing tremor bursting (51). The advantage of these models is that they are firmly linked to the primary pathological substrate in PD, which is dopaminergic dysfunction of the basal ganglia. Their disadvantage is that they do not explain the causal involvement of the cerebello-thalamo-cortical circuit in PD resting tremor, as evidenced by the strong tremor reduction after DBS of the VLp.

The dimmer-switch hypothesis

This hypothesis is based on a SPECT and EMG-fMRI study in tremor-dominant and non-tremor PD patients (35). It was found that:

a dopamine depletion in the pallidum, but not the striatum, correlated with tremor severity;

b cerebral activity time-locked to the onset of high-amplitude tremor episodes was localized to both the basal ganglia and the cerebello-thalamo-cortical circuit, while

c tremor amplitude-related activity was localized only to the cerebello-thalamo-cortical circuit, but not the basal ganglia;

d tremor-dominant PD patients had increased functional connectivity between the basal ganglia and the cerebello-thalamo-cortical circuit, as compared to non-tremor PD and healthy controls.

These data suggest that the basal ganglia trigger tremor episodes (analogous to a light switch), while the cerebello-thalamo-cortical circuit modulates tremor amplitude (analogous to a light dimmer). The depletion of pallidal dopamine in tremor-dominant PD fits with the specific degeneration of dopaminergic cells in the retrorubral area of the midbrain of tremor-dominant patients (25), which projects to the pallidum (29). This model explains why DBS in either the basal ganglia (STN or GPi) or the cerebello-thalamo-cortical circuit (VLp) can treat tremor. Within the cerebello-thalamo-cortical circuit, the thalamo-cortical axis may be crucially altered, as evidenced by data showing that changes in bidirectional connectivity explain differences between PD tremor and voluntary tremor (21). In contrast to the other models, which emphasize single oscillators, the dimmer-switch model emphasizes network parameters such as between-circuit coupling, while attributing specific contributions to different network nodes.

Parkinson's action tremor

Besides resting tremor, many PD patients also have action tremor, which is produced by voluntary contraction of muscle and includes postural, isometric, and kinetic tremor. Action tremor is probably an inherent symptom of PD. In 34-60% of PD patients, action tremor can be classified as re-emergent resting tremor. Re-emergent tremor occurs after a delay of 2 or more seconds after the limb affected by tremor has assumed a new posture, at the same frequency as the resting tremor, and it responds to levodopa. As such, re-emergent tremor most likely represents simple resting tremor, but now occurring in a new body position. Despite the commonly used term 're-emergent tremor', actually the most interesting phenomenon is the transient suppression of resting tremor during voluntary actions. It ranges from incomplete to complete suppression, and occurs only in PD patients but not in ET patients with resting tremor (52). In PD, resting tremor suppression by voluntary actions may be caused by interference between tremor- and action-related activity in the basal ganglia or the cerebello-thalamo-cortical circuit. Although this has never been tested, it is plausible that re-emergent tremor is caused by the same mechanisms as resting tremor. Action tremor that is not re-emergent tremor occurs at a higher frequency (6-15 Hz) and does not respond to levodopa. It may have different origins, such as enhanced physiological tremor, dystonic tremor, orthostatic tremor, or ET co-occurring in PD (53). Little is known about the pathophysiology of this type of action tremor.

Midbrain tremor

Midbrain tremor is a symptomatic tremor (sometimes accompanied by ipsilateral bradykinesia) with the following characteristics:
1 it is a rest and intention tremor, and sometimes also a postural tremor (the tremor is often not as rhythmic as other tremors);
2 the frequency of the tremor is mostly below 4.5 Hz; and
3 there is typically a variable delay (usually 4 weeks to 2 years) between the symptomatic lesion and the first occurrence of the tremor.

Midbrain tremor is also known as Holmes tremor, rubral tremor, or cerebellar overflow tremor. These names are confusing, because they suggest an exclusive relationship between a lesion in one of these structures and the occurrence of tremor. Instead, different brain lesions may cause midbrain tremor. It is thought that lesions in both the nigro-striatal system *and* the cerebello-thalamic circuit are required to produce midbrain tremor. This mostly occurs after a lesion (due to stroke, trauma, vascular malformations, or tumors) in the midbrain, but it may also occur in patients with PD who develop cerebellar pathology or vice versa (54). The different tremors that make up Holmes tremor may have a final common pathway in the VLp, since DBS in this area can abolish both resting and postural tremor in patients with Holmes tremor (55).

Orthostatic tremor

Orthostatic tremor is characterized by a feeling of unsteadiness that is accompanied by a high frequency (13-18 Hz) tremor of the legs when standing, and which is relieved by sitting or walking. In 75% of the cases orthostatic tremor is idiopathic, termed 'primary orthostatic tremor', whereas approximately 25% of cases have additional neurological features and have been referred to as having 'orthostatic tremor plus', including PD, cerebellar degeneration, dyskinesia, restless legs syndrome, peripheral neuropathy, pontine lesions, aqueduct stenosis and head trauma (56).

Dystonic tremor

Tremor occurs in ±17% of patients with dystonia, in a limb that may or may not be affected by dystonia (57). The tremor typically occurs during postural holding or actions, and may have an irregular appearance. Dystonic tremor can mimic PD resting tremor, especially when it precedes overt dystonia or when the dystonia is subtle, thereby leading to a misdiagnosis of PD. To confuse matters further, arm swing is often reduced in patients with dystonia, even in torticollis patients with no other arm involvement (58). People with dystonic tremor do not have true akinesia, however, and they also show normal dopamine transporter imaging (scans without evidence of dopaminergic deficit; SWEDDs), in contrast to patients with PD (59). Many dystonic tremors are also misclassified as essential tremor (2). The pathophysiology of dystonic tremor is largely unknown. However, the finding that DBS of either the GPi or the VLp are both effective in treating dystonic tremor suggests that both the basal ganglia *and* the cerebello-thalamo-cortical circuits are causally involved (60). This suggests that dystonic tremor and PD tremor may share some pathophysiological features.

Palatal tremor (PT)

Palatal tremor (PT), or palatal myoclonus, is characterized by rhythmic movements of the soft palate at 0.5 to 3 Hz (55). PT can be classified as essential when it is the only feature (with or without ear clicks) and all imaging and laboratory investigations are normal.

Essential palatal tremor

This tremor is mostly caused by contractions of the tensor veli palatini muscle, which inserts into the wall of the eustachian tube; hence there is an ear click. In a recent series of 10 patients with isolated PT, the diagnosis of psychogenic PT was made in 70% of the patients, while two patients had palatal tics and one patient had 'true' essential PT. The authors therefore suggested that psychogenic PT is a separate category besides essential and symptomatic PT (61).

Symptomatic palatal tremor

The symptomatic variant of PT is typically caused by a structural lesion in the Guillain-Mollaret triangle, which is the anatomical circuit connecting the red nucleus, inferior olivary nucleus, and contralateral dentate nucleus (Figure 25.6). The structural lesion may be caused by stroke, vascular malformations, neoplasms, or leukodystrophy in Alexander disease. In contrast to essential PT, the structural variant is associated with contractions of the levator veli palatini muscle, and hence there is no ear click. There is typically a delay of weeks to years between the lesion and the occurrence of PT. Symptomatic PT is explained as a loss of inhibitory projections between the cerebellar nuclei and the contralateral inferior olive. These two structures are connected though the superior cerebellar peduncle, red nucleus and central tegmental tract between the red nucleus

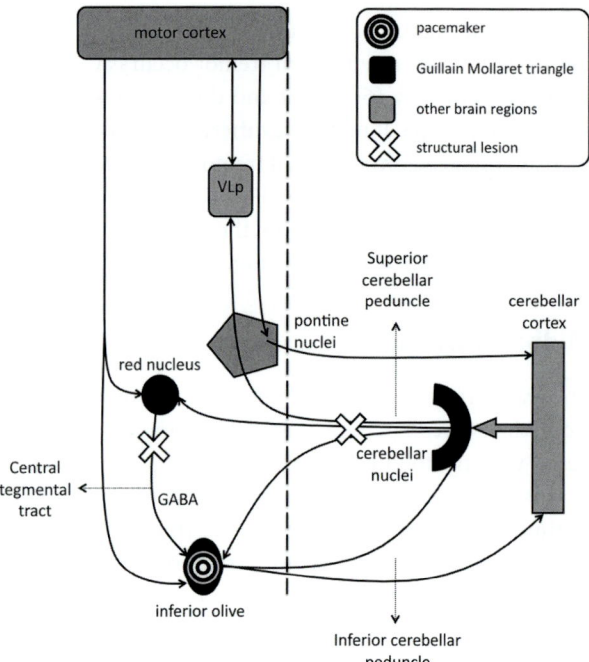

Figure 25.6 The pathophysiology of symptomatic palatal tremor. This figure summarizes the pathophysiology of symptomatic palatal tremor, which is caused by a structural lesion in the central tegmental tract or the cerebellar projections to the red nucleus or inferior olive. The Guillain-Mollaret triangle is shown in black. For abbreviations, see Figure 25.1.

and inferior olive. The rhythmic activity is explained by the pacemaker properties of the cells within the inferior olive. The gap junctions between olivary cells are thought to be important for synchronizing the rhythmic bursts. Magnetic resonance imaging (T2) shows olivary hypertrophy contralateral to the tremor, which is an unusual neurodegenerative response to the loss of inhibitory olivary afferents. In symptomatic PT, there are often accompanying symptoms such rhythmic movements of the eyes, the pharyngeal muscles or other body parts, and there may be ataxia. In oculopalatal tremor (OPT), patients have smooth ocular oscillations – besides PT. Based on a computational model and data from 15 OPT patients, it has been suggested that the hypertrophic inferior olive generates regular, pulsatile oscillations, while the cerebellum learns to contribute a smoothing and amplifying pulse (a form of maladaptive plasticity) (62).

References

1 Nieuwenhuys R, Voogd J, Van Huijzen C, van Huijzen C, Voogd J. The Human Central Nervous System. 2008.

2 Jain S, Lo SE, Louis ED. Common misdiagnosis of a common neurological disorder: how are we misdiagnosing essential tremor? Arch Neurol 2006;63:1100-1104.

3 Louis ED. Essential tremors: a family of neurodegenerative disorders? Arch Neurol 2009;66:1202-1208.

4 Deuschl G, Elble R. Essential tremor - Neurodegenerative or nondegenerative disease towards a working definition of ET. Mov Disord 2009;24:2033-2041.

5 Wilms H, Sievers J, Deuschl G. Animal models of tremor. Mov Disord. Wiley Online Library 1999;14:557-571.

6 Park YG, Park HY, Lee CJ, et al. CaV3.1 is a tremor rhythm pacemaker in the inferior olive. Proc Natl Acad Sci USA. National Acad Sciences 2010;107:10731-10736.

7 Louis ED, Babij R, Cortés E, Vonsattel J-PG, Faust PL. The inferior olivary nucleus: A postmortem study of essential tremor cases versus controls. Mov Disord 2013;28:779-786.

8 Louis ED. Essential tremor: evolving clinicopathological concepts in an era of intensive post-mortem enquiry. The Lancet Neurology 2010;9:613-622.

9 Rajput AH, Adler CH, Shill HA, Rajput A. Essential tremor is not a neurodegenerative disease. Neurodegenerative Disease Management 2012;2:259-268.

10 Louis ED, Faust PL, Vonsattel JPG, et al. Neuropathological changes in essential tremor: 33 cases compared with 21 controls. Brain 2007;130:3297-3307.

11 Shill HA, Adler CH, Sabbagh MN, et al. Pathologic findings in prospectively ascertained essential tremor subjects. Neurology 2008;70:1452-1455.

12 Helmich RC, Toni I, Deuschl G, Bloem BR. The pathophysiology of essential and Parkinson's tremor. Curr Neurol Neurosci Rep 2013;13:378.

13 Pagan FL, Butman JA, Dambrosia JM, Hallett M. Evaluation of essential tremor with multi-voxel magnetic resonance spectroscopy. Neurology 2003;60:1344-1347.

14 Málly J, Baranyi M, Vizi ES. Change in the concentrations of amino acids in CSF and serum of patients with essential tremor. J Neural Transm 1996;103:555-560.

15 Boecker H, Weindl A, Brooks DJ, et al. GABAergic Dysfunction in Essential Tremor: An 11C-Flumazenil PET Study. J Nucl Med 2010;51:1030-1035.

16 Paris-Robidas S, Brochu E, Sintes M, et al. Defective dentate nucleus GABA receptors in essential tremor. Brain 2012;135:105-116.

17 Shill HA, Adler CH, Beach TG, et al. Brain biochemistry in autopsied patients with essential tremor. Mov Disord 2011;27:113-117.

18 Schnitzler A, Münks C, Butz M, Timmermann L, Gross J. Synchronized brain network associated with essential tremor as revealed by magnetoencephalography. Mov Disord 2009;24:1629-1635.

19 Raethjen J, Govindan RB, Kopper F, Muthuraman M, Deuschl G. Cortical Involvement in the Generation of Essential Tremor. J Neurophysiol 2007;97:3219-3228.

20 Pedrosa DJ, Reck C, Florin E, et al. Essential tremor and tremor in Parkinson's disease are associated with distinct 'tremor clusters' in the ventral thalamus. Exp Neurol 2012;237:435-443.

21 Muthuraman M, Heute U, Arning K, et al. Oscillating central motor networks in pathological tremors and voluntary movements. What makes the difference? NeuroImage 2012;60:1331-1339.

22 Dupuis MJ-M, Evrard FL, Jacquerye PG, Picard GR, Lermen OG. Disappearance of essential tremor after stroke. Mov Disord 2010;25:2884-2887.

23 Jiménez-Jiménez FJ, Alonso-Navarro H, García-Martín E, Lorenzo-Betancor O, Pastor P, Agúndez JAG. Update on genetics of essential tremor. Acta Neurologica Scandinavica 2013; doi: 10.1111/ane.12148.

24 Jellinger KA. Neuropathology of sporadic Parkinson's disease: Evaluation and changes of concepts. Mov Disord 2012;27:8-30.

25 Hirsch EC, Mouatt A, Faucheux B, et al. Dopamine, tremor, and Parkinson's disease. Lancet. 1992;340:125-126.

26 Bergman H, Raz A, Feingold A, et al. Physiology of MPTP tremor. Mov Disord 1998;13S3:29-34.

27 Deutch AY, Elsworth JD, Goldstein M, et al. Preferential vulnerability of A8 dopamine neurons in the primate to the neurotoxin 1-methyl-4-phenyl-1,2,3,6-tetrahydropyridine. Neurosci Lett 1986;68:51-56.

28 German DC, Dubach M, Askari S, Speciale SG, Bowden DM. 1-Methyl-4-phenyl-1,2,3,6-tetrahydropyridine-induced parkinsonian syndrome in Macaca fascicularis: which midbrain dopaminergic neurons are lost? Neuroscience 1988;24:161-174.

29 Jan C, François C, Tandé D, et al. Dopaminergic innervation of the pallidum in the normal state, in MPTP-treated monkeys and in parkinsonian patients. Eur J Neurosci 2000;12:4525-4535.

30 Mounayar S, Boulet S, Tande D, et al. A new model to study compensatory mechanisms in MPTP-treated monkeys exhibiting recovery. Brain 2007;130:2898-2914.

31 Bernheimer H, Birkmayer W, Hornykiewicz O, Jellinger K, Seitelberger F. Brain dopamine and the syndromes of Parkinson and Huntington. Clinical, morphological and neurochemical correlations. J Neurol Sci 1973;20:415-455.

32 Rajput AH, Sitte HH, Rajput A, Fenton ME, Pifl C, Hornykiewicz O. Globus pallidus dopamine and Parkinson motor subtypes: clinical and brain biochemical correlation. Neurology 2008 Apr 15;70:1403-1410.

33 Spiegel J, Hellwig D, Samnick S, et al. Striatal FP-CIT uptake differs in the subtypes of early Parkinson's disease. J Neural Transm 2007;114:331-335.

34 Pirker W. Correlation of dopamine transporter imaging with parkinsonian motor handicap: How close is it? Mov Disord 2003;18:S43-S51.

35 Helmich RC, Janssen MJR, Oyen WJG, Bloem BR, Toni I. Pallidal dysfunction drives a cerebellothalamic circuit into Parkinson tremor. Ann Neurol 2011;69:269-281.

36 Isaias IU, Marzegan A, Pezzoli G, et al. A role for locus coeruleus in Parkinson tremor. Front Hum Neurosci 2011;5:179.

37 Doder M, Rabiner EA, Turjanski N, Lees AJ, Brooks DJ, 11C-WAY 100635 PET study. Tremor in Parkinson's disease and serotonergic dysfunction: an 11C-WAY 100635 PET study. Neurology 2003;60:601-605.

38 Caretti V, Stoffers D, Winogrodzka A, et al. Loss of thalamic serotonin transporters in early drug-naïve Parkinson's disease patients is associated with tremor: an [123I]β-CIT SPECT study. J Neural Transm 2008;115:721-729.

39 Levy R, Hutchison WD, Lozano AM, Dostrovsky JO. High-frequency synchronization of neuronal activity in the subthalamic nucleus of parkinsonian patients with limb tremor. J Neurosci 2000;20:7766-7775.

40 Raz A, vaadia E, Bergman H. Firing patterns and correlations of spontaneous discharge of pallidal neurons in the normal and the tremulous 1-methyl-4-phenyl-1,2,3,6-tetrahydropyridine vervet model of parkinsonism. J Neurosci 2000;20:8559-8571.

41 Lenz FA, Kwan HC, Martin RL, Tasker RR, Dostrovsky JO, Lenz YE. Single unit analysis of the human ventral thalamic nuclear group. Tremor-related activity in functionally identified cells. Brain 1994;117:531-543.

42 Reck C, Florin E, Wojtecki L, et al. Characterisation of tremor-associated local field potentials in the subthalamic nucleus in Parkinson's disease. Eur J Neurosci 2009;29:599-612.

43 Hurtado JM, Gray CM, Tamas LB, Sigvardt KA. Dynamics of tremor-related oscillations in the human globus pallidus: a single case study. Proc Natl Acad Sci USA 1999;96:1674-1679.

44 Timmermann L, Gross J, Dirks M, Volkmann J, Freund H-J, Schnitzler A. The cerebral oscillatory network of parkinsonian resting tremor. Brain 2003;126:199-212.

45 Fukuda M. Thalamic stimulation for parkinsonian tremor: correlation between regional cerebral blood flow and physiological tremor characteristics. NeuroImage 2004;21:608-615.

46 Antonini A, Moeller JR, Nakamura T, Spetsieris P, Dhawan V, Eidelberg D. The metabolic anatomy of tremor in Parkinson's disease. Neurology 1998;51:803-810.

47 Mure H, Hirano S, Tang CC, et al. Parkinson's disease tremor-related metabolic network: Characterization, progression, and treatment effects. NeuroImage 2011;54:1244-1253.

48 Helmich RC, Hallett M, Deuschl G, Toni I, Bloem BR. Cerebral causes and consequences of parkinsonian resting tremor: a tale of two circuits? Brain 2012;135:3206-3226.

49 Bergman H, Feingold A, Nini A, et al. Physiological aspects of information processing in the basal ganglia of normal and parkinsonian primates. Trends Neurosci 1998;21:32-38.

50 Plenz D, Kital ST. A basal ganglia pacemaker formed by the subthalamic nucleus and external globus pallidus. Nature 1999;400:677-682.

51 Dovzhenok A, Rubchinsky LL. On the Origin of Tremor in Parkinson's Disease. Cymbalyuk G, editor. PLoS ONE 2012;7:e41598.

52 Muthuraman M, Hossen A, Heute U, Deuschl G, Raethjen J. A new diagnostic test to distinguish tremulous Parkinson's disease from advanced essential tremor. Mov Disord 2011;26:1548-1552.

53 Hallett M, Deuschl G. Are we making progress in the understanding of tremor in Parkinson's disease? Ann Neurol 2010;68:780-781.

54 Deuschl G, Wilms H, Krack P, Würker M, Heiss WD. Function of the cerebellum in Parkinsonian rest tremor and Holmes' tremor. Ann Neurol 1999;46:126-128.

55 Zeuner KE, Deuschl G. An update on tremors. Curr Opin Neurol 2012;25:475-482.

56 Jones L, Bain PG. Orthostatic tremor. Pract Neurol 2011,11.240-243.

57 Defazio G, Gigante AF, Abbruzzese G, et al. Tremor in primary adult-onset dystonia: prevalence and associated clinical features. J Neurol Neurosurg Psychiatr 2013;84:404-408.

58 Abdo WF, Warrenburg BPCV de, Burn DJ, Quinn NP, Bloem BR. The clinical approach to movement disorders. Nature Reviews Neurology 2010;6:29-37.

59 Schneider SA, Edwards MJ, Mir P, et al. Patients with adult-onset dystonic tremor resembling parkinsonian tremor have scans without evidence of dopaminergic deficit (SWEDDs). Mov Disord 2007;22:2210-2215.

60 Hedera P, Phibbs FT, Dolhun R, et al. Surgical targets for dystonic tremor: Considerations between the globus pallidus and ventral intermediate thalamic nucleus. Parkinsonism Relat Disord 2013;19:684-686.

61 Stamelou M, Saifee TA, Edwards MJ, Bhatia KP. Psychogenic palatal tremor may be underrecognized: Reappraisal of a large series of cases. Mov Disord 2012;27:1164-1168.

62 Shaikh AG, Hong S, Liao K, et al. Oculopalatal tremor explained by a model of inferior olivary hypertrophy and cerebellar plasticity. Brain 2010;133:923-940.

63 Lenz FA, Tasker RR, Kwan HC, et al. Single unit analysis of the human ventral thalamic nuclear group: correlation of thalamic 'tremor cells' with the 3-6 Hz component of parkinsonian tremor. J Neurosci 1988;8:754-764.

26
Tremor in Neurological Diseases

Alex Rajput

Tremor is defined as a rhythmic movement about an axis. It is the most common movement disorder in adults. This chapter will review the clinical features of various primary tremor conditions.

Assessing tremors

A detailed history in addition to a careful neurological exam is essential. Onset of tremor, precipitating and relieving factors, general medical history, family history, medication use, alcohol and caffeine intake, and how the tremor interferes with daily functions should be noted. People tend to report tremor onset when it becomes bothersome, but a more probing history about whether tremor was present at a younger age or under other circumstances is essential.

There are six things to report when describing tremor: distribution, behavioural setting, amplitude, frequency, constancy and regularity.

Distribution

The first thing to note is the distribution: head/neck, face, upper or lower limbs, and whether it is more proximal or distal.

Behavioural setting

The next is the behavioural setting. If a particular activity or posture makes the tremor better or worse, the patient should reproduce it during the examination. Video recording the movements or having patients bring their own videos can be quite helpful.

Amplitude

Tremor amplitude describes the excursion of the body part. This can be described numerically on a five-point scale (0 to 4) with 0 as none and 4 as marked. Scales have been developed to assess tremor (1). The amplitude of tremor is much more variable than the frequency, and worsens with physical or mental stress. It is the amplitude of the tremor that is associated with impairment; for example, a fine 12 Hz tremor in the hands is much better tolerated than a coarse 3 Hz tremor. With stress and distraction, tremor amplitude tends to worsen. While tremors are involuntary movements, people may be able to suppress them to some degree, particularly if they are mild. As a rule, tremors improve or resolve with sleep.

Frequency

Tremor frequency can be measured at the bedside by counting the number of oscillations over a 5 second period and dividing by 5. While tremors are mostly rhythmic with a relatively fixed frequency, dystonic tremors have a more variable frequency and amplitude.

Constancy

Another thing to note is the constancy of the tremor (i.e. moderate amplitude all the time vs minimally present but intermittently severe with stress).

Regularity

Its regularity is also important (i.e. whether it is regular or irregular). The description of jerky, irregular tremor in the hands can signify what some call 'minipolymyoclonus': a cortically based, small-amplitude myoclonus that appears to be a tremor. It is seen in conditions such as Alzheimer's and multiple system atrophy, and some have called it a 'cortical tremor' (2).

Defining tremors

Action tremor or kinetic tremor

Action or kinetic tremor presents with activity. This may be evident with finger-nose-finger testing or with movements such as holding a cup, doing up buttons or shoelaces, etc. This type of tremor is typically seen with essential tremor.

Intention tremor or terminal tremor

Intention or terminal tremor accentuates as the limb reaches the target (as in finger-nose-finger testing). It is classically seen with cerebellar disease but is associated with ataxia. It is not uncommon in essential tremor, but in contrast to cerebellar disease, the underlying trajectory of the movement appears relatively smooth (i.e. not ataxic).

Postural tremor

Postural tremor is noted in a body part held against gravity. This is tested in the upper limbs by holding the hands out in front with the fingers outstretched and then with the hands underneath the chin. When testing the lower limbs, ask the subject to lift the leg off the floor (if seated) or the examining table (if supine). The head tremor of essential tremor is a postural tremor as antigravity muscles in the neck are actively keeping the head upright; this often resolves when the patient lies supine on the examining table. Postural tremor of the limbs may be seen in essential tremor, enhanced physiological tremor or drug-induced tremor.

Resting tremor

Resting tremor presents when the body part is fully supported or at rest. This is the classic tremor seen in Parkinson's disease (PD). The individual should be examined fully supine wherever possible. Having the arms on the armrest of a chair may produce a type of positional tremor; there are multiple patients whose tremor is present when seated but minimal or absent when lying supine with the limbs fully supported. By standing at the foot of the bed and having the patient dorsiflex the feet against resistance, the examiner gets a good look at the upper limbs, the head and face. Counting aloud as a distraction technique activates the facial muscles and improves any resting tremor of the jaw, lip or chin that may be seen in Parkinson's disease. Squeezing the examiner's hand allows one to observe tremor in the lower limbs.

Dystonic tremor

Dystonic tremor is an irregular, directionally preponderant tremor, seen in a body part affected by dystonia. It is typically a mix of postural/action tremor and is rarely seen with the body part completely at rest. The tremor and position are often improved with a sensory trick (geste antagoniste).

Orthostatic tremor

Orthostatic tremor is a fine rapid tremor (13-18 Hz) noted in the lower limbs upon standing which improves with walking. A similar tremor may involve the trunk and upper limbs.

Task-specific tremor

Task-specific tremor is a tremor occurring with a specific task. The most common task-specific tremor reported is primary writing tremor.

Isometric tremor

Isometric tremors occur with muscle contraction but not shortening (literally muscles being of fixed length). Examples of this include tremor while pushing against a wall (fixed object) or tremor of the hand that is squeezing the examiner's finger (3).

Table 26.1
Tremor syndromes with their typical activation condition and their frequency range as defined in the 1998 Consensus Statement of the Movement Disorder Society.

Diagnoses	Frequency range	Activity by		
		rest	posture	goal-directed movement
Enhanced physiologic tremor			necessary	may occur
Essential tremor syndromes				
Classical essential tremor		may occur	necessary	may occur
Primary orthostatic tremor			necessary	may occur
Task and position specific tremor			may occur	may occur
Unclassified tremor				
Dystonic tremor		may occur	necessary	necessary
Parkinsonian tremor		necessary	may occur	may occur
Cerebellar tremor			necessary	necessary
Holmes tremor		necessary	may occur	necessary
Palatal tremor		necessary		
Neuropathic tremor			necessary	may occur
Toxic and drug-induced tremor		may occur	may occur	may occur
Psychogenic tremor		may occur	may occur	may occur

Frequency axis: 0   5   10   15   Hz

Legend: ■ typical frequencies   □ rare frequencies   ▣ necessary for diagnoses   ☐ may occur

Classifying tremors

A syndromic classification of tremor is provided in Table 26.1 (4).

Essential Tremor (ET)

Epidemiology

Tremor is the most common movement disorder in adults, and the most common neurological cause of tremor is essential tremor (ET) (5). ET affects 0.4% - 0.9% of the general population

(6) and at least 5% of those aged 65 and older worldwide (5,7). Individual studies may report quite different results, depending on the population studied and methods used. While studies using medical records can underestimate the true prevalence of ET, door-to-door reporting may include a number of individuals evaluated only once with mild but non-bothersome tremor. The majority of cases have never been diagnosed by a physician.

ET affects people of all ages and races, though it becomes more common with advancing age. In general, there is no significant difference in the risk of males or females developing ET, though in a meta-analysis of ET prevalence, one-third of studies had a male preponderance (7). While a bimodal peak in the second and sixth decades has been reported (8,9), many other studies from various populations do not support this (7).

ET has an onset in childhood in 5-16% of cases, with males outnumbering females by at least a 2:1 ratio (10,11,12). A similar proportion of both boys and girls reported a positive family history of tremor (11), with the majority of studies reporting a positive family history of between 53% (10) and 91% (13). Childhood onset head tremor has been reported as uncommon (10,11), while others note a similar prevalence to adults (12).

Etiology

Pathology

The cause of ET is unknown. Early cases reported in the literature noted no significant or specific abnormalities in brain pathology. In 2004, the largest study to date reported on 20 ET autopsy cases from a single centre; six were noted to have ET in combination with rest tremor, and another six had ET plus parkinsonism (with all three features of bradykinesia, rigidity and resting tremor). Of these six ET plus parkinsonism cases, only one had incidental Lewy body disease (iLBD) pathology. There were no obvious pathological findings (14). In 2007, in a study of

33 ET and 21 control brains from several centres, mean Purkinje cell (PC) numbers were reduced in ET (15). While the PC count was reduced in a group of ET without Lewy bodies, the majority of ET had values at or above the lowest level reported in control brains (16). The presence of cerebellar torpedoes was also reported to occur more frequently in ET (15).

In another study comparing 11 ET and 11 controls, no consistent pathology was found. While a formal PC count was not done, 'there was no difference in Purkinje cell loss between the two groups' based on the neuropathologist's observations (17). Another group reported on 24 ET and 21 control brains and observed cerebellar atrophy in one, superior vermis atrophy in three, and dentate nucleus abnormality in one. Formal cell counting was not done (18).

Rajput and colleagues reported on 15 cases (7 ET, 6 PD and 2 normal controls) in 2011, counting Purkinje cells using three different methods (through the nucleus, through the nucleolus, and through any part of the PC (19)) and found no difference in the PC count between groups. It was criticized because of its small sample size; a subsequent report on 59 subjects, including 12 ET, 41 PD and 6 normal controls (20,21) found no significant difference between the groups, and if anything, the PC count was slightly higher in ET.

Pathological findings in ET are heterogenous (18), and no consistent pathology is identified. Purkinje cell loss and the presence of torpedoes are non-specific findings, and while noted in some ET cases, they cannot be used as markers to indicate cerebellar pathology in ET. PC counts also decline with age (20,22). The PC counts do not correlate with the duration or severity of ET, age of onset, distribution of tremor, response to treatment, and no critical threshold has been determined beyond which there is manifestation of tremor. In addition, significant and selective loss of PC does not result in an ET phenotype (23,24). Cerebellar lesions (e.g. stroke) can improve the postural tremor of ET (25,26).

Biochemistry

Gamma-amino butyric acid (GABA) is the primary inhibitory neurotransmitter in the brain. As GABAergic therapies (e.g. primidone, benzodiazepines, alcohol) are effective in treating ET, GABAergic dysfunction has been postulated to be involved in the pathophysiology of ET.

Boecker et al. compared ET (n = 8) with healthy controls (n = 11) using ^{11}C-flumazenil, a ligand for the ionotropic GABA-A benzodiazepine receptor. Significant increases in binding were noted in the dentate nucleus (but not cerebellar cortex), VL (ventrolateral) nucleus of the thalamus, and the lateral premotor cortex, implying receptor upregulation (27). Paris-Robidas reported on postmortem tissue from 10 ET, 10 PD and 16 controls. They noted a reduction in both GABA-A (ionotropic) and GABA-B (metabotropic) receptors in the dentate compared with controls and PD, but no such changes in the cerebellar cortex (28). In addition, concentrations of GABA-B receptors were inversely proportional to the duration of ET. The results support the idea that decreased GABA receptors in the dentate allow for overexcitation of the cerebellar-thalamocortical circuit. The results of decreased GABA binding in the dentate in postmortem studies conflict with the functional imaging studies of increased GABA receptor expression. Perhaps these discordant results could be reconciled by theorizing that the GABA receptors are initially upregulated in ET before being downregulated. Both studies (27,28) implicate the GABAergic system with involvement of the dentate (but not the cerebellar cortex) in the expression of essential tremor.

Genetics

Many ET cases are considered to be dominantly inherited with variable penetrance, but the genetics is still not well understood. A positive family history of tremor has been reported in 17-100% in ET (29). Expression in monozygotic twins is at least double that of dizygotic twins (30), and bilineal transmission has been report-ed to cause severer expression than in the parents (31).

Family-based, genome-wide linkage studies have identified three loci for ET: hereditary essential tremor-1 (ETM1) on chromosome 3q13, ETM2 (chromosome 2p), and ETM3 (6p23) – but no causal mutations in these genes were identified (6,32). The first GWAS (genome-wide association study) in ET found an association with increased risk of ET and two single nucleotide polymorphisms (SNPs) (rs9652490 and rs11856808) of the *LINGO1* (leucine-rich repeat and Ig domain containing 1 gene) on chromosome 15q; this has been confirmed by some not but other investigators (6,32). Five additional polymorphisms in *LINGO1* and one in its paralog *LINGO2* were identified by Vilariño-Güell (33) and colleagues to be associated with increased ET risk; one *LINGO1* variant was associated with risk of both ET and Parkinson's disease, while one SNP in *LINGO2* was associated with Parkinson's disease. One SNP variant in *LINGO1* and two in *LINGO2* influenced the mean age of onset of ET expression (6,32,33). *LINGO1* is a CNS-specific component of the Nogo-66 receptor (NgR1)/ p75/*LINGO1* signaling complex; this complex is involved in the inhibition of axonal myelination and regeneration, oligodendrocyte differentiation and neuronal survival (33). *LINGO1* expression is higher in the substantia nigra of PD than controls, and cell culture and in vivo models have noted improved survival, growth, and function of dopaminergic neurons when *LINGO1* activity was reduced (33). There is a biologic plausibility in the role of *LINGO1* being involved in both ET and PD.

Recently, novel gene variants in the *FUS* (fused in sarcoma) gene have been reported to be associated with ET (34). While genetic risk factors have been identified, identifying reproducible pathologic variants in ET has been elusive thus far.

ET and PD

While there has been a longstanding debate as to whether essential tremor increases the risk of

Parkinson's disease, there is no evidence of a definitive link between the two (35). Patients with incidental Lewy bodies do not have a greater risk of ET or action tremor, and those with ET are not at greater risk of having iLBD. There is also no evidence of a similar biochemical abnormality, with striatal tyrosine hydroxylase levels in ET being similar to controls (and not reduced as one would find in PD) (35,36). While genetic variants of alpha-synuclein are associated with Parkinson's disease, there is no such association in ET (37).

Pathophysiology

The pathophysiology of tremor seems to be related to a 'network' problem affecting the cerebellum, thalamus, and motor cortex, with a potential role of the inferior olive as a 'pacemaker'. A recent study shows no evidence of structural pathology in the inferior olive of ET cases compared with controls, however (38). Please see Chapter 25 for a more detailed explanation of tremor pathophysiology.

Clinical Presentation

The tremor of ET is a postural tremor of the upper limbs, with or without an accompanying action tremor (see Video fragment 26.1). It is noted when the hands are holding something such as a cup or a newspaper. There may be difficulty writing, eating and drinking, threading a needle, doing up buttons or zippers, or performing personal grooming (brushing teeth, applying make-up, etc.). Carrying food on a tray can be challenging, and eating soup out in public or drinking from a full cup should be avoided altogether. As the tremor is of similar frequency but generally out of phase between the upper limbs, drinking from a cup with two hands will improve as opposed to worsen the tremor. Holding a cup or spoon in a certain way for that individual may also improve the tremor somewhat. Persons requiring steady hands for their occupation can be significantly impaired.

ET is generally regarded as symmetric, though minor side-to-side differences are common. While those seen in the clinic setting with asymmetry tend to have greater severity (amplitude) in the dominant hand, community-based studies have noted that the non-dominant side is more severely affected (39).

Head tremor and voice tremor occur in 30 - 60% of all ET cases (40,41,42). Head tremor may be either vertical ('yes/yes' tremor) or horizontal ('no/no' tremor). Occasionally, there is both a vertical and horizontal component. Head tremor may go unnoticed until pointed out by a friend or family member. Head tremor is two to six times more frequent in women (42,43), and voice tremor also occurs more commonly in women (42). Voice tremor may be observed during conversational speech, but if it is only mild, it may not be detected until the patient is asked to sustain a vowel. ET patients may also exhibit rest tremor without other parkinsonian findings, and this is thought to represent a natural late stage evolution (44). No significant pathological differences exist between those with ET plus rest tremor and those without (44), and the rest tremor cannot be attributed to Lewy body pathology (45).

The remainder of the neurological exam in ET should be unremarkable. Tandem gait abnormalities have been reported in ET (46) and oculomotor abnormalities detected using electro-oculography (47), suggesting cerebellar dysfunction. The association of non-motor features such as personality or mood symptoms is controversial (48); these features are generally not thought to be present in ET.

Clinical scales have been developed to assess ET (1,49). Spiral tracing and copying, and drinking or pouring water from one cup to another can be easily tested at the bedside to quantify tremor severity. Pegboard testing and maze drawing can be performed when more detailed clinical testing is desired. More precise quantification of tremors can be conducted with accelerometry, but its availability is limited to research settings.

Table 26.2
Diagnostic criteria for classic (definite) essential tremor (50).

Tremor investigation group criteria	Movement disorder society consensus critera
Inclusion criteria:	Inclusion criteria:
1 Bilateral postural tremor, with of without kinetic tremor, in the hands that is visible and persistent	1 Bilateral, largely symmetric postural or kinetic tremor of the hands that is visible and persistent
2 Duration longer than 5 years	2 Additional or isolated head tremor in the absence of abnormal posturing
Exclusion criteria:	Exclusion criteria:
1 Other abnormal neurologic signs (with the exception of the presence of tremor and Froment's sign. The full neurologic examination should normal for age)	1 Other abnormal neurologic signs, especially dystonia
2 Presence of known causes of enhanced physiologic tremor	2 The presence of known causes of enhanced physiologic tremor, including current or recent exposure to tremorogenic drugs or the presence of a drug withdrawal state
3 Concurrent or recent exposure to tremorogenic drugs or the presence of a druk withdrawal stage	3 Historic of clinical evidence of psychogenic tremor
4 Direct or indirect trauma to the nervous system within 3 months preceding the onset of tremor	4 Convincing evidence of sudden onset or evidence of stepwise deterioration
5 Historic or clinical evidence of psychogenic origins of tremor	5 Primary orthostatic tremor
6 Convincing evidence of sudden onset or evidence of stepwise deterioration	6 Isolated voice tremor
	7 Isolated position-specific or tast-specific tremors including occupational tremors and primary writing tremor
	8 Isolated tongue or chin tremor
	9 Isolated leg tremor

Diagnosis

ET remains a clinical diagnosis. There are no biomarkers available to diagnose it or monitor its progression. In the past, two main diagnostic criteria have been used for essential tremor: TRIG (tremor investigation group) criteria and the MDS (Movement Disorder Society) consensus criteria (1,50) (see Table 26.2). MDS criteria incorporated the TRIG definite and probable criteria for ET, but did not require a specified duration. The two criteria are very similar. As there was concern that those criteria might be too restrictive and would hinder treatment and research into tremor, new criteria for the diagnosis of essential tremor were recently proposed (51). The various criteria are briefly as follows:

New Criteria

Hereditary ET
- fulfills consensus criteria for definite or classic ET and also has an unequivocal family history of at least one first-degree affected relative;
- onset for both subject and family member must be before age 65.

Sporadic ET
- fulfills published criteria but does not have an immediate family member with ET;
- onset is before age 65.

Senile ET
- fulfills criteria for definite or classic ET but develops tremor after age 65;
- family history may or may not be present.

Differential diagnosis

Parkinson's disease

The primary neurologic consideration in the differential diagnosis of essential tremor is Parkinson's disease (PD) (see Table 26.3). The tremor of ET is a postural and/or action tremor while the classic parkinsonian tremor is a resting tremor (see Video fragment 26.2). However, some ET patients have resting tremor, and both postural and action tremor are not uncommon in PD. The tremor frequency in ET is greater than that of PD, typically in the 8-12 Hz range for ET and classically in the 4-6 Hz range for PD. The distribution of tremor also differs between the two conditions. ET affects the upper limbs, and sometimes the head and voice, while PD affects both the upper and lower limbs, and sometimes the lips and chin. Asymmetric tremor favors PD over ET, though this is not absolute. Unilateral rest tremor of the leg can be considered PD until proven otherwise.

Tremor characteristics alone may be insufficient to differentiate ET from PD. Subjects with ET do not have bradykinesia or rigidity. However, tremor can interfere with the assessment of bradykinesia involving e.g. finger tapping; assessment using another method such as pronation/supination or hand opening and closing can yield better results. Tremor should not interfere with the assessment of heel tapping in ET, and the performance should be normal, without evidence of fatigue. There may be resistance to passive movement at the wrist when assessing for rigidity during voluntary movement of a distal body part (Froment's sign) in ET subjects, particularly in those with moderate to severe tremor. If Froment's sign is positive at the wrist, check the tone at the elbow or lower limbs (where tremor should be absent in ET).

Handwriting is affected in both ET and PD. The writing of ET is tremulous (sometimes to the point of being unable to put the pen to paper), while the handwriting of PD is micrographic. Speech can be affected in ET and is almost always involved in PD. The speech of ET, when affected, is tremulous; the speech of PD on the other hand is often hypophonic, hoarse, and

Table 26.3
Differentiating ET from PD.

	ET	PD
Tremor	Presenting feature	May be absent, especially in akinetic-rigid
Distribution	Upper limbs (usually symmetric); head, voice	Upper and lower limbs (usually asymmetric); jaw, libs
Behavioural setting	Postural +/− kinetic tremor	Resting tremor
Frequency	8-12 Hz	4-6 Hz
Amplitude	Worsens ET progresses	May lessen or disappear altogether with advanced PD
Age	Any age, but more common with advancing age	Uncommon before age 40; typically onset in 6th or 7th decade
Family history	Often positive	May have positive FH, but usually negative
Associated features	Absent as a rule	Bradykinesia, rigidity, shuffling gait and postural instability, dysarthria, dysphagia; nonmotor features (depression, dementia, bowel/bladder involvement, sleep disturbance including REM behaviour disorder, anosmia)

Table 26.4
Overview of therapeutic options for the different tremor syndromes (X* marks first choice treatment).

	Essential tremor	Ortho-static tremor	Task-specific tremor	Dystonic tremor	Parkinson tremor	Cere-bellar tremor	Holmes tremor	Neuro-pathic tremor
Propranolol	X*	X	X	X	X	X	X	X
Primidone	X*	X	X	X		X		
Gabapentin	X	X						
Alprazolam	X							
Topiramate	X							
Clozapine	X				X		X	
Botulinum toxin	X		X	X*				
Carbamazepine					X	X		
Clonazepam		X*		X		X	X	X
Phenobarbital		X						
Valproic acid		X						
Levodopa		X		X	X*		X*	
Dopamine agonist		X			X*		X*	
Anticholinergics			X	X	X		X	
Tetrabenazine				X				
Neurosurgery	X			X	X	X	X	X

may be either fast (tachyphemic) or slow, and sometimes stuttering.

The gait should be normal in ET, while in PD there may be early findings of asymmetric reduction in arm-swing and slightly flexed posture. Subjects with more advanced PD classically have an obviously flexed posture with marked reduction or absence of arm-swing, a slow, shuffling gait with difficulty changing directions and gait freezing.

Non-motor findings are generally not considered to be part of ET; non-motor findings associated with PD include depression, dementia, bowel and bladder dysfunction, dysphagia, and sleep disturbances including REM sleep behaviour disorder (RBD).

Both conditions are more common with increasing age, and it is not unheard of for persons to have both ET and PD. There may be longstanding ET with subsequent PD, simultaneous on-

set of PD and ET, or PD followed by ET. Those in the first category are the easiest to diagnose, while those in the second and third categories may require multiple subsequent visits to confirm clinically. The presence of all three cardinal features of parkinsonism (bradykinesia, rigidity, and resting tremor) is required when making the additional diagnosis of PD for someone with ET (14). For those with PD who subsequently develop ET, progressively worsening postural tremor in an upper limb with or without action tremor, and out of proportion to the degree of resting tremor, is needed to diagnose ET.

Differentiating advanced stage PD from ET should not be problematic, but it can be challenging early in the course. Benign tremulous parkinsonism (BTP) is an uncommon form of parkinsonism with rest tremor as an early and prominent sign accompanied by only mild non-tremor components (bradykinesia, rigidity, gait involvement), no disability aside from that related to tremor, and minimal progression eight years after onset (52). Subjects may develop both action and postural tremor as well (52,53,54). More than half of BTP have only a minimal response to levodopa (52,53), and some cases do not have pathologically verified PD (53,54); it has been argued that BTP may represent ET in some instances (54). Between 4% and 15% of patients with clinical PD studied in clinical trial settings have SWEDDs (Scans Without Evidence of Dopaminergic Dysfunction); there is little data on the pathology of SWEDD cases (53). The use of DaT (dopamine transporter) SPECT imaging to distinguish BTP from ET in challenging diagnostic cases may be helpful but is not readily available at many sites.

Other conditions

Included in the differential diagnosis of essential tremor are enhanced physiological tremor, dystonia (particularly as it relates to head tremor), cerebellar disease, and drug-induced tremor. Each of them is addressed in a separate section following the discussion of ET.

While improvement of tremor following alcohol ingestion has been reported as 'diagnostic' of ET, not every ET case improves with alcohol, and other types of tremor (including parkinsonian and cerebellar tremor) may also improve following alcohol ingestion (55).

Treatment

The two mainstays of pharmacologic treatment are propranolol, a non-selective beta-antagonist, and primidone, an anticonvulsant. Beta-blockers aside from propranolol have been used but are less effective. Benzodiazepines, topiramate, and gabapentin have each been shown to benefit some cases. For head or voice tremor, botulinum toxin injections can be useful. For severe tremor, deep brain stimulation (DBS) of the Vim thalamic nucleus can be very effective for contralateral upper limb tremor. Alcohol can also suppress the tremor and can be used in settings where it is socially acceptable. Therapy of tremor will be discussed in more detail in Chapter 27.

Prognosis

While ET used to be called 'benign essential tremor', this term is no longer used. Mild or greater functional impairment in at least 60% of subjects with ET has been reported in two community-based studies (56). Some individuals are so impaired that even personal care tasks such as feeding and dressing are difficult to perform. ET tends to progress fairly slowly. With time, the tremor amplitude increases and its frequency decreases. Increased tremor severity after the initial clinic visit has been associated with asymmetrical tremor, unilateral tremor onset and longer follow-up duration (57).

The 'benign' in the term 'benign essential tremor' referred to life expectancy. There are conflicting reports regarding mortality in ET (48), but overall the risk of death is not considered to be greater in ET.

Physiological tremor

Physiological tremor is present in all persons and is usually in the 8-12Hz range (58). While physiological tremor is typically associated with posture and/or action, it may be present with isometric contraction (and even at times with the limb at rest). When easily visible, it is called *enhanced physiological tremor* (see Video fragment 26.3). Contributing factors to physiological tremor include central oscillatory mechanisms, the mechanical properties of the limb, and spinal stretch reflex. While external loading can reduce the stretch-mediated oscillation frequency in physiological tremor (58), it does not alter the tremor frequency in ET (3). The amplitude of both physiological tremor and essential tremor is reduced with external loading.

Enhanced physiological tremor is believed to be due to increased beta-adrenergic stimulation (58). Causes of enhanced physiological tremor include stress/anxiety, fatigue, sleep deprivation, strenuous exercise, hypoglycemia, thyrotoxicosis, pheochromocytoma, and various medications. By definition, there is no underlying neurological cause. The association with a precipitating factor(s), lack of family history, and reduction of tremor frequency with weight loading all point to enhanced physiological tremor as opposed to ET. The two conditions can be difficult to differentiate at times.

Dystonic tremor (DT)

The association of tremor and dystonia is well known. It is encountered most commonly in cervical dystonia (CD), the most common primary dystonia affecting adults. Tremor can be classified as either dystonic tremor (DT) or tremor associated with dystonia (TAWD) (59). Dystonic tremor is tremor in a body part affected by dystonia. This is typically a postural and/or kinetic tremor of variable frequency (usually <7 Hz) typically not seen during complete rest (1). The tremor is often irregular, and the amplitude increases when the body part moves away from the direction of dystonia. For example, in a patient with cervical dystonia and torticollis with the head rotating to the left, asking the subject to rotate the head to the right will worsen the tremor, while the tremor will improve with head rotation to the left. There may be a 'null point' in CD when the person can position the head in such a way that there is minimal or no head tremor. A sensory trick (geste antagoniste) often improves the tremor and dystonia (see Video fragment 26.4). For subjects with voice tremor, trying to differentiate between spasmodic dysphonia and essential tremor may be difficult. The sensory 'trick' of singing or changing pitch when speaking can improve a dystonic voice tremor but should not alter the voice tremor of essential tremor (1).

Dystonic head tremor
Isolated head tremor may be due to essential tremor or cervical dystonia. Essential tremor may be either a 'yes/yes' (vertical) or 'no/no'

(horizontal) tremor. Head tremor due to cervical dystonia is typically irregular with a directional preponderance and improvement with sensory trick. Lying supine may improve both the head tremor of ET and cervical dystonia. In ET there are no antigravity muscles at work keeping the head up when lying supine, while in cervical dystonia, touching the head to the back of the pillow can act as a sensory trick, with some improvement of head position and tremor. Resolution of head tremor with lying supine has been reported to be more suggestive of ET than cervical dystonia (60). Some patients with cervical dystonia and dystonic head tremor also have ET-like head tremor; the ET-like tremor is of a higher frequency (>7 Hz) and usually more regular than dystonic head tremor, which has a lower frequency (3-7Hz) and is more irregular (61).

Dystonic cervical tremor
Persons with CD often complain of neck pain, tightness and/or associated headache (usually in the cervico-occipital region) while it would be highly unusual for ET patients to report such symptoms. ET patients may be unaware of their head tremor until it is pointed out by someone else, while those with CD and associated head tremor are often aware of their head movements. Pal and colleagues prospectively evaluated 114 consecutive patients with CD (62). More than two-thirds had head tremor, and more than one-third of those with head tremor reported tremor as one of the first symptoms. CD age at onset was similar in those with and without tremor. In the group with CD and head tremor, there was a higher prevalence of women, more frequent positive family history of essential-like hand/head tremor, and presence of essential-like hand tremor.

Dystonic limb tremor
The association of upper limb tremor with cervical dystonia is known, but its significance is controversial. In a sample of 429 primary adult-onset dystonia patients from Italian movement disorders centres, one in six had tremor (59).

Of those with tremor, nearly 60% had dystonic tremor (DT), over 30% had tremor associated with dystonia (TAWD), and the remainder had both types of tremor. All of the clinical features were similar between the DT and TAWD groups except for the tendency for the dystonia to spread, which was greater in the DT group (59). Shaikh and colleagues quantified limb tremor in 19 patients with CD and 35 patients with ET using a three-axis accelerometer (63). While the amplitude of limb tremor was higher in the CD group, the mean tremor frequency did not differ significantly between the groups. The postural tremor irregularity (quantified using cycle-to-cycle variability), however, was nearly 50% greater in the CD group.

Münchau et al. reported on upper extremity (UE) tremor in 11 ET and 19 CD plus UE tremor subjects (64). No group difference in reciprocal inhibition was noted between the two groups, but the data were more variable in the CD group. When the CD were divided into those with normal presynaptic inhibition and those with reduced or absent inhibition, the former had onset of UE tremor simultaneous to CD onset, while the latter had UE tremor preceding CD by a mean of 21 years (64). The clinical symptoms were otherwise similar. Schiebler and colleagues recently reported on 57 definite CD cases with or without arm tremor and concluded that there likely exists a subgroup of CD patients with early-onset UE tremor and later CD development with a male preponderance (65).

Dystonia may present with isolated action tremor (50). While there is certainly an overlap with an appearance of dystonia in tremor patients and vice versa, subtle findings may be overlooked (such as a mild head tilt or slightly irregular tremor) and observations skewed by the perspective of the examiner.

Primary tremor

A new classification scheme for dystonic tremor has been suggested (50): primary tremor is the term for patients in whom tremor is the sole or primary abnormality, allowing for better characterization of all the associated signs and symptoms. The distribution and behavioural setting of all tremors present would be described. The diagnosis of primary tremor acknowledges that a specific diagnosis or aetiology is still lacking and will facilitate research into the clinical phenomenology, aetiology, pathophysiology, genetics, and treatment of these conditions (50).

Cerebellar tremor

Cerebellar cortical lesions alone do not cause tremor (66). Cerebellar lesions causing tremor include the deep cerebellar nuclei (e.g. dentate) and the superior cerebellar peduncle/cerebellar outflow tract. A lesion proximal to the decussation of the cerebellar outflow tract would cause ipsilateral tremor, while a lesion after the decussation would cause contralateral tremor (66). The classic tremor seen is a terminal tremor with associated ataxia, though sometimes the ataxia may be mild if the patient volitionally slows the finger-nose-finger testing to improve accuracy. There should be no true postural tremor, though there may be the appearance of such as it can be difficult to get the limb to maintain a stable posture.

Other findings including dysarthria, nystagmus, and gait ataxia are found to a varying extent, depending on the extent of cerebellar involvement. Titubation is an oscillatory movement of the head and trunk possibly due to hypotonia of axial muscles (67) (see Video fragment 26.5). It does not localize well to any particular part of the cerebellum.

While the action tremor component can be treated with medications typically used for essential tremor, there is no good therapy for the associated ataxia.

Focal lesions such as stroke, mass lesions and demyelinating plaques should be considered in the appropriate clinical setting. It is beyond the scope of this chapter to discuss the differential diagnosis of degenerative cerebellar diseases, which as a rule cause pancerebellar involvement. Fragile X Tremor Associated Syndrome (FXTAS) has major features of ataxia and intention tremor, each being present in approximately 90% of cases. Parkinsonism is a minor feature of FXTAS, and resting tremor (usually symmetric) is reported in 30-40% (68).

Iatrogenic and metabolic tremors

While not a primary neurological cause, this category is the most common cause of tremor overall and therefore warrants mention. The typical tremor induced by medications and metabolic conditions is an enhanced physiological tremor (8-12 Hz), mainly postural, though there may be a kinetic component.

Medications that may cause tremor include antiseizure drugs (valproate, phenytoin, carbamazepine), psychiatric medications (lithium, neuroleptics, antidepressants), cardiac medications (amiodarone), asthma therapies (inhaled beta-agonists, steroids, aminophylline), and immunosuppressants (cyclosporine). Neuroleptic medications and other D2 dopaminergic blocking agents (such as metoclopramide) may cause a drug-induced parkinsonism and, rarely, a tardive tremor.

Metabolic conditions such as hyperthyroidism, hypoglycemia and, rarely, pheochromocytoma may cause tremor. Wilson disease causes neurologic, hepatic and psychiatric symptoms due to disordered copper metabolism and copper accumulation in the liver and brain. It can cause almost any movement disorder, though most commonly tremor, dystonia and/or parkinsonian features. The classic tremor associated with Wilson disease is a 'wing beating' tremor seen with shoulders abducted and arms flexed at the elbow (see Chapter 23).

Less common tremors/tremor syndromes

Task-specific tremor

The most commonly reported task-specific tremor is primary writing tremor (see Video fragment 26.6). Tremors with other activities such as playing a musical instrument, golfing, shooting a rifle and even bricklaying have been reported (69).

Pathophysiology
The pathophysiology of primary writing tremor (PWT) is unknown. Patients can be characterized as having a task-specific tremor - tremor only with writing - or having a positionally sensitive tremor, with hand tremor also occurring when assuming a similar posture to writing (70). Patients may have a minimal associated postural tremor with the hands outstretched, but by definition it is a task-specific tremor. PWT is generally considered a non-progressive condition and can be sporadic or dominantly inherited. The prevalence of PWT is not known, though it would be expected to be less common than writer's cramp. It has been viewed as a variant of essential tremor, a variant of writer's cramp (task-specific focal dystonia), or its own unique entity. There are points in support of each hypothesis (71).

Therapy
There have been no randomized, double-blind, controlled trials of therapy in PWT. Medical therapy can benefit approximately one-half to two-thirds of individuals with PWT. While some claim more success with anticholinergics and other treatments used for dystonia as a point favouring a dystonic aetiology to PWT, benefit has also been achieved with beta-blockers (such as propranolol) and primidone. Other treatments include levodopa/carbidopa, topiramate, benzodiazepines, and botulinum toxin injections. Surgical therapy with either thalamotomy or deep brain stimulation of the Vim nucleus has also been of benefit (71).

Orthostatic tremor

Orthostatic tremor (OT) is a rare form of primary tremor characterized by 13-18 Hz tremor in the legs appearing shortly (often within several seconds) upon standing and promptly relieved upon sitting. Patients report unsteadiness and tremor in the legs which may spread to the trunk (see Video fragment 26.7). The fine rapid tremor may be seen or felt in the thighs and calves, and patients may report that their legs feel like they are 'cramping' while they stand (67). Examination reveals a wide-based stance with inability to tandem because of the extra time spent on each leg compared to a normal gait. Some individuals may flex their toes ('claw') in an attempt to get a better grip. Auscultation with the diaphragm of a stethoscope over the thighs while the subject is standing reveals a repetitive thumping sound like a 'helicopter' (72).

Lumbar paraspinal and upper limb muscles contract at a similar frequency to the lower limb tremor (73). Alternating patterns of muscle contraction as well as co-contraction of agonist and antagonist muscles can be seen in OT (73).

Etiology and Pathophysiology

As the muscle contractions in OT are time locked (73), a central generator for the tremor has been postulated (74), most likely located in the brainstem (75). A study by Wu et al. noted that the tremor was reset by electrical stimulation over the posterior fossa, but not by stimulating the motor cortex or the limbs (74).

SPECT imaging revealed decreased ligand binding to striatal dopamine transporters in OT, consistent with a presynaptic dopaminergic deficiency. The values for OT cases were intermediate between normal controls and PD, and there was more symmetric striatal involvement in the OT group compared to PD cases (76).

Associated conditions

OT has been associated in some cases with action tremor or other neurological conditions. Orthostatic tremor has also been reported with cerebellar degeneration, pontine lesions, or even after head trauma (77).

Two large series of OT have been reported (77,78). Selected patients had clinical features

of OT and met the supporting EMG criteria (1). Both groups divided their cases into primary OT (consisting of OT alone), or OT-AT (OT and action tremor), and OT Plus, with other neurological conditions or features associated with OT. While Gerschlager et al. (77) noted the mean age of onset to be a decade younger in primary OT compared with OT Plus, Mestre and colleagues (78) did not find such a distinction. Onset in the vast majority occurred in the 6th and 7th decades. OT Plus was found in 25-30%, and concomitant neurological conditions included parkinsonism (PD, PSP, vascular parkinsonism), restless legs syndrome, dementia with Lewy bodies, focal dystonia, and multifocal action tremor. While patients with OT-AT were much more likely to be female (3:1 to 6:1 ratio), no gender predominance was observed in the OT alone and OT Plus groups. In addition, the OT-AT group had a family history of tremor more often and were more likely to respond to alcohol (77).

Differential Diagnosis

While OT has been postulated to represent a variant of essential tremor, it is its own distinct condition. ET may rarely display lower limb involvement; the tremor is a postural tremor and/or action tremor and may occur with walking and other activities such as maintaining the limb against gravity or with heel/shin testing, and also resolves with sitting (73). Similar symptoms of unsteadiness, tremor and/or twitching in the legs may be seen in patients with myoclonus, cerebellar ataxia or clonus (73).

Treatment

Clonazepam is the most commonly used medication in OT. Its benefit is modest, however, with only about 30% of patients tried on clonazepam noting improvement in two case series (77,78); improvement was sustained in 50-75%, however. Other treatments noted to improve OT include primidone, propranolol, levodopa, gabapentin, acetazolamide, valproic acid and mirtazapine (77,78).

Prognosis

Symptoms may progress to involve the trunk and arms, and severity may also worsen (77). Of the 25 cases with available follow-up reported by Mestre and colleagues, 72% had a progressive course, with an increased intensity, decreased latency of standing until the appearance of tremor, spread to other body regions (trunk, arms), and the need for a walking aid (78).

Peripheral tremor or neuropathy-associated tremor

Tremor associated with neuropathy was recognized in association with Charcot-Marie Tooth (CMT) disease, and the combination of tremor and CMT is known as Roussy-Levy syndrome. The frequency of tremor in hereditary sensori-motor neuropathies has varied from 10-40%, while that in inflammatory neuropathies has been reported as 40-90% (79). It is a postural tremor at 3-6 Hz, and a kinetic tremor may be seen (80). It has been reported as disabling and poorly responsive to medication.

Two recent studies have shed further light on inflammatory neuropathies and tremor. In the first epidemiologic case-control study, Ahlskog and colleagues identified 207 cases with neuropathy associated with IgM-monoclonal gammopathy of undetermined significance (IgM-MGUS) from medical records and compared them with 414 cases with non-IgM neuropathy (81). Tremor was documented in a significantly higher proportion of those with IgM-MGUS neuropathy (29%) compared to controls with another neuropathy (9%). The IgM-MGUS group was more likely to have a demyelinating neuropathy, and patients with tremor were even more likely to have a demyelinating than axonal neuropathy (82% vs 18%). Of the non-IgM MGUS neuropathy controls, only 25% had demyelinating neuropathy, and only 10% of the non-IGM MGUS with tremor had a demyelinating neuropathy. Postural-kinetic upper limb tremor was seen in over 80% of the IgM-MGUS neuropathy trem-

or cases, with resting upper limb tremor in 14% and mixed rest/action upper limb tremor in 5%. Of the 60 IgM-MGUS patients with tremor, more than 40% had an alternate explanation for their tremor, and only 25% were referred for movement disorders consultation. Four cases (7%) had major tremor-related disability (81).

Saifee et al. reported on 43 consecutive patients with inflammatory neuropathy receiving IVIG therapy who were referred for further evaluation (82); particular attention was paid to signs of tremor and parkinsonism. They noted tremor in 27 cases (63%). Mean age of onset of tremor was 58 years, and mean duration of disease prior to tremor was 6 years. Tremor was most common in IgM neuropathy, but more than 50% of patients with CIDP and multifocal motor neuropathy with conduction block had tremor. Tremor was always seen with posture and/or action (except for rest tremor in one case of anti-MAG associated neuropathy). The mean tremor frequency was 6 Hz, and it did not change with weight loading (82).

Only 5/27 reported improvement in their tremor with treatment for their neuropathy; 7/27 tried various medications specifically for their tremor, all without benefit (82).

Pathophysiology

The pathophysiology of neuropathy-associated tremor has not yet been determined, though the current theory involves altered feedback with abnormal central processing (83). However, while altered proprioceptive feedback has been thought to be a contributing feature to neuropathy-associated tremor, proprioceptive loss was not increased in those IgM-MGUS patients with tremor compared with non-tremulous IgM-MGUS (81). The authors theorized that IgM-MGUS may cause expression of tremor in those patients with subclinical impairment that eventually could cause tremor (81).

That tremor frequency does not change with weight loading (82) supports the role of a central generator. Successful treatment with thalamic DBS has been reported (81).

Holmes (midbrain) tremor

A series of nine cases was reported by Holmes in 1904 with both a resting tremor and an irregular action tremor. Involvement of the red nucleus and cerebellar outflow tract were felt to be essential to its production, hence the general acceptance of the term midbrain or 'rubral' tremor though Holmes never used those terms himself (84). Isolated lesions of the red nucleus alone do not produce such a tremor, however, and the term 'rubral tremor' has been replaced by midbrain or 'Holmes tremor'. Some prefer to call it a 'resting cerebellar' or 'severe postural cerebellar' tremor (85).

Holmes tremor has a slow frequency (<4.5 Hz) and is not as regular as other tremors. Rest and intention tremor must be present, and many patients have a postural tremor as well (see Video fragment 26.8). Regarding the amplitude, the rest tremor is of smaller amplitude than postural tremor, which is less severe than the intention tremor (1,84). The tremor is usually more of a proximal tremor, and sometimes the lower limb may also be affected with a similar tremor (86). There are often other accompanying features including cranial nerve findings, nystagmus, dysarthria, sensory findings, corticospinal tract involvement, dystonia, and sometimes parkinsonian symptoms.

The tremor is contralateral to the lesion, and evidence points to cerebellothalamic involvement (producing the intention tremor) and nigrostriatal denervation (producing the resting tremor). Holmes tremor is usually caused by either an ischemic or hemorrhagic insult, though mass lesions (such as abscess or tumour) and post-traumatic causes have been identified as well. A variable delay of 4 weeks to 2 years after the insult is generally accepted (1); in a case series of ten patients, 80% experienced onset within 6 months (86). Lesion sites producing Holmes tremor include the midbrain tegmentum, superior cerebellar peduncle, substantia nigra and thalamus (86).

Treatment

The treatment is challenging; while Remy and colleagues reported a good response to dopaminergic therapy for all aspects of tremor (85), others have not found such a response (86). Only 2/6 cases tried on levodopa improved in the series reported by Gajos et al. (86). No significant abnormality on DaT-SCAN imaging was found for dopamine transporter in six cases (not necessarily the same six that were tried on levodopa), but one of the two who improved modestly on levodopa had mild asymmetry in striatal uptake (reduced on the side contralateral to the tremor) (86). In cases responding well to dopaminergic therapy, dopaminergic striatal denervation on functional imaging studies has been documented (85,87).

Palatal tremor (PT)

Originally called palatal myoclonus, the rhythmic nature is mostly in keeping with a slow (1-3Hz) tremor. There are two types, *essential* and *symptomatic*. Rare cases of psychogenic palatal tremor have also been reported in the literature.

Essential PT

Essential palatal tremor is found in about 25% of palatal tremor cases. Rhythmic contractions of tensor veli palatini (innervated by V3) results in elevation of the roof of the soft palate at a mean frequency of under 2 Hz. Contraction of this muscle results in opening/closing of the Eustachian tube and the symptom of ear clicking (see Video fragment 26.9). The tremor disappears with sleep, and there are no other associated findings. Neuroimaging for essential palatal tremor is unremarkable. Its onset is often at a younger age than symptomatic palatal tremor (88,89).

Symptomatic PT

Symptomatic palatal tremor makes up the majority (~75%) of cases (88). A focal brainstem lesion is often identified. Symptomatic palatal tremor can be seen following stroke, encephalitis, demyelinating disease, mass lesion, or degenerative disease (89). Contractions of the levator veli palatini muscle (variably innervated by nn. IX, X or VII depending on the source) results in elevation of the corners of the soft palate. The frequency of contraction is reportedly a bit faster than essential palatal tremor (up to 3 Hz). There are often other associated findings including movements of the eyes (such as pendular nystagmus), face, tongue, neck and even the diaphragm. The movements are synchronous with the palatal tremor and may be subtle. Symptomatic palatal tremor can persist in sleep. There is often a latency (weeks to months) between the insult and the development of symptomatic palatal tremor. The pathway involved is the dentato-rubral-olivary tract (otherwise known as Mollaret's triangle). Fibers from the dentate nucleus in the cerebellum project to the contralateral red nucleus via the superior cerebellar peduncle; the fibers from the red nucleus travel in the central tegmental tract to the ipsilateral inferior olive; the inferior olivary fibers then project to the contralateral dentate via the inferior cerebellar peduncle. In unilateral palatal myoclonus, the lesion localizes to the ipsilateral dentate, with contralateral olivary hypertrophy. A lesion in the dentate would be expected also to cause ipsilateral limb ataxia. While much is made about unilateral lesions and the palatal movements being ipsilateral to the side of the dentate lesion, many cases and videos demonstrate bilateral palatal movements.

Diagnosis

Imaging has revealed signal changes in the olive evident even prior to the clinical appearance of the palatal tremor. Meta-analysis of MRI findings of the inferior olive noted increased T2 signal first appearing at 1 month and persisting for at least 3-4 years, while olivary hypertrophy appeared at 6 months and had resolved by 3-4 years (90). Shaikh and colleagues developed a mathematical model to account for the persistence of palatal tremor years after degeneration of the inferior olive; the oscillator (inferior olive) has its signals modulated (amplified) by the cerebellum, with the tremor persisting as long as the strength of the coupling remains (91).

Treatment

Various treatments have been used for palatal tremor including anticholinergic and dopaminergic agents, benzodiazepines, anticonvulsants, 5-hydroxytryptophan, sumatriptan, and even botulinum toxin injections into the palatal muscles (88), however without consistent effects.

Posttraumatic tremor

Both peripheral and central trauma have been associated with the development of tremor. The tremor may be isolated or not uncommonly occur with dystonia (92).

Peripheral trauma

Cardoso and Jankovic reported on 28 cases identified by medical records with significant peripheral injury associated with the development of tremor (93). The mean interval between injury and tremor onset was just over six weeks; 11 cases had other parkinsonian features; and in 20 of 28 the tremor spread beyond the initial site of involvement. Nine cases had ET or a family history of ET. The proposed pathophysiology is that peripheral trauma may cause central reorganization leading to tremor, particularly in those predisposed to develop tremor (94).

While the cause of peripherally induced tremor is uncertain (and its existence debated by some), there is much stronger evidence for posttraumatic central causes of tremor.

Central trauma

The most common tremor following severe head trauma is a combination of action and rest tremor, likely due to involvement of cerebellar outflow tracts and/or deep cerebellar nuclei and the substantia nigra (95). Krauss and

colleagues reported on 19 cases with severe kinetic post-traumatic tremor; 18/19 had severe
head trauma with diffuse axonal injury on MRI.
All 19 had postural and kinetic appendicular
tremor (13-unilateral, 6-bilateral), and 14 also
had accompanying rest tremor. Lesions of the
dentatothalamic tract were found in 22 instances in these 19 cases (96). Samie et al. reported
on three patients who developed posttraumatic
tremor involving midbrain damage developing
after more than 10 months post-injury (mean).
Postural, kinetic and rest tremor were accompanied by ocular dysmotility, palatal myoclonus,
dysarthria and corticospinal tract findings.
They noted a significant benefit with antricholin-
ergic or dopaminergic therapy (97).

Significant head trauma, however, is not required to develop posttraumatic tremor. Biary
and colleagues reported on seven patients with
either no or transient loss of consciousness who
developed tremor within 1-4 weeks of head trauma. The tremor was postural and kinetic hand
tremor, sometimes involving the head, legs and
trunk, and often with a myoclonic component.
The remaining neurological examination and
cranial imaging were unremarkable. Benefit was
noted in only 1/7 tried on propranolol and 3/6
treated with clonazepam (98).

Tremor associated with posttraumatic parkinsonism is well known to occur as part of the
'punch drunk syndrome' in boxers receiving
repeated blows to the head. Motor vehicle accidents are the most common cause of severe head
trauma and may result in tremor in addition to
other neurological problems. There is often a
latency of several weeks to months required for
posttraumatic movement disorders to develop,
and theories about axonal sprouting, resolution
of edema, oxidative damage or possibly development of a second lesion have been postulated
(95).

Therapies already tried include dopaminergic
medications, anticholinergics, beta-blockers,
benzodiazepines and even anti-seizure medications. Refractory cases may be considered for
surgery, but it is recommended to wait one year
after onset (95).

Video fragments

Fragment 26.1
Essential tremor
Here you might appreciate the clinical expression of a patient suffering a mild, (asymmetric
postural and accompanying action) tremor of
both hands.

Fragment 26.2
Parkinson tremor
Unilateral resting tremor with a short-lasting
suppression of the tremor amplitude after positioning of the hands.

Fragment 26.3
Enhanced physiological tremor
This patient shows a distal, high-frequency
tremor with small amplitude, especially in the
left hand/thumb.

Fragment 26.4
Tremor associated with dystonia (TAWD)
Young woman suffering from cervical dystonia
and torticollis, with an irregular, jerky, postural
tremor of the head with a directional preponderance, using a sensory trick to reduce the
tremor amplitude.

Fragment 26.5
Cerebellar tremor
Woman diagnosed with MS, showing titubation of the head, cerebellar ataxia, and an
intention tremor of both hands.

Treatment

The treatment of posttraumatic tremor is often
challenging. Occasionally, it resolves on its own.

Fragment 26.6
Task-specific tremor
Patient with a task-specific tremor of the right hand, only when writing (primary writing tremor).

Fragment 26.7
Orthostatic tremor
Patient without tremor in the sitting position, showing continuous movements of both legs, starting directly after rising. EMG showed a high-frequency tremor (17 Hz) in the standing position, which disappeared immediately upon sitting.

Fragment 26.8
Midbrain ('Holmes' or 'rubral') tremor
Young man with a posttraumatic midbrain tremor, consisting of a low-frequency position, rest and intention tremor of his left arm.

Fragment 26.9
Essential palatal tremor
Young-onset, rhythmic, low-frequency contractions of the tensor veli palatine resulting in elevations of the roof of the soft palate, with opening/closing of the Eustachian tube and the symptom of ear-clicking (which, unfortunately, cannot be appreciated in this video).

References

1 Deuschl G, Bain P, Brin M, et al. Consensus statement of the Movement Disorder Society. Mov Disord 1998;13:2-23.
2 Defebvre L. Myoclonus and extrapyramidal diseases. Neurophysiologie Clinique 2006;36:319-325.
3 Elble RJ. Differential diagnosis and clinical characteristics of essential tremor. In Lyons KE, Pahwa R, eds. Handbook of essential tremor and other tremor disorders. Boca Raton, FL. Taylor & Francis Group. 2005;77-91.
4 Elble R, Deuschl G. Milestones in tremor research. Mov Disord 2011;26:1096-1105.
5 Elble RJ. Tremor: Clinical features, pathophysiology, and treatment. Neurol Clin 2009;27:679-695.
6 Zeuner KE, Deuschl G. An update on tremors. Curr Opin Neurol 2012;25:475-482.
7 Louis ED, Ferreira JJ. How common is the most common adult movement disorder? Update on the worldwide prevalence of essential tremor. Mov Disord 2010;25(5):534-541.
8 Lou JS, Jankovic J. Essential tremor: clinical correlates in 350 patients. Neurology 1991;41:234-238.
9 Bain PG, Findley LJ, Thompson PD et al. A study of hereditary essential tremor. Brain 1994;117:805-824.
10 Tan EK, Lum SY, Prakash KM. Clinical features of childhood onset essential tremor. Eur J Neurol 2006;13:1302-1305.
11 Louis ED, Fernandez-Alvarez E, Dure LS 4th, et al. Association between male gender and pediatric essential tremor. Mov Disord 2005;20:904-906.
12 Jankovic J, Madisetty J, Vuong KD. Essential tremor among children. Pediatrics 2004;114:1203-1205.
13 Louis ED, Ottman R. Study of Possible Factors Associated With Age of Onset in Essential Tremor. Mov Disord 2006;21:1980-1986.
14 Rajput A, Robinson CA, Rajput AH. Essential tremor course and disability: a clinicopathological study of 20 cases. Neurology 2004;62:932-936.
15 Louis ED, Faust PL, Vonsattel JP, et al. Neuropathological changes in essential tremor: 33 cases compared with 21 controls. Brain 2007; 130: 3297-3307.
16 Rajput AH, Rajput A. Significance of cerebellar Purkinje cell loss to pathogenesis of essential tremor. Parkinsonism Relat Disord 2011;17:410-412.
17 Ross GW, Dickson D, Cersosimo M, et al. Pathological investigation of essential tremor. Neurology 2004;62:A537-A538.
18 Shill HA, Adler CH, Sabbagh MN, et al. Pathologic findings in prospectively ascertained essential tremor subjects. Neurology 2008;70:1452-1455.
19 Rajput AH, Robinson CA, Rajput ML, et al. Cerebellar Purkinje cell loss is not pathognomonic of essential tremor. Parkinsonism Relat Disord 2011;17:16-21.
20 Rajput AH, Robinson CA, Rajput ML, et al. Essential tremor is not dependent upon cerebellar Purkinje cell loss. Parkinsonism Relat Disord 2012;18:626-628.

21 Rajput AH, Robinson CA, Rajput A. Purkinje cell loss is neither pathological basis nor characteristic of essential tremor. Parkinsonism Relat Disord 2013;19:490-491.

22 Axelrad JE, Louis ED, Honig LS et al. Reduced Purkinje cell number in essential tremor: a postmortem study. Arch Neurol 2008;65:101-107.

23 Verschuuren J, Chuang L, Rosenblum MK, et al. Inflammatory infiltrates and complete absence of Purkinje cells in anti-Yo-associated paraneoplastic cerebellar degeneration. Acta Neuropathol 1996;91:519-525.

24 Ishida K, Mitoma H, Wada Y, et al. Selective loss of Purkinje cells in a patient with anti-glutamatic acid decarboxylase antibody-associated cerebellar ataxia. J Neurol Neurosurg Psychiatry 2007;78:190-192.

25 Rajput AH, Maxood K, Rajput A. Classic essential tremor changes following cerebellar hemorrhage. Neurology 2008;71:1739-1740.

26 Dupuis MJM, Evrad FLA, Jacquerye PG, et al. Disappearance of essential tremor after stroke. Mov Disord 2010;25:2884-2887.

27 Boecker H, Weindl A, Brooks DJ, et al. GABAergic dysfunction in essential tremor: an 11C-flumazenil PET study. J Nucl Med 2010;51:1030-1035.

28 Paris-Robidas S, Brochu E, Sintes M, et al. Defective dentate nucleus GABA receptors in essential tremor. Brain 2012;135:105-116.

29 Louis ED, Ottman RD. How familial is familial tremor? The genetic epidemiology of essential tremor. Neurology 1996;46:1200-1205.

30 Tanner CM, Goldman SM, Lyons KE, et al. Essential tremor in twins. An assessment of genetic vs environmental determinants of etiology. Neurology 2001;57:1389-1391.

31 Rajput AH, Rajput A. Increased tremor severity in bilineal essential tremor: a report of two families. Parkinsonism Relat Disord 2006;12:323-326.

32 Jasinska-Myga B, Wider C. Genetics of essential tremor. Parkinsonism Relat Disord 2012;18S1: S138-139.

33 Vilariño-Güell C, Wider C, Ross OA, et al. LINGO1 and LINGO2 variants are associated with essential tremor and Parkinson disease. Neurogenetics 2010;11:401-408.

34 Wood H. Novel FUS gene variants linked to essential tremor. Nat Rev Neurol 2013;9:418.

35 Adler CH, Shill HA, Beach TG. Essential tremor and Parkinson's disease: lack of a link. Mov Disord 2011;26:372-377.

36 Shill HA, Adler CH, Beach TG, et al. Brain biochemistry in autopsied patients with essential tremor. Mov Disord 2012;27:113-117.

37 Ross OA, Conneely KN, Wang T, et al. Genetic variants of α-synuclein are not associated with essential tremor. Mov Disord 2011;26:2552-2556.

38 Louis ED, Babij R, Cortés E, et al. The inferior olivary nucleus: a postmortem study of essential tremor cases versus controls. Mov Disord 2013;28:779-786.

39 Louis ED, Wendt KJ, Pullman SL. Is essential tremor symmetric? Observational data from a community-based study of essential tremor. Arch Neurol 1998;55:1553-1559.

40 Whaley NR, Putzke JD, Baba Y. Essential tremor: phenotypic expression in a clinical cohort. Parkinsonism Relat Disord 2007;13:333-339.

41 Koller WC, Busenbark K, Miner K. The relationship of essential tremor to other movement disorders: report on 678 patients. Essential Tremor Study Group. Ann Neurol 1994;35:717-723.

42 Hubble JP, Busenbark KL, Pahwa R, et al. Clinical expression of essential tremor: effects of gender and age. Mov Disord 1997;12:969-972.

43 Hardesty DE, Maraganore DM, Matsumoto JY, et al. Increased risk of head tremor in women with essential tremor: longitudinal data from the Rochester Epidemiology Project. Mov Disord 2004;19:529-533.

44 Rajput AH, Rozdilsky B, Ang L, et al. Significance of parkinsonian manifestations in essential tremor. Can J Neurol Sci 1993;20:114-117.

45 Louis ED, Asabere N, Agnew A, et al. Rest tremor in advanced essential tremor: a post-mortem study of nine cases. J Neurol Neurosurg Psychiatry 2011;82:261-265.

46 Singer C, Sanchez RJ, Weiner WJ. Gait abnormality in essential tremor. Mov Disord 1994;9:193-196.

47 Helmchen C, Hagenow A, Miesner J, et al. Eye movement abnormalities in essential tremor may indicate cerebellar dysfunction. Brain 2003;126:1319-1332.

48 Teive HAG. Essential tremor: phenotypes. Parkinsonism Relat Disord 2012;18S1:140-142.

49 Bain PG. The clinical assessment of essential tremor. In Lyons KE, Pahwa R, eds. Handbook of essential tremor and other tremor disorders. Boca Raton, FL. Taylor & Francis Group. 2005;93-115.

50 Elble R. Defining dystonic tremor. Curr Neuropharmacol 2013;11:48-52.

51 Deuschl G, Elble R. Essential tremor – neurodegenerative or nondegenerative disease towards a working definition of ET. Mov Disord 2009;24:2033-2041.

52 Josephs KA, Matsumoto JY, Ahlskog JE. Benign tremulous parkinsonism. Arch Neurol 2006;63:354-357.

53 Selikhova M, Kempster PA, Revesz T, et al. Neuropathological findings in benign tremulous parkinsonism. Mov Disord 2013;28:145-152.

54 Rajput AH, Robinson CA, Rajput A. Benign tremulous parkinsonism: a clinicopathological study. Mov Disord 2008;23:311-312.

55 Rajput AH, Jamieson H, Hirsh S, et al. Relative efficacy of alcohol and propranolol in action tremor. Can J Neurol Sci. 1975;2:31-35.

56 Deuschl G, Raethjen J, Hellriegel H, et al. Treatment of patients with essential tremor. Lancet Neurol 2011;10:148-161.

57 Putzke JD, Whaley NR, Baba Y, et al. Essential tremor: predictors of disease progression in a clinical cohort. J Neurol Neurosurg Psychiatry 2006;77:1235-1237.

58 Huang N, Tetrud J. Physiological Tremor. In Lyons KE, Pahwa R, eds. Handbook of essential tremor and other tremor disorders. Boca Raton, FL. Taylor & Francis Group. 2005;361-368.

59 Defazio G, Gigante AF, Abbruzzese G, et al. Tremor in primary adult-onset dystonia: prevalence and associated clinical features. J Neurol Neurosurg Psychiatry 2013;84:404-408.

60 Agnew A, Frucht SJ, Louis ED. Supine head tremor: a clinical comparison of essential tremor and spasmodic torticollis patients. J Neurol Neurosurg Psychiatry 2012;83:179-181.

61 Jankovic J, Mejia NI. Dystonic tremor. In Lyons KE, Pahwa R, eds. Handbook of essential tremor and other tremor disorders. Boca Raton, FL. Taylor & Francis Group. 2005;221-225.

62 Pal PK, Samii A, Schulzer M, et al. Head tremor in cervical dystonia. Can J Neurol Sci 2000;27:137-142.

63 Shaikh AG, Jinnah HA, Tripp RM, et al. Irregularity distinguishes limb tremor in cervical dystonia from essential tremor. J Neurol Neurosurg Psychiatry 2008;79:187-189.

64 Münchau A, Schrag A, Chuang C, et al. Arm tremor in cervical dystonia differs from essential tremor and can be classified by onset age and spread of symptoms. Brain 2001;124:1765-1776.

65 Schiebler S, Schmidt A, Zittel S, et al. Arm tremor in cervical dystonia – is it a manifestation of dystonia or essential tremor? Mov Disord 2011;26:1789-1792.

66 Seeberger LC, Hauser RA. Cerebellar tremor. In Lyons KE, Pahwa R, eds. Handbook of essential tremor and other tremor disorders. Boca Raton, FL. Taylor & Francis Group. 2005;227-241.

67 Fahn S, Jankovic J, Hallett M. Chapter 18: Tremors. In: Principles and practice of movement disorders, 2nd edition. Elsevier Saunders 2011;389-414.

68 Baba Y, Uitti RJ. Fragile X-associated tremor/ataxia syndrome and movement disorders. Curr Opin Neurol 2005;18:393-398.

69 Soland VL, Bhatia KP, Volonte MA, et al. Focal task-specific tremors. Mov Disord 1996;11:665-670.

70 Bain PG, Findley LJ, Britton TC, et al. Primary writing tremor. Brain 1995;118:1461-1472.

71 Hai C, Yu-ping W, Hua W, et al. Advances in primary writing tremor. Parkinsonism Relat Disord 2010;16:561-565.

72 Brown P. New clinical sign for orthostatic tremor. Lancet 1995;346:306-307.

73 Britton TC, Thompson PD, van der Kamp W, et al. Primary orthostatic tremor: further observations in six cases. J Neurol 1992;239:209-217.

74 Wu YR, Ashby P, Lang AE. Orthostatic tremor arises from an oscillator in the posterior fossa. Mov Disord 2001;16:272-279.

75 Piboolnurak P, Yu QP, Pullman SL. Clinical and neurophysiologic spectrum of orthostatic tremor: case series of 26 subjects. Mov Disord 2005;20:1455-1461.

76 Katzenschlager R, Costa D, Gerschlager W, et al. (123I)-FP-CIT-SPECT demonstrates dopamin-

ergic deficit in orthostatic tremor. Ann Neurol 2003;53:489-496.

77 Gerschlager W, Münchau A, Katzenschlager R, et al. Natural history and syndrome associations of orthostatic tremor: a review of 41 patients. Mov Disord 2004;19:788-795.

78 Mestre TA, Lang AE, Ferreira JJ, et al. Associated movement disorders in orthostatic tremor. J Neurol Neurosurg Psychiatry 2012;83:725-729.

79 Alonso-Navarro H, Fernández-Díaz A, Martín-Prieto M, et al. Tremor associated with chronic inflammatory demyelinating peripheral neuropathy: treatment with pregabalin. Clin Neuropharmacol 2008;31:241-244.

80 Saperstein DS, Barohn RJ. Neuropathic tremor. In Lyons KE, Pahwa R, eds. Handbook of essential tremor and other tremor disorders. Boca Raton, FL. Taylor & Francis Group. 2005;275-281.

81 Ahlskog MC, Kumar N, Mauermann ML, et al. IgM-monoclonal gammopathy neuropathy and tremor: a first epidemiologic case control study. Parkinsonism Relat Disord 2012;18:748-752.

82 Saifee TA, Schwingenschuh P, Reilly MM, et al. Tremor in inflammatory neuropathies. J Neurol Neurosurg Psychiatry 2013;84:1282-1287.

83 Deuschl G, Bergman H. Pathophysiology of nonparkinsonian tremors. Mov Disord 2002;17:S41-S48.

84 Dalvi A. Holmes tremor. In Lyons KE, Pahwa R, eds. Handbook of essential tremor and other tremor disorders. Boca Raton, FL. Taylor & Francis Group. 2005;243-250.

85 Remy P, de Recondo A, Defer G et al. Peduncular 'rubral' tremor and dopaminergic denervation: a PET study. Neurology 1995;45:472-477.

86 Gajos A, Bogucki A, Schinwelski M et al. The clinical and neuroimaging studies in Holmes tremor. Acta Neurol Scand 2010;122:360-366.

87 Seidel S, Kasprian G, Leutmezer F et al. Disruption of nigrostriatal and cerebellothalamic pathways in dopamine responsive Holmes' tremor. J Neurol Neurosurg Psychiatry 2009;80:921-923.

88 Goldman JG. Ear clicking after a stroke. In Reich SG, ed. Movement disorders: 100 instructive cases. Informa UK Ltd. 2008;57-60.

89 Fahn S, Jankovic J, Hallett M. Chapter 20: Myoclonus. In: Principles and practice of movement disorders, 2nd edition. Elsevier Saunders 2011;447-464.

90 Goyal M, Versnick E, Tuite P et al. Hypertrophic olivary degeneration: metaanalysis of the temporal evolution of MR findings. AJNR Am J Neuroradiol 2000;21:1073-1077.

91 Shaikh AG, Hong S, Liao K et al. Oculopalatal tremor explained by a model of inferior olivary hypertrophy and cerebellar plasticity. Brain 2010;133:923-940.

92 Jankovic J. Post-traumatic movement disorders: central and peripheral mechanisms. Neurology 1994;44:2006-2014.

93 Cardoso F, Jankovic J. Peripherally induced tremor and parkinsonism. Arch Neurol 1995;52:263-270.

94 Jankovic J. Can peripheral trauma induce dystonia and other movement disorders? Yes! Mov Disord 2001;16:7-12.

95 Hui JS, Lew MF. Posttraumatic tremor. In Lyons KE, Pahwa R, eds. Handbook of essential tremor and other tremor disorders. Boca Raton, FL. Taylor & Francis Group. 2005;283-296.

96 Krauss JK, Wakhloo AK, Nobbe F, et al. Lesion of dentatothalamic pathways in severe post-traumatic tremor. Neurol Res 1995;17:409-416.

97 Samie MR, Selhorst JB, Koller WC. Post-traumatic midbrain tremors. Neurology 1990;40:62-66.

98 Biary N, Cleeves L, Findley L, et al. Post-traumatic tremor. Neurology 1989;39:103-106.

27

Tremor Treatment

Deepa Pothalil & Francois J.G. Vingerhoets

Tremor is one of the most common movement disorders and includes a broad spectrum of entities. Essential tremor (ET) and Parkinson's disease (PD) tremor (see Chapter 26) are the most frequent ones and therefore most thoroughly studied. This review describes the latest recommendations regarding the treatment of different types of tremor, including pharmacological and surgical approaches.

Pharmacotherapeutical approaches

In this section, we will discuss the current therapies of the different types of tremor (1) (see Table 27.1).

Enhanced physiologic tremor

This physiologic tremor is characterized by a high-frequency (>6 Hz), mainly postural tremor without evidence of an underlying neurological disease (1). The cause of enhanced physiological tremor should be identified and corrected (see Table 27.2). In the absence of an evident cause and/or a significant disability induced by the tremor, propanolol (30-320 mg/d) may be administered. Other beta-blockers may be used if there are contra-indications to the use of propanolol (advanced atrioventricular block, severe bradycardia, congestive heart failure, asthma, chronic pulmonary disease and diabetes mellitus): atenolol (200mg/d), metoprolol (200mg/d), acebutolol (400mg/d), oxprenolol (160mg/d), nadolol (80mg/d), timolol (20mg/d) (2). However, selective beta-blockers (such as atenolol, metoprolol (200mg/d) and acebutolol) are known to be less effective in controlling tremor than non-selective ones such as propanolol, oxprenolol, nadolol. In case of a refractory tremor with severe disability, surgical strategies might be considered (see later).

Drug-induced tremor

Some drugs can induce rest, postural, action tremor or different combinations of them (see Table 27.3). If possible the responsible drug has to be stopped, reduced, or replaced. If the condition doesn't allow this or in case of persisting tremor, different therapies may be considered, depending on the type of tremor. For drug-induced parkinsonian and rest tremor, anticholinergics such as trihexylphenidyl (8 to 20 mg/d) or bornaprine (8 mg/d) may be administered (3). For predominant postural tremor, propanolol (30-120 mg/d) may be tried. In valproate-induced postural tremor, acetazolamide (100-150 mg/d) and propanolol have been reported to be effective (4). In lithium-induced postural tremor, beta-blockers (propanolol 60-320 mg/d, nadolol 40- 80 mg/d) and primidone (250 mg/d) are recommended (5). Tetrabenazine (25-200 mg /d) may be used for tardive (post-neuroleptic) tremor (6).

Essential tremor

ET is one of the most common movement disorders. Its overall prevalence is about 0.4%-0.9% in the general population and 4-6% in people aged 65 years and older (7). ET is defined according to the Movement Disorder Society (MDS) consensus statement (1) as a 4-12Hz, bilateral, mostly symmetric, postural or kinetic trem-

Table 27.1
Main pharmacological approaches in the treatment of tremors.

Type of tremor	Medication
Enhanced physiologic tremor	Propanolol (30-320 mg/d) (2)
Drug-induced tremor	Stop or reduce the medication Propanolol (30-120 mg/d) (4,5) Nadolol (40-80 mg/d) (4,5) Primidone (250 mg/d) (4,5) Tetrabenazine (25-200 mg/d) (6)
ET	Propanolol (30-320 mg/d) (7,8) Primidone (30-500 mg/d) (7,8) Association of PRP PRM (7,8) Gabapentin (1200-1400 mg/d) (7) or Topiramate (400-800 mg/d) (7)
PD tremor	L-dopa, Dopaminergic agonists IMAO-B (Anticholinergic drugs) (3) Clozapine (11)
Primary orthostatic tremor	Clonazepam (1.5-2mg/d) (13), Gabapentin (300-1800 mg/d) (14), Primidone (100-300 mg/d) (13)
Task and position-specific tremors	Propanolol (30-320 mg/d) (16), Primidone (62.5 mg/d) (16) Anticholinergic (trihexylphenidyl, up to 6 mg/d) (16), botulinum toxin (17)
Dystonic tremor	Trihexylphenidyl, (3-15 mg/d), Propanolol (120-240 mg/d), Lioresal (15-60 mg/d), Clonazepam (2-6 mg/d)
Cerebellar tremor	Clonazepam (1.5-6 mg) (20), Carbamazepine (400-600 mg/d) (19), Propanolol (30-180 mg/d), topiramate (25-100 mg/d)
Holmes tremor	Levetiracetam (2000-4000 mg/d) (21,22), L-dopa (300 mg/d) (23,24), anticholinergics (single cases)
Palatal tremor	Phenytoin, Carbamazepine, 5-HTP and Sumatriptan (25), Botulinum toxin (26,27)
Neuropathic tremor	Propranolol (80-120 mg /d) (28,29), Primidone (250-500 mg/d) (29,30), Pregabalin (150 mg/d) (31)

or of the hands and forearms, but also including other locations, which persists for 3-5 years without additional signs of neurological disease. Additional or isolated tremor of the head might occur but without abnormal posturing. Other causes for tremor must be excluded first.

First-line (level A) options
Propanolol (30-320 mg/d) or primidone (30-500 mg/d) should be administred as first-line therapy alone or together (level A), taking their

side effects into consideration (7,8). The side effects of propanolol include: bradycardia, hypotension, syncope, depression, apathy, dizziness, sleepiness, fatigue, dryness of the mouth and erectile dysfunction. Because of these side effects, the treatment has to be started at low doses and increased slowly over weeks in order to avoid quick intolerance and discontinuation. Other beta-blockers (arotinolol, sotalol) are also effective, but propanolol has the most potent anti-tremor effect. However, it is ineffective on

Table 27.2
Causes of enhanced physiological tremor.

Metabolic disorders
Hyperthyroidism
Hyperparathyroidism
Cushing syndrome
Hypocalcemia, hypoglycemia
Renal failure
Anxiety
Cold
Fatigue
Alcohol or drug withdrawal

head and voice tremor (7). Primidone's main side effects include sedation, confusion, vertigo, nausea, vomiting, and ataxia. Furthermore, numerous interactions with other medications (tricyclic antidepressants, benzodiazepine, beta-blockers, carbamazepine, cyclosporin, cyclophosphamide, dicoumarin, digitoxin, oral contraceptives, steroids, lamotrigine, losartan, valproic acid, phenytoin, topiramate, paracetamol) are reported.

Both propanolol and primidone tend to lose effectiveness over time; generally speaking, a good response is maintained in only 50% of the patients.

Second-line (level B) options
As second-line therapy, topiramate (400-800 mg/d) and gabapentine (1200-2400 mg/d), in monotherapy, are considered as probably effective (level B). However, there is a 30% drop-out rate because of side effects or ineffectiveness of treatment (7).

Other options
Many other drugs have been used or are in trials for ET (9). Among neuroleptics drugs, there is insufficient evidence to support or refute the use of clozapine as treatment for ET (level U), taking into account the well-known risk of agranulocytosis and cardiac toxicity (8). Among antiepileptic drugs, the use of lacosamide and carisbamate has not been shown to have significant clinical efficacy. Zonisamide showed contradictory re-

Table 27.3
Pharmacotherapeutic approaches for iatrogenic tremor (modified from (9)).

Group	Medication	Type of tremor
Antiarrythmic	Amiodarone, Procainamide	Action tremor
Antidepressant	Tricyclic, SSRI, IMAO A	Action tremor
Beta-adrenergic agents	Terbutaline, adrenaline, Epinephrine	Rest and action tremor
H2 antagonist	Cimetidine	Action tremor
Calcineurine inhibitor	Cyclosporine A	Action tremor
Anticonvulsant	Lamotrigine Valproate sodium	Postural and action tremor Rest and postural tremor
Antipsychotics	Haloperidol, Clozapine Lithium	Rest and postural tremor
Beta-adrenergic inhibitors	Pindolol	Postural tremor
Anti-obstructive agents	Theophylline, steroids	Postural tremor
Triazole antifungal agent	Itraconazole	Heterogeneous rest tremor
Vesicular monoamine transporter type 2 inhibitor	Tetrabenazine	Rest tremor

sults but seems clinically ineffective overall (9). Levetiracetam, 3,4-diaminopyridine and pregabalin do not seem to reduce limb tremor significantly in ET and should not be considered for treatment (9). Botulinum toxin type A injections may be considered in patients with head ET and voice ET refractory to medical therapies (weak recommendation) (7).

Parkinsonian tremor

Tremor in Parkinson's disease (PD) is variable. It is classified into the following three different subtypes (1):

- *Type I, the classic parkinsonian tremor: rest tremor or rest and postural/kinetic tremor with the same frequency.* The pure rest tremor frequency is higher than 4 Hz, while the upper limit can be as high as 9 Hz (in the early stages). The frequency of rest and postural/kinetic tremor is considered the same if their difference is less than 1.5 Hz.
- *Type II, rest and postural/kinetic tremor of different frequencies.* The frequency of the postural/kinetic tremor is higher (>1.5 Hz) than the rest tremor, and they are non-harmonically related. In PD, as a rule, most patients suffer from a rest tremor, along with a mild form of kinetic tremor. Some patients display a combination of a predominant postural tremor and a rest tremor. This specific type of tremor is considered to be related to an essential tremor.
- *Type III, pure postural/kinetic tremor.* This tremor, which is not present at rest, is characterized by a frequency that varies between 4 and 9 Hz.

Dopaminomimetic strategies

Current antiparkinonsian, dopaminomimetic pharmacological agents primarily target bradykinesia, akinesia and rigidity, which are often considered the most disabling symptoms in PD (10). Routinely, dopaminomimetics, both levodopa and dopamine agonists, are introduced first, because of their effects on the other motor signs of PD. The levodopa responsiveness of tremor is unpredictable, though usually the benefits are marginal. Adequate control of tremor in PD might only be achieved at higher doses, but with the risk of inducing fluctuations and dyskinesia. Combining levodopa and dopamine agonists may reduce the L-dopa refractory rest tremor in patients with fluctuations (6). Also, adding selective inhibitors of monoamine oxidase B (selegiline 10 mg/d or rasagiline 0.5 mg and 1 mg/d) to levodopa may improve tremor.

Anticholinergic strategies

Despite earlier assumptions, anticholinergics have not been proved superior to levodopa for the treatment of tremor, and unfortunately also have more side effects, especially the development of cognitive deficits in PD patients (including dementia). Therefore, as a rule, anticholinergics should be avoided, particularly in elderly PD patients. Their application as monotherapy in younger patients with early tremor-dominant PD, however, may be considered under close neuropsychological supervision.

Other strategies

In severe, treatment-refractory rest and postural PD tremor, a low dose of clozapine may be tried before resorting to a surgical approach (11). Also, budipine can be considered as a third-line option, keeping in mind its cardiac side effect (tachyarrythmia) (12).

For PD patients with mixed forms of tremor (type II and III), an association with ET may be suspected. In these patients, propanolol and primidone (level A for ET tremor) should be tried, as monotherapy or adjuvant therapy. Topiramate may also be considered, based on its effectiveness on ET. Zonisamide may also be tried when associated ET is suspected, but the available evidence for its efficacy is contradictory.

Primary orthostatic tremor

Orthostatic tremor is characterized by a subjective feeling of unsteadiness during stance that disappears when the patient walks, sits or lies.

Neurological examination is normal except for a mostly invisible and often only palpable, fine amplitude rippling of the leg muscles (quadriceps or gastrocnemius) when standing. An EMG recording of the leg muscles can confirm the diagnosis by revealing a typical 13-18 Hz tremor (1). The treatment is a challenge, though. Clonazepam (1.5-2mg) (13), gabapentin (300-1800 mg/d) (14,15) and primidone (100-300 mg/d) may be considered (13). Levetiracetam seems ineffective.

Task and position-specific tremors

These tremors are activated by specific situations. Primary writing tremor (PWT) is the most common and occurs only or predominantly during writing but not during other tasks in the active hand. Type A PWT (task-specific tremor) appears only during writing, while type B (position-sensitive tremor) occurs also during pronation of the hand in other tasks (1). Pharmacological treatment is rarely successful and includes propanolol (30-320 mg/d), primidone (62.5 mg/d) (16), anticholinergic (trihexylphenidyl, up to 6 mg/d) (16), or botulinum toxin injections (17).

Dystonic tremor

Different definitions have been proposed for dystonic tremor. It was initially defined as a tremor occuring in a patient with dystonia, but it may appear years before dystonia. Dystonic tremor can consist of (1) tremor in an extremity or body part, which has at least minimal signs of dystonia, (2) focal tremor, usually with irregular amplitudes or a variable frequency (mainly less than 7 Hz), (3) mainly postural/kinetic tremor and usually not seen during complete rest (1). Tremulous spasmodic torticollis (or dystonic head tremor) is a typical example of dystonic tremor. The presence of a *geste antagoniste* leading to a reduction of the tremor amplitude helps differentiate dystonic tremor from essential head tremor.

There is no established therapy. Various treatments have been tried and may be effective

such as: trihexylphenidyl (3-15 mg/d), propanolol (120-240 mg/d), baclofen (15- 60 mg/d) and clonazepam (2-6 mg/d). Botulinum toxin type A injections have also been reported to be effective in some cases (head and voice tremors) (18).

Cerebellar tremor

Cerebellar tremor is a pure or dominant, uni- or bilateral intention tremor with a frequency mainly below 5 Hz, which may be associated with postural tremor but not with rest tremor (1).

There is no established therapy. Small series have shown the efficacy of the following drugs: clonazepam (1.5-6 mg/d), carbamazepine (400-600 mg/d), propanolol (30-180 mg/d), isoniazide, ondansetron and topiramate (25-100 mg/d) (19-20).

Midbrain tremor (Holmes tremor, midbrain tremor, cerebellar overflow tremor, rubral tremor)

Midbrain tremor is a low-frequency (usually less than 4.5 Hz), large-amplitude tremor (proximal rest and sometimes intention though mostly postural) resulting from combined lesions of the nigrostriatal, cerebellothalamic and cerebello-olivary pathways. Adequate treatment is a challenge. In two cases, levetiracetam (2000-4000 mg/d) has led to remarkable improvement (21,22), and occasionally dopaminomimetics are reported to be effective (23,24).

Palatal tremor

Palatal tremor has two forms:

- *Essential palatal tremor*: this is a rhythmic palatal tremor (or myoclonus) accompanied by a rhythmic ear click, acknowledged by the patient. It is caused by an isolated brainstem lesion.
- *Symptomatic palatal tremor*: this is a rhythmic contraction of the levator veli palatini muscle, which might be associated with rhythmic movements of the eyes and/or other body parts. This tremor usually results from a brainstem or cerebellar lesion with subsequent olivary

hypertrophy (1). There are few treatment options. Phenytoin, carbamazepine, 5-HTP and sumatriptan may be effective (25). Botulinum toxin can be injected in the levator and tensor veli palatini muscles for severe cases (26,27).

Neuropathic tremor

This postural and kinetic tremor might be seen in patients with a peripheral neuropathy, predominantly a demyelinating neuropathy, particularly in association with dysgammaglobulinemia. The frequency of this tremor in the arm is often higher proximally than distally in patients with gammopathies (1). If the tremor persists after the treatment of the underlying peripheral neuropathy, propranolol (80-120 mg /d) (28,29), primidone (250-500 mg/d) (29,30), or pregabalin (150 mg/d) (31) might be effective.

Psychogenic tremor

Psychogenic tremors have a very heterogeneous clinical presentation. They might be suspected in the presence of one or more of the following criteria: (1) sudden onset and/or sudden remission of the condition; (2) unusual clinical combination of rest and postural/intention tremors; (3) decrease of tremor amplitude during distraction; (4) variation of tremor frequency during distraction or during voluntary movements of the contralateral hand; (5) coactivation of flexors and extensors digitorum about 300 msec prior to tremor onset in electromyographic recordings; (6) somatization in the past history; and (7) appearance of additional, unrelated neurological signs (1) (see Video fragment 27.1). Unfortunately, there is no established treatment for psychogenic tremor, but early diagnosis and an adequate multidisciplinary approach including psychotherapy are recommended (32,33).

Surgical approaches

In the case of severe, treatment-refractory tremor (defined as a tremor refractory to adequate trials of at least two medications, at a therapeutic dose, for more than 1 month), surgical approaches might be considered, such as high-frequency deep brain stimulation and lesional surgery. These approaches have been particularly well studied for patients with ET and PD tremor. Alternatives include stereotactic radiofrequency thalamotomy as well as the still experimental stereotactic radiosurgical thalamotomy (gammaknife) and MR-guided focused ultrasound thalamotomy (34) (see Table 27.4).

Deep brain stimulation (DBS)

Essential tremor

Between 25% and 55% of patients with ET will develop a disabling pharmaco-resistant tremor (35). The main neurosurgical target to treat ET is the ventro-intermediate thalamic nucleus (Vim) (see Video fragment 27.2). High-frequency deep brain stimulation offers advantages over classical lesioning surgery: the reversibility of the procedure, the post- surgical modulation, the possibility of bilateral procedures, the milder and less frequent adverse events (36,37). However, DBS implies an invasive procedure and relies on permanently implanted materials. Although DBS is rather safe and effective for tremor, there is still not enough evidence to fully support this strategy (level C) (8).

DBS-related complications are both device-related (lead breakage in 2.5% and electrode migration in 2%) or surgery-related (such as wound infection in 2% or intracranial hemorrhage in 1-4%) (37,38).

Over time, one-quarter of patients treated by Vim-DBS for ET may progressively lose the benefit of DBS. They will need continuous adjustments of stimulation parameters and may even need intermittent stimulation to regain the benefit initially obtained. DBS in the subthalamic nucleus (STN) has also been proposed as a target for long-term treatment of ET, but only very few studies support it (39) as it can be associated with severer adverse events in elderly patients (>70 years), for whom the Vim-DBS remains a preferable target (7).

Table 27.4
Overview of pros and cons of surgical therapeutic approaches.

	Advantages	Disadvantages
Deep brain stimulation (35,36,37,38,40)	▪ Good functional outcome ▪ Electrophysiological confirmation of the target ▪ Reversibility, post-surgical modulation ▪ Fewer adverse events than lesional surgery	▪ Invasive ▪ Lead breakage, wound infection ▪ Electrode migration ▪ Intracranial hemorrhage
Stereotactic radio-frequency thalamotomy (36,37,38)	▪ Good functional outcome	▪ Invasive ▪ Frequent major side effects contraindicating bilateral application (dysarthria, paresthesia, hemiparesis, abulia)
Stereotactic radiosurgical thalamotomy (gammaknife) (44,45,46)	▪ Less invasive ▪ Suitable for elderly patients, under anticoagulants, with coagulopathy or serious medical comorbidities contraindicating neurosurgical procedure	▪ No electrophysiological confirmation of the target ▪ Dependance on anatomical imaging ▪ Delay until clinical results Risks of delayed neurological deficits ▪ Outcome of bilateral procedure unknown
Focused, high-energy US (34)	▪ Good functional outcome ▪ Less invasive	▪ Side effects (dysarthria, paresthesia, hemiparesis ataxia, dystonia, speech disturbance, memory loss) ▪ No electrophysiological confirmation of the target ▪ Dependance on anatomical imaging ▪ Outcome of bilateral procedure unknown

It has been proposed that DBS of the posterior subthalamic area (with prelemniscal radiation and the caudal zona incerta) might be more effective in some patients (40), although this is still controversial. Vim and/or prelemniscal radiation DBS may be also useful for cerebellar, dystonic, orthostatic, and Holmes tremor, but to a lesser extent than for ET and PD tremors (41). DBS has also been suggested for disabling secondary tremors in multiple sclerosis and neuropathy. Its efficacy has been shown in open-labelled studies, but the benefits seem to disappear over time, emphasizing the need to stabilise the underlying disease before surgery (42).

PD tremor

In contrast to bradykinesia and rigidity, PD tremor responds better to surgical approaches than to medication. Therefore, while levodopa responsiveness of parkinsonism is mandatory for each indication for surgical approaches in advanced PD, this is not required for an indication aiming to treat parkinsonian tremor.

There are three main surgical targets which have proven effective in controlling PD rest and postural tremor: the ventro-intermediate nucleus (Vim), globus pallidus internus (GPi), and subthalamic nucleus (STN). Other targets also offering an adequate control of tremor include the posterior subthalamic area (zona incerta and prelemniscal radiation) (43).

Thalamic Vim stimulation is effective in treating pharmaco-resistant tremor in PD. In most patients, however, it is not the preferable target because of its lack of efficacy on other major signs of PD.

Both GPi and STN targets have the advantage of being effective for tremor and other motor symptoms of PD, and are the targets of choice even in a tremor-dominant case as disease progression will lead these motor signs to worsen (see Video fragment 27.3). As the evolution of PD implies the development of bilateral symptoms, bilateral procedures have to be considered. Although STN is the better documented target, the choice between the two targets is still being debated and mainly based upon associated comorbities, such as behaviour and neuropsychologic side effects that seem to occur less frequently with GPi stimulation.

Thalamotomies (Vim)

Used for decades to treat tremor, this neurosurgical procedure comprises a steretotactic operation to produce a localized coagulative lesion within the physiologically identified thalamic ventro-intermediate nucleus (Vim). More recently, such thalamotomies have also been realized by radiofrequency and/or radiation (gammaknife) (44-46).

Thalamotomy and high-frequency thalamic DBS appear to be equally effective for the suppression of drug-resisting tremor, but 6 months after the treatment there is greater improvement in function with thalamic stimulation. As the adverse events in classical thalamotomies are severer and more frequent than with DBS, particularly bilateral lesioning (47,48), lesional surgery is only considered for unilateral procedures in case of contraindication to DBS (44).

The recently introduced, radiosurgical thalamotomy appears to be as effective as Vim-DBS for refractory tremors, but there is not yet enough information to encourage its application (level

C) (8). In gammaknife thalamotomy, the lesion of the lateral part of the Vim nucleus is accomplished with a very focused, single shot of irradiation (130 Gy) on the isocenter of the target localized by MRI. Although unilateral, gammaknife-induced lesions are considered as effective in controlling the tremor as Vim DBS (success rate of 73-93%), its more frequent adverse events (hemiparesis/hemiplegia, aphasia, dysphagia, visual field defects, dystonia, tremor or other movement disorders) (46) prevent its routine application. As there is no electrophysiological confirmation of the target site, and as no definite optimal radiation dose has been defined, an unpredictable larger lesion than expected might occur, leading to those persisting neurological deficits. Because of the delay of weeks to months to achieve the final clinical results and/or delayed progressive neurological deficits, the application of the gammaknife in the treatment of refractory essential tremors is still being debated (level U) (5). It must be taken into consideration, though, that this method is less invasive, as it does not require penetration of the brain, and does not need implantation of devices. So, this strategy might be considered only in patients ineligible for invasive surgery (advanced age, use of anticoagulants, coagulopathy, serious medical comorbidities) (45,46). MR-guided, focused ultrasound thalamotomy offers the same advantages as gammaknife thalamotomy as it also depends on anatomical imaging, and may lead to serious side effects (dysarthria, paresthesia, hemiparesis ataxia, dystonia) (34). Thus, the same restrictions as with the gammaknife apply to its use: its unilateral approach might only be considered in research protocols for patients with a contraindication to DBS.

Conclusion

The treatment of each tremor has to be adapted to its specific type as well as its related functional disability. First and second lines of pharmacotherapeutical strategies should be tried before eventually considering surgical approaches. Surgical strategies should only be considered in disabling refractory tremors when the clinical benefits outweigh the potential risks. If bilateral surgery is required, DBS is the only acceptable option at the moment. Unilateral lesions are only an option when DBS is contraindicated. New approaches (gammaknife, high-density ultrasounds) should be considered in research protocols.

Video fragments

Fragment 27.1
Psychogenic tremor
Inconsistent distal tremor of the right hand, with variable frequency and amplitude. This tremor originally had the characteristics of a position tremor, but later on, there were also aspects of a resting tremor. The tremor is suppressed by entrainment.

Fragment 27.2
Bilateral Vim-DBS in essential tremor PD
(segments 1-2)
In this video you might see the significant effects of bilateral thalamic Vim-DBS in a 70 yr old lady with a disabling essential tremor before (segment 1) and after (segment 2) Vim-DBS.

Fragment 27.3
STN-DBS in tremor-dominant PD
In this video you might appreciate the quick response of rest tremor to STN-DBS macrostimulation during operative implantation of bilateral subthalamic electrodes in a 68-year-old patient with tremor-dominant idiopathic Parkinson's disease.

References

1 Deuschl G, Bain P, Brin M, . Consensus statement of the Movement Disorder Society on tremor. Ad hoc scientific committee. Mov Dis 1998;13S3:2-23.

2 Feely J, Peden N. Use of beta-adrenoceptor blocking drugs in hyperthyroidism. Drugs. 1984;27:425-446.

3 Katzenschlager R, Sampaio C, Costa J, Lees A. Anticholinergics for symptomatic management of Parkinson's disease. Cochrane Database Syst Rev. 2003;2:CD003735.

4 Perucca E. Pharmacological and therapeutic properties of valproate: a summary after 35 years of clinical experience. CNS Drugs 2002;16:695-714.

5 Arbaizar B, Gómez-Acebo I, Llorca J. Postural induced-tremor in psychiatry. Psychiatry Clin Neurosci. 2008;62:638-645.

6 Fernandez HH, Friedman JH. Classification and treatment of tardive syndromes. Neurologist. 2003;9:16-27.

7 Zappia M, Albanese A, Bruno E, et al. Treatment of essential tremor : a systematic review of evidence and recommendations from the Italian Movement Disorders Association. J Neurol 2013;260:714-740.

8 Zesiewicz TA, Elble RJ, Louis ED, et al. Evidence-based guideline update: treatment of essential tremor: report of the Quality Standards subcommittee of the American Academy of Neurology.Neurology 2011;77:1752-1755.

9 Zeuner KE, Deuschl G. An update on tremors Curr Opin Neurol 2012;25:475-482.

10 Jiménez MC, Vingerhocts FJ. Tremor revisited: treatment of PD tremor. Parkinsonism Relat Disord. 2012;18S1:93-95.

11 Thomas AA, Friedman JH. Current use of clozapine in Parkinson disease and related disorders. Clin Neuropharmacol 2010;33:14-16.

12 Reichmann H. Budipine in Parkinson's tremor. J Neurol Sci. 2006;248:53-55.

13 Gerschlager W, Münchau A, Katzenschlager R, et al. Natural history and syndromic associations of orthostatic tremor: a review of 41 patients. Mov Disord. 2004;19:788-795.

14 Evidente VG, Adler CH, Caviness JN, Gwinn KA. Effective treatment of orthostatic tremor with gabapentin. Mov Disord. 1998;13:829-831.

15 Rodrigues JP, Edwards DJ, Walters SE, et al. Blinded placebo crossover study of gabapentin in primary orthostatic tremor. Mov Disord. 2006;21:900-905.

16 Hai C, Yu-ping W, Hua W, Ying S. Advances in primary writing tremor. Parkinsonism Relat Disord. 2010;16:561-565.

17 Papapetropoulos S, Singer C. Treatment of primary writing tremor with botulinum toxin type a injections: report of a case series. Clin Neuropharmacol. 2006;29:364-367.

18 Brin MF, Lyons KE, Doucette J, et al. A randomized, double masked, controlled trial of botulinum toxin type A in essential hand tremor. Neurology. 2001;56:1523-1528.

19 Sechi GP, Zuddas M, Piredda M, et al. Treatment of cerebellar tremors with carbamazepine: a controlled trial with long-term follow-up. Neurology. 1989;39:1113-1115.

20 Gbadamosi J, Buhmann C, Moench A, Heesen C. Failure of ondansetron in treating cerebellar tremor in MS patients - an open-label pilot study. Acta Neurol Scand. 2001;104:308-311.

21 Ferlazzo E, Morgante F, Rizzo V,et al. Successful treatment of Holmes tremor by levetiracetam. Mov Disord. 2008;23:2101-2103

22 Striano P, Elefante A, Coppola A, Tortora F, Zara F, Minetti C. Dramatic response to levetiracetam in post-ischaemic Holmes' tremor. BMJ Case Rep. 2009:438-439.

23 Boelmans K, Gerloff C, Münchau A. Long-lasting effect of levodopa on holmes' tremor. Mov Disord. 2012;27:1097-1098.

24 Strecker K, Schneider JP, Sabri O, et al. Responsiveness to a dopamine agent in Holmes tremor--case report. Eur J Neurol. 2007;14:9-10.

25 Pakiam AS, Lang AE. Essential palatal tremor: evidence of heterogeneity based on clinical features and response to Sumatriptan. Mov Disord. 1999;14:179-180.

26 Carman KB, Ozkan S, Yarar C, Yakut A. Essential palatal tremor treated with botulinum toxin. Pediatr Neurol. 2013;48:415-417.

27 Penney SE, Bruce IA, Saeed SR. Botulinum toxin is effective and safe for palatal tremor: a report of five cases and a review of the literature. J Neurol. 2006;253:857-860.

28 Delwaide PJ, Schoenen J. Non-hypertrophic familial neuropathy associated with intention tremor. A variety of Charcot-Marie-Tooth disease? J Neurol Sci. 1976;27:59-69.

29 Bain PG, Britton TC, Jenkins IH, et al. Tremor associated with benign IgM paraproteinaemic neuropathy. Brain. 1996;119:789-799.

30 Budak F, Alemdar M, Kamaci S, Selekler M. Tremor in idiopathic distal acquired demyelinating symmetric neuropathy. Mov Disord. 2005;20:1529-1530.

31 Alonso-Navarro H, Fernández-Díaz A, Martín-Prieto M, et al. Tremor associated with chronic inflammatory demyelinating peripheral neuropathy: treatment with pregabalin. Clin Neuropharmacol. 2008;31:241-244.

32 Ellenstein A, Kranick SM, Hallett M. An update on psychogenic movement disorders. Curr Neurol Neurosci Rep. 2011;11:396-403.

33 Hinson VK, Weinstein S, Bernard B, Leurgans SE, Goetz CG. Single-blind clinical trial of psychotherapy for treatment of psychogenic movement disorders. Parkinsonism Relat Disord. 2006;12:177-180.

34 Lipsman N, Schwartz ML, Huang Y, et al. MR-guided focused ultrasound thalamotomy for essential tremor: a proof-of-concept study. Lancet Neurol. 2013;12:462-468.

35 Flora ED, Perera CL, Cameron AL, Maddern GJ. Deep brain stimulation for essential tremor: a systematic review. Mov Disord 2010;25:1550-1559.

36 Pahwa R, Lyons KE, Wilkinson SB, et al. Comparison of thalamotomy to deep brain stimulation of the thalamus in essential tremor. Mov Disord 2001;16:140-143.

37 Schuurman PR, Bosch DA, Bossuyt PM, et al. A comparison of continuous thalamic stimulation and thalamotomy for suppression of severe tremor. N Engl J Med. 2000;342:461-468.

38 Bahgat D, Magill ST, Berk C, McCartney S, Burchiel KJ. Thalamotomy as a treatment option for tremor after ineffective deep brain stimulation. Stereotact Funct Neurosurg 2013;91:18-23.

39 Lind G, Schechtmann G, Lind C, Winter J, Meyerson BA, Linderoth B. Subthalamic stimulation for essential tremor. Short- and long-term results and critical target area. Stereotact Funct Neurosurg. 2008;86:253-258.

40 Blomstedt P, Sandvik U, Fytagoridis A, Tisch S. The posterior subthalamic area in the treatment of movement disorders: past, present, and future. Neurosurgery 2009;64:1029-1042.

41 Elble R, Deuschl G. Milestones in tremor research. Mov Disord 2011;26:1096-1105.

42 Torres CV, Moro E, Lopez-Rios AL, et al. Deep brain stimulation of the ventral intermediate nucleus of the thalamus for tremor in patients with multiple sclerosis. Neurosurgery. 2010;67:646-651.

43 Blomstedt P, Sandvik U, Fytagoridis A, Tisch S. The posterior subthalamic area in the treatment of movement disorders: past, present, and future. Neurosurgery 2009;64:1029-1038.

44 Lim SY, Hodaie M, Fallis M, Poon YY, Mazzella F, Moro E. Gamma knife thalamotomy for disabling tremor: a blinded evaluation. Arch Neurol 2010;67:584-588.

45 Ohye C, Higuchi Y, Shibazaki T, et al. Gamma knife thalamotomy for Parkinson disease and essential tremor: a prospective multicenter study. Neurosurgery 2012;70:526-536.

46 Kondziolka D, Ong JG, Lee JY, Moore RY, Flickinger JC, Lunsford LD. Gamma Knife thalamotomy for essential tremor. J Neurosurg 2008;108:111-117.

47 Schuurman PR, Bosch DA, Bossuyt PM, et al. A comparison of continuous thalamic stimulation and thalamotomy for suppression of severe tremor. N Engl J Med 2000;342:461-468.

48 Schuurman PR, Bosch DA, Merkus MP, Speelman JD. Long-term follow-up of thalamic stimulation versus thalamotomy for tremor suppression. Mov Disord. 2008;23:1146-1153.

28
Myoclonus

Rodi Zutt, Jan Willem Elting & Marina A.J. Tijssen

Myoclonus is characterized by sudden, brief, involuntary jerks of a muscle or a group of muscles. It can be caused by muscle contraction (*positive myoclonus*) or by interruptions of tonic muscle activity (*negative myoclonus*). The symptom was first described in 1881 by Friedreich using the term 'paramyoclonus multiplex' in a patient with essential myoclonus (1). Negative myoclonus was first described in 1963 by Lance and Adams in patients with post-hypoxic myoclonus (2).

Classifications

There are three generally accepted ways to categorize myoclonus: anatomically, clinically, and etiologically. The most common classification is by anatomic origin of the myoclonic jerks. It can be generated from the cortex, subcortical areas (including brainstem), spinal cord or peripheral nerves. The second classification is based on clinical signs, including the relation to motor activity, the distribution and the temporal pattern. The third classification is based on aetiology and was first described by Marsden in 1982 (3). The numerous causes of myoclonus can be divided into 4 groups: physiological myoclonus, essential myoclonus (myoclonus dystonia), epileptic myoclonus and symptomatic myoclonus.

Because of its usefulness in daily practice, we will use the anatomical classification as the basis in this chapter. Each category has its own clinical and electrophysiological characteristics, aetiology and treatment options.

Epidemiology

Little is known about the epidemiology of myoclonus, mainly because it has a wide clinical spectrum with numerous causes. People with mild myoclonus may not consult a physician, physicians will not always recognize myoclonic jerks, and most importantly, myoclonus can be overshadowed by other neurological features. There is one study, carried out in a defined population in Olmsted Country from 1976 to 1990, showing a lifetime prevalence of persistent and pathological myoclonus of 8.6 cases per 100,000. In 72%, the cause of myoclonus was symptomatic, followed by 17% with an epileptic origin, and 11% essential myoclonus (4,5). In patients presenting at the emergency room with movement disorders, 27.6% suffered from myoclonus, mostly provoked by metabolic disturbance or drugs (6).

Clinical presentation

The clinical presentation of myoclonus has different aspects, including the relation to motor activity, the distribution, the temporal pattern, and the division into positive and negative myoclonus. The relation to motor activity can be classified as myoclonus at rest or during voluntary activity such as action or intention. *Action myoclonus* is frequently seen in patients with cortical myoclonus (CM). *Reflex myoclonus* can be provoked by unexpected tactile, visual or auditory stimuli. Usually, the fingers and toes are the most sensitive areas to a tactile stimulus, which can induce a series of myoclonus (7).

Reflex myoclonus is an important feature of CM and brainstem myoclonus.

The distribution of myoclonus can be focal, segmental, axial or generalized. In focal myoclonus the jerks are restricted to a defined body part. Jerks can originate from different levels of the central nervous system, but are most frequently generated in the cortex. Segmental myoclonus involves adjacent areas of one segment of the body (for example one limb or part of the face) and usually reflects spinal myoclonus. Multifocal myoclonus involves 2 or more nonadjacent areas of the body. Multifocal myoclonus can be part of subcortical myoclonus or CM as in progressive and static myoclonus encephalopathy or metabolic disorders. Generalized myoclonus involves synchronous jerks of multiple segments and is usually an expression of (propio-)spinal or brainstem myoclonus such as reticular reflex myoclonus or excessive startle reflexes.

The temporal pattern of myoclonus is generally arrhythmic, but it can be rhythmic (in segmental myoclonus or palatal myoclonus – therefore, the latter is also referred to as palatal tremor). In rare cases, the pattern is oscillatory and resembles fast tremor. Myoclonus can be synchronized (in brainstem reticular reflex myoclonus) or non-synchronized.

Myoclonus can be based on muscular contractions (positive myoclonus) or on an interruption of a muscle contraction (negative myoclonus). Both cortical and subcortical mechanisms may be involved in the generation of negative myoclonus (8). Two forms of negative myoclonus have been described (9). First, 'asterixis', also called flapping tremor, probably has a subcortical generator and can be seen in patients with a

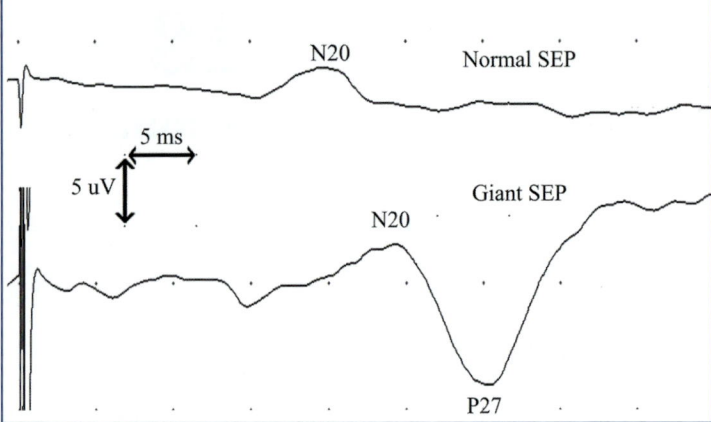

Figure 28.1 Giant SEP
Example of a giant somatosensory evoked potential (SEP). Upper trace: a normal SEP response showing a normal voltage N20 response at appropriate latency. Lower trace: Giant SEP response in a patient with mitochondrial encephalopathy and cortical myoclonus. The N20 is slightly delayed, and the late potential complex (P27/N30) is enlarged.

toxic-metabolic encephalopathy (10). This negative myoclonus is caused by a sudden interruption of ongoing muscle contraction and a brief lapse in limb posture (see Video fragment 28.1). It is usually bilateral and rhythmic. Unilateral asterixis can be seen in patients with thalamic lesions (11). The second form of negative myoclonus involves the axial and proximal lower limbs, resulting in patients losing their posture. For example in Lance–Adams syndrome, this can cause a person to fall.

Myoclonus assigned to anatomical classification

Cortical myoclonus (CM)

Pathophysiology
Cortical myoclonus is the result of abnormal firing of the sensorimotor cortex. This generated activity travels through the fast corticospinal pathways, resulting in short-lasting myoclonic jerks in muscles (13,14). Neuropathological studies show involvement of the cerebellum, fronto-temporal cortex, hippocampus, and thalamus, among other areas (15,16). The exact

mechanisms that induce cortical hyperexcitability and their localization in the brain are not fully known. A generator in the primary motor cortex is suggested by cortical lesions inducing myoclonus and supported by magnetoencephalography (MEG) studies (17). An alternative hypothesis includes functional cortical changes due to a channelopathy. Channelopathies are recognized in the inherited epilepsy syndromes. Finally, changes in sensory input may also be an important factor in the generation of CM, as suggested by its stimulus sensitivity and the giant somatosensory evoked potentials (SEPs) found on electrophysiological examination. Based on the cerebellar changes in patients with celiac disease and those with familial cortical myoclonic tremor and epilepsy (FCMTE), both with CM, it has been hypothesized that decreased cortical inhibition via the cerebello-thalamo-cortical loop is a principle cause of CM (15).

Clinical presentation
Jerks manifest predominantly (multi)focally and are often exacerbated by voluntary movements, although they can also occur spontaneously. Myoclonus can often be auditory, somasthetic, or provoked by an verbal stimulus (reflex myoclonus) (18,19). Because of the somatotopic distribution of the cortex, body parts with large cortical presentation, like mouth, face and hands, are more affected than other parts (19,20) (see Video fragment 28.2).

Electrophysiological examination
Electromyography in CM reveals short EMG bursts (usually < 50ms) (21,22). On the SEP, enlarged (giant) cortical amplitude reflects a decreased intra-cortical inhibition (see Figure 28.1). Hereby, the P27 and N35 peaks have large amplitudes (> 5mV) (17). In patients with CM, a C-reflex can be present. It can be seen in the ipsilateral thenar muscle with a latency of around

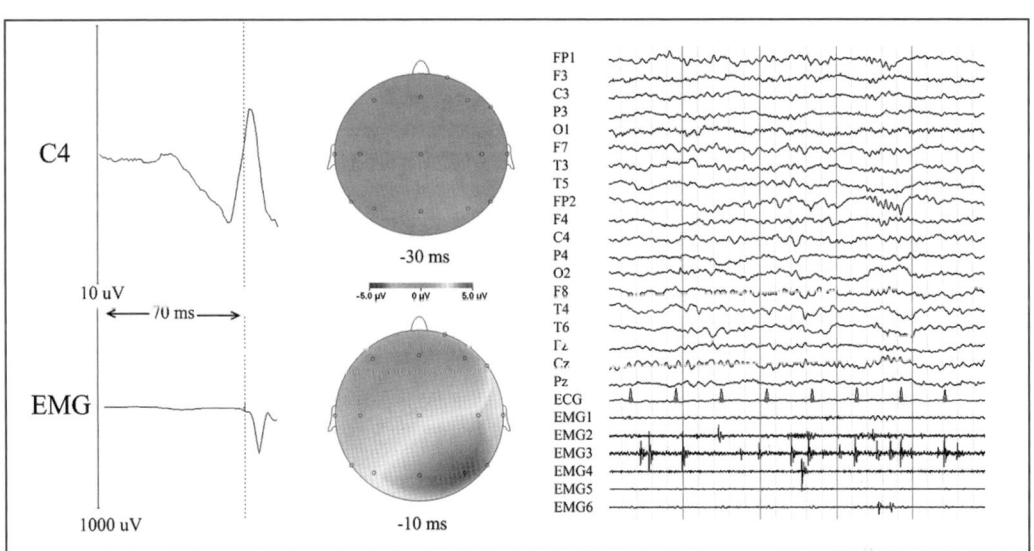

Figure 28.2 Cortical myoclonus
Example of a cortical potential preceding the myoclonus in a patient with cortical myoclonus due to encephalitis associated with anti-voltage-gated potassium channel (VGKC) antibodies. Right panel: 5 seconds of raw EEG and EMG data of muscles of the left arm. Note the short duration of the EMG bursts. The EEG shows generalized slowing but no epileptic abnormalities. Left panel: after backaveraging of 162 epochs of myoclonus, a clear positive-negative potential can be seen in the right centroparietal electrodes which starts at approximately 25 ms before myoclonus onset. Middle panel: Topographic mapping: at 30 ms before myoclonus onset, no cortical potential is visible, while at 10 ms before myoclonus onset, the right centroparietal field distribution can be appreciated.

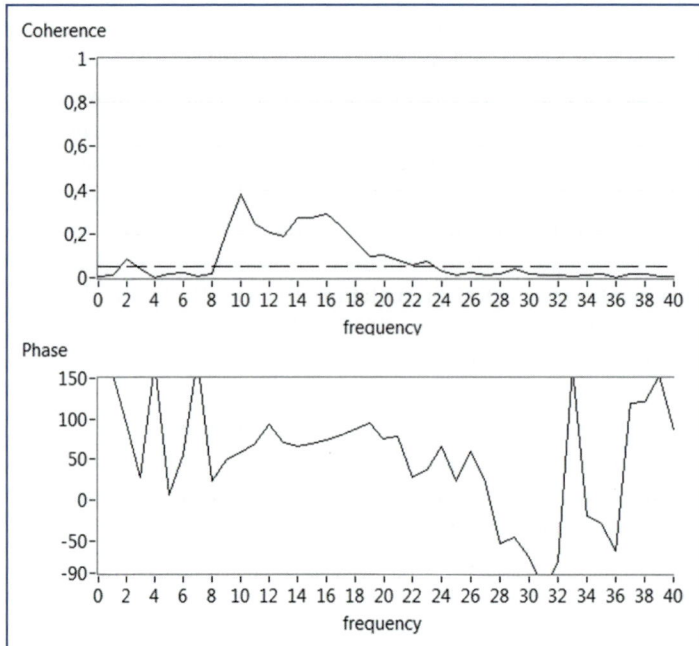

Figure 28.3 EEG-EMG coherence analysis in cortical myclonus
Example of coherence analysis in a patient with high frequency cortical myoclonus. EEG channel: C3 EMG channel: first dorsal interosseus muscle on the right side (raw data not shown). Analysis of a 60 seconds duration epoch in which high frequency myoclonus of 7-10 Hz was present. Averaging of 60 epochs of 1000 ms duration. Upper panel: Coherence vs frequency plot. The dotted line indicates the level above which coherence can be considered significant. Significant coherence is present in the 9-23 Hz frequency range. Lower panel: Phase plot which shows an increasing phase difference with increasing frequency. According to the 'constant phase shift plus constant time lag' model (74), this means that EEG leads EMG with a calculated lead time 19 ms, compatible with the expected cortico-muscular conduction time.

45 ms, and sometimes contralateral with a delay of 10-15 ms pointing to interhemispheric spread (22). With the use of EEG back-averaging, a 'time-locked' biphasic potential can be revealed on the contralateral sensory cortex preceding the jerks seen on the EMG (21) (see Figure 28.2). The biphasic potential precedes the EMG activity by 15-25 ms for jerks in the arms and by 40 ms for jerks in the legs (21). In high-frequency or continuous myoclonus, back-averaging is technically not possible, and coherence analysis can be performed to reveal the correlation between cortical and muscle activity and between muscles (23) (see Figure 28.3). In CM, an exagger-

ated corticomuscular and intermuscular coherence in the alpha and beta band can be detected with a phase difference consistent with a cortical drive (23-26).

All the described electrophysiological findings support the clinical diagnosis of CM. The sensitivity and specificity of the electrophysiological tests in clinical practice are unknown, however.

Etiology
CM is the most frequent form of myoclonus and can be induced by numerous underlying disorders. Causes of CM can roughly be divided into two different categories, i.e. as part of epilepsy syndromes and symptomatic due to a long list of causes (see Figure 28.4). Although symptomatic, the neurodegenerative, genetic or prion-induced progressive myoclonic encephalopathies (with epilepsy and/or dementia, with dementia or with parkinsonism) and the static (post-anoxic) myoclonic encephalopathies will be described separately.

Epileptic myoclonus
CM jerks can be part of different kinds of epilepsy syndromes such as isolated epileptic myoclonic jerks, photosensitive myoclonus, myoclonic absences with petit mal and progressive myoclonus epilepsy (PME). One of the most frequent forms is *juvenile myoclonus epilepsy* (JME), characterized by primary generalized epilepsy and myoclonic jerks which occur in-

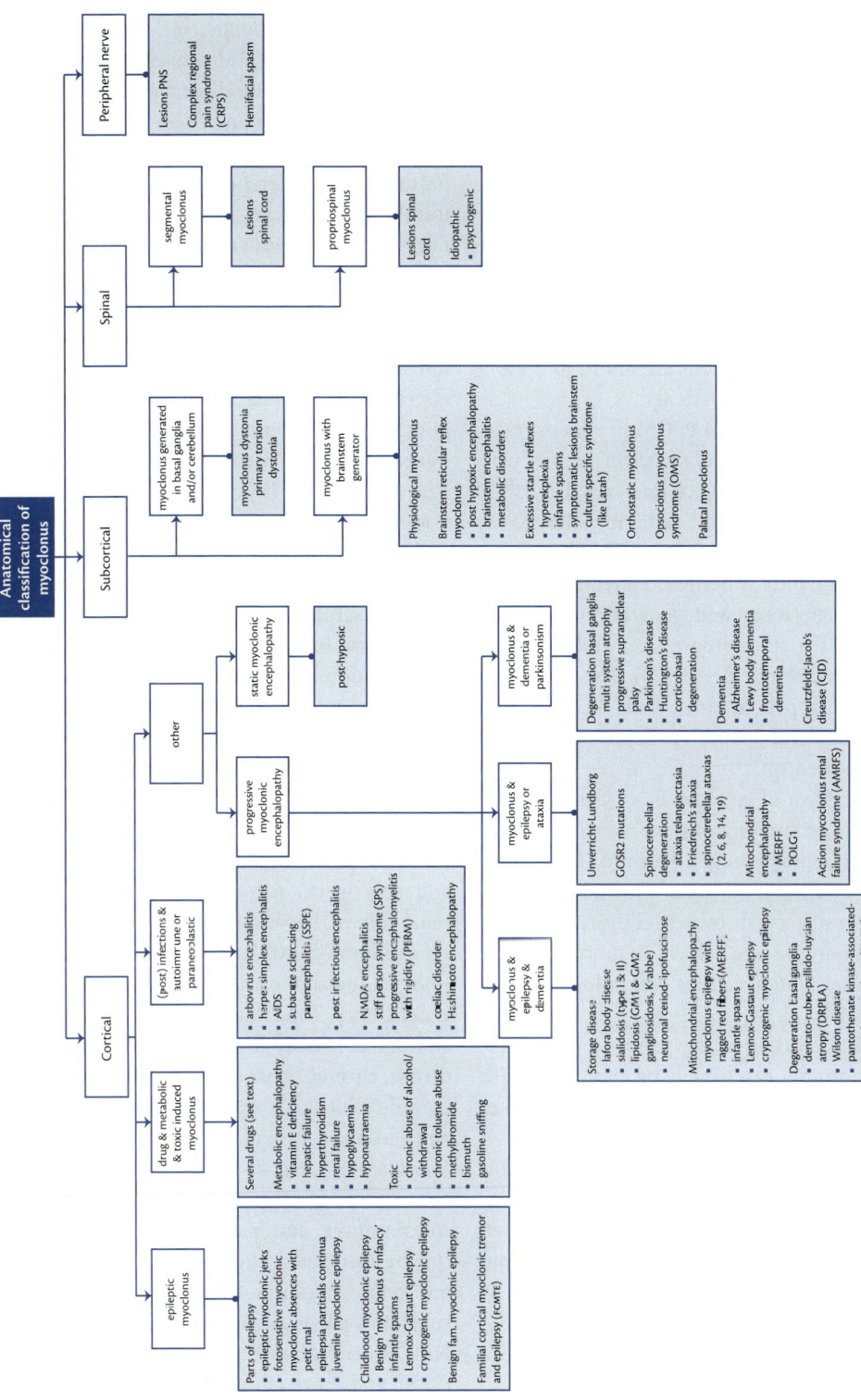

Figure 28.4 Aetiology based on anatomical classification of myoclonus.
Based on the anatomical classification a flowchart was constructed to help determination of aetiology of the myoclonus in clinical practice.

dependently of seizures, particularly on awakening. The genetic mechanisms causing JME are not fully understood yet, but it is probably caused by multifactorial mechanisms in most cases. Fifteen chromosomal loci are suspected of playing a central role in JME, with three putative genes: two mutation-containing ion channel genes, alfa1-subunit of the GABAa receptor (GABRA1), chloride channel 2 gene (CLCN2), as well as one non-ion channel gene, myoclonin1/EF-hand domain-containing protein 1 (EFHC1). These mutations are found in up to 9 percent of classic JME patients.

A relatively benign form of CM in epilepsy syndromes is *familial cortical myoclonic tremor with epilepsy* (FCMTE) (27), characterized by fine, shivering-like tremor and distal myoclonus, resembling an essential tremor. FCMTE is autosomal dominantly inherited. Patients may suffer from myoclonic and generalized seizures. FCMTE has a slow progression and responds well to anti-epileptic drugs (28). This condition has been mapped to three loci: 8q23.3-q24.1, 2p11.1-q12.2 and 5p15.31-p15, but no gene has been identified yet.

A specific form of epilepsy is '*epilepsia partialis continua*', consisting of continuous focal CM lasting for hours or longer. This is usually symptomatic, and the main causes include Rasmussen's syndrome, cerebrovascular disease, and the Alpers syndrome (see below). In more than 50% of the cases, abnormalities can be detected on imaging (29).

The epileptic origin of myoclonic jerks in epilepsy syndromes can usually be confirmed with EEG abnormalities such as spikes, polyspikes and slow wave complexes.

Movement disorders are the main issue of this book, and therefore, epileptic myoclonus in epilepsy syndromes will not be discussed further. For detailed information about this subject and its treatment, see Andrade et al (30).

Symptomatic myoclonus

The largest group of CM consists of symptomatic myoclonus. In daily clinical practice, drug-induced myoclonus is one of the most important causes. Alternative acquired causes include toxins or metabolic derangements, infections or autoimmune disorders.

Drug-induced myoclonus is one of the 'curable' causes of myoclonus. Therefore, the use of medication must be checked in every single patient. After discontinuation of medication, the symptoms usually vanish. The two neurotransmitter systems most frequently involved in the pathophysiology of different causes of medication-induced myoclonus are the serotonergic and GABA-ergic systems. Psychiatric medication is most notorious, but several drugs can be responsible, including levodopa, bismuth salts, benzodiazepines, antidepressants (cyclic antidepressants, selective serotonin uptake inhibitors, monoamine oxidase inhibitors), lithium, anti-infectious agents (quinolone antibiotics, cephalosporines), clozapine, opioids, anticonvulsants (particularly gabapentin, pregabalin, lamotrigine, phenytoin, phenobarbital), anesthetic propofol, cardiac medications (calcium channel blockers, antiarrhythmics) and contrast media (31).

Metabolic and toxic derangements cause both CM and subcortical myoclonus. Examples include renal failure, hepatic failure, respiratory failure, glycemic and electrolytic disturbances, hyperthyroidism, metabolic acidosis or alkalosis, vitamin E deficiency. Toxic causes of myoclonus include aluminum toxicity in patients with dialysis syndrome, chronic abuse of alcohol and withdrawal, chronic toluene abuse, methylbromide, bismuth, and gasoline sniffing (32).

Immune-mediated disorders of the central nervous system can cause CM with an acute onset. Autoimmune and paraneoplastic encephalitis can be associated with myoclonus. In the last few years, autoimmune disorders have been a subject of particular interest. Examples include NMDA encephalitis, stiff person syndrome (SPS), and *progressive encephalomyelitis with ri-*

gidity (PERM). Patients with PERM present with SPS symptoms and a combination of inflammatory cerebrospinal fluid (CSF), myoclonus, brainstem symptoms, long tract signs, cognitive involvement and rarely seizures. A significant number of PERM and SPS cases are associated with glutamic acid decarboxylase (GAD) antibodies, amphiphysin and glycine receptor (GlyR). The duration of PERM ranges from weeks to several years. Treatment includes immuno-modulatory therapies (33).

Another autoimmune disorder is coeliac disease, a disorder of the small intestine which can be accompanied by a combination of progressive ataxia and (action or stimulus-sensitive) myoclonus with occasional seizures. One should be aware that gastrointestinal symptoms may not be prominent. Age at onset is usually in the fifth decade of life (34). Diagnostic tests include measurement of anti-endomysial antibodies (EMA), anti-tissue transglutaminase (tTG), anti-reticulin (ARA), anti-gliadin (AGA) antibodies. Tissue biopsy of the small intestine is still considered the gold standard in the diagnosis of coeliac disease. Hashimoto encephalopathy is another autoimmune disorder, which can be accompanied by CM.

Different kinds of *infections of the central nervous system* can be accompanied by CM, for example arbovirus or herpes simplex encephalitis, AIDS, and subacute sclerosing panencephalitis (SSPE).

If the drug-induced, toxic, immune-mediated, metabolic or infectious, i.e. acquired causes of CM are unlikely, we apply a more detailed classification to a certain group of symptomatic myoclonus, i.e. *progressive myoclonic and static myoclonic encephalopathies*. In patients with progressive myoclonic encephalopathies, it is usually difficult to make the exact diagnosis, but by using subgroups based on associated neurological symptoms such as the presence or absence of epilepsy, ataxia and/or dementia (41), a more focused diagnostic strategy is possible. In clinical practice it is therefore important to determine the most prominent clinical symptom. Static, i.e.non-progressive myoclonic encephalopathy mainly occurs in patients with post-anoxic encephalopathy.

Progressive myoclonic encephalopathy
Patients with this category of CM suffer from progressive, action-induced, stimulus-sensitive, multifocal or generalized myoclonus. The combination of progressive myoclonic encephalopathy and prominent generalized epilepsy and progressive dementia occurs in different disorders. Differential diagnosis includes: Lafora body's disease, myoclonus epilepsy with ragged red fibers (MERRF), sialidosis, lipofuscinosis, and dentate-rubro-pallido-luysian atrophy (DRPLA) (35,36).

Lafora body disease patients suffer from a progressively worsening myoclonus combined with seizures, visual hallucinations and cognitive decline. Death occurs usually within 10 years of onset. Lafora disease is caused by mutations in the 'epilepsy, progressive myoclonus type 2A' (EPM2A) or 'epilepsy, progressive myoclonus type 2B' (EPM2B) genes and is inherited in an autosomal recessive fashion (37).

Myoclonic Epilepsy with Ragged Red Fibers (MERRF) is characterized by myoclonus and mitochondrial myopathy. Other features are seizures, deafness, ataxia, neuropathy and dementia. Symptoms vary widely among patients. MERRF is maternally inherited, and mutations in the mitochondrially encoded tRNA lysine (MTTK) gene are the most common cause of MERRF (80% of patients) (37).

Sialidosis type I (cherry-red spot myoclonus syndrome) features intention and action myoclonus in combination with ataxia, epilepsy and visual disturbances. Myoclonus also occurs in sialidosis type II. Sialidoses are autosomal recessive disorders.

Neuronal ceroid lipofuscinoses are characterized by the accumulation of abnormal amounts of lipopigment in lysosomes. Patients may suffer from progressive myoclonus and visual failure, sometimes accompanied by ataxia. The disease is inherited in an autosomal recessive mode, except for the adult form (*Kuff's disease*), which may have autosomal dominant inheritance (35) (37).

Dentate-rubro-pallido-luysian atrophy (DRPLA) is a rare, autosomal-dominant, neurodegenerative disorder, first described in Japan where it is most prevalent. There are three clinical forms, and in one form, progressive myoclonic epilepsy is the predominant phenotype. Patients with onset before 20 years often suffer from the PME form, characterized by ataxia, seizures, myoclonus, and cognitive decline. The affected phenotype of DRPLA is related to an abnormal CAG repeat expansion within the exon 5 of ATN-1 gene (35).

The combination of progressive myodonic encephalopathy with epilepsy or ataxia, without prominent decline in cognitive function, points towards another differential diagnosis: PME and progressive myoclonus ataxia (PMA). PMA was previously known as Ramsay-Hunt syndrome. *Unverricht Lundberg* (UL) is an important disorder in the group of PME. The disease starts around ten years of age. Patients suffer from progressive and disabling myoclonus. Other features include seizures, ataxia, depression and sometimes mild decline in cognitive function. UL is caused by mutations in the CSTB gene on chromosome 21q22.3.

Recently, mutations in the golgi SNAP receptor complex member 2 (GOSR2) gene were identified as a cause in patients with PME or PMA. All patients had a similar phenotype with progressive cortical reflex myoclonus, ataxia, generalized seizures, preserved cognition and areflexia. EMG demonstrates both sensory neuropathy and chronic anterior horn cell involvement (van Egmond et al, unpublished data), suggesting abnormalities in the central as well as the peripheral nervous system (see Video fragment 28.2). Differential diagnosis of PMA further includes:

mitochondrial disorders (e.g. MERFF, and polymerase-γ 1 -POLG1), *vitamin E deficiency* and *coeliac disease*. Mitochondrial DNA polymerase-γ (*POLG*) mutations can cause *Alpers syndrome*. Patients with Alpers syndrome suffer from a progressive neurological disorder usually starting in early childhood and characterized by developmental regression and refractory focal motor or myoclonic seizures. Liver dysfunction is a late symptom. Other signs include ataxia, visual disturbance, motor paresis, and tremor. This diagnosis must be kept in mind in young patients presenting with epilepsia partialis continua (38). Also, patients with *progressive spinocerebellar ataxia* (SCA) - like Friedreich ataxia or ataxia telangiectasia - can suffer from myoclonus. Myoclonus is reported in SCA2, 6, 8, 14 and 19. *Action myoclonus-renal failure syndrome* (AMRFS) is a distinct type of progressive myoclonic encephalopathy associated with renal impairment. Proteinuria is present in all cases and will progress to renal failure. Mutation of the LIMP-2 gene is found in patients with AMRFS (39). Approximately 40% of patients with PMA remain undiagnosed, even after detailed evaluation (40).

In *late-onset, progressive myoclonic encephalopathy with dementia or parkinsonism*, one must consider a neurodegenerative disorder. The differential diagnosis includes *Alzheimer's disease, Parkinson's disease, multiple system atrophy* (MSA), and less commonly dementia with *Lewy bodies, Huntington's disease*, and *corticobasal degeneration* (CBD) (41-43). In Alzheimer's disease, up to 50% of patients eventually develop myoclonus, and in case of early onset or familial Alzheimer's disease, myoclonus appears earlier and with a higher incidence (40). Patients with MSA often have irregular, small amplitude myoclonic movements of the fingers when holding arms in an outstretched posture (poly-mini-myoclonus). This phenomenon has also been described in patients with Parkinson's disease. Poly-mini-myoclonus is stimulus-sensitive and aggravated during voluntary movements. In CBD, myoclonus appears focally in the affected arm as irregular continuous jerks increasing with movement and can be provoked by an external stimulus. Approximately 50% of patients with CBD develop myoclonus during the course of their disease. After the age of 65 years, asymmetric CM can also appear without other clinical features suggestive of a neurodegenerative disorder. This syndrome is called '*primary progressive myoclonus of ageing*' and consists of asymmetric symptomatic cortical action myoclonus. Usually, there is an initial period of progression, followed by a static disease course (plateau period).

In case of myoclonic encephalopathy with a rapidly progressive dementia, a prion disease must be considered. *Creutzfeldt-Jakob's disease* (CJD) is a rare, degenerative, invariably fatal brain disorder. CJD is caused by prions and can be acquired by transmission due to exposure to contaminated brain or nervous system tissue. About 10-15% of CJD cases are inherited through a mutation of the gene that codes for the prion protein (PRNP). Symptoms commonly start in the fifth to seventh decade of age, showing a rapidly progressive, multi-domain cognitive impairment and confusion, occasionally accompanied by cortical visual disturbances, ataxia, and spontaneous or action-induced myoclonus. Occasionally, negative myoclonus can also be seen in CJD (40).

Static myoclonic encephalopathy

Post-anoxic myoclonus can be divided into early myoclonus developing within 72 hours after the event, and late onset (>72 hours) myoclonus.

Acute *post-anoxic myoclonus* occurs in about 19-37% of patients after cardiopulmonary resuscitation. Post-anoxic myoclonus is often suppressed during the first 24 hours in the period of artificial hypothermia induced by sedative drugs or neuromuscular blocking agents. Myoclonus can have a cortical or subcortical substrate ('or both') with their own characterizing features. Both types can be stimulus-sensitive. The origin of myoclonus might be important in the determination of treatment options and prognosis. Levetiracetam (or piracetam) is the first choice of treatment in CM, while subcortical myoclonus is usually treated with clonazepam. A recent study revealed that the outcome in patients with myoclonus after cardiopulmonary resuscitation may not be invariably correlated with poor outcome as previously described (44).

In the chronic phase after resuscitation, *Lance-Adams syndrome* can develop in patients who survived severe cerebral hypoxia. Myoclonus is multifocal, usually stimulus-sensitive and often consists of positive and negative myoclonus. Sudden falls secondary to negative myoclonus can occur (45).

Treatment

Because of the pathophysiological relationship between CM and epilepsy, many drugs which are beneficial in epilepsy are traditionally used in patients with CM. In a cross-over trial in 21 patients with different kinds of CM, piracetam significantly improved myoclonus (46). It improved myoclonus in patients with post-anoxic myoclonus (mostly add-on therapy) (46) and in patients with PME. However, a high daily dose is required (up to 24 g/day) (46). Because of its similarity to piracetam, the better tolerated levetiracetam is now considered the standard initial treatment of CM (daily dose up to 3000mg). Levetiracetam may be effective in both epileptic myoclonus and non-epileptic CM (46). There is a long clinical experience of CM treatment with valproic acid and clonazepam (46). In a very small trial, milacemide seemed beneficial. Treatment of CM generally necessitates polytherapy, consisting of clonazepam, valproic acid and levetiracetam (46).

Subcortical myoclonus

Subcortical myoclonus is generated between the cortex and spinal cord. Important areas are the basal ganglia and the brainstem. We will describe: 1) essential myoclonus (myoclonus dystonia, MD), considered a subcortical myoclonus arising from the basal ganglia and/or cerebellum, and 2) myoclonus with a brainstem generator.

Essential myoclonus (myoclonus dystonia)

MD is characterized by myoclonic jerks predominantly of the upper body, often combined with mild to moderate dystonia. Myoclonus predominantly appears in the arms and axial muscles. It is exacerbated by posture, action or stress. The myoclonic jerks are multifocal and have a variable amplitude. Myoclonus often has a highly positive relation to alcohol ingestion (47). Dystonia commonly manifests as cervical dystonia or writer's cramp. The disorder usually manifests in the first or second decade of life with myoclonus as the presenting symptom. In about 20% of cases, dystonia is the initial manifestation (see Video fragment 28.3). Normally, patients with MD have a normal lifespan. Patients with MD are supposed to be susceptible to psychiatric disorders including depression, anxiety disorder, and obsessive-compulsive disorder (OCD) (48).

Myoclonus in MD is hypothesized to be generated in the basal ganglia. Polymyographic recordings show arrhythmic or less frequently rhythmic jerks with a frequency not exceeding 10 Hz. Duration of EMG bursts ranges from 40 to 250 ms, with longer jerks being probably part of dystonic jerks. Local field potential recordings from the globus pallidus internus (GPi) in MD patients showed significant coherence between GPi and dystonic muscle activity in the 4-7 Hz 'dystonic band'. The cerebellum also seems to play an important part in the pathogenesis. In an eye movement study, impaired saccadic adaptation in patients with MD was associated with cerebellar dysfunction. Another clue in this regard is the fact that a major brain-specific SGCE isoform has a high expression in the cerebellum (49). Electrophysiological studies including (EMG-) EEG, and SSEP reveal no changes in cortical excitability. Cortical functional changes as detected in a transcranial magnetic stimulation study are thought to be secondary to basal ganglia pathology (47,50).

MD is autosomal dominantly inherited, mostly caused by mutations in the epsilon-sarcoglycan gene (DYT 11) on chromosome 7q21. A second locus has been discovered in a large MD family (DYT 15, 18p11), but the disease gene has not been identified. MD is typically inherited from the father due to maternal genomic imprinting. In many patients with the MD phenotype, no DYT 11 and 15 mutations have been found, suggesting the involvement of other genes or environmental factors. Other disorders presenting with a MD phenotype are benign hereditary chorea due to thyroid transcription factor-1 mutations, tyrosine hydroxylase deficiency (THD), GTP cyclohydrolase I (GTPCH1), vitamin E deficiency mitochondrial or neurometabolic disorders (51). There is no causal treatment for MD, and symptomatic drug treatment is disappointing. High doses of L-5-HTP (a serotonin precursor) were effective in a few patients, but often had to be stopped because of side effects (46). A few patients described benefitting from sodium oxybate, levodopa, and zolpidem. The effect of clonazepam, piracetam, levetiracetam and trihexyphenidyl is limited (46). Dystonia can be treated by botulinum toxin injections. In case of severe myoclonus and dystonia, a good response to deep brain stimulation of the globus pallidus interna (GPi) or ventralis intermedius nucleus (Vim) of the thalamus has been described (46).

Myoclonus with a brainstem generator

Here we will describe different kinds of myoclonus with a brainstem generator. The etiological diagnosis of brainstem myoclonus is diverse. An innocent form of brainstem myoclonus is physiological myoclonus, including sleep jerks (hypnagogic myoclonus) and hiccups. Others include brainstem reticular reflex myoclonus and startle syndromes, opsoclonus myoclonus syndrome (OMS), palatal myoclonus and orthostatic myoclonus.

Brainstem reticular reflex myoclonus is characterized by generalized, synchronized, predominantly axial stimulus-sensitive jerks (20,31). It is hypothesized that jerks in brainstem reticular reflex myoclonus originate from the reticular formation and subsequently spread in both rostral and caudal directions. Electrophysiological studies including (EMG-) EEG, and SSEP reveal no changes in cortical excitability. Polymyographic recordings show rostral and caudal activation of muscles (18,52). The muscles that are first activated are usually those innervated by the caudal brainstem, i.e. sternocleidomastoideus and the trapezius muscles. Brainstem reticular reflex myoclonus can be caused by post-hypoxic encephalopathy, brainstem encephalitis and metabolic disturbances (uraemia). In the treatment of brainstem reticular reflex myoclonus, L-5-HTP may be effective, but this compound is often not well tolerated.

Startle syndromes are also accompanied by generalized, synchronized, predominantly axial, stimulus-sensitive jerks (20,31). The pattern of muscle activation is resembles that of brainstem reticular reflex myoclonus. In contrast to reticular myoclonus, the EMG responses in the intrinsic hand and foot muscles during startle reflex are relatively delayed. Furthermore, the latencies of muscle activity after the auditory stimulus in reticular reflex myoclonus are compatible with the pyramidal tract, while the startle reflex latencies take longer travelling through the slower corticospinal tracts. Excessive startle reflexes can be part of *hyperekplexia* (HPX), an autosomal dominant disorder (mainly) characterized by pathologically exaggerated startle responses to unexpected, in particular auditory stimuli. The startle reaction is followed by a short period of general stiffness, during which voluntary movement is impossible. This short-lasting stiffness (not more than a few seconds) may cause falls during full consciousness. The third cardinal feature, after startling from birth and startle-induced stiff falls, is generalized stiffness at birth. Stiffness usually normalizes during the first years of life. Disorders with an excessive startle reflex but without stiffness were previously considered a minor form of HPX. This is confusing as there is no genetic background for the minor form of HPX. These patients are better described as 'excessive startle reflexes'. The cause, possibly learned behaviour, is still under debate (53). HPX is caused by mutations in different parts of the inhibitory glycine receptor (GlyR). In 80%, the alfa1 subunit of the glycine receptor (GLRA1) is the affected gene. In about 20% of cases, the GlyT2 (SCL6A5) gene is affected (usually recessive cases). Recently, the Glycine receptor β subunit (GLRB) gene has been described as the third major gene for HPX. Genetic heterogeneity has been described in very rare sporadic cases of HPX with mutations affecting gephyrin (GPHN) and collybistin (ARHGEF9). As the glycine receptor modulates inhibitory effects, it is hypothesized that a lack of inhibition in HPX results in a higher sensitivity to external stimuli. HPX can occasionally also be symptomatic due to a lesion in the brainstem (vascular lesion, brainstem encephalitis, multiple sclerosis) (52). Exaggerated startle response can be part of a culture-specific syndrome, for example Latah in Indonesia and Malaysia. Latah is characterized by an exaggerated startle response followed by various behavioural responses, including echolalia, echopraxia, coprolalia and 'forced obedience'. In a study of 12 Latah patients, significantly increased early motor startle reflexes as well as late orienting startle responses were found. The early response was insignificant compared to the late stereotyped behavioural responses, pointing towards a neuropsychiatric startle syndrome (54). Patients with HPX are treated with clonazepam, and the stiffness may be more responsive than the startle reflexes.

Opsoclonus myoclonus syndrome (OMS) is characterized by involuntary, arrhythmic, chaotic, multidirectional, fast eye movements combined with myoclonus, cerebellar ataxia and encephalopathy. Myoclonus is located in the axial and limb muscles, and triggered by muscle contraction and during movement. OMS may be associated with a paraneoplastic syndrome (breast carcinoma, small-cell lung carcinoma) (55), toxic-metabolic, or a post-infectious syndrome. Acute cocaine overdose can also result in a combination of opsoclonus myoclonus, dystonia and chorea ("crack dancing"). In children, most cases are associated with neuroblastoma (56). In OMS, myoclonus can respond to clonazepam. If appropriate, treatment of the underlying disease with rituximab, ACTH or intravenous immunoglobulin therapy should be considered.

Palatal myoclonus (also referred to as palatal tremor) is characterized by ear clicking, caused by spasmodic contractions of the levator (or tensor) veli palatine part with its origin from the cartilaginous auditory tube (57). The syndrome is occasionally accompanied by other features like ocular myoclonus, dysarthria or ataxia. Palatal myoclonus has been classified into essential and symptomatic groups. Symptomatic palatal myoclonus is caused by a lesion in Guillain-Mollaret triangle and associated with olivary hypertrophy. In about 70% of cases, the lesion is caused by an ischemic lesion. Less frequent causes are multiple sclerosis, tumors or traumatic lesions. Palatal myoclonus is difficult to treat. Clonazepam, carbamazepine, phenytoin, barbiturates and valproic acid can be tried. Other treatments include botulinum toxin and a tinnitus masking device.

Orthostatic myoclonus is a disorder of elderly patients. Myoclonic jerks occur in the upright position. Patients complain of leg jerking (shaky legs) or gait problems. The disease is slowly progressive and eventually disables the patients' gait. This type of myoclonus has not been formally anatomically classified yet, but is most likely of subcortical origin. Electrophysiological examination shows irregular, short bursts (<100ms) in the legs, occurring in the standing position and not present while sitting. Orthostatic myoclonus can be part of a neurodegenerative disease including

dementia disorders or Parkinson's disease (58). In 2011, in a 3-generation pedigree with autosomal dominant MD, orthostatic action myoclonus in the lower extremities provoked by upright posture resulting in instability was described (59). Regarding the treatment of orthostatic myoclonus, some beneficial effect was reported with clonazepam and gabapentin (46).

Spinal myoclonus

Spinal myoclonus is generated in the spinal cord. Spinal jerks can be subdivided into segmental or propriospinal myoclonus.

Segmental myoclonus

Segmental myoclonus is characterized by continuous, rhythmic jerks, unaffected by voluntary movement. The jerks are not stimulus-sensitive. Segmental myoclonus often persists during sleep. The myoclonus results from abnormal discharges from one or two contiguous spinal segments. It is hypothesized that spinal segmental systems become hyperexcitable, resulting in jerks in muscles innervated by the particular segment(s). Polymyographic recordings show jerks with a frequency ranging from 1 to 200 per minute, and burst duration up to 1000 ms. Segmental myoclonus is mostly caused by a lesion in the spinal cord, such as a neoplasia, syringomyelia, myelitis or ischemia. If possible, the underlying cause must be treated. Otherwise, clonazepam is the first drug of choice in the symptomatic treatment of segmental myoclonus (60). Other options for treatment are carbamazepine, tetrabenazine and botulinum toxin (46).

Propriospinal myoclonus

Propriospinal myoclonus is characterized by rhythmic, spontaneous and sometimes stimulus-sensitive jerks (61,62). Lying down often provokes propriospinal myoclonus. These jerks mainly affect the axial muscles (trunk and abdominal muscles), sometimes expanding to the distal limbs but excluding the cranially innervated muscles (61,62) (see Video fragment 28.4).

Propriospinal myoclonus is presumed to be caused by a spinal generator that induces muscle activity spreading up and down the spinal cord. Polymyographic recordings show initially bursts in the midthoracic segments followed by distribution up and down the spinal cord via propriospinal pathways (62). There is a fixed pattern of muscle activation with slow spreading of activity with repetitive bursts (frequency 1-7 Hz) with a long duration (up to several 100 ms). In some patients with propriospinal myoclonus, lesions of the spinal cord have been reported, but usually no cause can be detected (60). In the last few years, psychogenic-induced propriospinal myoclonus is being increasingly recognized. In a study of 20 patients with idiopathic propriospinal myoclonus, a definite Bereitschaftspotential (BP) was detected in 6 patients and a possible BP in 9 patients, suggesting a psychogenic origin (63).

Clonazepam is the first drug of choice (60), while an alternative treatment is zonisamide (46).

Peripheral myoclonus

Peripheral myoclonus is characterized by jerks limited to one segment of the body, usually the proximal part of a limb or the trunk. Myoclonus can be triggered by voluntary movement (64). In most cases peripheral myoclonus is caused by damage to the peripheral nerve system (PNS), and the EMG shows varied burst duration (64).

Hemifacial spasm is often considered to be an example of peripheral myoclonus, although the nomenclature and jerk duration fits more with the term spasm. Hemifacial spasm is characterized by ipsilateral facial nerve-generated jerks or tonic contractions of the muscles. It is mostly caused by vascular compression of the facial nerve at the exit zone. In hemifacial spasm, botulinum toxin is the treatment of choice (46). An alternative therapy is microsurgical vascular decompression.

Any peripheral nerve lesion that is accompanied by fasciculations or myokymia may result in small myoclonic movements, especially if enlarged motor units are involved, since this will result in an increase in the mechanical effect of axonal discharges. Often, clear signs of peripheral nerve dysfunction are present, and the diagnosis of peripheral myoclonus is evident. With more complex nerve lesions such as multiple radiculopathy, the diagnosis may be more difficult, and EMG may be required to confirm the presence of a chronic neurogenic lesion. Other examples of causes of damage of the peripheral nervous system (PNS) inducing peripheral myoclonus include lesions of the brachial plexus (65), spinal root (66), the long thoracic nerve or after amputation ("jumping stump") (64,67). In these forms, botulinum toxin can also be considered as symptomatic treatment.

In patients with complex regional pain syndrome (CRPS), myoclonus appears to be induced by peripheral trauma, although a peripheral nerve lesion cannot be detected with EMG. A psychogenic cause cannot be ruled out (68).

A special case of peripheral myoclonus due to damage of the PNS is *mini-poly-myoclonus*. In 1938, Denny-Brown and Pennybacker first described tremor-like movements in patients with chronic denervation. These movements were caused by the discharge of very large motor units in a muscle with a decreased number of motor units, resulting in a non-smooth contraction, resembling tremor-like movements. The low-amplitude jerks are mostly visible in the distal joints and the head. Stress, fatigue and fright intensify the rate and amplitude of the mini-poly-myoclonus. The jerks are absent during complete relaxation and sleep. In 1970, Spiro used the term mini-poly-myoclonus to describe these movements. This mini-poly-myoclonus was considered to be a good bedside sign of chronic denervation and reinnervation with large motor units. Mini-poly-myoclonus was observed in children with a benign form of childhood spinal muscular atrophy (69). Later, the term mini-poly-myoclonus was used for small-amplitude myoclonic movements of the hands of

Table 28.1
Clinical and electrophysiological features of myoclonus.

	Clinical presentation	Distribution	Temporal pattern	Electrophysiological examination	
				EMG / Polymyography	Other
Cortical myoclonus	Spontaneous Action induced Stimulus sensitive *also negative myoclonus*	(Multi) focal/ generalized: *Face, distal limbs*	Irregulair (rhythmic)	▪ Short bursts (usually <50ms) ▪ Backaveraging: time-locked contralateral cortical spike preceding myoclonus ▪ Coherence analysis: cortico-muscular and intermuscular coherence in alpha and beta band with a phase difference compatible with cortical drive	SSEP: giant potential (P25/P30/N35) Cortical reflex (C-reflex)
Brainstem myoclonus	Spontaneous Stimulus sensitive	Generalized/ synchronous *Axial/proximal limbs*	Irregulair	▪ Burst duration variable ▪ Simultaneous rostral and caudal activation of muscles	SSEP: normal No C-reflex
Myoclonus dystonia	Spontaneous Action induced	(Multi) focal *Axial/proximal limbs*	Irregulair	▪ Burst duration variable (25-256 ms)	SSEP: normal No C-reflex
Segmental myoclonus	Spontaneous (Action induced)	Focal or segmental	Irregulair	▪ Burst frequency from 1-200 per minute burst duration up to 1000ms ▪ Simultaneous rostral and caudal activation of muscles	SSEP: normal No C-reflex
Propriospinal myoclonus	Spontaneous Stimulus sensitive	Generalized/ synchronous	Irregulair	▪ Slow spreading of activity with repetitive bursts (frequency 1-7Hz) and long duration (up to several 100 ms)	SSEP: normal No C-reflex
Peripheral myoclonus	Spontaneous	Focal	Irregulair	▪ Burst duration variable ▪ *Large MUPs* ▪ *Fasciculations/myokymia*	SSEP: normal No C-reflex

cortical origin (see also the subchapter of CM in MSA) (70). Therefore, currently the concept of mini-poly-myoclonus is that of multiple, small myoclonic movements, which may be of peripheral or central origin (see Video fragment 28.5).

Diagnosis and differential diagnosis

The diagnostic procedure in patients with myoclonus starts with a history, neurological examination and determination of the anatomical classification (see Table 28.1).

History consists of age at onset and mode of myoclonus, associated symptoms (epilepsy, ataxia, and cognitive decline), progression of myoclonus, current and past drugs or toxin exposure, and family history. During physical examination, the physician takes notice of the features described under the section on clinical presentation. The history and physical examination determine the anatomical localization of the myoclonus. If the origin of myoclonus is still uncertain or requires confirmation, electrophysiological testing can be helpful. Electrophysiological studies include electromyography (EMG), electroencephalography-electromyography (EEG-EMG) with back-averaging, somatosensory evoked potential (SSEP), cortical reflex (C-reflex) and coherence analysis of EEG-EMG or EMG-EMG registrations.

Metabolic disturbance can be exposed by simple blood testing such as electrolytes, glucose, renal and hepatic function tests, thyroid function, and if necessary drug and toxin screen (12). If a focal lesion in the brain or spinal cord is suspected, imaging (MRI) should be performed. Advanced testing can consist of genetic testing, specific metabolic screening, lumbar puncture, antibody measurement including paraneoplastic antibodies.

Myoclonus should be differentiated from other hyperkinetic movement disorders. Alternative diagnoses include tremor, dystonia, tics, chorea, simple partial seizures, and psychogenic jerks. Differentiating symptoms should be sought. For example, CM or brainstem myoclonus is char-acterized by its stimulus sensitivity, not noticed in other movement disorders. In contrast to tics, myoclonus is not suppressible, often interferes with voluntary movements and increases with muscle activation. In case of a tremor, there is a rhythmic oscillatory movement, while myoclonus is generally arrhythmic. In dystonic jerks, the dystonic posture can often be relieved by a sensory trick, not occurring in myoclonus. In chorea the movements are more fluent and show usually a more random-like pattern. It should be noted that myoclonic jerks often occur in patients together with other movement disorders. Differential diagnoses of clinical syndromes are described in the section on 'myoclonus assigned to anatomical classification'.

Psychogenic myoclonus

About 10-20% of psychogenic movement disorder patients suffer from psychogenic myoclonus (71,72). In a study of 212 patients with myoclonus, 8.5% were defined as psychogenic (72). Psychogenic myoclonus is often variable and distractible. Patients have myoclonic jerks at rest, and in most patients the jerks increase with movement. Frequently, there is an abrupt onset and fast progression, improvement of motor function by distraction and suggestibility of symptoms (63,71). Entrainment is often present; when executing a repetitive movement with a different body part, the psychogenic myoclonus adopts the same frequency. Psychogenic myoclonus is mostly segmental, but can be focal or generalized. Patients often suffer from a coexisting psychiatric disease like depression, anxiety or panic disorders. In case of diagnostic uncertainty, electrophysiological testing can be useful to differentiate from alternative diagnoses. In case of psychogenic myoclonus, a consistent characteristic pre-movement potential (BP) can be detected in the EEG on back-averaging (see Figure 28.5). However, it has been demonstrated that tics can also be preceded by a BP, and the absence of this potential does not exclude a psychogenic origin (63,73).

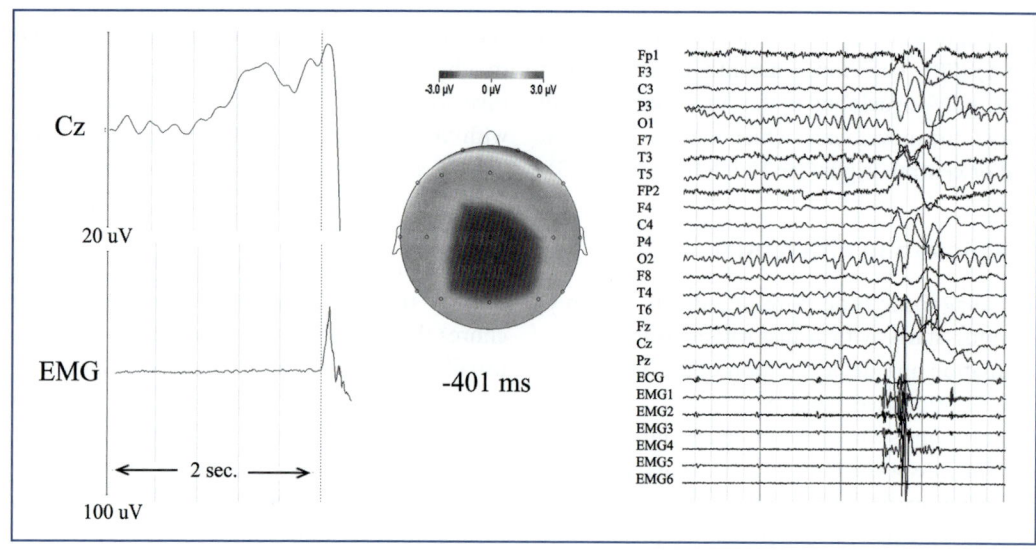

Figure 28.5 Bereitschaftpotential
Example of a Bereitschaftpotential (BP) in a young woman with generalized myoclonic jerks of functional origin.
Right panel: 4 seconds of raw EEG and EMG data. Note the long duration EMG bursts (+/- 500 ms), and the artefact in the EEG as the consequence of the jerks. Prior to the jerk, no EEG abnormalities can be seen. Left panel: After
back-averaging of 63 epochs of jerks, a BP can be seen, which starts approximately 1 second before jerk onset. Middle panel: Topographic mapping of the BP at 401 ms prior the fucntional myoclonic jerk onset. View from the top.
Note the centroparietal field distribution.

In case of generalized psychogenic myoclonus, the recruitment order of the affected muscle is highly variable. In a recently published study, the inter-rater agreement among 39 experts on movement disorders was determined in 60 patients with psychogenic jerks, myoclonus or tics. An absolute agreement on the diagnosis was found in 12 (20%) and reasonable agreement in 43 (75%) patients, demonstrating a moderate inter-rater agreement among clinical experts. The diagnosis of psychogenic jerking must be made with caution (63), When the diagnosis of psychogenic myoclonus is made, treatment must be initiated because a longer duration of the syndrome is related to poor outcome (71). Treatment consists of psychotherapy and pharmacological treatment of comorbid psychiatric disorders (71).

Treatment

The first focus of therapy of myoclonus is to treat the underlying cause, like removal of cer-tain drugs or toxin, or stabilization of metabolic disturbances (18). In the majority of cases, treatment of the underlying disorder is not possible, and symptomatic treatment is required. Symptomatic treatment can also be difficult. The drugs are effective in only a small proportion of patients. Therapy is often limited by side effects. For this reason, initial low doses with a slow increase are recommended. Several drugs may be tried to find the best treatment in an individual patient (see Table 28.2). Polytherapy is generally more effective than monotherapy, especially in CM (46). The choice of treatment is based on the classification of the anatomical origin of the myoclonus, and therefore specific treatment options are described in the corresponding section. Unfortunately, in general, therapeutic options are mainly based on small observational studies and expert opinions. Hopefully, future blind-randomized controlled trials on symptomatic therapies for myoclonus will be performed. Future treatments may include gene

Table 28.2
Treatment of myoclonus (46).

	First choice of treatment	Alternative treatment	Other therapy
Cortical myoclonus			
In general	Levetiracetam Piracetam	Valproic acid, Clonazepam	*Add on therapy with:* Primidone, Phenobarbital
Posthypoxic cortical reflex myoclonus	Clonazepam Valproic acid		
Subcortical myoclonus			
Myoclonus dystonia	Clonazepam Trihexyphenidyl	Levodopa, L-5-HTTP*, Sodium oxybate	Deep brain stimulation
Opsoclonus myoclonus syndrome	Clonazepam		*Treatment of underlying syndrome:* Rituximab, ACTH, iv immuno-globulin
Hyperekplexia	Clonazepam		
Reticular reflex myoclonus	L-5-HTTP*		
Palatal myoclonus	Clonazepam, Carbamazepine Botulinum toxin		Tinnitus masking device
Orthostatic myoclonus	Clonazepam	Gabapentin	
Spinal myoclonus			
Segmental myoclonus	Clonazepam	Carbamazepine, Tetrabenazin, Botulinum toxin	
Propiospinal myoclonus	Clonazepam	Zonisamide	
Peripheral myoclonus			
Hemifacial spasm	Botulinum toxin	Carbamazepine Clonazepam	Microsurgical vascular decompression
Others	Botulinum toxin		

* = in combination with a decarboxylase inhibitor

therapy and enzyme replacement in order to modify and improve the course of some of the progressive disorders.

Video fragments

Fragment 28.1
Negative myoclonus
This video fragment shows a patient with renal failure. While keeping his wrists actively extended, negative myoclonus (asterixis) can be seen due to muscular inhibition.

Fragment 28.2
Cortical myoclonus
This 7-year-old patient suffers from cortical myoclonus and ataxia. Genetic analysis revealed a mutation in the GOSR2 gene. The video shows multifocal myoclonus of muscles in the head, face and distal upper limbs. Myoclonus is provoked by somasthetic stimulus (reflex myoclonus).

Fragment 28.3
Subcortical myoclonus
The video shows a patient with myoclonus dystonia (with a mutation in the SGCE gene). Myoclonic jerks are seen in the upper part of the body. During action the myoclonus is exacerbated and also appears in the upper limbs. The patient suffers from a mild dystonia of the neck. Writer's cramp is shown on the video.

Fragment 28.4
Spinal myoclonus
The video shows a patient with propriospinal myoclonus. The bilaterally synchronised jerks are mainly located in the axial muscles. Electromyographic examination shows the fixed pattern of muscle activation on left side, starting in the lumbar spinal muscles and travelling cranially. A 'bereitschaft potential' (BP) was absent.

Fragment 28.5
Peripheral myoclonus
This patient suffers from peripheral nerve damage due to HMSN type II. Notice the atrophy of the hand muscles. Myoclonus is absent at rest, but during posture, peripheral mini-polymyoclonus is seen.

References

1 Friedreich N. Paramyoclonus multiplex. Neuropathologische Beobachtungen. Arch Path Anat (Virchow Arch) 1881;86:421-434.

2 Lance,J.W., Adams, R.D. The syndrome of intention or action myoclonus as a sequel to hypoxic encephalopathy. 1963;86:111-136.

3 Marsden,C.D. Hallett, M Fahn S. The nosology and patho-physiology of myoclonus. Movement disorders : official journal of the Movement Disorder Society 1982;3:196-248.

4 Caviness JN, Alving LI, Maraganore DM, Black RA, McDonnell SK, Rocca WA. The incidence and prevalence of myoclonus in Olmsted County, Minnesota. Mayo Clin Proc 1999;74:565-569.

5 Caviness JN. Epidemiology of myoclonus. Adv Neurol 2002;89:19-22.

6 Yoon JH, Lee PH, Yong SW, Park HY, Lim TS, Choi JY. Movement disorders at a university hospital emergency room. An analysis of clinical pattern and etiology. J Neurol 2008;255:745-749.

7 Obeso JA, Rothwell JC, Marsden CD. The spectrum of cortical myoclonus. From focal reflex jerks to spontaneous motor epilepsy. Brain 1985;108:193-124.

8 Rubboli G, Tassinari CA. Negative myoclonus. An overview of its clinical features, pathophysiological mechanisms, and management. Neurophysiol Clin 2006;36:337-343.

9 Obeso JA, Artieda J, Burleigh A. Clinical aspects of negative myoclonus. Adv Neurol 1995;67:1-7.

10 Fahn S, Marsden CD, Van Woert MH. Definition and classification of myoclonus. Adv Neurol 1986;43:1-5.

11 Tatu L, Moulin T, Martin V, Monnier G, Rumbach L. Unilateral pure thalamic asterixis: clinical, elec-

tromyographic, and topographic patterns. Neurology 2000;54:2339-2342.

12 Caviness JN, Brown P. Myoclonus: current concepts and recent advances. Lancet Neurol 2004;3:598-607.

13 Hallett M, Chadwick D, Marsden CD. Cortical reflex myoclonus. Neurology 1979;29:1107-1125.

14 Tassinari CA, Rubboli G, Shibasaki H. Neurophysiology of positive and negative myoclonus. Electroencephalogr Clin Neurophysiol 1998;107:181-195.

15 van Rootselaar AF, van der Salm SM, Bour LJ, Edwards MJ, Brown P, Aronica E, et al. Decreased cortical inhibition and yet cerebellar pathology in 'familial cortical myoclonic tremor with epilepsy'. Mov Disord 2007;22:2378-2385.

16 Cohen NR, Hammans SR, Macpherson J, Nicoll JA. New neuropathological findings in Unverricht-Lundborg disease: neuronal intranuclear and cytoplasmic inclusions. Acta Neuropathol 2011;121:421-427.

17 Mima T, Nagamine T, Ikeda A, Yazawa S, Kimura J, Shibasaki H. Pathogenesis of cortical myoclonus studied by magnetoencephalography. Ann Neurol 1998;43:598-607.

18 Caviness JN. Pathophysiology and treatment of myoclonus. Neurol Clin 2009;27:757-77.

19 Obeso JA. Therapy of myoclonus. Clin Neurosci 1995 -1996;3:253-257.

20 Caviness JN. Pathophysiology and treatment of myoclonus. Neurol Clin 2009;27:757-77.

21 Shibasaki H, Yamashita Y, Kuroiwa Y. Electroencephalographic studies myoclonus. Brain 1978;101:447-460.

22 Shibasaki H, Yamashita Y, Neshige R, Tobimatsu S, Fukui R. Pathogenesis of giant somatosensory evoked potentials in progressive myoclonic epilepsy. Brain 1985;108:225-240.

23 Grosse P, Cassidy MJ, Brown P. EEG-EMG, MEG-EMG and EMG-EMG frequency analysis: physiological principles and clinical applications. Clin Neurophysiol 2002;113:1523-1531.

24 Brown P, Farmer SF, Halliday DM, Marsden J, Rosenberg JR. Coherent cortical and muscle discharge in cortical myoclonus. Brain 1999;122:461-472.

25 Grosse P, Guerrini R, Parmeggiani L, Bonanni P, Pogosyan A, Brown P. Abnormal corticomuscular and intermuscular coupling in high-frequency rhythmic myoclonus. Brain 2003;126:326-342.

26 van Rootselaar AF, Maurits NM, Koelman JH, van der Hoeven JH, Bour LJ, Leenders KL, et al. Coherence analysis differentiates between cortical myoclonic tremor and essential tremor. Mov Disord 2006;21:215-222.

27 van Rootselaar AF, van Schaik IN, van den Maagdenberg AM, Koelman JH, Callenbach PM, Tijssen MA. Familial cortical myoclonic tremor with epilepsy: a single syndromic classification for a group of pedigrees bearing common features. Mov Disord 2005;20:665-673.

28 van Rootselaar AF, van Schaik IN, van den Maagdenberg AM, Koelman JH, Callenbach PM, Tijssen MA. Familial cortical myoclonic tremor with epilepsy: a single syndromic classification for a group of pedigrees bearing common features. Mov Disord 2005;20:665-673.

29 Cockerell OC, Rothwell J, Thompson PD, Marsden CD, Shorvon SD. Clinical and physiological features of epilepsia partialis continua. Cases ascertained in the UK. Brain 1996;119:393-407.

30 Andrade DM, Hamani C, Minassian BA. Treatment options for epileptic myoclonus and epilepsy syndromes associated with myoclonus. Expert Opin Pharmacother 2009;10:1549-1560.

31 Caviness JN, Brown P. Myoclonus: current concepts and recent advances. Lancet Neurol 2004 ;3:598-607.

32 Gordon MF. Toxin and drug-induced myoclonus. Adv Neurol 2002;89:49-76.

33 Shugaiv E, Leite IM, Sehitoglu E, Woodhall M, Cavus F, Waters P, et al. Progressive Encephalomyelitis with Rigidity and Myoclonus: A Syndrome with Diverse Clinical Features and Antibody Responses. Eur Neurol 2013;69:257-262.

34 Baizabal-Carvallo JF, Jankovic J. Movement disorders in autoimmune diseases. Mov Disord 2012;27:935-946.

35 Shahwan A, Farrell M, Delanty N. Progressive myoclonic epilepsies: a review of genetic and therapeutic aspects. Lancet Neurol 2005;4:239-248.

36 Shibasaki H, Thompson PD. Milestones in myoclonus. Mov Disord 2011;26:1142-1148.

37 Satishchandra P, Sinha S. Progressive myoclonic epilepsy. Neurol India 2010;58:514-522.

38 Wolf NI, Rahman S, Schmitt B, Taanman JW, Duncan AJ, Harting I, et al. Status epilepticus in children with Alpers' disease caused by POLG1 mutations: EEG and MRI features. Epilepsia 2009;50:1596-1607.

39 Badhwar A, Berkovic SF, Dowling JP, Gonzales M, Narayanan S, Brodtmann A, et al. Action myoclonus-renal failure syndrome: characterization of a unique cerebro-renal disorder. Brain 2004;127:2173-2182.

40 Borg M. Symptomatic myoclonus. Neurophysiol Clin 2006;36:309-318.

41 Caviness JN, Adler CH, Beach TG, Wetjen KL, Caselli RJ. Small-amplitude cortical myoclonus in Parkinson's disease: physiology and clinical observations. Mov Disord 2002;17:657-662.

42 Caviness JN, Adler CH, Caselli RJ, Hernandez JL. Electrophysiology of the myoclonus in dementia with Lewy bodies. Neurology 2003;60:523-524.

43 Salazar G, Valls-Sole J, Marti MJ, Chang H, Tolosa ES. Postural and action myoclonus in patients with parkinsonian type multiple system atrophy. Mov Disord 2000;15:77-83.

44 Bouwes A, van Poppelen D, Koelman JH, Kuiper MA, Zandstra DF, Weinstein HC, et al. Acute post-hypoxic myoclonus after cardiopulmonary resuscitation. BMC Neurol 2012;12:63-2377-12-63.

45 Frucht S, Fahn S. The clinical spectrum of posthypoxic myoclonus. Mov Disord 2000;15S1:2-7.

46 Dijk JM, Tijssen MA. Management of patients with myoclonus: available therapies and the need for an evidence-based approach. Lancet Neurol 2010;9:1028-1036.

47 Kinugawa K, Vidailhet M, Clot F, Apartis E, Grabli D, Roze E. Myoclonus-dystonia: an update. Mov Disord 2009;24:479-489.

48 Foncke EM, Cath D, Zwinderman K, Smit J, Schmand B, Tijssen M. Is psychopathology part of the phenotypic spectrum of myoclonus-dystonia?: a study of a large Dutch M-D family. Cogn Behav Neurol 2009;22:127-133.

49 Ritz K, van Schaik BD, Jakobs ME, van Kampen AH, Aronica E, Tijssen MA, et al. SGCE isoform characterization and expression in human brain:

50 Beukers RJ, Foncke EM, van der Meer JN, Nederveen AJ, de Ruiter MB, Bour LJ, et al. Disorganized sensorimotor integration in mutation-positive myoclonus-dystonia: a functional magnetic resonance imaging study. Arch Neurol 2010;67:469-474.

51 Stamelou M, Mencacci NE, Cordivari C, Batla A, Wood NW, Houlden H, et al. Myoclonus-dystonia syndrome due to tyrosine hydroxylase deficiency. Neurology 2012;79:435-441.

52 Bakker MJ, van Dijk JG, van den Maagdenberg AM, Tijssen MA. Startle syndromes. Lancet Neurol 2006;5:513-524.

53 Dreissen YE, Tijssen MA. The startle syndromes: physiology and treatment. Epilepsia 2012;53S7:3-11.

54 Bakker MJ, van Dijk JG, Pramono A, Sutarni S, Tijssen MA. Latah: An Indonesian Startle Syndrome. Mov Disord 2013;5:513-524.

55 Borg M. Symptomatic myoclonus. Neurophysiol Clin 2006;36:309-318.

56 Krug P, Schleiermacher G, Michon J, Valteau-Couanet D, Brisse H, Peuchmaur M, et al. Opsoclonus-myoclonus in children associated or not with neuroblastoma. Eur J Paediatr Neurol 2010;14:400-409.

57 Pearce JM. Palatal Myoclonus (syn. Palatal Tremor). Eur Neurol 2008;60:312-315.

58 Glass GA, Ahlskog JE, Matsumoto JY. Orthostatic myoclonus: a contributor to gait decline in selected elderly. Neurology 2007;68:1826-1830.

59 Groen J, van Rootselaar AF, van der Salm SM, Bloem BR, Tijssen M. A new familial syndrome with dystonia and lower limb action myoclonus. Mov Disord 2011;26:896-900.

60 Roze E, Bounolleau P, Ducreux D, Cochen V, Leu-Semenescu S, Beaugendre Y, et al. Propriospinal myoclonus revisited: Clinical, neurophysiologic, and neuroradiologic findings. Neurology 2009;72:1301-1309.

61 Brown P, Thompson PD, Rothwell JC, Day BL, Marsden CD. Axial myoclonus of propriospinal origin. Brain 1991;114:197-214.

62 Brown P, Rothwell JC, Thompson PD, Marsden CD. Propriospinal myoclonus: evidence for spi-

implications for myoclonus-dystonia pathogenesis? Eur J Hum Genet 2011;19:438-444.

nal "pattern" generators in humans. Mov Disord 1994;9:571-576.

63 van der Salm SM, de Haan RJ, Cath DC, van Rootselaar AF, Tijssen MA. The eye of the beholder: inter-rater agreement among experts on psychogenic jerky movement disorders. J Neurol Neurosurg Psychiatry 2013 Feb 14. (64 Jankovic J. Peripherally induced movement disorders. Neurol Clin 2009;27:821-832.

65 Banks G, Nielsen VK, Short MP, Kowal CD. Brachial plexus myoclonus. J Neurol Neurosurg Psychiatry 1985;48:582-584.

66 Seidel G, Vieregge P, Wessel K, Kompf D. Peripheral myoclonus due to spinal root lesion. Muscle Nerve 1997;20:1602-1603.

67 Tyvaert L, Krystkowiak P, Cassim F, Houdayer E, Kreisler A, Destee A, et al. Myoclonus of peripheral origin: two case reports. Mov Disord 2009;24:274-277.

68 Munts AG, Van Rootselaar AF, Van Der Meer JN, Koelman JH, Van Hilten JJ, Tijssen MA. Clinical and neurophysiological characterization of myoclonus in complex regional pain syndrome. Mov Disord 2008;23:581-587.

69 Spiro AJ. Minipolymyoclonus: A negelected sign in childhood spinal muscular atrophy. Neurology 1970;20:1124-1126.

70 Wilkins DE, Hallett M, Erba G. Primary generalised epileptic myoclonus: a frequent manifestation of minipolymyoclonus of central origin. J Neurol Neurosurg Psychiatry 1985;48:506-516.

71 Hinson VK, Haren WB. Psychogenic movement disorders. Lancet Neurol 2006;5:695-700.

72 Monday K, Jankovic J. Psychogenic myoclonus. Neurology 1993;43:349-352.

73 Shibasaki H, Hallett M. What is the Bereitschaftspotential? Clin Neurophysiol 2006;117:2341-2356.

74 Mina T, Steger J, Schulman AE, Gerloff C, Hallett M. Electroencephalographic measurement of motor cortex control of muscle activity in humans. Clin Neurophysiol 2000;111:326-337.

29
Chorea

Jan Roth

Chorea is a state of excessive, spontaneous movement, irregularly timed, non-repetitive, randomly distributed and abrupt in character, which might primarily occur in some genetic disorders and secondary to various (para)infectious, auto-immune and structural conditions and some toxic, iatrogenic and metabolic encephalopathies. These movements may vary in severity from restlessness with mild, intermittent exaggeration of gestures and expression, fidgeting movements of the hands, unstable dance-like gait to a continuous flow of disabling, violent movements. The word chorea is derived from the Greek word *khoreia*, which means dance. The term chorea was introduced in the 16th century by Paracelsus, who described bizarre motor and mental manifestations (deliriant trance, dancing mania) of medieval pilgrims during religious ceremonies (chorea sancti viti, Saint Vitus dance) (see Figure 29.1). It is now considered that the ingestion of the ergot alkaloids growing on corn likely played some role in these trances. Paracelsus also introduced the concept of chorea naturalis, caused by organic disease, and chorea lasciva, currently termed psychogenic. Another very important person in the history of chorea was a famous physician from London, Thomas Sydenham. At the end of 17th century he described a choreatic disease of childhood, chorea minor, currently termed Sydenham's chorea. George Huntington was another eminent physician, who in 1872 described hereditary choreic disease in three generations of a family living in East Hampton. The disease was later named Huntington's disease (HD).

Epidemiology

There are no valid data regarding the incidence of chorea in the population, however epidemiological data about a number of diseases that are, or might be, accompanied by chorea are available (e.g. Huntington's disease 4-10 / 100,000, benign hereditary chorea 0.2 / 100,000, and Wilson's disease 3 / 100,000).

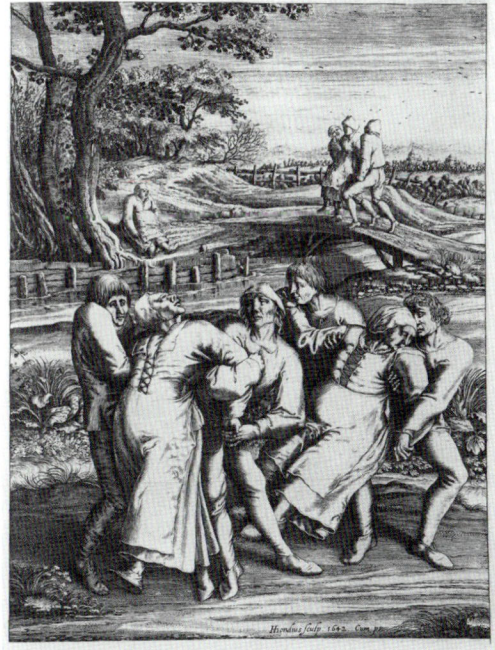

Figure 29.1
Saint Vitus dance.

Pathophysiology

Chorea results from pathological changes in the basal ganglia. For a better understanding, it is necessary to characterize the basal ganglia network in more detail. The interconnections in the basal ganglia may be (simplified) divided into two pathways: direct and indirect.

The direct pathway begins in the putamen. Its neurons (containing GABA, substantia P and dynorphin, and expressing NMDA and D1 dopamine receptors) project to the internal globus pallidus. The neurons from this nucleus (containing GABA) project to the ventral thalamus. The thalamic neurons (containing glutamate) project to the cerebral cortex. The projection from the thalamus to the cortex is thus excitatory (1,2) (see Figure 29.2). The indirect pathway starts from the medium-size spiny neurons of the striatum (containing GABA/encephalin and expressing NMDA and D2 dopamine receptors). These neurons project to the external globus pallidus. Neurons from the external globus pallidus (containing GABA) project to the subthalamic nucleus. Neurons from the subthalamic nucleus (containing glutamate) project to the internal globus pallidus and from that nucle-

us (containing GABA) to the ventral thalamus (containing glutamate) (1,2) (see also Chapters 1 and 2). According to many studies, the indirect pathway inhibits unwanted movements, and therefore the impairment of this pathway plays a significant role in the generation of involuntary movements (see Figure 29.2). The loss of subthalamic inhibition from the external globus pallidus leads to hyperactivity of the thalamocortical connection and results in dyskinesia (1,2).

Clinical presentation

Incipient, subtle chorea might be misinterpreted for anxiety, physiological grimacing or restlessness, as these movements may be camouflaged or masked as semi-purposeful gestures such as ruffling the hair, crossing the legs, adjusting clothing, etc.. However, higher degrees of chorea are prominent and undoubtedly recognized as involuntary movements. Chorea usually fluctuates according to stress as well as mental and physical activity, and initially dominate in the face and on the acral parts of the extremities. The fingers bend and stretch as if playing a piano, the feet scrape against the floor while seated. Typically, the big toe suddenly extends dorsally and quickly moves back (known as pseudo-Babinski sign). Grimacing is another typical finding in chorea; facial expressions change quickly from a frown to an angry expression, a smile, astonishment and disgust. Moreover, a protruding tongue (harlequin sign) or blepharospasm may be observed. Audible phenomena such as sighing, grinding or gnashing of teeth may be present. So, the clinical hallmark is motor impersistence, the inability to sustain posture or simple voluntary acts, and there are simple signs to rec-

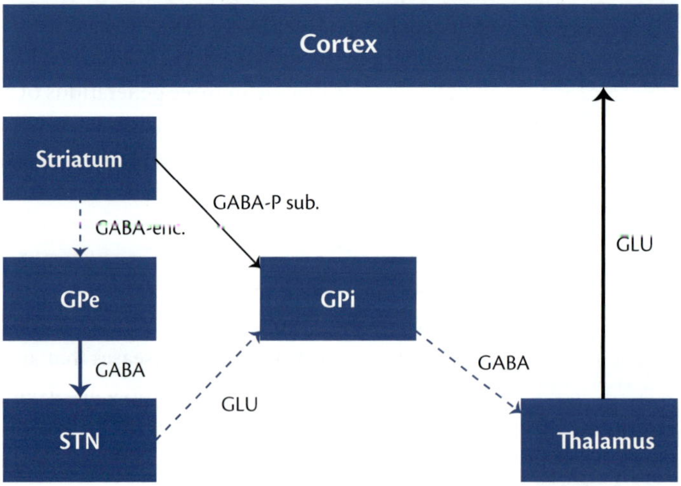

Figure 29.2
The basal ganglia network with the direct and indirecht connections between the striatum and GPi.

Table 29.1
Signs of motor impersistence.

Tongue protrusion sign:
patient cannot hold the tongue protruded, and moves the tongue irregularly around and back into the mouth (Video Fragment 29.2).

Grasp sign (milkmaid grip):
while grasping the examiner fingers, the patient involuntary relaxes and grips the hand, contracting and relaxing the hand muscles

ognize this impersistence, such as sometimes reflected in subtle, incipient chorea (see Table 29.1)

In later stages, choreatic dyskinesias affect the trunk, the proximal parts of the extremities and the neck. Patients nod their heads, wiggle and extend their shoulders and kick their feet. While standing or walking, a dance-like stance and gait are striking. Consequently, the harmony and interplay of movements worsens, movements are clumsy and injuries may even occur. Articulation worsens, explosive hyperkinetic dysarthria with dysrhythmic phonation is remarkable. Moreover, dyskinesias could affect swallowing, especially in the oral phase. An integral part of chorea are brisk tendon reflexes and muscle hypotonus. Otherwise, there are no additional phenomena. Patients suffer socially, as they are often assumed to be intoxicated. This may lead to a loss of employment, among other things.

Differential diagnosis: Chorea-like dyskinesias

Athetosis

Athetosis may be characterized as a slow form of chorea. Movements are snakelike, writhing or twisting. The only difference between chorea and athetosis is the speed of the movements; the pattern and other characteristics are the same. Thus, the word choreoathetosis means somewhat slower movement then chorea and somewhat faster than typical athetosis.

Pseudoathetosis

Pseudoathetosis arises as a consequence of impaired proprioceptive pathways. Finger movements are writhing, similar to athetosis.

Ballism

Ballism is a severe and violent form of chorea predominantly affecting proximal muscles, usually involving one side of the body (hemiballism). Biballism (bilateral ballism) appears only rarely. Hemiballism is due not only to lesions of the contralateral subthalamic nucleus (as is generally known), but also arises as a consequence of lesions in other contralateral basal ganglia structures, i.e., the striatum or even the thalamus (see chapter 30).

Stereotypies

Stereotypies are involuntary movements that occur in consistent patterns in certain regions, typically perioral in tardive stereotypies or in senile chorea. This type of dyskinesia is erroneously classified by many experts as a specific subgroup of choreatic dyskinesias, although most agree that stereotypies should be classified as an independent subtype of behavioural motor disorders due to the unwavering motor pattern that contrasts with the definition of chorea as random, irregular, and non-repetitive movement (see also Chapter 38).

Akathisia

Akathisia means inner-restlessness, and the urge to move manifests as the inability to remain motionless. Akathisia is often drug-induced. Motor restlessness may be misinterpreted as choreatic movement (crossing and uncrossing the legs, stamping the feet, etc.), however the inner urge, discomfort and anxiety in akathisia are exclusion criteria for chorea. For example, in Huntington's disease we can observe both types of movement disorder occurring at the same time: disease-related chorea and iatrogenic akathisia.

Table 29.2
The classification of choreas, adapted from (3,4).

Genetic chorea	<ul><li>HD and phenocopies</li><li>Ataxia telangiectasia</li><li>Benign hereditary chorea</li><li>Spinocerebellar ataxia (esp. SCA-2, SCA-3, SCA-12, Friedreich's ataxia)</li><li>Paroxysmal kinesiogenic choreoathetosis</li><li>Childhood metabolic disorders (e.g., gangliosidosis, galactosemia, phenylketonuria, homocystinuria, Lesch-Nyhan disease, neuronal ceroid-lipofuscinosis)</li></ul>
Structural basal ganglia lesions	<ul><li>Vascular and space-occupying lesions</li><li>Extrapontine myelinolysis</li><li>Multiple sclerosis</li></ul>
Infectious chorea	<ul><li>Syphilis, HIV, Diphtheria,</li><li>Toxoplasmosis, Cystercicosis</li><li>Bacterial endocarditis</li><li>Viral encephalitis (mumps, measles, varicella)</li></ul>
Parainfectious and autoimmune disorders	<ul><li>Sydenham's chorea</li><li>Systemic lupus erythematosus</li><li>Antiphospholipid antibody syndrome</li><li>Postinfectious/ postvaccinal encephalitis</li><li>Chorea gravidarum</li></ul>
Metabolic encephalopathies	<ul><li>Acute intermittent porphyria</li><li>Hypo/hypernatriaemia, Hypocalcemia</li><li>Hyperthyreoidism, Hypoparathyroidism</li><li>Hepatic and/or renal failure</li></ul>
Toxic encepalopathies	<ul><li>Carbon monoxide</li><li>Manganese</li><li>Mercury</li><li>Organophosphates</li></ul>
Iatrogenic encepalopathies	<ul><li>Dopamine receptor blocking agents</li><li>Antiparkinsonian drugs, Psychostimulants</li><li>Antiepileptic drugs</li><li>Calcium channel blockers</li><li>Tricyclic antidepressants, Lithium</li><li>Baclofen, Theophylline</li><li>Cyclosporine, Digoxin</li><li>Steroids, Oral contraceptives</li></ul>

HD: Huntington's disease; SCS: spino-cerebellar ataxia.

Choreatic disorders

In Table 29.2, the classification of the various choreatic diseases and disorders according to the various causes might be appreciated.

Choreatic disorders of childhood

Sydenham's chorea

Sydenham's chorea (SC) is a neuropsychiatric disease that arises as a complication of Group A β-hemolytic streptococcal infection, mediated by an autoimmune, anti-neuronal antibody mechanism that cross reacts with striatal neurons (5,6). According to the new Jones' criteria, the presence of SC alone is sufficient to make the diagnosis of acute rheumatic fever. The prevalence of acute rheumatic fever ranges from 5-35 per 1000, with the lowest rates in Europe and the highest in Africa (5,6). SC is present in nearly 50% of all cases of rheumatic fever. The prevalence of SC in Europe and North America has decreased dramatically in the last decades due to the accessibility and early use of antibiotics. SC affects individuals under 18 years of age, with girls being somewhat more affected. The occurrence of SC in adulthood is exceptional. The first manifestations of SC generally begin 3–6 months after streptococcal infection, laboratory markers (increased ESR, C-reactive protein, antistreptolysin, anti-DNAase-B) are thus negative in many patients. The most eminent manifestations are choreatic dyskinesias, i.e., grimacing, clumsiness, explosive dysarthria, gait disturbances, respiratory dysrhythmia and occasionally epileptic seizures. Problems with drawing and writing are usually the first signs of SC. Obsessive-compulsive disorders and anxiety or the attention deficit hyperactivity disorder (see Chapters 39, 40) are frequently observed. SC is a benign and self-limiting disorder. Manifestations usually develop within a few days, progress over several weeks with the tendency to resolve spontaneously in several months. However, recurrence is observed in approximately 20% of cases.

The primary therapy for SC is penicillin, amoxicillin or erythromycin i.m. for 10 days, followed by a prophylactic treatment until the age of 18 years. Secondary treatment includes immunomodulatory interventions, i.e., steroids or intravenous immunoglobulins (6). Additional treatment is purely symptomatic; anticonvulsants (e.g., valproate) for epilepsy and antipsychotics for chorea.

Non-ketotic hyperglycemia

In diabetes mellitus, in some cases, both hypo- and hyperglycaemia might be accompanied by chorea or ballism. These dyskinesias usually resolve spontaneously when normal levels of glucose are stabilized. In non-ketotic hyperglycaemia, on MRI-T1-weighted images, a typical hyperintense signal in the putamen might be seen.

Ataxia telangiectasia or Louis-Bar syndrome (AT)

Ataxia telangiectasia, or Louis-Bar syndrome, is a rare, autosomal recessive neurodegenerative disease due to a mutation in the ATM gene located on chromosome 11. Ataxia is the first manifestation, beginning in the toddler years (7). Children have problems while sitting or standing and tend to sway and fall. Later, in the pre-school years (generally between ages 3 and 5), oculomotor apraxia and slurred dysarthria develop and telangiectasias occur (small, dilated blood vessels over the sclera). At school age, chorea, dystonia or myoclonus appear and overall motor impairment worsens. Adolescent patients, as a rule, are confined to a wheelchair. AT patients have immune abnormalities with low levels of immunoglobulins and thus, are at higher risk for respiratory tract infections. AT patients also have an increased incidence of cancer (especially lymphomas) and are extremely sensitive to radiation. Many laboratory abnormalities occur in AT, such as elevated α-fetoprotein, lymphocytopenia and decreased levels of IgE and IgA immunoglobulins. Homozygosity of ATM genes may be detected. No effective treatment is available.

Benign hereditary chorea (BHC)

BHC is a non-progressive, autosomal dominant disorder due to a mutation in the thyroid transcription factor 1 gene (TITF-1) located on chromosome 14 (8). TITF-1 is essential for the development of the brain, thyroid and lung. Currently, BHC is frequently designated as brain-thyroid-lung syndrome, as BHC also manifests variable degrees of hypothyroidism and respiratory abnormalities (8). Non-progressive chorea is present from early infancy. Dystonia, myoclonus or tics are observable in some cases, as well as subtle mental manifestations (attention deficit hyperactivity disorder, learning difficulties, etc.). Intellect is normal. The treatment is purely symptomatic.

Postpump chorea

Postpump chorea is the development of choreatic dyskinesias in children following cardiac surgery (cardiopulmonary bypass). Most cases are mild and spontaneously resolve. It is not known whether chorea results from hypoxia or hypothermia in this condition.

Paroxysmal dyskinesias

Paroxysmal dyskinesias are rare, hereditary disorders (channelopathies) that manifest in childhood by sudden attacks of dyskinesias, usually provoked by various stimuli or triggers. Consciousness is preserved. Currently, no single mutations responsible for paroxysmal dyskinesias have been detected, although some loci on chromosomes 2, 16 and 22 have been established (9). *Paroxysmal kinesigenic dyskinesia* is manifested by choreodystonic attacks that are provoked by sudden movements (stretching after awakening, shaking hands, etc.), and also while walking. Abnormal sensations, termed aura, precede the attacks quite frequently. Dyskinesias are asymmetric, frequently affecting just one limb. The attacks may be enhanced by stress, discomfort or anxiety and last for seconds, usually not exceeding one minute. The frequency during the day may be high, patients may experience tens or even hundreds of events (9). Paroxysmal exercise-induced dyskinesia manifests as bilateral, long-lasting, sometimes painful dystonia. The attacks are provoked by physical exertion and exercise, and last for several minutes (9). Between attacks, patients are completely normal. Carbamazepine is highly effective. *Paroxysmal nonkinesigenic dyskinesias* last much longer, many minutes or even hours, but their frequency is low (9). The choreodystonic attacks are not provoked by exertion but by triggers such as caffeine or alcohol consumption. As in the kinesigenic type, the manifestation is asymmetric. Clonazepam has been found to be effective in some cases.

Main choreatic disorders of adulthood

Iatrogenic chorea

Drug-induced chorea is probably one of the most common causes of an isolated choreic syndrome. Neuroleptic-induced chorea develops after chronic exposure to typical neuroleptic agents and their derivatives, and manifests as a stereotypic oro-buccal-lingual dyskinesia (see Chapter 38). Other widely used dopamine-receptor antagonists also include the prokinetic metoclopramide, the antiemetic thiethylperazine, or the antihistamine prothazine. The typical manifestation is orofacial movements that are choreic in nature. Muscles of the upper face are much less commonly involved. A frequent initial presentation includes tongue impersistence, smacking and chewing movements (see Video fragment 38.4). Dyskinesias are characteristically exacerbated by anticholinergic treatment. The need for neuroleptic treatment should always be carefully considered, as the management of drug induced chorea is very difficult. There are no guidelines and various treatment strategies have been reported, however many patients are never well compensated. Slow reduction of the inducing drug and switching to an atypical neuroleptic agent is recommended, beta-blockers, benzodiazepines or tetrabenazine may be added. Botulinum toxin can be used for symptomatic focal treatment.

Lupus erythematosus

A choreic syndrome may develop in approximately 2% of patients suffering from lupus erythematosus or in patients with antiphospholipid antibodies and various clinical symptomatology not fulfilling the clinical and laboratory criteria for lupus erythematosus, such as lupus like-syndrome and antiphospholipid antibody syndrome (10). Children may also be affected. Chorea may be the first manifestation of disease; it is often asymmetric (hemichorea), of fluctuating intensity and may be recurrent. Treatment of the underlying disorder leads to amelioration of the dyskinesia. Neuroleptics may be used as well.

Chorea gravidarum

Chorea manifesting during the first trimester of pregnancy is very rare and generally simply coincidental, or a recurrence of Sydenham's chorea in very young patients during their first pregnancy. Systemic lupus erythematosus and antiphospholipid antibody syndrome must be ruled out. In females over 30 years of age with no history of chorea during previous pregnancies, HD must always be considered. The manifestation of chorea after the first trimester, almost always in the third trimester, is a sign of pre-eclampsia. This disorder is probably underlined by a hormonal imbalance in pregnancy. Chorea may also rarely occur with oral contraceptive use. The manifestations are typically unilateral, with the onset 8-10 weeks after initiation of contraceptive use. After withdrawal of the drug, the disorder resolves without further treatment.

Vascular chorea

Ischemic lesions of the basal ganglia (lenticulostriate artery; lesion of the head of the caudate nuclei, anterior part of the internal capsule and putamen) are the most common cause of chorea or choreodystonia in vascular brain lesions. Patients typically present with an acute or subacute onset of marked chorea or ballistic movements of one side of the body. The intensity of manifestations usually decreases, sometimes resulting in dystonia and only rarely persisting with high intensity (see Video fragment 29.1).

Idiopathic (senile) chorea

Senile, idiopathic and non-hereditary chorea in the elderly characteristically presents with oro-buccal-lingual dyskinesia, indistinquishable from tardive chorea. Stereotypic lip movements like lip-smacking, chewing and tongue protrusion are present. There may be a history of a new prosthetic device or extensive dental intervention. In retrospective series, as a rule many cases are recognized as iatrogenic and/or vascular chorea. Neuroleptics are usually effective but often not tolerated (Video fragment 29.1).

Huntington's disease

Huntington's disease

Huntington's disease (HD) is an autosomal dominant, incurable and devastating neurodegenerative disease with an incidence of 0.38 per 100,000 per year, and in Europe with a prevalence 5.70 per 100,000 inhabitants. The prevalence is higher in Europe, North America, and Australia than in Asia (11). Sometimes, HD centers are found, such as in Venezuela, where in an isolated community of approximately ten thousand inhabitants near Maracaibo Lake more than 100 HD-affected persons were identified. There are three clinical variants of HD: classical, juvenile and late onset, as well as several HD-like syndromes (HD phenocopies), which will be discussed later.

In 1993, the genetic mutation responsible for HD was discovered; multiplication of a cytosine-adenine-guanine (CAG) trinucleotide (triplet) at chromosome 4 (4p16.3) exceeding 39 repeats (12). One CAG triplet codes for one molecule of the amino acid glutamine. Thus,

HD is monogenic disease with a dosage effect. (CAG)n is generally unstable; the longer the repetition in the normal (wild-type) allele, the greater the tendency to multiply. The same, of course, applies to the mutated allele, with the tendency for further multiplication, especially in cases with paternal transmission; CAG triplets are more prone to expand during spermatogenesis than in oogenesis. The concept of anticipation means that the onset of HD may occur earlier in successive generations. Repetitions in the range of 6 to 26 triplets are physiological and stable. Repeats in the range of 27 to 35 are not accompanied with a risk of developing HD, but with the tendency to expand in the successive generations (15). CAG repetitions from 36 to 39 results in reduced penetrance, which does not allow prediction. This reduced penetrance or premutation is likely responsible for rare, *de novo* mutations. Repeats of 40 and more result in full penetrance (see Figure 29.3).

In HD, an inverse relationship between the number of CAG repeats and the age-at-onset has been shown (the greater the number of triplets, the sooner the disease manifests) (13). However, this relationship primarily applies to cases with more that 60 CAG repeats.

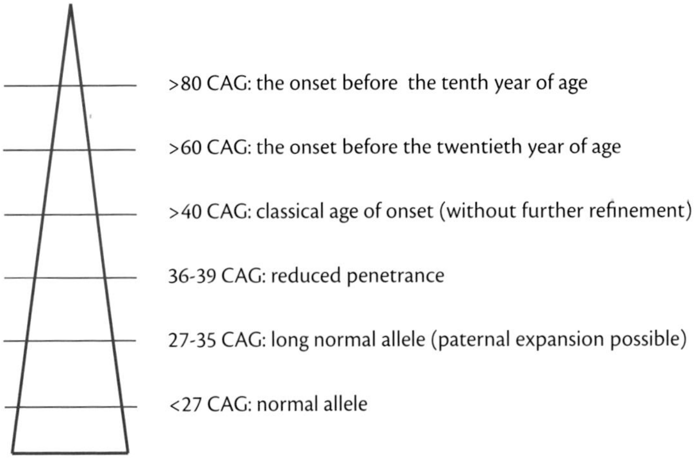

The multiplication of the CAG triplet is not the only factor that determines the age at which HD manifests, it is considered to account for approximately 70% of the variability (14). Other genetic and environmental factors that have yet to be elucidated may also play a significant role in the onset of HD.

The product of the gene is the huntingtin protein (htt).

Physiological htt (wild-type) is a cytoplasmic protein containing a polyglutamine chain at the N-terminus. The number of glutamine repetitions is equal to the number of CAG repetitions. Htt is an ubiquitous protein, present in all mammalian cells, with the highest expression in the brain. Htt has multiple physiological functions. It plays an essential role in the embryological development of the brain, and severe impairment of neurogenesis has been observed in htt knockout mice, incompatible with postnatal life (16). Furthermore, htt affects transcription, axonal transport, and upregulates the expression of various neurotrophic factors, primarily brain-derived neurotrophic factor (BDNF), which is essential for adequate neuroplasticity (17).

Pathological htt has an enlarged polyglutamine chain, designated as polyQ, with more CAG repetitions corresponding to a larger polyglutamine tract. PolyQ affects the structure of htt and leads to pathological conformation. Presumably, the pathogenesis of HD is mediated by pathological gain-of-function, with toxic consequences due to htt misfolding. Misfolded htt is not degraded by the ubiquitin-proteasomal and lysosomal proteolytic systems; its (toxic) protofibrils and fibrils will be neutralized in aggregates and inclusions (18,19). Aggregates are accu-

>80 CAG: the onset before the tenth year of age

>60 CAG: the onset before the twentieth year of age

>40 CAG: classical age of onset (without further refinement)

36-39 CAG: reduced penetrance

27-35 CAG: long normal allele (paternal expansion possible)

<27 CAG: normal allele

Figure 29.3
The relation between (CAG)n and age at the onset.

mulated in both the cytoplasm and the nucleus. This process is not specific to HD, as all neurodegenerative diseases share a common pathophysiology; the aggregation of mis-folded proteins (19,20).

The expression of pathological htt in the brain is not uniform, with the highest amount found in the striatum (21). The pathogenic mechanisms of htt have been extensively studied but are not yet fully understood. All of them show its relevance; excitotoxicity, oxidative stress, mitochondrial dysfunction, apoptosis, protein aggregation, impaired axonal transport, neurogenesis, synaptic dysfunction, microglial activation, etc. (19). Mutated htt is ubiquitous, not only in the brain but also in other tissues, with different pathological sequelae in various cellular subsystems. The principal, incipient neuropathological change in HD consists of a loss of GABA-ergic, medium-sized spiny neurons in the striatum, which are part of the indirect pathway of the striato-thalamo-cortical loop. Further progression manifests with atrophy of the globus pallidus, degenerative changes in the cortex, and later general atrophy of the brain (22).

As of now, a fascinating therapeutic approach in HD is to target the pathogenic problem at its roots; suppressing or silencing the mutation, thereby limiting the expression of the mutant htt. Several techniques exist: 1. at the level of DNA: zinc finger DNA protein (23), and 2. at the level of messenger RNA: antisense oligonucleotides, single stranded or duplex RNA interference (24). In order not to silence the wild-type htt, various allele-specific strategies have to be tested. Another approach is to influence the aggregation of synthesized, mutated htt by applying trehalose, geldanamycin or rapamycin, to inhibit transglutaminases, or histone deacetylase (mithramycin), or to develop antiapoptotic substances (e.g., minocycline) (18,25). Unfortunately, recent clinical trials to investigate the eventual symptomatic effects of ethyl-eicosapentaenoic acid, dimebon, nabilone or pridopidine, and other trials exploring the enhancement of mi-

tochondrial functions using creatine, coenzyme Q10 or remacemide, did not show any consistent robust effect (26,27). As of yet, a few preclinical studies aiming to deliver BDNF into the brain in order to protect the remaining striatal neurons have been initiated (28), and several transplant studies with stem cells are underway (29).

Classical form

The classical form of HD, with the onset of clinical manifestations between 35 and 50 years of age, is by far the most frequent form (approximately 90% of all patients). The phenoconversion of HD from the preclinical stage, detectable only by specific tools such as MRI-based morphometry or neuropsychology, to the stage of obvious clinical manifestation is poorly demarcated, thus resulting in remarkable bias in studies dealing with the exact age of HD onset.

Behavioural manifestations

Behavioural and personality changes are usually the first manifestation of HD. Two scenarios are often observed. In some families, the same scenario repeats uniformly in subsequent generations, so HD is easily recognized by other members of the family.

The first scenario manifests very gradually as a lack of interest in the family, partner, children and their needs. The affected person begins to be apathetic, emotionally flattened, losing interest in any hobbies. The HD patient has difficulty with work-related activities, partly due to the early appearance of executive dysfunction, and partly due to apathy and lack of concern. Global cognitive deterioration appears relatively early. The consequences of this scenario are usually repeated job loss and descent in the social hierarchy, especially in cases without family support, where even homelessness could easily be reached. Therapy of the above-mentioned manifestations does not exist. Psycho-social support and counseling is of great importance. Many years can pass until the first signs of subtle choreatic dyskinesias appear and at this time the proper diagnosis is first provided, especially in people with a negative family history.

The second scenario also begins with behavioural and personality abnormalities, but the manifestations are different. The first signs are usually irritability or even aggression (30). Anxiety and/or depression are the other frequent manifestations. Depression is present in nearly 50% of HD patients and the occurrence of bipolar affective disorder is not exceptional (30). The suicide rate for these patients is higher than in the healthy population (31). Anxiety is often reported by patients as somatoform symptoms (headache, gastrointestinal problems, neck pain, etc.), and could surprisingly present as the subjectively-dominant trouble, even in patients with very severe chorea to which they are anosognostic.

The first behavioural manifestations, often resulting in divorce and/or loss of child custody, may include jealousy, paranoid suspicions, obsessive thoughts and compulsive acts (30). Hypersexuality, promiscuity or sexually provocative behaviour is occasionally present, as well as alcohol abuse and a predisposition to petty criminality (32).

Psychotic manifestations may appear anytime during the progression of HD, mostly generalized paranoia or delusions. Hallucinations are quite rare (30). Aggression may be acutely mitigated or abolished using benzodiazepines (e.g., clonazepam) and antipsychotics (e.g., risperidone or haloperidol). In cases with dominant sexual aggression antiandrogenic treatment (medroxyprogesterone) is useful. In the prevention of aggression, SSRI's (especially sertraline) or mood stabilizers (preferentially valproate) are of great importance. The same applies for irritability. In the treatment of depression, SSRI's are the first choice. In the treatment of bipolar affective disorders, caution should be exercised in the use of lithium as there is a risk of intoxication due to lack of fluid intake. In psychotic depression, augmentation with antipsychotics is highly recommended. As a last option, electroconvulsive therapy may be applied.

Cognitive manifestations

In HD patients, cognitive decline is neither global nor equally progressive. Isolated cognitive deficits, particularly executive dysfunction, attention deficit, learning and memory dysfunction and changes of psycho-motor speed predominate in the early stages of HD (33). The degree of cognitive decline may not be directly proportional to behavioural or neurological manifestations. Working and short-term memory are impaired the most, while long-term memory is relatively well preserved. In general, the impairment of procedural memory (unconscious learning of motor skills, i.e., driving, walking, etc.) is a characteristic sign of basal ganglia disorder (and thus of HD). Information retrieval, but not information storage, is significantly disturbed, however it can be facilitated by recognition, cueing or creating associations. Memory disturbances are caused by executive dysfunction (degraded ability to plan and to generate strategies, impaired self-control and reduced set-shifting capacity in response to external requirements).

Executive dysfunction predominates from the early stages of HD. Patients are severely disabled and incapable of working shortly after disease onset. Dementia, a significant loss of global cognitive ability, interfering with activities of daily living, manifests as HD progresses. Subcortical dementia with predominate executive dysfunction, slowing of psycho-motor speed, memory disturbances, behavioural disorders (irritability, apathy, obsessive-compulsive manifestations, etc.), disturbances of mood (depression) and anxiety are characteristic in HD. Unlike in cortical dementia (such as Alzheimer's disease), aphasia, agnosia, and apraxia are rare, and cortical dysfunctions only develop in more severe cognitive decline. There is no therapy for HD-related cognitive manifestations.

Motor manifestations

Chorea is considered as an essential sign of HD and often leads to the diagnosis. Nevertheless, considering the time course of HD, in the diagnostic procedure, too much weight is allocated to chorea as an essential component of the diagnosis, as choreatic manifestations mostly become evident after several years after onset of the disease. Therefore, the correct diagnosis is usually established with great delay.

Although chorea is not the most disabling motor manifestation, in some cases, the intensity of chorea may result in severe disability (Video fragment 29.2). During the course of the disease, chorea might both progress or decline while being replaced by dystonia, and finally akinesia. In the Westphal HD variant, patients do not show choreatic movements because of a significant akinesia.

More significant motor manifestations of HD, developing in line with both disease duration and cognitive regression, comprise the loss of coordination and the development of motor parkinsonism, initially manifesting with bradykinesia and the loss of dexterity. In the intermediate stage of the disease, progressive postural instability with dysbasia and occasional falls may occurr due to the complex of discoordination, motor parkinsonism and chorea, as well as the first signs of dystonia (trunk dystonia). Apart from chorea and dystonia, myoclonus may be also observed in some patients. Later on, rigidity (sometimes more pronounced due to side-effects of antipsychotics and finally akinesia might develop. Patients then are completely immobile, and secondary complications such as decubitus and infections may develop.

Speech disorders (dysarthria), mostly an explosive speech (hyperkinetic dysarthria), sometimes speech with interrupting involuntary sounds such as groaning, may be observed, in the end resulting in an entirely unintelligible speech. may be present from the early stage. Due to the progressive course of the disease, speech therapy only has a limited impact (34).

Dysphagia represents a serious problem that can have fatal consequences, particularly in the later stages of the disease. Swallowing disturbances (both solid and liquid food) as well as postprandial cough or vomiting, fever and recurrent respiratory infections must be actively sought. There is a risk of aspiration, including clinically asymptomatic (silent) aspirations, without coughing or vomiting. Hyperphagia, the swallowing of large non-masticated mouthfuls, may rarely be observed. Hyperphagia may be due to an uncontrolled sense of hunger and presents an imminent risk of suffocation. Dysphagia can be influenced by small doses of prokinetic agents and, above all, by feeding the patient with the head upright. The consistency of liquid yoghurt is easiest to swallow. Swallowing therapy is of transitory benefit, being partially effective (34).

Advancing cachexia is a characteristic feature in the advanced stages of the disease and may not be related to the obvious loss of appetite and common difficulty with food intake. Degeneration of lateral thalamic nuclei with the subsequent need of increased caloric intake (approximately 4000Kcal/day) is thought to be responsible (35). Sipping is often helpful, but in the advanced stages percutaneous endoscopic gastrostomy should be employed.

In HD, there is also a typical facial expression with emotional flatness, empty gaze and the expression of subtle displeasure or disgust. As a rule, after 10-15 years, although the course of disease is highly individual, patients are fully dependent and will die marasmic after approximately 20 years of disease duration, largely due to complications such as infections, decubitus sores, etc.

Juvenile form

Juvenile HD (JHD) presents before 20 years of age and is rare, representing approximately 5% of all cases (36). Very rarely JHD begins even before the 10th year and exceptional cases manifest in the pre-school age. JHD results when the number of CAG triplets exceeds 60 (36). The first clinical manifestations are extremely diverse, as JHD occurs in the developing brain.

Typically, the first signs are difficulties with school activities related to psychomotor retardation, motor dyscoordination, motor parkinsonism and cognitive deterioration. Behavioural changes are characteristic for JHD: outbursts of anger, aggression, antisocial tendencies as well as obsessive thoughts and compulsive acts. Depression is frequent, but often hard to diagnose. Psychotic manifestations are more common than in adults with HD.

What is striking at first are the motor manifestations of JHD in contrast to classical HD. Chorea is rare, dystonia and/or rigidity with akinesia (the primary Westphal variant of HD) is much more common (see Video fragment 29.3). Gait disorder with postural instability and frequent falls arises rapidly.

Titubations or myoclonus of the head and trunk, postural and kinetic tremor of the upper extremities as well as supranuclear gaze palsy are frequently present in the middle stages. Epileptic seizures appear at any stage of JHD. Severe dysarthria or even mutism and dysphagia are relatively early signs. Dysphagia severely affects food-intake, being a cause of suffocation, postprandial vomiting and coughing. As a consequence of aspiration, recurrent pneumonia appears. Cachexy, frequently independent of dysphagia, is another extremely unfavorable sign requiring percutaneous gastrostomy. The progression is rapid and patients die approximately ten years after onset (37).

Amantadine is partially effective in the treatment of dystonia. Anticholinergics are more dangerous, as they might provoke delirious states and/or psychosis, and intensify cognitive impairment. L-DOPA and dopamine agonists are sometimes helpful in the amelioration of parkinsonian manifestations. Antipsychotics worsen motor abilities; when psychotic manifestations are present, atypical antipsychotics are thus strictly recommended.

Late onset form

The late onset form of HD manifests in persons over the age of 60 and represents approximately 5% of all cases. This form of the disease has a relatively benign course and most patients live to the average age of the healthy population. The principal and incipient manifestation is chorea, whose distribution and character do not differ from the classical form of the disease, but is less intensive and progresses more slowly. Apathy, depression or irritability are frequent behavioural manifestations. Isolated cognitive deficits, but not severe dementia, are usually present (especially dysexecutive syndrome, attention and short-term memory impairments), but to a lesser degree than in the classical form.

Huntington disease-like syndromes (HD phenocopies)

Approximately 1% of patients with typical HD-like manifestations lack the causative mutation (38). Such cases are considered Huntington's disease-like syndromes or Huntington's disease phenocopies (HDP). HDP are clinically and genetically heterogeneous, and the etiological diagnosis of the respective HDP is usually difficult to establish. Both, typical and atypical phenocopies are displayed in Table 29.3

Dentato-rubro-pallido-Luysian atrophy (DRPLA)

DRPLA is inherited in an autosomal dominant manner due to a mutation in the atrophin-1 gene on chromosome 12p13.3. The prevalence is highest in Japan, while in other populations DRPLA is rare (39,40). Ataxia, choreoathetosis and cognitive decline are common at the onset of disease after 40 years of age. Adolescents and young adults present with ataxia and signs of progressive myoclonic epilepsy; myoclonus, various forms of epileptic seizures, and cognitive decline. Diffuse cerebral atrophy and atrophy of the caudate nuclei are typical MRI findings.

Table 29.3
Huntington's disease-like syndromes (HD phenocopies).

Typical HD phenocopies	Atypical HD phenocopies
▪ Dentato-rubro-pallido-Luysian atrophy (DRPLA) ▪ Spinocerebellar ataxia type 17 (SCA-17) or Huntington's disease-like 4 (HDL-4) ▪ Choreoacanthocytosis (ChA) ▪ McLeod syndrome (MLS) ▪ Neuroferritinopathy (NFP) ▪ Huntington's disease-like 1+ (HDL-1) ▪ Huntington's disease-like 2+ (HDL-2) ▪ Huntington's disease-like 3+ (HDL-3) (onset at preschool age)	▪ Spinocerebellar ataxia type 2 (SCA-2) ▪ Spinocerebellar ataxia type 3 (SCA-3) ▪ Friedreich's ataxia (FRDA) ▪ Pantothenate kinase-associated neurodegeneration (PKAN) (onset in childhood and adolescence) ▪ Wilson's disease (WD)

+ extremely rare in Europe

Spinocerebellar ataxia type 17 (SCA-17)

SCA17, or Huntington's disease-like 4 (HDL4), is inherited in an autosomal dominant manner and is probably the most frequent HDP in Europe. It is caused by the expansion of a CAG/CAA repeat in the coding region of the TATA box binding protein gene l on chromosome 6q27 (41). Ataxia, cognitive deterioration and chorea usually manifest in adulthood. Other manifestations may include dystonia or parkinsonism. Brain MRI shows cerebellar and cortical atrophy. The intensity and combination of manifestations is highly variable.

Chorea-acanthocytosis (ChA)

Chorea-acanthocytosis, also named Levine-Critchley syndrome, is inherited in an autosomal recessive manner by a mutation in the gene that encodes chorein, localized on chromosome 9 (42). Manifestations typically begin in adulthood and are characterized by a combination of choreodystonia, dementia and epileptic seizures. Orofacial dyskinesia, buccolingual mutilation, dysarthria, dysphagia, respiratory disturbances and vocal tics are suggestive of ChA. Protrusion dystonia of the tongue (feeding dystonia) that causes the tongue to push food out of mouth is a feature of advanced disease. Bizarre gait with trunk dystonia is present. Neuropathic changes and areflexia are frequent findings. MRI reveals atrophy of the caudate nuclei. Acanthocytes are found in blood smears. Increased serum concentrations of muscle creatine kinase, aspartate aminotransferase, alanine aminotransferase, gamma-glutamyltransferase and reduced haptoglobin (hemolysis of acanthocytes) are present.

McLeod syndrome (MLS)

In MLS acanthocytosis is typical, but not invariable. MLS is a rare disorder inherited in an X-linked manner (43). Decreased expression of Kell antigens on erythrocytes is caused by a mutation of the XK gene. Adult males develop the disease. Clinical manifestations are similar to ChA, and cardiac manifestations include congestive or dilated cardiomyopathy, and atrial fibrillation or tachyarrhythmia. Hepatosplenomegaly may be present. Brain MRI shows atrophy of the caput nuclei caudati.

Neuroferritinopathy (NFP)

Neuroferritinopathy is a rare, autosomal dominant neurodegenerative disorder characterized by the deposition of ferritin in the brain and a decreased or normal level of serum ferritin. The disease is caused by a mutation in the ferritin light chain gene localized on chromosome 19 (44). The disorder presents with adult-onset motor manifestations and cognitive decline that is less prominent than in HD. Brain MRI shows excess iron storage (hypontensity on T2-weighted images in the basal ganglia), followed by cystic degeneration in the caudate and putamen nuclei in more advanced cases.

Friedreich's ataxia (FRDA)

FRDA is one of the most frequent hereditary ataxias due to an expanded GAA triplet repeat on chromosome 9. According to the Quebec cooperative study (QCS) criteria (45) (approximately 25% of patients not fulfilling these criteria have been reported), the disorder manifests with gait and limb ataxia, dysarthria, loss of vibration sense and eye movement abnormalities. Chorea rarely manifest, and sometimes also cerebellar manifestations are absent (46). Typical disease onset is in childhood, but adult onset has been reported as well.

Pantothenate kinase-associated neurodegeneration (PKAN)

PKAN belongs to the small group of neurodegenerative diseases with brain iron accumulation. PKAN is an autosomal recessive disease due to a mutation in the PANK 2 gene at chromosome 20, generally manifesting before 10 years of age (47). Severe disability in PKAN progresses quickly and patients usually die within ten years after onset. Atypical cases, with an onset in adolescence or even adulthood, have been observed. With a later onset, the prognosis is usually better. Dystonia, dysphagia, dysarthria and dementia are the most frequent manifestations. Retinitis pigmentosa is frequently present and epileptic seizures only occasionally occur. In PKAN patients with a proven mutation, the eye-of-the-tiger sign in the globus pallidus is found on MRI (central hyperintensity due to gliosis with surrounding hypointensity due to iron accumulation on T2-weighted images). There is no effective treatment available. Dystonia in PKAN may be controlled using deep brain stimulation of the internal globus pallidus.

Wilson's disease

Wilson's disease (see also Chapter 5, 23) is an autosomal recessive metabolic disorder predominantly affecting the liver and brain. The affected gene is located on chromosome 13 and encodes the copper-transporting ATP7B protein (48). Absent or reduced function leads to decreased hepatocellular excretion of copper into bile. This results in hepatic copper accumulation and injury. Eventually, copper is released into the bloodstream and deposited in other organs, notably the brain, kidneys, and cornea. Copper deposits are most likely toxic due to its ability to promote free radical formation.

Clinical manifestations of WD usually begin in childhood or early adulthood. The hepatic form usually begins at a younger age and may present only as asymptomatic abnormal serum aminotransferase levels, as chronic liver disease (cirrhosis) or even acute liver failure. Neuropsychiatric manifestations such as irritability, fatigability, decreased school performance, and clumsiness rarely appear in childhood.

In the third decade, WD manifests with virtually any neurological (tremor, parkinsonism, dysarthria, dystonia, postural instability or chorea) (see Video fragment 23.1) or psychiatric (anxiety, depression, psychosis) presentation. The vast majority of patients with the neuropsychiatric form of WD have detectable Kayser-Fleischer rings; gold-brown deposition of copper in Descemet's membrane of the cornea (see Figure 5.7).

The diagnosis of WD is based on clinical signs and symptoms, biochemical markers of liver disease and impaired copper metabolism (serum free copper and ceruloplasmin concentrations, 24-hour urinary copper excretion), MRI findings, the presence of Kayser-Fleischer rings, liver copper content and molecular genetic testing. A fast and accurate diagnosis is crucial as effective treatment is available and the sooner it is initiated, the better the outcome. Patients should avoid food rich in copper. Chelating agents, such as penicillamine or trientine, bind plasma and tissue copper and increase its urinary excretion.

Table 29.4
Routine information for the diagnosis of chorea.

- Family history
- Previous illnesses
- Age at onset of first manifestation (childhood, adolescence, adulthood, elderly)
- Speed and dynamics (acute, slowly progressive, fluctuating, paroxysmal)
- Underlying factors (i.e., preceding infections, exposure to drugs or toxins)
- Modifying factors (effects of previous treatment, psychological factors, startle reflex, etc.)
- Additional not chorea-related signs or symptoms

Zinc and tetrathiomolybdate prevent intestinal absorption of copper. Liver transplantation has also been shown to improve neurological signs in several patients.

Diagnosis and differential diagnosis

There are nearly 150 clinical entities that may be considered in the work-up of chorea. The following text focuses on pragmatic, useful clues that may serve as a practical guide for clinical practice. The most important factors for establishing the diagnosis of the diseases accompanied by chorea are outlined in Table 29.4. Those factors comprise, among others, age of onset, onset and dynamics of the disease, frequency, distribution, the presence of not chorea related signs and symptoms, neurophysiological and genetic tests, laboratory tests and neuro-imaging.

Age of onset

Some choreatic syndromes do appear mainly in childhood and adolescence (such as Sydenham's chorea, PANDAS, ataxia teleangectasia, PKAN), and others in adults and elderly (such as idiopathic, vascular and senile chorea) (see Tables 29.5 and 29.6).

Onset

Some choreatic disorders display an acute, sudden onset, others are insidious, slowly progressive. The type of onset, of course, is dependent of the underlying disorder (see Tables 29.5 and 29.6).

Frequency

As stated above, there are no valid data regarding the incidence of chorea in the population. However, choreatic dyskinesias do not appear as often in our population as restless legs syndrome, tics, or focal, primary dystonias. Choreatic dyskinesia likely occurs most frequently in association with advanced Parkinson's disease. The frequency of drug-induced tardive stereotypies has been decreasing in the last several decades. This is related to the wide-spread use of atypical antipsychotics as the first choice of treatment. The most common hereditary chorea (in Europe and North America) is Huntington's disease. Tables 29.5 and 29.6 display less sophis-

Table 29.5
Most common causes of chorea in childhood and adolescence.

Sudden onset	Slowly progressive (rare)
- Autoimmune Sydenham's chorea, PANDAS, Systemic lupus erythematosus, antiphospholipid antibody syndrome, postinfectious, postvaccinal, paraneoplastic disorders - Iatrogenic (more likely choreodystonia) - Vascular chorea (cerebral palsy) - Hypo/hyperglycemia in diabetes - Hyperthyreosis - Postpump chorea	- Benign hereditary chorea - Ataxia telangiectasia (Louis Bar disease) - PKAN - Metabolic disorders Lesch-Nyhan syndrome, mitochondrial diseases, lysosomal storage diseases, aminoacidopathies, glutaric aciduria

Table 29.6
Most common causes of chorea in adulthood and in the elderly.

Sudden onset	Slowly progressive (rare)

■ Stroke
■ Autoimmune
  vasculitis, systemic lupus erythematosus, antiphospholipid antibody syndrome, para-neoplastic
■ Iatrogenic (more likely choreodystonia)
■ Hypo/hyperglycemia in diabetes
■ Hyperthyreosis
■ Chorea gravidarum
	■ Iatrogenic
	  Levodopa and dopamine agonists in PD Anti-psychotics- and their derivatives-induced stereo-typies
	■ Neurodegenerative disorders
	  HD and phenocopies
	  SCA2, SCA3, Friedreich's ataxia
	■ Senile chorea

ticated clues based on the frequency of various choreatic syndromes with an onset in childhood or the adulthood.

Distribution

The localization or predominance of manifestations in various bodily regions may also help in the differential diagnosis of the various choreatic syndromes. Focal circumoral dyskinesias are typical for drug-induced stereotypies or senile chorea. Hemichorea is typically present in vascular chorea. Marked asymmetry may often be observed in Sydenham's chorea, chorea gravidarum, vascular chorea and chorea induced by contraceptive hormones.

Not chorea-related signs and symptoms

The presence of any additional manifestation is of particular value in the differential diagnosis (see Table 29.7), especially cerebellar signs, polyneuropathy, myopathy or amyotrophy, or behavioural changes and dementia.

Genetic tests

In HD, a genetic test can be performed from blood, amniotic fluid or other tissues. Finding the mutation in the absence of clinical presentation is not sufficient to establish a diagnosis of HD. A confirmative test is pursued in persons where the suspicion of HD is based on clinical findings. A presymptomatic predictive test can be carried out in people at risk, i.e., clinically

healthy persons at 25-50% risk of developing HD and willing to know their genetic status. A prenatal predictive test can be executed by request during the pregnancy of a woman that has HD or has tested positive, or whose partner is ill or has tested positive.

Predictive testing in HD is a unique example of an ethical dilemma in medicine; HD is a fatal, incurable and devastating disease appearing at the zenith of the productive life with a 50% risk of heredity for the subsequent generation (49). The person deciding to be tested or not bears

Table 29.7
Additional features in the various choreatic disorders.

Dystonia, rigidity, akinesia	Primary Westphal variant in Juvenile HD Wilson's disease
Dementia	HD and HDP Wilson's disease
Behavioural disturbances	HD and HDP Sydenham's chorea
Polyneuropathy	Choreoacanthocytosis McLeod syndrome
Cerebellar signs Spinocerebellar atrophy (SCA) types 2, 3, and 17	Friedreich's ataxia Ataxia telangiectasia
Epilepsia	Dentato-rubro-pal-lido-Luysian atrophy (DRPLA)

the full responsibility for their decision, which will affect their entire life. Therefore, predictive testing is prohibited in children and adolescents, and in persons that have not explicitly expressed their wish to be tested. Furthermore, it is recommended that the test be postponed in persons with uncertain motivation, under apparent influence from others or in the presence of factors that complicate responsible decision making (acute depression, etc.). The official international predictive guidelines are accessible (50). The role of experts involved in the predictive protocol is to provide maximum information, to accompany people at risk during their decision-making, and to offer support. It is absolutely necessary to abstain from any kind of eugenics. Pre-implantation genetic diagnosis has become available in the last decade, allowing people at risk that do not want to know their genetic status to have children without passing on the HD mutation (51). In HD phenocopies, genetic tests for HD are typically negative. A diagnostic algorithm for these Huntington's disease-like syndromes might be appreciated in Table 29.8.

Table 29.8
Diagnostic algorithm of Huntington's disease phenocopies (HDP).

1 Clinical manifestations fulfill HDP criteria; negative HD genetic tests

2 Genetic testing for *SCA 17 and DRPLA* (in older adults)

3 In case of negative SCA-17 and DRPLA genetic tests:

  a Males with polyneuropathy, elevated creatine-kinase, myoglobin, weak expression of Kell antigen, acanthocytes, caudate atrophy: *McLeod syndrome*

  b Both genders with polyneuropathy, elevated CK, myoglobin, acanthocytes, epilepsy, feeding dystonia, self-mutilation, caudate atrophy: *choreoacanthocytosis*

  c Cerebellar signs, cerebellar atrophy: *SCA 1,2,3,6,7,8,12, Friedreich's ataxia*

  d Myoclonus, epilepsy, caudate atrophy: *DRPLA in adolescents or young adults*

Additional clinical and neurophysiological investigations, laboratory tests and neuro-imaging findings

The value of additional clinical and neurophysiological investigations, laboratory tests and neuro-imaging studies in the differential diagnosis of choreatic syndromes is outlined in Table 29.9.

Therapy of chorea

Chorea can be suppressed by symptomatic pharmacological treatment. Dyskinesias are regularly accentuated under stress and therefore the severity of manifestations during the clinical examination may not correspond to the commonplace situation. Only chorea that causes disability to the patient should be treated. There are no double-blind, randomized, placebo-controlled clinical trials (evidence-based class I studies) for chorea as a general entity. There are studies that have assessed, apart from other parameters, the anti-choreatic effect of various drugs in HD, but only a few of them can be classified as class I. Meta-analysis published by Bonelli and Wenning (26) in 2006 and Cochrane Database analysis done by Mestre (27) reviewed and analyzed the results of all studies on pharmacological interventions in HD. The current treatment algorithm of motor manifestations in HD is presented in the review by Burgunder (52).

Antipsychotics (neuroleptics)

Postsynaptic blockade of dopamine receptors in the striatum can suppress dyskinesia. Typical neuroleptics are more effective than atypical, but they have a higher incidence of adverse events that may be severe, including sedation, apathy, decline of psychomotor speed, falls, dysphagia, dysarthria and even a drug induced parkinsonian syndrome or acute tardive dyskinesia. Furthermore, irritability, aggression and psychotic manifestations in HD can be positively influenced. According to a review by Bonelli, only haloperidol, fluphenazine and olanzapine have

Table 29.9
Important clinical, laboratory and neuro-imaging findings.

Blood
- Acanthocytes: choreoacanthocytosis, McLeod syndrome
- Erythrocyte Kx and Kell antigens: McLeod syndrome
- Abnormal liver tests: Wilson's disease, toxins, drugs, metabolic disorders
- Hyperglycemia/hypoglycemia: diabetes mellitus
- Elevated C-reactive protein: parainfectious disorders
- Elevated creatine kinase: choreoacanthocytosis, McLeod syndrome
- Decreased ferritin: neuroferritinopathy
- Sedimentation rate, antinuclear, anti-neuronal, antiphospholipid antibodies: systemic lupus erythematosus, antiphospholipid antibody syndrome, paraneoplastic syndromes
- Elevated thyroid gland hormones: hyperthyroidism
- Elevated free copper and urinary copper excretion, decreased ceruloplasmin: Wilson's disease
- Elevated antistreptolysin O, anti-DNase B: Sydenham's chorea (often negative), PANDAS
- Elevated alpha-fetoprotein: Ataxia-telangiectasia

Neuro-imaging (CT, MRI)
- Caudate nucleus atrophy: HD, choreoacanthocytosis, McLeod syndrome, DRPLA, SCA-3
- Panda sign in mesencephalon and changes in the lentiform nucleus: Wilson's disease
- Focal lesions: ischemic, traumatic, tumor changes
- Cerebellar atrophy: spinocerebellar atrophy
- Eye-of-the-tiger sign: PKAN
- Iron deposits: neuroferritinopathy

Electromyography
- Neurogenic lesion: DRPLA, choreoacanthocytosis
- Myogenic lesion: McLeod syndrome

Electroencephalography
- Epileptic grapho-elements: DRPLA, choreoacanthocytosis, HD Westphal variant

Ophthalmologic (slit-lamp) examination
- Kayser-Fleischer ring: Wilson's disease

Neuropsychological testing
- Dementia: HD, DRPLA, choreoacanthocytosis, McLeod syndrome, etc.

Genetic testing
- HD, SCAs, Wilson's disease, PKAN, benign hereditary chorea, McLeod syndrome, DRPLA, ataxia telangiectasia

Cardiac examination
- Cardiomyopathy in McLeod syndrome, Friedreich's ataxia

been considered "possibly useful" in the treatment of chorea by class I studies (26).

Presynaptic dopamine-depleting agents (reserpine and tetrabenazine) are effective in chorea (52). Therapeutic doses of tetrabenazine (up to 150–200 mg/day) does not cause the adverse events common with antipsychotics, but can induce depression.

GABAergic agents

Benzodiazepines can effectively suppress dyskinesias, but the dose needs to be increased during the course of treatment and side effects including addiction, postural instability and sedation may develop. An open-label clinical trial has been conducted for clonazepam (35).

Glutamate receptor antagonists
Riluzole, amantadine, lamotrigine have been tested in chorea, and none of these agents had a convincing effect (26,27). Remacemide has also been shown to be ineffective (26,27). However, amantadine appears to have a good clinical effect in dystonia.

Specific treatment options
Deep brain stimulation of the internal pallidum in chorea has been tested, but there are only occasional case reports with inconsistent outcomes available (53). Deep brain stimulation of the subthalamic nucleus or internal pallidum has became already an established treatment for drug induced dyskinesias in late motor complications in Parkinson's disease. Intensity of paroxysmal choreoathetosis can be influenced by valproate or carbamazepine. Drug induced chorea may be ceased by withdrawal of inducing agent, however this might not always be feasible if antipsychotic treatment is necessary. Tardive drug-induced stereotypies may persist chronically even after the withdrawal of inducing drug. Chorea of Sydenham may be a self-limiting condition but recurrence is common. Adequate antibiotic treatment is necessary, corticosteroids, intravenous immunoglobulines or plasmapheresis may help. Symptoms of chorea gravidarum disappear in the days after the child birth, in case of a severe clinical course, labor must be induced earlier.

Specific therapy with chelating agents or zinc is indicated for a rare chorea in Wilson's disease. Chorea in the autoimmune disorders can be considerably influenced by treatment of underlying disease, corticosteroids and other immunosuppressive or immunomodulating therapy, and compensation of hyperthyroidism or thyreotoxicosis brings rapid suppression of hormonally induced chorea.

Video fragments

Fragment 29.1
Chorea (Segments 1-4)
This videotape shows a senile chorea (segment 1), followed by hemichorea (ballism) after a striatal haemorrhage (segment 2) and hemichorea after stenting the left medial carotid artery (segment 3), and posttraumatic dystonic hemichorea (segment 4).

Fragment 29.2
Chorea (Huntington's disease)
(Segments 1-5)
Here are two patients suffering Huntington's disease (segments 1 and 2), followed by the tongue protrusion test in an HD patient (segment 3), the typical choreatic gait in HD patients (segment 4), and the impaired voluntary movements in these patients (segment 5).

Fragment 29.3
Chorea (young-onset Huntington's disease)
(Segments 1-3)
This tape demonstrates a parkinsonian phenotype in a young-onset HD patient (segment 1), as well as a bradykinetic dystonic phenotype (segment 2) and a clinical manifestation of young-onset HD with myoclonus, tics, and stereotypies (segment 3).

References

1   Albin RL, Young AB, Penney JB. The functional anatomy of basal ganglia. Trends Neurosci 1989;12:366–375.

2   Obeso JA, Rodríguez-Oroz MC, Benitez-Temino B, et al..Functional organization of the basal ganglia: therapeutic implications for Parkinson's disease. Mov Disord. 2008;23 Suppl 3:548-559.

3   Burgunder JM. Recent advances in the management of choreas. Ther Adv Neurol Disord. 2013 Mar;6:1171-1127.

4   Walker RH. Differential diagnosis of chorea. Curr Neurol Neurosci Rep. 2011;11:385-395.

5   Walker KG. An update on the treatment of Sydenham's chorea: the evidence for established and evolving interventions. Ther Adv Neurol Disord. 2010;3:301–309.

6   Church AJ, Cardoso F, Dale RC, Lees AJ, Thompson EJ, Giovannoni G. Anti–basal ganglia antibodies in acute and persistent Sydenham's chorea. Neurology 2002:59:227-231.

7   Perlman S, Becker-Catania S, Gatti RA. Ataxia-telangiectasia: diagnosis and treatment. Semin Pediatr Neurol. 2003;10:173-182.

8   Kleiner-Fisman G. Benign hereditary chorea. Handb Clin Neurol. 2011;100:199–212.

9   Unterberger I, Trinka E. Diagnosis and Treatment of Paroxysmal Dyskinesias Revisited.Ther Adv Neurol Disord. 2008;1:4–11.

10 Baizabal-Carvallo JF, Jankovic J. Movement disorders in autoimmune diseases. Mov Disord. 2012;27:935-946.

11 Pringsheim T, Wiltshire K, Day L, Dykeman J, Steeves T, Jette N. The incidence and prevalence of Huntington's disease: a systematic review and meta-analysis. Mov Disord. 2012;27:1083-1091.

12 The Huntington´s Disease Collaborative Research Group. A novel gene containing a trinucleotide repeat that is expanded and unstable on Huntington´s disease chromosomes. Cell 1993;2:971-983.

13 Semaka A, Collins JA, Hayden MR. Unstable familial transmissions of Huntington disease alleles with 27–35 CAG repeats (intermediate alleles). Am J Med Genet B Neuropsychiatr Genet. 2010;153B:314–320.

14 Andrew SE, Goldberg YP, Kremer B et al. The relationship between trinucleotide (CAG) repeat length and clinical features of Huntington's disease. Nature Genet 1993;4:398-403.

15 Langbehn DR, Hayden MR, Paulsen JS; PREDICT-HD Investigators of the Huntington Study Group. CAG-repeat length and the age of onset in Huntington disease (HD): a review and validation study of statistical approaches. Am J Med Genet B Neuropsychiatr Genet. 2010;153B:397-408.

16 Zeitlin S, Liu JP, Chapman DL, Papaioannou VE, Efstratiadis A. Increased apoptosis and early embryonic lethality in mice nullizygous for the Huntington's disease gene homologue. Nat Genet 1995;11:155-163.

17 Zuccato C, Cattaneo E. Brain-derived neurotrophic factor in neurodegenerative diseases. Nat Rev Neurol 2009;5:311-322.

18 Borrell-Pagès M, Zala D, Humbert S, Saudou F. Huntington's disease: from huntingtin function and dysfunction to therapeutic strategies. Cell Mol Life Sci 2006;63:2642-2660.

19 Gil JM, Rego AC. Mechanisms of neurodegeneration in Huntington´s dinase. Eur J Neurosci 2008;27:2803-2820.

20 Lehman NL. The ubiquitin proteasome system in neuropathology. Acta Neuropathol 2009;118:329-347.

21 Saudou F, Finkbeiner S, Devys D, Greenberg ME. Huntingtin acts in the nucleus to induce apoptosis but death does not correlate with the formation of intranuclear inclusions. Cell 1998;95:55-66.

22 Vonsattel JP, Meyers RH, Stevens TJ et al.: Neuropathological classification of Huntington´s disease. J Neuropathol and Exp Neurol 1985;44:559-577.

23 Garriga-Canut M, Agustín-Pavón C, Herrmann F, et al. Synthetic zinc finger repressors reduce mutant huntingtin expression in the brain of R6/2 mice. Proc Natl Acad Sci USA. 2012;109:E3136-3145.

24 Yu D, Pendergraff H, Liu J, et al. Single-stranded RNAs use RNAi to potently and allele-selectively inhibit mutant huntingtin expression. Cell. 2012;150:895-908.

25 Kordasiewicz HB, Stanek LM, Wancewicz EV, et al. Sustained therapeutic reversal of Huntington's dis-

ease by transient repression of huntingtin synthesis. Neuron 2012;74:1031-4104.

26 Bonelli RM, Wenning GK Pharmacological management of Huntington's disease: an evidence-based review. Curr Pharm 2006;12:2701-2720.

27 Mestre T, Ferreira J, Coelho MM, et al. Therapeutic interventions for symptomatic treatment in Huntington's disease. Cochrane Database Syst Rev 2009:CD006456.

28 Gallina P, Paganini M, Lombardini L, Giordano G, Mascalchi M, Romoli AM, Ghelli E, Porfirio B, Vannelli GB, Di Lorenzo N. Progress in restorative neurosurgery: human fetal striatal transplantation in Huntington's disease. J Neurosurg Sci. 2011;55:371-381.

29 Olson SD, Pollock K, Kambal A, et al. Genetically engineered mesenchymal stem cells as a proposed therapeutic for Huntington'sdisease. Mol Neurobiol 2012;45:87-98.

30 Paulsen JS, Ready RE, Hamilton JM et al. Neuropsychiatric aspects of Huntington's disease. J Neurol Neurosurg Psychiatry 2001;71:310–314.

31 Hubers AA, Reedeker N, Giltay EJ, Roos RA, van Duijn E, van der Mast RC.Suicidality in Huntington's disease. J Affect Disord. 2012;136:550-557.

32 Jensen P, Fenger K, Bolwig T, Sørensen SA. Crime in Huntington´s disease: a study of registered offences among patients, relatives, and controls. J Neurol Neurosurg Psychiatry 1998;65:467–471.

33 Paulsen JS.Cognitive impairment in Huntington disease: diagnosis and treatment. Curr Neurol Neurosci Rep. 2011;11:474-483.

34 Bilney B, Morris ME, Perry A. Effectiveness of physiotherapy, occupational therapy, and speech pathology for people with Huntington's disease: a systematic review. Neurorehabil Neural Repair 2003;17:12-24.

35 Trejo A, Boll MC, Alonso ME, et al. Use of oral nutritional supplements in patients with Huntington's disease. Nutrition. 2005;21:889–894.

36 Rasmussen A, Macias R, Yescas P, Ochoa A, Davila G, Alonso E. Huntington disease in children: genotype-phenotype correlation. Neuropediatrics. 2000;31:190-194.

37 Ribaï P, Nguyen K, Hahn-Barma V, et al. Psychiatric and cognitive difficulties as indicators of juvenile huntington disease onset in 29 patients. Arch Neurol 2007;64:813-819.

38 Wild EJ, Mudanohwo EE, Sweeney MG, et al. Huntington's disease phenocopies are clinically and genetically heterogeneous Mov Disord. 2008;23:716-720.

39 Tsuji S. Dentatorubral-pallidoluysian atrophy: clinical aspects and molecular genetics. Ad Neurol 2002;89:231-239.

40 Wardle M, Morris H, Robertson N. Clinical and genetic characteristics of non-Asian dentatorubral-pallidoluysian atrophy: A systematic review. Mov Disord 2009;24:1636–1640.

41 Schneider SA, van de Warrenburg BP, Hughes TD, et al. Phenotypic homogeneity of the Huntington disease-like presentation in a SCA17 family. Neurology 2006;67:1701–1703.

42 Rubio JP, Danek A, Stone C, et al. halmers R, Wood N, Verellen C, Ferrer X, Chorea–acanthocytosis: genetic linkage to chromosome 9q21. Am J Hum Genet 1997;61:899–908.

43 Danek A, Rubio JP, Rampoldi L, et al. McLeod neuroacanthocytosis: genotype and phenotype. Ann Neurol 2001;50:755–764.

44 Curtis AR, Fey C, Morris CM, et al. Mutation in the gene encoding ferritin light polypeptide causes dominant adult-onset basal ganglia disease. Nat Genet 2001;28: 350–354.

45 Filla A, De Michele G, Coppola G, et al. Accuracy of clinical diagnostic criteria for Friedreich's ataxia. Mov Disord. 2000;15:1255-1258.

46 Bhidayasiri R, Perlman SL, Pulst SM, Geschwind DH. Late-onset Friedreich ataxia: phenotypic analysis, magnetic resonance imaging findings, and review of the literature. Arch Neurol 2005;62:1865-1869.

47 Hartig MB, Prokisch H, Meitinger T, Klopstock T. Pantothenate kinase-associated neurodegeneration. Curr Drug Targets. 2012;13:1182-1189.

48 Rosencrantz R., Schilsky M. Wilson disease: pathogenesis and clinical considerations in diagnosis and treatment. Semin Liver Dis 2011;31:245–259.

49 Tibben A. Predictive testing for Huntington's disease. Brain Res Bull. 2007;30:165–171.

50 International Huntington Association (IHA) and the World Federation of Neurology (WFN) Research Group on Huntington´s Chorea. Guidelines for the molecular genetics predictive test in Huntington´s disease. Neurology 1994;44:1533-1536.

51 Van Rij MC, De Rademaeker M, Moutou C, et al. Preimplantation genetic diagnosis (PGD) for Huntington's disease: the experience of three European centres. Eur J Hum Genet 2012; 20:368–375.

52 Burgunder JM, Guttman M, Perlman S, et al. An international survey-based algorithm for the pharmacological treatment of chorea in Huntington's disease. PLoS Curr. 2011;3:RRN1260.

53 Biolsi B, Cif L, Fertit HE, Robles SG, Coubes P. Long-term follow-up of Huntington disease treated by bilateral deep brain stimulation of the internal globus pallidus. J Neurosurg 2008;109:130-132.

Supported by the Czech Ministry of Education, Research Program MSM 0021620849 and PRVOUK-P26/LF1/4

30

Ballism

Daniel Waldvogel

Ballism is defined as a movement disorder characterized by involuntary, forceful, flinging, high-amplitude 'throwing' movements. Ballism is often accompanied by choreatic movements, the latter being more distal while ballism describes the proximal movements. With time, the proximal ballistic movements may become less pronounced, and the distal choreatic movements predominate. Ballism increases with action and is absent during sleep. The movements can be so violent that patients injure themselves. Ballism usually affects one side of the body, and it is then referred to as hemiballism. Older terms are hardly ever used anymore, i.e. monoballism if only one limb is affected, biballism if both extremities on one side of the body but not the head or face are affected, or paraballism if both sides of the body are affected.

Epidemiology

Ballism is a rare movement disorder, and thus there are hardly any epidemiological data available. In a busy movement disorders clinic in Houston, only 0.7% of patients suffered from hemiballism (1). In a large stroke dataset from Lausanne, hemiballism was seen in 0.5% of all stroke patients (2), while in Belgrade, the incidence of hemiballism was estimated to be 0.45/100,000/year (3) .

Etiology

Most cases of hemiballism are due to a basal ganglia stroke. The second most important cause may be hyperglycemia (4), which can cause hemiballism despite being a metabolic disorder, i.e. it affects only one side of the body. There are reports of many other etiologies(see Table 30.1); common to all of them is disruption of the basal ganglia network. Focal lesions that have been reported include neoplasms (5), vascular mal-

Table 30.1
Different causes of hemiballism.

Frequent causes	
Vascular	▪ Basal-Ganglia Stroke
Metabolic	▪ Hyperglycemia
Rare causes	
Vascular	▪ Malformation
Metabolic	▪ Hypocalcemia ▪ Hypoclycemia
Drug induced	▪ Levodopa ▪ Anticonvulsants ▪ Contraceptives
Infectious	▪ AIDS ▪ Tuberculosis ▪ Toxoplasmosis ▪ Cysticercosis
Others	▪ Neoplasm ▪ Multiple Sclerosis ▪ Tuberous Sclerosis ▪ Trauma ▪ Ventriculoperitoneal shunting ▪ Sydenham's chorea ▪ Systemic lupus erythematodes
Iatrogenic	▪ Subthalamotomy ▪ Deep brain stimulation of STN

formations (6), demyelinating plaques, abscess, tuberculomas (7) and more recently AIDS-associated lesions (1). Single case reports mention head trauma, ventriculoperitoneal shunting, hypocalcemia or influenza, and last but not least surgical lesions, particularly subthalamotomy, as the underlying cause of hemiballism (8). The most prominent view is that ballism is caused by a lesion in the subthalamic nucleus. However, the largest published series of patients with hemiballism found that this applies only to 30% of patients (1,2,9-11). More commonly, the lesion was outside the subthalamic nucleus, or there was no lesion at all that could be detected. It must be mentioned, however, that CT scanning was used in some series, which may not be sensitive enough to detect a small lesion in a small nucleus. However, in patients with hemiballism due to hyperglycemia, the detectable MRI lesions are mostly in the striatum, with only one report of a pathological signal in the subthalamic nucleus (12).

Pathophysiology

Our understanding of the function of the basal ganglia has been advanced by the description of the basal ganglia circuitry. The classic model of the motor loop describes a direct pathway from the striatum through the globus pallidus internus to the thalamus and an indirect pathway from the striatum through the globus pallidus externus, the subthalamic nucleus and then through the globus pallidus internus to the thalamus and back to the cortex (see Chapter 2). Since the connection from the subthalamic nucleus to the globus pallidus internus is excitatory, the globus pallidus internus itself inhibits the thalamus, i.e. the outflow of the basal ganglia, and a lesion of the subthalamic nucleus can diminish the inhibitory drive of the globus pallidus internus, and therefore facilitate motor outflow. In other words, a lesion of the subthalamic nucleus resulting in a hyperkinetic movement disorder like ballism is entirely compatible with

the classic model of the basal ganglia circuitry. This has also been shown experimentally, e.g. by Whittier, Mettler, and Carpenter in animal models and many times since, more recently in patients who underwent surgical lesioning of the subthalamic nucleus to treat Parkinson's disease (8). It is more difficult to explain the pathophysiology for lesions outside the subthalamic nucleus, as the classical model does not account for it. Even more difficult to explain is the effect of pallidotomy on hemiballism patients with unremitting hemiballism, pallidotomy of the globus pallidus internus is a therapeutic option. However, according to the classical basal ganglia model, pallidotomy should worsen ballism, since it 're-leases' the thalamus, thereby increasing the outflow of the basal ganglia even further. This has been elegantly discussed in a seminal paper by Marsden and Obeso, titled 'The function of the basal ganglia and the paradox of stereotaxic surgery in Parkinson's disease' (13).

A possible insight towards solving this paradox is the notion that the firing pattern of the globus pallidus internus is disturbed in both hypokinetic (increased (14)) and hyperkinetic (decreased (15)) movement disorders, and that a lesion or deep brain stimulation of the globus pallidus internus shields the target structures of the basal ganglia output from the disturbed pattern, restoring a more physiological function (16). Although, recent advances in the understanding of basal ganglia physiology revealed that the connections and interactions between the different nuclei are far more complex than given in the classic model, so that we may be able to explain the inconsistencies in the future.

Clinical presentation and diagnosis

Most cases of hemiballism present acutely or subacutely, due to the underlying vascular or metabolic nature of the disorder. The diagnosis of hemiballism is clinical, based on the typical phenomenology of the movement disorder. A metabolic work-up (hyperglycemia being the most urgent question to be answered) as well as imaging, preferentially MRI, are mandatory. It should be highlighted again that hyperglycemia, being a metabolic disturbance, can manifest with hemi-ballism and that therefore a one-sided symptomatology is not a valid argument against a metabolic cause.

Differential diagnosis

If the aetiology of hemiballism remains unclear after the initial work-up, rare causes should be considered, like drug intoxication (lamotrigine and phenytoin have been reported to cause ballism) or an immunological cause such as Sydenham's disease, central systemic lupus erythematodes, or Fisher's syndrome.

In terms of phenomenology, other stroke-associated hyperkinetic movement disorders have been reported, such as dystonia or myoclonus, mostly after thalamic strokes (2,17).

Treatment

Due to the rarity of the disorder, there are no controlled studies for the treatment of hemiballism. Since many patients show remission with time, it is difficult to assess the effectiveness of a therapeutic approach versus natural history. In the acute phase, patients may need padding and cushioning since they may hurt themselves. The drugs most commonly prescribed are dopamine receptor blockers or dopamine-depleting drugs like tetrabenazine. Tetrabenazine carries little or no risk for the development of tardive symptoms and may therefore be the preferred option. A particular problem with dopamine-blocking or -depleting drugs may be that patients develop parkinsonism on the unaffected side. Other drugs reported to be beneficial in some cases are valproic acid, clonazepam or topiramate (18).

For patients who do not respond to medical therapy and show no spontaneous amelioration of symptoms, functional neurosurgery may be an option. The largest series so far performed

thalamotomy (19), while more recent case reports suggest pallidotomy as an alternative (14,15,20). The therapeutic significance of deep brain stimulation has yet to be determined.

Prognosis

In most cases, hemiballism resolves with time. In many patients, the proximal flinging movements of ballism lessen and the more distal choreatic movements become more apparent and persist longer. The overall prognosis is determined by the underlying pathology. Since the most common cause of hemiballism is vascular, an interdisciplinary work-up of the patient seems prudent.

Video fragment

Fragment 30.1 (24.1)
Hemiballism
This elderly woman shows continuous, irregular, flinging movements over the left side of her body, induced by a cerebral infarction involving the subthalamic nucleus.

References

1 Dewey RB, Jankovic J. Hemiballism-hemichorea. Clinical and pharmacologic findings in 21 patients. Arch Neurol 1989;46:862–867.

2 Ghika-Schmid F, Ghika J, Regli F, Bogousslavsky J. Hyperkinetic movement disorders during and after acute stroke: the Lausanne Stroke Registry. J Neurol Sci 1997;146:109–116.

3 Pekmezovi T, Svetel M, Risti A, et al. Incidence of vascular hemiballism in the population of Belgrade. Mov Disord 2004;19:1469–1472.

4 Bedwell SF. Some observations on hemiballismus. Neurology 1960;10:619–622.

5 Lemmen LJ, Davis JS, Fisher ER. Hemiballismus secondary to metastatic carcinoma of the gall bladder. Neurology 1957;7:873–874.

6 Lobo-Antunes J, Yahr MD, Hilal SK. Extrapyramidal dysfunction with cerebral arteriovenous malformations. J Neurol Neurosurg Psychiatry 1974; 37:259–268.

7 Dierssen GG, Gioino GG. Anatomic correlation of hemiballism. Rev Clin Esp 1961;82:283–305.

8 Chen CC, Lee ST, Wu T, Chen CJ, Huang CC, Lu CS. Hemiballism after subthalamotomy in patients with Parkinson's disease: Report of 2 cases. Mov Disord 2002;17:1367–1371.

9 Chung S, Im J-H, Lee M, Kim J. Hemichorea after stroke: Clinical-radiological correlation. J Neurol 2004;251:725-729.

10 Vidakovic A, Dragasevic N, Kostic VS. Hemiballism: report of 25 cases. J Neurol Neurosurg Psychiatry 1994;57:945-949.

11 Postuma RB, Lang AE. Hemiballism: revisiting a classic disorder. Lancet Neurol 2003;2:661–668.

12 Kim HJ, Moon WJ, Oh J, Lee IK, Kim HY, Han SH. Subthalamic lesion on MR imaging in a patient with nonketotic hyperglycemia-induced hemiballism. Am J Neurorad 2008;29:526–527.

13 Marsden CD, Obeso JA. The functions of the basal ganglia and the paradox of stereotaxic surgery in Parkinson's disease. Brain 1994;117:877–897.

14 Suarez JI, Metman LV, Reich SG, Dougherty PM, Hallett M, Lenz FA. Pallidotomy for hemiballismus: efficacy and characteristics of neuronal activity. Ann Neurol 1997;42:807–811.

15 Vitek JL, Chockkan V, Zhang JY, et al. Neuronal activity in the basal ganglia in patients with generalized dystonia and hemiballismus. Ann Neurol 1999;46:22–35.

16 Brown P, Eusebio A. Paradoxes of functional neurosurgery: Clues from basal ganglia recordings. Mov Disord 2008;23:12–20.

17 Lehericy S, Grand S, Pollak P, et al. Clinical characteristics and topography of lesions in movement disorders due to thalamic lesions. Neurology 2001;57:1055–1066.

18 Zesiewicz TA, Sullivan KL, Hauser RA. Vascular hemichorea/hemiballismus and topiramate. Mov Disord 2006;21:581–582.

19 Krauss JK, Mundinger F. Functional stereotactic surgery for hemiballism. J Neurosurg 1996;85:278–286.

20 Yamada K, Harada M, Goto S. Response of postapoplectic hemichorea/ballism to GPi pallidotomy: progressive improvement resulting in complete relief. Mov Disord 2004;19:1111–1114.

31
Tics

Andreas Hartmann

Tics are brief, sudden, non-rhythmical, repetitive and stereotyped movements. They can be motor or vocal. Both motor and vocal tics can be either simple or complex. *Simple tics* typically involve only one group of mucles and are brief and meaningless, whereas *complex tics* may last

longer and appear more purposeful (see also below). Tic disorders usually begin in childhood and are classified according to the *Diagnostic and Statistical Manual of Mental Disorders* (DSM IV-TR) (1) into four groups (see Table 31.1): (i) transient tic disorder, (ii) chronic motor or vocal tic disorder, (iii) Tourette syndrome (GTS), (iv) tic disorder not otherwise specified.

As tics can resemble almost any other movement disorder, phenotypic analysis alone is insufficient, and patients must be questioned about whether the execution is preceded by a premonitory sensation (*urge to do, urge to move*) and whether temporary control of the movement can be achieved. Also, relief following execution of the tic is frequently reported. There are no biomarkers available for tics, and the diagnosis therefore remains strictly clinical.

Epidemiology

The epidemiology of tics remains poorly understood. This is probably due to the variability and heterogeneity of tics, with large fluctuations depending on the age group studied. Transient tics are estimated to occur in 3% of children and adolescents, while Gilles de la Tourette syndrome (GTS) is estimated to occur in 0.3%-0.8% of the same population (2). A meta-analysis of two studies assessing adults for GTS suggested a prevalence of 0.05% (2), which reflects the favourable prognosis of tics after adolescence (see below).

Table 31.1
DSM IV-TR criteria for tic disorders.

Diagnostic criteria for Tourette syndrome (DSM-IV-TR 307.23):
Continuous or intermittent, daily, multiple motor and single or multiple vocal tics, not necessary concurrently, during >1 yr, without tic-free intervals >3 months, starting at age <18 yr, and not the effect of a substance and/or medical condition

Diagnostic criteria for chronic motor or vocal tic disorder (DSM-IV-TR 307.22):
Daily, single or multiple motor or vocal tics, starting at age <18yr, and not the effect of a substance or medical condition, and also not meeting the criteria of a Tourette syndrome

Diagnostic criteria for transient tic disorder (DSM-IV-TR 307.21):
One single or recurrent episodes with daily, single or multiple motor and/or vocal tics during a period > 4 weeks but <12 months, starting at age <18yr, and not the effect of a substance or medical condition, or meeting the criteria of a chronic motor or vocal tic disorder or Tourette syndrome

Tic disorder not otherwise specified (DSM-IV-TR 307.20):
Disorders characterized by tics that do not meet criteria for a specific tic disorder. Examples include tics lasting < 4 weeks or tics with an onset after age 18 years.

Etiology and pathophysiology

The focus of this review will be on GTS, as it is the most chronic and severe form of tic disease. Nonetheless, the etiologic and pathophysiologic mechanisms identified in GTS almost certainly apply to more common form of tics.

In his initial description in 1885, George Gilles de la Tourette had already proposed the hypothesis that tics were organic in origin with a strong hereditary component. Subsequently, however, psychodynamic interpretations of tics became prevalent. Since the 1970s, however, an increasing number of genetic, imaging and post-mortem studies have established the organic origin and cerebral structures implicated in the genesis of tics. This change of perspective has also been supported by animal models of tics, both in rodents (3) and non-human primates (4). Specifically, two structures and their respective connectivities have been implicated in the development of tics: the basal ganglia and the cortex. Inferences from various approaches support the hypothesis that GTS is a neurodevelopmental disorder associated with a dysfunction of cortico-striato-thalamo-cortical loops (5).

The basal ganglia are composed of the striatum (caudate nucleus and putamen), the pallidum (external segment – GPe, internal segment – GPi), the substantia nigra pars reticulata (SNr) and the subthalamic nucleus. They receive afferent inputs from the cortex. These cortical projections to the basal ganglia are functionally and topographically organized, leading to the concept of functional divisions of cortico-striato-thalamo-cortical loops into sensorimotor, associative and limbic circuits (see also Chapter 2) that are implicated in motor, cognitive and motivational aspects of behaviour, respectively (6) (see Figure 31.1).

It has been hypothesized in tics that an aberrant focus of striatal neurons becomes inappropriately active, causing unwanted inhibition of a group of basal ganglia output neurons (especially from the GPi), which in turn disinhibit particular movement programs, leading to an involuntary movement. Repetitive overactivity of a given specific set of striatal neurons could therefore result in involuntary and stereotyped movements such as tics (5).

Although the neural circuit hypothesis for tic production was developed specifically for the motor circuits of the cortico-striato-thalamo-cortical loops, it is likely that the fundamental principles of function in the limbic and cognitive basal ganglia circuits are similar. Malfunctions in these networks could lead to the emergence of the various behavioural problems occurring in GTS. This hypothesis is supported by several experimental data. In primate models, experiments inducing local inhibition of GABA-ergic transmission showed that dysfunction of premotor and sensorimotor circuits produced abnormal movements resembling simple motor tics, whereas dysfunction of associative and limbic circuits resulted in behavioural disorders resembling complex tics and compulsions, respectively (4).

What causes aberrant neuronal activity in GTS? Although there are several potential factors, decreased inhibitory function and/or abnormal dopamine neurotransmission probably play a major role. Neuropathological studies in GTS showed both decreased numbers and a deviant distribution of striatal GABAergic and cholinergic interneurons (7,8). These findings could be explained by a migration defect involving inhibitory interneurons originating in the ganglionic eminence. As cortical and basal ganglia interneurons originate from the same structures during brain development (9), reduced numbers of inhibitory interneurons may also be present in the cortex, leading to both structural changes and functional cortical abnormalities. This assumption is in line with neurophysiological data (10) showing diminished intracortical inhibition and hyperactivity of premotor and sensorimotor cortex in GTS.

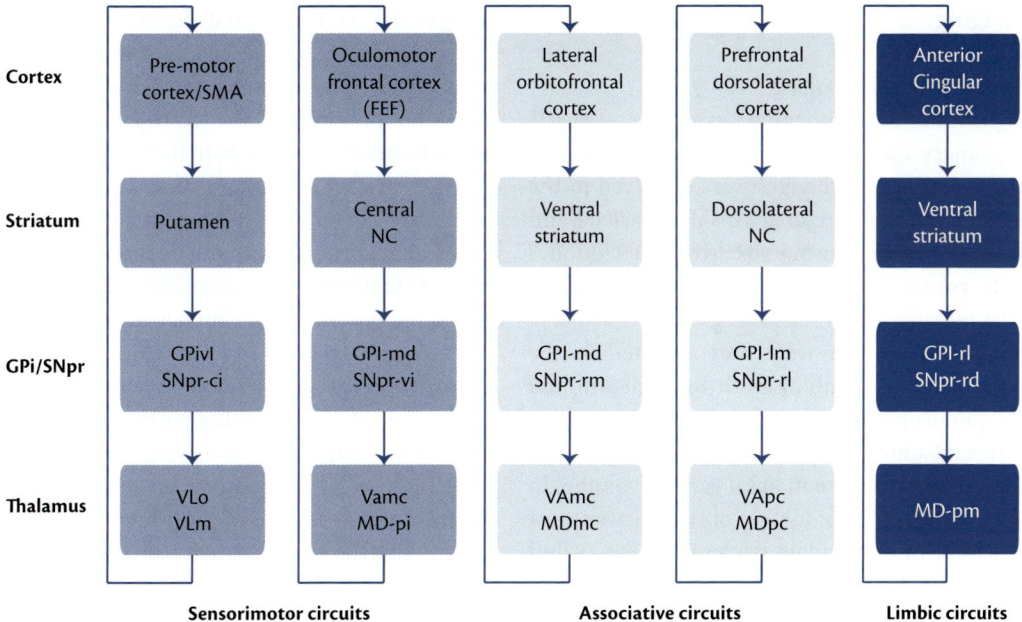

Figure 31.1

Segregated, parallel, corticobasal ganglia circuits. Abbreviations: CN, caudate nucleus; GPe, external segment of the globus pallidus; GPi, internal segment of the globus pallidus; mc, magnacellularis; MD, mediodrosal nucleus; pc, parvocellularis; SMA, supplementary motor area; SNpr, pars reticulate of the substantia nigra; VA, ventral anterior nucleus; VLo, ventrolateral oral nucleus; VLm, ventrolateral medial nucleus. Adapted from (6).

Other lines of evidence suggest that GTS is related to abnormal dopaminergic transmission. Notably, symptoms are markedly improved by classic antipsychotics (dopamine receptor antagonists), which remain the drugs of choice for the treatment of tics. Postmortem studies have also found increased concentrations of dopamine receptors and transporters in the frontal cortex and basal ganglia of GTS patients (11).

Taken together, these alterations could result in both structural changes and functional abnormalities in cortico-basal ganglia networks as shown in postmortem and imaging studies, which will be presented below.

Postmortem studies

Given the rarity of the condition and the patients' young age, there are very few postmortem studies of GTS. Two recent studies have opened an interesting perspective by observing a decrease in GABAergic parvalbumin-positive and cholinergic interneurons in the striatum, especially in the caudate nucleus, and an increase of density of these same neurons in the GPi (7,8). The authors explain the density variations of these interneurons by a tangential migration deficit during embryogenesis. Inhibitory interneurons are formed in the medial ganglionic eminence, which forms the pallidum and from which they migrate further to the lateral medial ganglionic eminence, eventually forming the striatum. As a consequence of this arrested migration, decreased striatal inhibition is plausible, which can assert pathological signaling output to the motor as well as to the associative and limbic territories. This corresponds well with the observed motor and behavioural abnormalities in GTS and underpins the neurodevelopmental deficit probably causing/facilitating tics within the basal ganglia.

Imaging

Structural neuroimaging

Significant neuroimaging evidence suggests a primary cortical dysfunction in GTS. In the cortex, structural changes were observed in the frontal, anterior cingulate, insular, parietal and temporal regions, using voxel-based techniques (12), region of interest (13) and cortical thickness measurements (14-16).

Structural changes were also reported in the basal ganglia, including both the striatum and the globus pallidus. In a large cohort of paediatric and adult GTS patients, Peterson et al. (17) identified a decrease in basal ganglia volume. In GTS children, the reduction of volume was most apparent in the caudate nucleus, whereas adult GTS patients showed volume reductions across all basal ganglia regions. Moreover, a smaller volume of the caudate nucleus head was predictive for persistence of tics in adulthood (18).

When correlating function with structural changes, analysis showed that tic severity (measured by the Yale global tic severity scale (YGTSS) is correlated with cortical thinning in the sensorimotor cortex and surrounding frontal and parietal areas (14,15). Finally, diffusion tensor imaging (DTI), which allows evaluation of white matter integrity, has revealed microstructural abnormalities in the white matter including a deficit in myelination involving the corpus callosum and anterior and posterior limb of the internal capsule in GTS patients (19,20).

Functional neuroimaging

Despite the numerous and extensive studies on structural abnormalities in GTS cited in the previous sections, it is not always obvious how these structural changes alter the functional activity of the brain and lead to heterogeneous clinical expressions of the syndrome. Several studies addressed the question of functional capacity of the brain in GTS patients using both task-specific and resting-state functional neuroimaging.

Wang et al. (21) investigated effective connectivity among the regions of sensorimotor networks and found stronger connectivity within the sensorimotor pathway in the GTS group during spontaneous tics compared to the control group, which expressed voluntary tics. Interestingly, connectivity from the primary somatosensory cortex to the primary motor cortex was stronger in the GTS group. This coincides with the expected temporal relationship between premonitory sensory urges and tics. Consequently, it can be suggested that greater activity within specific portions of sensorimotor pathways leads to premonitory urges, which drive tics within this same network in a feedforward manner. The results of this study are of great interest as they suggest that increased activity in the primary somatosensory cortex, putamen, and amygdala/hippocampus may represent activity associated with the premonitory urge and act as a trigger for tics. They also indicate that the primary sensory cortex exerts a causal influence on the putamen that is greater in GTS patients during spontaneous tics, confirming that a stronger generation of tics may be caused by a greater interaction between the motor cortices and striatum. A number of studies of tic suppression also pointed to the robust activity of the frontal cortex, which was thought to be related to a compensatory, neuroplastic hypertrophy of the frontal cortices that helps regulate activity within the motor circuit and consequently reduce tic symptoms (22).

Neurotransmission abnormalities

Evidence from pharmacological trials, particularly the fact that dopamine receptor blockers are the most effective treatment of tics to date, and postmortem analyses suggested that abnormalities of dopaminergic neurotransmission play a key role in the pathogenesis of GTS. However, most of the early analyses of striatal dopaminergic function in GTS using conventional positron emission tomography (PET) and single photon emission computerized tomography (SPECT) ligands have generated equivocal or contradictory results, indicating both increased and decreased dopaminergic function in GTS.

Interestingly, a recent study using baseline measurements and amphetamine challenge of dopaminergic function allowed evaluation of the specific affinity of subtypes of dopamine receptor in GTS patients (23). These results showed that compared to controls, patients with GTS had decreased binding potentials to D2/D3 receptors at baseline and an increased dopaminergic release after amphetamine challenge in the caudate nucleus and in many cortical regions, including the anterior cingulate, dorsolateral prefrontal, supplementary motor, premotor, and primary motor cortices as well as the superior temporal gyrus. All these regions, as already mentioned, have been postulated to play a primary role in the generation of tics.

Finally, a recent PET neuroimaging study in GTS patients using a ligand for $GABA_A$ receptors, ^{11}C-flumazenil, pointed to decreased GABAergic binding bilaterally in the ventral striatum, globus pallidus, thalamus, amygdala and right insula and to increased binding in the bilateral substantia nigra, left periaqueductal grey, right posterior cingulate cortex and bilateral cerebellum (24). These results are in agreement with neuropathological data that showed a diminished number and an aberrant distribution of GABAergic interneurons and support the hypothesis of cortico-striato-thalamo-cortical network hyperactivity in GTS (7,8).

In summary, animal models, postmortem and imaging studies in humans suggest that the cortex (motor and frontal/prefrontal) and particularly the basal ganglia are the two principal systems implicated in tic genesis and/or control. Accordingly, the following hypotheses can be formulated regarding the origin of tics and GTS:

- Tics are likely to be the result of neurodevelopmental abnormalities, which result in a dysfunction of the cortico-striato-thalamo-cortical loops. These deficits in basal ganglia and/or cortical maturation can express themselves in two ways: (i) by a loss of selectivity of projections from the cortex to the basal ganglia or (ii) by a quantitative shift of specific projections.
- With regard to GTS, the diversity of symptoms is probably related to the cortico-striato-thalamo-cortical loops involved, i.e. sensorimotor, associative and/or limbic. This dysfunction is most likely due to deficits in local inhibition within the basal ganglia, particularly the striatum.

Environmental factors

Tics can be provoked and/or exacerbated by stress hormones (cortisol, adrenaline, noradrenaline) and sex hormones (androgens), dopaminergic treatments, psychostimulants (cocaine, amphetamines) or caffeine without being, *sensu stricto*, causative (25). Furthermore, prenatal factors (maternal smoking) and perinatal factors (hypoxia/ischemia and low birth weight) might predispose to tics in later life. A complex interaction between genetic and environmental factors is probable and might also explain, at least partially, the great variability of phenotypes.

One of the most promising but also controversial hypotheses concerns the so-called 'pediatric autoimmune neuropsychiatric disorders associated with streptococcal infections' (PANDAS). According to this hypothesis, tic genesis might be due to the production of anti-neuronal antibodies directed against the basal ganglia resulting from a cross-reactivity with A group streptococci (26). Criteria required for the diagnosis of PANDAS are listed in Table 31.2. At present, the debate concerning the potential therapeutic value of plasmapheresis or intravenous immunoglobulins remains open. In any case, however, this hypothesis reinforces the notion that the basal ganglia play a major role in tic genesis and introduces an environmental factor that, depending on the patient's immune status, might help to explain fluctuation in tic severity and phenotype.

Table 31.2
Diagnostic criteria for PANDAS (pediatric auto-immune neuropsychiatric disorders associated with streptococcal infections).

1 The presence of a tic disorder and/or OCD consistent with DSM-IV
2 Prepubertal onset of neuropsychiatric symptoms
3 A history of a sudden onset of symptoms and/or an episodic course with abrupt symptom exacerbation interspersed with periods of partial or complete remission
4 Evidence of a temporal association between onset or exacerbation of symptoms and a prior streptococcal infection
5 Adventitious movements (e.g., motoric hyperactivity and choreiform movements) during symptom exacerbation

Genetics

The genetic component in GTS is beyond doubt: 50% of homozygous twins will develop GTS versus only 8% for first-degree relatives. These percentages increase to 77% and 23%, respectively, if only simple tics are taken into consideration (27). However, GTS genetics are probably very complex. Several transmission models have been proposed so far, either dominant with incomplete penetrance and variable expression, or a mixed, semi-dominant, semi-recessive transmission. Recent studies rather favour a polygenic transmission with several genes involved, which display additive effects. This later model does not preclude the existence of major genes in certain families (28).

Linkage analyses in families with a positive history for GTS have allowed the identification of several chromosomal regions. Recently, a linkage analysis has detected the L-histidine decarboxylase (HDC) gene in a large family with most members suffering from GTS (29). HDC codes for the rate-limiting enzyme in histamine synthesis. The mutation appears to be loss of function resulting in decreased histamine synthesis. However, the role of this mutation in larger cohorts remains to be verified. In this respect, a recent study suggests disruption of genes in the histaminergic and GABAergic pathways apart from HDC (30).

A second approach has consisted of characterizing chromosomal abnormalities visible on karyotype in sporadic forms of GTS; these studies also have allowed the identification of several chromosomal candidate regions. In 2005, Abelson et al. (31) proposed that mutations of the SLITRK-1 gene (SLIT and NTRK-like family, member 1) are responsible in a small number of GTS patients. SLITRK-1 is involved in dentritic growth and is abundant in the developing CNS, reinforcing the notion that tics and GTS are likely neurodevelopmental in nature and linked to abnormal contacts between different neuronal populations. However, the potential pathogenic role of SLITRK-1 in larger cohorts of GTS remains controversial.

A third approach lies with association studies to identify vulnerability genes in the hypothesis of polygenic heredity and/or the association of rare variants, which, individually, account for only small increments in risk for pathology. Candidate gene approaches have targeted the dopaminergic system and found significant associations with DRD2, DaT and MAO-A genes. Also, the LIM homeobox gene LHX6, which participates in the formation of striatal interneurons, was found to be affected in a tagging, single nucleotide polymorphism-based association study in a southern European sample (32). Finally, a genome-wide association study in 1285 GTS cases and 4964 ancestry-matched controls revealed no markers achieving a genome-wide threshold of significance, but those results await replication and extension in a larger sample (33).

Clinical presentation

Simple tics are brief, sudden, intermittent, repetitive, non-rhythmic and stereotyped movements (for instance, eye blinking or shoulder shrugs) or sounds (for instance, throat clearing or sniffing). *Complex* tics are characterized by normal motor or vocal sequences but occurring in an unadapted context. Examples include touching behaviour, copropraxia (showing the finger or touching one's genitals), or coprolalia (obscene language, often sexually tainted). Coprolalia also includes socially unacceptable phrases such as insults (ethnic, racial or religious). Finally, complex vocal tics also include repetition of one's own words or phrases (palilalia) or those of others (echolalia).

Tics can be distinguished from other abnormal movements by specific semiologic particularities. First, tics can be suppressed, at least temporarily; however, this control is achieved by a major mental effort and eventually results in the need to evacuate an increased number of tics during the post-suppression period (rebound phenomenon). Also, the suggestible character of tics (mimicking behaviour, tic production following specific environmental stimuli) reinforces the notion that tics are at the border between voluntary and involuntary movements.

Second, tics are often accompanied by premonitory sensations, which are mostly experienced as uncomfortable. These premonitory sensations can manifest as tension (local or generalized) or a burning sensation that is relieved by tic production. It is often called *urge to do* or *urge to move*. It is important to note that these sensations are usually experienced from the age of 10 onwards, but rarely before (34) (see Chapter 38).

Diagnosis and differential diagnosis

The diagnosis is entirely clinical and largely based on the patient's description of (i) partial movement or vocalisation control, (ii) premonitory sensations and (iii) relief following tic completion. These three criteria do not need to be simultaneously coexpressed at any time, but their complete absence suggests another aetiology (cf. differential diagnosis, Table 31.2). Tics usually appear between the age of 5 to 7 years with a severity peak around 9 to 11 years (35). In 50-70% of cases, tics are initially motor and predominate at the face, shoulder or neck level.

The differential diagnosis of tics includes all abnormal repetitive movements (Table 31.3). In these cases, complementary investigations such as MRI, EEG or electrophysiological recordings are often helpful.

Treatment

In 1959, the British psychiatrist Bockner treated two patients with tics with chlorpromazine, a recently introduced neuroleptic, one of them successfully. Two years later, the French psychiatrist Seignot treated one patient with severe GTS with haloperidol: the results were remarkable. These encouraging reports and subsequent ones inspired Shapiro and Shapiro, two American psychiatrists and pioneers in the field of GTS, to treat large series of patients with haloperidol, which thus became the drug of choice in the treatment of tics (36).

More than 50 years after these initial reports, neuroleptics still represent the first choice for the treatment of tics, at least in Europe. Many detailed and excellent reviews on the pharmacotherapy of tics and GTS are available (37,38).

Principles of treatment

The treatment of tics depends as much on common sense and clinical experience as on controlled, randomized and double-blind trials that are much too scarce in GTS due to the rarity of

Table 31.3
Differential diagnosis for tics.

- Myoclonus
- Dystonia
- Chorea
- Paroxysmal dyskinesia
- Hemiballism
- Hemifacial spasm
- Stereotypies
- Mannerisms
- Compulsions
- Akathisia
- Restless legs syndrome
- Epilepsy

the disease and the regrettable but somewhat understandable lack of interest from the pharmaceutical industry in this condition. Although the prevalence of GTS has been estimated to be around 0.3-0.8% (see above), the crucial but unanswered question is how many of these potential patients receive an accurate diagnosis and, if so, whether they require treatment beyond psychoeducation (see below).

Even if available, controlled trials in GTS are burdened with multiple methodological pitfalls. The most common one is duration of treatment, which is usually too short to accommodate the waxing and waning nature of tics, especially in children and adolescents (37). Another, more recent concern stems from the fact that apart from tic reduction *per se* (usually evaluated with the YTSS), quality of life is a major variable to be taken into account in future studies evaluating treatment efficacy, and for which the Gilles de la Tourette syndrome-quality of life scale (GTS-QOL) has recently become available (38).

The first step in treating GTS patients is usually referred to as psychoeducation: counsel and instruct the patient, the family as well as the school or work environment about the nature of tics, co-morbidities and overall prognosis. In a large number of cases, these simple measures, accompanied by regular follow-up, are remarkably effective and may prevent the need to introduce specific anti-tic therapy.

When psychoeducation is insufficient, a decision to initiate another strategy is based on four criteria:

- Tics cause sustained social problems for the patient (e.g., social isolation or bullying).
- Tics cause social and emotional problems for the patient (e.g., reactive depressive symptoms).
- Tics cause functional interference.
- Tics cause subjective discomfort (e.g. pain or injury).

Whereas the first three criteria are relatively subjective (although a sharp decline in school performance or impeding licensing are clear warning signs that action should be taken), the last criterion is rather objective, especially with regard to tic sequelae. For instance, violent neck tics can cause cervical myelopathies leading to tetraplegia or cause stroke through vertebral artery dissection (40). Automutilation (blindness through ocular enucleation, lacerations, fractures, burns, etc.) can be extremely severe and even life-threatening (41).

Furthermore, it is essential to take co-morbidities into account, including stereotypies (see Chapter 38), attention deficit with hyperactivity disorder (ADHD, see Chapter 39), obsessive-compulsive disorder (OCD, see Chapter 40), impulse control disorders (ICD, see Chapter 41), depression, anxiety, autism spectrum disorders and/or learning disabilities, present in more than 90% of GTS patients (42) and to prioritize the patients' needs accordingly. Several studies have shown that the patients' quality of life is often more extensively compromised by co-morbidities than by tics as such. Therefore, if possible and available, a multidisciplinary evaluation and follow-up is recommended (including neurologists, psychiatrists, psychologists, neuropsychologists, and social workers).

Pharmacotherapy

As discussed previously, many brain structures and neurotransmitters are implicated in the genesis of tics. Not surprisingly, the pharmacological treatment of tics is mostly empirical and dominated by case studies or series as well as open-label trials; very few studies fulfill class A evidence criteria (see Table 31.4). Also, even if based on rather solid evidence, treatment practices differ widely across countries and continents (to be discussed below).

Recent reviews have extensively listed all available evidence on tic treatment, in particular the recently published European society for the study of Tourette syndrome (ESSTS) guidelines (37), and we refer to this publication for anyone

Table 31.4
Pharmacologic treatment options for tics.

Neuroleptics	Empirical support	Starting doses (mg)	Therapeutic doses (mg)
Haloperidol	A	0,25-0,5	1-4
Pimozide	A	0,5-1,0	2-8
Risperidone	A	0,25-0,5	1-3
Fluphenazine	B	0,5-1,0	1,5-10
Tiapride	B	50-150	150-500
Olanzapine	C	2,5-5,0	2,5-12,5
Sulpiride	C	100-200	200-1000
Aripiprazole	C	2,5-5,0	2,5-15
Others			
Clonidine	B	0,0025-0,05	0,1-0,3
Guanfacine	B	0,5-1,0	1-3
Botulinum toxin	B	30-300U/injection site	
Tetrabenazine	C	12,5-25	25-150
Baclofen	C	10	40-60
Nicotine patch	C	7	7-21

Level of proof: (*Jobson KO, Potter WZ. Psychopharmacol Bull 1995;31:457-459*).

Category A = treatments with *good* supportive evidence for short-term safety and efficacy derived from at least two randomized placebo-controlled trials with positive results.

Category B = treatments with *fair* supportive data as evidenced by at least one positive placebo-controlled

Category C = treatments with *minimal* supportive evidence such as open-label studies and accumulated clinical experience.

seeking methodological details on case reports, case series and clinical trials. Interestingly, these guidelines revealed substantial differences in treatment recommendations between European and American centers. Besides obvious differences related to the varying availability of drugs, they also reflect different attitudes on the risks and benefits of certain classes of drugs, especially neuroleptics. In this line, the following treatment survey may reflect our personal approach of treating tics which is in agreement with European recommendations. A special mention is made of aripiprazole, which appears to us as the most promising drug for tic treatment to emerge over the last decade.

Neuroleptic drugs

Historically, the treatment of tics has been primarily based on the use of neuroleptics (dopamine receptor antagonists). Among 'typical' neuroleptics (which refers to their preferential affinity to D2 receptors), haloperidol and pimozide are the most commonly used, with a slightly better side-effect profile for the latter compared to the former, but also with slightly less efficacy (43). Common to both drugs as well as to most neuroleptics are sedation, weight gain and metabolic disturbances. Pimozide may prolong QT intervals, and patients therefore require ECG monitoring after introducing the drug. However, extrapyramidal side-effects (motor Parkinsonism and tardive dyskinesia) appear nowadays to be much less a concern than previously thought. In fact, a retrospective recent case series of 521 patients did not detect a single case of tardive dyskinesia in GTS patients treated with a variety of neuroleptics, including children and adolescents (n = 100 out of 521). The authors went so far as to question whether GTS 'protects' against neuroleptic-induced tardive dyskinesia (44). My own clinical experience supports this favorable side-effect profile of neuroleptics for treating tics. The reasons may include lower dosages and slower dose escalation in GTS than in classic antipsychotic indications, which lead to tardive dyskinesia in up to 30% of cases (see also Chapters 18 and 38). More speculatively, GTS patients, especially in younger age groups, might have an increased cerebral plasticity, rendering them more resistant to neuroleptic-induced extrapyramidal side-effects.

Nonetheless, in light of the fear of tardive dyskinesia, so-called 'atypical' neuroleptics have attracted great interest over the past two decades for treating tics. This class of compounds is characterized by a less potent blockade of D2 receptors as well as 5-HT_{2A} and 5-HT_{2C} receptor antagonism. Risperidone offers the best level of evidence in this group, and many consider it as first choice of treatment for tics. However, metabolic side-effects (increases in glucose, lipids, prolactin) occur frequently and must be closely monitored. Also, the risk of developing depression due to anti-serotoninergic activity, in addition to depression resulting from diminished dopaminergic transmission common to all neuroleptics, may be a concern. The benzamides (tiapride, sulpiride) are further selective D2 dopamine receptor antagonists but in contrast to the typical neuroleptics with low (sulpiride) or as good as no (tiapride) antipsychotic action which appear to result in less or no extrapyramidal side effects. Nonetheless, weight gain and sedation can occur and must be monitored (37).

Finally, among the atypical neuroleptics, tetrabenazine deserves special mention. As a monoamine depletor, it offers the potential advantage of not inducing tardive dyskinesia and is therefore especially favoured in North America (38). However, sedation is a major issue as well as rare but sometimes severe depressive reactions.

Aripiprazole is one of the most recently introduced neuroleptics and offers a particular mode of action: apart from its D2 antagonistic activity, it is also a partial D2 and 5-HT_{1A} receptor agonist as well as a 5-HT_{2A} antagonist. Over the past decade, it has become the favourite neuroleptic for treating tics in many centers despite a lack of controlled studies and a lack of approval for use in children. Many open-label studies and case series are now available which underline the remarkable efficacy of aripiprazole on tics while generally displaying its more favourable side-effect profile than most typical and atypical neuroleptics with regard to sedation and weight gain (45,46).

Non-neuroleptic drugs

Another group of compounds used for more than two decades in the treatment of tics is the alpha-2 receptor agonists, e.g. clonidine and guanfacine. Both compounds have been evaluated in controlled clinical trials and shown to be efficient for the treatment of tics, though their efficacy is usually lower than for neuroleptics with comparable sedation. They appear to be helpful in managing behavioural problems, especially ADHD (25).

Benzodiazepines, in particular clonazepam, are much less frequently used for treating tics since their efficacy seems to be limited and indirect. The same reasoning can be applied to antidepressants, particularly selective serotonin reuptake inhibitors, which can be helpful in reducing obsessive-compulsive disorders and/or anxiety, but seem devoid of intrinsic anti-tic activity. More recently, two antiepileptics, leviracetam and topiramate, have been suggested to be useful in the treatment of tics, but results remain preliminary and somewhat conflicting (47,48). Other interesting leads include the cannaboid system (49) and the GABAergic system (50).

Finally, the potential benefits of botulinum toxin to treat isolated tics should be mentioned. Botulinum toxin allows a targeted and limited intervention on localized, potentially dangerous tics, expecially those of the neck. Injections into the vocal cords can be considered in the presence of debilitating vocal tics (51). An interesting phenomenon is the observation that premonitory sensations sometimes diminish or even disappear after repeated injections of botulinum toxin into the affected muscle group (52).

Psychotherapy

Two types of cognitive-behavioural therapy for the treatment of tics have been investigated in controlled trials over the past decade: habit reversal training in order to prohibit tic realization by habit reversal, and exposure response prevention, prohibiting tic realization by suppressing negative reinforcement. They will be described in more detail thereafter.

Habit reversal training (HRT)
HRT as a treatment option for tics was proposed 40 years ago (53). It is a multicomponent therapy which can be divided into five phases: (i) tic description, (ii) tic awareness (self-management), (iii) the principal phase called habit reversal, (iv) motivational reinforcement and psychosocial support, and (v) a generalisation phase. The two major phases deal with tic awareness, especially the premonitory sensations that announce the tic(s) and habit reversal. The latter consists in defining and applying an antagonistic/competitive gesture that will make tic realization impossible. In other words, this means developing a muscular contraction incompatible with the tic: for instance, keeping your jaw clenched and your lips sealed for a tic involving mouth opening; or anterior neck flexion to prevent a neck extension tic. These antagonistic movements not only prevent tic realization but ultimately decrease the mostly unpleasant premonitory sensation preceding the tics. Therefore, this movement must be initiated as soon as the premonitory sensation appears and maintained for 1-3 minutes, or at least until the premonitory sensation disappears (24). In the long run and ideally, the *urge to do* should fade completely, and accordingly the tic should disappear. The precise physiological mechanisms underlying the technique's efficacy remain unknown to date but can probably be attributed to interruption of the stimulus-response association.

In general, 8-15 sessions are required, spaced weekly and lasting about one hour. It is important to note that HRT treats tics sequentially according to their level of nuisance. Therefore, it is primarily recommended for patients with a limited number of tics, a rather stable tic repertoire and the presence of clear premonitory sensations.

The two major studies on HRT were published recently, one in children (54) and the other in adults (55). In both studies, around 120 patients were randomized into each treatment arm (comprehensive behavioural intervention for tics (CBIT) versus supportive psychotherapy and psychoeducation) comprising 8 sessions over 10 weeks. Children benefitted slightly more than adults from CBIT, which was superior to the control condition in both studies. Some 53% of children and 38% of adults reported a significant improvement on the clinical global impression-improvement (CGII) scale. On the Yale global tic severity scale (YGTSS), 31% of children and 26% of adults displayed significant improvement. These scores were still maintained up to 6 months after therapy completion.

Exposure response prevention (ERP)
All cognitive behavioural strategies are based on the negative association between a discomforting sensation (*urge to do*) and the tic realisation that will alleviate discomfort. As tic realisation reactivates the urge to do, thus engaging a vicious, feedforward cycle, behavioural therapies aim to interrupt this negative re-inforcement by prohibiting tic realisation. ERP constrains

patients to gradually accept premonitory sensations while holding back tics. The underlying mechanism is thus one of extinction.

ERP comprises two initial training sessions during which the patient learns to refrain from giving in to the tic over longer time periods by applying relaxation techniques. During the following sessions, premonitory sensations are evoked (stress, divided attention) over prolongued periods (exposure) in order to increase the capacity to resist the urge to tic (response prevention). The patient learns to tolerate and handle the *urge to do* by a habituation phenomenon, which eventually results in a decreased need to tic or even its absence. Interestingly, no rebound phenomenon has been observed following ERP.

To date, the major controlled study on ERP (compared to HRT) in 43 patients, both children and adults, has shown a tic decrease of one-third in 58% of patients treated with ERP compared to 28% of patients treated by HRT (56). However, it must be noted that ERP sessions lasted for two hours while HRT sessions took one hour. Currently, trials are under way that include shortened session durations (one hour, as in HRT/CBIT). The main advantage of this technique is the possibility of treating all tics simultaneously. Also, the presence of premonitory sensation is not an absolute prerequisite as in HRT. Therefore, ERP appears most suited to patients with multiple tics and in children who have not yet experienced premonitory sensations. In contrast, HRT is better suited to patients who have few or no tics during training sessions as antagonistic movements can be trained and applied outside of training sessions.

An intriguing question pertains to the anatomical correlates of cognitive behavioural therapies such as HRT and ERP, in particular whether successful application of these techniques might induce morphological changes (thickening of the frontal and prefrontal cortex or reinforcement of cortico-striatal projections) with increasing inhibition of striato-pallido-thalamic pathways.

Neurosurgery (deep brain stimulation)

Over the past 20 years, deep brain stimulation (DBS) has been shown to be an efficient method to treat a variety of movement disorders, first and foremost Parkinson's disease, with an estimated 150,000 patients operated on worldwide. With tics, but not in neurodegenerative diseases such as Parkinson's disease, DBS might offer not only symptomatic but also disease-modifying effects, as tics are the consequence of neurodevelopmental disorders; therefore, a lasting improvement over time without readjusting the stimulation parameters during disease progression can be expected. Since the first DBS intervention into the central parafascicular nucleus of the thalamus (CM-Pf) in a tic patient, in 1999, about 100 patients have undergone this reversible intervention worldwide (57). Eventual targets for this indication include the GPi (sensorimotor and limbic territories), the thalamus (median and intralaminary nuclei), the capsula interna (anterior portion) and the nucleus accumbens.

So far, two small, controlled studies have shown encouraging results (58,59), though another study had universally disappointing results with regard to the side-effect profile when targeting the centromedian nucleus of the thalamus (60). Larger controlled, multicenter trials are under way and should help clarify the best targets and best age of intervention, selection criteria (co-morbidities) and impact on quality of life. As a majority of patients improve around the age of 18, and as clear prognostic criteria for individual patients are not available, determining the optimal age of this intervention seems crucial. The current consensus is to wait well into adulthood (>25 years of age) before proposing DBS to patients suffering from severe chronic tics (61). However, very severe juvenile tics can lead to complete desocialisation and removal from school, with an accordingly devastating impact on the patients' lives once they reach adulthood. Therefore, the question of DBS in adolescents remains open (57).

In summary, we propose an approach based on the recommendations adapted from the Tourette Practice Parameter Work Group (62):

1 Mild tics generally do not require treatment.
2 For moderate tics, cognitive-behavioural therapy (CBT) should be proposed, if available. If a pharmacologic treatment is the first option, aripiprazole is the compound of choice (2.5-5 mg/day).
3 For isolated tics, botulinum toxin injections should be considered.
4 For severe tics, first increase the ariprazole dose, then consider risperidone, pimozide, haloperidol or any other neuroleptic. Next, consider tetrabenazine and anticonvulsants.
5 Finally, in the case of pharmaco-resistance, deep brain stimulation can be considered.

Prognosis

Tics begin in childhood and often wane within a year (transient childhood tic disorder). In GTS or chronic tic disorder, tics tend to worsen during puberty but regress significantly around the age of 18: only 20% of GTS patients retain a moderate to severe degree of tics once they reach adulthood (63). This favorable prognosis must be emphasised when meeting children or adolescents with their parents.

Conclusions and further directions

Future pharmacologic studies in GTS should target two questions: (i) association of CBT with pharmacotherapy ; (ii) combination pharmacotherapy using substances with different modes of action. In both cases, the treatment periods should not be less than 3 months. We recommend forming sub-groups with regard to age and co-morbidity as far as possible. In addition, quality of life as an indicator of treatment response and success should be monitored. Regarding DBS, the indication for adolescents with severe tics or for adults with moderate tics but intolerance to pharmaceutical treatments will need to be evaluated in the future. Finally, the advent of biomarkers, most likely the definition of endophenotypes, may prove very helpful to assess and even predict the treatment response.

Video fragment

Fragment 31.1 (21.1)
Gilles de la Tourette syndrome
(Segments 1-2)
The first segment shows a mentally handicapped man with several stereotypic motor tics. The second segment shows a patient with a mild multiple tic syndrome, consisting of facial and phonic tics, with a good response on tetrabenazine.

References

1 Association AP. Diagnostic and statistical manual of mental disorders. (DSM-IV-TR). Washington: American Psychiatric Association; 2000.
2 Knight T, Steeves T, Day L, Lowerison M, Jette N, Pringsheim T. Prevalence of tic disorders: a systematic review and meta-analysis. Pediatr Neurol 2012;47:77-90.
3 Berridge KC, Aldridge JW, Houchard KR, Zhuang X. Sequential super-stereotypy of an instinctive fixed action pattern in hyper-dopaminergic mutant mice: a model of obsessive compulsive disorder and Tourette's. BMC Biol 2005;3:4.
4 Worbe Y, Sgambato-Faure V, Epinat J, et al. Towards a primate model of Gilles de la Tourette syndrome: Anatomo-behavioural correlation of disorders induced by striatal dysfunction. Cortex 2013;37:1157-1161.
5 Albin RL, Mink JW. Recent advances in Tourette syndrome research. Trends Neurosci 2006;29:175-182.
6 Alexander GE, DeLong MR, Strick PL. Parallel organization of functionally segregated circuits linking basal ganglia and cortex. Annu Rev Neurosci 1986;9:357-381.

7 Kalanithi PS, Zheng W, Kataoka Y, et al. Altered parvalbumin-positive neuron distribution in basal ganglia of individuals with Tourette syndrome. Proc Natl Acad Sci U S A 2005;102:13307-13312.

8 Kataoka Y, Kalanithi PS, Grantz H, et al. Decreased number of parvalbumin and cholinergic interneurons in the striatum of individuals with Tourette syndrome. J Comp Neurol 2010;518:277-291.

9 Marín O. Interneuron dysfunction in psychiatric disorders. Nat Rev Neurosci 2012;13:107-120.

10 Heise KF, Steven B, Liuzzi G, et al. Altered modulation of intracortical excitability during movement preparation in Gilles de la Tourette syndrome. Brain 2010;133:580-590.

11 Minzer K, Lee O, Hong JJ, Singer HS. Increased prefrontal D2 protein in Tourette syndrome: a postmortem analysis of frontal cortex and striatum. J Neurol Sci 2004;219:55-61.

12 Müller-Vahl KR, Kaufmann J, Grosskreutz J, Dengler R, Emrich HM, Peschel T. Prefrontal and anterior cingulate cortex abnormalities in Tourette Syndrome: evidence from voxel-based morphometry and magnetization transfer imaging. BMC Neurosci 2009;10:47.

13 Peterson BS, Staib L, Scahill L, et al. Regional brain and ventricular volumes in Tourette syndrome. Arch Gen Psychiatry 2001;58:427-440.

14 Sowell ER, Kan E, Yoshii J, et al. Thinning of sensorimotor cortices in children with Tourette syndrome. Nat Neurosci 2008;11:637-639.

15 Fahim C, Yoon U, Das S, et al. Somatosensory-motor bodily representation cortical thinning in Tourette: effects of tic severity, age and gender. Cortex 2010;46:750-760.

16 Worbe Y, Gerardin E, Hartmann A, et al. Distinct structural changes underpin clinical phenotypes in patients with Gilles de la Tourette syndrome. Brain 2010;133:3649-3660.

17 Peterson BS, Thomas P, Kane MJ, et al. Basal Ganglia volumes in patients with Gilles de la Tourette syndrome. Arch Gen Psychiatry 2003;60:415-424.

18 Bloch MH, Leckman JF, Zhu H, Peterson BS. Caudate volumes in childhood predict symptom severity in adults with Tourette syndrome. Neurology 2005;65:1253-1258.

19 Neuner I, Kupriyanova Y, Stöcker T, et al. White-matter abnormalities in Tourette syndrome extend beyond motor pathways. Neuroimage 2010;51:1184-1193.

20 Bäumer T, Thomalla G, Kroeger J, et al. Interhemispheric motor networks are abnormal in patients with Gilles de la Tourette syndrome. Mov Disord 2010;25:2828-2837.

21 Wang Z, Maia TV, Marsh R, Colibazzi T, Gerber A, Peterson BS. The neural circuits that generate tics in Tourette's syndrome. Am J Psychiatry 2011;168:1326-1337.

22 Mazzone L, Yu S, Blair C, Gunter BC, Wang Z, Marsh R, Peterson BS. An FMRI study of frontostriatal circuits during the inhibition of eye blinking in persons with Tourette syndrome. Am J Psychiatry 2010;167:341-349.

23 Steeves TD, Ko JH, Kideckel DM, et al. Extrastriatal dopaminergic dysfunction in tourette syndrome. Ann Neurol 2010;67:170-181.

24 Lerner A, Bagic A, Simmons JM, et al. Widespread abnormality of the γ-aminobutyric acid-ergic system in Tourette syndrome. Brain 2012;135:1926-1936.

25 Swain JE, Scahill L, Lombroso PJ, King RA, Leckman JF. Tourette syndrome and tic disorders: a decade of progress. J Am Acad Child Adolesc Psychiatry 2007;46:947-968.

26 Martino D, Dale RC, Gilbert DL, Giovannoni G, Leckman JF. Immunopathogenic mechanisms in tourette syndrome: A critical review. Mov Disord 2009;24:1267-1279.

27 Pauls DL, Raymond CL, Stevenson JM, Leckman JF. A family study of Gilles de la Tourette syndrome. Am J Hum Genet 1991;48:154-163.

28 State MW. The genetics of child psychiatric disorders: focus on autism and Tourette syndrome. Neuron 2010;68:254-269.

29 Ercan-Sencicek AG, Stillman AA, Ghosh AK, et al. L-histidine decarboxylase and Tourette's syndrome. N Engl J Med 2010;362:1901-1908.

30 Fernandez TV, Sanders SJ, Yurkiewicz IR, et al. Rare copy number variants in tourette syndrome disrupt genes in histaminergic pathways and overlap with autism. Biol Psychiatry 2012;71:392-402.

31 Abelson JF, Kwan KY, O'Roak BJ, et al. Sequence variants in SLITRK1 are associated with Tourette's syndrome. Science 2005;310:317-320.

32 Paschou P. The genetic basis of Gilles de la Tourette Syndrome. Neurosci Biobehav Rev 2013;37:1026-1039.

33 Scharf JM, Yu D, Mathews CA, et al. Genome-wide association study of Tourette's syndrome. Mol Psychiatry 2013;18:721-728.

34 Banaschewski T, Woerner W, Rothenberger A. Premonitory sensory phenomena and suppressibility of tics in Tourette syndrome: developmental aspects in children and adolescents. Dev Med Child Neurol 2003;45:700-703.

35 Leckman JF, Zhang H, Vitale A, et al. Course of tic severity in Tourette syndrome: the first two decades. Pediatrics 1998;102:14-19.

36 Kushner HI. A Cursing Brain? The Histories of Tourette Syndrome. Cambridge : Harvard University Press 2000.

37 Roessner V, Plessen KJ, Rothenberger A, et al. European clinical guidelines for Tourette syndrome and other tic disorders. Part II: pharmacological treatment. Eur Child Adolesc Psychiatry 2011;20:173-196.

38 Pringsheim T, Doja A, Gorman D, et al. Canadian guidelines for the evidence-based treatment of tic disorders: pharmacotherapy. Can J Psychiatry 2012;57:133-143.

39 Cavanna AE, Schrag A, Morley D, et al. The Gilles de la Tourette syndrome-quality of life scale (GTS-QOL): development and validation. Neurology 2008;71:1410-1416.

40 van Meerbeeck P, Behar C, Czernecki V, Roze E, Deniau E, Hartmann A. Motor tic of the neck: a probable cause of stroke in a child with Gilles de la Tourette syndrome. Mov Disord 2011;26:928-929.

41 Cheung MY, Shahed J, Jankovic J. Malignant Tourette syndrome. Mov Disord 2007;22:1743-1750.

42 Cavanna AE, Servo S, Monaco F, Robertson MM. The behavioral spectrum of Gilles de la Tourette syndrome. J Neuropsychiatry Clin Neurosci 2009;21:13-23.

43 Pringsheim T, Marras C. Pimozide for tics in Tourette's syndrome. Cochrane Database Syst Rev 2009;(2):CD006996.

44 Müller-Vahl KR, Krueger D. Does Tourette syndrome prevent tardive dyskinesia? Mov Disord 2011;26:2442-2443.

45 Neuner I, Nordt C, Schneider F, Kawohl W. Effectiveness of aripiprazole in the treatment of adult Tourette patients up to 56 months. Hum Psychopharmacol 2012;27:364-369.

46 Wenzel C, Kleimann A, Bokemeyer S, Müller-Vahl KR. Aripiprazole for the treatment of Tourette syndrome: a case series of 100 patients. J Clin Psychopharmacol 2012;32:548-550.

47 Hedderick EF, Morris CM, Singer HS. Double-blind, crossover study of clonidine and levetiracetam in Tourette syndrome. Pediatr Neurol 2009;40:420-425.

48 Jankovic J, Jimenez-Shahed J, Brown LW. A randomised, double-blind, placebo-controlled study of topiramate in the treatment of Tourette syndrome. J Neurol Neurosurg Psychiatry 2010;81:70-73.

49 Müller-Vahl KR. Treatment of Tourette syndrome with cannabinoids. Behav Neurol 2013;27:119-124.

50 Singer HS, Wendlandt J, Krieger M, Giuliano J. Baclofen treatment in Tourette syndrome: a double-blind, placebo-controlled, crossover trial. Neurology 2001;56:599-604.

51 Porta M, Maggioni G, Ottaviani F, Schindler A. Treatment of phonic tics in patients with Tourette's syndrome using botulinum toxin type A. Neurol Sci 2004;24:420-423.

52 Marras C, Andrews D, Sime E, Lang AE. Botulinum toxin for simple motor tics: a randomized, double-blind, controlled clinical trial. Neurology 2001;56:605-610

53 Azrin NH, Nunn RG. Habit-reversal: a method of eliminating nervous habits and tics. Behav Res Ther 1973;11:619-628.

54 Piacentini J, Woods DW, Scahill L, et al. Behavior therapy for children with Tourette disorder: a randomized controlled trial. JAMA 2010 May;303:1929-1937.

55 Wilhelm S, Peterson AL, Piacentini J, et al. Randomized trial of behavior therapy for adults

with Tourette syndrome. Arch Gen Psychiatry 2012;69:795-803.

56 Verdellen CW, Keijsers GP, Cath DC, Hoogduin CA. Exposure with response prevention versus habit reversal in Tourettes's syndrome: a controlled study. Behav Res Ther 2004;42:501-511.

57 Müller-Vahl KR, Cath DC, Cavanna AE, et al. European clinical guidelines for Tourette syndrome and other tic disorders. Part IV: deep brain stimulation. Eur Child Adolesc Psychiatry 2011;20:209-217.

58 Maciunas RJ, Maddux BN, Riley DE, et al. Prospective randomized double-blind trial of bilateral thalamic deep brain stimulation in adults with Tourette syndrome. J Neurosurg 2007;107:1004-1014.

59 Welter ML, Mallet L, Houeto JL, et al. Internal pallidal and thalamic stimulation in patients with Tourette syndrome. Arch Neurol 2008;65:952-957.

60 Ackermans L, Duits A, van der Linden C, et al. Double-blind clinical trial of thalamic stimulation in patients with Tourette syndrome. Brain 2011;134:832-844.

61 Mink JW, Walkup J, Frey KA, et al. Patient selection and assessment recommendations for deep brain stimulation in Tourette syndrome. Mov Disord 2006;21:1831-1838.

62 Scahill L, Erenberg G, Berlin CM Jr, et al. Contemporary assessment and pharmacotherapy of Tourette syndrome. NeuroRx 2006;3:192-206.

63 Bloch MH, Craiglow BG, Landeros-Weisenberger A, et al. Predictors of early adult outcomes in pediatric-onset obsessive-compulsive disorder. Pediatrics 2009;124:1085-1093.

32

Mitochondrial Movement Disorders

Erik Ch. Wolters, Hans H. Jung & Christian R. Baumann

In all human body cells, except in red blood cells, intracellular mitochondria play an essential role in their maintenance by synthesising adenosine triphosphate (ATP). These organelles convert the energy of food, mainly fat and glucose, in the respiratory chain (RC) via oxidative phosphorylation (OXPHOS) into ATP, which powers most cell functions. Indeed, their primary function is to support aerobic respiration and to provide energy and heat, though they also play other important roles, including cell signaling for apoptotic cell death.

Mitochondria are the only organelles in the cell (aside from the nucleus) that have their own genome and genetic machinery. About 850 polypeptides, all encoded by nuclear DNA (nDNA) and all synthesized in the cytoplasm, are required to produce and maintain this organelle, 75 of them being structural components of the respiratory complexes, and another 20 needed to assemble and maintain them in working order. The respiratory chain is the only metabolic pathway in the cell that is under the dual control of mitochondrial (mtDNA) and nuclear (nDNA) DNA.

mtDNA carries 37 genes encoding 22 transfer ribonucleic acid (tRNA), two ribosomal RNAs (12S and 16S) and 13 messenger RNAs (mRNA). Messenger mRNA is a large family of RNA molecules that convey genetic information from DNA to the ribosome, where they specify the amino acid sequence of the protein products of gene expression. These last 13 mtDNA-encoded mRNAs are part of the respiratory chain system and are assembled together with nuc-lear-encoded subunits. Seven of them belong to complex I or reduced nicotinamide adenine dinucleotide dehydrogenase (NADH) (ND1, ND2, ND3, ND4, ND4L, ND5, and ND6). One belongs to complex III or ubiquinol cytochrome c oxidoreductase, three to complex IV or cytochrome c oxidase (COX I, II and III), and the final two to complex V or ATP synthase (ATPase6 and 8). The remaining mitochondrial proteins, including all of the complex II subunits, are encoded by nDNA.

Mitochondriopathies

Mitochondriopathies (MCP) are a group of disorders caused by impairment of the mitochondrial respiratory chain (RC) protein complex. These mitochondrial diseases are a wide group of disorders resulting from mutations of the mitochondrial or nuclear genes encoding for OXPHOS proteins. Defects of mitochondrial OXPHOS activity not only cause energy insufficiency but also an increase of reactive oxygen species (ROS). Physiologically, the cell compensates for the excess of ROS production by enhancing the antioxidant defense system, including up-regulation of antioxidant enzymes such as superoxide dismutase and glutathione peroxidase. However, when there is an imbalance between ROS levels and antioxidant defense, oxidative stress will result, which may lead to cell death with both apoptotic and not apoptotic pathways.

As a rule, organs with a high dependency on oxidative metabolism for energy generation are affected in MCP. Thus, the skeletal muscles are frequently affected. Patients with mitochondrial myopathies (MM) often exhibit exercise intolerance, fatigue, lactic acidosis and muscle pain during low to moderate exercise activity. Exercise intolerance encourages a sedentary lifestyle that promotes further reduction of muscle aerobic capacity through physical deconditioning; this has been shown to benefit from aerobic training, although the mechanisms explaining this are not fully clear as of yet. The precocious activation of anaerobic metabolism in contractile activity leads to an increased production of lactate.

The estimated prevalence of MCPs is 1-2 in 10,000 (1). In about 15% of the cases, mitochondrial diseases are caused by spontaneous or inherited mtDNA mutations that affect mitochondrial function. Each cell contains multiple copies of mtDNA (polyplasmy), normally identical (homoplasmy), though sometimes with both normal and mutated mtDNA populations (heteroplasmy) (1,2). In case of cells with over 70% mutated mtDNA, maternally inherited mitochondriopathies may occur. Mostly, however, MCPs are the consequence of mutations in nDNA encoding for mitochondrial proteins involved in the mitochondrial respiratory chain (MRC), whether Mendelian inherited or sporadically induced by exogenous factors. MCPs might also result from primary mutations in gene products not targeted to mitochondria or from still unknown causes, often through ROS. These last MCPs are mostly involved in the development of neurodegenerative disorders. However, regardless of the cause, such neurodegenerative disorders with recognizable mitochondrial dysfunction, whether maternally or Mendelian inherited or a sporadic epiphenomenon, are mostly defined as neurodegenerative mitochondriopathies (3,4).

Mitochondriopathies usually present with multiorgan involvement, with varying onset between birth and late adulthood, and display a chronic, slowly progressive course (5). Mitochondria and their DNA are inherited exclusively from the mother, and pathogenic mtDNA mutations may thus cause maternally inherited syndromes, with phenotypic consequences when the ratio of mutated to normal mtDNA is above two (7:3) (6). Given that the mutational load, which can change from one cell generation to the next due to mitotic segregation, surpasses the clinical threshold, and given the varying pathogenic thresholds of each tissue due to its relative dependence on oxidative metabolism, the phenotypes show enormous heterogeneity (1). Because of their wide variation in presentation and course, mitochondriopathies therefore represent a diagnostic challenge.

Among the systems which are frequently affected in MCP because of their high dependence on oxidative metabolism for energy generation are the skeletal muscles and the central and peripheral nervous system, eyes and ears, endocrinium, cardiovascular, gastrointestinal and urogenital systems. Common (primary and/or secondary-induced) mitochondrial DNA mutation-induced phenotypes therefore often include signs and symptoms of progressive external ophthalmoplegia (PEO), encephalomyelopathy with stroke-like episodes, myoclonic epilepsy with ragged-red fibers, blindness and/or deafness, ataxia, (cardio)myopathy, pancreas insufficiency, diabetes and/or hypogonadism (7). A diagnostic work-up of suspected MCPs must comprise a careful history (negative family history does not exclude MRC) and neurological examination. There is also an extensive overlap of symptoms between different syndromes. Clinical assessments should be followed by blood and cerebrospinal measurements including CK and lactate (both at rest and during exercise) and lactate/pyruvate ratio (increased in case of respiratory chain defect), electromyography (to document myopathy and neuropathy), muscle biopsy and studying blood cells for nuclear genes and searching for mtDNA point mutations, preferably in affected tissues in particular muscles (8). MRI findings in mitochondrial disorders may be helpful but can be non-specific or change over time. Magnetic resonance spectroscopy can provide estimates of abnormal metabolite concentrations in different brain regions, e.g. by measuring the peaks of lactate, creatine, pyruvate, succinate, or N-acetyl-L-aspartate. The definitive diagnosis by identifying the causative mutations is difficult because of the large number of genes and the complex dual genome involvement.

Primary (mtDNA mutation-induced) mitochondriopathies

Primary MCP syndromes are the consequence of sporadic or inherited mutations in mtDNA, encoding the structure and content of mitochondrial proteins responsible for the RC-related energy supply. Maternally inherited mtDNA mutations with sequence changes in the mtDNA genome are a primary cause. These mutations may lead to the following phenotypes: *chronic progressive external ophthalmoplegia (PEO), Kearns-Sayre syndrome (KSS), mitochondrial encephalopathy, lactic acidosis and stroke-like episodes (MELAS), myoclonic epilepsy with ragged-red fibres (MERRF)*. A short clinical overview can be found in Table 32.1.

Mutations of mtDNA genes encoding respiratory chain subunits (complexes I-V) will induce RC dysfunction related MCPs by affecting OX-PHOS (7). These MCPs include *Leber hereditary optic neuropathy (LHON)* (9) or *LHON-plus syndromes* (in case of disturbed Complex I activity) and *neurogenic ataxia with retinitis pigmentosa (NARP)* or a subacute necrotizing encephalomyelopathy, known as *maternally inherited Leigh syndrome (MILS)* (in case of a Complex V dysfunction). Leigh syndrome initially starts with an inability to grow and gain weight due to vomiting and diarrhoea, followed later by ataxia, peripheral neuropathy with ophthalmoparesis and/or optic atrophy, loss of sensorimotor functions, dystonia and increased urine/serum/spinal fluid lactate levels.

In LHON, the ganglionic cell layer of the optic nerves is affected. The mitochondriopathic encephalomyelopathic KSS, MELAS, MERFF and NARP share degeneration of the cerebellar Purkinje cells with clinical signs of ataxia. This degeneration may also comprise cortical neurons (MELAS), caudate and sometimes also pallidoluysian, nigral, inferior olivary, cerulean, pontine tegmental and spinal neurons (MERFF), brainstem nuclei (KSS), olfactory, visual and auditory pathways and putamenal, inferior olivary and dentate degeneration (NARP) (10-14). In MILS, the optic nerves, basal ganglia, thalamus, brainstem and spinal cord neurons are involved (14). Secondary respiratory chain dysfunction might be reached by nuclear gene mutations encoding the assembly and maintenance of respiratory chain complexes (7).

These mitochondriopathies may phenotypically manifest with disorders of high energy-dependent organs (encephalomyopathies) (see Table 32.2). Thus, a diagnosis of mitochondrial parkinsonism might be considered in patients suffering from parkinsonism in combination with some of the other phenotypic mitochondriopathic manifestations.

Secondary, nDNA mutation-induced mitochondriopathies

Nuclear DNA mutation-derived MCPs might be caused by various mutations in the structural components or ancillary proteins of the RC, by defects of the membrane lipid milieu, co-enzyme Q10 biosynthesis and/or intergenomic signaling (1). Often mutations in the nDNA gene are involved, which encodes polymerase gamma (POLG), the only DNA polymerase in human mitochondria and essential for mtDNA replication and repair.

Mutations of the adenine nucleotide translocator 1 (ANT1), twinkle mitochondrial helicase and mitochondrial catalytic subunit of POLG1 result in mtDNA deletions with a *progressive external ophthalmoplegia (PEO)* (Orsucci) or *optic*

Table 32.1
Clinical characteristics of selected mitochondrial disorders.

	Movement abnormalities	Other clinical findings
MELAS		• stroke-like episodes with hemiparesis/cortical blindness • recurrent migraine headaches • sensorineural hearing loss • muscle weakness, exercise intolerance • epileptic seizures
MERFF	• myoclonic seizures • cerebellar ataxia	• mental deterioration • muscle weakness • sensorineural hearing loss • short stature • night blindness
LHON		• bilateral optic neuropathy, acute or subacute
Leigh's Syndrome	• dystonia, usually multifocal • potential other findings: parkinsonism, tremor, chorea, myoclonus, tics	• epileptic seizures • behavioural abnormalities • loss of appetite, vomiting • lactic acidosis
KSS	• cerebellar ataxia (in few patients)	• mild visual acuity loss • modest night blindness • ophthalmoplegia, ptosis • atrioventricular block • hearing loss
Alpers syndrome		• epileptic seizures • mental retardation, dementia • spasticity • early-onset progressive liver disease • blindness, deafness may occur
CPEO		• bilateral ptosis • ophthalmoplegia (downward gaze best spared)
NARP	• cerebellar ataxia	• sensorimotor neuropathy • night blindness • proximal muscle weakness • developmental delay • epileptic seizures • hearing loss

Abbreviations: MELAS: mitochondrial encephalomyopathy, lactic acidosis, and stroke-like episodes. MERFF: myoclonic epilepsy with ragged red fibers. LHON: Leber's hereditary optic neuropathy. KSS: Kearn-Sayre syndrome. CPEO: Chronic progressive external ophthalmoplegia. NARP: neuropathy, ataxia, and retinitis pigmentosa.

atrophy type 1 (OPA1) phenotype, or in mtDNA depletions with *Alpers' syndrome* phenotype (8). POLG1 mutations are sometimes associated with parkinsonism. Alpers' syndrome manifests with mental retardation and dementia, blind-ness, deafness, epilepsy and liver dysfunction manifesting after the first year of life, but so-metimes as late as the fifth year. Rarely, nuclear mutations in structural components of the RC, such as NDUFV2 (15), may also cause familial

Table 32.2
Phenotypical expression of primary and secondary, POLG-mediated mitochondriopathies.

Primary mitochondrial encephalomyopathies	Stroke-like episodes (Cardio)myopathy, WPW syndrome Polyneuropathy Blindness, deafness, sensorimotor deficits Migraine, depression, psychosis Hypothyreoidism Diabetes mellitus
Secondary (especially POLG-mediated) mitochondrial encephalomyopathies	Myopathy Polyneuropathy Blindness, deafness Ophthalmoplegia Epilepsy Ataxia Parkinsonism Dystonia Liver failure Hypogonadism

POLG: polymerase gamma; WPW syndrome: Wolff-Parkinson-White syndrome.

parkinsonism (16). In these patients, sodium valproate should be avoided because of the risk of liver failure.

Secondary MCPs might also be caused by exogenous mutations such as those induced by ROS-mediated damage of mitochondrial proteins (OXPHOS and non-OXPHOS). Some of these exogenous mitochondrial mutations are associated with specific phenotypes, such as parkin and PTEN-induced putative kinase 1 (PINK1) in *genetic parkinsonism*, huntingtin in autosomal dominant *Huntington's disease* (17), fraxatin (FXN) in autosomal recessive *Friedreich's ataxia* (18), and copper-mediated mitochondrial toxicity in autosomal recessive *hepatolenticular degeneration (Wilson's disease)* (WD) (19). As a matter of fact, applying selective inhibitors to selective RC components might provide an adequate animal model for

those diseases, as was the case with the succinate dehydrogenase (complex II) inhibitors malonate or 3-nitropropionic acid, providing an adequate mice model of Huntington's disease (20).

There is an increasing list of diseases in which mitochondria are implicated in Mendelian neurodegeneration. Along with OPA1 and PEO, PINK1, HD, FA, and Wilson's disease, *neurodegeneration with brain iron accumulation (NBIA)*, some variants of *hereditary spastic paraplegia (SP)*, and *Charcot-Marie-Tooth (CMT)* disease are the best known examples (12).
Secondary MCP phenotypes manifest in early infancy to late middle age (21,22) with signs of encephalopathy, optic atrophy and external ophthalmoplegia, deafness-dystonia syndrome (*Mohr-Tranebjaerg syndrome*), ataxia, myopathy, Leigh's syndrome, and/or neurogastrointestinal and hepatocerebral failure (Wilson's disease) (see Chapter 23).

Other non-mitochondrial protein mutation-induced mitochondriopathies

It has been speculated that mtDNA mutations accumulating with age might lead to impaired energy generation and to increased numbers of reactive oxygen species (ROS), both resulting in cell damage. Polymorphisms in mtDNA may cause subtle differences in the encoded proteins and, thus, minimal changes in mitochondrial respiratory chain activity and free radical overproduction, and predispose to an earlier onset of apoptotic processes, including somatic mtDNA mutations and mitochondrial impairment. Mitochondrial dysfunctions may also occur sporadically without any cause or when primary mutated gene products are not targeting mitochondria. These disorders could account for the vast majority of neurodegenerative disorders, including Alzheimer disease (AD), Parkinson's disease (PD) (23), Huntington's disease (HD), multiple system atrophy (MSA), progressive supranuclear palsy (PSP) and amyotrophic lateral sclerosis (ALS). As neurons are highly dependent on oxidative energy metabolism, a unified pathogenetic mechanism of neurodegeneration based on underlying dysfunction in the mitochondrial energy metabolism is suggested in these diseases (24). The rapidly increasing understanding of the pathophysiological background of MCPs may further facilitate the diagnostic approach and open perspectives to future, possibly causative therapies.

Mitochondrial movement disorders

Mitochondrial movement disorders include mitochondrial parkinsonism, dystonia, chorea, myoclonus and ataxia. Parkinsonism is the typical phenotype of idiopathic PD, genetic parkinsonism, vascular, posttraumatic, toxic and iatrogenic parkinsonism, MSA, PSP and CBD. While the aetiology of sporadic PD still remains unclear, there is accumulating evidence suggesting mitochondrial dysfunction in PD patients. Primarily mtDNA genetic abnormalities but more commonly secondary abnormalities and especially POLG1-related gene mutations have also been implicated in the etiopathophysiology of parkinsonism. Parkinsonism in these patients might be inherited or sporadic due to OXPHOS-related, disturbed gene-environmental factors. The treatment of mitochondrial movement disorders is not at variance with the treatment of the movement disorders per se, though mitochondrial disorders might require additional therapeutic support because of their multisystem nature.

Mitochondrial parkinsonism

In the majority of cases, mitochondrial disorders are multisystem conditions that most frequently affect the skeletal muscles, followed by the central nervous system. Incidentally, parkinsonism is seen in these disorders. There is increasing evidence that impaired mitochondrial functions and oxidative damage may indeed

induce parkinsonism. Such evidence comes from mitochondriopathic patients developing parkinsonism and from parkinsonistic patients who later on developed mitochondrial signs or symptoms, such as an elevated cerebrospinal fluid lactate level.

Mitochondrial dysfunctions with maternally inherited parkinsonism

Mitochondrial point mutations rarely manifest with maternally inherited parkinsonism (25), and if they do, parkinsonism is mostly part of parkinsonism with sensorideafness and neuropathy (26), MELAS (27), MERFF (28), POLG1-related mitochondrial encephalomyopathy including OPA and PEO and/or LHON (29). Mostly, however, mitochondrial parkinsonism is reported in POLG-1 CAG repeat-induced mtDNA point mutations with Mendelian inherited parkinsonism, also causing male infertility and testicular cancer (30-32).

Mendelian inherited parkinsonism with mitochondrial dysfunctions

Familial Mendelian transmitted parkinsonism might also be caused by mutations in genes, identified by linkage analyses. So far, linkage studies have shown 18 different parkinsonism-related genetic loci (PARK1-PARK18), and mutations in some of them such as PARK1/PARK4 (alpha-synuclein: SNCA), PARK2 (Parkin), PARK6 (PINK1), PARK7 (DJ1) and PARK8 (leucine-rich repeat kinase 2: LRRK2) have been linked to genetic parkinsonism (see Chapter 16). These mutations also cause mitochondrial dysfunction, which is one of the reasons why they are called mitochondrial nigropathies.

PARK1/PARK4 is a very rare, autosomal dominant form of early-onset, rapidly progressive, levodopa-responsive parkinsonism. During the course of their illness, patients may also manifest with cognitive impairment, dysautonomia and psychiatric symptoms (in the alpha-synuclein multiplications more than in the SNCA missense mutations), or myoclonus and other neurological symptoms.

PARK2 is a common cause of an autosomal recessive or sporadic form of early-onset, levodopa-responsive parkinsonism with levodopa-induced motor fluctuations and dyskinesias. Most patients develop leg dystonia in the early stages of their illness, as well as dysautonomia and psychiatric symptoms. PARK2 is caused by POLG-induced mutations in the parkin (PRKN) gene, increasing susceptibility to oxidative stress and mitochondrial toxins implicated in parkinsonism. In the case of the co-existence of parkinsonism and mutations in the mitochondrial polymerase gamma nDNA gene (POLG1), this gene could be responsible for part of the Mendelian transmission of parkinsonism.

PARK6 is a rare, autosomal recessive form of parkinsonism, caused by POLG mutation-induced mutations in the PINK1 gene, encoding mitochondrial phosphatase and tensin homolog-induced putative kinase 1 (PINK1), which is associated with protection against mitochondrial dysfunction and proteasome-induced apoptosis. Affected patients typically present with an early-onset, slowly progressive, levodopa-responsive parkinsonism with levodopa-induced motor fluctuations and dyskinesia (33).

PARK7 is also a rare, autosomal recessive form of early-onset, levodopa-responsive parkinsonism mostly in combination with blepharospasm, leg dystonia, and psychiatric symptoms in the early stage of the illness. It is caused by mutations in the DJ-1gene, associated with the modulation of transcription, chaperone-like functions, and maintenance of mitochondrial integrity.

PARK8 is the most common form of autosomal dominant parkinsonism. Patients typically present with a late-onset, slowly progressive form of levodopa-responsive parkinsonism, often in combination with psychiatric symptoms such as depression, anxiety, and hallucinations, sometimes also with cognitive impairment, dysautonomia, sleep problems, and anosmia. PARK8 is caused by mutations in the LRRK2 gene, encoding leucine-rich repeat kinase 2 (LRRK2), which is a protein that is widely expressed in human tissue, including the cerebral cortex and spinal cord, thought to be associated with signaling cascades and cytoskeletal dynamics (see Chapter 16).

Sporadic mitochondrial parkinsonism

As the MRC-I inhibitor 1-methyl-4-phenyl-1,2,3,6-tetrahydropyridine (MPTP) is an environmental factor that induces parkinsonism, parkinsonism might indeed be caused by an OXPHOS-related, abnormal interaction of gene-environmental factors (34). Sporadic PD is considered to be a complex neurodegenerative disease entity with both genetic susceptibility and environmental factors contributing to its etiopathogenesis. Recent genome-wide association studies have identified susceptibility loci, which overlap with classical PD genes, linking the aetiology of familial parkinsonism with that of sporadic PD. Both genetic and environmental factors influence various mitochondrial aspects, such as bioenergetics, dynamics, transport, and quality control.

Mitochondrial dystonia

MtDNA mutations, especially gene mutations encoding the various subunits of Complex I, are thought to induce dystonia. Complex I (NADH: ubiquinone oxidoreductase) is the largest enzyme complex of the mitochondrial oxidative phosphorylation system. It consists of 45 subunits, 7 of which are encoded by the mitochondrial genome, and the remainder by the nuclear genome. Mutations in one of the nuclear encoded structural or assembly genes of complex I have a dramatic effect on neurodevelopment and overall patient survival. The majority of the children with an isolated complex I deficiency (OMIM 252010) present with Leigh syndrome (35,36). These patients usually present within the first months of life with psychomotor retardation in combination with signs of brainstem or extrapyramidal dysfunction and lactic acidemia. The most prevalent symptoms include hypotonia, nystagmus, respiratory abnormalities, pyramidal signs, dystonia, psychomotor retardation or regression.

In the literature, mtND1 mutations may cause sporadic adult-onset dystonia (37), ND3 mutations cause dystonic features in Leber's hereditary optic neuropathy (38), and MtND6 mutations cause progressive generalized dystonia with bilateral striatal necrosis (39) or dystonia in Leigh's syndrome (35), all due to a decreased Complex I activity (39) (see also Chapters 22, 23).

Mitochondrial chorea

The expression of pathological huntingtin (htt) in the central nervous system, with relatively high striatal levels, is not uniform. The pathogenic mechanisms of htt have been extensively studied but are not yet fully understood, although all confirmed excitotoxicity, oxidative stress, mitochondrial dysfunction, apoptosis, protein aggregation, impaired axonal transport, disturbed neurogenesis, synaptic dysfunction, microglial activation, etc. Unfortunately, recent clinical trials to investigate the eventual symptomatic effects of ethyl-eicosapentaenoic acid, dimebon, nabilone or pridopidine, and other trials exploring the enhancement of mitochondrial functions using creatine, coenzyme Q10 or remacemide did not show any consistent robust effect (40).

Mitochondrial myoclonus

Myoclonic Epilepsy with Ragged Red Fibers (MERRF) is characterized by myoclonus and mitochondrial myopathy. Other features are seizures, deafness, ataxia, neuropathy and dementia. Symptoms vary widely among patients. MERRF is maternally inherited, and mutations in the mitochondrially encoded tRNA lysine (MTTK) gene are its most common cause (80% of patients) (41). Mitochondrial DNA polymerase-γ (POLG) mutations might cause the Alp-

ers' syndrome phenotype. These patients suffer from a progressive neurological disorder usually starting in early childhood and characterized by developmental regression and refractory focal motor and/or myoclonic seizures (42) (see also Chapter 28).

Mitochondrial ataxia

Many mitochondrial disorders have cerebellar ataxia as one of their multitude of clinical features. These MCPs include both disorders that are caused by an mtDNA mutation, such as MELAS, MERFF and NARP, and disorders in which a defect is caused by a mutated nDNA gene that affects mitochondrial function. The latter type of disorder usually manifests as classical recessive diseases. In particular, mutations in the POLG gene (polymerase gamma) may constitute a relatively frequent cause of ataxia in combination with neuropathy and progressive ophthalmoplegia, such as in sensory ataxic neuropathy with dysarthria and ophthalmoparesis (SANDO). Due to the many POLG mutations, though, there is a huge phenotypic heterogeneity. Other examples of such recessive diseases of which the causative mitochondrial genes are nuclear coded are Friedreich's ataxia, cerebellar ataxia with muscle Coenzyme Q deficiency (41) and the infantile onset spinocerebellar ataxia (IOSCA) exclusively seen in Finland (43) (see also Chapter 33).

Video fragment

Fragment 32.1

Kearns-Sayre syndrome

This patient suffers from Kearns-Sayre syndrome, with generalized cerebellar ataxia and progressive ophthalmoplegia due to a mitochondrial DNA mutation.

References

1 DiMauro S, Schon EA. Mitochondrial respiratory-chain diseases. N Engl J Med 2003;348:2656-2668.

2 Finsterer J. Inherited mitochondrial disorders. Adv Exp Med Biol2012;942:187-213.

3 Swerdlow RH. Treating neurodegeneration by modifying mitochondria: potential solutions to a 'complex' problem. Antooxid Redox Signal 2007;9:1591-1603.

4 Swerdlow RH. The neurodegenerative mitochondriopathies. J Alzheimers Dis 2009;17:737-751.

5 Finsterer J. Mitochondriopathies. Eur J Neurol. 2004;11:163-186.

6 Schon EA, Manfredi G. Neuronal degeneration and mitochondrial dysfunction. J Clin Invest 2003;111:303-312.

7 Schapira AHV. Mitochondrial diseases. Lancet 2012; 379:1825-1834

8 Orsucci D, Ienco EC, Mancuso M, Siciliano G. POLG1-related and other 'Mitochondrial Parkinsonisms': an overview. J Mol Neurosci 2011;44:17-24.

9 Mackey DA, Oostra RJ, Rosenberg T, et al. Primary pathogenic mtDNA mutations in multigeneration pedigrees with Leber hereditary optic neuropathy. Am J Hum Genet 1996;59:481-485.

10 Betts J, Lightowlers RN, Turnbull DM. Neuropathological apects of mitochondrial DNA disease. Neurochem Res 2004;29:505-511.

11 Takeda S, Wakabayashi F, Ohama E, Ikuta F. Neuropathology of myoclonus epilepsy associated with ragged-red fibers (Fukuhara's disease). Acta Neuropathol 1988;75:433-440.

12 Filosto M, Tomelleri G, Tonin P, et al. Neuropathology of mitochondrial diseases. Biosci Rep 2007;27:23-30.

13 Rojo A, Campos Y, Sanchez JM, et al. NARP-MILS syndrome caused by 8993 T>G mitochondrial DNA mutation: a clinical, genetic and neuropathological study. Acta Neuropathol 2006;111:610-616.

14 Rojo A, Campos Y, Sanchez JM, et al. NARP-MILS syndrome caused by 8993 T>G mitochondrial DNA mutation: a clinical, genetic and neuropathological study. Acta Neuropathol 2006;111:610-616.

15 Nishioka K, Cobb SA, et al. Genetic variation of the mitochondrial complex I subunit NDUFV2 and Parkinson's disease. Parkinsonism Relat Disord 2010;16:686-687.

16 Copeland WC. The mitochondrial DNA polymerase in health and disease. Subcell Biochem 2010;50:211-222.

17 Cui L, Jeong H, Borovecki F, et al. Transcriptional repression of PGC-1alpha by mutant huntingtin leads to mitochondrial dysfunction and neurodegeneration. Cell 2006;127:59-69.

18 Lodi R, Cooper JM, Bradley JL et al. Deficit of in vivo mitochondrial ATP production in patients with Friedreich ataxia. Proc Natl Acad Sci USA 1999;96:11492-11495.

19 Rossi L, Lombardo MF, Ciriolo MR, Rotilio G. Mitochondrial dysfunction in neurodegenerative diseases associated with copper imbalance. Neurochem Res 2004;29:493-504.

20 Kordasiewicz HB, Stanek LM, Wancewicz EV, et al. Sustained therapeutic reversal of Huntington's disease by transient repression of huntingtin synthesis. Neuron 2012;74:1031-4104.

21 Hudson G, Chinnery PF. Mitochondrial DNA polymerase-gamma and human disease. Hum Mol Genet 2006;15:244-252.

22 Chan SS, Copeland WC. DNA polymerase gamma and mitochondrial disease: understanding the consequences of POLG mutations. Biochim Biophys Acta 2009;1787:312-319.

23 Fukae J, Mizuno Y, Hattori N. Mitochondrial dysfunction in Parkinson's disease. Mitochondrion 2007;7:58-62.

24 Schon EA, Manfredi G. Neuronal degeneration and mitochondrial dysfunction. J Clin Invest 2003;111:303-312.

25 Manusco M, Filosto M, Orsucci D, Siciliano G. Mitochondrial DNA sequence variation and neurodegeneration. Hum Genomics 2008;3:71-78.

26 Thyagajaran D, Bressman S, Bruno C, et al. A novel mitochondrial 12SrRNA point mutation in parkinsonism, deafness, and neuropathy. Ann Neurol 2000;48:730-736.

27 Horvath R, Kley RA, Lochmuller H, Vorgerd M. Parkinson syndrome, neuropathy, and myopathy

caused by the mutation A8344G (MERFF) in tR-NAlys. Neurology 2007;68:56-58.

28 Horvath R, Kley RA, Lochmuller H, Vorgerd M. Parkinson syndrome, neuropathy, and myopathy caused by the mutation A8344G (MERRF) in tR-NALys. Neurology. 2007 Jan 2;68:56-58

29 Nikoskelainen EK, Martilla RJ, Huoponen K, et al. Leber's "plus" neurological abnormalities in patients with leber's hereditary optic neuropathy. J Neurol Neurosurg Psychiatry 1995;59:160-164.

30 Luoma PT, Eerola J, Ahola S,et al. Mitochondrial DNA polymerase gamma variants in idiopathic sporadic Parkinson disease. Neurology 2007;69:1152-1159.

31 Eerola J, Luoma PT, Peuralinna T, et al. POLG1 polyglutamine tract variants associated with Parkinson's disease. Neurosci Lett 2010;477:1-5.

32 Anvret A, Westerlund , Sydow O. Variations of the CAG trinucleotide repeat in DNA polymerase gamma (POLG1) is associated with Parkinson's disease in Sweden. Neurosci Lett 2010;485:117-120.

33 Synofzik M, Asmus F, Reimold M, Schols L, Berg D. Sustained dopaminergic response of parkinsonism and depression in POLG-associated parkinsonism. Mov Disord 2010;25:243-245.

34 Bueler H. Impaired mitochondrial dynamics and function in the pathogenesis of Parkinson's disease. Exp Neurol 2009;218:235-247.

35 Lera G, Bhatia K, Marsden CD. Dystonia as the major manifestation of Leigh's syndrome. Mov Disord 1994;9:642-649.

36 Koene S, Rodenburg RJ, van der Knaap MS, et al. Natural disease course and genotype-phenotype correlations in Complex I deficiency caused by nuclear gene defects: what we learned from 130 cases. J Inherit Metab Dis. 2012;35:737-747.

37 Simon DK, Friedman J, Breakefield XO, et al. A heteroplasmic mitochondrial complex I gene mutation in adult-onset dystonia. Neurogenetics 2003;4:199-205

38 Wang K, Takahashi Y, Gao ZL, et al. Mitochondrial ND3 as the novel causative gene for Leber hereditary optic neuropathy and dystonia. Neurogenetics. 2009;10:337-345

39 Solano A, Roig M, Vives-Bauza C, et al. Bilateral striatal necrosis associated with a novel mutation in the mitochondrial ND6 gene. Ann Neurol 2003;54:527-530.

40 Mestre T, Ferreira J, Coelho MM, et al. Therapeutic interventions for symptomatic treatment in Huntington's disease. Cochrane Database Syst Rev 2009:CD006456.

41 Emmanuele V, Lopez LC, Berardo A, et al. Heterogeneity of coenzyme Q10 deficiency: patient study and literature review. Arch Neurol 2012;69:978-983.

42 Satishchandra P, Sinha S. Progressive myoclonic epilepsy. Neurol India 2010;58:514-522.

43 Nikali K, Suomalainen A, Saharinen J, et al. Infantile onset spinocerebellar ataxia is caused by recessive mutations in mitochondrial proteins Twinkle and Twinky. Hum Mol Genet 2005;14:2981-2990.

PART IV

Dyskinetic Motor
Behavioural Disorders

33

Ataxia: Pathophysiology and Classification

Berry Kremer

'Ataxia' was derived from the Greek word αταξία, meaning 'failure to put in order' (Wikipedia) and 'without measure'. In clinical neurology the term is used in two ways. It describes the syndrome of motor coordination impairment. And often in its plural as 'ataxias', it designates a large and nosologically complex group of degenerative cerebellar and spinal cord diseases that have as their most prominent manifestation a slowly progressive symmetrical motor coordination impairment (over years). Many other neurological signs may accompany the evolution of the ataxias. Such additional neurological signs are often highly characteristic for a particular disease and therefore helpful in making a diagnosis. The current clinical challenges are to be aware of all the possible diseases that should be considered, and to select an appropriate diagnostic strategy. Recent progress in the molecular understanding and subsequent classification of this vast and often debilitating group of disorders has greatly helped the clinical diagnosis. At the same time we have come to appreciate their clinical and genetic heterogeneity, illustrated by a vastly expanding spectrum of phenotypes and genotypes. And while it was initially thought that the facilitation of the molecular diagnosis by next-generation sequencing methods would reduce the significance of clinical information, it turns out that in order to interpret interindividual genomic sequence variations, precise phenotypic descriptions and definitions have become more important than ever before.

Ataxia classification: history and current principles

The history of research into the cerebellar ataxias has been dominated by the search for a rational, a valid and a clinically relevant classification system. In this 150-year-old quest, three more or less distinct approaches have been pursued: clinical description and classification, structural (neuropathological) parcelation, and genetic ordering. All three, it turns out, are still important. Early clinical descriptions were presented by clinicians whose names are still eponymous: Nicolaus Friedreich (1825-1882), Pierre Marie (1853-1940), Gordon Holmes (1876-1965), Joseph Jules Dejerine (1849-1917) and André Thomas (1867-1963). Their approach was to describe the clinical details meticulously and hope that a classification could be based upon the differences found between the different patients. But as more data became available about patients and their families, the more bewildering became their clinical classification.

The second approach was neuropathological. Morphological differences in the brains of deceased patients would provide a superior, more fundamental approach towards classification than the clinical approach. This programme was worked out by the neuropathologists James G. Greenfield (1884-1958), author of a classic monograph on spinocerebellar degenerations, and Bruce W. Konigsmark (1928-1973) and Leslie P. Weiner, who published an influential paper on the olivopontocerebellar atrophies in 1970 (1). But again, their efforts foundered on the heterogeneity of clinical and pathological presentations. One commonly cited example of the limitations of their classification was the fact that within the famous Schut family (which later turned out to be a SCA1 family), members were included in at least two neuropathological categories.

Genetics ultimately provided the key to a modern classification system. To 19th-century clinicians, although they recognized heredity as an important principle, Gregor Johann Mendel's work was unknown, as it was conducted and published between 1856 and 1868. Only after its rediscovery by the botanists Hugo de Vries, Carl Correns and Erich Tschermak around 1900 did the principles and causes of the various forms of heredity become known to the medical community. In the field of ataxia classification, it was the British neurologist Anita Harding (1952-1995) who emphasized the potential value of a genetic classification system (2). Although her system owed much to her predecessors, she classified the various forms of degenerative ataxia primarily according to the mode of inheritance, arguing that the distinction between dominant, recessive and sporadic forms might offer the most workable approach towards rational classification, based upon the underlying molecular pathobiology. It paved the road to the identification of causative mutations. Thus, she singled out the Autosomal Dominant Cerebellar Ataxias (ADCAs) as a separate group. Her insights have yielded spectacular results in ataxia taxonomy. Examples of discoveries that resulted from this approach were the linkage of one form of autosomal dominant ataxia, SCA1, to HLA genes on chromosome 6 in 1977 and the subsequent discovery in 1993 of the gene itself with its causative mutation, an expanded CAG repeat (3,4). The Friedreich gene was linked to chromosome 9 and identified in 1996, 133 years after its original description (5).

The modern classification system is based upon the molecular (mutational) cause of the ataxia. For both the clinician and the molecular geneticist, the challenge has become to identify the causative mutation accurately and efficiently in an individual patient, and to understand the underlying molecular pathophysiology as a basis for ultimately developing rational treatments. While this last goal is currently still far off, the first is clearly within sight.

General clinical and diagnostic issues in ataxia patients

In making a diagnosis in a patient with a slowly progressive ataxia, a large number of underlying diseases should be considered. This requires taking a careful history and a comprehensive neurological examination. In the history, particular attention should be paid to the age of onset, the speed of clinical progression, the occurrence of similarly affected family members and the presence of consanguinity. The conceptually broadest approach is first to consider whether a patient suffers from a non-degenerative or degenerative ataxia (see Table 33.1). Table 33.2 lists a number of causes of non-degenerative ataxia. In general, non-degenerative diseases that lead to cerebellar ataxia have a much more rapid disease course than degenerative forms and often display asymmetrical signs on neurological examination (see Video fragment 33.1).

Age at onset offers a first approximation to the underlying genetic mechanism. In general, disease onset is much lower for recessive disorders (e.g. Friedreich's ataxia) than for dominant

Table 33.1
A broad conceptual diagnostic framework for slowly progressive cerebellar ataxia.

Slowly progressive ataxia
▪ Non-degenerative
▪ Degenerative
• Non-hereditary (MSA, ILOCA)
• Hereditary
Dominant (ADCA / SCAs)
Recessive
X-linked
(Mitochondrial)

Table 33.2
Some non-degenerative causes of cerebellar ataxia.

Multiple sclerosis

Diseases associated with neoplasms:
- primary or metastatic tumours
- paraneoplastic cerebellar degeneration
- Langerhans histiocytosis

Vascular disease of cerebellum, brainstem or hemispheres:
- hypertensive or arteriosclerotic small-vessel disease
- chronic lymphocytic inflammation with ponto-cerebellar perivascular enhancement responsive to steroids – CLIPPERS
- superficial hemosiderosis of the nervous system

Immune-mediated disorders:
- paraneoplastic cerebellar degeneration
- anti-GAD cerebellopathy
- celiac disease without vitamin E deficiency ?
- steroid-responsive encephalopathy associated with autoimmune thyroiditis – SREAT/Hashimoto
- autoimmune polyglandular syndrome type 2

Metabolic diseases / deficiencies:
- Wernicke encephalopathy
- acquired vitamin E deficiency
- hypoparathyroidism (with dentate nucleus calcifications)

Non-drug intoxications:
- Ethanol

Drug intoxications:
- Anti-epileptics: fenytoine, carbamazepine, valproate, topiramate, vigabatrin, clobazam, lamotrigine, levetiracetam, oxcarbamazepine, zonisamide
- Cytostatics / immunosuppressants: 5-FU, Ara-C, cytarabine, capecitabine, cyclosporine, fluorouracil, interferon, tacrolimus, irinotecan, paclitaxel
- Psychiatric drugs: clomipramine, lithium, maprotiline
- Antibiotics: metronidazole, trimethoprim, raltegravir, colistine
- Hormones: octreotide
- Analgesics: gabapentin, pregabaline, lidocaine, ziconotide

Source: Dutch ataxia protocol – Dutch Neurological Society, 2013

forms, while sporadic disorders such as multiple System Atrophy and idiopathic late-onset cerebellar ataxia (ILOCA) present late in life (6). The early debut of recessive disorders can be understood as the result of a decrease in gene product from dizygous alleles, which leads to a loss of function of the pertinent gene product already early in life. In contrast, many dominant ataxias are likely caused by a dominant negative or toxic effect of the single mutated allele, which only gradually takes effect over decades. Particularly for the repeat expansion diseases like SCA1 and SCA3, this mechanism has been suggested experimentally. As yet, there is no molecular explanation for the onset of the sporadic forms late in life – a situation which is similar to many other sporadic neurodegenerative diseases such as Parkinson's or Alzheimer's disease.

The speed of disease progression is probably the single most important feature that distinguishes degenerative ataxias from non-degenerative variants. Degenerative ataxias typically run a slowly progressive course over many years to decades, but again, the various forms have characteristic speeds of clinical deterioration (6).

The second crucial piece of information is the family history, necessitating the drawing of a pedigree. It should be stressed that if no similarly affected family members can be identified, a hereditary recessive disease still cannot be excluded. Parental consanguinity is a compelling finding in identifying hereditary recessive disease. In dominant disorders the occurrence of multiple affected individuals in subsequent generations is more or less standard, although the phenomenon of anticipation (earlier disease onset in younger generations) may complicate the interpretation of the family history. Postulating 'novel mutations' to support hereditary ataxia disease should be avoided.

A comprehensive neurological and general examination often reveals relevant features that may identify a specific diagnosis at best, but at least may delineate a phenotype that allows targeted (and thus restricted and efficient) molecular diagnostics. Prominent pyramidal tract involvement, axonal neuropathy, sensory impairment, or extrapyramidal involvement may suggest particular diagnoses. Other signs that occur more rarely, but are quite specific if present are: orthostatic hypotension in multiple system atrophy; retinal pigmentary alterations in mitochondrial disease or SCA7; and extrapyramidal features in SCA3, SCA17, ataxia telangiectasia or Niemann Pick type C. Non-neurological abnormalities such as cataract, skin abnormalities, scoliosis or cardiomyopathy may provide important clues to a correct diagnosis. The term 'spinocerebellar ataxia' was coined by neurologists to account for clinical signs of spinal tract pathology – pyramidal tract dysfunction with dorsal column and spinothalamic tract abnormalities – as part of the clinical manifestation. The designation in its abbreviated form, SCA, has been hijacked by geneticists to label all dominant ataxias.

Dominant ataxias

The number of hereditary, autosomal-dominant cerebellar ataxias as defined by genotype has rapidly increased over the past 20 years. The number of forms that are currently classified as SCAs (followed by a number) stands currently at 30 (mid-2013), with 'SCA36' being the latest addition to this list. The postfixed number simply reflects the order in which the various loci were identified. As it happens, the most common forms were discovered first, while rare forms with sometimes complicated clinical manifestations tended to be discovered later.

Over the years, novel forms were added to the list but certain designated genotypes were also weeded out. SCA9 was removed as this designation was published in 1997 for a family in whom neither linkage nor gene identity has ever been found. SCA19 and SCA22 turned out to be the same gene, KCND3, a potassium channel subunit (7,8). A similar situation exists for SCA 15/16/29. Families whose diseases cosegregated with markers linked to 3p26.1 all turned out have mutations

in the inositol 1,4,5-triphosphate receptor type 1 (9). The family that was initially designated as SCA24 turned out later to have a recessive disease (SCAR4, see online Mendelian inheritance in man OMIM, 607317), the locus of which was only reported in an abstract. Dentato-rubro-pallido-luysian atrophy (DRPLA) and the dominant episodic ataxias have never been assigned a SCA number, as their clinical features set them apart from the other dominant ataxias.

The status of SCA8 is still debated. After the initial description of an untranslated CTG-CTA repeat expansion in the Ataxin-8 gene, and in its complementary TAG-CAG repeat in a gene on the Ataxin-8 opposite strand (ATXN8OS), it was argued that this expansion must be pathogenic as it strongly segregates with ataxia in affected families, while a common haplotype has been described for a number of Northern European families with ataxia and a SCA8 repeat expansion (10). But such expansions were also found in ataxia patients with other proven ataxia genotypes such as vitamin E deficiency, SCA6 and SCA1, as well as in patients with other neurodegenerative diseases such as Multiple Systems Atrophy (11-14). A strong argument in favor of SCA8 pathogeneity is the ataxic phenotype in transgenic mice with a SCA8 mutation (15). Given these conflicting data, the current approach in many clinics is to assess SCA8 repeat length in patients with ataxia of unknown origin, but to discuss the remaining diagnostic uncertainties when finding a repeat expansion.

The phenotypic spectrum of dominant ataxias is very broad, ranging from a gradually evolving, isolated cerebellar ataxia over the whole course of the disease, as in SCA6 and SCA14, to ataxia with neuropathy (SCA2, SCA3), extrapyramidal features (SCA3, SCA17), motor neuron disease (SCA36), and many other neurological features, often at the same time. The clinical differences between the various genotypes offer clues to the diagnosis, but even within one family, patients with an identical genotype may display marked phenotypic variability, in terms of both systems affected and onset and disease progression. For example, in single families with SCA3 (the most common form of autosomal-dominant cerebellar ataxia worldwide), some members may suffer from a relatively late onset, mild ataxia with axonal peripheral neuropathy, while others may display the full spectrum of what was formerly known as Machado Joseph disease. While in these SCA3 families intrafamilial CAG repeat length polymorphism may explain phenotypic differences – smaller repeat lengths being primarily associated with axonal neuropathy (16) – other genetic, epigenetic or environmental factors must clearly be involved. Severe multisystem disease with the involvement of extracerebral structures has been described in SCA7 (with very long repeat expansions) (17). Isolated extracerebral features seem specific to some forms, like erythrokeratodermia in SCA34 or azoospermia in SCA32.

Acknowledging this phenotypic variability, dominant ataxia genotypes with additional phenotypes like dentato-rubro-pallido-luysian atrophy (DRPLA), episodic ataxia (EA1), spastic ataxia (SPAX1 (18), or 'deafness and narcolepsy' (ADCA-DN) (19) may then claim their place among the ADCAs. They are therefore included in Table 33.3, which provides an overview of currently established dominant genotypes.

Recessive ataxias: an ever expanding group

The recessive ataxias, even more so perhaps than the dominant ones, are a genetically and particularly clinically heterogeneous group of disorders. For many years genotyping these recessive ataxias lagged behind that for dominant forms. In the past years the number of different genotypes identified has expanded rapidly, due to the use of single-nucleotide polymorphism (SNP) arrays and whole exome sequencing that supported homozygosity mapping – techniques which have evolved over the past few decades. Finding such novel genotypes has increased diagnostic capabilities, particularly for isolated patients without affected siblings.

With the rapid increase in novel genotypes, recessive ataxias' nomenclature has become quite obfuscated. Initially, phenotype abbreviations were used, such as FRDA for Friedreich's ataxia, AT for ataxia teleangiectasia, or ARSACS for autosomal recessive spastic ataxia of Charlevoix Saguenay. Attempts were made to introduce the term ARCA for autosomal recessive cerebellar ataxia, followed by a suffixed number, for those forms without an established name and starting at ARCA1 (for SYNE1 mutations). A competing system to further formalize nomenclature is the designation SCAR (spinocerebellar ataxia, recessive) with a suffix that again reflects the temporal order of discovery for those novel genotypes that had not yet received an established name. This resulted, for example, in ANO10 ataxia having been designated as both ARCA3 and SCAR10 (20-22). Here, the nomenclature of the online MIM database (with 6-digit codes) will be used.

How many recessive ataxias have been identified so far? That question cannot be answered as we have no shared concept as to what delineates hereditary degenerative ataxias from other neurodegenerative diseases. Many recessively inherited metabolic diseases – i.e. diseases detectable by abnormal metabolites in the body fluids – that manifest in childhood have cerebellar atrophy and cerebellar ataxia as one of many clinical features, but they are not consistently being recognized in the literature as 'recessive ataxias'. For example, in late-onset GM_2 gangliosidosis (GM2G), cerebellar atrophy may be one of the features, and therefore it has been grouped under the recessive ataxias in a recent review (23), although many clinicians would not consider it as such, with other neurological signs being so much more prominent. Abetalipoproteinemia (Bassen-Kornzweig disease) and Refsum's disease are often considered in the differential diagnosis of childhood-onset ataxias although they have many features that distinguish them from the classical ataxias. The currently known forms of Joubert syndrome, about 20 different genotypes,

Table 33.3
Autosomal dominant ataxias.

Designation (MIM)	Affected gene	Locus	Mutational mechanism	Affected protein
SCA1 (164400)	ATXN1	6p22.3	translated CAG repeat expansion	Ataxin-1
SCA2 (183090)	ATXN2	12q24.12	translated CAG repeat expansion	Ataxin-2
SCA3 (109150)	ATXN3	14q32.12	translated CAG repeat expansion	Ataxin-3
SCA4 (600223)	?	16q22.1	?	?
SCA5 (600224)	SPTBN2	11q13.2	Inframe deletions; point mutation	Beta-III spectrin
SCA6 (183086)	CACNA1A	19p13.2	translated CAG repeat expansion; point mutations	Voltage-dependent, P/Q-type, calcium channel subunit alpha-1A
SCA7 (164500)	ATXN7	3p14.1	translated CAG repeat expansion	Ataxin-7
SCA8 (608768)	ATXN8 / ATXN8OS	13p21.33 / 13p21	CTG-CTA / TAG-CAG repeat expansion	Ataxin-8 / ATXN8OS (opposite strand)
SCA10 (603516)	ATN10	22q13.31	intronic ATTCT repeat	Ataxin-10
SCA11 (604432)	TTBK2	15q15.2	inframe insertion, deletion	Tau tubulin kinase 2
SCA12 (604326)	PPP2R2B	5q32	5'UTR CAG repeat expansion	(brain-specific) regulatory subunit of the protein phosphatase PP2A,
SCA13 (605259)	KCNC3	19q13.33	point mutations	Potassium channel, voltage-gated, Shwa-related subfamily, member 3
SCA14 (605361)	PRKCG	19q13.42	point mutations; inframe deletion	Protein kinase C, type gamma
SCA15 / 16 / 29 (606658)	ITPR1	3p26.1	large deletions; point mutations	inositol 1,4,5-triphosphate receptor type 1
SCA17 (607136)	TBP (TFIID)	6p27	translated CAG/CAA repeat expansion	TATA box binding protein (Transcription factor IID)
SCA18 (607458)	?	7q22-q32	?	?
SCA19 / 22 (607346)	KCND3	1p13	point mutations, inframe deletion	Potassium channel, voltage-gated, Shal-related subfamily, member 3
SCA20 (608687)	?	11p13-q11	genomic duplication	?

SCA21 (607454)	?	7p21.3-p15.1	?	?
SCA23 (610245)	PDYN	20p13	point mutations	Prodynorphin
SCA25 (608703)	?	2p21-p13	?	?
SCA26 (609306)	?	19p13.3	?	?
SCA27 (609307)	FGF14	13q33.1	point mutations, chromosomal translocation	Fibroblast growth factor 14
SCA28 (610246)	AFG3L2	18p11.21	point mutations	AFG3-like protein 2
SCA30 (613371)	?	4q34.3-q35.1	?	?
SCA31 (117210)	TK /BEAN	16q21	Intronic TGGAA repeat expansion	Intronic to two opposite strand genes
SCA32 (613909)	?	7q32-q33	?	?
SCA34 (133190)	?	6p12.3-q16.2	?	?
SCA35 (613908)	TMG6	20p13	point mutations	Transglutaminase 6
SCA36 (614153)	NOP56		Intronic CGCCTG repeat expansion	RNA processing protein
DRPLA (125370)	ATN1	12p13.31	translated CAG repeat expansion	Atrophin-1
ADCA-DN (604121)	DNMT1	19p13.2	point mutations	DNA Methyltransferase 1
EA1 (160120)	KCNA1	12p13,32	point mutations	Potassium voltage-gated, Shaker-related subfamily, member 1
EA2 (108500)	CACNA1A	19p13.2	Insertions, deletions, exonic and intronic point mutations	Voltage-dependent, P/Q-type, calcium channel subunit alpha-1A
EA3 (606554)	?	1q42	?	?
EA5 (613855)	CACNB4	2q23.3	point mutation	Voltage-dependent, calcium channel subunit beta-4
EA6 (612656)	SLC1A3 / EAAT	5p13.2	point mutations	Glial high-affinity glutamate transporter, member 3
EA7 (611907)	?	19p13	?	?
SPAX1 (108600)	VAMP1	12p13	point mutations	vesicle-associated membrane protein 1

are traditionally not considered in reviews on cerebellar ataxias. On the other hand, conditions that were previously categorized within other groups, such as spastic paraplegias and myoclonic epilepsies, may display such prominent cerebellar ataxia that they really should be considered when thinking about the differential diagnosis of a patient with recessive ataxia. Examples include SPG7 in the differential diagnosis of spastic ataxia and GOSR2-mutations in the differential diagnosis of ataxia with myoclonus (24,25). Table 32.4 lists a number of conditions that currently should be considered as recessive ataxias.

With the increasing number of recessive ataxias that can be diagnosed through mutation analysis, the number of patients drops for whom no specific molecular cause can be found. Prior to 1996, the year in which the causative Friedreich's disease mutation was identified (5), patients with a phenotype that differed from classical Friedreich's were labelled by descriptive diagnoses such as early-onset cerebellar ataxia with retained tendon reflexes, or simply early-onset cerebellar ataxia (EOCA) (6,26). The diagnosis 'EOCA' should now be considered as a provisional one, until a definite molecular diagnosis is available.

The vast majority of early-onset ataxias are probably recessive. In general, recessive ataxia starts early in life. In contrast, dominant ataxias usually have their onset in adulthood or even in later life. However, there are many exceptions to this rule, as the examples of ARCA1 (SYNE1) and SCAR4 illustrate: recessive diseases with late onset without many other features than cerebellar ataxia (27). In contrast, some dominant ataxias may also start in childhood. Examples are CAG repeat expansion diseases with very long repeat expansions, e.g. SCA7 and SCA2 (17). Rare dominant genotypes may also debut early in life, e.g. SCA28 (28). Yet, as a rule of the thumb and as a first approximation to a diagnosis, early-onset ataxias will probably be recessive, and later-onset ataxias will most likely be dominant ones.

X-Linked ataxias

Table 33.5 lists a few X-linked conditions that have ataxia as a prominent feature. This is not to say that X-linked conditions are rare in patients with ataxia. For example, many boys with X-linked mental retardation will display cerebellar ataxia or cerebellar atrophy on MRI as a feature of a complex phenotype, e.g. Pelizaeus Merzbacher disease. Combinations such as dystonia with ataxia and deafness with ataxia may represent underlying X-linked diseases (29,30). X-linked adrenoleukodystrophy and its variant adrenomyeloneuropathy rarely present ataxia as one of their features. The X-linked variant of the Joubert syndrome listed in Table 33.5, JBTS10, is caused by specific mutations in the OFD1 protein. Mutations in this protein display marked phenotypic heterogeneity, as can be appreciated from its full name: the oral-facial-digital syndrome 1 protein.

The only condition that should be considered quite prevalent among these X-linked ataxias is the Fragile-X associated tremor/ataxia syndrome. CGG trinucleotide repeats in the 5' untranslated region of the associated FMR1 gene that exceed 200 repeats are associated with the Fragile X mental retardation syndrome. Premutation repeat sizes, i.e. those between 55 and 200, are associated with premature ovarian failure in women and with the ataxia-tremor syndrome in men (31,32). Women may be affected as well, but not consistently and with much milder manifestations (33,34). MRI T2 signal hyperintensities in the middle cerebellar peduncles, the cerebellar white matter around the output nuclei and the periventricular and deep white matter of the hemispheres offer strong diagnostic clues (35).

Mitochondrial ataxias

As in X-linked neurological disorders, many mitochondrial disorders have cerebellar ataxia as one of their many clinical features, but often not the most prominent one. They include both disorders that are caused by a mitochondrial DNA mutation, such as mitochondrial myopathy, en-

Table 33.4
Some autosomal recessive ataxias.

Designation (MIM)	Affected gene	Locus	Mutational mechanism	Affected protein
Friedreich's ataxia / FRDA (229300)	FXN	9q13	intronic GAA repeat expansion; compound heterozygous point mutation	Frataxin
FRDA2 (601992)	?	9p23-p11	?	?
AVED (277460)	TTPA	18q12.3	point mutations	a-tocopherol transfer protein
SANDO / MIRAS (607459)	POLG1	15q25	specific point mutations	DNA polymerase subunit g-1
Cayman type cerebellar ataxia – (601238)	ATCAY	19p13.3	point mutation, intronic splice site mutation	caytaxin
SCAN1 (607250)	TDP1	14q31-q32	point mutation	Tyrosyl-DNA phosphodi-esterase 1 DNA repair enzyme
ARCA1/SCAR8 (610743)	SYNE1	6q25	point mutations; small deletions	Nuclear envelope spec-trin repeat protein 1 (Nesprin-1)
ARCA2/SCAR9 (612016)	ADCK3 / CABC1	1q42.2	point mutations, inser-tions, small deletions	Chaperone, ABC1 activi-ty of bc1 complex
SCAR10 (613728)	ANO10	3p22.1	point mutations	Anoctamin-10
SCAR13 (614831)	GRM1	6q24.3	deletion; point mutation	metabotropic glutamate receptor
Ataxia telangiectasia – AT (208900)	ATM	11q22.3	point mutations, inser-tions, deletions	AT mutated (DNA repair and/or cell cycle control)
AT-like (604391)	MRE11A	11q21	point mutations	(homologue of S. cerevi-siae) Meiotic recombina-tion 11A
AOA1 (208920)	APTX	9p21.1	point mutations, inser-tions, deletions	Aprataxin
AOA2/ SCAR1 (606002)	SETX	9q13.34	point mutations, dele-tions	Senataxin (DNA/RNA helicase)
Niemann-Pick type C (257220)	NPC1	18q11.2	point mutations, dele-tions	NPC1 protein
Niemann-Pick type C (607625)	NPC2	14q24.3	point mutations, dele-tions	HE1 (epididymal secreto-ry protein)

SCAR2 (213200)	?	9q34-qter	?	?
SCAR4 (607317)	?	1p36	?	(Formerly SCA24)
(Unnamed)	KIAA0226	3q28-qter	deletion	Rundataxin
IOSCA (271245)	C10ORF2	10q24.31	point mutations	Twinkle, Twinky
EAST syndrome (612780)	KCNJ10			
ARSACS / SPAX6 (270550)	SACS	13q12.12	point mutations, deletions, insertions	Sacsin
SPAX2 (611302)	?	17p13	?	?
SPAX3 / ARSAL (611390)	MARS2	2q33-q34	complex rearrangements	Mitochondrial methionyl-tRNA synthetase
SPAX4 (613672)	MTPAP	10p11	point mutation	Mitochondrial poly(A) polymerase
SPAX5 (614487)	AFG3L2	18p11	point mutation	ATPase family gene 3-like 2
'North Sea' myoclonic ataxia / EPM6 (614018)	GOSR2	17q21.32	point mutation	Golgi SNAP receptor complex member 2

cephalopathy, lactic acidosis and stroke-like episodes (MELAS), myoclonus epilepsy with ragged red fibers (MERFF) or neuropathy, ataxia and retinitis pigmentosa (NARP) syndromes, and disorders in which a defect is caused by a mutated nuclear gene that affects mitochondrial function (see Chapter 32). The latter type of disorders usually manifests as classical recessive diseases (see Table 33.4). In particular, mutations in the POLG1 gene (polymerase gamma-1) may constitute a relatively frequent cause of ataxia. Often the combination of ataxia, neuropathy and progressive ophthalmoplegia (such as in sensory ataxic neuropathy with dysarthria and ophthalmoparesis [SANDO] or MIRAS) points to POLG1 mutations. There is a high phenotypic heterogeneity of the many mutations described in this gene, with widely divergent phenotypes resulting from the various mutations. The number of mutations and their associated phenotypes are listed and updated in: http://tools.niehs.nih.gov/polg.

Other examples of such recessive diseases of which the causative genes are nuclear-coded and mitochondrially active are Friedreich's ataxia and *cerebellar ataxia with muscle Coenzyme Q deficiency*, a manifestation of a heterogeneous group of conditions with established mutations in the ADCK3/CABC1 gene in some families, at least (36,37). This recessive disease is listed in Table 33.4. Mitochondrial depletion syndromes may feature prominent ataxia, as in *infantile onset spinocerebellar ataxia* (IOSCA), a condition that has been described in Finland only (38).

Epidemiology

Ataxias are rare diseases with widely variable prevalences regionally. Knowledge of local ataxia prevalence helps in selecting rational and efficient diagnostic strategies. From a worldwide perspective the most prevalent, dominant ataxia appears to be SCA3. A comprehensive invento-

Table 33.5
X-linked ataxias.

Designation	Affected gene	Locus	Mutational mechanism	Affected protein
FXTAS (300623)	FMR1	Xq27.3	CGG-repeat expansion	FMRP
SCAX1 (302500)	ATP2B3	Xp11.21-q21.3	point mutations	ATPase, Ca++ transporting, plasma membrane 3
SCAX5 (300703)	?	Xq25-q27.1	?	?
ASAT (301310)	ABCB7	Xq13.3	point mutations	Mitochondrial ATP-binding cassette transporter
JBTS10 (300804)	OFD1	Xp22.2	inframe deletions; point mutations	Oral-facial-digital syndrome 1 protein

ry in the Netherlands using data from all DNA diagnostic labs that offered genotyping yielded a minimum prevalence of about 3 per 100,000 inhabitants (39). The actual prevalence may be somewhat higher. SCA3 was the most common genotype, accounting for one-third of all cases, while SCA6 was also quite prevalent, similar to Germany and Japan. In contrast, SCA1 and SCA2 were most prevalent in Italy (40). In Cuba, India and Korea, SCA2 may be the most prevalent, while SCA10 appears to have a Meso-American (Mexican) founder with mutations outside Mexico being rare (41-43). DRPLA is relatively common in Japan, but exceedingly rare outside that country. Such marked ethnographic differences must reflect founder effects as well as the vagaries of history.

The worldwide distribution of recessive ataxias reveals equally major regional and ethnic differences. Friedreich's ataxia is probably the single most prevalent recessive ataxia, with an overall prevalence of about 2 in 100,000, and an estimated gene carrier frequency of about 1:100. In contrast, it seems rare to absent in black Africans and Japanese (44). The incidence of ataxia telangiectasia has been estimated at about 0.3-1.0 per 100,000 live births, while the ATM mutated gene carrier frequencies may be about 0.5-1.0 in 100, although percentages as high as 3.5 have been suggested (45). In Europe, ataxia with

oculomotor apraxia type 2 (AOA2) or ARSACS may be the next most frequent recessive ataxias after Friedreich's (46,46-48).

Some very rare recessive ataxias occur only regionally. Examples are IOSCA in Finland, the ataxia found on the Cayman islands, and SCAR13 that, until now, has been found exclusively confined to Bulgarian bowlmaker Roma (49).

In contrast to these very rare recessive forms, the estimated frequency of FMR1/FXTAS premutations in the general population is quite high: 1 in about 150 females and 1 in about 400 males (32). Assessing FMR1 repeat sizes in men over age 50 with sporadic, late-onset ataxia may therefore be an appropriate strategy (50, 51).

When performing diagnostic mutation analysis in patients, epidemiological considerations are important in the prioritization of sequencing efforts. With novel molecular analytical methods, such epidemiological considerations may perhaps become less necessary.

Genetic and molecular diagnostic considerations

Finding a causative mutation is currently the ultimate diagnostic step in patients with degenerative ataxia. The easiest situation from a clinical diagnostic point of view would be one in which a particular phenotype would predict one known gene with at most a few, previously confirmed pathogenic mutations. The aim of molecular testing would then be to confirm the clinical diagnosis. This is the situation often encountered in movement disorders practice in patients with Huntington's disease, and it works in a similar way in patients with classical Friedreich's ataxia. In ataxia clinics, the diagnostic work-up is often much more complex and messy. The number of established causative genes/mutations is growing every year, and thus the number of genes to be tested expands in parallel. Having an updated list of potential genes is imperative (see Tables 33.3, 33.4 and 33.5).

Unfortunately, the 'one disease, one gene, one mutation' principle is not applicable.

Locus heterogeneity, the phenomenon that a single phenotype may be caused by mutations in genes at various loci, is the rule rather than the exception in ataxia patients. It implies that to identify one patient's molecular diagnosis, multiple genes will have to be sequenced, which is currently done by automated traditional and serial Sanger sequencing. Due to the current costs, a clear strategy and prioritization are required. As an example: in patients with autosomal-dominant cerebellar ataxia in whose family the mutation is still unknown, most labs and clinicians in the world would opt to first assess the CAG repeat in SCA1, SCA2, SCA3, SCA6 and perhaps SCA7, depending on the regional situation. Only after having excluded these would clinicians proceed with analysis of lower prevalence genotypes, such as SCA5, SCA12, SCA13, SCA14, SCA17, SCA23 and DRPLA. It should be pointed out that locus heterogeneity also provides guidance to the molecular diagnostics. Recognizing and delineating the phenotype limits the potential selection of genes to be sequenced.

Allelic heterogeneity, the phenomenon that various mutations within one gene may yield a similar phenotype, is in general well addressed by single gene sequencing. One example is the P/Q-type, voltage-dependent, calcium channel alpha-subunit 1A (CACNA1A)/SCA6 gene. Both expansion of the CAG repeat at the 3' translation product of the gene and point mutations in more upstream exons may cause a slowly progressive ataxia (52). Another example involves the large number of point mutations, insertions and deletions in POLG1 that may cause similar phenotypes. The major issue in allelic heterogeneity is how to interpret all the single nucleotide and oligonucleotide variations that is present in the human exome. In order to consider a polymorphism pathogenic, its pathogenicity has to be assessed, in population prevalence studies, in interspecies comparisons or in functional studies. This may become an issue in large genes, particularly when mutations dispersed all over the gene result in a uniform phenotype. One such example is the mutations in the autosomal-recessive spastic ataxia of Charlevoix-Saguenay (ARSACS). These mutations are dispersed all over the very large (> 11,000 basepair) SACS gene that consists of one gigantic exon as well as 8 small exons. Most mutations so far have resulted in a remarkably similar, highly recognizable, early-onset spastic-ataxic phenotype, although phenotypic variation has been described (48, 53).

Pleiotropy or *phenotypic heterogeneity* adds another layer of diagnostic complexity. It means that mutations in one single gene may lead to vastly different clinical manifestations or phenotypes. One of the best known examples, again, can be found in the CACNA1A, SCA6 gene. Apart from progressive dominant ataxia caused by CAG repeat expansion and point mutations, various missense and nonsense mutations may lead to episodic ataxia type 2 (EA2) and familial hemiplegic migraine (52,54). POLG1 not only demonstrates locus heterogeneity but also phenotypic heterogeneity. The various mutations described up to now are associated with various different phenotypes that range from progressive chronic external ophthalmoplegia to cerebellar ataxia with neuropathy to severe infantile hepatocerebral syndrome. Heterozygous mutations in the SPTBN2/beta-III spectrin gene have been found to cause dominant SCA5, which represents a relatively pure cerebellar ataxia. But recently, homozygous (bi-allelic) mutations in this gene have been found to be associated with recessive, early-onset, developmental ataxia with cognitive impairment (55,56). However, caution should be applied in interpreting the functional significance of allelic variation. It has been argued that recessive missense mutations in the senataxin/SETX (ataxia with oculomotor apraxia, AOA) type 2 gene that were previously considered to be associated with juvenile onset motor neuron disease ALS4 may in many instances represent harmless polymorphisms, rather than pathogenic mutations (57,58).

The classical approach towards diagnosing mutations in ataxia patients has been a sequential one: to try to match the patient's phenotype to established candidate genes, as a guidance for the prioritization of sequencing efforts. In other words: the patient's phenotype prioritizes the molecular sequencing efforts. As an example: in a patient with a clinical phenotype that resembles Friedreich's ataxia, the first molecular diagnostic step would be to assay the GAA repeat length on both alleles of the Frataxin gene. If that does not yield a mutation, subsequent analysis of potential point mutations in the FTDA and in other genes will be undertaken. When suspecting a genotype with known allelic heterogeneity, classical Sanger sequencing is still perfectly suitable to sequence all exons, as well as the exon-intron boundaries of the gene of interest, to come up with all sequence variants in that gene. The issue here would be to interpret the functional significance of the variant sequences. Classical Sanger sequencing also works when a few genes have to be analysed; even then, multiple sequencing is feasible in terms of time and costs. But such strategies become more and more problematic as the number of known ataxia genes increases,

and the phenotype is no longer able to predict the genotype accurately.

Next-generation sequencing (NGS) allows novel and efficient strategies for clinical diagnostic mutation detection in genetically and phenotypically heterogeneous diseases with many genes involved. Two approaches in particular have emerged: whole exome sequencing, and targeted NGS (59-61). Whole exome sequencing is an unbiased technique that is not only suitable for clinical diagnostics but also for research purposes, allowing the typing of variants for homozygosity mapping and linkage purposes, as well as the identification of novel mutations (62, 63). Its disadvantages are the huge amount of data that are generated and subsequently need to be analysed, and the number of reads required to obtain sufficient coverage. In addition, introns with pathogenic mutations, such as the expanded oligonucleotide repeat in Friedreich's ataxia, cannot be detected. The second method, targeted NGS, requires a preselection of genes (or genomic areas) of interest, to generate probes that capture the selected targeted genes. The advantages of targeted NGS are greater coverage and a much more restricted amount of sequence data being generated, thus simplifying the data analysis. Targeted NGS also allows the examination of the intronic sequence, thereby theoretically enabling the detection of intronic mutations. However, for technical reasons, both methods are currently experiencing major problems in sequencing and sizing repeats, both exonic and intronic. Targeted NGS has already been introduced as a diagnostic strategy for both hereditary spastic paraplegias and hereditary ataxias (64).

Whatever the method used for diagnostics, the issue will be how to interpret the sequence variations that are found. Which are the innocent polymorphisms, what are pathogenic variants, and which variant is to be held responsible for the patient's ataxia? Here again, careful consideration of the clinical phenotype becomes as important as ever before, requiring a comprehensive clinical description and classification.

Clinical presentation

Clinical phenotypes can be grouped into a number of broad categories. Establishing into which category the patient's clinical manifestations cluster remains a major step towards the diagnosis. The other major step is to determine the mode of inheritance. Although it is impossible to summarize all the clinical features according to genotype, the following broad categories can be delineated.

Pure cerebellar ataxia

This is the simplest and most recognizable phenotype: a gradually progressive cerebellar ataxia with no or hardly any other feature. A problem in interpretation may be that patients with various genotypes may present with this phenotype in the early stages of their disease, only to evolve more complex, and informative, phenotypes later. Information on other family members' features may therefore be helpful.

If the clinical manifestations remain purely cerebellar and the family history suggests autosomal dominant disease with onset in middle age, SCA6 caused by an expanded CAG repeat is the most likely diagnosis, although point mutations in that same gene, CACNA1A, are another possibility (52). SCA6 genotyping should also be done in sporadic, late-onset, slowly degenerative cases. The most prevalent dominant ataxia worldwide, SCA3, may present as a late-onset disease with restricted clinical features, particularly when the causative CAG expansion is relatively short. SCA5 has been described in only a few families worldwide and may be associated with downbeat nystagmus. Other low to very low prevalence candidates would be SCA10, SCA11, SCA13, SCA14, which may sometimes be associated with tremor, SCA23, SCA26 and SCA30. SCA31, another pure cerebellar syndrome, is caused by a TGGAA pentanucleotide repeat in a shared intron of two genes, TK2 and BEAN, on opposite strands. It appears to occur mainly in Japan, although cases in Eastern China have been described (65,66). Mild sensorineural hearing loss may be part of its disease spectrum.

When the family tree is not consistent with dominant disease, the following two recessive conditions should be considered: ARCA1 / SYNE1 and SCAR10/ANO10 (20, 27). In contrast to the general rule that recessive disease starts early, SYNE1 mutations may present as a late-onset, purely cerebellar syndrome, up to age 50.

Finally, in elderly men, rarely in elderly women, a purely cerebellar syndrome, particularly if accompanied by tremor, should raise a suspicion of FXTAS.

Ataxia with prominent neuro(no)pathy

Axonal neuropathy, either sensorimotor or only sensory, is a feature of many ataxias, both dominant and recessive. Neuropathy or neuronopathy (in which not only the distal axon but also the cell body in the dorsal root is affected) in dominant ataxias may be encountered prominently in SCA3, SCA1, SCA2 and SCA7 (67), in general as part of a much more complex phenotype, but in SCA3 sometimes as a major manifestation in gene carriers with relatively brief CAG repeat lengths. Neuropathy has also been described in rare genotypes such as SCA18 and in SCA25. As many other co-morbid causes may underlie neuropathy in a patient, only marked and consistent findings are helpful when using this feature as an indication for an underlying molecular diagnosis.

A sensory neuropathy is also a consistent feature of many recessive ataxias, such as Friedreich's ataxia (FRDA), ataxia with vitamin E deficiency (AVED), infantile-onset spinocerebellar ataxia (IOSCA) and the sensory ataxic neuropathy with dysarthria and ophthalmoparesis (SANDO) phenotype of certain POLG1 mutations, specifically W748S and A467T (68). Mixed, severe, axonal sensorimotor neuropathies are consistently found in ataxia telangiectasia, AOA type1 and AOA type 2, and in the very rare spinocerebellar ataxia with axonal neuropathy (SCAN1). In fact, neuropathy is a more frequent and consistent clinical finding in AOA2 than oculomotor apraxia (69).

Ataxias associated with metabolic diseases, such as abetalipoproteinemia (Bassen-Kornzweig disease), and Refsum's disease will cause demyelinating neuropathies rather than axonal forms. Thus, nerve conduction studies may be helpful in making a diagnosis.

Ataxia with lower motor neuron disease

Lower motor neuron abnormalities, notably muscle atrophy and fasciculations, are probably not common during the largest part of the disease course in SCA1, bulbar dysfunction starting to become prominent only in late stages of the disease (70). In contrast, fasciculations, muscle cramps and muscle atrophy may be prominent in SCA3 patients, not only in those with the Machado Joseph phenotype, but also in those with early disease or relatively brief repeat lengths, in whom muscle cramps may be an inconvenient symptom (70,71). The muscle weakness and atrophy in SCA18, with neurogenic atrophy demonstrated by muscle biopsy, are probably caused by axonal motor neuropathy (72). In SCA36, known by other names such as 'Costa da Morte' or 'Asidian' disease, tongue fasciculations early in the disease and generalized limb fasciculations later on appear to be true manifestations of lower motor neuron degeneration (73,74).

The relation between SCA2/ATN2 and motor neuron disease/amyotrophic lateral sclerosis (ALS) is more complex. Patients with SCA2 may have muscle cramps and facial fasciculations (75). But it also appears that intermediate repeat length alleles (>29) in ATXN2, the SCA2 disease gene, constitute a risk factor for sporadic ALS (76). In fact, recently a family with coexistent SCA2 ataxia and ALS was described, with a full pathological repeat expansion (77).

In ataxia telangiectasia, motor neuron disease may be a cardinal feature, not only in classical patients but also in late-onset 'variant' disease patients (78). Fasciculations and muscle wasting can also occasionally be observed in AOA1 and AOA2 patients, but this may be due to the motor neuropathy, rather than to spinal motor neuron disease.

As stated before, the previous claim that recessive missense mutations in the SETX/AOA2 gene that cause juvenile-onset motor neuron disease ALS4 has recently been challenged with the argument that many so-called pathogenic variants may be innocent variants instead (57, 58).

Ataxia with specific oculomotor abnormalities

Saccadic intrusions into smooth pursuit, overshoot and undershoot saccades, multistep saccades and nystagmus are non-specific findings in many degenerative as well as non-degenerative ataxias (see Video fragment 34.1). Moreover, oculomotor abnormalities tend to develop and change over the course of the disease. However, there are specific oculomotor abnormalities that may offer strong and specific clues to the underlying genotype, for both recessive and dominant diseases.

Oculomotor apraxia consists of initial saccadic slowing, head thrust on fast lateral gaze with gaze lag, difficulties in saccade initiation, and ultimately gaze paralysis. The phenomenon is associated with ataxia telangietasia (AT) and ataxia with oculomotor apraxia type 1 (AOA1) where it is encountered in all affected individuals. It is much less consistently present in AOA2; in these patients, oculomotor apraxia was found (occasionally!) in about 50% of the subjects (69). Also, in individuals with variant AT that presents later in life, oculomotor apraxia is rarely encountered (78). In the very rare AT-like disorder, caused by mutations in the MRE11A gene (79), oculomotor apraxia appears to be present in at least the majority of patients.

In Niemann-Pick type C (NPC) disease, caused by both NPC1 and NPC2 mutations, severe slowing of vertical saccades and vertical supranuclear gaze palsy (with less severe slowing of horizontal saccades) is a highly sensitive and specific clinical diagnostic disease marker, in both children and adults with this disease (80,81).

Severe saccadic slowing, supranuclear gaze palsies and even ophthalmoparesis in dominant ataxias are strongly indicative of SCA1 or SCA2. Often, such severe oculomotor phenotypes occur only late in the cause of the disease, as in SCA28 (28).

Congenital ataxia

Congenital ataxias present in infancy with hypotonia and delayed motor development, with or without intellectual disability later in life. On imaging, cerebellar hypoplasia is apparent and must reflect developmental impairment, rather than cerebellar degeneration as in many other ataxias. Some severe phenotypes are associated with it, such as Joubert syndrome, while other forms evolve as only mild and probably stationary cerebellar ataxia later in life without any cognitive problems. This phenotype represents a vastly heterogeneous group of diseases, in terms of both more detailed phenotypes and causative genotypes.

Some genotypes seem to present congenital ataxia as their core phenotype, such as perhaps SCAR2 and SCAR6 (82, 83). In others, congenital ataxia clearly represents phenotypic heterogeneity of existing ataxia genes. One form of recessive congenital ataxia with intellectual disability is caused by a homozygous deletion in the SPTBN2 gene, thus being allelic with the dominant SCA5 phenotype (56). Mutations in the sacsin (SACS) gene, best known for its association with spastic ataxia, may cause a congenital ataxia (63). Congenital ataxia not only occurs as a recessive condition; a missense mutation in the ITPR1 gene that is associated with SCA15/16/29 was found to cause SCA29 dominant congenital ataxia (62).

Given this locus heterogeneity as well as phenotypic heterogeneity, whole exome sequencing may be expected in the coming years to reveal many novel mutations that cause congenital ataxias.

Spastic ataxia

The spastic ataxias constitute a phenotype in which ataxia of the head and upper body (sometimes mild) is combined with a prominent spastic paraparesis of the legs. As such, it appears as an easily recognizable clinical phenotype intermediate between cerebellar ataxia and complex spastic paraplegia. Awareness of its genetic heterogeneity has expanded over the past few years, with both dominant and recessive mutations being described (84).

Of the recessive genotypes, autosomal recessive spastic ataxia of Charlevoix Saguenay (ARSACS; SPAX6) was originally considered to occur only in Quebec. It has since been diagnosed in many regions of the world, being by far the most prevalent spastic ataxia and indeed one of the most prevalent recessive ataxias in many regions. At least four other rare, recessive spastic ataxia genotypes with established genomic loci are listed in the MIM database: SPAX2, SPAX3 with focal white-matter changes, SPAX4 with optic atrophy in an old order Amish family, and SPAX5 with dystonia and myoclonic epilepsy. In addition, recessive spastic ataxia may occur in late-onset Friedreich's ataxia, in SPG7 (which usually manifests as a complex recessive spastic paraplegia), in adult-onset Alexander disease, in cerebrotendinous xanthomatosis, in adrenomyeloneuronopathy and in fatty acid hydroxylase-associated neurodegeneration (84).

Dominant spastic ataxia SPAX1 has been described in Newfoundland families and is caused by mutations in the VAMP1 protein that disrupt the splicing of at least one isoform, VAMP1A (18).

It should be stressed that although brisk reflexes and extensor toe responses may be a feature of many dominant as well as recessive cerebellar ataxias, the spasticity in spastic ataxia is much more than this, contributing significantly to the patient's disability.

Ataxia with chorea and/or dystonia

The combination of ataxia with chorea as an autosomal dominant disease should raise the suspicion of either dentate-rubro-pallido-luysian atrophy (DRPLA) or SCA17. DRPLA is very rare outside Japan. Apart from ataxia and chorea, myoclonus epilepsy in early-onset patients and progressive dementia are prominent manifestations. Likewise, SCA17 is rare and features focal dystonias and behavioural and cognitive deterioration along with ataxia and chorea. Both disorders may present with a Huntington's disease-like phenotype (see Video fragment 33.2). Dystonia, sometimes chorea, may also occur in other dominant ataxias with a severe phenotype such as SCA1, SCA2, and SCA3. Minor distal choreic movements have been observed in patients with SCA7, while dystonia may be a feature of SCA8, SCA12 (axial) and SCA14 (task induced).

In recessive ataxias, dystonia and chorea are very frequently encountered in ataxia telangiectasia, particularly in late-onset variant cases where they may be more prominent than ataxia (78). In AOA1 patients, chorea is present in many patients, while chorea and dystonia seem to occur only in a minority of AOA2 patients (69). Chorea rarely manifests in Friedreich's ataxia, but it may be severe (85). Axial or generalized dystonia is also a feature of Niemann-Pick type C (80).

Ataxia with myoclonus (Ramsay Hunt syndrome / phenotype)

This rare clinical syndrome, originally called dyssynergia cerebellaris myoclonica, consists of ataxia and myoclonus, without or with epilepsy, in which case overlap exists with the myoclonus epilepsies. Many different diseases may manifest as the Ramsay Hunt syndrome, such as POLG1 mutations, other mitochondrial disorders (e.g. MERFF), sialidosis type I, the various progressive myoclonus epilepsies (Unverricht-Lundborg disease, Lafora disease, myoclonus epilepsy type 4 [EPM4]), DRPLA or, rarely, Friedreich's ataxia. It may occur in celiac disease as well.

Recently, a homozygous loss of function mutation in the GOSR2 gene was described that is associated with this phenotype (25). Quite a few patients have been described with this particular mutation, all of them tracing their ancestry back to countries and areas around the North Sea (86). Although this form is classified as a myoclonus epilepsy (EPM6), epilepsy appears a minor feature; ataxia and myoclonus are the truly debilitating features of the disease.

In dominant diseases, myoclonus, including palatal myoclonus, may rarely be part of a much severer phenotype, such as SCA1, SCA2 and SCA3.

Ataxia with other extrapyramidal features

Parkinsonism is an infrequent feature of most ataxias, being primarily found in SCA3 patients as part of the Machado Joseph phenotype, and in the single French SCA21 family.

In SCA2 L-dopa-responsive parkinsonism has been described in a few families, mostly of Chinese and Indian descent, and in late-onset patients with mildly expanded or CAG/CAA interrupted repeats, some of them even without ataxia (87-89). As such, SCA2 should currently be considered in the differential diagnosis of familial parkinsonism.

Action and postural tremors, other than ataxia, have been described in many dominant forms, including SCA2, SCA3, SCA15, SCA17, SCA19/22, SCA21, SCA23, SCA31, and SCA35, while resting tremor has been noted in patients with SCA5, and deafness and narcolepsy in ADCA (ADCA-DN). Head tremor occurs in SCA14. Action and postural tremors may be a consistent feature of SCA27 (FGF-mutations). Palatal tremor has been described in the single reported SCA20 family (90).

In recessive disorders, irregular resting tremor has been described in ataxia telangiectasia, head tremor in AOA2, and late-onset resting tremor in Niemann-Pick type C1. And, of course, tremor is a major feature in FXTAS.

Given the descriptions of tremor in so many ataxias, although generally as minor and inconsistent clinical signs, they may go underreported, action tremor perhaps being mistaken for ataxia.

Ataxia with retinal or optic nerve pathology, or deafness

Retinal degeneration due to progressive cone-rod dystrophy, with resulting blindness, is a defining clinical feature of SCA7 (91). Retinal degeneration in dominant ataxia has also been described in a SCA2 patient with a very long repeat. The autosomal-dominantly inherited combination of ataxia, sensorineural deafness, narcolepsy and, later in the course of the disease, optic atrophy and dementia may be due to mutations in the DNMT1 gene (19). Optic atrophy may develop in SCA1 and SCA2 patients. Recently, OPA1 mutations have been described that cause early optic atrophy with late ataxia and even spastic paraparesis (92). This combination, both as dominant or recessive disease, has been labeled Behr's syndrome.

In ARSACS retinal striation ('retinal streaks') may be part of the clinical phenotype, without notable consequences for the patients (48). The rare combination of cerebellar ataxia, retinal degeneration and hypogonadotrophic hypogonadism has been labeled the Boucher-Neuhäuser syndrome.

It should be noted that combinations of ataxia with retinal, optic nerve or auditory nerve pathology occur in a wide variety of recessive metabolic and mitochondrial diseases. Thus, expert opthalmologic or audiologic examination may be an appropriate diagnostic approach.

Episodic ataxias

The episodic ataxias, as their name implies, develop and wane over time periods that may last from minutes to days. It may be difficult to di-
agnose them if they cannot be observed during the ictus. Interictal clinical phenomena may be helpful, although they may point to a more progressive degenerative disease that is punctuated by ataxia attacks. There is overlap with paroxysmal dyskinesias and epilepsies, and many are caused by ion channel mutations.

Dominant conditions include EA2, which is caused by mutations in the CACNA1A gene and is thus allelic with SCA6 progressive ataxia and familial hemiplegic migraine. Dominant heredity may be difficult to demonstrate as the disease transmits with incomplete penetrance. In between attacks that may last from one hour to days, eye movement abnormalities persist, particularly gaze-evoked nystagmus. In EA1 the episodes of ataxia are characteristically much briefer, lasting up to several minutes. The most characteristic feature of this condition is the continuous 'rippling' of the muscles (myokimia). This autosomal dominant disease is caused by mutations in the KCNA1 potassium voltage-gated channel subunit gene. Other dominant episodic ataxias currently include EA3 with tinnitus and vertigo, EA5 with interictal downbeat nystagmus and slowly progressive static ataxia, EA6 with slowly progressive truncal ataxia over the years, and EA7 without interictal phenomena. Episodic ataxias should be considered very rare disorders, having been described in only a few families.

Other recognizeable features and lab findings

In general, few additional features can be observed during the general examination of an ataxia patient, while biochemical or morphological lab findings are not very helpful in making a diagnosis. Exceptions are ocular telangiectasias in ataxia telangiectasia, narcolepsy in AD-CA-BN, or erythrokeratodermia in SCA34. A family history of male infertility would suggest azoospermia, and thus SCA32. In routine laboratory examinations, elevated levels of alpha-fetoprotein would strongly suggest AT, AOA1 or AOA2, while decreased levels of vitamin E would point to AVED and hypoalbuminemia and hypercholesterolemia would suggest AOA1. Sideroblastic anemia would suggest X-linked ataxia with sideroblastic anemia (ASAT). But in general, it is the genetic molecular diagnostics lab that should come up with a diagnosis.

Treatment

For the vast majority of the disorders discussed in this chapter, no causative treatment is available. Moreover, and unlike in Parkinson's disease, there is even no treatment available for ataxia as a symptom. Rarely and paradoxically, low doses of benzodiazepines may offer some relief for motor coordination impairment, particularly if overshoot and dysmetria are prominent. And if oscilloscopia due to oculomotor incoordination is troublesome, baclofen may be of benefit.

The basis of disease management is a thorough discussion with the patient and the family of the nature of the disorder and its resulting impairments, as well as paramedical support, primarily physiotherapy, speech therapy and occupational interventions. Speech therapy has such obvious short-term benefits in those with speech and swallowing impairment that no patient should be denied access to a speech therapist. Speech and swallowing can be improved by simple instructions such as slowing of articulation and specific postures during swallowing. The subjective benefit of physiotherapy seems less obvious than that of speech therapy, although many patients appreciate a regular visit to a physiotherapist. Finally, tips and interventions from an occupational therapist often yield straightforward and obvious benefits. Consultations by a rehabilitation specialist may be useful in complementing and coordinating the various paramedical interventions.

An important issue is genetic counseling early in the course of the disease. For many patients and their families, the hereditary nature of the disease imposes an important and extra burden, apart from the physical discomfort that is part of daily life. In many of the disorders discussed in this chapter, predictive molecular testing is possible, particularly in the dominant ataxias. But predictive testing is not a necessary step in the counseling of the family. The decision of an unaffected at-risk individual to undergo predictive testing is a very personal consideration that involves being fully informed and emotionally supported and that should be well considered. It is a personal decision by an autonomous individual, not a medical decision.

Video fragments

Fragment 33.1
Non-degenerative cerebellar ataxia
This videotape shows an MS patient with an atactic gait, axial titubation, and incoordinated volitional movements.

Fragment 33.2
Sporadic cerebellar atrophy
A case with SCA17, Huntington phenotype.

References

1 Koningsmark BW, Weiner LP. The olivopontocerebellar atrophies: a review.. Medicine (Baltimore) 1970;49:227-241.

2 Harding AE. The hereditary ataxias and related disorders.. Edinburgh: Churchill Livingstone; 1984.

3 Jackson JF, Currier RD, Terasaki PI, Morton NE. Spinocerebellar ataxia and HLA linkage: risk prediction by HLA typing. N Engl J Med 1977;296:1138-1141.

4 Orr HT, Chung MY, Banfi S, et al. Expansion of an unstable trinucleotide CAG repeat in spinocerebellar ataxia type 1. Nat Genet 1993;4:221-226.

5 Campuzano V, Montermini L, Molto MD, et al. Friedreich's ataxia: autosomal recessive disease caused by an intronic GAA triplet repeat expansion. Science 1996;271:1423-1427.

6   Klockgether T, Ludtke R, Kramer B, et al. The natural history of degenerative ataxia: a retrospective study in 466 patients. Brain 1998;121:589-600.

7   Duarri A, Jezierska J, Fokkens M, et al. Mutations in potassium channel kcnd3 cause spinocerebellar ataxia type 19. Ann Neurol 2012;72:870-880.

8   Lee YC, Durr A, Majczenko K, et al. Mutations in KCND3 cause spinocerebellar ataxia type 22. Ann Neurol 2012;72:859-869.

9   van de Leemput J, Chandran J, Knight MA, et al. Deletion at ITPR1 underlies ataxia in mice and spinocerebellar ataxia 15 in humans. PLoS Genet 2007;3:e108.

10 Koob MD, Moseley ML, Schut LJ, et al. An untranslated CTG expansion causes a novel form of spinocerebellar ataxia (SCA8). Nat Genet 1999;21:379-384.

11 Cellini E, Piacentini S, Nacmias B, et al. A family with spinocerebellar ataxia type 8 expansion and vitamin E deficiency ataxia. Arch Neurol 2002;59:1952-1953.

12 Izumi Y, Maruyama H, Oda M, et al. SCA8 repeat expansion: large CTA/CTG repeat alleles are more common in ataxic patients, including those with SCA6. Am J Hum Genet 2003;72:704-709.

13 Sulek A, Hoffman-Zacharska D, Zdzienicka E, Zaremba J. SCA8 repeat expansion coexists with SCA1--not only with SCA6. Am J Hum Genet 2003;73:972-974.

14 Factor SA, Qian J, Lava NS, Hubbard JD, Payami H. False-positive SCA8 gene test in a patient with pathologically proven multiple system atrophy. Ann Neurol 2005;57:462-463.

15 Moseley ML, Zu T, Ikeda Y, et al. Bidirectional expression of CUG and CAG expansion transcripts and intranuclear polyglutamine inclusions in spinocerebellar ataxia type 8. Nat Genet 2006;38:758-769.

16 van Alfen N, Sinke RJ, Zwarts MJ, et al. Intermediate CAG repeat lengths (53,54) for MJD/SCA3 are associated with an abnormal phenotype. Ann Neurol 2001;49:805-807.

17 van de Warrenburg BP, Frenken CW, Ausems MG, et al. Striking anticipation in spinocerebellar ataxia type 7: the infantile phenotype. J Neurol 2001;248:911-914.

18 Bourassa CV, Meijer IA, Merner ND, et al. VAMP1 mutation causes dominant hereditary spastic ataxia in Newfoundland families. Am J Hum Genet 2012;91:548-552.

19 Winkelmann J, Lin L, Schormair B, et al. Mutations in DNMT1 cause autosomal dominant cerebellar ataxia, deafness and narcolepsy. Hum Mol Genet 2012;21:2205-2210.

20 Vermeer S, Hoischen A, Meijer RP, et al. Targeted next-generation sequencing of a 12.5 Mb homozygous region reveals ANO10 mutations in patients with autosomal-recessive cerebellar ataxia. Am J Hum Genet 2010;87:813-819.

21 Vermeer S, van de Warrenburg BP, Willemsen MA, et al. Autosomal recessive cerebellar ataxias: the current state of affairs. J Med Genet 2011;48:651-659.

22 Sailer A, Houlden H. Recent advances in the genetics of cerebellar ataxias. Curr Neurol Neurosci Rep 2012;12:227-236.

23 Anheim M, Tranchant C, Koenig M. The autosomal recessive cerebellar ataxias. N Engl J Med 2012;366:636-646.

24 van Gassen KL, van der Heijden CD, de Bot ST, et al. Genotype-phenotype correlations in spastic paraplegia type 7: a study in a large Dutch cohort. Brain 2012;135:2994-3004.

25 Corbett MA, Schwake M, Bahlo M, et al. A mutation in the Golgi Qb-SNARE gene GOSR2 causes progressive myoclonus epilepsy with early ataxia. Am J Hum Genet 2011;88:657-663.

26 Harding AE. Early onset cerebellar ataxia with retained tendon reflexes: a clinical and genetic study of a disorder distinct from Friedreich's ataxia. J Neurol Neurosurg Psychiatry 1981;44:503-508.

27 Dupre N, Gros-Louis F, Christian N, et al. Clinical and genetic study of autosomal recessive cerebellar ataxia type 1. Ann Neurol 2007;62:93-98.

28 Cagnoli C, Mariotti C, Taroni F, et al. SCA28, a novel form of autosomal dominant cerebellar ataxia on chromosome 18p11.22-q11.2. Brain 2006;129:235-242.

29 Reardon W, Wilson J, Cavanagh N, Baraitser M. A new form of familial ataxia, deafness, and mental retardation. J Med Genet 1993;30:694-695.

30 Le Ber I, Clot F, Vercueil L, et al. Predominant dystonia with marked cerebellar atrophy: a rare phenotype
in familial dystonia. Neurology 2006;67:1769-1773.

31 Hagerman RJ, Leehey M, Heinrichs W, et al. Intention tremor, parkinsonism, and generalized brain
atrophy in male carriers of fragile X. Neurology
2001;57:127-130.

32 Hagerman R, Hagerman P. Advances in clinical and
molecular understanding of the FMR1 premutation
and fragile X-associated tremor/ataxia syndrome.
Lancet Neurol 2013;12:786-798.

33 Hagerman RJ, Leavitt BR, Farzin F, et al. Frag-
ile-X-associated tremor/ataxia syndrome (FXTAS)
in females with the FMR1 premutation. Am J Hum
Genet 2004;74:1051-1056.

34 Apartis E, Blancher A, Meissner WG, et al. FXTAS:
new insights and the need for revised diagnostic
criteria. Neurology 2012;79:1898-1907.

35 Brunberg JA, Jacquemont S, Hagerman RJ, et al.
Fragile X premutation carriers: characteristic MR
imaging findings of adult male patients with progressive cerebellar and cognitive dysfunction. AJNR
Am J Neuroradiol 2002;23):1757-1766.

36 Lagier-Tourenne C, Tazir M, Lopez LC, et al.
ADCK3, an ancestral kinase, is mutated in a form
of recessive ataxia associated with coenzyme Q10
deficiency. Am J Hum Genet 2008;82:661-672.

37 Emmanuele V, Lopez LC, Berardo A, et al. Heterogeneity of coenzyme Q10 deficiency: patient study
and literature review. Arch Neurol 2012;69:978-983.

38 Nikali K, Suomalainen A, Saharinen J, et al. Infantile onset spinocerebellar ataxia is caused by recessive mutations in mitochondrial proteins Twinkle
and Twinky. Hum Mol Genet 2005;14:2981-2990.

39 van de Warrenburg BP, Sinke RJ, Verschuuren-Bemelmans CC, et al. Spinocerebellar ataxias in the
Netherlands: prevalence and age at onset variance
analysis. Neurology 2002;58:702-708.

40 Pareyson D, Gellera C, Castellotti B, et al. Clinical
and molecular studies of 73 Italian families with
autosomal dominant cerebellar ataxia type I: SCA1
and SCA2 are the most common genotypes. J Neurol 1999;246:389-393.

41 Matsuura T, Ranum LP, Volpini V, et al. Spinocerebellar ataxia type 10 is rare in populations other
than Mexicans. Neurology 2002;58:983-984.

42 Lee WY, Jin DK, Oh MR, et al. Frequency analysis and clinical characterization of spinocerebellar
ataxia types 1, 2, 3, 6, and 7 in Korean patients. Arch
Neurol 200360:858-863.

43 Velazquez Perez L, Cruz GS, Santos Falcon N, et al.
Molecular epidemiology of spinocerebellar ataxias
in Cuba: insights into SCA2 founder effect in Hol-
guin. Neurosci Lett 2009;454:157-160.

44 Dürr A. Friedreich's ataxia: treatment within reach.
Lancet Neurol 2002;1:370-374.

45 Swift M, Morrell D, Cromartie E, Chamberlin AR,
Skolnick MH, Bishop DT. The incidence and gene
frequency of ataxia-telangiectasia in the United
States. Am J Hum Genet 1986;39:573-583.

46 Nanetti L, Cavalieri S, Pensato V, et al. SETX mutations are a frequent genetic cause of juvenile and
adult onset cerebellar ataxia with neuropathy and
elevated serum alpha-fetoprotein. Orphanet J Rare
Dis 2013;8:123.

47 Anheim M, Fleury M, Monga B, et al. Epidemiological, clinical, paraclinical and molecular study
of a cohort of 102 patients affected with autosomal
recessive progressive cerebellar ataxia from Alsace,
Eastern France: implications for clinical management. Neurogenetics 2010;11:1-12.

48 Vermeer S, Meijer RP, Pijl BJ, et al. ARSACS in the
Dutch population: a frequent cause of early-onset
cerebellar ataxia. Neurogenetics 2008;9:207-214.

49 Guergueltcheva V, Azmanov DN, Angelicheva D, et
al. Autosomal-recessive congenital cerebellar ataxia
is caused by mutations in metabotropic glutamate
receptor 1. Am J Hum Genet 2012;91:553-564.

50 Brussino A, Gellera C, Saluto A, et al. FMR1 gene
premutation is a frequent genetic cause of late-onset
sporadic cerebellar ataxia. Neurology 2005;64:145-
147.

51 Van Esch H, Dom R, Bex D, et al. Screening
for FMR-1 premutations in 122 older Flemish
males presenting with ataxia. Eur J Hum Genet
2005;13:121-123.

52 Yue Q, Jen JC, Nelson SF, Baloh RW. Progressive
ataxia due to a missense mutation in a calci-

um-channel gene. Am J Hum Genet 1997;61:1078-1087.

53 Baets J, Deconinck T, Smets K, et al. Mutations in SACS cause atypical and late-onset forms of AR-SACS. Neurology 2010;75:1181-1188.

54 Ophoff RA, Terwindt GM, Vergouwe MN, et al. Familial hemiplegic migraine and episodic ataxia type-2 are caused by mutations in the Ca2+ channel gene CACNL1A4. Cell 1996;87:543-552.

55 Lise S, Clarkson Y, Perkins E, et al. Recessive mutations in SPTBN2 implicate beta-III spectrin in both cognitive and motor development. PLoS Genet 2012;8:e1003074.

56 Elsayed SM, Heller R, Thoenes M, et al. Autosomal dominant SCA5 and autosomal recessive infantile SCA are allelic conditions resulting from SPTBN2 mutations. Eur J Hum Genet 2013;doi 10.10.1038/ejhg.

57 Chen YZ, Bennett CL, Huynh HM, et al. DNA/RNA helicase gene mutations in a form of juvenile amyotrophic lateral sclerosis (ALS4). Am J Hum Genet 2004;74:1128-1135.

58 Arning L, Epplen JT, Rahikkala E, Hendrich C, Ludolph AC, Sperfeld AD. The SETX missense variation spectrum as evaluated in patients with ALS4-like motor neuron diseases. Neurogenetics 2013;14:53-61.

59 Laing NG. Genetics of neuromuscular disorders. Crit Rev Clin Lab Sci 2012;49:33-48.

60 Foo JN, Liu J, Tan EK. Next-generation sequencing diagnostics for neurological diseases/disorders: from a clinical perspective. Hum Genet 2013;132:721-734.

61 Sikkema-Raddatz B, Johansson LF, de Boer EN, et al. Targeted next-generation sequencing can replace Sanger sequencing in clinical diagnostics. Hum Mutat 2013;34:1035-1042.

62 Huang L, Chardon JW, Carter MT, et al. Missense mutations in ITPR1 cause autosomal dominant congenital nonprogressive spinocerebellar ataxia. Orphanet J Rare Dis 2012;7:67-1172-7-67.

63 Liew WK, Ben-Omran T, Darras BT, et al. Clinical application of whole-exome sequencing: a novel autosomal recessive spastic ataxia of Charlevoix-Sa-guenay sequence variation in a child with ataxia. JAMA Neurol 2013;70:788-791.

64 Kumar KR, Blair NF, Vandebona H, et al. Targeted next generation sequencing in SPAST-negative hereditary spastic paraplegia. J Neurol 2013;260:2516-2522.

65 Sato N, Amino T, Kobayashi K, et al. Spinocerebellar ataxia type 31 is associated with "inserted" penta-nucleotide repeats containing (TGGAA)n. Am J Hum Genet 2009;85:544-557.

66 Ouyang Y, He Z, Li L, Qin X, Zhao Y, Yuan L. Spinocerebellar ataxia type 31 exists in northeast China. J Neurol Sci 2012;316:164-167.

67 van de Warrenburg BP, Notermans NC, Schelhaas HJ, et al. Peripheral nerve involvement in spinocerebellar ataxias. Arch Neurol 2004;61:257-261.

68 Schulte C, Synofzik M, Gasser T, Schols L. Ataxia with ophthalmoplegia or sensory neuropathy is frequently caused by POLG mutations. Neurology 2009;73:898-900.

69 Anheim M, Monga B, Fleury M, et al. Ataxia with oculomotor apraxia type 2: clinical, biological and genotype/phenotype correlation study of a cohort of 90 patients. Brain 2009;132:2688-2698.

70 van de Warrenburg BP, Notermans NC, Schelhaas HJ, et al. Peripheral nerve involvement in spinocerebellar ataxias. Arch Neurol 2004;61:257-261.

71 Franca MC,Jr, D'Abreu A, Nucci A, Lopes-Cendes I. Muscle excitability abnormalities in Machado-Joseph disease. Arch Neurol 2008;65:525-529.

72 Brkanac Z, Fernandez M, Matsushita M, et al. Autosomal dominant sensory/motor neuropathy with Ataxia (SMNA): Linkage to chromosome 7q22-q32. Am J Med Genet 2002;114:450-457.

73 Ikeda Y, Ohta Y, Kobayashi H, et al. Clinical features of SCA36: a novel spinocerebellar ataxia with motor neuron involvement (Asidan). Neurology 2012;79:333-341.

74 Garcia-Murias M, Quintans B, Arias M, et al. 'Costa da Morte' ataxia is spinocerebellar ataxia 36: clinical and genetic characterization. Brain 2012;135:1423-1435.

75 Geschwind DH, Perlman S, Figueroa CP, Treiman LJ, Pulst SM. The prevalence and wide clinical spectrum of the spinocerebellar ataxia type 2 trinucleotide re-

peat in patients with autosomal dominant cerebellar ataxia. Am J Hum Genet 1997;60:842-850.

76 Ross OA, Rutherford NJ, Baker M, et al. Ataxin-2 repeat-length variation and neurodegeneration. Hum Mol Genet 2011;20:3207-3212.

77 Tazen S, Figueroa K, Kwan JY, et al. Amyotrophic Lateral Sclerosis and Spinocerebellar Ataxia Type 2 in a Family With Full CAG Repeat Expansions of ATXN2. JAMA Neurol 2013;doi 10.1001 2013.443.

78 Verhagen MM, Abdo WF, Willemsen MA, et al. Clinical spectrum of ataxia-telangiectasia in adulthood. Neurology 2009;73:430-437.

79 Stewart GS, Maser RS, Stankovic T, et al. The DNA double-strand break repair gene hMRE11 is mutated in individuals with an ataxia-telangiectasia-like disorder. Cell 1999;99:577-587.

80 Vanier MT. Niemann-Pick disease type C. Orphanet J Rare Dis 2010;5:16-1172-5-16.

81 Klunemann HH, Elleder M, Kaminski WE, et al. Frontal lobe atrophy due to a mutation in the cholesterol binding protein HE1/NPC2. Ann Neurol 2002;52:743-749.

82 Delague V, Bareil C, Bouvagnet P, et al. Nonprogressive autosomal recessive ataxia maps to chromosome 9q34-9qter in a large consanguineous Lebanese family. Ann Neurol 2001;50:250-253.

83 Tranebjaerg L, Teslovich TM, Jones M, et al. Genome-wide homozygosity mapping localizes a gene for autosomal recessive non-progressive infantile ataxia to 20q11-q13. Hum Genet 2003;113:293-295.

84 de Bot ST, Willemsen MA, Vermeer S, Kremer HP, van de Warrenburg BP. Reviewing the genetic causes of spastic-ataxias. Neurology 2012;79:1507-1514.

85 Hanna MG, Davis MB, Sweeney MG, et al. Generalized chorea in two patients harboring the Friedreich's ataxia gene trinucleotide repeat expansion. Mov Disord 1998;13:339-340.

86 Boisse Lomax L, Bayly MA, Hjalgrim H, et al. 'North Sea' progressive myoclonus epilepsy: phenotype of subjects with GOSR2 mutation. Brain 2013;136:1146-1154.

87 Furtado S, Farrer M, Tsuboi Y, et al. SCA-2 presenting as parkinsonism in an Alberta family: clinical, genetic, and PET findings. Neurology 2002;59:1625-1627.

88 Ragothaman M, Sarangmath N, Chaudhary S, et al. Complex phenotypes in an Indian family with homozygous SCA2 mutations. Ann Neurol 2004;55:130-133.

89 Charles P, Camuzat A, Benammar N, et al. Are interrupted SCA2 CAG repeat expansions responsible for parkinsonism? Neurology 2007;69:1970-1975.

90 Knight MA, Gardner RJ, Bahlo M, et al. Dominantly inherited ataxia and dysphonia with dentate calcification: spinocerebellar ataxia type 20. Brain 2004;127:1172-1181.

91 Hugosson T, Granse L, Ponjavic V, Andreasson S. Macular dysfunction and morphology in spinocerebellar ataxia type 7 (SCA 7). Ophthalmic Genet 2009;30:1-6.

92 Yu-Wai-Man P, Griffiths PG, Gorman GS, et al. Multi-system neurological disease is common in patients with OPA1 mutations. Brain 2010 ;133:771 786.

34

Ataxia: Clinical Considerations, Diagnosis and Treatment

Alexander A. Tarnutzer

As discussed in Chapter 33, cerebellar ataxia can be divided into hereditary and non-hereditary (acquired and sporadic) forms. Ataxia of voluntary movements may involve several aspects: a) the movements are initiated more slowly, are broken into isolated subsequent steps, and lack ease and smoothness (dyssynergia), b) rapidly alternating movements are impaired (dysdiadochokinesia), c) amplitudes of movements are abnormal and accompanied by errors in reaching a precise target (dysmetria). Cerebellar ataxia must be distinguished from sensory ataxia resulting from lesions along the peripheral nerve fibers or within the spinal cord (affecting the posterior columns). Ataxic sensory gait is characterized by brisk leg movements, wide base of stance and gait, steps of variable length, and a need for carefully watching the ground (with gait becoming worse if visual cues are removed). Deep tendon reflexes may be reduced or abolished in peripheral neuropathy or increased if combined with other pyramidal tract signs in myelopathy. It is interesting that, in sensory ataxia, speech and eye movements are unaffected.

Table 34.1
Typical signs and symptoms in cerebellar ataxia (modified after (1)).

- Walking difficulties (gait ataxia) unrelated to muscle weakness
- Clumsiness (limb ataxia), leading to e.g. impaired handling of utensils, writing and dressing
- Dizziness and imbalance resulting in sway, falls and fall-related injuries
- Slurred speech (dysarthria)
- Reduced muscle tone (hypotonia) and slowness of movements
- Intentional hand tremor, i.e. oscillations that increase when approaching the target
- Delayed motor development (e.g. onset of walking not before the age of 18 months)
- Visual disturbances (i.e., blurred vision or oscillopsia) due to gaze-evoked nystagmus, downbeat nystagmus, impaired vestibulo-ocular reflex and abnormal saccades (being delayed, slow, and dysmetric)

General clinical aspects of cerebellar ataxia

The typical signs and symptoms in cerebellar ataxia are summarized in Table 34.1. Its key findings on clinical examination are disturbances of

a. stance and gait (wide base, imbalance with irregularity of steps and veering, difficulties with tandem walking, fast turns and stops),
b. limb movements,
c. muscle tone (reduced, referred to as 'hypotonia'),
d. speech (termed 'cerebellar dysarthria', characterized by altered word articulation like slurring or scanning dysarthria and abnormal fluency of speech), and
e. eye movements (including saccadic smooth pursuit, dysmetric saccades, impaired eccentric gaze holding and downbeat nystagmus).

Table 34.2
Classification of cerebellar ataxias (modified after (3,4)).

1 Hereditary cerebellar ataxias

  a Autosomal dominant cerebellar ataxias (ADCA)
  - Spino-cerebellar ataxias (SCA1-36)
  - Episodic ataxias (EA 1-7)
  - Dentatorubral-pallidoluysian atrophy (DRPLA)
  - Autosomal dominant mitochondrial disorders with ataxia (LS, AD-CPEO, AD-OAD)

  b Autosomal recessive cerebellar ataxias (ARCA)
  - Mitochondrial disorders (FRDA, SANDO, MIRAS, Alper's syndrome, CPEO)
  - Metabolic disorders (AVED, ABL, Refsum disease, CTX)
  - DNA-defect repair disorders (AT, AOA1, AOA2, ATLD, NBS, SCAN1)
  - Abnormal protein folding and degradation (ARSACS, MSS)
  - Others (e.g. CANVAS)

  c X-linked cerebellar ataxia
  - Fragile-X tremor ataxia syndrome (FXTAS)
  - Hereditary sideroblastic anaemia and ataxia
  - Other X-linked congenital and childhood ataxias

  d Mitochondrial cerebellar ataxia (CPEO, KSS, MELAS, MERFF, NARP)

2 Sporadic cerebellar ataxias

  a Acquired cerebellar ataxias
  - Autoimmune disorders
    - Demyelinating disorders (e.g. MS)
    - Gluten ataxia and anti-GAD ataxia
    - Paraneoplastic cerebellar degeneration
    - SREAT
  - Endocrine disorders (hypothyroidism)
  - Infectious disorders
    - Acute (viral) cerebellitis and post-viral cerebellar ataxia
    - HIV-related progressive ataxia (due to opportunistic infections or CNS lymphoma, rarely due to diffuse cerebellar damage)
    - Neurosyphillis, Lyme borreliosis
    - Sporadic Creutzfeldt-Jakob disease
    - Whipple's disease
  - Malabsorption
    - Wernicke encephalopathy (lack of vitamin B1)
    - Acquired vitamin B12 deficiency or vitamin E deficiency
  - Superficial siderosis
  - Structural lesions and malformations (Arnold-Chiari malformation, cerebellar neoplasms, NPH)
  - Toxic agents
    - Alcoholic cerebellar degeneration
    - Drugs (lithium, phenytoin, amiodarone, toluene, 5-fluorouracil, cytosine arabinoside)
    - Heavy metals and solvents

  b Idiopathic
  - Multiple system atrophy cerebellar type (MSA-C)
  - Sporadic adult-onset ataxia (SAOA)

Abbreviations Table 34.2-34.7:

ABL = abetalipoproteinaemia; ADCA = autosomal dominant cerebellar ataxia; ADOAD = autosomal-dominant optic atrophy and deafness; AOA = ataxia with ocular motor apraxia; AOA1 = ataxia with ocular motor apraxia type 1; AOA2 = ataxia with ocular motor apraxia type 2; ARCA= autosomal recessive cerebellar ataxia; ARSACS = autosomal-recessive, spastic ataxia of Charlevoix-Saguenay; AT = ataxia telangiectasia; ATLD = ataxia telangiectasia-like disorder; AVED = ataxia with vitamin E deficiency; CANVAS = cerebellar ataxia, neuropathy, vestibular areflexia syndrome; CPEO = chronic progressive external ophthalmoplegia; CTX = cerebrotendinous xanthomatosis; DRPLA = dentatorubro-pallidoluysian atrophy; EA = episodic ataxia; FRDA = Friedreich's ataxia; FXTAS = fragile X-tremor ataxia syndrome; GAD = glutamic acid decarboxylase; GRE = gradient-echo sequence; HIV= human immunodeficiency virus; IOSCA = infantile-onset spinocerebellar ataxia; KSS = Kearns Sayre syndrome; LS = Leigh syndrome; MELAS = myopathy, encephalopathy, lactate acidosis and stroke-like episodes; MERFF = myoclonic epilepsy and ragged red fibers, MIRAS = mitochondrial autosomal-recessive ataxia syndrome; MS = multiple sclerosis; MSA-C = multiple system atrophy of cerebellar type; MSS = Marinesco-Sjögren syndrome; NARP = neuropathy, ataxia and retinitis pigmentosa; NBS = Nijmegen breakage syndrome NPC = Niemann-Pick type C disease; NPH = normal pressure hydrocephalus; SANDO = sensory axonal neuropathy with dysarthria and ophthalmoplegia; SAOA= sporadic adult-onset ataxia; SCA = spinocerebellar ataxia; sCJD = sporadic Creutzfeldt-Jakob disease; SREAT = steroid-responsive encephalopathy associated with autoimmune thyroiditis; TPo = thyroid peroxidase; vLOFA = very late-onset Friedreich ataxia; WE = Wernicke encephalopathy.

Characteristically, ataxia becomes more evident in tasks that require rapid changes in muscle force and almost completely disappears if these force changes are applied slowly. Slowing of saccades and gaze palsies, on the other hand, indicate brainstem involvement.

The primary distinction to make is the differentiation between hereditary and non-hereditary ataxia, with the latter further separated into acquired and sporadic ataxia (see Table 34.2) (see also Chapter 33). The classification and correct diagnosis in patients with adult-onset progressive ataxia without an obvious familial background remain a challenge, as pointed out by Klockgether (2). In these cases, the whole spectrum of hereditary and non-hereditary causes of cerebellar degeneration must be considered. This includes acquired ataxias such as alcoholic cerebellar degeneration (ACD), immune-mediated inflammatory disorders, malnutrition, chronic central nervous system (CNS) infections and various toxic agents, and idiopathic ataxias like multiple system atrophy of cerebellar type (MSA-C) and sporadic adult-onset ataxia (SAOA) of unknown aetiology. It is interesting that MRI and genetic testing have greatly facilitated the early recognition and correct classification of cerebellar ataxia within the last decades.

Diagnostic considerations regarding disease onset and progression

Acute onset of ataxia is an emergency and demands an immediate diagnostic work-up, followed by appropriate treatment of the underlying cause. The most important differential diagnoses of acute-onset ataxia are cerebellar stroke or hemorrhage, cerebellar abscess, drug intoxication, Wernicke encephalopathy (due to vitamin B1 deficiency) and basilar meningitis (due to tuberculosis or listeriosis) (see Table 34.3). Symptom onset over a few days might suggest Miller-Fisher syndrome or para-infectious cerebellitis (especially in children) due to varicella (in children) or Epstein-Barr virus (in adults). Neurodegenerative disorders should be included in the differential diagnosis if the course of cerebellar ataxia is progressive and unremitting. First, however, acquired subacute causes need to be ruled out – in case of rapid deterioration and severe ataxia within weeks to a few months – such as the ataxic variant of sporadic Creutzfeldt-Jakob disease, paraneoplastic

Table 34.3
Onset of ataxia and its diagnostic value.

Acute
- Cerebellitis (mostly viral, e.g. varicella-zoster virus infection or Epstein-Barr virus)
- Cerebellar stroke (ischaemic or haemorrhagic)
- Cerebellar abscess
- Relapse in multiple sclerosis
- Basilar meningitis (due to tuberculosis or listeriosis)
- Toxic agents (mercury, toluene, pesticides and others)
- Drugs (carbamazepine, phenytoin, phenobarbital, metronidazole, amiodarone, chemotherapeutics including 5-FU and cytosine arabinoside)
- Alcohol intoxication
- Vitamin B1 deficiency (Wernicke encephalopathy)

Subacute
- Alcoholic cerebellar degeneration
- Paraneoplastic cerebellar disease
- Wernicke encephalopathy
- Steroid-responsive encephalopathy associated with autoimmune thyroiditis
- Structural (Arnold-Chiari malformation, cerebellar neoplasm, normal pressure hydrocephalus)
- HIV-associated ataxia
- Sporadic Creutzfeldt-Jakob disease

Chronic
- Autoimmune (gluten ataxia, anti-GAD ataxia)
- Neurodegenerative (MSA-C, SAOA)
- Hereditary (ADCAs, ARCAs, X-linked, mitochondrial)
- Inflammatory / infectious (tabetic neurosyphilis, Lyme borreliosis, Whipple's disease)
- Metabolic
- Paraneoplastic

Abbreviations: see legend of Table 34.2.

cerebellar disease, cerebellar tumor, steroid-responsive encephalopathy associated with autoimmune thyroiditis (SREAT), HIV-associated ataxia, Whipple's disease and chronic causes (celiac disease, cerebellar ataxia associated with au-

toantibodies related to glutamic acid decarboxylase, CNS infections, ACD, toxic agents).

Diagnostic approach to cerebellar ataxia

In the clinical work-up of patients presenting with signs of cerebellar ataxia, thorough history-taking and a comprehensive clinical neurological examination are important. The family history may provide clues to an underlying hereditary disorder and the manner of inheritance: affected family members in successive generations suggest an autosomal dominant course, while affected siblings with their parents being unaffected favors an autosomal recessive form. Maternal transfection is seen with mitochondrial disorders, and restriction to males may suggest an X-linked form of inheritance.

Frequently, cerebellar dysfunction is accompanied by non-cerebellar signs and symptoms. In the clinical examination, therefore, the clinician must search for signs of non-cerebellar involvement. They can be localized to the pyramidal tracts, the extrapyramidal system, the brainstem, the cerebral cortex (cognition), the autonomic system (especially orthostatic dysregulation, urinary incontinence and erectile dysfunction) and the spinal cord (see Table 34.4 for clinical signs helping in the differential diagnosis). In patients with ataxia due to mitochondrial disorders, both neurological and systemic disorders can often be found. Examples of accompanying neurological symptoms are seizures, muscle weakness and fatigue, while increased rates of diabetes mellitus, early cataract surgery and cardiomyopathy may underline the wide range of non-neurological symptoms.

To evaluate the clinical course of the disease, rating scales for cerebellar ataxia including the scale for the assessment and rating of ataxia (SARA) (5) or the more extensive international ataxia cooperative rating scale (ICARS) (6) have been developed.

Imaging of the brain (and preferentially also of the spinal cord) by use of MRI should be performed in every patient presenting with cerebellar ataxia (see Table 34.5 for MRI and CT findings that may help in the differential diagnosis). When a paraneoplastic disorder is considered in the differential diagnosis, the search for the primary tumor must be performed thoroughly, ideally including whole-body [18]fluoro-deoxyglucose positron emission tomography (FDG-PET) in combination with CT or MRI. The extent and distribution of cerebellar atrophy vary widely between different disorders presenting with cerebellar dysfunction including ataxia. Atrophy may be absent (as in fragile-X tremor ataxia syndrome (FXTAS) or Friedreich's ataxia), mild or severe, and may affect only midline (vermian) cerebellar structures or the hemispheres or the whole cerebellum.

A laboratory work-up with selected biomarkers based on the clinical presentation (see Table 34.6) is usually performed. In addition, lumbar puncture may be necessary to exclude an underlying inflammatory cause.

Nerve conduction studies and electromyography, visual evoked potentials, and cardiac investigations may be advised. While severe sensory neuropathy is observed in Friedreich's ataxia (FRDA), ataxia with vitamin E deficiency (AVED) and abetalipoproteinaemia (ABL), sensory neuropathy mostly restricted to the legs may be found in spinocerebellar ataxia (SCA) 1, 2, or 3. Myopathy may point to mitochondrial disorders and fasciculations, or myoclonus could be linked to SCA1, 2, or 3. If a heredoataxia is suspected based on clinical grounds, genetic testing should be ordered. Testing is available for various autosomal dominant cerebellar ataxias (ADCAs) (including SCA1, 2, 3, 6, 7, 17, dentatorubro-pallidoluysian atrophy, episodic ataxia type 2), autosomal recessive cerebellar ataxias (ARCAs) (FRDA, AVED, ABL, cerebrotendinous xanthomatosis, Refsum disease), X-linked disorders (FXTAS) and mitochondrial disorders.

Clinical description of specific disorders

Ataxias may be hereditary or non-hereditary, with the latter further classified into either acquired or sporadic (including symptomatic and idiopathic ones). A description of the most frequent hereditary ataxia syndromes is followed by an introduction to the most relevant causes of acquired ataxia.

Heredoataxias

Hereditary ataxias can be classified based on their pattern of inheritance: autosomal dominant, autosomal recessive, X-linked and mitochondrial. Another way to distinguish them is based on the underlying pathology. De Michele and colleagues proposed six different categories (7): 1) mitochondrial, 2) metabolic, 3) defective DNA repair, 4) abnormal protein folding and degradation, 5) channelopathies, 6) others.

Overall, heredoataxias are rare causes of cerebellar ataxia, with prevalences of about 1.6-5.5 per 100,000 people for autosomal dominant cerebellar ataxias (ADCAs) (8,9) and about 2.2-7/100,000 for autosomal recessive cerebellar ataxias (ARCAs) (10). It is interesting that most cases of cerebellar ataxia are sporadic. Taking an accurate family history is a key element in these disorders. However, a negative family history does not rule out hereditary ataxia. Possible explanations for seemingly sporadic disease can be *de novo* mutations, anticipation and incomplete penetrance. Therefore, a hereditary ataxia should always be excluded in patients younger than 50 years. In a first step, screening for ARCAs may be most promising, combined with testing for X-linked ataxia in male adults. Then screening for ADCAs (SCAs) is also advised, although the yield of screening is relatively low (2-19%) (11-13). Identification of a hereditary ataxia syndrome may be important for both genetic counseling and preventive screening (such as for diabetes or cardiomyopathy in FRDA). When all

Table 34.4
Clinical findings helpful in the differential diagnosis of cerebellar ataxia syndromes.

Associated neurological signs	Disorders
Chorea	• Acquired (Wilson's disease, gluten ataxia) • ARCA (late-onset Tay-Sachs, MIRAS, AT, AVED, ATLD, AOA1, AOA2, IOSCA) • ADCA (DRPLA, occasionally SCA1, SCA2, SCA14 and SCA17)
Cognitive impairments (mental retardation or cognitive decline)	• Acquired (HIV, NPH, WE, sCJD, SREAT) • ARCA (late-onset Tay-Sachs, CTX, MIRAS, AOA1, (AOA2), ARCA1, ARCA2, ARSACS, MSS, NPC, SANDO, IOSCA) • ADCA (SCA2, SCA3, SCA10, SCA12, SCA13, SCA15/16, SCA17, SCA19, SCA21, SCA27, DRPLA, occasionally SCA1, SCA14, SCA28) • X-linked (FXTAS)
Dystonia	• ARCA (late-onset Tay-Sachs, CTX, AVED, AT, AOA1, AOA2) • ADCA (SCA3, occasionally SCA14 and SCA17)
Fasciculations	• ADCA (SCA1-3)
Generalized areflexia	• ADCA (SCA2, SCA4, SCA3 with older adult-onset)
Hearing loss	• ARCA (FRDA, Refsum disease, mitochondrial disorders, IOSCA) • Acquired (superficial siderosis)
Hypotonia	• ARCA (late-onset Tay-Sachs, AOA1, IOSCA, MSS, Cayman ataxia)
Myoclonus	• Acquired (sCJD, SREAT, gluten ataxia) • ARCA (late-onset Tay-Sachs, CTX, MIRAS, AT, AOA2) • ADCA (SCA2, SCA14, DRPLA, occasionally SCA1, SCA3, SCA15/16, SCA19)
Myopathy	• MSS, various mitochondrial disorders
Ocular motor impairment	• Various, see Table 34.7
Oculocephalic dissociation	• ARCA (AOA1, AOA2, AT, ATLD)
Optic nerve atrophy	• ARCA (FRDA, AOA1, IOSCA)
Orthostatic hypotension	• Sporadic (MSA-C)
Parkinsonism	• Acquired (Wilson's disease, sCJD) • ARCA (CTX) • ADCA (SCA1, SCA2, SCA3, SCA12, sometimes SCA6, SCA14, SCA17 and SCA21) • Sporadic (MSA-C) • X-linked (FXTAS)
Peripheral neuropathy	• Acquired (WE, gluten ataxia, vitamin B12 deficiency, vitamin E deficiency) • ARCA: (FRDA, AVED, SANDO, AT, AOA1, AOA2, ARSACS, vLOFA) • ADCA: (SCA1, SCA2, SCA3, SCA4, SCA6, SCA8, SCA12, SCA18, SCA22, variable in SCA25, sometimes in SCA11 and SCA27) • Mitochondrial (NARP) • Sporadic (SAOA)

Psychiatric findings	▪ Acquired (WE) ▪ ARCA (late-onset Tay-Sachs, CTX, MIRAS) ▪ ADCA (SCA17, DRPLA) ▪ X-linked (FXTAS)
Pyramidal tract signs	▪ Acquired (superficial siderosis, sCJD) ▪ Sporadic (MSA-C, SAOA) ▪ ARCA (CTX, FRDA, ARSACS, AVED) ▪ ADCA (SCA1, SCA2, SCA3, SCA4, SCA12, sometimes SCA7, SCA8, SCA10, SCA11, SCA13, SCA15, and SCA23)
Pure sensory neuropathy	▪ ARCA (FRDA, AVED, ABL, SANDO) ▪ ADCAs (SCA24)
Seizures	▪ Acquired (WE) ▪ ARCA (late-onset Tay-Sachs, CTX, MIRAS, ARCA2, IOSCA) ▪ ADCA (SCA 7, 10 and 13, EAs (1,2,6), DRPLA, occasionally SCA14 and SCA17)
Spasticity	▪ ARCA (late-onset FA, CTX, ARSACS) ▪ ADCA (SCA3, SCA17, occasionally SCA6)
Tremor	▪ Acquired (SREAT) ▪ ARCA (AVED, late-onset Tay-Sachs, MIRAS, AT, AOA1, AOA2, Cayman ataxia, MSS) ▪ ADCA (SCA2, SCA8, SCA12, SCA16, SCA19, SCA20, SCA27) ▪ X-linked (FXTAS)
Associated non-neurological signs	
Cardiomyopathy	▪ ARCA (FRDA, AVED, ABL, Refsum disease) ▪ Mitochondrial (KSS)
Cataract	▪ ARCA (MSS, CTX) ▪ Mitochondrial (KSS)
Diarrhoea and abdominal pain	▪ Acquired (Whipple's disease)
Immunodeficiency	▪ ARCA (AT, ATLD)
Kayser-Fleischer ring	▪ ARCA (Wilson's disease)
Oculocutaneous telangiectasias	▪ ARCA (AT)
Organomegaly	▪ ARCA (NPC, Gaucher disease)
Pes cavus	▪ ARCA (FRDA, AVED, ABL, Refsum disease, CTX, MIRAS, SCAN1, AOA1, AOA2, ARSACS, IOSCA)
Pigmentary retinopathy	▪ ARCA (AVED, ABL) ▪ ADCA (SCA7)
Radiosensitivity	▪ ARCA (AT, ATLD)
Retinitis pigmentosa	▪ ARCA (AVED, ABL, Refsum disease) ▪ Mitochondrial (KSS, NARP)
Scoliosis / skeletal deformities	▪ ARCA (FRDA, AOA1, AOA2, MSS, Refsum disease, MSS)

Abbreviations: see legend of Table 34.2.

Table 34.5
Characteristic imaging findings in cerebellar ataxia.

CT	
Dentate calcification on CT	SCA20
MRI (sagittal sections preferred)	
Cerebral white-matter lesions	Metachromatic leukodystrophy, X-linked adrenoleukodystrophy, Krabbe disease, CTX, MS
Cervical spinal cord atrophy	FRDA, AVED,
DWI abnormalities cortically and in thalamus	sCJD
Hemosiderin deposits (black rim on GRE)	WE
'Hot-cross-bun' sign and putaminal rim sign	MSA-C
No obvious cerebellar atrophy	ARCA (FRDA, AVED, Refsum's disease, abetalipo-proteinemia)
Olivopontocerebellar atrophy	MSA-C
Prominent midline (vermian) cerebellar degeneration	ACD, AOA1/2, AT, SCAN, Cayman ataxia
T2-hyperintensities of the middle cerebellar peduncles	FXTAS Superficial siderosis
Tonsillar herniation	Arnold Chiari malformation type 1

Abbreviations: see legend of Table 34.2.

tests are negative, the term 'idiopathic late-onset cerebellar ataxia' (ILOCA) has been proposed. This includes symptomatic and sporadic adult-onset ataxia, as outlined further below.

Non-specific treatment approaches in patients with cerebellar ataxia include physical therapy (14) and occupational therapy for gait dysfunction, speech rehabilitation for dysarthria, psychological support and, if necessary, orthopedic surgery for foot deformities and scoliosis. Drug treatment in cerebellar ataxia is often based on expert opinion and case reports, as placebo-controlled, randomized and double-blind studies are frequently lacking.

Autosomal dominant cerebellar ataxias (ADCAs)

SCAs, EAs and DRPLA

Affected family members in consecutive generations or male-to-male inheritance is suggestive of an autosomal dominant inheritance. The au-

tosomal dominant hereditary ataxia syndromes include the large (and still growing) group of spinocerebellar ataxias (SCAs), episodic ataxias (EAs) and the dentatorubro-pallidoluysian atrophy (DRPLA). Other rare autosomal dominant disorders, which can present with ataxia as a prominent feature, include neuroferritinopathy, hereditary spastic ataxia, sensory motor neuropathy with ataxia, Alexander disease and adult-onset leukodystrophy.

SCAs are inherited neurodegenerative disorders that become symptomatic around the age of 35 years on average, albeit the age at onset may vary considerably (from early childhood in SCA2 and SCA7 to more than 60 years in SCA6). However, almost half of all ADCA cases cannot be assigned to a specific SCA type by the genetic testing currently available (15), as for example in the patient illustrated in Figure 34.1.

In the pre-genetic area, a classification of ADCAs was made based on the phenotype (16). While ADCA1 includes disorders with both cerebellar

Table 34.6
Biomarkers in cerebellar ataxia.

Biomarker	Abnormality	Disease
14-3-3 protein from CSF	Present	sCJD
Acanthocytes	Present	ABL
Albumin	Reduced	AOA1, SCAN1
Alpha-fetoprotein	Elevated	AT, AOA2
Anti-GAD antibodies	Present	Anti-GAD associated ataxia
Anti-gliadin antibodies	Present	Gliadin-associated ataxia
Anti-Gq1b antibodies	Present	Miller-Fisher syndrome
Co-enzyme Q10	Reduced	Mitochondrial disorders
Creatinine kinase	Elevated	Mitochondrial disease, AOA1, MSS
Cholestanol	Elevated	CTX
Cholesterol	Elevated	AOA1, AOA2, SCAN1
Copper / ceruloplasmin	Elevated	Wilson's disease
Hexosaminidase A	Reduced	Late-onset Tay-Sachs
Immunoglobulins	Reduced	AT, ATLD
Lactate	Elevated	Mitochondrial disease
Phytanic acid	Elevated	Refsum's disease
Paraneoplastic antibodies	Present	See separate Table 6
Radiosensitivity	Present	AT, ATLD
Thyroid antibodies (TPO, thyroglobulin-antibodies)	Present	SREAT
Very long chain fatty acids	Elevated	Peroxin-associated ataxias, Refsum disease
Vitamin E	Reduced	AVED, ABL

Abbreviations: see legend of Table 34.2.

and non-cerebellar symptoms (SCA1-4, 8, 10, 12-23, 25, 27-28, 32-36, DRPLA) (17), ADCA2 requires concomitant pigmentary maculopathy (SCA7), and ADCA3 is considered a purely cerebellar ataxia syndrome (SCA5, 6, 11, 26, 29-31) with occasional non-cerebellar symptoms such as pyramidal tract signs, ophthalmoplegia and tremor (18). The ADCA3 patients tend to have a better prognosis with slower progression and less impairment of quality of life than ADCA1. This clinical classification, however, is gradually being replaced by a genetic classification.

Spinocerebellar ataxias (SCAs)

Based on the genetic defect, SCAs can be divided into three groups: 1) polyglutamine expansion disorders in coding regions (SCA1, 2, 3, 6, 7, 17, DRPLA), 2) polyglutamine expansion disorders in non-coding regions (SCA 8, 10, 12, 31, 36) and 3) conventional mutations (5, 11, 13, 14, 15/16, 20, 23, 27, 28, 35). Currently, there are 30 separate SCA loci, with the associated genetic mutation identified in 21 (19). Overall, polyglutamine expansion disorders are more frequently observed than conventional mutations in SCAs.

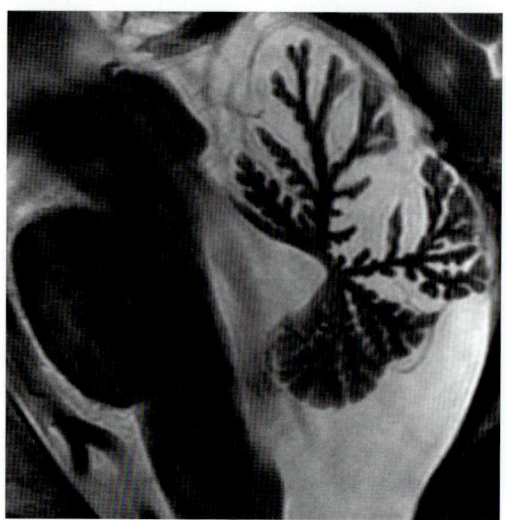

Figure 34.1
Sagittal MRI of the cerebellar vermis in a 41-year-old patient with progressive ataxia of stance and gait, moderate limb ataxia, dysarthria, ocular motor complaints (gaze-evoked nystagmus, rebound nystagmus and downbeat nystagmus, saccadic smooth pursuit and dysmetric saccades) since the age of 31 years. It demonstrates severe atrophy of the cerebellar lobules I-VII, while the inferior vermis (lobules VIII-X) and the brainstem are spared. Based on the positive family history (cerebellar ataxia syndrome in the patient's brother and mother), a hereditary, most likely autosomal dominant, cerebellar ataxia must be suspected. However, genetic testing for SCA 1, 2, 3, 6, 7, 10, 12, 17, DRPLA was negative (courtesy Dept Neuroradiology, University Hospital Zurich, Switzerland).

Based on the pathogenetic classification proposed by de Michele and colleagues (7), SCAs with polyglutamine expansion belong to group 4 (abnormal protein folding and degradation), while those with point mutations and other SCAs with identified loci belong to group 6.

With these repeat-expansion disorders, the concept of anticipation must be taken into account (i.e. unstable DNA in polynucleotide expansion disorders with the ability to expand the number of repeats from one generation to the next). An inverse relationship between the number of repeats and the onset and severity of disease has been described for many polyglutamine expansion disorders. The largest shifts in disease

onset from generation to generation have been observed for SCA2 and SCA7. This may result in the situation that the disorder becomes symptomatic in the child before the first signs can be found in the parents, suggesting a sporadic rather than an inherited disease. It is interesting that repeat instability is more pronounced in paternal inheritance. Overall, repeats become unstable only above a certain number of repeats (in the range of 37-40, but varying from gene to gene).

The best available evidence suggests a prevalence of SCAs of around 2-4/100,000 persons (20). Amongst the spinocerebellar ataxias, the relative prevalence of various SCA subtypes differs considerably due to founder effects. Worldwide, SCA3 is most frequently observed, followed by SCA1, SCA2, SCA6 and SCA7. These five subtypes account for about 50-65% of all ADCA cases (3,20). Founder effects have been described for SCA2 (Cuba) and SCA 3 (Portugal). On the other hand, for example, SCA3 is rare in India (15).

Gait disorders are the initial presenting symptom in two-thirds of all SCA patients (21), while other symptoms (diplopia, dysarthria, episodic vertigo and impaired handwriting) precede ataxia in 4% each. Long spinal tract involvement is frequently found in SCAs with signs of diminished vibration sense of the legs and hyperreflexia. Extrapyramidal signs, spasticity, cognitive impairment, PNP, ophthalmoplegia and seizures are also observed. The cognitive impairments often reported in SCAs might be explained by studies suggesting that the cerebellum also contributes to cognition and executive functions. Ataxia is usually of the cerebellar type, but sensory ataxia may strongly contribute (SCA3) or even predominate (SCA4).

While SCAs share many clinical signs and symptoms, some are specific to certain subtypes and therefore help to decide which genetic test should be done first. For example, pigmentary retinopathy is almost always associated with SCA7. Pure cerebellar syndromes and late-onset occurrence are linked to SCA6, 10-12. Anticipation is most profound in SCA2, 7 and 17, resulting in severe phenotypes in early childhood, while a childhood onset accompanied by tremor is characteristic of SCA27. The phenotype of ADCA may depend on the number of repeats (15), as observed in DRPLA (with longer repeats being associated with progressive myoclonus, epilepsy and dementia, while shorter repeats preferentially present with chorea and psychiatric symptoms) (22) and SCA3 (with pyramidal tract signs becoming more frequent with larger repeat numbers and altered vibration sense decreasing in frequency at the same time). Seizures are most frequently observed in SCA10, 17, and DRPLA; peripheral neuropathy in SCA1-4, 8, 18, 25; cognitive impairment and behavioural disturbances in SCA17 and DRPLA. Disease progression is slowest in SCA6 (when compared with SCA1, 2, and 3).

Abnormal eye movements (see Table 34.7) may help with the differential diagnosis of ataxia syndromes including SCAs (23): while saccadic hypermetria and choppy smooth pursuit are frequent in SCA1, very slow saccades are associated with SCA2, and hypometric saccades and gaze-evoked nystagmus (GEN) are often present in SCA3. Downbeat nystagmus (DBN) is often noted in SCA6, along with GEN, saccadic smooth pursuit and hypometric saccades of normal velocity.

MRI shows progressive cerebellar atrophy in all SCA syndromes over the course of the disease, sometimes combined with spinal cord atrophy and brainstem atrophy (pontine atrophy may predominate, as e.g. in SCA 1, 2, and 7). It is interesting that in polyglutamine expansion SCAs, cerebellar atrophy is often restricted to the vermis, and brainstem involvement is regularly found.

Noteworthy, the phenotype in SCAs varies depending on the underlying pathology: patients with conventional mutations often have disease onset in childhood (possibly with mental retardation but without cognitive deterioration), but the disease is not as severe as expected in a child or adolescent with polyglutamine expansion SCA, and there is no anticipation. The disease often presents as the pure cerebellar phenotype, progresses little if at all, and the lifespan is normal in patients with conventional mutation SCAs compared to the shortened lifespan with multisystem and substantial neurological dysfunction in polyglutamine expansion SCAs. This is also reflected on neuroimaging with pure and global cerebellar atrophy in conventional mutation SCAs vs. more diffuse (brainstem > cerebellum) atrophy in polyglutamine expansion SCAs (15). Amongst the polyglutamine expansion SCAs, SCA6 resembles the phenotype of conventional mutation SCAs as it lacks early death and brainstem atrophy and is less often associated with non-cerebellar features.

In the following, the most common SCAs will be described in more detail, while more extensive reviews of all SCAs can be found elsewhere (17,18,25).

SCA1

SCA1 is related to a CAG-repeat expansion in the ataxin-1 gene, and its onset is often late (21). Besides a cerebellar syndrome (gait ataxia, blurred vision or double vision, dysarthria), ophthalmoplegia, pyramidal and extrapyramidal signs as well as polyneuropathy may be found.

SCA2

Gait ataxia, dysarthria, double vision and Parkinsonism are often found in SCA2, which is the result of a CAG-repeat expansion in the ataxin-2 gene. Very slow saccades are a hallmark feature; other signs include hyporeflexia, postural or action tremor, and retinopathy. In SCA2, atrophy of the pons, the inferior olivary nucleus, the substantia nigra and the cerebellum is a key imaging feature. In some patients, Parkinsonism or an MSA-like pattern may dominate. Levodopa or dopamine agonists may be prescribed to alleviate extrapyramidal signs and symptoms.

Table 34.7
Ocular motor abnormalities in hereditary cerebellar ataxia (modified after 37).

Abnormality	ARCAs affected	ADCAs affected
Downbeat nystagmus	▪ none	▪ EA2 ▪ SCAs (SCA6 (65-100%), occasionally SCA5)
Fixation instability (SWJ, saccadic intrusions)	▪ FRDA ▪ AT (36%) ▪ AOA1 (100%)	▪ SCAs (SCA3 (SWJ in 43%), SCA6 (SWJ in 0-60%), SCA20, SCA24 (saccadic intrusions) ▪ DRPLA ▪ EA2
GEN	▪ FRDA (33%) ▪ AT (50%) ▪ AOA1 (100%) ▪ AOA2 (89%) ▪ ARSACS	▪ EA2 ▪ SCA1 (20-50%), SCA2 (38-40%), SCA3 (63-100%), SCA5, SCA6 (86-95%), SCA13, SCA19, occasionally in SCA11, SCA14 (20%), SCA15/16,SCA25, SCA28, SCA30 and SCA31 ▪ DRPLA
Hypermetric saccades	▪ FRDA	▪ SCAs (SCA1 (60-80%), SCA2 (26-40%), SCA3 (40-86%), SCA4 (57% vertical), SCA5, SCA6 (37-48%), SCA8, SCA20, SCA30) ▪ EA2
Hypometric saccades	▪ AT ▪ AOA1 ▪ AOA2	▪ SCAs ((SCA1), SCA2 (42%), SCA3 (30%), SCA5, SCA6 (26%), (SCA7, 14%), SCA8)
Impaired OKN	▪ FRDA ▪ AT ▪ AOA1	▪ SCAs (SCA1 (70-80%), SCA2 (86%), SCA3 (59%), SCA6 (69%)) ▪ EA2
Impaired VOR	▪ FRDA (31%) ▪ CANVAS	▪ SCAs (SCA1 (variable), SCA2 (71%), SCA3)
Impaired VOR-cancellation	▪ AT ▪ AOA1 ▪ AOA2	▪ SCAs (SCA1 ('often impaired'), SCA6 (50-100%), SCA7 (100%), SCA20) ▪ EA2
Increased saccadic latency	▪ AT ▪ AOA2 (~50%)	▪ SCA1
Ocular motor apraxia	▪ AT ▪ ATLD ▪ AOA1 ▪ AOA2	▪ none
Ophthalmo-paresis	▪ MIRAS ▪ AOA1 ▪ IOSCA	▪ SCAs (SCA2 (37-79%), SCA1 (30-69%), SCA3 (56-60%), SCA7 (71%), occasionally SCA5 and SCA6)
Rebound nystagmus	▪ FRDA (13%) ▪ AT	▪ SCAs (SCA1 (33%), SCA6 (60%)) ▪ EA2

Impaired (saccadic) smooth pursuit	• FRDA AVED • AT • AOA1 • AOA2 • late-onset Tay Sachs • MIRAS • ARSACS	• SCAs (SCA1 (50-80%), SCA2 (50-79%), SCA3 (94-100%), SCA4 (57%), SCA5, SCA6 (69-100%), SCA7 (100%), SCA8, SCA10, SCA11, SCA14 (80%), SCA17, SCA19, SCA20, SCA26, SCA27) • DRPLA • EA2
Slow saccades	• None	• SCAs (SCA1 (50-60%), SCA2 (80-100%), SCA3 (10-30%), SCA7 (79-86%), SCA14 (46%), SCA17, SCA23, SCA28) • DRPLA

Abbreviations: see legend of Table 34.2; SWJ = square-wave jerks; GEN = gaze-evoked nystagmus; OKN = optokinetic nystagmus; VoR = vestibulo-ocular reflex.

SCA3 (Machado-Joseph disease)

SCA3 is the most prevalent SCA worldwide and becomes manifest usually after 40 years of age. Key findings are gait disturbances, double vision, dysarthria, hypometric saccades, impaired vestibular function, frequent falls, Parkinsonism and axonal neuropathy. Fasciculations may be present in up to 25% of the patients, while muscle cramps are reported in almost every second patient. SCA3 is due to a CAG-repeat expansion in the ataxin-3 gene. In SCA3, lesions of the basal ganglia and the posterior spinal columns are severe. As in SCA2, levodopa or dopamine agonists may be prescribed to reduce extrapyramidal signs and symptoms. Muscle cramps (most disabling in SCA3) may be treated with magnesium or mexiteline.

SCA6

Slow progression and pure cerebellar ataxia combined with ocular motor disturbances (GEN, DBN, rebound nystagmus, saccadic smooth pursuit, slow and dysmetric saccades, impaired vestibulo-ocular reflex) and cognitive dysfunction are characteristic of SCA6, which is caused by a CAG-repeat expansion in the alpha-1A, voltage-dependent, calcium-channel subunit gene (CACNA1A). It is assumed that increased polyglutamine repeats in CACNA1A reduce Ca^{2+} influx, leading to cell death. SCA6 may make up 13% of all ADCA cases, being the second most common ADCA after SCA3. The age of disease onset varies greatly, ranging from 16 to 72 years, with approximately 60% of patients developing the disease after age of 50 years. Anticipation in SCA6 is lacking, disease penetrance is almost 100%. Most patients complain of ataxia as the first symptom, but in some, episodic vertigo, diplopia and dysarthria are noted prior to gait abnormalities (21). Occasionally, extrapyramidal symptoms are observed in SCA6, including pyramidal tract signs, polyneuropathy, Parkinsonism, cognitive impairment, tremor, depression and fatigue. MRI of the brain reveals severe cerebellar atrophy accompanied by mild atrophy of the middle cerebellar peduncle, the pons and the red nucleus (26). Drug treatment options include acetazolamide (250-500mg/d) (27), gabapentin (1200mg/d), 4-aminopyridine and 3,4-diaminopyridine (28). Intensive coordination training significantly improved the motor performance in patients with cerebellar degeneration of various causes, including SCA6 (14).

SCA7

A combination of severe cerebellar ataxia, achromatopsia with cone-rod retinal dystrophy and macular degeneration is characteristic of SCA7. Other symptoms include spastic paraparesis, cranio-cervical dystonia, dysarthria, pyramidal signs, parkinsonism, sensory deficits and cognitive impairment. SCA7 is due to a CAG-repeat expansion in the ataxin-7 gene.

Episodic ataxias

Episodic ataxias (EAs) are a group of rare auto-somal dominant diseases characterized by recurrent episodes of ataxia and vertigo (29). EA usually starts during childhood or early adulthood, although the first symptoms may occur as late as the fifth decade of life in EA2. EA1, EA2 and EA5 share a common pathomechanism: they are channelopathies associated with mutations in genes encoding either voltage-gated potassium (EA1) or calcium-channel (EA2, EA5) subunits (29). In EA6, mutations in a sodium-dependent transporter molecule regulating neurotransmitter concentrations have recently been described, while in EA3 only the genetic locus is known, and in EA4 no genetic defect has been identified yet. EA2 is the most common form (see Figure 34.2), followed by EA1. It is interesting that EA2 is allelic with SCA6 and familial hemiplegic migraine (phenotypes in CACNA1A mutations might be found in (29)).

On clinical grounds (especially with regard to the duration of attacks), a distinction between EA1 and EA2 is possible (see Table 34.8). EA5 presents with an EA2-phenotype and EA6 is associated with seizures. Triggers in EA include exercises, startle and changes in position in EA1 ('kinesiogenic attacks') and caffeine, alcohol and phenytoin in EA2 ('non-kinesiogenic attacks'). Emotional stress may trigger attacks in both EA1 and EA2. Although most patients with EA2 will develop mild interictal cerebellar signs like GEN or DBN, the episodic exacerbation of symptoms allows a distinction from the SCAs. Treatment options of EAs include acetazolamide (especially for EA2), while the same drug has also been reported to improve cerebellar signs in SCAs (see Table 34.8).

Dentatorubro-pallidoluysian atrophy (DRPLA)

DRPLA has the highest prevalence in Japan (0.2-0.7/100,000), while it is rarely observed in Europe and North America. It belongs to the polyglutamine repeat expansion disorders and

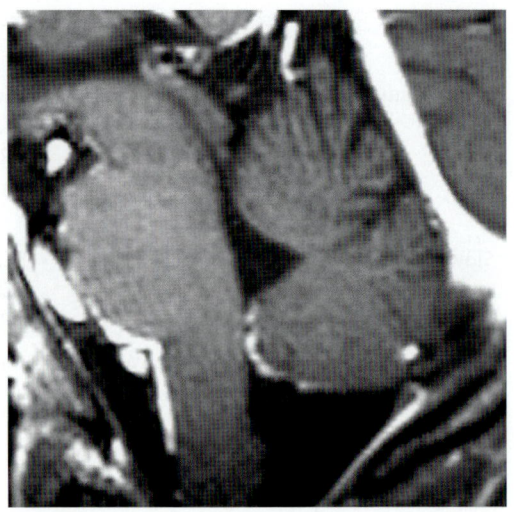

Figure 34.2
This 61-year-old female patient complained of recurring episodes of vertigo and dizziness, gait ataxia and vertical oscillations (suggesting downbeat nystagmus) lasting several hours to a whole day. Between attacks, slight downbeat nystagmus and gaze-evoked nystagmus are the only cerebellar signs evident. It is interesting that she has a positive history of mesial temporal lobe epilepsy related to temporal lobe sclerosis. On MRI (sagittal view), vermal atrophy is restricted to lobules IV and V; in addition, mild atrophy of the cerebellar hemispheres and the flocculus was reported (not shown here). Based on the duration of the episodes, EA2 is most likely, but genetic testing for EA2 (CACNA1A gene) and SCA6 was negative (courtesy Dept of Neuroradiology, University Hospital Zurich, Switzerland).

affects the protein atrophin-1. Its age of onset is variable, ranging between 1 and 80 years (mean 47.3 years) (30). The clinical features and age of onset are strongly correlated with the size of CAG repeats of DRPLA, and it is characterized by prominent anticipation (22). While myoclonus epilepsy and mental retardation are the most prominent features in patients with onset before the age of 20 years, late onset (aged 40 years or older) is associated with cerebellar ataxia, chorea and dementia. MRI may show atrophy in the cerebellum, brainstem and cerebrum accompanied by high-signal changes in the periventricular white matter.

Table 34.8
Autosomal-dominant episodic ataxias (modified after (4) and (42)).

	EA1	EA2	EA3	EA4	EA5	EA6	EA7
Mutation	KCNA1 gene	CACNA1A gene	Localized on 1q42, but genetic defect un-known	Unknown	CACNB4β4	SLC1A3	Unknown
Age of onset	2-15 y	2-20y	1-42y	23-60y	3y to teens	5y	Before age 20y
Triggers	Exercises, emotion-al stress, startle, positional changes	Emotion-al stress, exercises, caffeine, alcohol, phe-nytoin	Unknown	Unknown	Unknown	Unknown	Exertion, excitement
Duration of attacks	Less than 15 min	Variable: minutes to hours (days)	1 min to 6 hours	'brief'	Hours	Hours to days	Hours to days
Other neu-rological symptoms	Tremor, stiffening of extremities, muscle cramps	Migraneous headaches, nausea, (hemi)pare-sis, dystonia, diplopia, tin-nitus, DBN	Myokymia, migraine, tinnitus, vertigo, dysarthria	Late-onset vertigo, diplopia,	Vertigo	Alternating hemiplegia, seizures, cognitive impairment	Vertigo, weakness, slurring, dysarthria
Interictal signs	Myokymia	Nystagmus (DBN, GEN), limb ataxia	none	Nystag-mus, impaired smooth pursuit	Nystagmus, ataxia, epi-lepsy	Epilepsy, migraine, ataxia, delayed motor milestones	none
Treatment options	Aceta-zolamide, carba-mazepine, valproate, phenytoin	Aceta-zolamide, flunarizine, 4-aminopyri-dine	Acetazola-mide	Unknown	Aceta-zolamide (transient effect)	Unknown	Unknown
Associated disorders		Familial hemiplegic migraine, SCA6					

Abbreviations: DBN = downbeat nystagmus; EA = episodic ataxia; GEN = gaze-evoked nystagmus; SCA6 = spino-cerebellar ataxia type 6.

Autosomal recessive cerebellar ataxias (ARCAs)

Autosomal recessive hereditary ataxias typically become symptomatic in children or adults before the age of 25 years, allowing a distinction from most ADCAs based on the age of onset. ARCAs must therefore be included in the differential diagnosis of every patient up to age 25-30 years with a persistent and slowly progressive cerebellar syndrome including gait and balance impairments, excessive clumsiness, dysarthria or hypotonia (i.e. decreased muscle tone). Particularly suggestive of an autosomal-recessive trait of inheritance is the presence of affected siblings and parental consanguinity despite the fact that both parents are healthy. However, in countries where large families and parental consanguinity are rare, ARCAs most often present as seemingly sporadic cases. The most frequent causes of ARCA are Friedreich's ataxia (FRDA) and ataxia telangiectasia (AT). Other important syndromes with cerebellar ataxia and an autosomal-recessive inheritance are ataxia with ocular motor apraxia type 1 (AOA1) and 2 (AOA2). Clinically, ARCAs are heterogeneous, complex and often disabling disorders, often affecting both the central and peripheral nervous system and presenting with various systemic signs (see Table 34.1). The key feature in these disorders is spinocerebellar ataxia, involving the cerebellum, brainstem or the spinocerebellar long tracts. ARCAs are generally associated with peripheral polyneuropathy (sensory or sensorimotor), reflected mostly by loss of proprioception and vibration sense. Important neurological signs besides cerebellar ataxia are optic nerve atrophy, postural or kinetic tremor, movement disorders such as chorea or Parkinsonism, ocular motor disturbances, pyramidal tract dysfunction including excessive tendon reflexes, spasticity and extensor plantar responses, mental retardation, impaired cognition and epilepsy. Systemic (non-neurological) symptoms are more frequently observed than in ADCAs. Early onset in combination with cerebellar atrophy is characteristic of AT, ataxia with ocular motor apraxia types 1 & 2, autosomal recessive spastic ataxia of Charlevoix-Saguenay, and Marinesco-Sjögren syndrome. If the diagnostic approach to suspected ARCA remains negative, screening for SCA mutations should be considered in all patients, as an autosomal dominant pattern of inheritance cannot be ruled out (11).

A selection of ARCAs where ataxia is a leading complaint is described in detail below, with FRDA being the prototypic ARCA. A second group of ARCAs consists of disorders that can mimic the FRDA phenotype, but can be readily distinguished based on additional clinical neurological findings (epilepsy, cognitive impairment, psychiatric symptoms) typically not seen in FRDA, and initially manifest cerebellar atrophy on imaging. Representative disorders of this group are DNA polymerase-gamma ataxia (cerebellar ataxia, myoclonus, impaired cognition, psychiatric symptoms, migraine headaches and seizures), late-onset Tay-Sachs, and cerebrotendinous xanthomatosis (CTX). Late-onset Tay-Sachs is caused by a mutation in the hexosaminidase A gene impairing the ganglioside metabolism and presenting with extrapyramidal signs, cognitive decline and developmental delay, blindness associated with a characteristic cherry-red spot on fundoscopy, seizures, muscle weakness and proximal wasting, and mood disturbances. Other autosomal recessive disorders that may present with ataxia less commonly, such as coenzyme Q10 deficiency, hereditary spastic paraplegia type 7 (HSP7), Wilson's disease, aceruloplasminaemia or metachromatic leukodystrophy are not addressed here.

ARCAs with mitochondrial dysfunction

Friedreich's ataxia (FRDA)

With an estimated prevalence of 2-4.5/100,000 (and a carrier frequency of about 1:85-100) (31), FRDA is the most frequent ARCA worldwide – accounting for about 30-40% of all ARCAs (albeit being rare in Japan) – and the most common heredoataxia in Caucasian populations. A GAA trinucleotide repeat expansion (range 90–1300 repeats, normal range 6–33) in the frataxin (FRDA1) gene is the underlying cause in over 90% of cases, leading to reduced levels of frataxin (loss-of-function mutation) (32). Few patients are compound heterozygous, with point mutations on one allele and the expansion on the other. Frataxin is considered a mitochondrial protein involved in iron handling and respiratory chain function, and FRDA is believed to be a mitochondrial disorder related to oxidative damage (33). The expansion size is inversely correlated to the age of symptom onset and impairment of mobility and directly related to the frequency of cardiomyopathy. First signs usually occur between the ages of 7 and 25 years, but a late-onset variant (age of onset up to 40 years or more) is found in about 15% of patients, often with retained deep tendon reflexes and lower limb spasticity (34). Clinically, progressively worsening ataxia (gait, trunk and limbs) of both cerebellar and sensory (presenting as axonal sensory neuropathy) origin is observed in combination with dysarthria, dysphagia, areflexia, muscle hypotonia and distal muscle atrophy, optic atrophy, and pyramidal signs as extensor plantar reflexes (33). Common non-neurological signs include scoliosis (two-thirds of patients), left ventricular hypertrophy (60% of patients) progressing to end-stage cardiomyopathy, and diabetes mellitus (10%). Regular cardiac follow-up including ECG and echocardiography are recommended in patients with confirmed FRDA. Eye movement abnormalities are usually only subtle (such as fixation instability) or lacking, and rarely head tremor may develop. Early loss of large-diameter sensory neurons in the dorsal root ganglia may result in deterioration of the spinocerebellar tract, the pyramidal tract and the posterior columns. Although disease progression is variable, patients generally lose independent locomotion 10–15 years after disease onset and suffer from severe

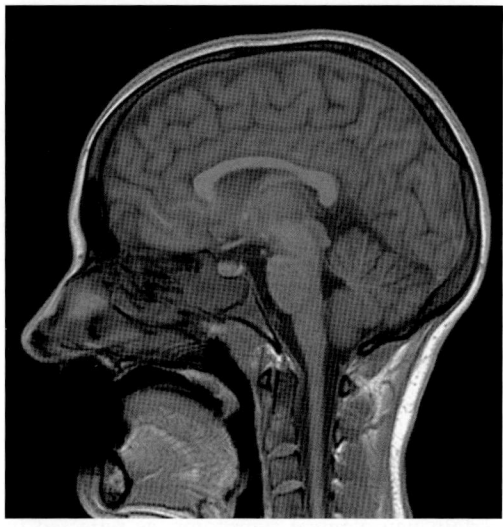

Figure 34.3
This 23-year-old female patient with genetically confirmed FRDA has a history of slowly progressive ataxia of gait since the age of 20 years, while her family history for gait problems was negative. On clinical examination, the deep tendon reflexes were reduced (arms) or lost (legs), her vibration sense was slightly impaired, and ataxia of stance worsened significantly on eye closure, suggesting sensory ataxia. On MRI, mild atrophy of the entire spinal cord was reported while no cerebellar or brainstem atrophy was found (courtesy d0ept of Neuroradiology, University Hospital Zurich, Switzerland).

dysarthria and dysphagia. For the late-onset variant a more slowly progressive phenotype without cardiomyopathy has been reported. On MRI no obvious cerebellar atrophy is usually found in the first years of the disease (marked cerebellar atrophy speaks against an initial diagnosis of FRDA), but later atrophy in the dorsal medulla, cerebellar hemispheres, rostral vermis and the dentate nucleus is seen (35) (see Figure 34.3 for MRI findings in a FRDA patient). FRDA therefore should be considered in all patients presenting with progressive ataxia with the exception of those with severe olivopontocerebellar atrophy demonstrated on MRI. Other ARCAs with a similar clinical presentation to FRDA and also little or no cerebellar atrophy on imaging include ataxia with vitamin E deficiency (AVED), abetalipoproteinaemia (ABL) and Refsum disease. A similar phenotype but cerebellar atrophy on MRI is characteristic of late-onset Tay-Sachs disease (LOTS), CTX, mitochondrial autosomal-recessive ataxia syndromes, and spinocerebellar ataxia with neuropathy type 1 (SCAN1). Therefore, in the clinical evaluation, it may be more suitable to describe the syndrome as Friedreich's ataxia phenotype until genetics confirm the diagnosis of FRDA.

Treatment trials in FRDA have aimed at antioxidant protection. In a pilot study with 10 patients, a combination of high-dose vitamin E and coenzyme Q10 led to improved cardiac function and possible stabilization or reduced decline of certain neurological symptoms, as reflected in increased kinetic scores and stable ocular motor and speech scores on ICARS (36). Studies with low-dose idebenone, a synthetic analogue to coenzyme Q10, have suggested a reduction of cardiac hypertrophy (37-40) but failed to demonstrate any improvement in cardiac function. In FRDA drug trials, no consistent improvement or even stabilization of ataxia has been found so far. While some studies reported improvement in ataxia (40) and other neurological symptoms (38, 41), others found neurological disease progression to be unaffected by the treatment (39, 42). Amantadine was reported to reduce functional disability in FRDA slightly in two case series (43, 44). Other potential treatment strategies include increasing frataxin expression by the application of recombinant human erythropoietin or histone deactylase inhibitors, but these approaches are still under investigation.

Other autosomal recessive mitochondrial disorders

Among the autosomal recessive mitochondrial heredoataxias (45) (see Chapter 32), POLG syndromes (based on nuclear mutations of the polymerase-gamma (POLG1) gene (4)) need to be considered as they may be the second most common cause of ARCAs. The POLG phenotype includes several syndromes such as Alper's

syndrome, chronic progressive external ophthalmoplegia (CPEO), mitochondrial autosomal recessive ataxia syndrome (MIRAS; cerebellar ataxia associated with polyneuropathy, dysarthria, mild cognitive impairment and psychiatric symptoms, seizures) and sensory ataxic neuropathy, dysarthria and ophthalmoparesis (SANDO; triad of cerebellar or sensory ataxia, dysarthria and progressive external ophthalmoplegia). Sequencing of POLG1 may be advised in ataxic patients negative for SCA and FRDA mutations when presenting with CPEO, psychiatric symptoms and/or axonal neuropathy.

ARCAs with metabolic dysfunction

Ataxia with vitamin E deficiency (AVED)

As a result of a mutation in the alpha-tocopherol transfer protein (46), vitamin E metabolism and transport are impaired in AVED, leading to very low serum vitamin E levels (but lack of intestinal fat malabsorption or abetalipoproteinaemia) and oxidative stress (47). Typical clinical signs are similar to those in FRDA (such as areflexia and loss of vibration sense in the legs, often combined with pyramidal tract signs), but include impaired vision and retinitis pigmentosa early on (48). Cardiomyopathy is the most common systemic finding (19-31%), although it is observed at lower rates than in FRDA. Diabetes is thought to be uncommon in AVED. Onset usually occurs before the age of 20 years (range 2-52 years), and most patients are from the Mediterranean area. Compared to FRDA the disease course progresses more slowly (49). Mild cerebellar atrophy is found in about half of patients. Early supplementation of vitamin E seems to stop disease progression (49) and may even mildly improve ataxia (50).

Abetalipoproteinaemia (ABL; previously called Bassen-Kornzweig disease)

This disorder is characterized by an impaired lipoprotein metabolism due to mutations of the microsomal triglyceride transfer protein (MTP) gene (51), ultimately leading to fat malabsorption with vitamin A, E, and K deficiency and hypocholesterolaemia. The first symptoms of ABL (intestinal celiac-like symptoms followed by ataxia) are noted in childhood or early teens, and the phenotype resembles FRDA and AVED. Pigmentary retinopathy (probably caused by vitamin A deficiency) is frequently observed, along with polyneuropathy with sensory loss, distal muscle atrophy and areflexia. Acantocytosis in the peripheral blood smear is characteristic. Treatment includes dietary modifications and supplementation of lipid-soluble vitamins (A, E, K), which may prevent neurological complications if initiated early.

Refsum disease

Refsum disease is a peroxisomal disorder caused either by a mutation in the phytanoyl-CoA hydroxylase gene (resulting in an accumulation of phytanic acid in the body fat and myelinated neurons) or less frequently by a mutation of the peroxin-7 gene (52). Retinitis pigmentosa (always present before the age of 28 years) combined with anosmia (this distinguishes it from FRDA which rarely presents with anosmia), polyneuropathy, cerebellar ataxia and sensorineural deafness are characteristic findings. Cardiomyopathy, skeletal abnormalities, ichthyosis and renal insufficiency are additional features. Disease onset is usually before the age of 20 years, but late-onset variants have been described (53). Rapid weight loss or illness can result in mobilization of phytanic acid from fat stores, leading to a sudden worsening of symptoms or even acute presentation similar to Guillain-Barré syndrome (53). Restriction of intake of phytanic acid halts disease progression and may prevent the onset of symptoms if initiated early. Plasmapheresis has been proposed in acutely ill patients to reduce phytanic acid levels rapidly (52).

Cerebrotendinous xanthomatosis (CTX)

CTX belongs to the leukodystrophies. It is caused by a mutation in the CYP27 gene encoding the mitochondrial sterol 27-hydroxylase (54) and becomes symptomatic around the age of 20 years. Juvenile cataracts represent a characteristic finding of this disorder along with tendon xanthomas, chronic diarrhea and progressive neurological symptoms (ataxia, pyramidal tract signs and extrapyramidal signs, dementia, seizures, sensorimotor axonal polyneuropathy). Elevated cholesterol and bile alcohols are typically found in the laboratory work-up, while MRI demonstrates generalized cerebral and cerebellar atrophy and diffuse white-matter hyperintense lesions. Early treatment with bile-acid replacement therapy (application of chenodeoxycholic acid and statins) should be considered in order to stabilize and even lessen the symptoms.

ARCA, with DNA-damage repair disorders

Ataxia telangiectasia (AT)

The first clinical signs of AT, the second most common ARCA after FRDA (incidence 1:40,000 to 1:100,000 in the USA), can usually be found by the age of 2-3 years (a late-onset variant, however, has been reported (55)) and include progressive hypotonia and clumsiness that lead to loss of independent ambulation about 10 years after disease onset and death about 20 years after onset. AT is the most frequent cause of progressive cerebellar ataxia presenting before the age of 5 years. Besides cerebellar ataxia, oculocutaneous telangiectasias (usually manifesting by the age of 6 years), oculocephalic dissociation, nystagmus (which may be treated with 4-aminopyridine (56)) and impaired vestibulo-ocular reflex, chorea or dystonia (up to 90% of patients) and sensorimotor axonal polyneuropathy are other frequent clinical findings. AT belongs to the DNA-damage repair disorders (with mutations in the ataxia telangiectasia mutated (ATM) gene leading to loss of function (57)), with a greatly increased risk of malignant conditions (especially leukemia and lymphoma), hypersensitivity to ionizing radiation, and recurrent infections due to immunoglobulin deficiencies.

Alpha-fetoprotein (AFP) levels are typically elevated. On MRI, extensive, diffuse, white-matter demyelination, focal lesions on T1 and T2 (hypo- or hyperintense), severe cerebellar atrophy and telangiectasias (with contrast-enhanced sequences) may be found (58).

Several disorders with clinical and biochemical similarities to AT have been reported, including ataxia telangiectasia-like disorder (ATLD) and Nijmegen breakage syndrome (NBS). In these disorders, patients have normal AFP and lack telangiectasias, but they are prone to malignancies and sensitive to ionizing radiation.

A number of disorders resemble the AT phenotype and share with AT their role in DNA-damage repair, including AOA1, AOA2 and SCAN1. However, these disorders have normal AFP levels, lack telangiectasias, and do not feature an increased risk of malignancies or infections. Furthermore, unlike AT and ATLD which are associated with damage in double-strand DNA, these disorders show single-strand DNA damage.

Ataxias with ocular motor apraxia (AOA1, AOA2)

Among the disorders resembling the AT phenotype, AOA1 (mutation in the aprataxin gene (59)) and AOA2 (mutation in the senataxin gene (60)) are characterized by ocular motor apraxia (i.e. an impaired ability to initiate voluntary saccades which is more prominent in AOA1), oculocephalic dissociation (i.e. an inability to coordinate eye-head movements on head turns with the head reaching the new target before the eyes), sensorimotor axonal neuropathy (more pronounced in AOA1), dystonia, chorea (in about 80% in AOA1 and in 10-22% in AOA2), and mild mental retardation (AOA1). Both are involved in the DNA repair of single-strand DNA damage. Whereas AOA1 becomes symptomatic in early childhood (on average around the age of 7 years), the first symptoms in AOA2 usually develop later (around the age of 15 years). While AFP serum levels are increased in 75-100% of patients and albumin levels are nor-

mal in AOA2 (61), the serum albumin levels are low, cholesterol levels are high, and AFP levels are normal in AOA1 (62). Coenzyme Q10 may be reduced in AOA1. In contrast to AT, patients suffering from AOA1 or AOA2 do not have an increased susceptibility to cancer. AOA2 may represent up to 8% of all non-FRDA ARCAs and therefore is one of the more common ARCAs (61). On MRI, marked cerebellar (vermian) atrophy can be observed in both disorders.

Spinocerebellar ataxia with axonal neuropathy (SCAN1)

SCAN1 is caused by a mutation in the DNA repair protein tyrosyl DNA phosphodiesterase and shares the AT phenotype, but is rare and lacks ocular motor apraxia (63). SCAN1 typically becomes manifest in childhood or teenage years, and presents with cerebellar atrophy, axonal sensorimotor polyneuropathy, distal muscle wasting and pes cavus.

ARCAs with protein misfolding and chaperone dysfunction

ARSACS and MSS

Autosomal recessive spastic ataxia of Charlevoix-Saguenay (ARSACS, mutation in the sacsin SACS gene (64)) and Marinesco-Sjögren syndrome (MSS, mutation in the SIL1 gene (64)) both show chaperone deficiency. The typical age of onset is 1-5 years in ARSACS (65), although adult-onset has been reported. Clinically, ARSACS is characterized by cerebellar dysfunction, pyramidal tract signs (most prominent in the lower legs), retained deep tendon reflexes, axonal sensorimotor neuropathy, and muscle wasting and presents with anterior vermal atrophy and spinal cord atrophy on MRI. MSS is a rare cerebellar ataxia syndrome becoming manifest in childhood. Characteristic clinical findings include mental retardation, seizures, cataracts, myopathy, neuropathy, skeletal abnormalities and hypergonadotropic hypogonadism. On MRI, cerebellar atrophy can be seen.

Other ARCAs

Cerebellar ataxia, neuropathy, vestibular areflexia syndrome (CANVAS)

The combination of cerebellar ataxia, bilateral vestibular hypofunction and axonal sensory neuropathy has been recently described as a probably late-onset, autosomal recessive disorder, although most cases reported so far were apparently sporadic (66). Cerebellar atrophy on MRI was described in most cases (located in the anterior and dorsal vermis and hemispheric crus I), while the inferior vermis and the brainstem were spared (see Figure 34.4). The differential diagnosis includes SCA3 (because of vestibular impairment), FRDA and other SCAs presenting with sensory neuropathy.

X-linked cerebellar ataxia

Cerebellar ataxia affecting only males in one or more generations in the maternal line favors an X-linked mode of inheritance. Few cerebellar ataxia syndromes have a confirmed X-linked inheritance: they include fragile-X tremor ataxia syndrome (FXTAS), X-linked sideroblastic anemia with ataxia (XLSA/A) and adrenomyeloneuropathy. The last one is an adult subtype of adrenoleukodystrophy, presenting with progressive spastic paraparesis with sphincter and sexual dysfunction. White matter lesions on brain MRI and increased blood levels of very long fatty acids are diagnostic. XLSA/A is a rare mitochondrial disorder presenting with mild sideroblastic anemia and cerebellar ataxia (with marked cerebellar atrophy on MRI).

FXTAS usually becomes manifest after the age of 50 years and is characterized by two core clinical features (see (67) for an extensive review of FXTAS): progressive intention tremor and gait ataxia. Besides these two major diagnostic criteria, minor criteria include Parkinsonism and cognitive decline with short-term memory deficits and executive function deficits (68). During the course of the disease, autonomic dysfunc-

tion and polyneuropathy may develop. FXTAS belongs to the trinucleotide expansion disorders and consists of a premutation in the fragile-X mental retardation I (FMR1) gene with 55-200 repeats. A full mutation with a repeat length of over 200 causes fragile-X syndrome, a relatively frequent cause of mental retardation in boys due to silencing of the FMR1 gene. In patients with the FRM1 premutation, increased levels of FRM1 messenger RNA are found. A toxic gain of function of the mRNA levels has been suspected

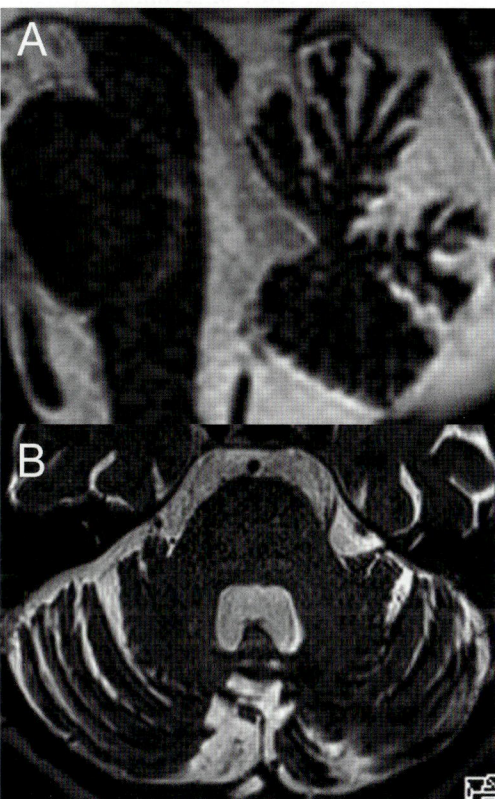

Figure 34.4
This 76-year-old female patient has a 15-year history of progressive gait imbalance and dizziness becoming worse in darkness. Along with severe atrophy of both the cerebellar vermis (panel A, sagittal view) and the hemispheres (panel B, axial view), bilateral vestibular loss and peripheral neuropathy were found. This combination is characteristic for CANVAS (cerebellar ataxia, neuropathy, vestibular areflexia syndrome) (courtesy of the Dept of Neuroradiology, University Hospital Zurich, Switzerland).

to be key to the pathogenesis of FXTAS (69). On brain MRI, characteristic symmetric, T2-hyperintense lesions in the middle cerebellar peduncles (and adjacent cerebellar white matter) are found in 60% of FXTAS patients (70) (see Figure 34.5). The current diagnostic criteria require the presence of MRI white-matter lesions in the middle cerebellar peduncle and one major clinical criteria or the presence of FXTAS inclusions on autopsy (67).

Epidemiologic studies suggest that FXTAS is a relatively frequent cause of seemingly sporadic ataxia in older adult males, therefore all males presenting with onset of ataxia after the age of 50 years or with Parkinsonism, action tremor or dementia in combination with either a positive family history of such complaints or hyperintensities in the middle cerebellar peduncles should be screened for FXTAS (67). In various studies reporting on genetic testing in male ataxic patients aged 50 years or more, FXTAS was identified in about 2%, as summarized by (71). It is interesting that the clinical phenotype of MSA-C and FXTAS may overlap. Prominent tremor and slowly progressive disease in patients that meet the diagnostic criteria of MSA-C should raise the suspicion of FXTAS (72). Few female permutation carriers of the FMR1-gene who become symptomatic with FXTAS have been described, but the rates are far too low to promote screening in women. Female carriers bear an increased risk of early ovarian failure (i.e. before the age of 40 years) and are intrinsically vulnerable to psychiatric problems with depression, anxiety or both occurring in about 40% of carriers (73). Treatment of the tremor includes the prescription of betablockers, primidone and topiramate.

Mitochondrial heredoataxias

Mitochondrial diseases leading to cerebellar ataxia may present with different modes of inheritance as genes coded in both the nuclear and mitochondrial DNA contribute to mitochondrial function. Mutations in mitochondrial DNA genes affect the respiratory chain only, while mutations in the nuclear DNA genes may impair various mitochondrial proteins. Furthermore, mitochondrial DNA mutations may mimic autosomal dominant, autosomal recessive and X-linked traits of inheritance, and point mutations in mitochondrial DNA are often sporadic. On clinical grounds, different subtypes of mitochondrial disorders are distinguished, often presenting as multisystem disorders with both neurological and non-neurological abnormalities. Cerebellar ataxia is a frequent finding (and sometimes even the presenting symptom) in Kearns-Sayre syndrome (KSS; chronic progressive external ophthalmoplegia, pigmentary retinopathy, cardiac conduction defects, ataxia), MELAS (myopathy, encephalopathy, lactate acidosis and stroke-like episodes), MERFF (myoclonic epilepsy and ragged red fibers, presenting with myopathy, ataxia, dementia, chronic progressive external ophthalmoplegia, deafness, seizures), and NARP (neuropathy, ataxia, retinitis pigmentosa) (see (45) for an extensive review).

Acquired ataxias

Various disorders may be accompanied by cerebellar ataxia (including toxins, specific drugs). Endocrine disorders (like hypothyroidism) and vitamin deficiencies due to malabsorption (e.g. of vitamin B12 or vitamin E) are other possible causes of symptomatic ataxia. Initially, the rate of progression is helpful in identifying those disorders that require urgent evaluation due to rapid progression. In a study with 500 patients with progressive ataxia, 404 were found to have sporadic ataxia (74). Amongst them, gluten ataxia (25%), clinically probable MSA-C (13%), alcohol-related ataxia (11%), paraneoplastic ataxia (4%) and anti-GAD-associated ataxia (2%) were the most common causes, while 28% were classified as idiopathic.

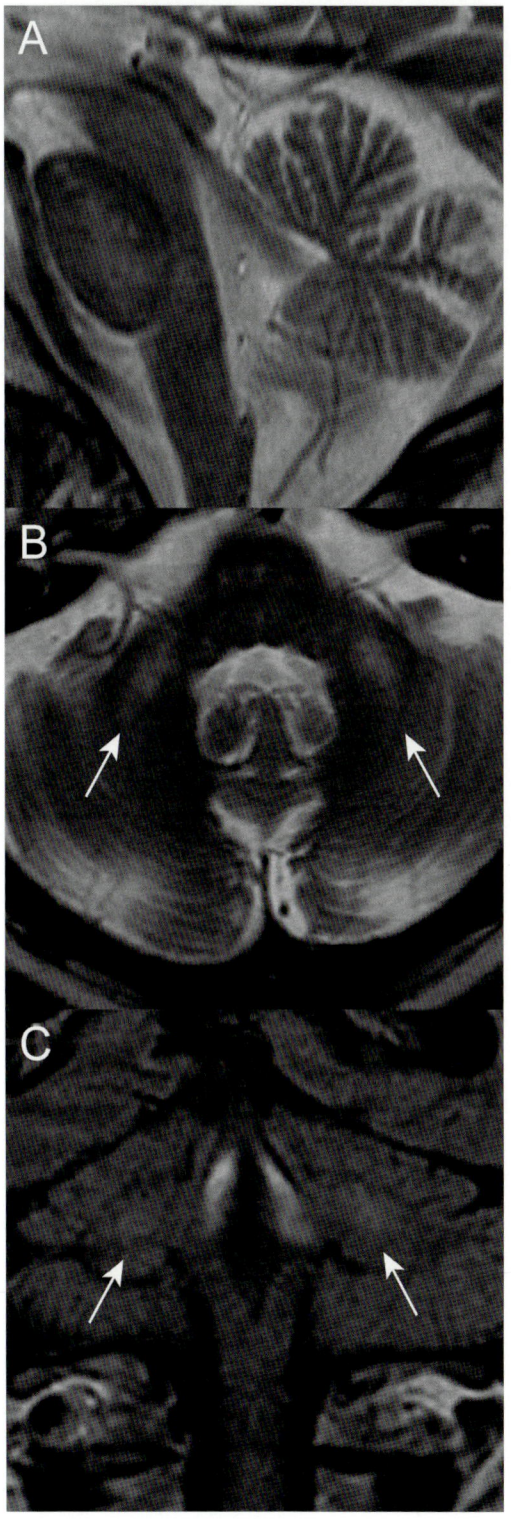

Wernicke's encephalopathy (WE)

Acute- or subacute-onset cerebellar ataxia related to severe vitamin B1 deficiency is known as Wernicke's encephalopathy (see (75) for an excellent in-depth review) and is related to hemorrhagic lesions around the third ventricle affecting the mammillary bodies and the thalamic nuclei. Clinically, ataxia, double vision, peripheral neuropathy, seizures and neuropsychological deficits are noted. While the classical teaching emphasizes the link between chronic alcohol abuse and WE, other conditions with impaired resorption of vitamin B1 may also lead to WE, such as hyperemesis gravidarum, critical illness, bulimia and bariatric surgery (76). On MRI, restrictions on diffusion weighted imaging (DWI) and T2-hyperintensities are found in the mammillary bodies and the thalamic nuclei that are potentially reversible with appropriate treatment. If WE is suspected, immediate high-dose supplementation of vitamin B1 is mandatory (ideally combined with drawing blood for serum vitamin B1 level estimates) (77). Guidelines for the diagnostic work-up and treatment have been provided by EFNS (77). Strict abstinence improves ataxia, while ongoing alcohol consumption will lead to deterioration.

Alcoholic cerebellar degeneration (ACD)

Expert opinion suggests that ACD is one of the most frequent causes of chronic cerebellar ataxia

Figure 34.5
This patient with genetically confirmed FXTAS had a 7-year history of slowly progressive gait ataxia and dysphagia. On clinical examination, ataxia of gait and stance, ocular motor abnormalities (saccadic smooth pursuit, gaze-evoked nystagmus, hypermetric saccades), dysphagia, intermittent resting tremor, extensor plantar response bilaterally, mild cognitive impairment and peripheral neuropathy were observed. Vermal atrophy (panel A) as well as atrophy of the cerebellar hemispheres were very mild and only punctual. Panels B (axial plane, T2-weighted) and C (frontal plane, FLAIR sequence) illustrate the characteristic signal hyperintensities in the middle cerebellar peduncle (white arrows) reported in FXTAS (courtesy of the Dept of Neuroradiology, University Hospital Zurich, Switzerland).

(2). Clinically, ACD is characterized by ataxia of gait and stance with minor involvement of the upper extremities, speech and eye movements. It typically occurs mainly in middle-aged male patients with a history of chronic alcohol abuse. This is reflected in cerebellar atrophy being most prominent on MRI in the dorsal cerebellar vermis and the anterior parts of the hemispheres – cerebellar areas that mainly receive spinal afferents. Disease progression can be rapid (weeks to a few months) or slow and steady over years. Symptoms tend to progress in those patients who continue to drink and may stabilize in those who stop alcohol consumption. There is an ongoing discussion as to the extent to which ACD is related to malnutrition of vitamin B1 (resembling the pathomechanism of WE) or to direct toxic effects of alcohol (such as depression of neuronal firing, increased lipid peroxidation and reduced antioxidants) or to a combination of both. The role of vitamin B1 in ACD is emphasized by the observation that reduced serum vitamin B1 levels and cerebellar volume loss on MRI in chronic alcoholics correlate well (78). ACD can therefore be considered a chronic variant of WE, again prompting vitamin B1 supplementation. However, a clear distinction between WE and ACD can be difficult in chronic alcohol users presenting with subacute ataxia.

While autopsy studies have reported cerebellar degeneration in up to 27% of patients with known chronic alcohol consumption, many patients with chronic alcohol abuse have cerebellar atrophy without ataxia (79).

Superficial siderosis – induced ataxia

Repeated subarachnoidal bleeding related to vascular abnormalities or tumors or secondary to neurosurgical procedures leads to the accumulation of hemoglobin and free iron on the surface of the brain and the spinal cord (80). Subsequent damage to cerebral, brainstem and cerebellar structures, cranial nerves and the spinal cord may result (see Figure 34.6). Clinical

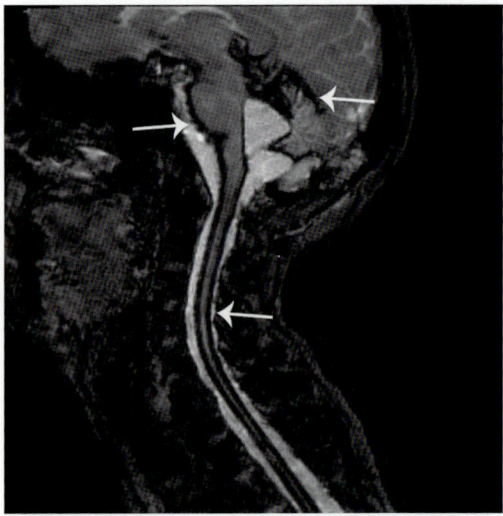

Figure 34.6
Superficial siderosis in a 64-year-old female patient with progressive cerebellar (gait ataxia, gaze-evoked nystagmus), pyramidal tract signs and hearing loss. On MRI, extensive haemosiderin deposits (in black, indicated by the white arrows) on the surface of the brainstem, cerebellum and the entire spinal cord are accompanied by severe atrophy of vestibulo-cerebellar structures including the nodulus, superior vermis, and the flocculus as well as enlargement of the fourth ventricle (courtesy of the Dept of Neuroradiology, University Hospital Zurich, Switzerland).

findings in patients with superficial siderosis include hearing loss and pyramidal tract signs along with progressive cerebellar ataxia. The key to the correct diagnosis is the demonstration of linear T2-hypointensities on the surface of the brain and the spinal cord along with xanthochromasia in the CSF (81). Removal of the source of bleeding may stop further progression.

Structural disorders – induced ataxia

Congenital Chiari malformations with caudal displacement of deformed cerebellar tonsils (see Figure 34.7), cerebellar neoplasms (primary or metastases) and traumatic brain injury including the cerebellum may lead to acute or episodic cerebellar ataxia and central positional vertigo. The diagnosis is readily made on sagittal MRI

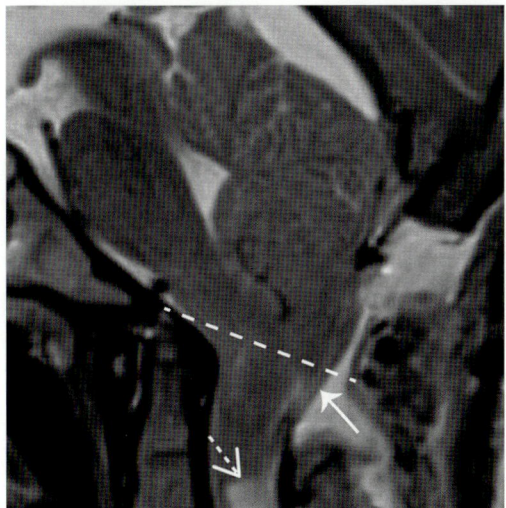

Figure 34.7
Arnold-Chiari malformation type 1. This 16-year-old patient presented with episodic vertigo and progressive gait ataxia. Sagittal MRI shows elongated and caudally displaced cerebellar tonsils (indicated by the white solid arrow), with the tips of the tonsils about 13 mm (normal range: < 3 mm) below the foramen magnum (indicated by the dashed white line). In addition, a cervical syrinx can be depicted (white dashed arrow) (courtesy of the Dept of Neuroradiology, University Hospital Zurich, Switzerland).

sequences, although more subtle tonsillar herniation related to Chiari malformations, cerebellar tumors or lumboperitoneal CSF-shunts may be missed on imaging. Normal pressure hydrocephalus (NPH) should be considered if the ataxic gait is accompanied by cognitive decline and urinary incontinence. Enlarged ventricles on CT or MRI with little or no cortical atrophy and improvement after large volume (30-40 ml) spinal taps further support a diagnosis of NPH. In these patients, the benefits and disadvantages of ventriculo-peritoneal shunting (shunt infections, overdrainage leading to subdural hematoma) need to be addressed before applying this procedure.

Toxic – induced ataxia

Various agents may cause ataxia, either acutely due to intoxication (e.g. lithium or phenytoin) or chronically due to cerebellar damage (e.g. phenytoin). For the clinician, lithium, phenytoin, amiodarone, toluene, heavy metals and anti-cancer drugs like 5-fluorouracil (by inactivation of vitamin B1) and cytosine arabinoside are the most relevant substances in this context.

Infection – induced ataxia

Cerebellitis / post-inflammatory cerebellar ataxia

Acute viral infections may trigger cerebellar inflammation, and post-viral ataxia can present as rather acute ataxia in children or as Miller-Fisher syndrome. The most common cause in children is varicella, while in adults mononucleosis is most frequently found. Unilateral cerebellar involvement, encephalitis, mutism and coma are unusual clinical findings in cerebellitis. The prognosis of ataxia related to acute viral infection is usually favorable, and the treatment is symptomatic (while immunotherapy is typically not prescribed). Rare complications reported are tonsillar herniation, hydrocephalus and cerebellar atrophy. The differential diagnosis includes demyelinating disorders, encephalitis, labyrinthitis, vestibular migraine, intoxication, Wernicke's encephalopathy, cerebellar stroke/haemorrhage (if unilateral signs dominate) and paraneoplastic syndromes.

Chronic CNS infections associated with ataxia

Progressive ataxia can be observed in various chronic CNS infections, including tabetic neurosyphilis due to infection with *Treponema pallidum* (presenting as purely sensory ataxia associated with pain, bladder dysfunction and abnormal pupillary reflexes), Lyme borreliosis (although cerebellar ataxia is rare), or Whipple's disease due to infection with *Tropheryma whipplei* (presenting with gastrointestinal problems like diarrhea, abdominal pain and weight loss along with arthritis and fever) (82). About half of all patients with neurological symptoms display cerebellar ataxia in Whipple's disease. The diagnosis is confirmed by positive PCR in a duodenal biopsy or the CSF. HIV may result in rapidly progressive ataxia due to opportunistic infections or CNS lymphoma, but rarely also due to diffuse cerebellar damage.

Sporadic Creutzfeldt-Jakob disease (sCJD)

New-onset cerebellar ataxia in combination with rapidly progressive dementia, myoclonus, pyramidal tract features and restricted diffusion on DWI may originate from sCJD (83). It is interesting that isolated cerebellar ataxia may be the first symptom in a minority of patients, with cognitive decline being delayed by weeks or even months. Initially, paraneoplastic cerebellar degeneration is an important differential diagnosis. Diagnostic clues are increased concentrations of 14-3-3 protein in the CSF and basal ganglia signal changes on DWI and FLAIR (fluid-attenuated inversion-recovery) (84), while characteristic EEG signs are absent or develop in the late stages only.

Immune-mediated ataxia

Demyelinating lesions related to multiple sclerosis (MS) within the cerebellum or the cerebellar peduncles may result in acute-onset ataxia. Other causes include Miller-Fisher syndrome, systemic lupus erythematodes, Sjögren syndrome and Cogan syndrome. Subacute to chronic cerebellar ataxia may be related to paraneoplastic syndromes, gluten sensitivity ('gluten ataxia') or anti-GAD-antibody ataxia.

Paraneoplastic cerebellar degeneration (PCD)

Paraneoplastic cerebellar degeneration (PCD) belongs to the immune-mediated causes of cerebellar degeneration and typically presents as subacute pancerebellar syndrome (with midline cerebellar structures being affected the most). Therefore, in the differential diagnosis of rapidly progressive cerebellar ataxia with severe ataxia in less than 12 weeks, a paraneoplastic phenomenon must be evaluated (85). Estimates have proposed that up to 50% of patients with subacute ataxia aged 50 years or older suffers from a malignancy. Usually, gait ataxia and dysarthria are severe, and vertigo is common. PCD may occur in association with almost every tumor (see Table 34.9 for details). Most frequently, small-cell lung cancer (SCLC), breast and gynaecological tumours, and lymphoma are reported. Typically, ataxia preceeds the diagnosis of the underlying tumour (except for lymphoma). Other paraneoplastic syndromes such as Lambert-Eaton myasthenic syndrome or opsoclonus-myoclonus syndrome may accompany PCD. Early on in PCD, cerebellar atrophy is mild or absent as depicted on MRI, but in the course of the disease, cerebellar atrophy usually develops as the correlate of Purkinje cell loss on histopathology (reflecting the irreversibility of cerebellar damage).

Patients with suspected PCD should be screened for anti-neuronal antibodies as antibodies found in the serum or cerebrospinal fluid (CSF) that react with antigens expressed by the tumour and the central nervous system are diagnostic (86). In one series with 137 patients with paraneoplastic neurological syndromes (50 with PCD) and anti-neuronal antibodies, all patients with anti-Yo, anti-Tr and anti-mGluR1 antibodies had PCD. Rates were lower for anti-Ri (86%) and anti-Hu (18%) (86). Furthermore, while the clinical presentation is similar in all types of PCD, anti-Ri antibodies may form an exception due to their characteristic association with opsoclonus, resulting in oscillopsia (87). However, the absence of antibodies does not rule out a diagnosis of PCD. If the suspicion of PCD remains high despite negative autoantibodies or if specific autoantibodies are found, a thorough search for an underlying tumour including imaging (whole-body FDG-PET-CT preferred, alternatively chest and abdominal CT), ultrasonography of the testes, and gynaecological evaluation is mandatory every six months for at least four years according to guidelines (88).

Table 34.9
Paraneoplastic cerebellar degeneration: most frequent antibodies associated with cerebellar ataxia (modified after (2) and (89)).

Antibody	Associated with PCD in [%] (86)	Underlying tumor	Other paraneoplastic syndromes
Anti-Hu (ANNA-1)	18%	SCLS, neuroblastoma, sarcoma	Paraneoplastic encephalitis, paraneoplastic sensory neuropathy, limbic encephalitis
Anti-Ri (ANNA-2)	86%	Breast, gynaecological, SCLC	Opsoclonus myoclonus syndrome, brainstem encephalitis
Anti-CV2/CRMP5		SCLC, thymoma	Paraneoplastic encephalitis, polyneuropathy
Anti-Tr	100%	Hodgkin's lymphoma	
Anti-VGCC		SCLC	Lambert-Eaton myasthenic syndrome
Anti-Yo (PCA-1)	100%	Gynaecological, breast	
mGlu1R1-alpha	100%	Hodgkin's lymphoma	
Anti-Ma		Breast	Limbic encephalitis, brainstem encephalitis, opsoclonus-myoclonus syndrome

Abbreviations: SCLC = small-cell lung carcinoma.

Treatment of the underlying tumour or immunosuppressive therapy rarely halts the progression of cerebellar degeneration; clinical remission has only been described for successfully treated lymphoma with associated anti-Tr and anti-mGluR1 antibodies. Current theories suggest that paraneoplastic syndromes reflect an effective autoimmune response to cancer. This is supported by the observation that for a given cancer and stage, patients with paraneoplastic symptoms have a more favourable outcome than those without paraneoplastic symptoms.

Gluten ataxia

Gluten ataxia may be one of the most common causes of idiopathic sporadic ataxia (74), making up 11.5-41% of all sporadic ataxia cases. On MRI, cerebellar atrophy may be found in up to 60% of cases. The mean age of onset is 53 years. Gluten sensitivity (as defined by the presence of antibodies against gliadin) or celiac disease may result in autoimmune-mediated cerebellar ataxia termed 'gluten ataxia' associated with sensorimotor axonal neuropathy in about half of the cases (74), although there is ongoing controversy about whether there is a causal relationship between asymptomatic celiac disease and sporadic ataxia (2). Anti-gliadin antibodies are found in 30-40% of patients with sporadic cerebellar ataxia, compared to 5-12% in the normal population (depending on the assay used), while the prevalence of celiac disease in the same population is at least 1% (74). Often, these patients do not have gastrointestinal symptoms, but intestinal biopsy may show the typical changes of celiac disease. While some studies have reported a strong association between cerebellar ataxia and asymptomatic celiac disease (as defined by the presence of anti-gliadin antibodies) (90, 91), others failed to document such a link (92, 93). It is interesting that increased frequencies of anti-gliadin antibodies have also been noted in hereditary ataxias like SCA2 and Huntington disease, suggesting that gluten sensitivity may be an epiphenomenon in neurodegenerative disorders rather than a pathogenic factor (94).

Nonetheless, a gluten-free diet may be recommended in cases of suspected gluten ataxia or asymptomatic celiac disease and should be discussed with the patient. Monitoring of anti-gliadin antibodies over the course of the diet may be used to evaluate the immunologic response. If a strict gluten-free diet for at least a year fails to improve the symptoms or the complaints become worse, treatment with immunosuppressants or immunoglobulins may be considered (74).

Anti-GAD-associated ataxia

Patients with polyglandular endocrine autoimmune syndrome (especially diabetes) and antibodies to glutamic acid decarboxylase (GAD) may present with ataxia (either in combination with stiff-person syndrome or in isolation). In case series, anti-GAD antibodies were found in patients with sporadic ataxia at rates varying between 0% and 25% (12, 74, 95). Slowly progressive cerebellar ataxia in combination with cerebellar atrophy was reported in about half the cases. No established treatment is available, although in single cases improvement after treatment with immunomodulatory substances including steroids and intravenous immunoglobulins has been reported.

The entity of anti-GAD-associated ataxia is still controversial as anti-GAD antibodies are found with increasing frequency in other hereditary and immune-mediated ataxia syndromes (up to 50% of patients with gluten ataxia have positive anti-GAD antibodies (96)). This suggests that anti-GAD antibodies could reflect an epiphenomenon, indicating the presence of a possible autoimmune pathogenesis and an association with other autoimmune diseases including gluten ataxia, stiff-person syndrome and type 1 diabetes (74).

Steroid-responsive encephalopathy associated with autoimmune thyroiditis (SREAT)

Subacute encephalopathy with predominantly cognitive changes, high serum levels of thyroperoxidase antibodies, and rapid clinical improvement on steroids are characteristic of SREAT, formerly known as Hashimoto encephalitis. In addition, various other neurological symptoms have been described, including ataxia, tremor and myoclonus (97). Important differential diagnoses are PCD and the ataxic variant of sCJD (98).

Women are diagnosed with SREAT about five times more frequently than men, and the mean age of onset is between 45 and 55 years. These patients often have other autoimmune-mediated disorders (like type 1 diabetes or Sjögren syndrome). The thyroid function remains normal in about half of the cases.

Vitamin deficiency – induced ataxia

Deficiency in various vitamins may result in acquired ataxia, including vitamin B1, B12 and E. Lack of vitamin B1 is well established in WE and ACD (see above). Sensorimotor polyneuropathy and subacute combined degeneration of the spinal cord resulting in sensory ataxia should prompt an evaluation for vitamin B12 deficiency (including testing of vitamin B12, holotranscobalamine, homocysteine and methylmalonic acid levels), and if confirmed, long-term supplementation should be initiated (see (99) for recent review of treatment guidelines).

Malabsorption in gastrointestinal disease may result in acquired vitamin E deficiency, as seen e.g. in celiac disease and short-bowel syndrome. Clinically, ataxia of stance and gait, dysarthria and sensory neuropathy with loss of deep tendon reflexes are characteristic (100). Long-term intramuscular supplementation of vitamin E (100-200 mg daily) may stop further progression. Autosomal recessive ataxia syndromes with low vitamin E levels like AVED and ABL typically become symptomatic in early life, but must be included in the differential diagnosis, especially if the family history is positive for vitamin E deficiency.

Idiopathic cerebellar ataxias

Even with an extensive work-up including a search for hereditary or acquired causes, no specific diagnosis can be made in many patients with cerebellar ataxia (2). These patients are then assumed to suffer from an idiopathic degenerative cerebellar disorder; however, they may eventually develop MSA-C as the underlying cause. For those patients who do not fulfill the diagnostic criteria of MSA-C, the term 'sporadic adult-onset ataxia or SAOA' has been coined.

Multiple system atrophy of cerebellar type (MSA-C)

While most patients with cerebellar ataxia do not meet the criteria for MSA-C early on and will be classified as having SAOA, up to 30% will later develop MSA (101). The prevalence of MSA is about 4.4/100,000 and the mean age of onset is around 55 years, with rapid progression, severe disability and death within 10 years (102). In Europe, the cerebellar variant makes up only 20% of all MSA cases, while higher proportions (70%) are observed in Japan. Besides cerebellar ataxia, orthostatic dysregulation, pyramidal tract signs and Parkinsonian features are reported in MSA (103). On imaging, the 'hot-cross-bun sign' – referring to a characteristic pontine signal hyperintensity – may be helpful in the differential diagnosis along with olivopontocerebellar atrophy (see Figure 34.8). The response to levodopa is poor. For a more detailed description of MSA, see Chapter 19 of this book.

Sporadic adult-onset ataxia (SAOA)

SAOA is a diagnosis of exclusion. It is defined as a slowly progressive ataxia with disease onset af-

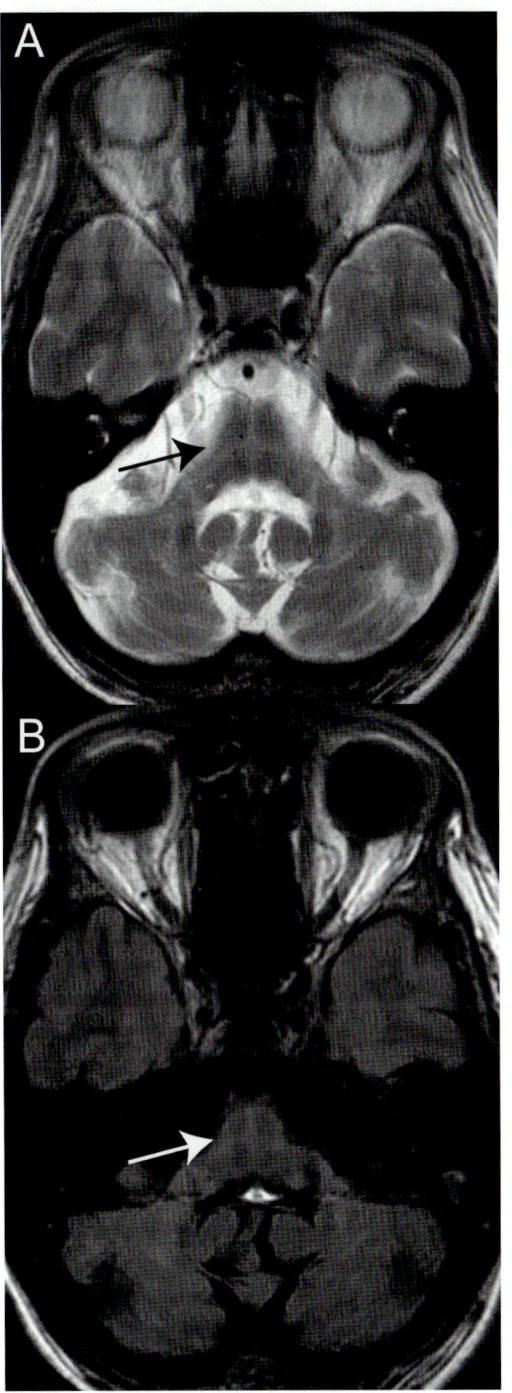

Figure 34.8
Axial MRIs in a 59-year-old female patient diagnosed with MSA illustrating the characteristic 'hot-cross-bun sign' both on T2-weighted (panel A) and FLAIR (panel B) sequences, as indicated by the arrow (courtesy of the Dept of Neuroradiology, University Hospital Zurich, Switzerland).

ter the age of 20 years and a lack of a causative gene mutation, symptomatic cause or possible/probable MSA-C according to diagnostic criteria. The onset of symptoms is around the age of 47 years in SAOA, and the life expectancy is almost normal. Estimates suggest that SAOA is about twice as frequent as MSA-C. The clinical course is more benign than in MSA-C as reflected in unimpaired walking rates of about 50% at 12 years after disease onset (2). Besides the dominant cerebellar signs, non-cerebellar abnormalities are often found, such as sensory neuropathy and extensor plantar responses. The essential difference from MSA-C is the continuing absence of severe autonomic failure in SAOA. In 2-22% of seemingly sporadic ataxia, an underlying genetic cause could be identified when applying a more in-depth examination (most frequently FRDA (5-8%) and SCA6) (11-13, 104). Therefore, in patients with a negative family history, molecular tests for FRDA, SCAs and FXTAS (only in men) are recommended if there is no evidence of an acquired ataxia or MSA-C (87). If the age of onset is already in the thirties, a more extensive investigation including genetic testing for ARCAs is needed. In most patients with SAOA, MRI of the brain reveals isolated cerebellar atrophy with little or no brainstem or spinal involvement (105) (see Figure 34.9 for a typical case of SAOA). Besides physical therapy with a focus on balance and gait, treatment with 4-aminopyridine or 3,4-diaminopyridine may improve the gait (106) and reduce oscillopsia due to downbeat nystagmus (107, 108) in patients with SAOA. Acetazolamide was found to be effective for EA2 (109) and SCA6 (27) and should also be evaluated in patients with SAOA.

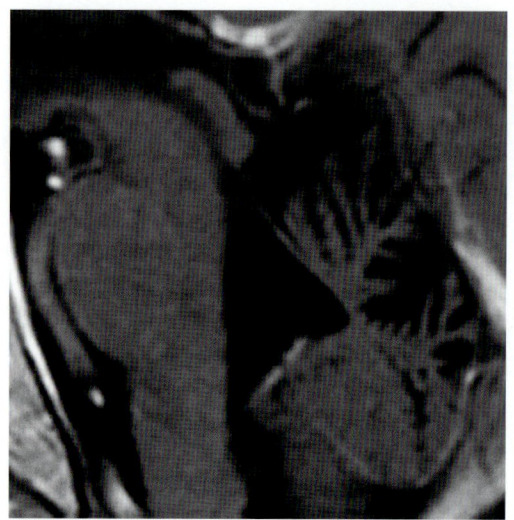

Figure 34.9
This 68-year-old female patient presented with a history of slowly progressive gait imbalance and episodic dizziness which started a few years ago. A family history for ataxia was negative. On clinical examination, her gait was ataxic, and ocular motor abnormalities (gaze-evoked nystagmus, downbeat nystagmus, saccadic smooth pursuit, impaired VOR-cancellation) were noted. MRI showed diffuse cerebellar atrophy, including the cerebellar vermis (mostly the anterior and cranial parts), while brainstem atrophy was very mild. A thorough evaluation for an acquired cause of ataxia including a laboratory work-up and whole-body FDG-PET remained negative, suggesting a possible sporadic adult-onset ataxia, although no genetic testing for late-onset hereditary cerebellar ataxia syndromes was performed due to lack of coverage by the health-insurance company. A treatment trial with 4-aminopyridine did not result in improvement of the ocular motor abnormalities or gait (courtesy of the Dept of Neuroradiology, University Hospital Zurich, Switzerland).

Sensory ataxia

Damage to the large-diameter sensory fibres or the central afferent tracts may result in a loss of proprioception and subsequent sensory ataxia. This includes lesions within the posterior (lemniscal) columns of the spinal cord and within the medial lemniscus while passing through the brainstem and thalamus, reaching the prima-ry somatosensory cortex. On clinical examination, loss of deep tendon reflexes in combination with reduced vibration and proprioception suggests large-fibre sensory neuropathy. Neuronopathies, i.e. degeneration primarily within the dorsal root ganglion cells, usually results in damage to both the peripheral nerves and the posterior columns, with the latter causing spasticity. Disorders presenting with sensory neuronopathy include paraneoplastic diseases, autoimmune-mediated ataxia syndromes like

Sjögren syndrome, CIDP, GBS or Miller-Fisher syndrome, toxic neuronopathies (secondary to pyridoxine deficiency/intoxication or chemotherapy with carboplatin, cisplatin or oxaloplatin) and FRDA amongst others.

Combined peripheral and central degeneration is found in vitamin B12 deficiency (with a focus on central myelinated fibres within the posterior and lateral columns of the spinal cord) and in copper deficiency. Sensory and cerebellar ataxia is usually also noticed in FRDA, AVED or acquired vitamin E deficiency while other ARCAs may present with predominantly sensory ataxia (SANDO). An in-depth review of sensory ataxia can be found elsewhere (110).

fragment, segment 3, shows a rebound nystagmus in the same patient, elicited after a prolonged (20 seconds) eccentric gaze. During this eccentric gaze (in darkness, looking at a briefly flashing red dot at 30 degrees eccentricity), a gaze-evoked nystagmus can be seen, although it lessens over time. Upon returning to the primary position, a strong drift towards the previous eccentric eye position followed by centripetal correction saccades (a so-called rebound nystagmus) can be appreciated. This phenomenon is thought to be the consequence of central compensation for the gaze-evoked nystagmus.

Acknowledgement

I would like to express my special thanks to Dominik Straumann, MD, for thoroughly reading and commenting on the manuscript.

Video fragment

Fragment 34.1

Nystagmus in cerebellar disorders

(segments 1-3)

In segment 1, a gaze-evoked nystagmus in a female patient presenting with cerebellar degeneration secondary to superficial siderosis is shown. Holding her eyes in an eccentric position (30 degrees to the left), her eyes drift slowly back to the primary position, which is then centrally compensated by an outwardly directed correction saccade. Note the absence of any downbeat nystagmus when looking eccentrically, and of any downbeat or rebound nystagmus after returning to the primary position. Segment 2 demonstrates a downbeat nystagmus in a young patient (aged 27 years) with presumably hereditary cerebellar degeneration. In the primary position his eyes drift slowly upwards, which is then followed by a downward correction saccades. The last

References

1 Anheim M, Tranchant C, Koenig M. The autosomal recessive cerebellar ataxias. N Engl J Med 2012;366:636-646.

2 Klockgether T. Sporadic ataxia with adult onset: classification and diagnostic criteria. Lancet Neurol 2010;9:94-104.

3 Brusse E, Maat-Kievit JA, van Swieten JC. Diagnosis and management of early- and late-onset cerebellar ataxia. Clin Genet 2007;71:12-24.

4 Finsterer J. Ataxias with autosomal, X-chromosomal or maternal inheritance. Can J Neurol Sci 2009;36:409-428.

5 Schmitz-Hubsch T, du Montcel ST, Baliko L, et al. Scale for the assessment and rating of ataxia: development of a new clinical scale. Neurology 2006;66:1717-1720.

6 Trouillas P, Takayanagi T, Hallett M, et al. International Cooperative Ataxia Rating Scale for pharmacological assessment of the cerebellar syndrome. The Ataxia Neuropharmacology Committee of the World Federation of Neurology. J Neurol Sci 1997;145:205-211.

7 De Michele G, Coppola G, Cocozza S, Filla A. A pathogenetic classification of hereditary ataxias: is the time ripe? J Neurol 2004;251:913-922.

8 Manto MU. The wide spectrum of spinocerebellar ataxias (SCAs). Cerebellum 2005;4:2-6.

9 Klockgether T. The clinical diagnosis of autosomal dominant spinocerebellar ataxias. Cerebellum 2008;7:101-105.

10 Koht J, Tallaksen CM. Cerebellar ataxia in the eastern and southern parts of Norway. Acta Neurol Scand 2007;187S:76-79.

11 Kerber KA, Jen JC, Perlman S, Baloh RW. Late-onset pure cerebellar ataxia: differentiating those with and without identifiable mutations. J Neurol Sci 2005;238:41-45.

12 Abele M, Burk K, Schols L, et al. The aetiology of sporadic adult-onset ataxia. Brain 2002;125:961-968.

13 Schols L, Szymanski S, Peters S, et al. Genetic background of apparently idiopathic sporadic cerebellar ataxia. Hum Genet 2000;107:132-137.

14 Ilg W, Brotz D, Burkard S, Giese MA, Schols L, Synofzik M. Long-term effects of coordinative training in degenerative cerebellar disease. Mov Disord 2010;25:2239-2246.

15 Durr A. Autosomal dominant cerebellar ataxias: polyglutamine expansions and beyond. Lancet Neurol 2010;9:885-894.

16 Harding AE. Classification of the hereditary ataxias and paraplegias. Lancet 1983;1:1151-1155.

17 Whaley NR, Fujioka S, Wszolek ZK. Autosomal dominant cerebellar ataxia type I: a review of the phenotypic and genotypic characteristics. Orphanet J Rare Dis 2011;6:33.

18 Fujioka S, Sundal C, Wszolek ZK. Autosomal dominant cerebellar ataxia type III: a review of the phenotypic and genotypic characteristics. Orphanet J Rare Dis 2013;8:14.

19 Hersheson J, Haworth A, Houlden H. The inherited ataxias: genetic heterogeneity, mutation databases, and future directions in research and clinical diagnostics. Hum Mutat 2012;33:1324-1332.

20 van de Warrenburg BP, Sinke RJ, Verschuuren-Bemelmans CC, et al. Spinocerebellar ataxias in the Netherlands: prevalence and age at onset variance analysis. Neurology 2002;58:702-708.

21 Globas C, du Montcel ST, Baliko L, et al. Early symptoms in spinocerebellar ataxia type 1, 2, 3, and 6. Mov Disord 2008;23:2232-2238.

22 Ikeuchi T, Koide R, Tanaka H, et al. Dentatorubral-pallidoluysian atrophy: clinical features are closely related to unstable expansions of trinucleotide (CAG) repeat. Ann Neurol 1995;37:769-775.

23 Rivaud-Pechoux S, Durr A, Gaymard B, et al. Eye movement abnormalities correlate with genotype in autosomal dominant cerebellar ataxia type I. Ann Neurol 1998;43:297-302.

24 Parker JL, Santiago M. Oculomotor aspects of the hereditary cerebellar ataxias. Handb Clin Neurol 2012;103:63-83.

25 Matilla-Duenas A, Corral-Juan M, Volpini V, Sanchez I. The spinocerebellar ataxias: clinical aspects and molecular genetics. Adv Exp Med Biol 2012;724:351-374.

26 Eichler L, Bellenberg B, Hahn HK, Koster O, Schols L, Lukas C. Quantitative assessment of brain stem and cerebellar atrophy in spinocerebellar ataxia types 3 and 6: impact on clinical status. AJNR Am J Neuroradiol 2011;32:890-897.

27 Yabe I, Sasaki H, Yamashita I, Takei A, Tashiro K. Clinical trial of acetazolamide in SCA6, with assessment using the Ataxia Rating Scale and body stabilometry. Acta Neurol Scand 2001;104:44-47.

28 Tsunemi T, Ishikawa K, Tsukui K, Sumi T, Kitamura K, Mizusawa H. The effect of 3,4-diaminopyridine on the patients with hereditary pure cerebellar ataxia. J Neurol Sci 2010;292:81-84.

29 Jen JC, Graves TD, Hess EJ, Hanna MG, Griggs RC, Baloh RW. Primary episodic ataxias: diagnosis, pathogenesis and treatment. Brain 2007;130:2484-2493.

30 Tsuji S. Dentatorubral-pallidoluysian atrophy. Handb Clin Neurol 2012;103:587-594.

31 Cossee M, Schmitt M, Campuzano V, et al. Evolution of the Friedreich's ataxia trinucleotide repeat expansion: founder effect and premutations. Proc Natl Acad Sci USA 1997;94:7452-7457.

32 Campuzano V, Montermini L, Molto MD, et al. Friedreich's ataxia: autosomal recessive disease caused by an intronic GAA triplet repeat expansion. Science 1996;271:1423-1427.

33 Di Donato S, Gellera C, Mariotti C. The complex clinical and genetic classification of inherited ataxias. II. Autosomal recessive ataxias. Neurol Sci 2001;22:219-228.

34 Bhidayasiri R, Perlman SL, Pulst SM, Geschwind DH. Late-onset Friedreich ataxia: phenotypic analy-

sis, magnetic resonance imaging findings, and review of the literature. Arch Neurol 2005;62:1865-1869.

35 Della Nave R, Ginestroni A, Tessa C, et al. Brain white matter tracts degeneration in Friedreich ataxia. An in vivo MRI study using tract-based spatial statistics and voxel-based morphometry. Neuroimage 2008;40:19-25.

36 Hart PE, Lodi R, Rajagopalan B, et al. Antioxidant treatment of patients with Friedreich ataxia: four-year follow-up. Arch Neurol 2005;62:621-626.

37 Buyse G, Mertens L, Di Salvo G, et al. Idebenone treatment in Friedreich's ataxia: neurological, cardiac, and biochemical monitoring. Neurology 2003;60:1679-1681.

38 Rustin P, von Kleist-Retzow JC, Chantrel-Groussard K, Sidi D, Munnich A, Rotig A. Effect of idebenone on cardiomyopathy in Friedreich's ataxia: a preliminary study. Lancet 1999;354:477-479.

39 Mariotti C, Solari A, Torta D, Marano L, Fiorentini C, Di Donato S. Idebenone treatment in Friedreich patients: one-year-long randomized placebo-controlled trial. Neurology 2003;60:1676-1679.

40 Artuch R, Aracil A, Mas A, et al. Friedreich's ataxia: idebenone treatment in early stage patients. Neuropediatrics 2002;33:190-193.

41 Di Prospero NA, Baker A, Jeffries N, Fischbeck KH. Neurological effects of high-dose idebenone in patients with Friedreich's ataxia: a randomised, placebo-controlled trial. Lancet Neurol 2007;6:878-886.

42 Lynch DR, Perlman SL, Meier T. A phase 3, double-blind, placebo-controlled trial of idebenone in friedreich ataxia. Arch Neurol 2010;67:941-947.

43 Peterson PL, Saad J, Nigro MA. The treatment of Friedreich's ataxia with amantadine hydrochloride. Neurology 1988;38:1478-1480.

44 Botez MI, Young SN, Rotez T, Courchesne Y. Treatment of Friedreich's ataxia with amantadine. Neurology 1989;39:749-750.

45 Finsterer J. Inherited mitochondrial disorders. Adv Exp Med Biol 2012;942:187-213.

46 Ouahchi K, Arita M, Kayden H, et al. Ataxia with isolated vitamin E deficiency is caused by mutations in the alpha-tocopherol transfer protein. Nat Genet 1995;9:141-145.

47 Cavalier L, Ouahchi K, Kayden HJ, et al. Ataxia with isolated vitamin E deficiency: heterogeneity of mutations and phenotypic variability in a large number of families. Am J Hum Genet 1998;62:301-310.

48 Benomar A, Yahyaoui M, Meggouh F, et al. Clinical comparison between AVED patients with 744 del A mutation and Friedreich ataxia with GAA expansion in 15 Moroccan families. J Neurol Sci 2002;198:25-29.

49 Marzouki N, Benomar A, Yahyaoui M, et al. Vitamin E deficiency ataxia with (744 del A) mutation on alpha-TTP gene: genetic and clinical peculiarities in Moroccan patients. Eur J Med Genet 2005;48:21-28.

50 Gabsi S, Gouider-Khouja N, Belal S, et al. Effect of vitamin E supplementation in patients with ataxia with vitamin E deficiency. Eur J Neurol 2001;8:477-481.

51 Narcisi TM, Shoulders CC, Chester SA, et al. Mutations of the microsomal triglyceride-transfer-protein gene in abetalipoproteinemia. Am J Hum Genet 1995;57:1298-1310.

52 Weinstein R. Phytanic acid storage disease (Refsum's disease): clinical characteristics, pathophysiology and the role of therapeutic apheresis in its management. J Clin Apher 1999;14:181-184.

53 Wills AJ, Manning NJ, Reilly MM. Refsum's disease. Qjm 2001;94:403-406.

54 Verrips A, Hoefsloot LH, Steenbergen GC, et al. Clinical and molecular genetic characteristics of patients with cerebrotendinous xanthomatosis. Brain 2000;123:908 919.

55 Verhagen MM, Abdo WF, Willemsen MA, et al. Clinical spectrum of ataxia-telangiectasia in adulthood. Neurology 2009;73:430-437.

56 Shaikh AG, Marti S, Tarnutzer AA, et al. Effects of 4-aminopyridine on nystagmus and vestibulo-ocular reflex in ataxia-telangiectasia. J Neurol 2013; Epub ahead of print

57 Savitsky K, Bar-Shira A, Gilad S, et al. A single ataxia telangiectasia gene with a product similar to PI-3 kinase. Science 1995;268:1749-1753.

58 Habek M, Brinar VV, Rados M, Zadro I, Zarkovic K. Brain MRI abnormalities in ataxia-telangiectasia. Neurologist 2008;14:192-195.

59 Le Ber I, Moreira MC, Rivaud-Pechoux S, et al. Cerebellar ataxia with oculomotor apraxia type 1: clinical and genetic studies. Brain 2003;126:2761-2772.

60 Moreira MC, Klur S, Watanabe M, et al. Senataxin, the ortholog of a yeast RNA helicase, is mutant in ataxia-ocular apraxia 2. Nat Genet 2004;36:225-227.

61 Le Ber I, Bouslam N, Rivaud-Pechoux S, et al. Frequency and phenotypic spectrum of ataxia with oculomotor apraxia 2: a clinical and genetic study in 18 patients. Brain 2004;127:759-767.

62 Date H, Onodera O, Tanaka H, et al. Early-onset ataxia with ocular motor apraxia and hypoalbuminemia is caused by mutations in a new HIT superfamily gene. Nat Genet 2001;29:184-188.

63 Takashima H, Boerkoel CF, John J, et al. Mutation of TDP1, encoding a topoisomerase I-dependent DNA damage repair enzyme, in spinocerebellar ataxia with axonal neuropathy. Nat Genet 2002;32:267-272.

64 Senderek J, Krieger M, Stendel C, et al. Mutations in SIL1 cause Marinesco-Sjogren syndrome, a cerebellar ataxia with cataract and myopathy. Nat Genet 2005;37:1312-1314.

65 Bouchard JP, Richter A, Mathieu J, et al. Autosomal recessive spastic ataxia of Charlevoix-Saguenay. Neuromuscul Disord 1998;8:474-479.

66 Szmulewicz DJ, Waterston JA, Halmagyi GM, et al. Sensory neuropathy as part of the cerebellar ataxia neuropathy vestibular areflexia syndrome. Neurology 2011;76:1903-1910.

67 Hagerman R, Hagerman P. Advances in clinical and molecular understanding of the FMR1 premutation and fragile X-associated tremor/ataxia syndrome. Lancet Neurol 2013;12:786-798.

68 Berry-Kravis E, Abrams L, Coffey SM, et al. Fragile X-associated tremor/ataxia syndrome: clinical features, genetics, and testing guidelines. Mov Disord 2007;22:2018-2030, quiz 140.

69 Apartis E, Blancher A, Meissner WG, et al. FXTAS: new insights and the need for revised diagnostic criteria. Neurology 2012;79:1898-1907.

70 Brunberg JA, Jacquemont S, Hagerman RJ, et al. Fragile X premutation carriers: characteristic MR imaging findings of adult male patients with progressive cerebellar and cognitive dysfunction. Am J Neuroradiol 2002;23:1757-1766.

71 Leehey MA, Hagerman PJ. Fragile X-associated tremor/ataxia syndrome. Handb Clin Neurol 2012;103:373-386.

72 Kamm C, Healy DG, Quinn NP, et al. The fragile X tremor ataxia syndrome in the differential diagnosis of multiple system atrophy: data from the EMSA Study Group. Brain 2005;128:1855-1860.

73 Roberts JE, Bailey DB, Jr., Mankowski J, et al. Mood and anxiety disorders in females with the FMR1 premutation. Am J Med Genet B Neuropsychiatr Genet 2009;150B:130-139.

74 Hadjivassiliou M. Immune-mediated acquired ataxias. Handb Clin Neurol 2012;103:189-199.

75 Sechi G, Serra A. Wernicke's encephalopathy: new clinical settings and recent advances in diagnosis and management. Lancet Neurol 2007;6:442-455.

76 Singh S, Kumar A. Wernicke encephalopathy after obesity surgery: a systematic review. Neurology 2007;68:807-811.

77 Galvin R, Brathen G, Ivashynka A, Hillbom M, Tanasescu R, Leone MA. EFNS guidelines for diagnosis, therapy and prevention of Wernicke encephalopathy. Eur J Neurol 2010;17:1408-1418.

78 Maschke M, Weber J, Bonnet U, et al. Vermal atrophy of alcoholics correlate with serum thiamine levels but not with dentate iron concentrations as estimated by MRI. J Neurol 2005;252:704-711.

79 Hillbom M, Muuronen A, Holm L, Hindmarsh T. The clinical versus radiological diagnosis of alcoholic cerebellar degeneration. J Neurol Sci 1986;73:45-53.

80 Posti JP, Juvela S, Parkkola R, Roine S. Three cases of superficial siderosis of the central nervous system and review of the literature. Acta Neurochir 2011;153:2067-2073.

81 Kumar N. Neuroimaging in superficial siderosis: an in-depth look. AJNR Am J Neuroradiol 2010;31:5-14.

82 Schneider T, Moos V, Loddenkemper C, Marth T, Fenollar F, Raoult D. Whipple's disease: new aspects of pathogenesis and treatment. Lancet Infect Dis 2008;8:179-190.

83 Zerr I, Kallenberg K, Summers DM, et al. Updated clinical diagnostic criteria for sporadic Creutzfeldt-Jakob disease. Brain 2009;132:2659-2668.

84 Meissner B, Kallenberg K, Sanchez-Juan P, et al. MRI lesion profiles in sporadic Creutzfeldt-Jakob disease. Neurology 2009;72:1994-2001.

85 Graus F, Delattre JY, Antoine JC, et al. Recommended diagnostic criteria for paraneoplastic neurological syndromes. J Neurol Neurosurg Psychiatry 2004;75:1135-1140.

86 Shams'ili S, Grefkens J, de Leeuw B, et al. Paraneoplastic cerebellar degeneration associated with antineuronal antibodies: analysis of 50 patients. Brain 2003;126:1409-1418.

87 Klockgether T. Parkinsonism & related disorders. Ataxias. Parkinsonism Relat Disord 2007;13S3:391-394.

88 Titulaer MJ, Soffietti R, Dalmau J, et al. Screening for tumours in paraneoplastic syndromes: report of an EFNS task force. Eur J Neurol 2011;18:19-e3.

89 Dalmau J, Rosenfeld MR. Paraneoplastic syndromes of the CNS. Lancet Neurol 2008;7:327-340.

90 Hadjivassiliou M, Grunewald RA, Chattopadhyay AK,et al. Clinical, radiological, neurophysiological, and neuropathological characteristics of gluten ataxia. Lancet 1998;352:1582-1585.

91 Pellecchia MT, Scala R, Filla A, De Michele G, Ciacci C, Barone P. Idiopathic cerebellar ataxia associated with celiac disease: lack of distinctive neurological features. J Neurol Neurosurg Psychiatry 1999;66:32-35.

92 Bushara KO, Goebel SU, Shill H, Goldfarb LG, Hallett M. Gluten sensitivity in sporadic and hereditary cerebellar ataxia. Ann Neurol 2001;49:540-543.

93 Abele M, Schols L, Schwartz S, Klockgether T. Prevalence of antigliadin antibodies in ataxia patients. Neurology 2003;60:1674-1675.

94 Bushara KO. Neurologic presentation of celiac disease. Gastroenterology 2005;128:S92-97.

95 Honnorat J, Saiz A, Giometto B, et al. Cerebellar ataxia with anti-glutamic acid decarboxylase antibodies: study of 14 patients. Arch Neurol 2001;58:225-230.

96 Hadjivassiliou M, Williamson CA, Woodroofe N. The immunology of gluten sensitivity: beyond the gut. Trends Immunol 2004;25:578-582.

97 Castillo P, Woodruff B, Caselli R, et al. Steroid-responsive encephalopathy associated with autoimmune thyroiditis. Arch Neurol 2006;63:197-202.

98 Seipelt M, Zerr I, Nau R, et al. Hashimoto's encephalitis as a differential diagnosis of Creutzfeldt-Jakob disease. J Neurol Neurosurg Psychiatry 1999;66:172-176.

99 Stabler SP. Clinical practice. Vitamin B12 deficiency. N Engl J Med 2013;368:149-160.

100 Harding AE, Muller DP, Thomas PK, Willison HJ. Spinocerebellar degeneration secondary to chronic intestinal malabsorption: a vitamin E deficiency syndrome. Ann Neurol 1982;12:419-424.

101 Gilman S, Little R, Johanns J, et al. Evolution of sporadic olivopontocerebellar atrophy into multiple system atrophy. Neurology 2000;55:527-532.

102 Schrag A, Ben-Shlomo Y, Quinn NP. Prevalence of progressive supranuclear palsy and multiple system atrophy: a cross-sectional study. Lancet 1999;354:1771-1775.

103 Stefanova N, Bucke P, Duerr S, Wenning GK. Multiple system atrophy: an update. Lancet Neurol 2009;8:1172-1178.

104 Moseley ML, Benzow KA, Schut LJ, et al. Incidence of dominant spinocerebellar and Friedreich triplet repeats among 361 ataxia families. Neurology 1998;51:1666-1671.

105 Abele M, Minnerop M, Urbach H, Specht K, Klockgether T. Sporadic adult onset ataxia of unknown etiology : a clinical, electrophysiological and imaging study. J Neurol 2007;254:1384-1389.

106 Schniepp R, Wuehr M, Neuhaeusser M, et al. 4-aminopyridine and cerebellar gait: a retrospective case series. J Neurol 2012;259:2491-2493.

107 Sprenger A, Rambold H, Sander T, et al. Treatment of the gravity dependence of downbeat nystagmus with 3,4-diaminopyridine. Neurology 2006;67:905-907.

108 Claassen J, Spiegel R, Kalla R, et al. A randomised double-blind, cross-over trial of 4-aminopyridine for downbeat nystagmus--effects on slowphase eye velocity, postural stability, locomotion and symptoms. J Neurol Neurosurg Psychiatry 2013; Epub ahead of print.

109 Griggs RC, Moxley RT, 3rd, Lafrance RA, McQuillen J. Hereditary paroxysmal ataxia: response to acetazolamide. Neurology 1978;28:1259-1264.

110 Riggins S, England JD. Ataxias related to sensory neuropathies. Handb Clin Neurol 2012;103:605-617.

PART V

Behavioural Motor Disorders

35

REM Sleep Behaviour Disorder

Ronald B. Postuma

Rapid eye movement (REM) sleep behaviour disorder is characterized by loss of the normal atonia that accompanies REM sleep (1). As a result, dream content is acted out; patients can talk, yell, thrash or punch in apparent response to the content of their dreams. REM sleep behaviour disorder (RBD) can be primary (termed idiopathic) or secondary (accompanied by other conditions). The most prominent association in secondary RBD is with neurodegenerative synucleinopathies, namely Parkinson's disease (PD), multiple system atrophy (MSA) and dementia with Lewy bodies (DLB).

Epidemiology

The prevalence of idiopathic RBD remains unclear. There have been two prevalence studies that screened for RBD in the general population, and then confirmed it with polysomnography (PSG) (2,3). They estimated a prevalence of 0.4-0.5%. However, they screened for sleep-related injury, and so they may have identified only severe cases; milder cases may be much more common. A recent population-based study found that approximately 6% of elderly subjects endorsed probable RBD (4); however, without PSG confirmation of this cohort, the true prevalence remains unclear. Most patients with idiopathic RBD are male, and most over 50 years old. The reasons for this demographic distribution remain unclear; the demographics do mimic Parkinson's disease (PD), which also occurs predominantly in male and older patients. However, selection biases due to prominent inclusion of aggressiveness of dream content or awareness/availability of spouses could explain some of the residual differences in the present studies. Of note, RBD is not clearly more predominant in men than women among PD patients (5,6).

Etiology

Idiopathic RBD

Risk factors for idiopathic RBD have not yet been fully established. A recent case-control study of 347 idiopathic RBD patients and 347 controls found that many factors for idiopathic RBD were similar to those for PD, in particular head trauma, farming, and pesticide use (7). Low level of education, a known risk factor for dementia, was also a risk factor for RBD. Patients with RBD were more likely to report a family history of dream enactment behaviour than controls, suggesting a possible genetic component (8). Of note, two extremely well-established risk factors for PD, caffeine non-use and non-smoking, were not associated with idiopathic RBD. In fact, the smoking relationship was the opposite; smoking was a risk factor for RBD. This may have implications for our understanding of the mechanism of action of these substances: if caffeine and nicotine 'prevent' clinical PD but do not prevent its prodromal syndrome, it may be that caffeine and nicotine act directly upon the substantia nigra and not on all regions prone to synucleinopathy. Studies measuring medication use and co-morbidities as risk factors for RBD are pending.

Secondary RBD

The most common secondary forms of RBD are related to synucleinopathies. Within PD, RBD is a relatively common manifestation. Although estimates vary, it appears that between 30-50% of PD patients have clinical RBD on cross-sectional analysis, with an additional 10-30% having asymptomatic REM atonia (5,9,10). There have been fewer studies of the prevalence of RBD in multiple system atrophy (MSA), although estimates as high as 100% (19/19) have been reported (11). One recent study documented that 76% of autopsy-confirmed dementia with Lewy bodies (DLB) patients had a history of dream-enactment behaviour (12).

Although the most prominent association in secondary RBD is with neurodegenerative synucleinopathies, RBD has also been associated with a wide array of other conditions, including narcolepsy, progressive supranuclear palsy, the Guam PD-dementia-amyotrophic lateral sclerosis (ALS) complex, spinocerebellar ataxias (particularly Type III), limbic encephalitis secondary to voltage-gated potassium channels, Guillain Barré syndrome, etc. (13). Most but not all of these conditions involve degeneration or damage to lower brainstem structures. RBD has also been reported as a side effect of medications, most notably antidepressants. Nearly all antidepressants, with the exception of bupropion, may cause this syndrome.

Pathophysiology

The essential anatomical structures for the normal generation of RBD atonia are mainly located in the lower pons and medulla (14-16). Of particular importance is the peri-locus ceruleus area (equivalent to the sublaterodorsal nucleus in rats). Neurons in this area consist of a flip-flop switch that, when activated, induce REM atonia by directly innervating spinal interneurons. They may also send an indirect pathway to the ventral gigantocellular nucleus in the medulla, which in turn sends inhibitory GABAergic innervation to spinal motor interneurons. According to the Braak staging system of PD, these lower brainstem neurons are predicted to be involved in Stage II disease before motor involvement (17); this therefore provides a pathologic substrate by which RBD can precede clinical synucleinopathies.

In general, duration of REM sleep, proportion of other sleep stages, and sleep efficiency are relatively preserved in idiopathic RBD, suggesting a specific loss of REM atonia neuronal groups. Hypocretin (orexin) neurons may also be important in some cases, as evidenced by the association between narcolepsy and RBD. In this case, RBD may be one manifestation of the generalized sleep-stage instability seen in narcolepsy. Hypocretin loss may also explain the link between RBD and Guillain-Barré syndrome, as RBD occurred mainly in those who also had a narcolepsy phenotype (18).

In addition, the limbic cortex may be important in the pathogenesis, as RBD has been linked to voltage-gated potassium-channel encephalitis without MRI evidence of brainstem involvement (19). Serotonergic neurons are also likely to be important in the generation of RBD, especially given the well-recognized propensity of antidepressants to trigger RBD. This may be related either to persistence of serotonergic activation of motor neurons (which is normally reduced during sleep) or to the cholinergic effects of some antidepressants (which may inactivate cholinergic nuclei that generate REM atonia) (14).

Clinical presentation

Typically, patients with RBD report apparent dream enactment behaviour. Idiopathic RBD can be dramatic and dangerous, which explains why patients have sought medical attention. However, screening for RBD in neurodegenerative disease often discloses much less dramatic manifestations, such as occasional sleep talking or minor motor movements, suggesting that many undiagnosed mild cases of idiopathic RBD exist in the community. It should also be noted that transitory myoclonic movements or even brief episodes of more complex movement can occasionally be seen in normal individuals, which is why documentation of REM atonia loss is essential (see diagnosis below). Eyes are typically closed during episodes, and there may be a spe-

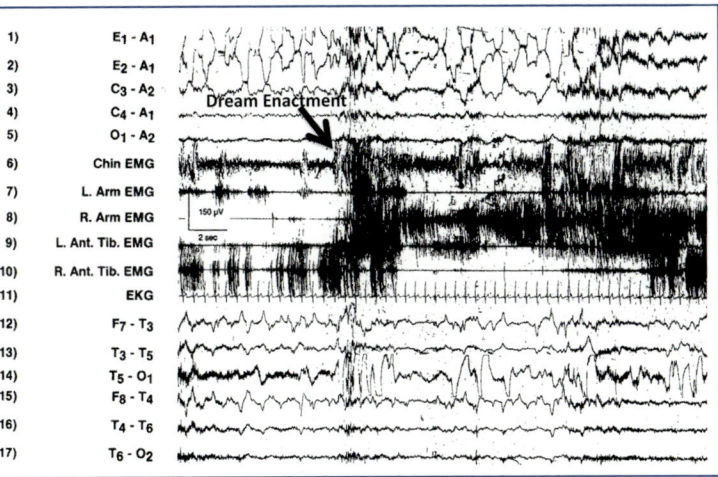

Figure 35.1 Diagnosis of RBD by Polysomnography.
Polysomnogram of RBD patient during REM sleep – baseline complete REM atonia loss is followed by full dream enactment, visible on all EMG leads.

cific 'motor signature' of RBD that is characterized by a slight dyscoordination/jerky character of movements, with a limp posture of the hand (14). Of note, movements can be rapid even in patients with advanced parkinsonism who are incapable of performing these movements during wakefulness (20). This is true even for MSA, which is typically not responsive to deep brain stimulation procedures; whether this may signal a potential, still-undiscovered surgical target remains unclear.

Diagnosis

According to the international classification of sleep disorders (ICSD) criteria, RBD diagnosis requires documentation of two features:

1 Loss of REM atonia during REM sleep, and
2 Clinical history of dream enactment or documentation of abnormal REM movements on polysomnogram (21).

Therefore, the gold standard diagnosis for RBD requires a polysomnogram (PSG). The ICSD criteria do not explicitly define how loss of REM atonia should be documented, though, and during REM sleep, even normal subjects will

demonstrate phasic twitching or even occasional epochs with increased tonic REM. Therefore, the diagnosis of RBD can be a challenge (see Figure 35.1), and various models have been suggested to define significant REM atonia loss (22, 23). Now, consensus is emerging that the presence of any tone (phasic and tonic combined) for >30% of the REM period can be used as a cutoff for abnormal tone. Most centers use the musculus mentalis as part of the standard montage, and this can provide reasonably good sensitivity; however, sensitivity probably will improve if musculus flexor digitorum superficialis is added to the montage (23).

In an effort to simplify diagnostic procedures, numerous screening questionnaires for RBD have been developed. The first, the 14-item Stiasny-Kolster RBD screening questionnaire, obtained 96% sensitivity for screening idiopathic RBD, but only 56% specificity when using sleep center patients as controls (specificity was 92% when using normal volunteers as a control group) (24). With PD patients, sensitivity and specificity may be better; one study of the Japanese version obtained 84% sensitivity and 96% specificity (25). The 13-item RBD-HK scale has

Mayo Sleep Questionnaire-*Informant*

Do you live with the patient? ☐ Yes ☐ No (If No, END FORM HERE)

Do you sleep in the same room as the patient? ☐ Yes ☐ No

If no, is it because of his/her sleep behaviors (i.e. snores too loud, acts out dreams, etc.)? ☐ Yes ☐ No

Please mark "Yes" if the described event has occurred at least 3 times.

1. Have you ever seen the patient appear to "act out his/her dreams" while sleeping? (punched or flailed arms in the air, shouted or screamed)

    ☐ 0 no
    ☐ 1 yes

    - **If Yes,**

      a. How many months or years has this been going on?

          ☐☐ year(s)
          ☐☐ months

      b. Has the patient ever been injured from these behaviors (bruises, cuts, broken bones?

          ☐ No
          ☐ Yes

      c. Has a bedpartner ever been injured from these behaviors (bruises, blows, pulled hair)?

          ☐ No
          ☐ Yes
          ☐ No bedpartner

      d. Has the patient told you about dreams of being chased, attacked or that involve defending himself/herself?

          ☐ No
          ☐ Yes
          ☐ Never told you about dreams

      e. If the patient woke up and told you about a dream, did the details of the dream match the movements made while sleeping?

          ☐ No
          ☐ Yes
          ☐ Never told you about dreams

2. Do the patient's legs repeatedly jerk or twitch during sleep (not just when falling asleep)?

    ☐ No
    ☐ Yes

3. Does the patient complain of a restless, nervous, tingly, or creepy-crawly feeling in his/her legs that disrupts his/her ability to fall or stay asleep?

    ☐ No
    ☐ Yes

    - **If Yes,**

      a. Does the patient tell you that these leg sensations decrease when he/she moves them or walks around?

          ☐ No
          ☐ Yes

      b. When do these sensations seem to be the worst?

          ☐ before 6 pm
          ☐ after 6 pm

4. Has the patient ever walked around the bedroom or house while asleep?

    ☐ No
    ☐ Yes

5. Has the patient ever snorted or choked him/herself awake?

    ☐ No
    ☐ Yes

6. Does the patient ever seem to stop breathing during sleep?

    ☐ No
    ☐ Yes

    - **If Yes,**

      a. Is the patient currently being treated for this (e.g., CPAP)?

          ☐ No
          ☐ Yes

7. Does the patient have leg cramps at night? (e.g., also called a "charlie horse" with intense pain in certain muscles in the leg)?

    ☐ No
    ☐ Yes

8. Rate the patient's general level of alertness for the past 3 weeks on a scale from 0 to 10.

    0   1   2   3   4   5   6   7   8   9   10
    Sleep   Fully &
    all day   normally
                                                       awake

Figure 35.2
The Mayo sleep questionnaire.

simply, suggesting that simpler screens could be used. A single question of dream enactment from the Mayo sleep questionnaire (the first question) asked of bed partners was able to detect RBD with 98% sensitivity and 74% specificity (26) (see Figure 35.2). A very similar question, the RBD single question (RBD1Q), was recently tested in 242 idiopathic RBD patients and controls and was found to have 94% sensitivity and 87% specificity (27). It is free for clinical or research use, has been translated into 8 languages, and consists of the following question:

> Have you ever been told, or suspected yourself, that you seem to 'act out your dreams' while asleep (for example, punching, flailing your arms in the air, making running movements, etc.)!

Given that questionnaires can obtain up to 90% sensitivity and specificity, is PSG still required for the diagnosis of RBD in clinical care? The answer to this question depends very much on the clinical context, patterns of health care utilization, availability of PSG, etc. In the authors' personal view, the answer hinges upon the pre-test probability in different clinical situations. In PD itself, with an

demonstrated 82% sensitivity and 87% specificity using predominantly sleep-center controls; this scale has the advantage of grading severity of dream enactment, and therefore may serve as the severity scale in clinical trials. One practical limitation of these scales is their length (≥13 questions each). Yet RBD can be summarized quite

approximately 50% baseline likelihood of having RBD, a questionnaire specificity of 90% translates into a 90% chance of having RBD. In this case, it may be prudent in a clinical setting to treat empirically (assuming symptoms are severe enough to warrant treatment), and follow-up with PSG if the response is atypical or further problems arise. The situation is different in idiopathic RBD. If one were to assume a 2% prevalence of RBD, using a test with 90% specificity would translate into a positive predictive value of only 18%, which is clearly insufficient for the clinical diagnosis. In addition, the diagnosis of idiopathic RBD has much more profound implications than a diagnosis of RBD in PD; a diagnosis of idiopathic RBD indicates for the first time a very high risk of developing a serious neurological disease, whereas diagnosis in PD identifies a single manifestation of already established disease. This implies that the clinical diagnosis of idiopathic RBD probably necessitates PSG confirmation.

Beyond the diagnosis of RBD itself, there is increasing recognition that documenting RBD in neurodegenerative disease can improve the accuracy of the clinical diagnosis. Whereas RBD can occur in diverse syndromes, it is abundantly clear that the large majority of cases of secondary RBD have an underlying synucleinopathy. In a recent comprehensive autopsy study, Boeve et al. found that 94% of autopsy samples from patients with both neurodegenerative disease and a clinical history of RBD had synuclein deposition on pathological examination (28). When the analysis was restricted to PSG-confirmed cases (i.e. a higher standard of evidence, removing potential false-positive RBD diagnoses), this proportion increased to 98%. Of note, despite the fact that Alzheimer's disease is at least 4 times more common than DLB and PD combined, only 1/82 autopsy cases had pure Alzheimer's disease without synuclein deposition. A second paper, restricted to samples from the Mayo Clinic, demonstrated that not only did RBD increase the sensitivity for DLB diagnosis, but defining DLB based upon

the presence of RBD alone actually provided better diagnostic accuracy than all of the remaining clinical DLB consensus criteria features combined (12). Moreover, with DLB, the presence of RBD is associated with more classic features of the disease and a 'purer' synuclein pathology (i.e. fewer alternate pathologies such as amyloid deposition) (29). *This suggests that among dementia patients, RBD is such a strong sign of DLB that it essentially suffices to make a clinical diagnosis.* Among patients with parkinsonism, the diagnostic utility is less clear, but RBD can be considered a relative indication of PD or MSA rather than PSP or vascular parkinsonism.

Differential Diagnosis

The main differential diagnoses of RBD are nonREM parasomnias, obstructive sleep apnea, and epilepsy.

Non-REM parasomnias

NonREM parasomnias are relatively common and generally occur upon arousal from slow wave sleep. Although manifestations can overlap, the clinical history can usually distinguish the two conditions. NonREM parasomnias often occur in younger patients and manifest predominantly in the first half of the night; many patients have a family history (although some cases of nonREM parasomnia can occur late in life, particularly as a component of parasomnia overlap disorder). Critically, RBD patients rarely interact with their environment unless it is in their immediate vicinity, whereas nonREM parasomnia patients may walk to or reach out and handle objects or people. NonREM parasomnia patients can engage in an often-confused conversation, which is a rare feature of RBD. RBD patients may respond to conversation, but generally only after they waken, in which case conversation is generally relatively normal. Unlike nonREM parasomnia patients, RBD patients almost never walk during episodes. Whereas nonREM parasomnias have gradual offset (often terminated by returning to sleep), RBD patients usually emerge suddenly from an episode when wakened, with relatively normal alertness. Whereas sleep talking is common in both conditions, the presence of prolonged screaming or yelling, long conversation episodes without interaction with the bed partner, and a characteristic 'one-half of a conversation' are features more associated with RBD.

Obstructive sleep apnea

The ability of obstructive sleep apnea to mimic symptoms of RBD is well documented (Iranzo and Santamaria, 2005). In many cases, this represents a form of 'confusional arousal', in which patients waken from an apneic episode, often hypoxic or with some sleep inertia, and act in ways that can resemble RBD. Note that documentation of obstructive apnea need not rule out the diagnosis of RBD; many patients can have co-existing apnea and RBD, and will then continue to have dream enactment even with successful use of CPAP.

Epilepsy

Nocturnal epilepsy (particularly frontal lobe seizures) can occasionally cause symptoms suggestive of RBD; for this reason, in the ICSD criteria, idiopathic RBD cannot be definitively diagnosed in the presence of epileptiform activity on the EEG.

Treatment

So far, there has been no definitive, randomized, controlled trial evidence clearly documenting the benefit of any treatment for RBD. Nevertheless, observational studies and one small randomized trial have identified two medications of particular utility: clonazepam and melatonin.

Clonazepam

Clonazepam was the first medication described as effective for RBD. Initial reports found that it helped up to 90% of patients (1). In a recent, sys-

tematic, observational study, clonazepam treatment was associated with a moderate or greater improvement in 78% of patients, with a mean reduction of 2.4 points on a visual analogue scale (30). The mechanism of action of clonazepam is unclear. It appears to have no effect on tonic REM, but may reduce phasic EMG activity and aggressiveness of dream content (1). Doses can be started at 0.5 mg at h.s. and increased to a maximum of approximately 2 mg. As a long-acting benzodiazepine, clonazepam has the potential to cause daytime somnolence, cognitive impairment, and falls. Therefore, it should be used with caution in vulnerable populations.

Melatonin

The second major option of treatment of RBD is melatonin. Although the mechanism of action is not fully defined, melatonin appears to directly increase the proportion of atonic REM. Dosing typically starts with 3 mg and can be increased to 6 or 9 mg if partially effective. Early reports of effectiveness demonstrated efficacy in up to 80%, with a possibly slightly lowered efficacy compared to clonazepam. In the same observational study cited above, melatonin provided moderate or greater improvement in 48% (i.e. lower than clonazepam), but with a mean reduction in the visual analogue scale similar to clonazepam (i.e. 2.5). The effectiveness of melatonin was also confirmed in a small, preliminary, randomized controlled trial (31). Side effects can include daytime sedation and depression, particularly in individuals with cognitive impairment. Melatonin may have less cognitive or gait side effects than clonazepam; 61% of patients on clonazepam reported side effects compared to 33% of those on melatonin, with significant differences in the occurrence of unsteadiness (39% vs. 14%) and dizziness (22% vs. 4%). Therefore, it may be the treatment of initial choice in patients prone to these side effects.

Other strategies

Other treatment options are less well-established. One paradoxical therapy in resistant cases may be antidepressants. Although antidepressants can trigger RBD, they also can reduce or abolish REM sleep, thereby reducing episode frequency. There are inconsistent reports as to the utility of pramipexole for RBD. One prospective study suggested a benefit, but others have found none. This variability accords with the author's personal experience in treating PD patients, in which dopaminergic therapy (regardless of type) can be associated with either reduction or exacerbation of dream enactment, without a clear, predictable pattern visible. Other potential options, generally supported only by case studies or small series, include donepezil, sodium oxybate, levodopa, and zopiclone.

Finally, the critical issue in the treatment of idiopathic RBD is the prevention of underlying neurodegeneration. One could speculate as to the utility of aerobic exercise, caffeine, creatine, inosine, calcium channel blockers, nicotine, and NSAIDs, which are all agents potentially associated with a lower risk of PD in epidemiologic surveys. In addition, one can hope for the future potential of growth factors, mitochondrial agents, synuclein blockers, immunotherapy, etc. However, given the plurality of potential options, one particular therapy does not clearly distinguish itself from the others, and at the current time no neuroprotective therapy can clearly be recommended,.

Prognosis

In general, the prognosis of the dream enactment of RBD is relatively benign. Treatment is successful in 80-90% of cases. Treatment resistance can certainly occur and can rarely be associated with a substantial impact on the quality of life. On the other hand, the prognosis for RBD in general is more worrying, since patients with idiopathic RBD are at a very substantial risk of developing neurodegenerative disease. The original report of a link between RBD and neuro-

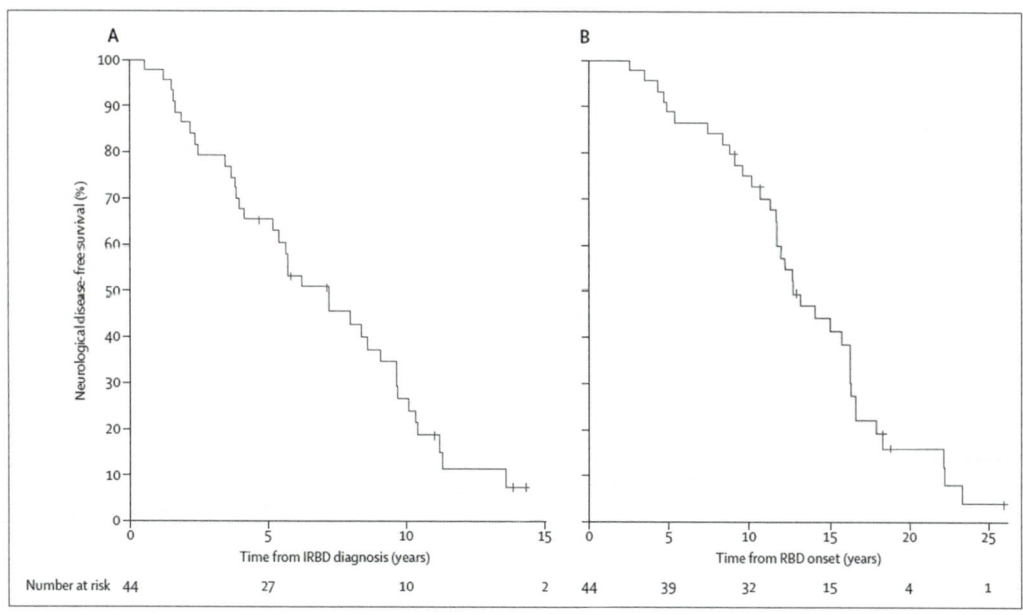

Figure 35.3
Rates of neurogical disease-free survival according to the time of (A) diagnosis of idiopathic RBD, and (B) estimated RBD onset (43). n = 49 patients.

degeneration came from the landmark paper by Schenck et al., who found that 11 (38%) of their 29 original cohort patients developed a parkinsonian disorder after a median follow-up of 5 years (32). Subsequently, three prospective cohort studies confirmed that RBD patients have a profoundly elevated risk of developing PD and DLB. The five-year risk of developing a neurodegenerative syndrome is 28-45% (see Figure 35.3), a percentage that continues to rise as follow-up duration increases (33-35). The most recent reports of the original Schenck cohort found that 81% of these original patients have subsequently developed disease (36). In the two series which included serial motor examination and neuropsychological assessment (33,34), approximately half of the patients developed parkinsonism, and half developed DLB. A recent population-based study also confirmed the elevated risk of developing MCI or PD after a mean follow-up of 3.8 years (4), although in this elderly cohort, cognitive impairment was more common than PD.

This profoundly elevated risk of neurodegenerative disease is by far the highest of any clinical predictive (or prodromal) marker of PD. This has major implications for the study of PD in general. First, patients with RBD may help evaluate other potential prodromal markers of PD, by providing a high-risk group that can be tested before developing disease. Prospective studies have suggested that the severity of REM atonia (37), olfaction dysfunction (38) (see Figure 35.4), impaired color vision (38), dopaminergic neuroimaging (39), transcranial ultrasound, and whole-brain glucose utili-

zation SPECT (40) can identify which RBD patients will develop neurodegenerative disease. These studies therefore provide direct evidence that these markers can 'predict' PD and DLB, suggesting that screening programs for neuroprotective therapy in a future age of neuroprotection are possible. In some cases (e.g. olfaction and color vision), abnormality of these measures can identify 5-year disease risks of 65-70%.

Second, the study of idiopathic RBD offers a rare opportunity to directly witness the emergence of a disease from its prodromal stages. For example, tracking changes in quantitative motor testing in patients who were ultimately destined to develop disease revealed that motor abnormalities deviate from normal between 5 and 9 years before disease (see Figure 35.5), and that motor testing can detect prodromal parkinsonism with approximately 80% sensitivity and specificity up to three years before disease diagnosis (41). Progression of dopaminergic abnormalities on B-CIT SPECT has also been measured in RBD, paving the way towards biomarkers of progres-

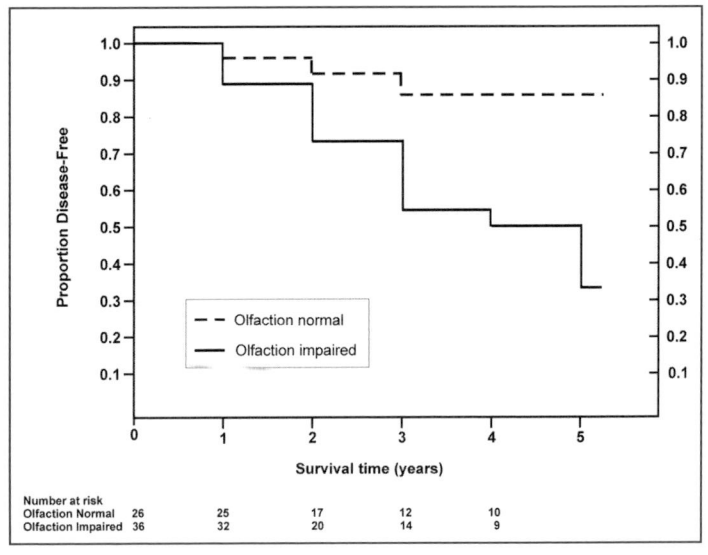

Figure 35.4

Kaplan-Meier plot of disease risk according to olfactory function at baseline examination in patients with idiopathic RBD. For illustration, values are dichotomized. Olfaction is defined as abnormal if UPSIT scores are <80% expected for age and sex (38).

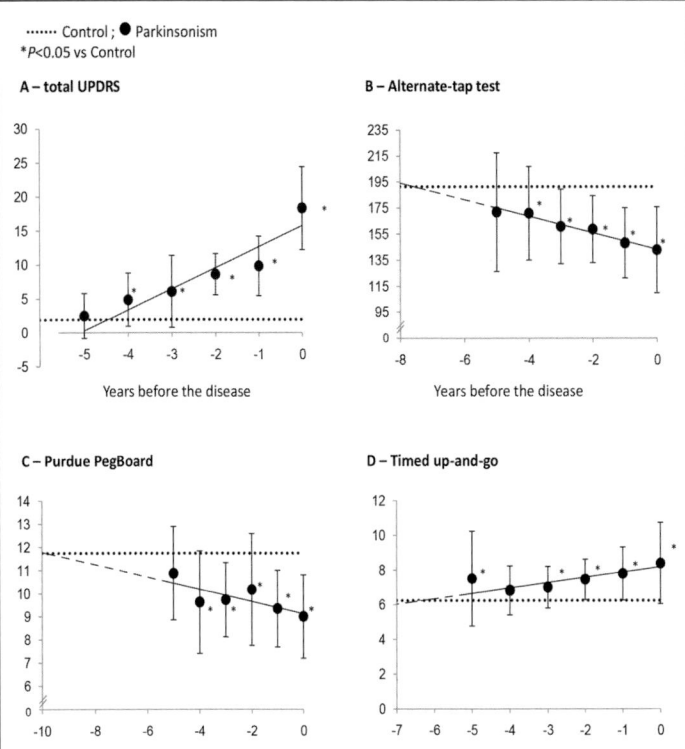

...... Control ; ● Parkinsonism
*P<0.05 vs Control

A – total UPDRS

B – Alternate-tap test

C – Purdue PegBoard

D – Timed up-and-go

Years before the disease

Years before the disease

Figure 35.5
Progression of quantitative motor markers in the five years before diagnosis of parkinsonism in patients who had idiopathic RBD but then developed clinical parkinsonism. Year 0 is set at the year parkinsonism was diagnosed. Results of measures in the years before disease are set as years -1 to -5. Error bars represent standard deviation. 90% confidence intervals of the slope are represented by the thin dashed lines. Reference value is the mean control value (horizontal line). The number beside each point represents the number of observations at this time interval (41).
*= significantly different from control values on the non-parametric Mann-Whitney U-test.
1a: UPDRS; 1b: Alternate-tap test; 1c: Purdue Pegboard; 1d: Timed Up-and-go.

jor barrier to the development and use of neuroprotective therapy is that the disease process of PD is well-established by the time patients present for medical attention. Being able to treat a disease in its prodromal stages could dramatically increase the effectiveness of neuroprotective therapy. Other than being high-priority candidates for neuroprotective therapy once it becomes available, RBD patients may be the ideal subjects for testing neuroprotective strategies in prodromal stages; disease risk is high enough so that the trial size would not be prohibitively large, and the latency between RBD and established PD is long enough that there is a sufficient window of opportunity to intervene.

Given the profound risk of neurodegenerative disease, what should patients be told? Obviously, a major (and perhaps overriding) principle is autonomy; patients have a right to know about their medical condition. Therefore, withholding information from a patient who wants full details about their condition cannot be defended. However, this may not always be simple, as autonomy also includes the right 'not to know'. The desire not to know is very difficult to communicate, and eliciting the level of information that patients wish to be provided is a skill, requiring a subtle approach. Moreover, autonomy is not the only consideration, and beneficence must be considered. At the current time, there is no treatment that can be given to forestall the neurodegenerative process; therefore, pro-

sion in prodromal PD (24). A similar analysis of autonomic dysfunction has suggested that autonomic symptoms and signs can become abnormal as long as 10-20 years before the clinical disease, consistent with predictions of the Braak staging system that proposes onset of synuclein deposition in autonomic structures at Stage I disease (26).

Third, and most critically, RBD opens a potential pathway to neuroprotective therapy. A ma-

viding information may cause patient stress with no clear benefit on the course of their illness. To further complicate the issue, manifestations of neurodegenerative disorders, although not preventable, are treatable - often patients in PD clinics have been suffering from numerous untreated symptoms for some years, which could have been mitigated if recognized. Therefore, periodic follow-up of these patients with neurological specialty support is strongly recommended, and so enough information must be provided that patients will engage in this. Due to the complexity and individual differences, universal blanket recommendations cannot be made - information must be provided according to the needs and values of each individual.

Another aspect is the recent documentation that in PD, the presence of RBD may be a poor prognostic sign. Many cross-sectional studies have examined the relationship between RBD status and PD manifestations. Many of them are limited by the absence of PSG confirmation of disease (introducing misclassification bias that tends to wash out true differences), low sample size (with resultant low power), or examination of a limited number of disease features. Results vary considerably across studies, but many have associated RBD with an akinetic-rigid subtype, more symmetric disease, increased motor severity, falls, freezing, increased autonomic dysfunction, and visual hallucinations (5,6). Perhaps the most consistent associations with RBD in cross-sectional studies are severer autonomic dysfunction, impaired cognition (although this requires cognitive tests that are sensitive to domains affected in PD), and motor subtype to a lesser extent. Of special clinical importance, two recent prospective studies have independently found that the presence of RBD was a risk factor for the eventual development of PD dementia (25, 42). Additionally, RBD may also have prognostic significance in DLB; in an study of autopsy-confirmed DLB, parkinsonism occurred earlier and survival was shorter in those who

had associated RBD (29). Therefore, aside from being a treatable condition and a prodromal feature of disease, RBD may indicate important differences in disease prognosis in secondary cases.

Conclusion

RBD is an under-recognized syndrome that nonetheless has a characteristic phenotype. Symptomatic treatment is almost always successful, although exceptions can occur. The identification of RBD as a prodromal marker for neurodegenerative synucleinopathy has profound implications for the study of early neurodegeneration, and perhaps its eventual prevention.

References

1 Schenck CH, Mahowald MW. REM sleep behavior disorder: clinical, developmental, and neuroscience perspectives 16 years after its formal identification in SLEEP. Sleep 2002;25:120-138.

2 Chiu HF, Wing YK, Lam LC, et al. Sleep-related injury in the elderly--an epidemiological study in Hong Kong. Sleep 2000;23:513-517.

3 Ohayon MM, Caulet M, Priest RG. Violent behavior during sleep. J ClinPsychiatry 1997;58:369-376.

4 Boot BP, Boeve BF, Roberts RO, et al. Probable rapid eye movement sleep behavior disorder increases risk for mild cognitive impairment and Parkinson disease: a population-based study. Ann Neurol 2012;71:49-56.

5 Sixel-Doring F, Trautmann E, Mollenhauer B, Trenkwalder C. Associated factors for REM sleep behavior disorder in Parkinson disease. Neurology 2011;77:1048-1052.

6 Romenets SR, Gagnon JF, Latreille V, et al. Rapid eye movement sleep behavior disorder and subtypes of Parkinson's disease. Mov Disord 2012;27:996-1003.

7 Postuma RB, Montplaisir JY, Pelletier A, et al. Environmental risk factors for REM sleep behavior disorder: A multicenter case-control study. Neurology 2012;79:428-434.

8 Dauvilliers Y, Postuma RB, Ferini-Strambi L, et al. 2013. Family history of idiopathic REM behavior

disorder: A multicenter case-control study. Neurology 2013;80:2233-2235.

9 Gagnon JF, Bedard MA, Fantini ML, et al. REM sleep behavior disorder and REM sleep without atonia in Parkinson's disease. Neurology 2002;59:585-589.

10 Nomura T, Inoue Y, Kagimura T, Nakashima K. Clinical significance of REM sleep behavior disorder in Parkinson's disease. Sleep Med 2013;14:131-135.

11 Vetrugno R, Provini F, Cortelli P, et al. Sleep disorders in multiple system atrophy: a correlative video-polysomnographic study. Sleep Med 2004;5:21-30.

12 Ferman TJ, Boeve BF, Smith GE, et al. Inclusion of RBD improves the diagnostic classification of dementia with Lewy bodies. Neurology 2011;77:875-882.

13 Gagnon JF, Postuma RB, Mazza S, Doyon J, Montplaisir J. Rapid-eye-movement sleep behaviour disorder and neurodegenerative diseases. Lancet Neurol 2006;5:424-432.

14 Arnulf I. REM sleep behavior disorder: motor manifestations and pathophysiology. Mov Disord 2012;27:677-689.

15 Boeve BF, Silber MH, Saper CB, et al. Pathophysiology of REM sleep behaviour disorder and relevance to neurodegenerative disease. Brain 2007;130:2770-2788.

16 Luppi PH, Clement O, Sapin E, et al. The neuronal network responsible for paradoxical sleep and its dysfunctions causing narcolepsy and rapid eye movement (REM) behavior disorder. Sleep MedRev 2011;15:153-163.

17 Braak H, Del TK. Nervous system pathology in sporadic Parkinson disease. Neurology 2008;70: 1916-1925.

18 Cochen V, Arnulf I, Demeret S, et al. Vivid dreams, hallucinations, psychosis and REM sleep in Guillain-Barre syndrome. Brain 2005;128:2535-2545.

19 Iranzo A, Graus F, Clover L, et al. Rapid eye movement sleep behavior disorder and potassium channel antibody-associated limbic encephalitis. Ann Neurol 2006;59:178-181.

20 De Cock VC, Debs R, Oudiette D, et al. The improvement of movement and speech during rapid eye movement sleep behaviour disorder in multiple system atrophy. Brain 2011;134:856-862.

21 American Sleep Disorders Association. International classification of sleep disorders, revised: diagnostic and coding manual. Rochester, MN: American Sleep Disorders Association; 1997:177-180.

22 Montplaisir J, Gagnon JF, Fantini ML, et al. Polysomnographic diagnosis of idiopathic REM sleep behavior disorder. Mov Disord 2010;25:2044-2051.

23 Frauscher B, Iranzo A, Gaig C, et al. Normative EMG values during REM sleep for the diagnosis of REM sleep behavior disorder. Sleep 2012;35:835-847.

24 Iranzo A, Valldeoriola F, Lomena F, et al. Serial dopamine transporter imaging of nigrostriatal function in patients with idiopathic rapid-eye-movement sleep behaviour disorder: a prospective study. Lancet Neurol 2011;10:797-805.

25 Nomura T, Inoue Y, Kagimura T, Uemura Y, Nakashima K. Utility of the REM sleep behavior disorder screening questionnaire (RBDSQ) in Parkinson's disease patients. Sleep Med 2011;12: 711-713.

26 Postuma RB, Gagnon JF, Pelletier A, Montplaisir J. Prodromal autonomic symptoms and signs in Parkinson's disease and dementia with Lewy bodies. Mov Disord 2013;28:597-604.

27 Postuma RB, Arnulf I, Hogl B, et al. A single-question screen for rapid eye movement sleep behavior disorder: A multicenter validation study. Mov Disord 2012;27:913-916.

28 Boeve BF, Silber MH, Ferman TJ, et al. Clinicopathologic correlations in 172 cases of rapid eye movement sleep behavior disorder with or without a coexisting neurologic disorder. Sleep Med 2013;14:754-762.

29 Dugger BN, Boeve BF, Murray ME, et al. Rapid eye movement sleep behavior disorder and subtypes in autopsy-confirmed dementia with Lewy bodies. Mov Disord 2013;27:72-78.

30 McCarter SJ, Boswell CL, St Louis EK, et al. Treatment outcomes in REM sleep behavior disorder. Sleep Med 2013;14:237-242.

31 Kunz D, Mahlberg R. A two-part, double-blind, placebo-controlled trial of exogenous melatonin

in REM sleep behaviour disorder. J Sleep Res 2010;19:591-596.

32 Schenck CH, Bundlie SR, Mahowald MW. Delayed emergence of a parkinsonian disorder in 38% of 29 older men initially diagnosed with idiopathic rapid eye movement sleep behaviour disorder. Neurology 1996;46:388-393.

33 Iranzo A, Molinuevo JL, Santamaria J, et al. Rapid-eye-movement sleep behaviour disorder as an early marker for a neurodegenerative disorder: a descriptive study. Lancet Neurol 2006;5:572-577.

34 Postuma RB, Gagnon JF, Vendette M, Fantini ML, Massicotte-Marquez J, Montplaisir J. Quantifying the risk of Neurodegenerative Disease in Idiopathic REM sleep behavior disorder. Neurology 2009;72:1296-1300.

35 Wing YK, Li SX, Mok V, et al. Prospective outcome of rapid eye movement sleep behaviour disorder: psychiatric disorders as a potential early marker of Parkinson's disease. J Neurol Neurosurg Psychiatry 2012;83:470-472.

36 Schenck CH, Boeve BF, Mahowald MW. Delayed emergence of a parkinsonian disorder or dementia in 81% of older males initially diagnosed with idiopathic REM sleep behavior disorder (RBD): 16year update on a previously reported series. Sleep Med 2013;14:744-748.

37 Postuma RB, Gagnon JF, Rompre S, Montplaisir J. Severity of REM Atonia Loss in Idiopathic REM Sleep Behavior Disorder Predicts Parkinson Disease. Neurology 2010;74:239-244.

38 Postuma RB, Gagnon JF, Vendette M, Desjardins C, Montplaisir J. Olfaction and Color Vision Identify Impending Neurodegeneration in REM behavior disorder. AnnNeurol 2011;69:811-818.

39 Iranzo A, Lomena F, Stockner H, et al. Decreased striatal dopamine transporters uptake and substantia nigra hyperechogenicity as risk markers of synucleinopathy in patients with idiopathic rapid-eye-movement sleep behaviour disorder: a prospective study. Lancet Neurol 2010;9:1070-107.

40 Dang-Vu TT, Gagnon JF, Vendette M, Soucy JP, Postuma RB, Montplaisir J. Hippocampal perfusion predicts impending neurodegeneration in REM sleep behavior disorder. Neurology 2012;79:2302-2306.

41 Postuma RB, Lang AE, Gagnon JF, Pelletier A, Montplaisir JY. How does parkinsonism start? Prodromal parkinsonism motor changes in idiopathic REM sleep behaviour disorder. Brain 2012;135:1860-1870.

42 Postuma RB, Bertrand JA, Montplaisir J, et al. Rapid eye movement sleep behavior disorder and risk of dementia in Parkinson's disease: a prospective study. Mov Disord 2012;27:720-726.

43 Iranzo A, Tolosa E, Gelpi E, et al. Neurodegenerative disease status and post-mortem pathology in idiopathic rapid-eye-movement sleep behavior disorder: an observational cohort study. Lancet Neurol 2013;12:443-453.

36

Sleep-related Movement Disorders

Claudio L.A. Bassetti

Non-rapid eye movement (NREM) and REM sleep are associated with profound neurophysiological and neurochemical changes in the brain, which alter the control of motor functions (1). This explains why movement disorders and disturbances of motor control sometimes appear only or preferentially during sleep.

Sleep-related movement disorders and disturbances of motor control are of clinical relevance because they are very common and may lead to a significant sleep disturbances (e.g. sleep fragmentation/insomnia, sleep-associated injuries and violence) and consequent daytime symptoms (e.g. fatigue, sleepiness). Also, they can represent the first or main manifestation of an underlying disorder of the brain (e.g. epilepsy, neurodegenerative disease) which requires a specific work-up and treatment.

Definition and classification

Movement disorders occurring during sleep are typically characterized, with the exception of sleep paralysis, by involuntary, excessive motor activities (hyperkinesias), i.e. positive motor symptoms. On rare occasions (e.g. in the context of REM sleep behaviour disorder, RBD) voluntary movements during sleep can be different from those seen during the day (2). Finally, changes in muscle tone are, not a relevant feature of sleep-related movement disorders, with the exception of RBD.

Motor activities during sleep can be classified according to their clinical features, the sleep stages in which they occur, and their aetiology. Table 36.1 presents a possible classification of motor activities during sleep which take into account:

- clinical features:
  - simple vs complex (i.e. those leading to behavioural manifestations)
- aetiology:
  - physiological vs pathological
  - movements disorders (sensu strictu)
  - epileptic disorders
  - psychiatric disorders
  - others
- sleep stage of occurrence (when pertinent)

Epidemiology

Sleep-related movements disorders and disturbances of motor control are common and often age-dependent (1). The frequencies of the most relevant disorder/disturbances are summarized in Table 36.2.

Aetiology

Several factors have been identified as contributing to sleep-related movement disorders and disturbances of motor control, not uncommonly in combination.

- Genetic factors are known to be involved in several disorders including restless legs syndrome (RLS, familial in 50% of cases), sleepwalking (SW, 25-50%), bruxism, nocturnal frontal lobe epilepsy (NFLE, 25% of cases), and Rolandic epilepsy (3-5).
- Neurodegeneration is relevant in RBD. Over 50% of patients with idiopathic RBD devel-

Table 36.1
Classification of motor activities during sleep.

A	Physiological activities

- Hypnic jerks/sleep starts
- Hypnagogic (sleep onset) foot tremor
- Alternating leg muscle activation
- NREM myoclonus (physiologic fragmentary myoclonus)
- REM myoclonus/twitches
- Postural shifts
- Sleeptalking

B	Pathological activities (disorders of nocturnal/sleep-related motor control)

B1 *Simple motor activities*

- Diurnal movement disorders
  - Frequently persisting during sleep
    Palatal myoclonus/tremor
    Hemifacial spasm
    Spinal myoclonus
    Tics
  - Sometimes persisting during sleep
    Tremor
    Chorea
    Dystonia
    Hemiballism
- Nocturnal (sleep-related) movement disorders
  - Sleep-related bruxism
  - Nocturnal groaning (catathrenia)
  - Faciomandibular myoclonus
  - Neck myoclonus during REM sleep
  - Sleep-related leg cramps
  - Excessive NREM (fragmentary) myoclonus/ benign neonatal myoclonus
  - Excessive REM myoclonus (twitches)
  - Restless legs/limbs syndrome (RLS)
  - Periodic limb movements in sleep (PLMS)
  - Propriospinal myoclonus at sleep onset
  - Sleep paralysis
- Nocturnal (sleep-related) epileptic disorders
  - Nocturnal epilepsy with simple motor manifestations
    Idiopathic focal epilepsy with centrotemporal spikes and variants (benign Rolandic seizure, Landau-Kleffner syndrome, epilepsy with continuous spike waves during slow wave sleep (CSWS))
    Nocturnal frontal lobe epilepsy with paroxysmal arousals (NFLE)
    Panayatopoulos syndrome
    Others (e.g. temporal lobe seizures)
  - Epilepsy with diurnal and nocturnal simple motor manifestations
- Others
  - Arousal reactions secondary to sleep-disordered breathing

B2 *Complex motor activities/behaviours*

- Nocturnal (sleep-related) movement disorders
  - Sleep-related rhythmic movement disorders
  - NREM parasomnias (arousal disorders)
    Confusional arousals
    Sleep terror (pavor nocturnus)
    Sleepwalking
  - REM sleep behaviour disorder/overlap parasomnia/status dissociatus
- Nocturnal (sleep-related) epileptic disorders
  - Nocturnal frontal lobe epilepsy (NFLE) with complex motor manifestations
    Paroxysmal dystonic seizures
    Epileptic wandering
    Hypermotor seizures (occasionally also of non-frontal origin)
  - Epilepsy with diurnal and nocturnal complex motor manifestations
- Nocturnal (sleep-related) psychiatric disorders
  - Nocturnal panic attacks
  - Posttraumatic stress disorder
  - Sleep-related dissociative disorders
  - Sleep-related psychogenic non-epileptic seizures

op a neurodegenerative Parkinsonian disorder (typically Lewy body disease) within 5-10 years (6). Idiopathic RBD may precede onset of neurodegenerative disorders by up to 20-40 years.

- Focal brain damage is critical in a multitude of syndromes. Nocturnal epilepsy (e.g. in the context of cortical dysplasia), RBD (e.g. brainstem stroke, demyelinating disorders), and RLS (e.g. spinal cord demyelination, subcortical stroke) have been shown to be occasionally related to a developmental or acquired focal brain damage. Sleepwalking has been observed to appear secondary to traumatic brain injury or stroke.

Table 36.2
Frequency of sleep-related movement disorders/ disturbances of motor control in the general population.

10-50%	Nocturnal leg cramps • highest frequency in the elderly • rare below the age of 10
10-20%	Sleep-related bruxism • highest frequency in children
5-20%	Periodic limb movements in sleep (PLMS) • rare below the age of 30-40 • more common in sleep disordered breathing, narcolepsy • very common (70-90%) in restless legs syndrome
5-15%	Sleep paralysis • more common in narcolepsy (50%), psychiatric patients
5-15%	Sleepwalking • highest frequency in children below the age of 10 • lower frequency (1-5%) in adults
1-10%	Restless legs/limbs syndrome • rare in children • more common in uraemia, iron deficiency, pregnancy (10-30%)
1-5%	Sleep terrors • lower frequency in adults
1%	REM sleep behaviour disorder • more common (25-50%) in Parkinsonian syndromes
1%	Sleep-related (nocturnal) eating disorders • more common in patients with RLS/ PLMS, sleepwalking

• **Psychiatric factors/disorders** should be evaluated in many patients. An underlying stress or psychiatric disorder is often found in (particularly adult) patients with sleepwalking, bruxism, sleep related rhythmic disorders, and nocturnal eating disorder. Patients with RLS and sleep paralysis present psychiatric disturbances more commonly than the normal population (7).

• **Drug effects** including those related to benzodiazepine and antidepressants may exacerbate (trigger) sleepwalking; antidepressants may exacerbate RBD, RLS and bruxism; neuroleptics can exacerbate RLS and bruxism.

• **Other factors** alcohol has been shown to exacerbate RBD, PLMS, bruxism and sleepwalking (8). A deficient iron transport/metabolism may underlie RLS

Pathophysiology

Motor control requires afferent, integrating, and efferent systems involving the spinal cord, the brainstem, the cerebellum, the basal ganglia and the cerebral cortex.

Nocturnal/sleep-related motor manifestations arise from a disruption of such mechanisms, often in form of the abnormal activation and/or disinhibition of motor circuits. The exact contribution of afferent or efferent systems (and corresponding neurotransmitters) in most sleep-related movement disorders/disturbances of motor control remains essentially speculative (9,10). For instance, in sleepwalking, autosomal dominant nocturnal frontal lobe epilepsy, and nocturnal (sleep-related) panic attacks, a primary dysfunction of *ascending, activating systems* may prevail (10,11). In RBD, on the other hand, a primary dysfunction of *descending, inhibitory systems* is currently favoured (see also Chapter 35) (9). In most situations, a dysfunction of both systems is likely to be involved (12).

Complex nocturnal/sleep-related motor manifestations/behaviours eventually arise from the abnormal (non-epileptic and epileptic) activation of innate (genetically determined) or learned motor patterns (central pattern generators) that are essential for survival (13,14). The term of 'state dissociation' has been used to describe the co-existence of abnormally activated brain areas with others that exhibits features of normal sleep (15). By means of neuroimaging and neurophysiological methods, such dissociation has been documented in a few patients with parasomnias and sleep-related epilepsy (11,16,17).

Clinical presentation

The clinical phenomenology of sleep-related movement disorders and disturbances of motor control is very broad and its detailed presentation exceeds the scope of this chapter. The readers are referred to a recent monograph on this topic for detailed information (10).

Generally speaking, clinical manifestations are usually classified according to the body part(s) involved and the type of motor activity involved (simple vs complex, where complex implies those activities leading to behavioural correlates). The manifestations of the different disorders/disturbances are often suggested by the name used to describe them (e.g. sleeptalking, nocturnal groaning, sleep-related eating disorder). Complex motor activities such as laughing/crying, locomotion, sex, eating, aggressive behaviour are observed in the context of a variety of sleep-related conditions (e.g. parasomnias, epilepsy, dissociative disorders) and can eventually lead to injuries of the patients or their bed partners (18). The key-features of the main sleep-related movement disorders and disturbances of motor control are presented in the following sections.

Hypnic jerks

Hypnic jerks (sleep starts, predormital myoclonus) are sudden, brief contractions of the body or limbs at sleep onset which occur spontaneously or after a stimulus (19). The contractions can be accompanied by a cry and hallucinations (flashes, feeling of falling, dreams). The diagnosis usually does not require any ancillary tests (20).

Sleep-related bruxism

Bruxism consists of rhythmic tooth grinding or tapping. It typically occurs in light NREM and REM sleep. Masseter hypertrophy can be observed and jaw muscle discomfort is often reported during the day. Primary and secondary forms (associated with sleep disorders, movements disorders, neurologic or psychiatric disorders) are known. Diagnosis is suspected clinically and can be confirmed by typical EMG artifacts during polysomnography (20).

Nocturnal groaning (catathrenia)

This consists of repetitive expiratory respiratory (groaning, moaning) monotonous sounds occurring in clusters (mainly but not exclusively in REM sleep) and lasting for up to 30-50 seconds (21). There is an association with other parasomnias.

Facio-mandibular myoclonus

This refers to nocturnal myoclonic jerks involving the jaw and facial musculature which can lead to diurnal jaw discomfort and even a loss of teeth (22).

Excessive NREM (fragmentary) myoclonus/ benign neonatal myoclonus

This involves excessive, non-rhythmic and non-periodic limb twitches with no or only minimal movement effect in NREM sleep (23). The term benign neonatal myoclonus refers to repetitive, rhythmic myoclonic jerks that occur during sleep. The condition typically resolves by 3 months of age without sequelae (24).

Restless legs/limbs syndrome (RLS)

The restless legs/limbs syndrome (RLS) is a common, often still underdiagnosed, sensorimotor disorder characterized by uncomfortable and disagreeable sensations in the limbs, especially in the lower legs, which induce a strong desire to move (25). The urge to move the legs can be present without the uncomfortable sensations. Sensory discomfort may involve the arms (30 to 50% of patients) or other body parts as well (Figure 36.1) (26). Around one-third of patients describe their sensations as painful. The symptoms appear or get worse during rest and are partially or completely alleviated by movement. The unpleasant feeling follows a circadian trend, occurring or worsening

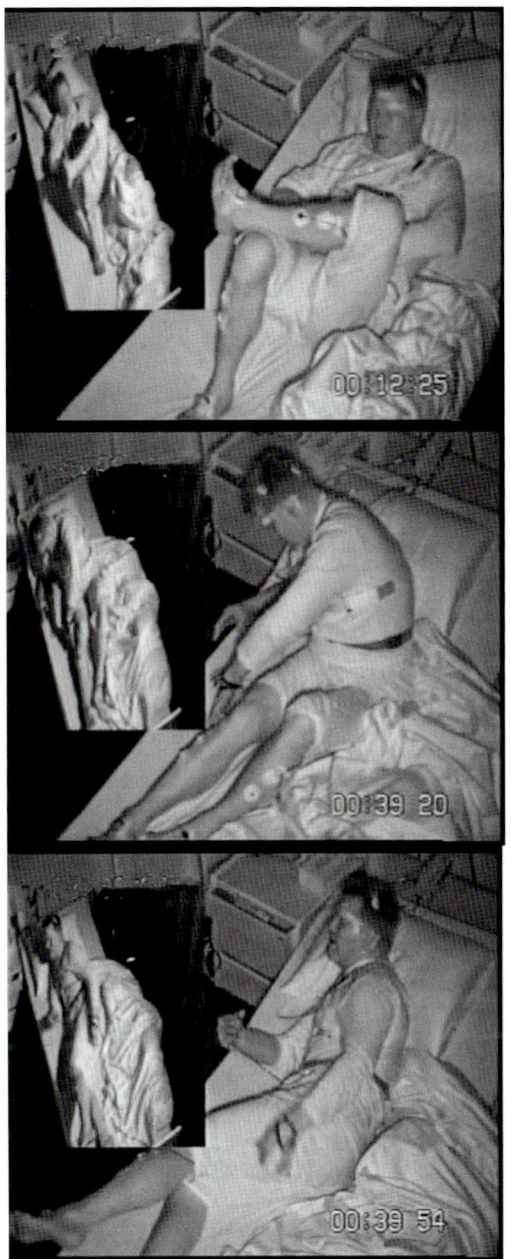

Figure 36.1
Restless limbs syndrome: clinical features.
Pictures taken from a video-polysomnography of a
30-year-old man with severe, familial RLS showing restlessness of the patient while trying to fall asleep.

during the evening or night. As a consequence, patients often present with insomnia, and occasionally with daytime fatigue and even excessive daytime sleepiness (27). They may also present psychiatric symptoms and/or a co-morbidity with psychiatric disorders. The disease can appear in childhood, its course is usually chronic, with rare periods of remission. The severity of symptoms varies largely but usually enhances with age.

Primary and secondary forms (associated with pregnancy, iron deficiency, uremia, spinal cord diseases, Parkinsonian disorders, spinocerebellar atrophies, amongst others) are known (28). Several medications including neuroleptics and antidepressants can exacerbate or trigger RLS. The diagnosis is usually made clinically. Essential and supportive criteria are summarized in Table 36.3. Supportive criteria include the detection of periodic limb movements in sleep (PLMS, by polysomnography or leg actigraphy, see Video fragment 36.1), which are present in 70-90% of RLS patients (29,30). Supportive criteria may be helpful to differentiate RLS from RLS-mimics (31).

Periodic limbs movements in sleep (PLMS)

These are repetitive, periodic-pseudoperiodic, stereotyped movements, usually consisting of

Table 36.3
Criteria for the diagnosis of restless legs syndrome (RLS).

Essential criteria for the diagnosis
1   Symptoms: urge to move, usually accompanied by unpleasant sensations in the legs (limbs)
2   Symptoms begin or worsen during periods of rest or inactivity such as sitting or lying down
3   Symptoms are partially or totally relieved by movements (including walking, stretching) (Figure 36.1)
4   Symptoms are worse or occur only in the evening or at night

Supportive criteria for the diagnosis
1   Response to dopaminergic treatment (present in about 90% of patients)
2   Positive family history (present in about 50% of patients)
3   Periodic limb movements in sleep (PLMS, present in 70-90% of patients)

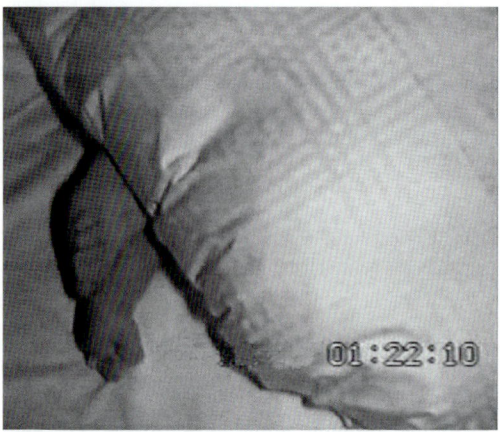

Figure 36.2 Periodic limb movements during sleep (PLMS).
Pictures taken from a video-polysomnography of a 45-year-old man with RLS and PLMS showing dorsiflexion of the left great toe during PLMS (resembling the Babinski sign).

a toe extension with a dorsiflexion of the ankle and a flexion of the knee and hip (Figure 36.2, Video fragment 36.1). The contractions last 0.5-10 seconds, the episodes consist of at least 4 consecutive contractions/movements, the intervals between the episodes ranges from 5 to 90 seconds (on average 20-40 seconds) (Figure 36.3). The detection of PLMS can be made by polysomnography, and an estimation can be made by leg actigraphy.

Propriospinal myoclonus at sleep onset

This refers to repetitive axial jerks slowly spreading rostrally and downward in the process of falling sleep and may leading to falls out of the bed (32).

Sleep paralysis

The term refers to the inability and struggle to move and speak while in the process of falling asleep or awakening (33). Sleep paralysis usually last less than 10 minutes, although episodes of up to 30 minutes have been reported (34). Its frequency can vary from a few life events to daily episodes. Stress, excessive sleepiness, irregular sleep-wake cycle, jet lag, and sleeping in an uncomfortable may increase its frequency. Anxiety is often experienced. Sleep paralysis is commonly associated with hallucinations including sensed presence, sensation of a pressure on the chest with shortness of breath (incubus) (Figure 36.4), or sensation of floating/flying (out-of-body experience). Primary (sporadic and familial) and secondary forms (associated with narcolepsy, other sleep disorders, nor psychiatric disorders) are known. The diagnosis is usually made clinically.

Nocturnal epilepsy with simple motor manifestations

The most common syndrome is that of Rolandic epilepsy (also called benign epilepsy with centrotemporal spikes, BECTS). This is an idiopathic focal epilepsy which typically starts around the age of 10 years and presents with in-

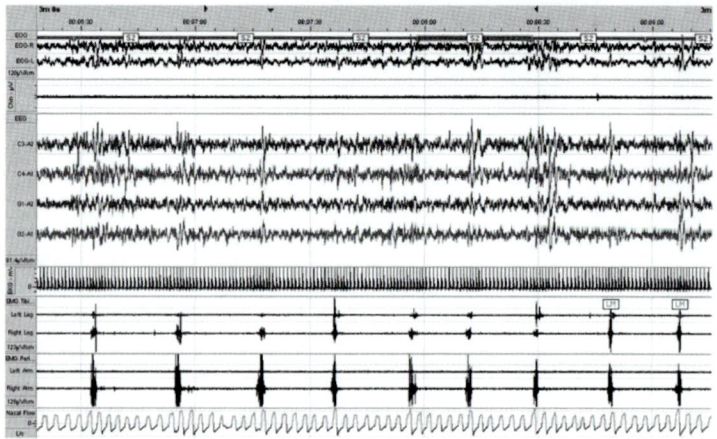

Figure 36.3 Periodic limb movements during sleep.
Pictures taken from a video-polysomnography of a 60-year-old man with RLS and PLMS showing periodic EMG activities in the four limbs occurring at intervals of about 15 seconds.

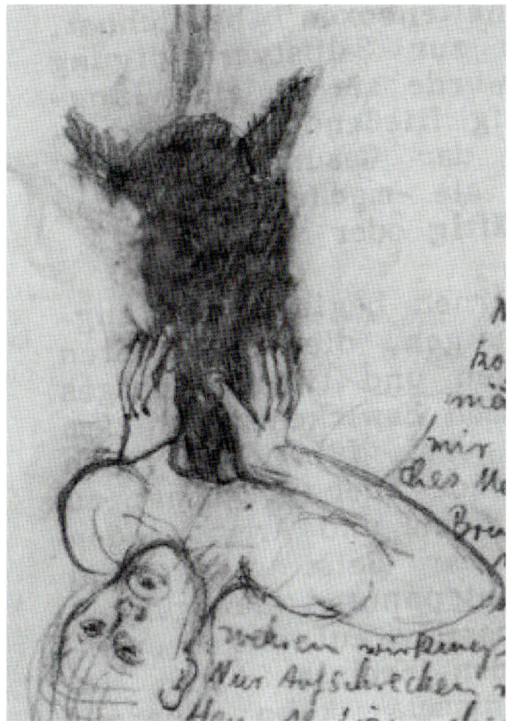

Figure 36.4 Sleep paralysis.
Drawing of a 32-year-old patient with sleep paralysis, depicting his experience of frightening visual hallucinations accompanying his episodes.

frequent nocturnal seizures (often at sleep onset or before awakening), lasting 1-3 minutes. The seizures consist of brief, simple, hemifacial motor seizures, often associated with somatosensory symptoms and occasionally evolving into generalized tonic-clonic seizures. Postictal amnesia is not always present. Variants of BECTS are the epilepsy syndrome with continuous spike waves during slow wave sleep (CSWS) and the Landau-Kleffner syndrome (also called acquired epileptic aphasia). These epileptic syndromes appear to belong to the same spectrum of disorders as suggested also by a similar genetic background (5).

Nocturnal frontal lobe epilepsy with paroxysmal arousals

Nocturnal frontal lobe epilepsy (NFLE) typically presents with complex nocturnal motor manifestations (so-called hypermotor seizures). Patients may present, however, also with simple nocturnal manifestations (e.g. paroxysmal arousals) that are often overlooked or interpreted as non-epileptic in origin (22).

Panyatopoulos syndrome

This syndrome refers to an idiopathic epileptic syndrome which typically starts around the age of 5 with episodes of disturbed autonomic functions (most commonly nausea, retching, vomiting but also pallor, mydriasis, apneas, incontinence) (35). Syncope-like epileptic seizures can also be observed, seizures may end with brief convulsions. Seizures appear mostly but not only during sleep, last typically for several minutes, and may end with brief convulsions.

Other epileptic syndromes

Other epileptic syndromes may manifest with nocturnal simple motor spells, including temporal lobe epilepsy (36).

Sleep-related rhythmic movement disorders

These are stereotyped, repetitive movements such as head rolling, had banging, body rolling, and body rocking occurring at sleep onset but also in other sleep stages, with a frequency of 0.5-2 Hz and lasting for seconds up to several minutes. These movements typically first appear in early infancy, can however be observed also in later ages, particularly in patients with a positive family history, mental retardation or associated sleep disorders (37).

The diagnosis is suspected clinically and confirmed by videography or video-polysomnography.

Sleep terror (pavor nocturnus)

It consists of spells characterized by sudden onset of fear, loud screaming, and autonomic symptoms arising from deep NREM sleep and usually lasting only few minutes. Patients are difficult to be awaken and have no recall of the episodes (20). These episodes typically first appear at the age of 5-10 years, can however be observed also in later ages in patients with a positive family history. Patients with sleep terrors often also present sleepwalking/other NREM parasomnias. The diagnosis is suspected clinically and confirmed by video-polysomnography.

Sleepwalking (somnambulism)

Sleepwalking (SW) refers to an ambulatory activity arising (in most cases) from deep NREM sleep (10,20,38). Patients wake up suddenly, sit up, look around with a confused stare, leave the bed and ambulate. Movements can be repetitive and purposeless, whereas on other occasions, they may appear complex and meaningful (39). Autonomic activation (sweating, tachycardia, tachypnea) is more common in confusional arousals and sleep terrors than in SW. Patients are difficult to awaken and when awakened appear confused. There is usually no recall of SW episodes, dream-like experiences and some recall are however possible particularly reported in adult SW. Self-injuries are possible. Reports of homicidal, filicidal and suicidal SW also occur rarely (18). Nocturnal eating (somnophagia) and abnormal sexual behaviour during sleep have been reported in association with SW (40). Typically, SW occurs once per night and in the first third of the night. The frequency can range from few episodes in a lifetime up to several (5-6) episodes per night (41). The duration of SW ranges from 1-3 to 7-10 minutes, rarely longer. More often, SW appears between the age of 5 and 15 years. Earlier and later onset (including 'de novo' in adulthood) are possible (41).

Patients with SW have a higher frequency of sleep terrors (pavor nocturnus), confusional arousals, enuresis, sleeptalking, and bruxism. Sleepwalking usually appears in the context of a sporadic or familial NREM parasomnia. Still, nocturnal, sleep-related ambulatory activity can occur also in the context of a more complex NREM-REM (overlap) parasomnia (e.g. in the course of a neurodegenerative disease), of nocturnal epilepsy ('epileptic wandering'), or of

dissociative disorders (Table 36.4) (42-44). Diagnosis is usually made clinically. In adult SW, video-polysomnography may be needed for the correct interpretation of reported nocturnal ambulatory activities. Sleep restriction before polysomnography can help trigger events.

Table 36.4
Differential diagnosis of nocturnal (sleep-related) complex behaviours.

- NREM parasomnias (sleepwalking, sleep terrors, confusional arousals)
- REM sleep behaviour disorder
- overlap parasomnia
- nocturnal frontal lobe epilepsy/hypermotor seizures
- dissociative disorders

REM sleep behaviour disorder

REM sleep behaviour disorder (RBD) is a disorder characterized by an abnormal behaviour arising from REM sleep which is accompanied by (oft frightening) vivid dreaming (Figure 36.5) (20,45). The patients 'act out their dreams', exhibiting a variety of motor activities ranging from talking and twitching of the limbs to screaming, kicking, punching, reaching, grabbing, kicking and even complex violent and non-violent behaviours (2). Injuries are not infrequent and may involve both the patients and their bed partners. Autonomic activation is limited/absent. Typically, RBD occurs repeatedly in the second part of the night. More often, RBD appears in elderly males. Patients with RBD often present also PLMS. RBD usually appears in the context of neurodegenerative disease (most commonly with Parkinson's disease, multiple system atrophy, and Lewy body dementia) and narcolepsy. The onset of RBD may precede the appearance of daytime (e.g. cognitive, motor) manifestations by decades (46). During REM sleep with RBD, Parkinsonian patients may exhibit a paradoxical improvement of motor function in comparison to speech, facial and limb motor functions during wakefulness. In addition, RBD in Parkinsonian patients is more commonly associated with psychiatric abnormal-

extreme form of overlap parasomnia in which a breakdown of wake-sleep state boundaries appear and features of NREM, REM sleep, and wakefulness, coexist (50,51). Diagnosis of RBD is confirmed by video-polysomnography, by documenting a loss of motor atonia, an increase of phasic muscle activity during REM sleep and corresponding behaviours (Figure 36.6).

Nocturnal epilepsy with complex motor manifestations

Nocturnal frontal lobe epilepsy (NFLE)

This is a seizure disorder characterized by a wide spectrum of stereotyped, repetitive motor manifestations, mostly occurring during NREM sleep. Episodes are characterized by sudden onset of motor behaviours including repetitive hand clenching, arm raising/lowering, knee bending, but also more complex patterns such as body rocking, kicking, pedaling, hitting, boxing, screaming and even walking/running (episodic nocturnal/epileptic wandering) (4,22,52-54) (Figure 36.7). The term hypermotor/hyperkinetic seizure has been suggested for these very complex motor presentations (55). Occasionally, spells are characterized by asymmetric tonic posturing of the extremities (nocturnal paroxysmal dystonic seizures). The duration of the spells is typically short (10-30 seconds, less commonly 1-2 minutes), the amnesia can be incomplete.

In most cases with hypermotor seizures, a frontal origin is found, but in about one third of cases, seizures originate from the insula, the temporal or the occipital cortex (hypermotor seizures of non-frontal origin).

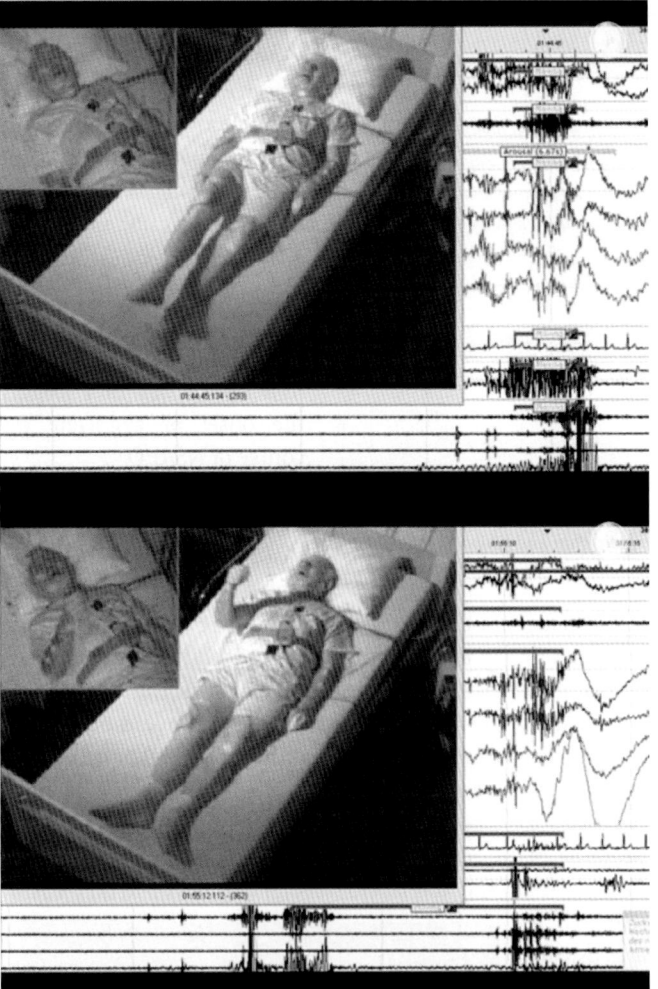

Figure 36.5 REM sleep behaviour disorder (RBD).
Pictures taken from a video-polysomnography of a 76-year-old man with RBD in the context of a Parkinsonian syndrome (multiple system atrophy).

ities, hallucinations, cognitive decline, and sleepwalking (*overlap parasomnia*), when compared to Parkinsonian patients without the syndrome (2,12). Acute and transient RBD can be seen with focal brain lesions (limbic encephalitis, brainstem stroke, demyelinating disorders) (47,48). Medication (e.g. antidepressants) and alcohol can also lead to acute RBD. Rarely, RBD occurs also in the context of a NREM-REM (overlap) parasomnia (49). In advance stages of neurodegeneration, a so-called *status dissociatus* can be observed, an

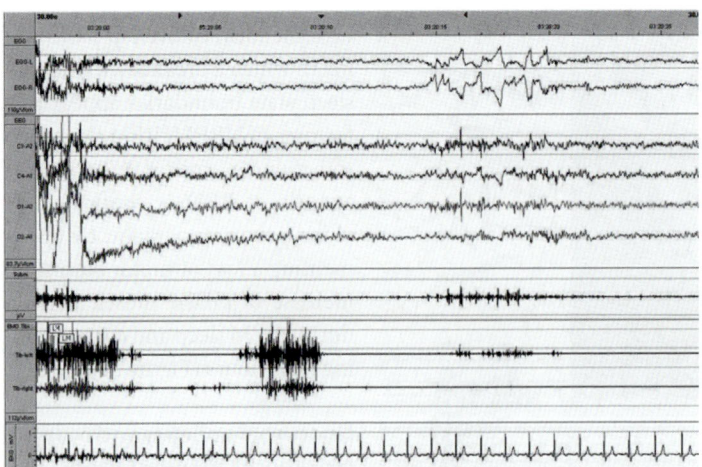

Figure 36.6 REM sleep behaviour disorder (RBD), polysomnographic findings. Pictures taken from a video-polysomnography of a 60-year-old man with RBD showing increased tonic and even more so phasic chin and tibialis anterior EMG activities during REM sleep.

NFLE is underdiagnosed because clinical manifestations are similar to those of motor parasomnias and sleep-related dissociative disorders. Also, nocturnal seizures and parasomnias can co-exist in a single patient (22,56).

A family history of possible NFLE is found in about one fourth of cases. The genetic bases of the disease have been identified in a minority of cases (mutations causing increased function of the neuronal nicotinic acetylcholine receptors). A focal cortical dysplasia of Taylor-type was usually found in surgically treated cases (57).

For the diagnosis of NFLE, video-polysomnography is required. The features differentiating NFLE from motor parasomnias and dissociative sleep-related disorders are: (a) several attacks per night at any time during the night; (b) brief duration of the attacks; (c) stereotyped motor pattern (52,53).

Nocturnal sleep-related eating disorders

Nocturnal sleep-related eating disorders (NSRED) are characterized by evening hyperphagia and/or nocturnal awakening and ingestion of food two or more times per week. Awareness of nocturnal eating is inconstant or completely absent. When awareness is present,

the term of night eating syndrome (NES) is preferred.

The age of onset is typically in adulthood, women are more frequently affected than men. Patients with NSRED have higher scores for depression and typically also present insomnia, RLS, or sleepwalking (58,59). Occasionally, intake of benzodiazepines or dopaminergic drugs may trigger the onset or aggravate the course of NSRED.

Sleep-related dissociative disorders and psychogenic non-epileptic seizures

These are disorders typically appearing in patients with known underlying psychiatric disorders which manifest with nocturnal episodes of complex motor behaviours (e.g. vocalization, screaming, crying, ambulation, sleepwalking, violence, self-mutilation) (44,60). Episodes appear typically after awakening from sleep, are variable in their clinical presentation and may last for several minutes up to hours. Am-

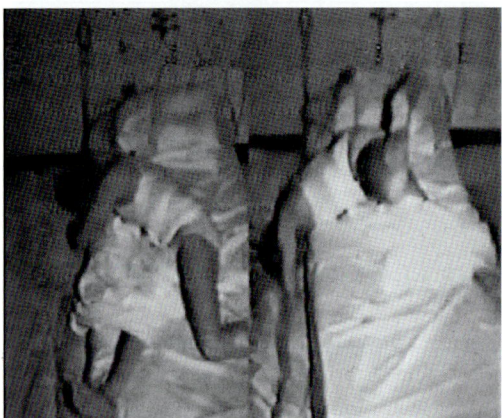

Figure 36.7 Nocturnal frontal lobe epilepsy (NFLE). Pictures taken from a video-polysomnography in a 24-year-old man with non-familial NFLE manifesting with hypermotor seizures. The two pictures show the similarity of motor patterns of two different episodes recorded in the same night.

nesia for the episodes is typically present. A co-existence of 'true' epileptic seizures and parasomnias in a single patient is possible and can hinder the correct diagnosis. The latter can be made only by video-polysomnography or EEG telemetry.

Diagnosis, differential diagnosis and diagnostic work up

The aetiological differential diagnosis is sometimes difficult. In the literature, several examples of disorders that were initially misdiagnosed can be found (e.g. as parasomnia instead of nocturnal epilepsy) (4). From a clinical perspective, it is important to stress that the clinical phenomenology *per se* is not diagnostic because same manifestations can be observed in the context of sleep disorders of different aetiology. International diagnostic criteria exist only for a few disorders including RLS and RBD (30,61). A few scales have been proposed to estimate the severity of some of these disorders (e.g. RLS and RBD), others to differentiate between epileptic and non-epileptic disorders (see Chapter 43) (12,62,63).

The diagnostic work-up of sleep-related movement disorders and disturbances of motor control include the following steps and tools:
- detailed history, whenever possible including an interview with bed partners
- questionnaires
- homevideo may be helpful and suggested as a first step before regular sleep or telemetric investigations (22)
- video-polysomnography including multiple EEG and EMG derivations

In some situations (e.g. NREM parasomnias, nocturnal epilepsy), sleep deprivation prior to polysomnography may be used to trigger motor events. Neuroimaging is mandatory in patients with nocturnal epilepsy RBD, and adult onset, frequent NREM parasomnias. Daytime neurophysiological studies (e.g. EEG, electroneuromyography, vigilance tests), genetic tests, detailed cognitive and psychiatric assessments should be obtained based on specific diagnostic hypotheses.

Treatment and prognosis

For most sleep-related movement disorders and motor disturbances, only anecdotal reports or small series on treatment have been published. The prognosis is very variable and depends in particular on the presence of an underlying brain disorder, progressive or not.

International treatment guidelines have been published only for RLS (64). They include level A recommendations for rotigotine, ropinirole, pramipexole, gabapentin and pregabalin, which are all considered effective for the short-term treatment for RLS. For the long-term treatment of RLS, rotigotine is considered effective, gabapentin is probably effective, and ropinirole, pramipexole and gabapentin are considered possibly effective (64).

Generally speaking treatment options for sleep-related movement disorders include the following:
- avoidance of triggering/exacerbating situations: sleep deprivation, fever in NREM parasomnias and nocturnal epilepsy, and drugs (see above)
- treatment of co-morbid sleep disorders (e.g. sleep-disordered breathing) may have a positive impact also on sleep-related movement disorders/motor disturbances
- non-pharmacological interventions: e.g. stress-reducing techniques and cognitive-behavioural treatment for NREM parasomnias, bruxism and nocturnal psychiatric disorders; safe sleep environment for sleepwalkers; oral appliances (splints) for bruxism
- pharmacological treatments (see Table 36.5)
- surgery (e.g. in severe nocturnal frontal lobe epilepsy, parasomnias in the context of Parkinson's disease).

Table 36.5
Pharmacological interventions in sleep-related movement disorders.

Interventions	Sleep-related movement disorders
clonazepam/ benzodiazepines	▪ NREM parasomnias, RBD, intermittent RLS ▪ sleep-related rhythmic movement disorders, excessive NREM and REM myoclonus, and nocturnal eating disorders
dopaminergic drugs	▪ RLS, PLMS, RBD, and nocturnal eating disorders
melatonin	▪ RBD (up to 12-16mg)
antiepileptic drugs carbamazepin, gabapentin or topiramate	▪ nocturnal epilepsy, RLS, and nocturnal eating disorder
antidepressants	▪ sleep paralysis, nocturnal panic attacks ▪ sleep-related rhythmic movement disorders ▪ may aggravate RLS
opioids	▪ RLS

Video fragment

Fragment 36.1
PMLS in RLS
52-year-old patient with restless legs syndrome. Nocturnal polysomnography with (from top to bottom) electro-oculography, chin electromyography, electro-encephalography, electrocardiography, and tibial electromyography (EMG) reveals periodic limb movements of sleep (PLMS) which can be seen both clinically and in EMG recordings.

References

1 Chokroverty S, Allen RP, Walters AS, Montagna P. Sleep and movement disorders: Oxford University Press, 2013.

2 De Cock Cochen VC, Vidaihlet M, Leu S, et al. Restoration of normal motor control in Parkinson's disease during REM sleep. Brain 2007;130:450-456.

3 Xiong L, Montplaisir J, Desautels A, et al. Family study of restless legs syndrome in Quebec, Canada: clinical characterization of 671 familial cases. Arch Neurol 2010;67:617-622.

4 Scheffer IE, Bhatia KP, Lopes-Cendes I, et al. Autosomal dominant nocturnal frontal lobe epilepsy misdiagnosed as sleep disorder. Lancet 1995;343:515-517.

5 Lemke JR, Lal D, Reinthaler EM, et al. Mutations in GRIN2A cause idiopathic focal epilepsy with rolandic spikes. Nature Genet 2013;45:1067-1072.

6 Iranzo A, Tllosa E, Gelpi E, et al. Neurodegenerative disease status and post-mortem pathology in idiopathic rapid-eye-movement sleep behaviour disorder: an observational cohort study. Lancet Neurol 2013;12:443-453.

7 Ohayon MM, Zulley J, Guilleminault C, Smirne S. Prevalence and pathologic associations of sleep paralysis in the general population. Neurology 1999;52:1194-1200.

8 Pressmann MR. Factors that predispose, prime and precipitate NREM parasomnias in adults: Clinical and forensic implications. Sleep Med Rev 2007;11:5-30.

9 Boeve BF. Pathophysiology of REM sleep behaviour disorder and relevance to neurodegenerative disease. Brain 2007;130:2770-2788.

10 Zadra A, Desautels A, Petit D, Montplaisir J. Somnambulism: clinical aspects and pathophysiological hypotheses. Lancet Neurol 2013;12:285-294.

11 Bassetti C, Vella S, Donati F, Wielepp P, Weder B. SPECT during sleepwalking. Lancet 2000;356:484-485.

12 Poryazova R, Oberholzer M, Baumann CR, Bassetti C. REM sleep behaviour disorder in Parkinson's disease: a Questionnaire-based Survey. J Clin Sleep Med 2013;9:55-59.

13 Katz PS. Neurons, networks, and motor behaviour. Neuron 1996;16:245-253.

14 Tassinari CA, Rubboli G, Gardella E, et al. Central pattern generators for a common semiology in fronto-limbic seizures and in parasomnias. A neuro-othologic approach. Neurol Sci 2005;26:225-232.

15 Mahowald MK, Schenck CH. Dissociated states of wakefulness and sleep. Neurology 1992;42S6:44-52.

16 Schindler K, Gast H, Bassetti C, et al. Hyperperfusion of anterior cingulate gyrus in a case of paroxysmal nocturnal dystonia. Neurology 2001;57:917-920.

17 Terzaghi M, Sartori I, Tassi L, et al. Evidence of dissociated arousal states during NREM parasomnia from an intracerebral neurophysiological study. Sleep 2009;32:409-412.

18 Siclari F, Khatami R, Urbaniok F, et al. Violence in sleep. Brain 2010;133:3494-3509.

19 Oswald I. Sudden bodily jerks on falling asleep. Brain 1959;82:92-103.

20 American Academy of Sleep Medicine (AASM). The International Classification of Sleep Disorders, Second Edition ed. Westchester, IL, 2005.

21 De Roeck J, van Hoof E, Cluydts R. Sleep-related expiratory groaning: a case report. Sleep 1983;12:237.

22 Tinuper P, Provini F, Bisulli F, et al. Movement disorders in sleep: Guidelines differentiating epileptic from non-epileptic motor phenomena arising from sleep. Sleep Med Rev 2007;11:255-267.

23 Broughton R, Tolentino MA, Krelina M. Excessive fragmentary myoclonus in NREM sleep: a report of 38 cases. Electroencephal Clin Neurophysiol 1985;61:123-133.

24 Resnick TJ, Moshé SL, Perotta L, Chambers HJ. Benign neonatal myoclonus. Arch Neurol 1986;43:266-268.

25. Ekbom KA. Restless legs: A clinical study. Acta Med Scand 1945;158S:1-124.

26 Bassetti C, Mauerhofer D, Mathis J, Gugger M, Hess CW. Restless legs syndrome: A clinical study of 55 patients. Eur Neurol 2001;45:67-74.

27 Kallweit U, Siccoli M, Poryazova R, Werth E, Bassetti CL. Excessive daytime sleepiness in idiopathic restless legs syndrome: Characteristics and evolution under dopaminergic treatment. Eur Neurol 2009; 62:176-917.

28 Hübner A, Krafft A, Gadient S, Werth E, Zimmermann R, Bassetti CL. Characteristics and determinants of restless legs syndrome in pregnancy: A prospective study. Neurology 2013;80:738-742.

29 Montplaisir J, Boucher S, Poirier G, Lavigne G, Lapierre O, Léspérance P. Clinical, polysomnographic and genetic characteristics of restless legs syndrome: A study of 133 patients diagnosed with standard criteria. Mov Disord 1997;12:61-65.

30 Allen RP, Picchietti D, Hening WA, Trenkwalder C, Walters AS, Montplaisir J. Restless legs syndrome: diagnostic criteria, special considerations, and epidemiology. A report from the restless legs syndrome diagnosis and epidemiology workshop of the National Institute of Health. Sleep Med 2003;4:101-119.

31 Baumann C, Marti I, Bassetti CL. Restless legs symptoms without periodic limb movements in sleep and without response to dopaminergic agents: a restless legs-like syndrome? Eur J Neurol 2007;14:1369-72.

32 Vetrugno R, Provini F, Meletti S, et al. Propriospinal myoclonus at the sleep-wake transition: A new-type of parasomnia. Sleep 2001;24:835-843.

33 Dahlitz M, Parkes JD. Sleep paralysis. Lancet 1993;341:406-407.

34 Passouant P, Billiard M. The evolution of narcolepsy with age. In: Guilleminault C, Dement WC, Passouant P, eds. Narcolepsy. New York: Spectrum Publications Inc., 1976: 179-200.

35 Panayiotopoulos CP, Michale M, Sanders S, et al. Benign childhood focal epilepsies: assessment of established and newly recognized syndromes. Brain 2008;131:2264-2286.

36 Bernasconi A, Andermann F, Cendes F, Dubeau F, Andermann E, Olivier A. Nocturnal temporal lobe epilepsy. Neurology 1998;50:1772-1777.

37 Mayer G, Tracik F, Wilde F. Rhythmic movement disorder revisited. J Sleep Res 2000;9S1:127.

38 Bassetti CL. Sleepwalking (Somnambulism). In: Laures S, Tononi G, eds. The Neurology of Consciousness: Cognitive Neuroscience and Neuropathology: Academic Press, 2009.

39 Schenck CH, Mahowald MW. A polysomnographically documented case of adult somnambulism with long-distance automobile driving and frequent nocturnal violence: Parasomnia with continuing danger as a noninsane automatism. Sleep 1995;18:765-772.

40 Andersen ML, Poyares D, Alves RSC, Skomro R, Tufik S. Sexsomnia: Abnormal sexual behaviour during sleep. Brain Res Reviews 2007;56:271-282.

41 Kavey NB, Whyte J, Resor SR, Gidro-Frank S. Somnambulism in adults. Neurology 1990;40:749-752.

42 Pedley TA, Guilleminault C. Episodic nocturnal wanderings responsive to anticonvulsant drug therapy. Ann Neurol 1977;2:30-35.

43 Oberholzer M, Poryazova R, Bassetti CL. Sleepwalking in Parkinson's disease: A questionnaire-based survey. J Neurol 2011;258:1261-1267.

44 Schenck CH, Milner DM, Hurwitz TD, et al. Dissociative disorders presenting as somnambulism: Polysomnographic, video and clinical documentation. Dissociation 1989;2:194-204.

45 Schenck CH, Bundlie SR, Patterson AL, Mahowald MW. Rapid eye movement sleep behaviour disorder. JAMA 1987;257:1786-1789.

46 Iranzo A, Molinuevo JL, Santamaria J, et al. Rapid-eye movement sleep behaviour disorder as an early marker for a neurodegenerative disorder: a descriptive study. Lancet Neurol 2006;5:572-577.

47 Mathis J, Hess CW, Bassetti C. Isolated mediotegmental lesion causing narcolepsy and rapid eye movement sleep behaviour disorder: a case evidencing a common pathway in narcolepsy and rapid eye movement sleep behaviour disorder. J Neurol Neurosurg Psychiatry 2007;78:427-429.

48 Iranzo A, Graus F, Clover L, et al. Rapid eye movement sleep behaviour disorder and potassium channel antibody-associated limbic encephalitis. Ann Neurol 2006;59:178-81.

49 Di Fabio N, Poryazova R, Oberholazer M, Baumann CR, Bassetti CL. Sleepwalking, REM sleep behaviour disorder and overlap parasomnia in patients with Parkinson's disease. Eur Neurol 2013;70:297-303.

50 Mahowald MW, Schenck CH. Status dissociatus - a perspective on states of being. Sleep 1991;14:69-79.

51 Provini F, Vetrugno R, Pastorelli F, Lombardi C, Plazzi G, et al. Status dissociatus after surgery for tegmental ponto-mesencephalic cavernoma: A state-dependent disorder of motor control during sleep. Mov Disord 2004;19:719.

52 Provini F, Plazzi G, Tinuper P, Vandi S, Lugaresi E, Montagna P. Nocturnal frontal lobe epilepsy. A clinical and polygraphic overview of 100 consecutive patients. Brain 1999;122:1017-1022.

53 Plazzi G, Provini F, Tinuper P, et al. Nocturnal frontal lobe epilepsy: Clinical, video- polysomno-

graphic, and genetic data in 100 cases. Neurology 1998;50:A67.

54 Tinuper P, Provini F, Bisulli F, Lugaresi E. Hyperkinetic manifestations in nocturnal frontal lobe epilepsy. Semiological features and physiopathological hypothesis. Neurol Sci 2005;26:210-214.

55 Siclari F, Nobili L, Lo Russo G, al. e. Stimulus-induced, sleep-bound, focal seizures: A case report. Sleep 2011;34:1727-1730.

56 Tinuper P, Bisulli F, Provini F. The parasomnias: mechanisms and treatment. Epilepsia 2012;S7:12-19.

57 Nobili L, Francione S, Mai R, et al. Surgical treatment of drug-resistant nocturnal frontal lobe epilepsy. Brain 2007;130:561-573.

58 Vetrugno R, Manconi M, Ferini-Strambi L, Provini E, Plazzi G, Montagna P. Nocturnal eating: Sleep-related eating disorder or night eating syndrome ? A video-polysomnographic study. Sleep 2006;29:949-954.

59 Auger RR. Sleep-related eating disorders. Psychiatry 2006;3:64-70.

60 Thacker K, Devinsky O, Perrine K, Alper K, Luciano D. Non-epileptic seizures during apparent sleep. Ann Neurol 1993;33:414-418.

61 Schenck CH, Montplaisir JY, Frauscher B, al. e. Rapid eye movement sleep behaviour disorder: devising controlled active treatment studies for symptomatic and neuroprotective therapy-a consensus statement from the International Rapid Eye Movement Sleep Behaviour Disorder Study Group. Sleep Med 2013;14:795-806.

62 The International Restless Legs Syndrome Study Group. Validation of the International Restless Legs Syndrome Study Group rating scale for restless legs syndrome. Sleep Med 2003;4:121-132.

63 Manni R, Terzaghi M, Repetto A. The FLEP scale in diagnosis nocturnal frontal lobe from epilepsy, NREM and REM parasomnias: Data from tertiary sleep and epilepsy unit. Epilepsia 2008;49:1581-1585.

64 Garcia-Borreguero D, Ferini-Strambi L, Kohnen R, et al. European guidelines on management of restless legs syndrome: report of a joint task force by the European Federation of Neurological Societies, the European Neurological Society and the European Sleep Research Society. Eur J Neurol 2012;19:1385-1396.

37

Psychogenic (Functional) Movement Disorders

Isabel Parees & Mark J. Edwards

Psychogenic movement disorders (PMD) are part of the broad spectrum of 'functional' neurological symptoms which together account for 16% of new patients attending neurology outpatient clinics (1). Patients can present with the whole range of abnormal movements, which are defined as incongruous and inconsistent with movement disorders in typical neurological diseases. Different terms have been used over time to describe these patients (functional, hysteria, psychogenic, psychosomatic, conversion disorder, somatisation disorder, non-organic, medically unexplained), many of which reflect different theories relating to aetiology, particularly with regard to the importance placed on psychological triggering and maintaining factors. Recently, more neurobiologically focussed models of the pathophysiology of these symptoms have been developed within the framework provided by modern cognitive neuroscience. This chapter covers the current state of knowledge regarding the diagnosis, pathophysiology and management of this group of patients.

Epidemiology

The prevalence of PMD is uncertain due to the lack of consensus on diagnostic criteria and the different methodologies used to ascertain cases. It has been estimated at between 1% and 9% of patients in general neurological clinics (2-4). In adult movement disorders clinics, this ranges between 2% and 20% (5). The mean age at onset

is reported to be between 37 and 50 years (6), and women are more commonly affected. In approximately 70% of the cases, patients present with tremor or dystonia. Although PMD usually occur as a single neurological diagnosis, they have been reported to be associated with organic neurological disorders in 10-15% of the patients (7,8). This association has been called 'functional overlay' and has been the topic of recent studies (7,9-11). PMD are thought to be uncommon in the elderly, but one recent study has reported that 21% of a large cohort of patients with PMD had an onset of symptoms after the age of 60 years, which highlights the importance of considering this diagnosis in older people (12). PMD are also reported in children, but not commonly, with gait disorder and tremor being the most common manifestations.

Aetiology

Classically, psychogenic neurological symptoms, including PMD, have been explained as resulting from psychological stressors which lead to unconsciously produced physical symptoms. In keeping with this theory, several authors have reported psychogenic symptoms to be associated with early childhood trauma (13-15) or have stressed the aetiological importance of emotional stress or recent life events (16,17). Indeed, it was not possible to make a diagnosis of conversion disorder according to DSM IV criteria without the presence of a psychological stressor that preceded the onset of physical symptoms. However, pure psychological explanations are not well implemented in the brain. Also, recent epidemiological data do not support the hypothesis that childhood or recent traumatic events are common in patients with PMD (18). It is not uncommon to see patients who do not report recent life events and in whom 'stress' cannot easily be related to their symptoms. Such patients are particularly vulnerable to the neurology-psychiatry 'merry-go-round' where they are referred from neurology to psychiatry and then back again as there is no sign of psychopathology. Such patients can become lost in the gap between psychiatry and neurology or simply start a cycle of diagnostic tests again with a different neurologist. The lack of a psychological stressor in many patients has been reflected in the DSM V criteria, in which its presence is no longer part of the diagnostic criteria for conversion disorders.

More recently, physical events have been emphasised as playing a potentially key role in symptom development (19). Injuries, infections, surgery, etc. are commonly reported to precede the onset of PMD (12,19-23). Indeed, having an organic neurological disease has been recognized as one of the most powerful risk factors for developing psychogenic symptoms (24).

Pathophysiology

The notion of psychogenic symptoms can be traced to ancient times. The first works that aimed to reach a scientific understanding of the underlying mechanisms come from the late 19th and early 20th centuries. Initial formulations from Charcot and Janet were primarily related to explaining sensory loss and are based on the idea of dissociation. Here, psychogenic symptoms are thought to be the result of a spontaneous narrowing of attention when individuals with a pathologically weak mental state are exposed to traumatic events (25). This narrowing of attention restricts the number of sensory

channels that can be attended to simultaneously, and over time, the individual may develop a habitual tendency to concentrate on some sensory channels and neglect others, leading to the loss of deliberate attentional control over neglected channels (25). The impairment of attention over the neglected body part may result in negative somatic symptoms such as unexplained sensory loss. One shortcoming of this theory is the difficulty it has in explaining positive motor symptoms such as PMD as a result of an abnormal attentional process. Later on, influential Freudian theories of conversion disorder proposed that psychogenic symptoms were the result of repressing memories associated with emotional trauma. Within this framework, the negative affect of the trauma is 'converted' into a somatic symptom that either was present at the time of the original trauma or is some symbolic representation of it (25).

Recently, there has been a shift away from pure psychodynamic formulations, and a burst of research within modern cognitive neuroscience has aimed to understand psychogenic symptoms from a more neurobiological perspective. Over the past few years, different models have been suggested to explain PMD. For instance, Hallett (5), based on a number of functional imaging studies, has proposed a model which has 'a previously mapped conversion motor representation' as a key concept, i.e. a (conditioned) pattern of movement established perhaps by a previous triggering event. The presence of physical precipitating factors at the onset of the abnormal movement reported by many patients (e.g. injury) could provide a relevant trigger for the development of a 'conversion motor representation'. The additional emotional arousal that is often reported in the background and/or at the time of onset could certainly increase the salience of sensory information arising during a physical trigger and facilitate this process. Edwards et al. aimed to explain functional motor and sensory psychogenic symptoms by employing well-established Bayesian theories of brain function (active inference) (26). Within this framework, the brain is understood as an inference machine that actively predicts and explains its sensations. Perception arises from integrating sensory information from the environment with internal predictions about the expected data (priors). A mismatch between sensory information and priors is known as prediction error. In physiological states, neuronal systems are hypothesised to try to minimize prediction error through interactions between multiple levels of a cortical hierarchy. The minimization of prediction error can occur via a variable combination of modifications to priors so that they better fit the sensory data and by actively adjusting the precision which is assigned to sensory data to better conform to priors. Attention plays an important role here as 'attended' priors or sensations are granted high precision. It is proposed that physical triggering events, combined with many other factors, including past illness experiences and beliefs, cognitive and affective biases, can lead to new priors whose content is an abnormal movement or sensation. When combined with self-directed attention, the precision of these priors is high enough to overwhelm contrary sensory data from lower levels and clinically produce the abnormal movement or sensations consistent with the high-level prior. Irrespective of the framework used, it seems reasonable to incorporate three key concepts that clinically define PMD in any model seeking to explain the underlying mechanisms: attention, symptom-related beliefs and agency.

Attention

A key feature that distinguishes patients with PMD from those with 'organic' movement disorders is that the PMD requires attention to manifest: when attention is distracted, there is typically a reduction, even disappearance of the movement disorder. The role of attention in PMD has been demonstrated in different studies. For instance, patients with psychogenic tremor (PT) have been shown to spend significantly

more time looking directly at their affected limb during clinical examination compared to patients with 'organic' tremor, suggesting a role for self-directed visual attention in the generation of motor symptoms (27). Also, it has been reported that they overestimate the amount of time with tremor during the day and that when attention is turned towards the symptom an increase in tremor occurs (28). Reaction and movement times have been assessed in a group of patients with PMD in different paradigms designed to manipulate the degree of predictability of the movement (and hence its capacity for pre-planning). Movement impairment was restricted to tasks where conscious movement control in the setting of explicit movement production was possible, and not where movement occurred in a more automatic, implicit fashion (29). Finally, a recent study that compared positron emission tomography of regional cerebral blood flow in a small cohort of patients with 'fixed' psychogenic dystonia and genetically characterised primary dystonia as well as healthy controls showed that fixed dystonia patients had reduced blood flow in the primary motor cortex and increased blood flow in the basal ganglia and cerebellum, which was contrary to that seen in patients with genetic primary dystonia. The authors suggested that the abnormal subcortical activation in psychogenic patients could reflect problems with self-directed attention/monitoring, perhaps related to fronto-subcortical circuits mediating motor attention (30).

Symptom-related beliefs/expectations

Some features seen in PMD reveal that beliefs about the symptoms play an important role in symptom generation. These beliefs are often at odds with the constraints of anatomy and physiology. For instance, the 'tubular' visual field defect is characterised by a central visual field defect of the same diameter, whether it is mapped close to them or far away. This challenges the laws of optics, but fits with personal beliefs about the nature of vision. An important effect of beliefs altering sensory experience in PMD has been demonstrated in a study assessing the duration of PT under real-life conditions (28). Patients with psychogenic and 'organic' tremor were asked to wear an ambulatory actigraph which constantly recorded and stored data on tremor duration over 5 days. During this time patients also completed diaries rating how much of the time they felt they had tremor. Patients with PT had on average 30 minutes of tremor a day, but rated themselves affected by tremor 80-90% of the waking day. It was suggested that very strong top-down prediction of constant tremor overwhelmed real sensory data in this group, and periods without tremor were simply ignored (28).

Agency

The key clinical feature that separates patients with PMD from those with typical movement disorders is that the movements resemble ones that are made voluntarily but patients report them as being involuntary and not under their control. We have already mentioned that malingering is an unlikely explanation for most patients with psychogenic symptoms. Then why do patients with PMD experience a voluntary movement as involuntary? Cognitive neuroscience has revealed the existence of mechanisms within the brain that confer a sense of agency to movement (that one is the cause of one's own actions). In the field of movement disorders, an important study using fMRI to understand PT showed a relative reduction in activation of the right inferior parietal lobule in patients when comparing activation patterns while they experienced functional tremor and when they voluntarily produced tremor (31). This brain area is thought to be a comparator of internal sensory prediction and the actual sensory state and is considered to be important in processes such as self-agency (see Chapter 1). Edwards et al. assessed the conscious experience of volition for movement in patients with PT (32). Based on Libet's paradigm, patients judged the feeling

of intention to move significantly closer to the action of moving compared to control participants. They concluded that the sense of volition prior to movement is impaired in patients with PMD, and this might help to explain why they experience the abnormal movement as involuntary (32). Another study has used the phenomenon of action-effect binding as an implicit measure of agency in patients with PMD (33). A decreased action-effect binding when making normal voluntary movements compared with healthy volunteers was found, suggesting a reduced sense of agency in this group of patients.

Clinical presentation

Different features from the clinical history and examination findings are commonly noted in patients with PMD irrespective of the type of movement disorder that they display. None of these features is entirely specific for PMD, and the diagnosis should not be based on these features alone, though they can be helpful as part of the diagnostic process.

PMD often have a sudden onset with rapid progression to maximum severity; they can present with spontaneous remissions, paroxysmal exacerbations, and relapses. Patients may experience a shift in phenomenology over time (tremor turning to abnormal posture, for example) and may have a history of previously unexplained medical symptoms (see Video fragment 37.1). General clues on clinical examination include the co-existence of other psychogenic signs such as 'give-way' weakness, 'false' weakness (e.g. positive Hoover's sign) or non-physiological patterns of sensory loss. Fekete et al. has recently drawn attention to the frequent presence of convergence spasm (34).

Psychogenic tremor

PT is the most common form of PMD (4,6). A combination of rest, postural and intention tremor is commonly seen, which is an unusual pattern for organic tremor (see also Chapters

25,26). Arms are the most common body part affected, usually sparing the fingers. A sudden onset of the symptoms is common in many patients, and this is often preceded by a physical injury (35).

Distracting the patient's attention away from the tremor during examination usually makes the PT significantly change in frequency or even stop (see Video fragment 37.1, segment 2). Cognitive distracters (serial subtraction), tapping with an unaffected limb at a different frequency to the tremor and making a sudden ballistic movement with the other hand, are often used. With clinical assessment alone (without supplementation with tremor recordings), tapping tasks are the most sensitive and specific means for distinguishing essential tremor from PT (see Box 37.1). Self-paced cognitive tasks are not very effective. Also, tapping with the hands may not be a good distractor for tremors affecting the legs or head. In these cases, tapping with one foot or moving the tongue side to side, respectively, can be of help. Using tremor recordings, tapping tasks have again been shown to be helpful in distinguishing PT from organic tremors. Here patients with PT may 'entrain' to the tapping frequency, may show a shift in tremor frequency towards the tapping frequency, or may instead be inexplicably unable to perform the tapping task correctly with their normal hand. This illustrates an important point with distractor tasks, which is that the performance of the task must draw sufficient attention away from the tremoring limb. Ballistic movements of the non-tremoring limb cause a small pause in the tremor in patients with PT. Additional electrophysiological characteristics include a paradoxical worsening of the tremor with loading (which typically damps organic tremor) and co-contraction at the onset of tremor. A recent study aimed to differentiate psychogenic and organic tremors by comparing all these tests in a group of patients with PT and a mixed group of patients with typical tremors (PD, dystonic tremor, essential tremor, or neuropathic tremor (36). No single test was found to be of sufficient sensitivity and specificity to distinguish PT from typical tremor. However, a cut-off score was devised by combining several of these measures, and PT could be successfully distinguished from organic tremor. Nevertheless, these preliminary results need confirmation in a prospective study.

Psychogenic dystonia

Psychogenic dystonia is the second most common PMD after tremor (4). Patients with functional dystonia are usually women who present with fixed abnormal postures (see Figure 37.1)

Box 37.1

Main Features to look for in the examination of a patient with suspected psychogenic tremor.

Distractibility of Tremor

This comprises variable combinations of brief pauses in tremor, complete cessation of tremor, fluctuations in tremor frequency that occur in response to externally paced tasks, such as finger taps to a rhythm set by the examiner.

Entrainability of Tremor

A particular type of distractibility where the frequency of the patient's tremor shifts to exactly match that set by the examiner. This is not a common finding, but when it occurs, it is pathognomic of functional tremor.

Poor Task Performance

This is where the patient is unable to perform a simple rhythmic tapping movement to the frequency set by the examiner. The explanation for this sign is that attention is so focused on the production of the functional tremor that it interferes with any other task (dual task effect).

Pause with Ballistic Movement

The patient experiences a pause in their tremor when performing a quick, externally paced, ballistic movement with the other hand. It is important to monitor task performance here: slow movements with a delayed reaction time will not cause a pause in functional tremor.

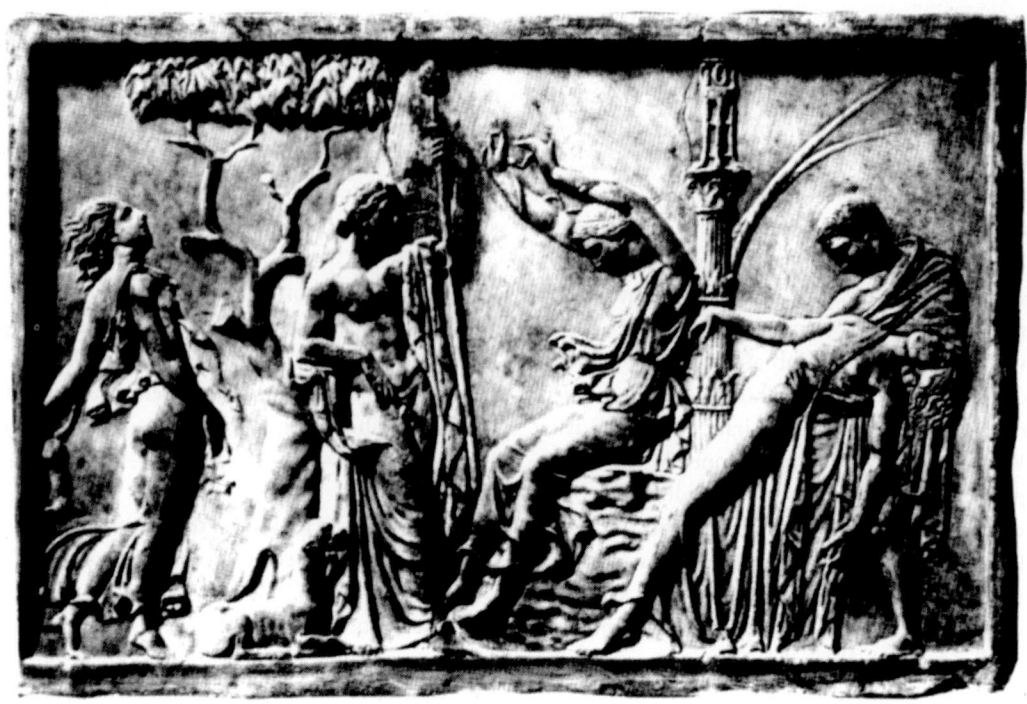

Figuur 37.1
In this statue, 'the dying bacchant', the female on the right shows a classical dystonic 'arc de cercle'.

typically triggered by an apparently minor injury, accompanied by severe pain similar to that noted in chronic regional pain syndrome type 1 (CRPS1). The nature of fixed dystonia continues to be debated, and lack of consensus exists as to whether it is best considered an organic or psychogenic movement disorder. Recently, it has been proposed that abnormalities in central body schema may be present in these patients, which might contribute to pain and other unusual features, such as the searching for an amputated limb seen in this condition (37). Clinically, psychogenic dystonia predominantly affects the limbs and less commonly the neck/shoulder region, jaw or face (22). Psychogenic blepharospasm has been recently reported to have different electrophysiological features compared with typical blepharospasm (38). An unusual distribution of dystonia given the age of onset can be a further clue that points toward psychogenic dystonia. For instance, primary generalized dystonia (with classic limb onset) occurs in individuals younger than 25 years, focal upper limb dystonia in individuals between 25-45 years and focal dystonia involving the craniocervical area usually occurs in individuals over the age of 45-50 years (see also Chapter 22). An unusual distribution given the age of onset can also be seen in secondary/neurodegenerative dystonia (see also Chapter 23), and such conditions should be taking into account in the differential diagnosis. In psychogenic dystonia there is typically an absence of task/position specificity commonly seen in organic dystonia, and patients often do not have sensory tricks. It can be difficult to demonstrate distractibility in fixed dystonia. Indeed, some patients do develop limb contractures demonstrating maintenance of postures even when unobserved. However, a brief give way of muscle activity in the affected limb can be felt with distraction in a number of patients.

It has recently been reported that some patients with fixed dystonia can respond immediately (within minutes) to botulinum toxin injections (see also Chapter 24) (39). This is in contrast to the known physiological effects of botulinum toxin, which usually take 36-72 hours to begin to become apparent. The dramatic response seen in these patients is therefore likely to be due to placebo effect and may help to confirm that such patients are different from those with typical dystonia.

Psychogenic myoclonus
Functional myoclonus is reported in about 20% of patients with PMD (4). Psychogenic myoclonus can be difficult to differentiate from typical myoclonus (see also Chapter 28) as it is difficult to demonstrate distractibility in patients with intermittent movements. Electrophysiological tests can be particularly helpful in supporting the clinical diagnosis (see Box 37.2). Simple recording of the duration of the jerks can be useful, particularly to demonstrate variability in duration and recruitment pattern of EMG burst, suggestive of a psychogenic cause. Bursts of less than 75 ms duration are unlikely to be psychogenic. However, bursts of more than 75 ms do not prove psychogenicity as some forms of organic myoclonus (e.g. brainstem myoclonus, spinal segmental myoclonus) may have EMG burst lengths longer than 75ms. The most definitive test to confirm the psychogenic origin of the myoclonus is detection of the readiness potential or Bereitschaftspotential (BP). This EEG potential starts around 1.5 seconds before voluntary self-paced movement and reflects activity in areas associated with movement preparation. It can be found in patients with psychogenic myoclonus, but has never been reported in patients with typical myoclonus. Two studies assessing the presence of BP have confirmed that most patients diagnosed with idiopathic spinal myoclonus or propriospinal myoclonus had in fact a psychogenic origin (40,41).

Box 37.2
Useful Electrophysiological tests in distinguishing organic from psychogenic myoclonus.

Favours Organic Myoclonus
Presence of a cortical spike ~20ms before jerk (seen in some patients with cortical myoclonus) Short duration of EMG burst (<75ms). However, burst length above this is seen in various forms of non-cortical myoclonus including sub-cortical myoclonus, reflex reticular myoclonus. Presence of giant somatosensory evoked potential (SEP)
Favours Functional Myoclonus
Presence of a pre-movement potential (Bereitschaftspotential) before jerk. Note that in patients with very frequent jerks (>1 per 2-5 seconds) the premovement potential may be difficult to record due to artefact in the EEG recording. Conversely, pre-movement potentials may be absent in patients with very infrequent jerks, as often a number of jerks need to be averaged to detect the pre-movement potential.

Psychogenic gait disorder
Abnormal gait can be an isolated phenomenon in patients with PMD or mixed with other clinical manifestations. In the classical manifestation of psychogenic gait disturbance, patients veer from side to side when walking, often waving their arms at the same time. They seem to be about to lose their balance, but tend not to. This ability to shift their centre of gravity from one side to the other without losing balance is actually a demonstration of good balance in direct contrast to the patient's subjective report of poor balance. This pattern has been termed the 'walking on ice' gait. Other features include: narrow base, hesitation, dramatic response to Romberg's test and tests of postural stability, 'uneconomic' postures or excessive slowness. Some patients with typical neurological conditions such as Huntington's disease or generalised dystonia

can exhibit bizarre patterns of gait, and clinical experience in both psychogenic and organic disorders can be required to make a clear diagnosis.

Psychogenic parkinsonism

The diagnosis of psychogenic parkinsonism is not always easy. Rigidity may be present but feels similar to voluntary oppositional resistance against passive movements rather than true cogwheel rigidity. Movements may appear to require great effort and be slow, but true bradykinesia with decreasing amplitude with rapid repetitive movements is not seen. When patients are distracted, the velocity of the movements can normalize. When tremor is present, features such as distractibility, entrainment, and stopping of the tremor with ballistic movements of the contralateral hand are often seen. Postural stability testing may lead to a dramatic loss of balance and falls. It is established that patients with Parkinson's disease have a strong response to placebo (42), so caution needs to be taken in interpreting the response to placebo in patients with suspected psychogenic parkinsonism. Dopamine transporter (DaT) SPECT scanning is a useful test to investigate the integrity of the nigrostriatal system and discriminate psychogenic parkinsonism from Parkinson's disease (see also Chapter 5). However, it is worth noting that the diagnosis of Parkinson's disease does not exclude the presence of psychogenic symptoms or vice versa. Indeed, it has been suggested that patients with Parkinson's disease are more prone to develop psychogenic symptoms than other neurodegenerative disorders (9, 10).

Psychogenic paroxysmal movement disorders

Although a 'paroxysmal' component is one of the most important clinical presentations of PMD, psychogenic paroxysmal disorders have been rarely mentioned in the literature. Because organic paroxysmal disorders such as paroxysmal kinesogenic dyskinesia, paroxysmal non-kinesogenic dyskinesia, and paroxysmal exercise-induced dyskinesia or even focal seizures are by definition brief and reversible, the clinical diagnosis can be very difficult. However, they have typical precipitating factors, and the length of the episodes is also well defined. Incongruous features can therefore raise suspicions of a psychogenic cause, and on examination such patients will often have other signs consistent with PMD. Often, ictal-EEG and video recording of the episode are very useful to reach the diagnosis (see Video fragment 37.1, segment 3, 4).

Diagnosis

Over the past few years, movement disorder specialists have placed a marked emphasis on using positive physical signs and investigation findings to support the diagnosis of PMD rather than make a diagnosis based on exclusion or the presence of psychological distress. The most widely used criteria were developed by Fahn and Williams in 1989 (43). PMD are divided into four categories of diagnostic certainty: documented, clinically established, probable and possible. These criteria were in fact first developed for psychogenic dystonia alone, but were later expanded to cover all PMD. Gupta and Lang have suggested revisions to these criteria which delete the 'possible' category as being not sufficiently specific for PMD, and also introduce the concept of a laboratory-supported level of certainty (44). Shill and Gerber proposed alternative criteria, but they have been criticised for relying too heavily on historical factors such as 'disease modelling' without reference to the movement disorder phenomenology (15).

Recently, these criteria have been assessed with regard to inter-rater reliability, and have been found to demonstrate moderate to poor reliability for the probable and possible categories. Therefore, new criteria, which perhaps include more specific emphasis on the positive physical signs that predict PMD rather than the unspecified 'incongruency' with typical movement disorders, is urgently needed to improve reliability.

Giving the diagnosis of a PMD to patients can be sometimes even more challenging than making the diagnosis itself. A poor explanation such as 'all the tests have come back normal, so it's all because of stress' often causes incredulity and sometimes hostility (mainly because many patients are not stressed, and this explanation is often interpreted as meaning that there is nothing wrong and the symptoms are 'not real'. Explaining what they do have, what they do not have and why (for example, Parkinson's disease), how you have reached the diagnosis (for example, explaining the positive signs in the examination), stating that the diagnosis is very common and that you believe them (you do not think that it is all in their mind or they are faking the symptoms) are often helpful (24). It is also important to explain that a potential for reversibility does exist and that treating psychological issues (when relevant) can also help to treat the condition. Many patients find written information about the symptoms useful, such as the information at www.neurosymptoms.org (24).

Differential diagnosis

Many clinicians do not feel confident during the diagnostic process and frequently worry about erroneously labelling a patient as psychogenic. A systematic review of studies of misdiagnosis in functional neurological symptoms found, however, that only 5% of patients had a change in diagnosis after an average of five years (46). This is the same rate of misdiagnosis as for most neurological and psychiatric conditions. However, the diagnosis is not always easy, and it is usually prudent to ask for a second opinion if uncertainty persists.

There are detailed general clues in the history and positive signs in the examination for each type of PMD that may help to differentiate them from their 'organic' counterparts. Additionally, Stone et al. have recently discussed general pitfalls in approaching patients with psychogenic symptoms, those that can lead erroneously to a diagnosis of neurological disease as psychogenic ('mimics') as well as those that can lead to the diagnosis of psychogenic patients as having a typical neurological disease ('chameleons') (24). Putting too much emphasis on the presence of psychiatric disorders and life events, failure to consider that patients may have an overlay of psychogenic symptoms on typical neurological diseases, being reassured by normal imaging results or the presence of 'la belle indifference' can lead to a misdiagnosis of patients with neurological disease as having psychogenic symptoms. In contrast, relying on the sense that the patient is too 'nice, normal, or not stressed' or too old to have psychogenic symptoms, or that symptoms came on after injury or other illness can be associated with a misdiagnosis of psychogenic symptoms as due to organic neurological disease (24). Because PMD resemble movements that are voluntarily produced, there is often a question as to whether patients are deliberately producing symptoms in order to gain psychological or financial benefits. It is generally acknowledged to be very difficult to distinguish malingering from 'true' PMD, but the consensus of opinion is that malingering is likely to be rare and is not a satisfying explanation for the disorder in the majority of patients. Data arguing against the idea that malingering is the most likely explanation for PMD comes from functional imaging studies in PT and fixed dystonia (30,31). Here, patterns of brain activation in patients were different to those seen in subjects feigning symptoms. Another study that argues against malingering used ambulatory actigraphy to monitor PT (28). Although patients were aware of being monitored, they failed to perceive how bad their symptoms were and they reported tremor to be present 83% of the time, when in fact it was only present 4% of the time.

Treatment

There are no official guidelines for the treatment of PMD. However, effective communication of the diagnosis that allows patients to understand their symptoms seems a good start. The benefit of simply explaining the diagnosis, at least in the early stages, has been found to lead to long-term improvement of symptoms in some patients with non-epileptic seizures (47), and it seems likely that this would extend to patients with PMD, too.

Referral of patients with PMD to physiotherapy is common practice by neurologists. However, in a recent survey, most physiotherapists reported that although they are interested in this group of patients, they have little knowledge (self-estimation) about how to treat them (48). Preliminary evidence for regular, low to medium intensity walking exercise has been found in a single-blind study which assessed patients with PMD after a 12-week program (49). In a study of 60 patients from the Mayo clinic with functional motor symptoms, a 5-day, inpatient, physical rehabilitation program produced benefits in over 60% of patients, which were sustained in most for over 2 years (50). Such work encourages the development of further studies to provide evidence for how physiotherapy could best be structured to design and deliver successful treatments to patients with PMD.

Psychological intervention can be helpful in patients who consider psychological factors as relevant in symptom development or maintenance. Indeed, a small study provided preliminary evidence for a positive effect of antidepressant treatment in those patients diagnosed with primary conversion disorder but not in those with somatisation disorder (51). Recently, a community-based study of psychogenic neurological symptoms demonstrated that patients receiving cognitive behavioural therapy (CBT)-based guided self-help combined with the standard care benefitted more than those who received just the standard care (52).

The use of placebo as a treatment strategy for PMD is still under debate. Because the prognosis and successful treatment of PMD may be highly dependent on the patients' belief that they will get better, some neurologists support the use of placebo in this group of patients. Indeed, dramatic therapeutic benefits mediated through placebo therapy have been described (39). However, the loss of patient autonomy and the erosion of the doctor-patient relationship are important ethical concerns that should be taken into account. Recently, the need for clinical trials to define optimal regimes for placebo therapy in these patients as well as guidelines for the education of health professionals in the use of placebos has been stressed (53).

Additional treatments have been suggested to be effective in PMD. For example, intrathecal baclofen was reported to be effective in fixed dystonia compared to placebo (54). However, it is unclear whether there was systematic unblinding of the participant by the systematic effects of the baclofen. Low-frequency, repetitive transcranial magnetic stimulation (TMS) has been used as a therapeutic tool in PMD with some promising results (long-lasting clinical improvement immediately after the TMS session was seen in many patients) (55,56). However, the unmasked nature of the intervention in most of these studies makes the placebo effect a likely explanation for the results.

There is limited controlled trial data to guide treatment in PMD, but the evidence that is available suggests that a multidisciplinary approach gives the best chance of benefit. A recent study that retrospectively evaluated a multidisciplinary inpatient programme suggested that this approach can provide long-lasting benefit for some patients with treatment-refractory PMD, at least as measured by retrospective self-reporting (57). However, similar to other studies, most patients failed to return to work, and the health-related financial benefits generally continued despite the reported clinical benefits.

Prognosis

Long-term follow-up studies have shown a high percentage of PMD patients with persistence of abnormal movements and the development of additional, unexplained medical symptoms. In one study, 90% of a group of 80 patients with a range of PMD still had abnormal movements after a mean of 3.2 years since their initial assessment (58). In another study, a third of patients was employed at the time of follow-up, while 11.5% was on disability and 1.3% was involved in litigation (59). In contrast, other studies of the long-term outcome in PMD have revealed that half of the patients report some improvement in their symptoms at the last follow-up (3-5 years after presentation) (35). Predictors of a favorable outcome were a short duration of illness, patient's perception of effective treatment by the physician, and the presence of a comorbid psychiatric diagnosis of depression or anxiety (amenable to treatment).

Conclusions

PMD are common and disabling, and represent a major social problem and huge financial burden to the health system. After being neglected for many years, a burst of research interest in the topic has recently occurred which, hopefully, will lead to improved biological understanding of these disorders. Because the potential for reversibility exists, there is an urgent need to find the best way to structure and deliver successful treatments to patients with PMD.

Video fragment

Fragment 37.1
Somatoform Disorders (Segments 1-4)
In this fragment some somatoform movement disorders are shown: a pseudo-paresis of the non-dominant body-half in a young woman (segment 1), a rather inconsistent tremor in the left arm of a right-handed young man (segment 2), a generalized, bizarre, hyperkinetic disorder, probably to be diagnosed as malingering (segment 3), and a man with bizarre posturing (segment 4).

References

1 Stone J, Carson A, Duncan R, et al. Who is referred to neurology clinics? The diagnoses made in 3781 new patients. Clin Neurol Neurosurg 2010;112:747-751.

2 Lempert T, Dieterich M, Huppert D, Brandt T. Psychogenic disorders in neurology: frequency and clinical spectrum. Acta Neurol Scand 1990;82:335-340.

3 Marsden CD. Hysteria - a neurologist's view. Psychol Med 1986;16:277-288.

4 Factor SA, Podskalny GD, Molho ES. Psychogenic movement disorders: frequency, clinical profile, and characteristics. J Neurol Neurosurg Psychiatry 1995;59:406-412.

5 Hallett M. Psychogenic movement disorders: a crisis for neurology. Curr Neurol Neurosci Rep 2006;6:269-271.

6 Hinson VK, Haren WB. Psychogenic movement disorders. Lancet Neurol 2006;5:695-700.

7 Stone J, Carson A, Duncan R, et al. Which neurological diseases are most likely to be associated with 'symptoms unexplained by organic disease'. J Neurol 2012;259:33-38.

8 Ranawaya R, Riley D, Lang A. Psychogenic dyskinesias in patients with organic movement disorders. Mov Disord 1990;5:127-133.

9 Onofrj M, Bonanni L, Manzoli L, Thomas A. Cohort study on somatoform disorders in Parkinson

disease and dementia with Lewy bodies. Neurology 2010;74:1598-1606.

10 Onofrj M, Thomas A, Tiraboschi P, et al. Updates on Somatoform Disorders (SFMD) in Parkinson's Disease and Dementia with Lewy Bodies and discussion of phenomenology. J Neurol Sci 2011;310:166-171.

11 Parees I, Saifee TA, Kojovic M, et al. Functional (psychogenic) symptoms in Parkinson's disease. Mov Disord 2013.

12 Batla A, Stamelou M, Edwards MJ, et al. Functional movement disorders are not uncommon in the elderly. Mov Disord 2013;28:540-543.

13 Alper K, Devinsky O, Perrine K, Vazquez B, Luciano D. Nonepileptic seizures and childhood sexual and physical abuse. Neurology 1993;43:1950-1953.

14 Bowman ES, Markand ON. Psychodynamics and psychiatric diagnoses of pseudoseizure subjects. Am J Psychiatry 1996;153:57-63.

15 Roelofs K, Keijsers GP, Hoogduin KA, Naring GW, Moene FC. Childhood abuse in patients with conversion disorder. Am J Psychiatry 2002;159:1908-1913.

16 Binzer M, Andersen PM, Kullgren G. Clinical characteristics of patients with motor disability due to conversion disorder: a prospective control group study. J Neurol Neurosurg Psychiatry 1997;63:83-88.

17 Irfan N, Badar A. Top ten stressors in the hysterical subjects of Peshawar. J Ayub Med Coll Abbottabad 2002;14:38-41.

18 Kranick S, Ekanayake V, Martinez V, Ameli R, Hallett M, Voon V. Psychopathology and psychogenic movement disorders. Mov Disord 2011;26:1844-1850.

19 Stone J, Carson A, Aditya H, et al. The role of physical injury in motor and sensory conversion symptoms: a systematic and narrative review. J Psychosom Res 2009;66:383-390.

20 Koller W, Lang A, Vetere-Overfield B, et al. Psychogenic tremors. Neurology 1989;39:1094-1099.

21 Stamelou M, Saifee TA, Edwards MJ, Bhatia KP. Psychogenic palatal tremor may be underrecognized: reappraisal of a large series of cases. Mov Disord 2012;27:1164-1168.

22 Schrag A, Trimble M, Quinn N, Bhatia K. The syndrome of fixed dystonia: an evaluation of 103 patients. Brain 2004;127:2360-2372.

23 Deuschl G, Koster B, Lucking CH, Scheidt C. Diagnostic and pathophysiological aspects of psychogenic tremors. Mov Disord 1998;13:294-302.

24 Stone J, Reuber M, Carson A. Functional symptoms in neurology: mimics and chameleons. Pract Neurol 2013;13:104-113.

25 Brown RJ. Psychological mechanisms of medically unexplained symptoms: an integrative conceptual model. Psychol Bull 2004;130:793-812.

26 Edwards MJ, Adams RA, Brown H, Parees I, Friston KJ. A Bayesian account of 'hysteria'. Brain 2012;135:3495-3512.

27 van Poppelen D, Saifee TA, Schwingenschuh P, et al. Attention to self in psychogenic tremor. Mov Disord 2011;26:2575-2576.

28 Parees I, Saifee TA, Kassavetis P, et al. Believing is perceiving: mismatch between self-report and actigraphy in psychogenic tremor. Brain 2012;135:117-123.

29 Parees I, Kassavetis P, Saifee TA, et al. Failure of explicit movement control in patients with functional motor symptoms. Mov Disord 2013;28:517-523.

30 Schrag AE, Mehta AR, Bhatia KP, et al. The functional neuroimaging correlates of psychogenic versus organic dystonia. Brain 2013;136:770-781.

31 Voon V, Gallea C, Hattori N, Bruno M, Ekanayake V, Hallett M. The involuntary nature of conversion disorder. Neurology 2010;74:223-228.

32 Edwards MJ, Moretto G, Schwingenschuh P, Katschnig P, Bhatia KP, Haggard P. Abnormal sense of intention preceding voluntary movement in patients with psychogenic tremor. Neuropsychologia 2011;49:2791-2793.

33 Kranick SM, Moore JW, Yusuf N, et al. Action-effect binding is decreased in motor conversion disorder: Implications for sense of agency. Mov Disord 2013;28:1110-1116.

34 Fekete R, Baizabal-Carvallo JF, Ha AD, Davidson A, Jankovic J. Convergence spasm in conversion disorders: prevalence in psychogenic and other movement disorders compared with controls. J Neurol Neurosurg Psychiatry 2012;83:202-204.

35 Jankovic J, Vuong KD, Thomas M. Psychogenic tremor: long-term outcome. CNS Spectr 2006;11:501-508.

36 Schwingenschuh P, Katschnig P, Seiler S, et al. Moving toward 'laboratory-supported' criteria for psychogenic tremor. Mov Disord 2011;26:2509-2515.

37 Edwards MJ, Alonso-Canovas A, Schrag A, Bloem BR, Thompson PD, Bhatia K. Limb amputations in fixed dystonia: A form of body integrity identity disorder? Mov Disord 2011;26:1410-1414.

38 Schwingenschuh P, Katschnig P, Edwards MJ, et al. The blink reflex recovery cycle differs between essential and presumed psychogenic blepharospasm. Neurology 2011;76:610-614.

39 Edwards MJ, Bhatia KP, Cordivari C. Immediate response to botulinum toxin injections in patients with fixed dystonia. Mov Disord 2011;26:917-918.

40 van der Salm SM, Koelman JH, Henneke S, van Rootselaar AF, Tijssen MA. Axial jerks: a clinical spectrum ranging from propriospinal to psychogenic myoclonus. J Neurol 2010;257:1349-1355.

41 Esposito M, Edwards MJ, Bhatia KP, Brown P, Cordivari C. Idiopathic spinal myoclonus: a clinical and neurophysiological assessment of a movement disorder of uncertain origin. Mov Disord 2009;24:2344-2349.

42 de la Fuente-Fernandez R, Ruth TJ, Sossi V, Schulzer M, Calne DB, Stoessl AJ. Expectation and dopamine release: mechanism of the placebo effect in Parkinson's disease. Science 2001;293:1164-1166.

43 Fahn S, Williams DT. Psychogenic dystonia. Adv Neurol 1988;50:431-455.

44 Gupta A, Lang AE. Psychogenic movement disorders. Curr Opin Neurol 2009;22:430-436.

45 Shill II, Gerber P. Evaluation of clinical diagnostic criteria for psychogenic movement disorders. Mov Disord 2006;21:1163-1168.

46 Stone J, Smyth R, Carson A, et al. Systematic review of misdiagnosis of conversion symptoms and 'hysteria'. BMJ 2005;331:989.

47 Hall-Patch L, Brown R, House A, et al. Acceptability and effectiveness of a strategy for the communication of the diagnosis of psychogenic nonepileptic seizures. Epilepsia 2010;51:70-78.

48 Edwards MJ, Stone J, Nielsen G. Physiotherapists and patients with functional (psychogenic) motor symptoms: a survey of attitudes and interest. J Neurol Neurosurg Psychiatry 2012;83:655-658.

49 Dallocchio C, Arbasino C, Klersy C, Marchioni E. The effects of physical activity on psychogenic movement disorders. Mov Disord 2010;25:421-425.

50 Czarnecki K, Thompson JM, Seime R, Geda YE, Duffy JR, Ahlskog JE. Functional movement disorders: successful treatment with a physical therapy rehabilitation protocol. Parkinsonism Relat Disord 2012;18:247-251.

51 Voon V, Lang AE. Antidepressant treatment outcomes of psychogenic movement disorder. J Clin Psychiatry 2005;66:1529-1534.

52 Sharpe M, Walker J, Williams C, et al. Guided self-help for functional (psychogenic) symptoms: a randomized controlled efficacy trial. Neurology 2011;77:564-572.

53 Rommelfanger KS. Opinion: A role for placebo therapy in psychogenic movement disorders. Nat Rev Neurol 2013;9:351-356.

54 van Hilten BJ, van de Beek WJ, Hoff JI, Voormolen JH, Delhaas EM. Intrathecal baclofen for the treatment of dystonia in patients with reflex sympathetic dystrophy. N Engl J Med 2000;343:625-630.

55 Garcin B, Roze E, Mesrati F, et al. Transcranial magnetic stimulation as an efficient treatment for psychogenic movement disorders. J Neurol Neurosurg Psychiatry 2013;84:1043-1046.

56 Dafotakis M, Ameli M, Vitinius F, et al. Transcranial magnetic stimulation for psychogenic tremor – a pilot study. Fortschr Neurol Psychiatr 2011;79:226-233.

57 Saifee TA, Kassavetis P, Parees I, et al. Inpatient treatment of functional motor symptoms: a long-term follow-up study. J Neurol 2012;259:1958-1963.

58 Feinstein A, Stergiopoulos V, Fine J, Lang AE. Psychiatric outcome in patients with a psychogenic movement disorder: a prospective study. Neuropsychiatry Neuropsychol Behav Neurol 2001;14:169-176.

59 Thomas M, Vuong KD, Jankovic J. Long-term prognosis of patients with psychogenic movement disorders. Parkinsonism Relat Disord 2006;12:382-387.

38
Movement Disorders in Psychiatry

Marie-An C.J. de Letter & Erik Ch. Wolters

This chapter deals with abnormal, spontaneous and reactive motor behaviour in combination with psychiatric behaviour in psychiatric but not psychogenic conditions, including abnormal motility, locomotion, gestures, mimic, and speech. Such disorders may be seen in chronic psychosis, depression, and stereotyped behaviour in childhood as well in some other conditions such as REM sleep behaviour disorder (RBD), choreatic disorders, attention-deficit hyperactivity disorder (ADHD), obsessive-compulsive disorders (OCD), tic syndromes (TS) and impulse control disorders (ICD). In this chapter, early-onset (neuroleptic-induced) and late-onset (tardive) dyskinesia and the dopamine receptor agonist- and/or antagonist-induced malignant neuroleptic syndrome will also be discussed. Psychogenic (somatoform) motor behavioural abnormalities, the result of conversion, somatisation and/or factious disorders (malingering) are described in chapter 37.

Chronic psychosis

Chronic psychosis or schizophrenia manifests with both perceptional and behavioural abnormalities.

Epidemiology
Schizophrenia has a yearly incidence of 1/10,000 and a lifetime prevalence of 1%, in line with its chronic character. The onset in women, as a rule in their twenties/early thirties, is later than in men, in which this disease mainly manifests in their teens or twenties. The female to male ratio is 1:1 (1-3).

Clinical expression

Positive symptoms
Symptoms in schizophrenia are classified as 'positive' or 'negative'. Positive symptoms reflect active, abnormal behaviour due to an excess or distortion of normal processing functions in the orchestration of behaviour. Those symptoms comprise hallucinations, delusions, thought disorders and disorganized behaviour.

Hallucinations are false sensory perceptions with or without loss of reality-testing. They are acoustical and/or visual. Delusions are misinterpreted perceptions or experiences leading to unrealistic beliefs. Thought disorders are the result of an inadequate organization of thoughts and manifest with the loss of adequate verbal expression of thoughts (word salad) or stopping speech mid-sentence, and disorganized behaviour may range from unpredictable agitation to childlike silliness.

Negative symptoms
Negative symptoms reflect the lack of specific emotivational and cognitive behavioural modalities, leading to anhedonia (in which patients do not experience pleasure), alogia (a marked poverty of speech due to a reduced content of speech or affective flattening), asociality, apathy (lack of interest), and avolition (lack of motivation).

Motor behavioural disorders
Movement disorders in chronic psychosis manifest as hypokinesia or hyperkinesia in volition, activity and/or mobility as well as repeated, non-goal-directed behaviour. Catatonia is a

term that describes such movement disorders with a psychiatric background, varying from catatonic excitement with uncontrolled aimless motor activity to catatonic stupor, in which patients are immobile, mute yet conscious. Stuporous patients show waxy flexibility of their limbs, which they keep in the posture in which the examiner positions them, like a wax doll (see Video fragment 38.1).

Stereotypy is another movement disorder in which patients perform repeated, typically non-goal-directed movements. In psychosis stereotypies include mannerisms, echopraxia, 'mitgehen', automatic obedience and negativism. Mannerisms (such as grimacing or repeatedly running one's hand through one's hair) suggest social significance and include goal-directed activities, but are out of context or odd in appearance. Echopraxia is the imitation of another person's movements. Mitgehen is moving a limb in response to light pressure despite being told not to do so, and automatic obedience is carrying out commands in a robot-like fashion. Negativism is refusing to cooperate with simple requests for no reason.

Etiology

The concordance rates of schizophrenia in relatives are remarkably high: approximately 50% in monozygotic and 12-15% in dizygotic twins, 40% if both parents and 12% if one parent suffers from schizophrenia, and 8% in non-twin siblings (compared to approximately 1% in the general population). Thus, an individual with a schizophrenic first degree relative has a ten-fold increased risk for this disorder. These figures suggest that the disorder is heritable, though with an incomplete penetrance, or that it is multifactorial. The most widely accepted theory is that schizophrenia is triggered by environmental insults in genetically predisposed, vulnerable persons (4-7). Such insults may include prenatal exposure to fluoramines, obstetric complications, early childhood CNS infections, and serious psychosocial stress in childhood and/or early adulthood.

Pathophysiology

The fine-tuning of the cerebral procession of sensory input necessary to orchestrate adequate behaviour is modulated by dopamine through the various dopaminergic receptors. In the striatum, mainly D1 and D2 dopamine receptors are expressed, while D3 receptors are mostly found in the nucleus accumbens, and D4 receptors in the frontal cortex and limbic areas. Postmortem studies in schizophrenics have provided evidence for an overall increased number of striatal dopaminergic neurons and a decreased number of nucleus accumbens dopaminergic neurons, with a change in the striatal synaptic organization. In schizophrenics, striatal D1 receptor-mediated activities correlate with the severity of 'negative' symptoms and dysexecution of frontal executive tasks, while striatal D2 activities correlate with 'positive' symptoms. Antipsychotic pharmaceuticals act primarily as D2 receptor blockers and only to a lesser extent as D1 receptor blockers. During the treatment of schizophrenia with typical and to a lesser extent atypical antipsychotics, antipsychotic effects are mainly achieved through downregulation of D2 receptor-mediated activities. By reducing this activity, those antipsychotics reduce regional dopamine hyperactivity, which manifests as the positive symptoms of schizophrenia. There is a significant correlation between the D2 receptor blockade and the clinical efficacy of antipsychotics in treating positive symptoms. Complementary downregulation of D1 receptor-mediated activity in the frontal cortex will reduce dopaminomimetic activity in the mesocortical pathway, which manifests as the negative symptoms (8). Atypical antipsychotics also block D4 and maybe D3 receptors.

Depression

In depressive disorders, patients can suffer from both bradykinetic and agitated hyperkinetic behaviour, implying that not only purely physically derived motor behaviour (somatomotorics) but also mentally/psychiatrically derived movements (psychomotorics) are part of our daily behaviour (adapted or not). Differentiating between somat-omotoric and psychomotoric behaviour is not that easy, however. In Parkinson's disease, for instance, motor behaviour might change quantitatively due to both motor parkinsonism and emotions, while depression might change behaviour in a more qualitative way (9-11).

Clinical expression

In depression, the gait is slowed and the posture slightly bent over. As a consequence, locomotion will also be mildly impaired (12). Voluntary and involuntary movements of the upper extremities, so-called gestic movements, are slightly different in depressed patients; they tend to touch their head, body and hands more frequently (13,14). Psychomotor slowing in depression manifests with reduced eye contact and facial expressions when analyzed with kinematics. Speech is mainly soft, monotone and monosyllabic, with a decreased word fluency (15). In ~10% of depressed patients, tricyclic antidepressants such as imipramine may induce an iatrogenic tremor, mostly a high-frequency, 7-14 Hz, postural or action tremor (16).

Pathophysiology

In depressive syndromes there is a slowing down of normal motor behaviour. This motor slowing might be explained by functional changes in the dorsolateral prefrontal cortex (17). The orchestration of movements in the primary (area 4) and secondary motor cortex (area 6) is modulated not only by sensorimotor but also by emotivational and cognitive input (18,19). In apathy, anhedonia and/depression, emotivational modulation, which is supposedly serotinergic- (raphe nucleus) and/or noradrenergic-mediated (locus coeruleus), changes are the result of functional/metabolic changes within the various basal ganglia-thalamocortical circuits in these conditions. Indeed, traumatic, infectious or vascular lesions in these frontal, striatal and/or pal-

lidal regions (such as in encephalitis lethargica and carbon monoxide intoxication) also result in both motor (bradykinesia) and mental (apathy, anhedonia) behavioural abnormalities.

During depressive periods, the increased parasympathetic (cholinergic) tonus and, in mania, an increased sympathetic (adrenergic) tonus will also play a significant role. Along with the dopaminergic balance, the cholinergic balance will play a relevant role in the final orchestration of both motor and non-motor behaviour. Thus, in depression, a multi-transmitter deficit presumably underlies the behavioural abnormalities, including at least the dopaminergic, cholinergic, serotinergic, and adrenergic/noradrenergic central neurotransmitter systems.

Stereotypies

A stereotypy is a repetitive or ritualistic, non-functional movement, posture, or utterance, which lasts more than four weeks, interferes strongly with normal activity, causes bodily injury, and is not necessarily due to a medical condition or substance (20). Stereotyped behaviour is typically seen in captive animals, particularly those held in small enclosures with little opportunity to engage in more normal behaviours. These behaviours may be maladaptive, involving self-injury or reduced reproductive success. Examples of those stereotypies include pacing, rocking, swimming in circles, excessive sleeping, self-mutilation, and mouthing cage bars. In humans, manifestations in childhood include 'compulsive' behaviour such as rocking or headbanging, in adolescence and adulthood rather 'disinhibited' behaviours such as self-caressing, crossing and uncrossing of legs, marching in place. Also, more inappropriate behaviours such as masturbating-like behaviour or coitus-like pelvic thrusting, humming, whistling, etc. might been seen. When these behaviours are mild and/or sporadic, non-violent and not inducing distress or dysfunctioning, they could be considered non-pathological and aberrant though still within the 'normal' non-patho-

693

logical range of behaviour of the general population. Such behaviours become pathological when they induce distress or dysfunctioning. Related terms include levodopa-induced punding to describe repetitive behaviour that is a side effect of some drugs. Stereotype behaviour might be seen in childhood, mental retardation, autism spectrum disorders, choreatic disorders (see Chapter 29), attention deficit and hyperactivity disorder (ADHD) (see Chapter 39), REM sleep behaviour disorder (RBD) (see Chapter 35), and/or psychosis. More specifically, stereotype movement disorders are the clinical hallmarks in the spectrum of obsessive-compulsive disorders, characterized by abnormal operant conditioning (see Chapter 1). Here, stereotypies are repetitive activities, undesirable habits which, similar to addiction, patients continue to do even though recognizing that it might not be the best thing to do. They may manifest as obsessions or impulses coupled with maladaptive impulsive behaviours, for instance in tic disorders, impulse control disorders (trichotillomania), and the body dysmorphic disorder (BDD) with overemphasised body image, body sensitization, and body weight concerns. In these OCD spectrum disorders, stereotype behaviour is induced by abnormal operant conditioning. In compulsive behaviours with aversive obsessions (see Chapter 40) they typically reduce anxiety or distress, while these behaviours with impulsive obsessions do increase gratification or stimulation (see Chapter 41).

Stereotypies in childhood

Typical examples of these stereotypies comprise nose-picking, nailbiting, thumbsucking, breath-holding, bruxism, self-biting, headbanging, rocking, self-hitting, skin-picking, mouthing of objects and hair pulling (trichotillomania). They can fit the criteria of a compulsion, a stereotypy in a developmental disorder, a tic disorder or an impulse control disorder. Although these habits can be seriously self-injuring, most are relatively benign, innocent, self-limiting 'habits' during development, and do not require any treatment.

However, when they cause impairment of functioning or self-injury, a stereotypic movement disorder should be suspected. Stereotypies in childhood start before the age of two, while tics mostly become overt around the age of seven. These stereotypies, but not tics, are mainly bilateral and continue for a longer time (21). A child suffering from a tic is mostly bothered more by it than children with a stereotypical movement disorder.

When stereotypies occur with coexisting conditions (see Table 38.1), or when they are severely restricting or include self-injurious behaviours, then it may be appropriate to employ a pharmacological strategy. The coexisting conditions will require management first. The prognosis depends on the severity of the disorder, and early recognition reduces the risk of self-injury.

Table 38.1
Coexisting conditions with stereotypies in childhood.

Learning difficulties
Language or motor developmental delay
Attention-deficit hyperactivity disorder
Obsessive-compulsive disorder spectrum
Tic disorder, Gilles de la Tourette syndrome

Stereotypies in choreatic disorders

Chorea is a state of excessive, spontaneous movement, irregularly timed, non-repetitive, randomly distributed and abrupt in character. It primarily occurs in some genetic disorders and secondary to various (para)infectious, auto-immune and structural conditions as well as some toxic, iatrogenic and metabolic encephalopathies. These movements vary in severity from restlessness with mild, intermittent exaggeration of gestures and expression, fidgeting movements of the hands, unstable dance-like gait to a continuous flow of stereotypic, disabling, and violent movements. The best recognized choreatic syndromes are Sydenham's chorea (SC) and Huntington's disease (HD).

Sydenham's chorea (SC)

SC is a neuropsychiatric disease that arises as a complication of Group A β-hemolytic streptococcal infection, mediated by an autoimmune, anti-neuronal antibody mechanism that cross-reacts with striatal neurons (22), affecting mainly children and young adults. This disorder is sufficient in itself to diagnose acute rheumatic fever, and half of patients suffering this disorder also suffer SC. The most prominent manifestations in SC are choreatic dyskinesias, including repetitive, non-functional, sometimes stereotypic behaviours with grimacing and typical gait disturbances, sometimes resembling manifestations of obsessive-compulsive and/or attention-deficit hyperactivity disorders. SC is a benign and self-limiting disorder. Manifestations usually develop within a few days and will progress over several weeks with the tendency to resolve spontaneously in several months, although recurrence is observed in about 20% (see Chapter 29). The primary therapy for SC is penicillin, amoxicillin or erythromycin i.m. for 10 days, followed by a prophylactic treatment until the age of 18 years. Secondary treatment includes steroids or intravenous immunoglobulins (22).

Huntington's disease (HD)

In HD behavioural changes and personality changes are usually the first manifestations. Behavioural changes manifest as jealousy, paranoid suspicions, obsessive thoughts and sometimes stereotypic compulsive acts. Personality changes mainly manifest as apathy, lack of concern, global cognitive deterioration, executive dysfunction, and sometimes irritability, aggression, anxiety and depression. Hypersexuality, promiscuity or sexually provocative behaviour is occasionally present, as well as alcohol abuse and a predisposition to criminality (23). At any time, psychotic manifestations with paranoia or delusions may appear, but no hallucinations (24). As

a rule, motor manifestations such as chorea, followed by motor parkinsonism and/or dystonia and finally akinesia, proceed to an immobile, cachectic, dysarthric and dysphagic endstage, normally within 10 years, and often with secondary complications such as decubitus and infections (25). In the juvenile Westphal variant, predominant akinesia masks choreatic movements (see also Chapter 29).

Stereotypies in attention-deficit hyperactivity disorder (ADHD)

One of the most common and probably overdiagnosed disorders in child and adolescent psychiatry, attention-deficit/hyperactivity disorder (ADHD), is a clinically heterogeneous, neurodevelopmental syndrome with onset in childhood, persisting into adulthood in up to 60% (28). ADHD is characterized by the inability to allocate and sustain attention, modulate activity level, and moderate impulsive actions. Such stereotypic, maladaptive behaviour, inconsistent with age and developmental level, causes substantial difficulties, especially in highly structured situations, and thus often results in a wide range of symptoms from poor social functioning to unemployment and substance abuse (32), as these children cannot comply with the requirements of their social context. Many of them manage to adapt to their problems and develop compensation strategies, facilitating psychosocial adaptation (see Chapter 39). ADHD is thought to be caused by a combination of genetic and environmental factors. Due to exposure to maternal smoking and/or alcohol use in pregnancy (29,30), ADHD is hypothesised to be the result of dysfunctional connections between the basal ganglia and both the associative prefrontal cortex and the secondary motor cortical areas, resulting in disturbances in attention processing and motor planning (31).

Stereotypies in the spectrum of obsessive-compulsive disorders

OCD-like stereotypies are seen in OCD, tic disorders, impulse control disorders (trichotillomania), and the body dysmorphic disorder (BDD) with overemphasised body image, body sensitization, and body weight concerns. In these OCD spectrum disorders, compulsive behaviours with aversive obsessions will typically reduce anxiety or distress, while these behaviours with impulsive obsessions function to increase gratification or stimulation (see chapter 41).

Obsessive compulsive disorders

Obsessive-compulsive disorders (OCD), as well as other disorders in the OCD spectrum, are defined by recurrent obsessions, isolated or in combination with compulsions, that result in clinically significant distress and impaired functioning. Obsessions (obsessive thinking) are persisting, intrusive and ego-dystonic ideas, thoughts, impulses, or images (about contamination, aggressiveness, sexuality, religion or somatic contents, symmetry and hoarding) that cause marked anxiety or distress.

Compulsions are repetitive stereotyped behaviours or mental acts (cleaning, checking, ordering, arranging, counting, repeating, hoarding and collecting) to prevent or reduce obsession-induced anxiety or distress (33), as the patients are unable to control the experience of these obsessions they produce, which are not excessive worries about real-life issues. The negative effects of OCD include time spent on compulsive rituals, disrupted family and social relationships, impaired work or academic performance, and an overall decrease in quality of life (see Chapter 40).

Although the etiology of OCD has not been established, the functional relationship between obsessions and compulsions might be explained by the fear response after fear acquisition. The fear response will then be reinforced by attempts to escape, avoid, or reduce the fear (34).

Tic syndromes

Stereotypies in childhood mainly appear before the age of 2. Tics usually appear after that age, mostly non-violent, simple, motor and/or vocal tics which might be suppressed for a brief peri-

od, such as blinking and throat clearing, and do not result in any distress and/or impaired functioning. Fortunately, the majority of these children outgrow these tics by 16-18 years of age. More complex, stereotypic tics appear between 4 and 10 years of age, are preceded by premonitory sensations and followed by post-executional relief, and are likely to be part of a more serious tic syndrome (TS) such as Gilles de la Tourette syndrome (GTS). These stereotypies typically do not have the ever-changing, waxing and waning nature of tics, and usually remain constant for years. Transient tics are estimated to occur in about 3% of children and adolescents, while tic syndromes including Gilles de la Tourette syndrome (GTS) develop in only 0.3% - 0.8% of the same population (26).

Gilles de la Tourette syndrome

In GTS, patients might display brief, non-rhythmic, stereotypic, repetitive behaviours which are fully inappropriate, such as copropraxia (showing the finger or touching one's genitals), coprolalia (obscene, often sexually tinted language), palilalia (repeating words or phrases) and echolalia (repeating someone else's words or phrases). The mimicking behaviour reinforces the idea that these tics are involuntary movements. Regarding its pathophysiology, it is suggested that an aberrant focus of striatal neurons is repetitively and inappropriately active and causes unwanted inhibition of basal ganglia output neurons (the neural circuit hypothesis). GTS is thought to have a genetic basis, but so far, no genes have been identified. Many patients cope with their disease without the use of therapeutic strategies such as physical and occupational therapy, pharmacotherapy including botulinum toxin and/or intrathecal baclofen therapy (ITB), and/or deep brain stimulation (27) (see Chapter 31).

Impulse control disorders (ICD)

In ICD, stereotyped behaviours include pathological gambling, hypersexuality, binge eating,

compulsive shopping, punding, hoarding, kleptomania and substance use disorders.
They can be broadly defined as repeated urges and compulsive actions with associated negative consequences (see Chapter 41). Stereotypic behaviours with impulsive obsessions function to increase gratification or stimulation. ICDs are thought to be more common in patients treated with dopaminomimetics, including those suffering from Parkinson's disease (PD), multiple system atrophy (MSA), progressive supranuclear palsy (PSP) and restless legs syndrome (RLS), as compared to the general population. Levodopa-induced punding, with typical, more or less continuous, non-functional, stereotypic behaviour, is also an example of repetitive stereotypic behaviour that is a side-effect of some drugs.

Neuroleptic-induced early-onset and late-onset ('tardive') dyskinesia

Iatrogenic movement disorders comprise both early- and late-onset dyskinesia as well as the malignant neuroleptic syndrome. Of course, drug-induced parkinsonism (see Chapter 18) and dopaminomimetic-induced dyskinesias and impulse control disorders (see Chapter 12, 41) including punding (see above) are examples of iatrogenic dyskinesia, though in this section only psychiatric (mainly neuroleptic) medication-induced dyskinesia will be dealt with. Vulnerability to late-onset dyskinesia is higher in cases of early-onset dyskinesia with rigidity, tremor, and bradykinesia following the initial administration of an antipsychotic, and there is abundant evidence that the older the patient, the more vulnerable he or she is to develop late-onset dyskinesia. Patients ≥60 years of age have a four- to ten-fold greater risk of developing these dyskinesia than young or middle-aged adults. Gender is also a factor, as postmenopausal females tend to be more prone to it. Also, patients suffering from a bipolar disorder are more at risk (35,36).

Clinical expression

Early-onset dyskinesia

The most common, iatrogenic, neuroleptic-induced, early-onset dyskinesias present with hypokinetic parkinsonism (see Chapter 18), acute dystonic reactions including oculogyric crises (see Video 38.2), and akathisia (described as inner restlessness, restless limbs or agitation). Sporadically, with an estimated incidence of 0.2%, an acute neuroleptic malignant syndrome may also develop (see below).

Late-onset dyskinesia

The term late-onset (tardive) dyskinesia is the term used for persistent iatrogenic symptoms, mainly arising during long-term treatment with an offending agent. 'Tardive' means late onset, a term applied earlier to describe abnormal, oro-buccal-lingual, facial dyskinesias (tardive dyskinesias) and/or dystonias (tardive dystonia) that appeared as a late side-effect of mostly neuroleptic medications and that tended to persist or worsen with the removal of the drugs (37). Late-onset dyskinesia mainly presents with rapid, involuntary, choreo-athetoid, and occasionally dystonic and/or tic-like movements of the fingers, toes, hands, as well as tongue or lips (see Video 38.3, 38.4 and 38.5). In exceptional cases, dystonic posturing of the neck and trunk might be seen, or dystonic contractions of the diaphragm, affecting respiration and speech. Late-onset dyskinesia, although usually mild and not disabling, often reduces the quality of life, is distressing and stigmatizing.

Etiology

Early-onset dyskinesia

Acute iatrogenic dyskinesia, both parkinsonistic and dystonic, is temporally related to the administration of the offending drug. As a rule, it responds quickly to intravenous anticholinergic medication, in combination with drug withdrawal of course.

697

Late-onset dyskinesia

Attributing a medication-related etiology to the chronic, iatrogenic (tardive) dyskinesia is not that simple. An etiological understanding of tardive dyskinesia comprises not only chronic application of the offending drug but also the underlying illness (often psychotic) and patient's age (38). Late-onset dyskinesias, mostly caused by chronic administration of antipsychotic drugs, are thought to be caused by iatrogenic changes in neuromuscular function. While acute iatrogenic dyskinesia is self-limiting and short-lived, resolving immediately after the agent is withdrawn, late-onset dyskinesia may last for many years if not a lifetime after drug withdrawal.

Late-onset dystonia

Although a mutation of the DYT1 gene on band 9q34 has been identified in familiar idiopathic torsion dystonia, there is no clear evidence for any genetic predisposition in iatrogenic, late-onset dystonia. For late-onset dyskinesia, but not dystonia, predictive factors have been defined, including the dopamine receptor 3 (D3R)-Ser-9Gly polymorphism, which could not be identified in late-onset dystonia patients (39). To date, no genetic markers have been identified that predict the development of late-onset dystonia.

Pathophysiology

It is still not clear why neuroleptics sometimes manifest with parkinsonism and sometimes with chorea or dystonia. Of course, it was suggested that tardive dystonia may develop in individuals at risk for dystonia, when the offending drugs activate the latent predisposition (40), but convincing evidence for such a mechanism has not been found. Primary and tardive dystonias are different entities although they share many similarities, and it cannot be concluded that they exist on a continuum. The pathophysiology of tardive dystonia is still not well understood.

Diagnosis

To diagnose acute and tardive dyskinesia, observation of the patient's body parts, extremities, tongue, and mouth under resting conditions as well as in response to a motor or cognitive task (counting backwards from 100 by sevens) and applying clinical rating scales are essential.

Treatment

Unfortunately, there is still no adequate therapy for tardive dyskinesia. Cholinergic agents are inconsistently effective. The best treatment is simply reducing or, if possible, withdrawing the offending D2 antagonists or switching patients to a very low-potency D2 antagonist. Indeed, some patients with tardive dystonia experienced a dramatic improvement after switching to clozapine (41).

Neuroleptic malignant syndrome

The neuroleptic malignant syndrome (NMS) is a neurological emergency, mainly but not exclusively associated with the use of neuroleptic agents and characterized by changes in mental status in combination with high fever, motor parkinsonism and dysautonomia.

Epidemiology

The incidence rates for NMS range from 0.02% to 3% among patients taking neuroleptic agents. This wide range probably reflects differences in the populations sampled, for example, inpatient versus outpatient psychiatric populations, as well as differences in the surveillance methods and definitions of disease used. While most patients with NMS are young adults, the syndrome has been described in all age groups from 9 to 78 years (42). Age is not a risk factor. In most studies, men outnumber women twofold. Both age and gender distributions correspond to the distribution of the exposure to neuroleptic agents. Reported mortality rates for NMS are 5-20% (43,44). The disease severity and the occurrence of medical complications are the strongest predictors of mortality (45).

Etiology

The etiology of NMS is unknown, and thus the clinical manifestations and therapeutic interventions are not fully understood. Unfortunately, animal models do not fully correspond with the clinical condition.

Although every class of neuroleptic drugs has been implicated, including chlorpromazine and the newer atypical antipsychotic drugs clozapine, rispiridone and olanzapine, typical high-potency neuroleptic agents such as haloperidol and fluphenazine mostly cause NMS (46-48). NMS may occur after a single dose or after long-term treatment with the same agent at the same dose. Symptoms usually develop during the first two weeks of neuroleptic therapy, but the association of the syndrome with drug use is idiosyncratic. It is not a dose-dependent condition, although higher doses do increase the risk. Case-control studies implicate recent or rapid dose escalation, a switch from one agent to another, and parenteral administration as risk factors.

NMS is also seen in patients treated with the antiemetics metoclopramide and promethazine, as well as in PD patients after reductions and/or withdrawal of levodopa or dopamine agonists, or after switching from one agent to another (49). Cofactors include infections and/or surgery. Although NMS occurring in such specific conditions is preferably labelled as neuroleptic malignant-like syndrome, other terms including parkinsonism hyperpyrexia syndrome, acute akinesia or the malignant syndrome in Parkinson disease are also used in the literature (50,51). These last conditions are generally milder, the laboratory findings less specific and the prognosis better (52), though some severe cases and even fatalities have been reported (50,53).

Pathophysiology

As NMS-eliciting drugs share dopaminomimetic activity, dopamine receptor blockade is central in most theories concerning its pathogenesis. Hypothalamic dopamine receptor blockade can cause hyperthermia and other signs of dysautonomia (54), and nigrostriatal blockade can cause motor parkinsonism (55). Other neurotransmitter systems (gamma-aminobutyric acid, epinephrine, serotonin, and acetylcholine) might also be involved, either directly or indirectly (56).

Alternative theories comprise a direct toxic effect of neuroleptics, inducing rigidity and muscle damage-inducing mitochondrial dysfunctions (55,57) as well as dopaminergic agonist-induced destabilization of the efferent sympathetic activity, leading to dysautonomia with metabolic, sudomotor, and cardiovascular dysfunction resulting in ineffective heat dissipation, labile blood pressure and heart rate (57).

Familial NMS clusters suggest a genetic predisposition, and indeed, a specific allele of the dopamine D2 receptor gene associated with reduced density and activity of this dopamine receptor is found to be over-represented in NMS patients (58).

Clinical expression

NMS can be a life-threatening neurologic emergency characterized by a distinctive clinical syndrome of (sub)acute changes in mental status (>80%) in combination with a defining high fever (38°C - 40 °C), motor parkinsonism and dysautonomia. Motor parkinsonism mainly manifests with generalized muscular 'lead pipe' rigidity and tremor (in about 75% of the patients). Superimposed tremor may lead to a cogwheel phenomenon. Less commonly, dystonia with opisthotonus and/or trismus, chorea and other dyskinesias may be expressed. Patients can also suffer from prominent sialorrhea, dysarthria, and dysphagia. Autonomic failure comprises labile or high blood pressure (~70%), tachypnea (~75%) and tachycardia (~90%), as well as dysrhythmias and a profuse diaphoresis. The underlying disorder is an agitated delirium with confusion rather than a psychosis, although sometimes catatonic signs and mutism can be prominent. NMS as a rule will progress into a serious encephalopathy with stupor and eventual coma (59), and about 15% of the patients ultimately might die because of their dysautonomia and/or systemic complications.

Diagnosis

Except for a higher creatine kinase (CK) level as characteristically induced by rigidity, the laboratory abnormalities are nonspecific. Already in the earliest phase of NMS, CK is typically raised above 1,000 IU/L and can, in correlation with disease severity and prognosis, increase further up to 100,000 IU/L (55,60).

In patients with possible NMS, brain imaging studies and lumbar puncture are required to exclude structural brain disease and infection. Magnetic resonance imaging (MRI) and computed tomography (CT) results are typically normal, although in isolated cases, diffuse cerebral edema in the setting of severe metabolic derangements, as well as cerebellar and basal ganglia signal abnormalities similar to those seen in malignant hyperthermia, might be noticed (61). The cerebrospinal fluid is usually normal, but a nonspecific elevation in protein is reported in ~35% of cases. Electroencephalography screening rules out an eventual nonconvulsive status epilepticus; in NMS patients, generalized slow wave activity might be seen.

Differential diagnosis

The differential diagnosis of NMS can be broadly defined in two categories: conditions that are related to NMS and conditions that are unrelated but commonly considered in the differential diagnosis.

NMS-related disorders

NMS-related disorders comprise malignant hyperthermia, malignant catatonia, intrathecal baclofen withdrawal syndrome, and the heroin and ecstasy syndromes. Malignant hyperthermia, a rather rare genetic disorder, can be dis-

tinguished from NMS by its clinical setting, as it only occurs after application of a potent, inhalational, halogenated anesthetic agent and/or succinylcholine. Malignant catatonia is more difficult to differentiate from NMS, as both disorders share the clinical features of hyperthermia and rigidity. However, in malignant catatonia there is usually a typical behavioural prodrome lasting some weeks, characterized by psychosis, agitation, and catatonic excitement. Motor behaviour in this disorder is also characterized by more positive phenomena (dystonic posturing, waxy flexibility, and stereotyped repetitive movements) as normally seen in NMS, and laboratory values are typically normal.

The intrathecal baclofen withdrawal syndrome also may display NMS-like symptoms (62), as is also the case in acute intoxications with street drugs such as cocaine and ecstasy (3,4-methylene-dioxy-meth-amphetamine) (MDMA). These drugs do not induce rigidity; rather, their CNS-stimulating activities produce a higher state of vigilance, energy, and euphoria (although these effects may also manifest as psychomotor agitation), delirium, and even psychosis. Only in combination with acute stressful conditions, increased physical activity or high temperature, can acute intoxications with these drugs also induce hyperthermia and rhabdomyolysis. Of course, MDMA abuse might also cause a serotonin syndrome.

Non NMS-related disorders

Alternative, serious, neurologic and medical disorders which should be excluded in NMS, particularly in patients suffering the extrapyramidal side-effects of concomitant neuroleptic use (47), are displayed in Table 38.2.

Therapy

As NMS may be associated with life-threatening conditions, as a rule, admission to intensive care facilities is mandatory. The best therapy in NMS is to withdraw the causative agent, as well as eventual, potentially contributing, psycho-

Table 38.2
Non-NMS-related conditions with NMS-like symptomatology.

Infections	Meningitis, encephalitis, neurovasculitis systemic infections (pneumonia, sepsis)
Seizures	Epileptic seizures
Hydrocephalus	Acute hydrocephalus
Spinal cord injury	Acute spinal cord injury
Heat stroke	Predisposed by neuroleptic drug-induced impaired thermoregulation
Dystonia	Acute dystonia
Tetanus	
Thyrotoxicosis	
Withdrawal states	Neuroleptic drugs, dopaminomimetic drugs
Toxic syndromes	Amphetamines, cocaine, ecstasy, phencyclidine, lithium
Pheochromocytoma	
Porphyria	Acute porphyria

tropic agents such as lithium, anticholinergic and serotonergic agents. In the case of dopaminomimetic withdrawal-induced NMS, dopaminomimetics should be reinstituted. Of course, further supportive care in NMS is essential and uncontroversial. Recommendations for other specific medical treatments are only based upon anecdotal evidence, as stated in case reports, and clinical experience. The high morbidity and mortality of NMS urge the application of these strategies, although there are no data from controlled clinical trials, and although their efficacy in NMS is unclear and disputed (63). Commonly used agents are dantrolene, a direct-acting skeletal muscle relaxant, and bromocriptine, a dopamine agonist (to restore lost dopaminergic tone) or amantadine (to restore lost dopaminergic and anticholinergic tones).

Although there are also no prospective, randomized, controlled data supporting its efficacy, electroconvulsive therapy (ECT) might offer another strategy. Its rationale is based on its efficacy in the treatment of malignant catatonia, and on anecdotal reports of parkinsonism improving with ECT. A further impetus for ECT comes from the frequent need for psychotropic therapy in a setting in which neuroleptics cannot be used. In one review, lower mortality rates in ECT-treated NMS patients were found compared with those receiving supportive care alone (~10% versus 21%) (64), and in another review, a clinical response was established after an average of 4.1 treatments (65). However, the interpretation of these findings is complicated by the variable timing of ECT in relation to symptom onset. Methodological issues, including publication bias and lack of randomization, preclude conclusions about the suggested efficacy of ECT, and adverse events such as cardiovascular complications (in 4 out of 55 patients, including 2 patients with ventricular fibrillation and cardiac arrest with permanent anoxic brain injury) and, rarely, status epilepticus, as well as the requirement for anesthesia prevent its common use. As of yet, ECT is generally reserved for patients not responding to other treatments. Because of concerns for associated malignant hyperthermia, some authors suggest the use of nondepolarizing agents.

Video fragments

Fragment 38.1 Catatonia
This video displays an akinetic-mutistic young man with typical posturing (note his catalepsy: the tonic maintenance for a long period of time of a limb in a potentially uncomfortable posture, where it has been placed by the examiner) and staring. His catatonia was diagnosed as manifestation of an acute psychotic condition, and he responded well to treatment with neuroleptics.

Fragment 38.2
Iatrogenic acute dystonia (Segments 1-2)
The dramatic presentation of a young man with a frightening, obviously painful, generalized dystonic storm (segment 1). Dystonic features include characteristic orofacial and axial dystonia with cervical and/or thoracic hyperextension, lateroflexion, and torsion. After intravenous application of anticholinergics, this dystonic storm disappeared within minutes (segment 2).

Fragment 38.3
Tardive tremor
A patient with a tardive tremor.

Fragment 38.4
Tardive dyskinesia
A patient with haloperidol-induced, tardive blepharospasm and typical perioral dyskinesia (stereotypies).

Fragment 38.5
Tardive chorea
A patient with lamotrigine-induced tardive chorea with stereotypies.

References

1 McGrath J, Saha S, Chant D, Welham J. Schizophrenia: a concise overview of incidence, prevalence, and mortality. Epidemiol Rev 2008;30:67-76.

2 Abel KM, Drake R, Goldstein JM. Sex differences in schizophrenia. Int Rev Psychiatry 2010;22:417-428.

3 Grossman LS, Harrow M, Rosen C, et al. Sex differences in schizophrenia and other psychotic disorders: a 20-year longitudinal study of psychosis and recovery. Compr Psychiatry 2008;49:523-529.

4 Usall J, Ochoa S, Araya S, et al. Gender differences and outcome in schizophrenia: a 2-year follow-up study in a large community sample. Eur Psychiatry 2003;18:282-284.

5 Krabbenda L, van Os J. Schizophrenia and urbanicity: a major environmental influence-conditional on genetic risk. Schizophr Bull 2005;31:795-799.

6 Pedersen CB, Mortensen PB. Evidence of a dose-response relationship between urbanicity during upbringing and schizophrenia risk. Arch Gen Psychiatry 2001;58:1039-1046.

7 Werbeloff N, Levine SZ, Rabinowitz J. Elaboration on the association between immigration and schizophrenia: a population-based national study disaggregating annual trends, country of origin and sex over 15 years. Soc Psychiatr Epidemiol 2012;47:303-311.

8 Goldman-Rakic PS, Castner SA, Svensson TH, et al. Targeting the dopamine D1 receptor in schizophrenia: insights for cognitive dysfunction. Psychopharmacology (Berl) 2004; 174:3-16.

9 Sloman L, Berridge M, Homatidis S, Hunter D, Duck T. Gait pattern of depressed patients and normal subjects. Am J Psychiatry 1989;139:94-97.

10 Winkler T, Buhl K, Linnemann M, Mieth B, Stolze H, Lemke MR. Alterartions of gait parameters in depression. Eur Arch Psychiat Cli Neursci 1998;248:S126.

11 Marsden CD, Owen DAL. Mechanisms underlying emotional variation in Parkinsonian tremor. Neurology 1967;17:711-715.

12 Woolacott MH, Jensen JL. Haltung und Fortbewegung. In: Heuer H, Keele SW (Hrsg) Psychomotorik. Hofgrefe, Göttingen, 1994:413-496.

13 Jones IH, Pansa M. Some non-verbal aspect of depression and schizofrenia occuring during th interview. J Nerv Ment Dis 1979;167:402-409.

14 Ulrich G, Harms K. A videoanalysis of the nonverbal behaviour of depressed patients before and after treatment. J Affective Disord 1985;63-67.

15 Widlöcher DJ. Psychomotor retardation: clinical theoretical, and psychometric aspect. Psychiatr Clin North Am 1983;6:27-40.

16 Kronfol Z, Greden JF, Zis AP. Imipramine-Induced tremor: effects of a beta-adrenergic blocking agent. J Clin Psychiatry 1983;44:225-226.

17 Bech CJ, Friston KJ, Brown RG, Frackowiak RS, Dolan RJ. Regional cerebral blood flow in depression measured by positron emission tomography: the relationship with clinical dimensions. Psychol Med 1993;23:579-590.

18 Alexander GE, DeLong MR, Strick PL. Parallel organisation of functionally segregated circuits linking basal ganglia and cortex. Ann Rev Neurosci 1986;9:357-381.

19 Dum RP, Strick PL. The origin of corticospinal projections from the premotor areas in the frontal lobe. J Neurosci 1991;11:667-689.

20 Jankovic J. Tics and Stereotypies. Oxford: Oxford University Press, 2005.

21 Harris KM, Mahone EM, Singer HS. Nonautistic motor stereotypies: clinical features and longitudinal follow-up. Pediatr Neurol 2008;38:267-272.

22 Church AJ, Cardoso F, Dale RC, Lees AJ, Thompson EJ, Giovannoni G. Anti–basal ganglia antibodies in acute and persistent Sydenham's chorea. Neurology 2002;59:227-231.

23 Jensen P, Fenger K, Bolwig T, Sørensen SA. Crime in Huntington´s disease: a study of registered offences among patients, relatives, and controls. J Neurol Neurosurg Psychiatry 1998;65:467-471.

24 Paulsen JS, Ready RE, Hamilton JM et al. Neuropsychiatric aspects of Huntington's disease. J Neurol Neurosurg Psychiatry 2001;71:310–314.

25 Ribaï P, Nguyen K, Hahn-Barma V, et al. Psychiatric and cognitive difficulties as indicators of juvenile huntington disease onset in 29 patients. Arch Neurol 2007;64:813-819.

26 Knight T, Steeves T, Day L, Lowerison M, Jette N, Pringsheim T. Prevalence of tic disorders: a systematic review and meta-analysis. Pediatr Neurol 2012;47:77-90.

27 Gilbert D. Treatment of children and adolescents with tics and Tourette syndrome. J Child Neurol 2006;21:690-700.

28 Rizzo P, Steinhausen H-C, Drechsler R. Self-perception of self-regulatory skills in children with attention-deficit/hyperactivity disorder ages 8-10 years. ADHD Attent Def Hyp Disord 2010;2:171-183.

29 Zhu JM, Zhang X, Yu YH, Spencer TJ, Biederman J, Bhide PG. Prenatal nicotine exposure mouse model showing hyperactivity, reduced cingulate cortex volume, reduced dopamine turnover, and responsiveness to oral methylphenidate treatment. J Neurosci 2012;32:9410-9418.

30 Biederman J, Faraone SV. Attention-deficit hyperactivity disorder. Lancet 2005;366:237-248.

31 Sullivan RM, Brake WG. What the rodent prefrontal cortex can teach us about attention-deficit/hyperactivity disorder: the critical role of early developmental events on prefrontal function. Behav Brain Res 2003;146:43-55.

32 Lara C, Fayyad J, de Graaf R, et al. Childhood predictors of adult attention-deficit/hyperactivity disorder: results from the World Health Organization World Mental Health Survey. Initiative Biol Psychiatr 2009;65:46-54.

33 Franklin ME, Foa EB. Cognitive behavioral treatment of obsessive-compulsive disorder. In: Nathan PE, Gorman JM, eds. A guide to treatments that work. New York: Oxford, 2007:431-446.

34 Franklin ME, Foa EB. Cognitive behavioral treatment of obsessive-compulsive disorder. In: Nathan PE, Gorman JM, eds. A guide to treatments that work. New York: Oxford, 2007:431-446.

35 Glazer WM. Expected incidence of tardive dyskinesia associated with atypical antipsychotics. J Clin Psychiatry 2000;61(S4):21-26.

36 Kane JM. Tardive dyskinesia rates with atypical antipsychotics in adults: prevalence and incidence. Clin Psychiatry. 2004;65(S9):16-20.

37 Burke RE, Fahn S, Jankovic J, et al. Tardive dystonia: late-onset and persistent dystonia caused by anti-psychotic drugs. Neurology 1982;32:1335-1346.

38 Burke RE. Neuroleptic-induced tardive dyskinesia variants. In: Lang AE, Weiner WJ, eds. Drug-Induced Movement Disorders. Futu, New York1992:168-198

39 Mihara K, Kondo T, Higuchi H, Takahashi H, Yoshida K, Shimizu T. Tardive dystonia and genetic polymorphisms pf cytochrome P4502D6 and Dopamine D2 and D3 receptors: a preliminary finding. Am J Med Genet. 2002;114:693-695.

40 Sachdev P. Risk factors for tardive dystonia: a case-control comparison with tardive dyskinesia. Acta Psychiatr Scand. 1993;88:98-103.

41 Blake LM, Marks RC, Nierman P, Luchins DJ. Clozapin and clonazepam in tardive dystonia. J Clin Psychopharmacol. 1991;11:268-269.

42 Margetic B, Aukst-Margetic B. Neuroleptic malignant syndrome and its controversies. Pharmacoepidemiol Drug Saf 2010;19:429-435

43 Tural U, Onder E. Clinical and pharmacologic risk factors for neuroleptic malignant syndrome and their association with death. Psychiatry Clin Neurosci 2010;64:79-87.

44 Nakamura M, Yasunaga H, Miyata H, et al. Mortality of neuroleptic malignant syndrome induced by typical and atypical antipsychotic drugs: a propensity matched analysis from the Japanese Diagnosis Procedure Combination Database. J Clin Psychiatry 2012;73:427-430.

45 Carbone JR. The neuroleptic malignant and serotonin syndromes. Emerg Med Clin North Am 2000;18:317-325.

46 Chandran GJ, Mikler JR, Keegan DL. Neuroleptic malignant syndrome: case report and discussion. CMAJ 2003;169:439-442.

47 Strawn JR, Keck PE jr, Caroff SN. Neuroleptic malignant syndrome. Am J Psychiatry 2007;164:870-876.

48 Seitz DP, Gill SS. Neuroleptic malignant syndrome complicating antipsychotic treatment of delirium or agitation in medical and surgical patients: case reports and a review of the literature. Psychosomatics 2009;50:8-15.

49 Wu YF, Kan YS, Yang CH. Neuroleptic malignant syndrome associated with bromocriptin withdrawal in Parkinson's disease: a case report. Gen Hosp Psychiatry 2011;33:301.e7-e8.

50 Onofrj M, Thomas A. Acute akinesia in Parkinson disease. Neurology 2005;64:1162-1169.

51 Mizuno Y, Takubo H, Mizuta E, Kuno S. Malignant syndrome in Parkinson's disease: concept and review of the literature. Parkinsonism Relat Disord 2003;9(S1):3-9.

52 Serrano-Duenas M. Neuroleptic malignant syndrome like, or dopaminergic malignant syndrome due to levodopa therapy withdrawal. Clinical features in 11 patients. Parkinsonism Relat Disord 2003;9:175-178.

53 Newman EJ, Grosset DG, Kennedy PG. The parkinsonism-hyperpyrexia syndrome. Neurocrit Care 2009;10:136-140.

54 Boulant JA. Role of the preoptic-anterior thalamus in thermoregulation and fever. Clin Infect Dis 2000;31(S5):157-161.

55 Adnet P, Lestavel P, Krivosic-Horber R. Neuroleptic malignant syndrome. Br J Anaeasth 2000;85:129-135.

56 Spivak B, Maline DI, Vered Y, et al. Prospective evaluation of circulatory levels of catecholamines and serotonin in neuroleptic malignant syndrome. Acta psychiatry Scand 2000;102:226-230.

57 Gurrera RJ. Is neuroleptic malignant syndrome a neurogenic form of malignant hyperthermia? Clin Neuropharmacol 2002;25:183-193.

58 Mihara K, Kondo T, Suzuki A, et al. Relationship between functional D2 and D3 receptors gene polymorphisms and neuroleptic malignant syndrome. Am J Med Genet B Neuropsychiatr Genet 2003;117B:57-60.

59 Koch M, Chandragiri S, Rizvi S, et al. Catatonic signs in neuroleptic malignant syndrome. Compr Psychiatry 2000;41:73-75.

60 Hermesh H, Manor I, Siloh R, et al. High serum creatinekinase level: possible risk factor for neuroleptic malignant syndrome. J Clin Psychopharmacol 2002;22:252-256.

61 Lyons JL, Cohen AB. Selective cerebellar and basal ganglia injury in neuroleptic malignant syndroms. J Neuroimaging 2013;23:240-241.

62 Coffey RJ, Edgar TS, Fransisco GE, et al. Abrupt withdrawal from baclofen: recognition and management of a potentially life-threatening syndrome. Arch Phys Med Rehabil 2002;83:735-741.

63 Reulbach U, Dütsch C, Biermann T, et al. Managing an effective treatment for neuroleptic malignant syndrome. Crit Care 2007;11:R4.

64 Davis JM, Janicak PG, Sakkas P, et al. Electroconvulsive treatment in the therapy of neuroleptic malignant syndrome. Convuls Ther 1991;7:111-120.

65 Trollor JN, Sachdev PS. Electroconvulsive treatment of neuroleptic malignant syndrome: a review and report of cases. Aust N Z J Psychiatry 1999;33:650-659.

39

Attention-Deficit/Hyperactivity Disorder

Manfred Gerlach & Marcel Romanos

Among the most common disorders in child and adolescent psychiatry, attention-deficit/hyperactivity disorder (ADHD) is a clinically heterogeneous neurodevelopmental syndrome with onset in childhood, which persists into adulthood in up to 60% of those afflicted (at least partially) (1-3). ADHD is associated with a wide range of functional impairments throughout the life span, including deficits in psychological, social, family-related, academic and occupational functions. ADHD-like symptoms were first described by Heinrich Hoffmann as early as 1864 (see Figure 39.1), although it took several decades before the behavioural phenomena were recognized as a medical condition (4-6).

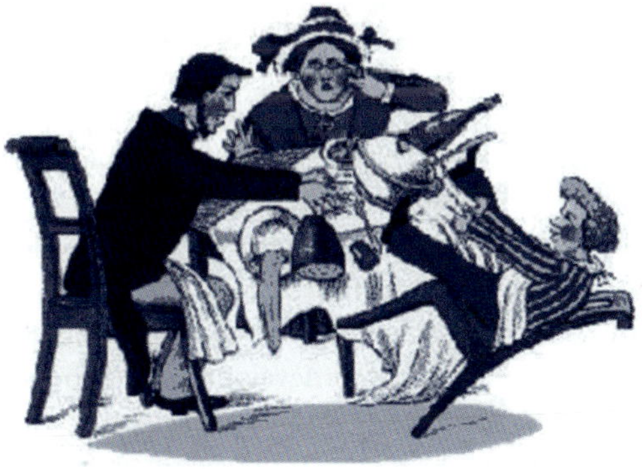

Figure 39.1
An illustration from 'Der Struwelpeter' by Heinrich Hoffman (1809-1894). The picture is in the 'Die Geschichte vom Zappel-Philipp' and shows Fidgety Phil who cannot keep still; indeed he creates a mess and upset his parents (from Taylor 2011).

Patients with ADHD show characteristic, age-inappropriate symptoms of inattention, impulsiveness, and hyperactivity. The European diagnostic criteria defined by the international classification of diseases (10th edition, ICD-10) (7) and the Diagnostic and statistical manual of mental disorders, fourth edition-text revision (DSM-IV-TR) (8) differ in regard to the definition of ADHD subtypes. ICD-10 considers the full syndrome ('hyperkinetic disorder') with the comorbid condition of hyperkinetic conduct disorder. DSM-IV, however, makes a distinction between the combined subtype, the inattentive and the hyperactive–impulsive subtype, although this distinction is still being debated and is expected to be refined in the upcoming DSM-V.

Epidemiology

ADHD is the most prevalent mental disorder in children, affecting approximately 5.29% of children and adolescents worldwide (9). The prevalence rates vary, depending on the study, and may be overestimated if the diagnosis does not adequately incorporate functional impairment. In addition, the figures often depend on the (sub)type investigated. Epidemiological studies have demonstrated that male sex, low socio-economic status, and young age are associated with an increased prevalence of ADHD (10). In clinical samples, an average male-to-female ratio of 5:1 has been found, but in epidemiological samples, ratios of 3:1 or 2:1 have been reported (11), which indicates that female individuals with the disorder are less likely to be referred for services than male individuals. For the inattentive subtype, however, gender differences are less pronounced or even absent.

Prevalence rates in adults have been less thoroughly investigated. The persistence from childhood into adulthood with an age-dependent decline in symptoms ranges between 33% and up to 70%, while the prevalence in the general adult population is around 4.4% and 5%, respectively (3,12-14). However, there are several population subgroups with a significantly increased prevalence, for example, prison inmates or people suffering from alcoholism (15). In a cross-national survey (16), an average prevalence rate of 3.4% has been reported, with the lowest rate in lower-income countries (1.9%) compared to higher-income countries (4.2%).

ADHD is highly comorbid with many mental health disorders, including depression and anxiety, or disruptive behaviour disorders (17). The rate of comorbid mental health disorders among children with ADHD is reported to be over 80%, with reading disorder also commonly reported (18). Among adults presenting for treatment of ADHD, approximately 25% of clinically referred patients also have a history of conduct disorders, and 7-14% have a history of antisocial personality disorder (19). Children with ADHD and conduct disorder vs. ADHD alone had a much higher risk (30% vs. 6%) of developing substance use disorder in adolescence (20), and elevated risky behaviours as adults (21).

Etiology

Although the aetiology of ADHD is elusive, emerging evidence documents its strong neurobiological basis. Family, twin and adoption studies have demonstrated that ADHD is a highly heritable disorder, and heritability estimates are consistently around 0.8 (10,22,23). However, neither genome-wide association studies (GWAS) nor large-scale meta-analyses of GWAS have so far unequivocally identified specific genes conferring major risk (24). Genome-wide analysis of rare (frequency ≤ 1%) copy number variations (CNVs), which are, by definition, chromosomal deletions or duplications of at least 1kb up to several Mb and are variable in size among carriers, have revealed neurodevelopmental genes, the neuropeptide Y gene, the CHRNA7 gene, and metabotropic glutamate receptor genes as candidates genes for ADHD (see for a review 25). Interestingly, it was shown that copy number variants at the PARK-2 locus contribute to the genetic susceptibility of ADHD (25). Mutation and CNVs in PARK-2, which encodes parkin, are known to be associated with Parkinson´s disease.

There is increasing evidence that genetic factors interact with environmental risk factors in complex ways. For example, a risk haplotype of dopamine transporter (DaT)-1 in combination with maternal alcohol consumption in pregnancy was associated with increased ADHD symptoms in the offspring (26). The same risk factors that influence the origins of ADHD may play a role in the developmental course of the disorder, although it is also possible that a different set of risk and protective factors influence the course and outcome of ADHD (27).

ADHD and its subsequent developmental course can not entirely be explained by genes. There are a number of environmental factors that also appear to be associated with ADHD, two of which have withstood meta-analysis or pooled analyses (27): exposure to maternal smoking in pregnancy (estimated odds ratio 2.39) and low birth weight/prematurity (odds ratio 2.64). With exposure of the foetus to nicotine, maternal smoking can damage the brain at critical points in the developmental process. Indeed, a recent study in mice showed that prenatal nicotine exposure produces behavioural, neurochemical and structural features of human ADHD (28). Delivery complications associated with ADHD frequently lead to hypoxia and tend to include chronic exposures to the foetus (such as toxaemia) rather than acute, traumatic events (such as delivery complications). Notably, the basal ganglia, which are commonly implicated in ADHD (see pathophysiology), are also one of the most metabolically active structures in the brain and are particularly sensitive to hypoxic insults, which have been shown to cause persistent effects on dopaminergic functioning in animals (10). Prospective studies of infants show that foetal exposure to maternal alcohol use also leads to behavioural, cognitive, and learning problems that could present as ADHD, and studies of children with the disorder show an increased likelihood of having been exposed to alcohol as a foetus (10).

Particular foods or food additives have been suggested to cause ADHD, but systematic studies have shown that this assumption provides a relevant explanation for only the largest part of phenotypic variance (10). Thus, dietary procedures may only be effective in a small subset of children sensitive to certain food components (29). Lead exposure during early childhood has also been discussed as a risk factor of the disorder; however, most affected children do not show lead contamination, and many children with high lead exposure do not become affected with the disorder (30). Cross-sectional and longitudinal studies have identified psychosocial adversity as a predisposing risk factor (10). For example, the aggregate of risk factors in the family such as severe marital discord, low social class, large family size, paternal criminality, maternal mental disorder, and foster placement is associated with ADHD, measures of ADHD-associated psychopathology, impaired cognition, and psychosocial dysfunction. Taylor (5) hypothesized that there are also strong cultural influences, not as to the neurobiological variation but to the extent in which it leads to impairment or to disability and especially to diagnosis.

Pathophysiology

The pathophysiology of ADHD has not been fully characterized, although structural and functional imaging studies consistently suggest dysfunction in cortico-basal ganglia-thalamo-cortical circuits and imbalances in dopaminergic systems as the origin of the core symptoms (31,32). However, there is also evidence for dysfunction of other neurotransmitters including noradrenaline, serotonin and glutamate. There is much debate about what core neuropsychological deficit might cause both ADHD symptoms and neuropsychological impairments. Candidates for core deficits include failure of inhibitory control; dysregulation of brain systems mediating reward and response cost; and deficits in arousal, activation, and effortful control (10).

Structural neuroimaging studies have shown small volume reductions in the basal ganglia of ADHD patients. Other studies have also implicated structures such as the cerebellum and corpus callosum (10), which are outside the cortico-basal ganglia-thalamo-cortical circuits. Functional neuroimaging studies that assessed the degree of brain activation associated with neuropsychological tasks of attention and disinhibition are consistent with the structural studies locating abnormalities of brain activation in patients with ADHD. For example, in drug-naive ADHD children, a functional magnetic resonance study revealed reduced striatal activity during stimulus-controlled tasks, which was normalized by methylphenidate treatment (33). Dopamine has long been known to be a crucial modulator of the striatal processing of cortical and thalamic signals mediated through glutamatergic synapses on the principal striatal neurons (medium spiny). Regulation of these neurons by dopamine is important for a wide array of psychomotor functions ascribed to the basal ganglia, including motor, cognitive and motivational functions. Recent studies have strongly suggested that disturbance of the dopaminergic system is also involved in the pathophysiology of ADHD (32). The most convincing evidence comes from the demonstration of the efficacy of psychostimulants such as the dopamine transporter (DaT) re-uptake blocker methylphenidate in the symptomatic treatment of ADHD. Genetic studies have shown an association between ADHD and genes involved in dopaminergic neurotransmission (for example, the dopamine receptor genes DRD-4 and DRD-5, and the DaT gene DaT-1). DaT knockout mice display a phenotype with increased locomotor activity, which is normalized by psychostimulant treatment. Finally, neuroimaging studies demonstrated an increased density of DaT in the striatum of ADHD patients.

Failing dopaminergic neurotransmission results in dysregulation of dopamine-modulated cortico-basal ganglia-thalamo-cortical neurocircuits including frontal, striatal and limbic regions. Based on what is known about the physiological brain function of dopamine, ADHD may result in part from disturbances in the dopaminergic system in cortical brain structures like the prefrontal cortex and subcortical areas such as the nucleus accumbens and the striatum. However, there is an ongoing debate on whether there is a hyper- or a hypodopaminergic dysfunction in ADHD.

Recent studies have strongly suggested that ADHD represents a deficiency in parts of the basal ganglia linked to the associative prefrontal cortex and to secondary motor cortical areas involved in attention processes and motor planning. For example, rodent studies demonstrated that the core processes, which are deficient in ADHD, are mediated by the right prefrontal cortex, and that the mesocortical dopamine system plays a central role in the modulation of these functions (34). Dyskinesia, attention deficit with or without hyperactivity, and stereotyped behaviour can be induced by microinjections of a GABAergic antagonist into different parts of the external globus pallidus, and pharmacological studies in non-human primates using axonal tracer injections have shown that the pallidal sites related to dyskinesia, attention deficit with or without hyperactivity, and stereotyped behaviour was associated with distinct motor, associative and limbic circuits (35). Using functional magnetic resonance imaging, drug-naive ADHD adolescents differed from healthy comparison subjects in the activation of the left ventral aspects of the basal ganglia during the performance of a divided attention task (36). As soon as ADHD adolescents were given a challenge dose of methylphenidate before scanning, they recruited this region of the basal ganglia to a similar degree as normal subjects. These findings of reduced striatal activation for adolescents with ADHD are consistent with previous neuroimaging studies showing that ADHD subjects exhibit less activity in basal ganglia structures both at rest and during the performance of cognitive tasks (see for a review 32). Moreover, the finding that methylphenidate normalizes striatal activation is consistent with previous reports that methylphenidate preferentially modulates striatal activity in ADHD patients (32,37) and increases extracellular striatal dopamine levels in healthy adults (38).

Clinical presentation

ADHD is characterized by the inability to allocate and sustain attention, modulate activity levels, and moderate impulsive actions. The result is maladaptive behaviour that is inconsistent with age and the developmental level, causing substantial difficulties for affected children, their families and/or the environment. Children with ADHD have consistently been found to demonstrate a large variety of difficulties in everyday life, such as academic underachievement, social deficits and behavioural problems (39).

In the story of Fidgety Phil that gives a first hint of the presence of an underlying persistent disorder (4,6), Hoffmann illustrates a family conflict at dinner caused by the fidgety behaviour of the son and culminating in his falling over together with the food on the table (see Figure 39.1). The story of Fidgety Phil illustrates the difficulties of affected children whenever the social context requires what is most difficult for them: sitting still, controlling themselves, paying attention. Thus, it becomes obvious that highly structured situations such as school or homework are generally considered to be the most difficult ones. The children fail to comply with expectations, and a cycle of criticism and negative feedback further fuels a developmental trajectory characterized by poor psychosocial adaptation and comorbid development. These difficulties continue in adolescence and adulthood, resulting in a wide range of symptoms from poor social functioning to unemployment and substance abuse. On the other hand, several patients adapt to their problems and develop compensation strategies facilitating a high psychosocial adaptation (17).

Diagnosis

The ability to direct and sustain attention, regulate activity, and control impulses emerges for all children in a developmental process. Therefore, the cornerstone of the diagnosis is the anamnestic history of symptom development specific to the diagnosis, the context in which these symptoms occur, and the degree to which they are inconsistent with age and persist to cause impairment (40). The diagnosis of ADHD requires the identification of specific behaviours that meet the criteria of DSM-IV or ICD-10 (7,8). DSM-IV and ICD-10 have adopted almost identical criteria for the identification of inattentive, hyperactive, and impulsive symptoms (Table 39.1). However, significant differences are still evident in the number of criteria in each domain required for a diagnosis, the importance of inattention, and the handling of comorbidity. In comparison with DSM-IV (7), ICD-10 (8) is more demanding about cross-situational pervasiveness and requires that all necessary criteria be present, both at home and at school or oth-

er situations. The upcoming DSM-V will refine the subtype concept of DSM-IV and is expected to introduce a further subtype referring to those children with attention problems but without hyperactive-impulsive symptoms, in contrast to the full syndrome and those with more or less difficulty in the attention or hyperactive/impulsive domain.

The diagnosis of ADHD is based on validated ratings and clinical interviews. Although widely used, neuropsychological measurements of impulsivity or attention may be supportive of a diagnosis, but are not suitable as the sole diagnostic marker. Furthermore, no objective biological markers exist that may determine a diagnosis. Differences found in neuroimaging (see above) and electrophysiological studies, cognitive performance, olfaction as well as genotyping are all subjects of thorough examination, yet far from being potentially used as valid diagnostic markers.

The diagnosis in adults is currently still based on the diagnostic criteria for children, although the upcoming DSM-V will probably provide some adaptations for the diagnosis in adult patients relating to the observation that some symptoms of childhood are attenuated in adulthood despite persisting impairment (14). Nevertheless, in order to diagnose ADHD in adulthood, it is imperative that ADHD was already present in childhood (41). And complicating the diagnosis, comorbidity in adulthood is even higher compared to childhood (42).

Differential diagnosis

Apart from the heterogeneity of ADHD, the overlap between comorbidity and differential diagnoses renders the clinical diagnosis very difficult. Conduct disorders, emotional disorders or tic disorders, autism spectrum disorders, bipolar disorders or specific developmental disorders may be comorbidities of ADHD, but all these psychiatric conditions also have to be considered in the diagnostic process as differential

Table 39.1
Diagnostic criteria for ADHD: DSM-IV and ICD-10 research criteria (41).

	DSM-IV	ICD-10
Symptom criteria	Two domains: • Inattention: 9 symptoms (e.g. difficulty organizing tasks and activities, easily distracted by extraneous stimuli); 6 or more symptoms necessary (criterion A1) • Hyperactivity-impulsivity: 9 symptoms, for instance: hyperactivity: 6 symptoms: (e.g. talks excessively) and impulsivity: 3 symptoms: (e.g. difficulty awaiting turn); 6 or more symptoms necessary (criterion A2)	Three domains: • Attention: 9 symptoms (e.g. often impaired in organizing tasks and activities; often fails to sustain attention during tasks); 6 or more symptoms necessary • Hyperactivity: 5 symptoms (e.g. often fidgets with hands or feet or squirms on seat: exhibits a persistent pattern of excessive motor activity); 3 or more symptoms necessary • Impulsivity: 4 symptoms (e.g. often blurts out answers before questions have been completed; often fails to wait in line); 1 or more symptoms necessary
Onset and duration	Before age of 7 years: at least 6 months	Before age of 7 years: at least 6 months
Impairments	In 2 or more settings (e.g. at school/work or at home) Clinically significant impairment in social, academic, or occupational functioning	Clinically significant distress or impairment in social, academic, or occupational functioning
Exclusion criteria	Symptoms do not occur exclusively during the course of other psychiatric disorders (e.g. schizophrenia) or not better accounted for by another mental disorder (e.g. mood disorder)	Several other psychiatric disorders (e.g. mood disorder, anxiety disorder)
Diagnostic algorithm and diagnosis	Attention-deficit hyperactivity disorders, combined type (criteria A1 and A2) Attention-deficit hyperactivity disorders, predominantly inattentive type (criterion A1) Attention-deficit hyperactivity disorders, predominantly hyper-active-impulsive type (criterion A2) 314.9 Attention-deficit hyperactivity disorders, disorder not otherwise specified	F90 Hyperkinetic disorders F90.0 Disturbance of activity and attention F90.1 Hyperkinetic conduct disorder F90.8 Other hyperkinetic disorder
Comments	'In partial remission': symptoms are present, but not full criteria	No subtypes available

diagnoses (17). Comorbid disorders of ADHD may result in ADHD-like symptoms: depressive syndromes, for example, may comprise inattention, distractibility, aggression and irritability, symptoms that could mimic the phenotype of ADHD. On the other hand, ADHD may be accompanied by a depressive disorder or result in a depressive mood due to constant and repeated psychosocial failure and discouragement.

According to the 'guideline on the clinical investigation of medicinal products for the treatment of attention deficit hyperactivity disorder' (43), ADHD should be differentiated from otherwise 'normal' behaviour in active children, but also from disruptive behaviour in children due to low intelligence (mental retardation) or high intelligence (gifted children) when there is no 'match' between demands and capabilities. ADHD should also be differentiated from oppositional behaviour due to repeated failure in performance and the inability of living up to expectations. Furthermore, differentiation should be made between ADHD and stereotypic movement disorders such as tic disorders (see Chapter 31, 38), where the hyperactivity is more focussed on specific body parts. In addition, ADHD, if not co-morbid, should be discriminated from other mental disorders that share similar symptoms, e.g. mood and anxiety and personality disorders. Although rarely diagnosed before adulthood in Europe, bipolar disorders in children and adolescents may be another differential diagnosis. The age of onset of first symptoms (younger than 7 years) should be kept as one of the hallmarks for differentiation. Finally, ADHD should not be diagnosed if symptoms present in the context of a pervasive developmental or psychotic disorder. Nor should the presence of symptoms be due to the use of medication. For adults, ADHD should be discriminated from disorders where inattention or other cognitive impairments are present, such as bipolar disorder, depression and anxiety disorders or another condition with cognitive impairment.

Treatment

The treatment of ADHD is directed towards improvement of attention and reduction of hyperactivity/impulsivity in order to be able to focus on tasks and performance, and improve associated behavioural and psychosocial problems. Various guidelines exist that show a great degree of overlap (44). Psycho-education alone and in combination with pharmacotherapy is usually the standard of care in Europe. Behavioural treatment is often provided in order to sustain the eventual success of pharmacotherapy and to modify conduct problems. In the context of other non-pharmacological interventions such as cognitive treatment, neurofeedback training and dietary measures, a recent meta-analysis concluded that better evidence of efficacy from blinded assessments is required before they can be supported as adequate interventions for core ADHD symptoms (29). Those interventions may nevertheless be helpful in regard to comorbidity or psychosocial difficulties.

For more than 50 years, psychostimulant drugs, such as methylphenidate and amphetamine, have been the golden pharmacotherapeutical standard in the treatment ADHD. These drugs consistently showed efficacy and safety when compared with placebo in randomized, controlled trials (45,46). Other medications used in the pharmacological treatment of ADHD are summarized in Table 39.2.

Despite many decades of clinical use, psychostimulant drugs have been controversial because of concerns that they might cause tics, kindle substance abuse, delay growth, and have potential adverse effects on the developing brain, specifically as related to dopamine brain function. However, results obtained in healthy animals provided evidence that the administration of amphetamine and methylphenidate using procedures that adequately simulate clinical treatment conditions do not lead to long-term adverse developmental, neurobiological, or be-

Table 39.2
Drug treatment for ADHD.

Psychostimulants
- Methylphenidate: immediate-release and long-acting (sustained, osmotic, modified, extended release) formulations
- Amphetamine: immediate-release and long-acting (extended release and lisdexamphetamine, a pro-drug of amphetamine) formulations

Non-psychostimulants
- Atomoxetine
- Modafinil
- Pemoline (hepatotoxic effects!)

Others
- α2-Adrenoreceptor agonists = α-agonists (clonidine, guanfacine)
- Tricyclic antidepressants (amitriptyline, desipramine, imipramine, clomipramine, nortriptyline)
- Bupropion (efficacious for controlling cigarette smoking, which is increased in ADHD patients)
- Monoamine oxidase inhibitors (phenelzine, selegiline)
- Memantine

havioural consequences of the dopaminergic system in non-human primates (47). It has also been discussed that psychostimulants increase the cardiovascular risk and risk of genetic damage in ADHD patients. However, no evidence for a negative impact of methylphenidate on heart rate variability in ADHD children has been demonstrated (48). In contrast, it was found that methylphenidate treatment does increase the decreased vagal tone with diminished heart rate variability in drug-naive children (48,49). Prospective follow-up studies, fortunately, did not establish any mutagenicity of methylphenidate therapy in ADHD-affected children (50)

Prognosis

ADHD is a highly impairing, neurodevelopmental condition that manifests in childhood and is characterized by increasing rates of psychiatric and non-psychiatric comorbidity in the course of the disorder (17). Comorbid disorders sig-

nificantly contribute to ADHD-associated morbidity and further decrease the patient's overall quality of life. Some studies suggest that ADHD increases the risk of personality disorders and, if untreated, is associated with functional impairments such as dysfunction within the school environment, peer problems, family conflict, poor occupational performance, injuries, antisocial behaviour, traffic violations, and traffic accidents (10, 42). A recent long-term prospective study found further evidence for high morbidity associated with ADHD across the life cycle, stressing the importance of early recognition of this disorder for prevention and early intervention strategies (51).

References

1 Mannuzza S, Klein RG, Moulton JL. Persistence of attention-deficit/hyperactivity disorder into adulthood: what have we learned from the prospective follow-up studies? J Attention Dis 2003;7:93–100.

2 Biederman J, Monuteaux MC, Mick E, et al. Young adult outcome of attention deficit hyperactivity disorder: a controlled 10-year follow-up study. Psychol Med 2006;36:167–179.

3 Lara C, Fayyad J, de Graaf R, et al. Childhood predictors of adult attention-deficit/hyperactivity disorder: results from the World Health Organization World Mental Health Survey. Initiative Biol Psychiatr 2009;65:46–54.

4 Lange KW, Reichl S, Lange KM, Tucha L, Tucha O. The history of attention deficit hyperactivity disorder. ADHD Attent Def Hyp Disord 2010;2:241-255.

5 Taylor E. Antecedents of ADHD: a historical account of diagnostic concepts. ADHD Attent Def Hyp Disord 2011;3:69-75.

6 Thome J, Jacobs K. Attention deficit hyperactivity disorder (ADHD) in a 19th century children's book. Eur Psychiatr 2004;19:303–306.

7 World Health Organization: The ICD-10 classification of mental and behavioural disorders. Diagnostic criteria for research. Geneva: WHO,1994.

8 American Psychiatric Association. Diagnostic and statistical manual of mental disorders, 4th ed. Text

Revision. Washington DC: American Psychiatric Association, 2000.

9 Polanczyk G, de Lima MS, Horta BL, Biederman J, Rohde LA. The worldwide prevalence of ADHD: a systematic review and metaregression analysis Am J Psychiatr 2007;164:942–948.

10 Biederman J, Faraone SV. Attention-deficit hyperactivity disorder. Lancet 2005;366:237-248.

11 Staller J, Farone SV. Attention-deficit hyperactivity disorder in girls: epidemiology and management. CNS Drugs 2006;20:107-123.

12 Franke B, Faraone SV, Asherson P, et al. The genetics of attention deficit/hyperactivity disorder in adults, a review. Mol Psychiatr 2012;17:960-987.

13 Polanczyk G, Rohde LA. Epidemiology of attention-deficit/hyperactivity disorder across the lifepan. Curr Opin Psychiatr 2007;20:386-392.

14 Biederman J, Petty CR, Evans M, Small J, Faraone SV. How persistent is ADHD? A controlled 10-year follow-up study of boys with ADHD. Psychiat Res 2010;177: 299–304.

15 Retz W, Retz-Junginger P, Hengesch G, et al. Psychometric and psychopathological characterization of young male prison inmates with and without attention deficit/hyperactivity disorder. Eur Arch Psychiatr Clin Neurosci 2004;254:201–208.

16 Fayyad J, De Graaf R, Kessler R, et al. Cross-national prevalence and correlates of adult attention-deficit hyperactivity disorder. Brit J Psychiatr 2007;190:402-409.

17 Taurines R, Schmitt J, Renner T, Conner AC, Warnke A, Romanos M. Developmental comorbidity in attention-deficit/hyperactivity disorder. ADHD Attent Def Hyp Disord 2010;2:276-289.

18 Levy F, Young D, Bennett KS, Martin NC, Hay DA. Comorbid ADHD and mental health disorders: are these children more likely to develop reading disorders? ADHD Attent Def Hyp Disord 2013;5:21-28.

19 Murphy K, Barkley RA. Attention deficit disorders adults: Comorbidity and adaptive impairments. Compr Psychiatr 1996:37:393-401.

20 Klein RG, Mannuzza S. Long-term outcome of hyperactice-children – A review. J Am Acad Child Adoles Psychiatr 1991;30:383-387.

21 Olazagasti MAR, Klein RG, Mannuzza S, et al. Does childhood attention-deficit/hyperactivity disorder predict risk-taking and medical illnesses in adulthood? J Am Acad of Child Adolesc Psychiatr 2013;52:153-162.

22 Faraone SV, Mick E. Molecular genetics of attention hyperactivity disorders. Psychiatr Clin North Am 2010;33:159-180.

23 Freitag CM, Rohde LA. Lempp T, Romanos M. Phenotypic and measurement influences on heritability estimates in childhood ADHD. Eur Child Adoles Psychiatr 2010;19:311-323.

24 Gizer IR. Ficks C, Waldman ID. Candidate gene studies of ADHD: a meta-analytic review. Hum Genet 2009;126:51–90.

25 Jarick I, Volckmar A-L, Pütter C, et al. Genome-wide analysis of rare copy number variations reveals *PARK2* as a candidate gene for attention-deficit/hyperactivity disorder. Mol Psychiatr 2012;doi:10.1038/mp.2012.161.

26 Brookes K, Mill J, Guindalini C, et al. A common haplotype of the dopamine transporter gene associated with attention-deficit/hyperactivity disorder and interacting with maternal use of alcohol during pregnaXncy, Arch Gen Psychiatr 2006:63:74-81

27 Thapar A, Langley K, Asherson P, Gill M. Gene-environment interplay in attention-deficit hyperactivity disorder and the importance of a developmental perspective. Brit J Psychiatr 2007;190:1-3.

28 Zhu JM, Zhang X, Yu YH, Spencer TJ, Biederman J, Bhide PG. Prenatal nicotine exposure mouse model showing hyperactivity, reduced cingulate cortex volume, reduced dopamine turnover, and responsiveness to oral methylphenidate treatment. J Neurosci 2012;32:9410-9418.

29 Sonuga-Barke EJS, Brandeis D, Cortese S,et al. European ADHD Guidelines Group (2013). Nonpharmacological interventions for ADHD: Systematic review and meta-analyses of randomized controlled trials of dietary and psychological treatments. Am J Psychiat 2013;170:275-289.

30 Williams JHG, Ross L. Consequences of prenatal toxin exposure for mental health in children and adolescents. Eur Child Adoles Psychiatr 2007;16:243-253.

31 Chamberlain SR, Robbins TW, Sahakian B. The neurobiology of attention-deficit/ hyperactivity disorder. Biol Psychiatry 2007;61:1317-1319.

32 Mehler-Wex C, Riederer P, Gerlach M. Dopaminergic dysbalance in distinct basal ganglia neurocircuits: implications for the pathophysiology of Parkinson´s disease, schizophrenia and attention deficit hyperactivity disorder. Neurotox Res 2006;10:167-179.

33 Vaidya CJ, Austin G, Kirkorian G, et al. Selective effects of methylphenidate in attention deficit hyperactivity disorder: A functional magnetic resonance study. Proc Natl Acad Sci USA. 1998;95:14494-14499.

34 Sullivan RM, Brake WG. What the rodent prefrontal cortex can teach us about attention-deficit/hyperactivity disorder: the critical role of early developmental events on prefrontal function. Behav Brain Res 2003;146:43-55.

35 Francois C, Grabli D, McCairn K, et al. Behavioural disorders induced by external globus pallidus dysfunction in primates - II. Anatomical study. Brain 2004;127:2055-2070.

36 Shafritz KM, Marchione KE, Gore JC, Shaywitz SE, Shaywitz BA. The effects of methylphenidate on neural systems of attention in attention deficit hyperactivity disorder. Am J Psychiatr 2004;161:1990-1997.

37 Lou HC, Henriksen L, Bruhn P, Borner H, Nielsen JB. Striatal dysfunction in attention deficit and hyperkinetic disorder. Arch Neurol 1989;46:48-52.

38 Volkow ND, Wang GJ, Fowler JS, et al. Therapeutic doses of oral methylphenidate significantly increase extracellular dopamine in the human brain. J Neurosci 2001;21:121-125.

39 Rizzo P, Steinhausen H-C, Drechsler R. Self perception of self-regulatory skills in children with attention-deficit/hyperactivity disorder ages 8-10 years. ADHD Attent Def Hyp Disord 2010;2:171-183.

40 Rappley MD. Attention deficit-hyperactivity disorder. N Engl J Med. 2005;352:165-173.

41 Stieglitz R-D. Attention-deficit hyperactivity disorder in adults: diagnosis and prevalence. In: Retz W, Klein RG, eds. Attention-deficit hyperactivity disorder (ADHD) in adults. Key Issues in Mental Health. Basel: Karger, 2010;176:105-125.

42 Jacob CP, Romanos J, Dempfle A, et al. Co-morbidity of adult attention-deficit/hyperactivity disorder with focus on personality traits and related disorders in a tertiary referral center. Eur Arch Psychiatr Clin Neurosci 2007;257:309-317.

43 European Medicines Agency. Guidelines on the clinical investigation of medicinal products for the treatment of attention deficit hyperactivity disorder (ADHD). 2010

44 Kendall T, Taylor E, Perez A, Taylor C. Guideline Development Group. Diagnosis and management of attention-deficit/hyperactivity disorder in children, young people, and adults: summary of NICE guidance. Brit Med J 2008;337:1239.

45 AACCP Official Action. Practice parameter for the use of stimulant medications in the treatment of children, adolescents, and adults. J Am Acad Child Adolesc Psychiatr 2002;41(S2):26-49.

46 Huang YS, Tsai MH. Long-Term outcomes with medications for attention-deficit hyperactivity disorder. Current status of knowledge. CNS Drugs 2011;25:539-554.

47 Gerlach M, Grünblatt E, Lange KW. Is the treatment with psychostimulants in children and adolescents with attention deficit hyperactivity disorder harmful for the dopaminergic system? ADHD Attent Def Hyp Disord 2013;5:71-81.

48 Buchhorn R, Conzelmann A, Willaschek C, Störk D, Taurines R, Renner T. Heart rate variability and methylphenidate in children with ADHD. ADHD Attent Def Hyp Disord 2012;4:85-91.

49 Rash JA, Aguirre-Camacho A. Attention-deficit hyperactivity disorder and cardiac vagal control: a systematic review. ADHD Attent Def Hyp Disord 2012;4:167-177.

50 Walitza S, Kämpf K, Oli R, Warnke A, Gerlach M, Stopper H. Commentary. Prospective follow up studies found no mutagenicity of methylphenidate therapy in ADHD affected children. Toxicol Lett 2010;193:4-8.

51 Biederman J, Petty CR. Woodworth KY, Lomedico A, Hyder LL, Faraone SV. Adult outcome of attention-deficit/hyperactivity disorder: A controlled 16-year follow-up study. J Clin Psychiatr 2012;73:941-950.

40

Obsessive-Compulsive Disorder

Jesse M. Crosby & Thröstur Björgvinsson

Obsessive-compulsive disorder (OCD) is defined by recurrent obsessions and/or compulsions that result in clinically significant distress and impaired functioning (1). Obsessions are described as 'persistent ideas, thoughts, impulses, or images that are experienced as intrusive and inappropriate and cause marked anxiety or distress'. The idea that obsessions are intrusive suggests the individual is unable to control the experience of the obsessions, and the idea that they are inappropriate refers to their ego-dystonic nature (in opposition to personal values, goals, preferences). It is also important to note that these are not just excessive worries about real-life issues, and that they are the product of the individual's own mind, not imposed from the outside as with thought insertion. Compulsions are described as 'repetitive behaviours… or mental acts… the goal of which is to prevent or reduce anxiety or distress'. They can be overt (behavioural) or covert (mental) actions (2).

While obsessive thinking and compulsive behaviours can be observed in the general population, these phenomena become pathological for individuals with OCD as they can result in significant distress and impaired functioning. The negative effects of the disorder can include excessive amounts of time spent performing compulsive rituals, disrupted family and social relationships, impaired work or academic performance, and an overall decrease in quality of life. OCD is considered a severe psychiatric disorder that can have a significant and pervasive impact on the individual and society.

The characteristic symptoms of OCD have been recognized in several different cultures for centuries (3). The content or theme of the obsessions and compulsions has been grouped into four basic symptom clusters (4). For obsessions, they are: 1) contamination; 2) aggressive, sexual, religious, and somatic; 3) symmetry; and 4) hoarding. Table 40.1 provides a list of common obsessions. The four symptoms clusters of compulsions are: 1) cleaning, 2) checking, 3) ordering, arranging, counting, and repeating, and 4) hoarding and collecting. Table 40.2 provides a list of common compulsions.

It is important to note the functional relationship between obsessions and compulsions as the compulsions serve to reduce the anxiety or distress associated with the obsessions. In one study, 90% of the participants reported that their compulsions were associated with their obsessions, while the other 10% reported that the compulsions and obsessions were unrelated (5). In that case, the compulsions may function to reduce distress according to other rigid rules (2). While the presentation of behavioural and mental compulsions may differ, they are equivalent in their functional relationship to obsessions. There are also cases of obsessions only. In the study mentioned above, 90% of participants reported experiencing both obsessions and behavioural compulsions, 8% reported obsessions and mental compulsions, with the other 2% experiencing only obsessions (5).

Table 40.1
List of common obsessions.

Obsession	Examples
Contamination	Concern or disgust with bodily fluids; concern with dirt or germs; excessive concern with environmental contaminants; excessive concern with household cleaners; excessive concern with animals; bothered by sticky substances; concern of contracting or spreading disease caused by contaminant
Aggression	Fear might harm self; fear might harm others; violent or horrific images; fear of blurting out obscenities; fear of doing something embarrassing; fear will act on unwanted impulses; fear will steal things; fear will harm others because not careful; fear will be responsible for something terrible happening
Sexual	Forbidden or perverse thoughts, images, or impulses; content involves children or incest; content involves homosexuality; aggressive sexual behaviour toward others
Religious	Concerned with sacrilege or blasphemy; excessive concern with morality
Somatic	Concerns with illness of disease; excessive concern with body part or aspect of appearance
Symmetry	Need for symmetry or proper alignment
Hoarding	Obsessions about hoarding or saving things
Miscellaneous	Need to know or remember things; fear of saying certain things; fear of not saying just the right thing; fear of losing things; intrusive images; intrusive sounds, words, or music; bothered by certain sounds or noises; lucky or unlucky numbers; colors with special significance; superstitious fears

Adapted from Goodman WK, Price LH, Rasmussem SA, et al. The Yale-Brown Obsessive Compulsive Scale. Arch Gen Psychitary 1989;46:1006-1011.

A variety of disorders share similar characteristics with OCD and have been conceptualized as OCD spectrum disorders (see Chapter 38). Three categories of OCD spectrum disorders have been suggested (6): 1) neurological disorders with repetitive behaviours (e.g., tic disorders) (see also Chapter 41); 2) impulse control disorders (trichotillomania) (see also Chapter 41); and 3) body image, body sensitization, and body weight concerns (e.g., Body Dysmorphic Disorder). The shared OCD characteristic is the presence of obsessions or impulses coupled with maladaptive impulsive behaviours that are difficult to control. For the OCD spectrum disorders, it is important to note that the compulsive behaviours associated with basic OCD function to reduce anxiety or distress and are typically experienced as aversive, whereas the impulsive OCD spectrum behaviours function to increase gratification or stimulation and are typically experienced as appetitive.

Epidemiology

Historically, the occurrence of OCD was thought to be rare, with early studies suggesting that it made up a small proportion of psychiatric patients. This was likely due to patient underreporting and lack of symptom recognition by clinicians. Current estimates of the prevalence of OCD are much higher. The lifetime prevalence of OCD in adults has been estimated at 1.9%-3.3% (7). In the USA, the national epidemiological catchment area study found OCD to be the fourth most common mental disorder, with a six-month point prevalence of 1.6% (8) and lifetime prevalence of 2.5% (9). International cross-cultural studies have found similar esti-

Table 40.2
List of common compulsions.

Compulsion	Examples
Cleaning/washing	Excessive or ritualized hand washing; excessive or ritualized showering, bathing, tooth brushing, grooming, or toilet routine; excessive or ritualized cleaning of household items or other inanimate objects; other measures to prevent or remove contact with contaminants
Checking	Checking locks, stove, appliances; checking that did not or will not harm others; checking that did not or will not harm self; checking that nothing terrible did or will happen; checking for mistakes; checking related to somatic obsessions
Ordering/Arranging	Need to order and reorder; need to arrange and rearrange items
Counting	Need to count and recount objects, events, or experiences
Repeating	Rereading or rewriting; need to repeat routine activities
Hoarding/Collecting	Compulsion to hoard or collect things
Miscellaneous	Mental rituals; need to ask, tell, or confess; need to touch, tap or rub; measures to prevent harm or terrible consequences to self or others; ritualized eating behaviours; superstitious behaviours; hair pulling/trichotillomania

Adapted from Goodman WK, Price LH, Rasmussem SA, et al. The Yale-Brown Obsessive Compulsive Scale. Arch Gen Psychitary 1989;46:1006-1011.

mates with a one-year point prevalence of 1.1% - 1.8% and a lifetime prevalence of 1.9% - 2.5% (10). In adolescents, estimates have varied with one-year point prevalence estimates ranging from 0.7% (11) to 4% (12). There has been some concern that these estimates are high because of methodological assessment issues, so it is possible that the actual prevalence rates are lower.

In adult populations, OCD is found among women more than men by a slight margin. In the DSM-IV field trial, 51% of the participants was female (5), and another study reporting results from a clinical population of individuals with OCD found 55% of the participants were female (13). In adolescent populations of individuals with OCD, a larger proportion of males (67%) has been observed (14), and several studies have estimated a 2:1 male to female ratio for adolescents with OCD (2). The age of onset differs for males and females with an earlier modal onset in males (13-15 years old); the female modal onset is 20-24 years (15). It is estimated that 50- 60% of individuals with OCD experience at least one additional mental disorder (16), with depression and substance abuse as the most common co-morbid disorders.

Etiology

The aetiology of OCD has not been established, but behavioural, cognitive, environmental, genetic, and neurobiological factors have been implicated in the onset and maintenance of its symptoms. Several behavioural and cognitive models of OCD have been proposed. A two-stage behavioural theory of fear acquisition and maintenance served as the basis of earlier behavioural accounts of the aetiology of OCD, where a neutral event is experienced in association with an event that inherently provokes fear so that the neutral event now evokes a fear response (17). This fear response is reinforced by attempts to escape, avoid, or reduce the fear. These behaviours are then maintained through the process of negative reinforcement as the fear response is reduced. It has been argued that this theory does not provide an adequate account for the initial process of fear acquisition (18), but it does explain the functional relationship between obsessions and compulsions.

To account for the complex phenomenology of OCD, several cognitive conceptualizations have been proposed. It has been suggested that obsessions are caused by catastrophic misinterpretations of thoughts, images, or impulses and are maintained as long as the misinterpretations persist (19). This is supported by evidence that much of the general population without a psychiatric diagnosis experiences intrusive thoughts similar to those experienced by an individual with OCD (20), suggesting that it is the interpretation of the importance, relevance, and potential consequences of the thought that results in an anxiety response. Inflated responsibility to cope with the possible consequences of an intrusive thought has also been suggested as a cognitive conceptualization of OCD (21). In this theory, the individual's perception of responsibility to prevent a negative outcome is influenced by distorted assumptions, beliefs, and appraisals of the thoughts. Related to this is the metacognitive model that suggests that distorted beliefs about the importance, meaning, and power of thoughts result in the need to control obsessions with the performance of compulsions (22). This model includes the role of fusion beliefs in which thoughts are experienced as the moral equivalent of the actual behaviour (e.g., thinking about harming someone is as bad as actually harming someone).

Environmental experiences have also been implicated in the development of OCD symptoms. Experiences characterized by heightened arousal or stress have been linked to the development of OCD. Traumatic experiences have been implicated where the risk of OCD has been reported to be 10 times greater in individuals with posttraumatic stress disorder (23). OCD has been linked to pregnancy and childbirth where first-time parents, especially mothers, develop OCD symptoms related to the care of the child

(24). Family environments with strict parental controlling and interfering attitudes have also been associated with OCD (25).

Pathophysiology

While it is clear that OCD is linked to significant cognitive and behavioural learning processes that contribute to the development and maintenance of the disorder, there is also evidence that OCD is a biological disorder. The genetic understanding of OCD is growing, with sufficient evidence of a genetic component in OCD. Twin studies have shown that OCD is heritable, with a greater genetic influence in childhood-onset OCD (45%-65%) than in adult-onset OCD (27%-47%) (26). First-degree relatives of individuals with OCD have been found to be 3-12 times more likely to have OCD than the general population (27). Genetic linkage studies using the genome-wide association study approach are encouraging, but have yet to find any associations with genome-wide significance (28).

Neuroimaging research has implicated the cortico-striatal-thalamo-cortical (CSTC) circuit as a primary focus in the pathophysiology of OCD (29). Multiple studies have shown that the key nodes in this circuit (the orbitofrontal cortex, anterior cingulate cortex, and striatum) are hyperactive in resting state scans. This hyperactivity is increased when symptoms are provoked, and it attenuates after successful treatment (30). Other studies have implicated other brain regions in the pathophysiology of OCD, including the amygdala (31) and the hippocampus (32), but the CSTC circuit remains of primary interest in the neurobiology of OCD.

Increasing attention is being paid to the role of infection in the sudden onset of OCD symptoms, as seen in a syndrome of emerging concern, pediatric autoimmune neuropsychiatric disorders associated with streptococcus (PANDAS) such as in Sydenham's chorea (see also

Chapter 29) (33). This syndrome is characterized by the sudden onset of OCD symptoms in a pediatric population after infection with streptococcus, although current research has expanded the investigation to include more than just streptococcus as possible precipitants to the sudden onset of symptoms (34). The research is just beginning, but identifying the neuropsychological systems associated with the immunobiological pathology may open new doors to the understanding of the pathophysiology of OCD.

Clinical presentation

To illustrate the clinical presentation of OCD, the following de-identified case shows a typical symptom presentation observable at intake. Bill was a married male in his 40s who had a successful law career prior to the worsening of his OCD symptoms. He sought treatment after he was unable to work due to the nature of his intrusive obsessions. He described a normal childhood, one of four siblings, and reported that he was close to his parents and siblings. He married his high school sweetheart, and she was encouraging him to seek treatment. His symptoms began to emerge about 10 years prior to seeking treatment when he first noticed intrusive and disturbing thoughts that he could not avoid.

He reported four types of obsessions: 1) religious, 2) intrusive sexual thoughts, 3) fear that he might harm or had harmed someone, and 4) fear of contamination. His religious obsessions were mostly associated with the devil. For example, any numbers that were remotely similar to '666' had to be neutralized or they would lead to something horrible. This included going to hell or harm coming to him, his wife, or his family. He had to neutralize it (this was his compulsion) by changing the number 6 to the number 7, such as adding a 1 to each number and making it '777' as a way to neutralize the intrusive association with the devil. His intrusive sexual thoughts involved a flickering thought of sexually abusing his nieces and nephews, something that he found

abhorrent and very difficult to tolerate. His way of coping with these obsessions was to avoid going to family gatherings, something that he used to enjoy in the past, and avoid places where he might run into children. His harming obsessions included intrusive images of him killing his two dogs with a shovel. This caused him tremendous distress, and he would insist on removing all tools when he was close to the dogs and not be left alone with the dogs. His fear of contamination involved contact with bodily fluids and contracting a communicable disease. He worried that he might contract the disease himself, or that he might spread the contaminant/disease to his family members. He avoided all contact with anything that might have been contacted directly by a bodily fluid (e.g., toilet seat) or by hands that may not have been washed after contact with a bodily fluid (bathroom door handle). He used paper towels or tissues as barriers when he had to touch a feared stimulus. His symptoms were enabled by his wife and children as they did the best they could to reduce his distress in the hopes that he could improve his functioning. At the intake interview, Bill reported that his obsessions and compulsions were all consuming and that he could do little else during the day except use his energy to make sure that he would neutralize these obsessions. He reported spending over 12 hours per day struggling with his OCD.

Diagnosis

The *Diagnostic and Statistical Manual of Mental Disorders* (*DSM-IV-TR*) (1) classifies OCD as an anxiety disorder. Five diagnostic criteria must be met to receive a diagnosis:

A The first criterion is the presence of obsessions or compulsions. Obsessions are defined by: 1) recurrent and persistent thoughts, impulses, or images that are experienced, at some point during the disturbance, as intrusive and inappropriate and that cause marked anxiety or distress, 2) the thoughts, impulses, or images are not simply excessive worries about real-life problems, 3) the person attempts to ignore or suppress such thoughts, impulses, or images, or to neutralize them with some other thought or action, and 4) the person recognizes that the obsessional thoughts, impulses, or images are a product of his or her own mind (not imposed from without as in thought insertion). Compulsions are defined by: 1) repetitive behaviours or mental acts that the person feels driven to perform in response to an obsession, or according to rules that must be applied rigidly, and 2) the behaviours or mental acts are aimed at preventing or reducing distress or preventing some dreaded event or situation; however, these behaviours or mental acts either are not connected in a realistic way with what they are designed to neutralize or prevent or are clearly excessive.

B   Recognition by the person at some point during the course of the disorder that the obsessions or compulsions are excessive or unreasonable (this does not apply to children).

C   The obsessions or compulsions cause marked distress, are time-consuming (take more than 1 hour a day), or significantly interfere with the person's normal routine, occupational (or academic) functioning, or usual social activities or relationships.

D   The content of the obsessions or compulsions is not better explained by another Axis I disorder.

E   The disturbance is not due to the direct physiological effects of a substance or general medical condition

It is possible to specify if the person has poor insight, i.e. if the person does not recognize that the obsessions or compulsions are excessive or unreasonable for most of the time during the current episode (see criterion B). It has been suggested that insight falls on a continuum based on the strength of belief in the obsessions (35).

To arrive at a diagnosis, structured interviews, semi-structured interviews, and self-report assessments can be used to evaluate a symptom presentation. There are two empirically validated, structured interviews based on *DSM-IV-TR* criteria, the anxiety disorder interview schedule for *DSM-IV* (36) and the structured clinical interview for *DSM-IV* (37). There are two well-validated, semi-structured interviews that can be very useful in indentifying the symptom clusters, specific symptoms, and symptom insight of OCD. The Yale-Brown obsessive compulsive scale (Y-BOCS) (38) has both a symptom checklist and a scale to rate the severity of each symptom. The checklist can be a useful tool to establish a diagnosis and also inform treatment planning, and the severity scale can provide an indication of the seriousness of the disorder. The Brown assessment of beliefs scale (BABS) (39) is a measure of the level of insight into how excessive or unreasonable the obsessions are. There are also multiple self-report assessments that provide an indication of symptom type and severity, in addition to providing a more detailed assessment of symptom subtypes or underlying issues, two of which are highlighted here. The obsessive-compulsive inventory-revised (OCI-R) (40) is a useful measure as it provides a brief self-report assessment of general OCD symptoms and impairment. The obsessive beliefs questionnaire (OBQ) (41) can provide an assessment of the primary beliefs and appraisals underlying the obsessions.

So far, diagnostic criteria presented herein were taken from the DSM-IV-TR. In the new fifth edition (*DSM-5*), some changes are anticipated in how OCD is conceptualized and diagnosed (42). OCD was previously listed in the Anxiety Disorder category, but will now be moved to a new category dedicated to 'Obsessive Compulsive and Related Disorders', which will include the OCD spectrum disorders: body dysmorphic disorder, hoarding, skin picking, and trichotillomania. This change recognizes the unique symptom presentation of OCD, as compared to general anxiety disorders, and provides a conceptual home for the OCD spectrum disorders (43). In the *DSM-5*, there will be three changes to the diagnostic criteria. First, expanded options will be available for specifying the level of insight. Instead of just 'poor insight,' the options will now include 'good insight', 'poor insight', and 'absent insight/delusional OCD beliefs'. This allows for a better differential diagnosis between OCD and the psychotic disorders, and recognizes the range of insight levels in individuals with OCD. Second, a new specifier will be added to designate a past or current tic disorder, as this has important medication considerations in treatment. And, third, in the definition of obsessions, the word 'impulse' will be changed to 'urge' to avoid confusion with the impulse control disorders.

Differential diagnosis

The OCD diagnostic criteria provide important guidance in the process of differential diagnosis. It is important to clarify whether the content of the obsessions and/or compulsions is not restricted to another disorder. For example, obsessive thinking about eating, weight, or dieting would be better explained as an eating disorder; preoccupation with a substance or compulsive use of a substance would be better explained as a substance use disorder; or ruminative/obsessive guilt might be better explained as a depressive disorder.

Obsessive thinking / worrying

Obsessions in OCD will be within the OCD themes/categories and not just excessive worries about real-life problems. This can include non-clinical issues, such as obsessive thinking about an important life decision, as well as other mental disorders. For example, excessive worries about multiple life concerns would likely be part of a generalized anxiety disorder, while recurrent and persistent worries about being judged negatively by others in social situations is more likely part of a social phobia.

Psychosis

The level of insight is an important part of the differential diagnosis. Two of the diagnostic criteria refer to the level of insight: 1) recognition that the obsessions are a product of his or her mind and not the result of external thought insertion, and 2) recognition that the obsessions or compulsions are excessive or unreasonable. Both of these criteria help differentiate between OCD and a psychotic episode or disorder. Even bizarre obsessions may not be psychotic in nature. It is important to remember that insight is thought to occur on a continuum, but in severe cases of OCD, the obsessions can appear delusional in nature, and the compulsions can be similar to the bizarre stereotyped behaviours observed in schizophrenia. In these cases, it is important to examine the entire clinical picture, especially the history and course of the disorder. It is also helpful to remember that OCD obsessions and compulsions are typically ego-dystonic in nature.

OCD spectrum disorders

While the OCD spectrum disorders are similar to OCD, it is important to identify the correct diagnosis as different treatments may be recommended (e.g., habit reversal may be a more effective treatment for the impulse control disorders). A process of comparing and contrasting the symptom presentation can be useful in making a differential diagnosis.

- To differentiate between OCD and a *tic disorder*, both will involve repetitive physical or vocal behaviours, but individuals with a tic disorder will engage in a tic in response to a sense of discomfort or physical need to feel right whereas individuals with OCD will engage in repetitive behaviours in response to an obsession.
- To differentiate between OCD and *trichotillomania*, both involving repetitive behaviours in response to feeling uncomfortable, individuals with trichotillomania will derive a good feeling from hair pulling whereas individuals with OCD will engage in a repetitive behaviour to escape unwanted emotions such as anxiety.

- To differentiate between OCD and *body dysmorphic disorder*, both involving the repetitive checking of body image concerns, individuals with body dysmorphic disorder will engage in obsessions and compulsions that only focus on body appearance whereas individuals with OCD will report additional obsessions and compulsions.
- To differentiate between OCD and *obsessive-compulsive personality disorder* (OCPD), both involving making excessive lists, perfectionism, and hoarding, individuals with OCPD will typically experience impairment as a result of their perfectionism and experience their symptoms as ego-syntonic whereas individuals with OCD may experience symptoms as ego-dystonic and typically experience greater anxiety.
- To differentiate between OCD and the *impulse control disorders* (e.g., gambling, impulsive sexual behaviours, impulsive shopping), both involving strong urges to repeat certain behaviours and problems with attention, individuals with an impulse control disorder will engage in the behaviour to increase arousal or excitement and take risks to engage in the behaviour whereas individuals with OCD repeat behaviours to escape unwanted emotion and are typically risk-averse.
- To differentiate between OCD and *autism spectrum disorders*, both involving obsessive interests or stereotyped behaviours, individuals with an autism spectrum disorder will usually only have thoughts or feelings focused on repeating things, do not try to prevent thoughts, and may have severe social impairment whereas individuals with OCD have thoughts focused on one of the symptom categories and try to stop obsessions.

Treatment

OCD was once considered to be refractory to treatment, but there is now an established body of evidence for successful treatment as the last four decades saw the emergence of effective behavioural and pharmacological therapies (2). This section will describe the established first- and second-line behavioural, cognitive and pharmacological interventions for OCD.

Exposure and response prevention (ERP)

Behaviour therapy, specifically exposure and response prevention (ERP), has been clearly established as an effective treatment for OCD (2). ERP involves deliberate and prolonged exposure to stimuli that trigger obsessions and/or compulsions along with the strict prevention of compulsions in response to the obsessions. It is estimated that 60-80% of individuals who complete the treatment get significantly better. The treatment response is usually evaluated by reductions in scores on the Y-BOCS, with a 35% or more score reduction indicating improvement (44). The ERP treatment procedures are focused and time-limited, with a standard length of 12-20 sessions (45).

Trigger identification

The treatment process is established through assessment of the individual symptoms and symptom triggers. If several symptoms are present, decide in what order the symptoms will be addressed and then identify the symptoms triggers or stimuli. Both external stimuli (e.g., seeing or touching something dirty or leaving a room without checking the stove) and internal stimuli (thoughts, images, or impulses) can be used for exposure. It is important to also include any avoidance behaviours, safety behaviours, and covert or mental rituals when developing an exposure plan. The symptom trigger information is then used to create a list of situations or experiences that will provide exposure to the intended stimuli. This list is organized into a hierarchy where each experience is ranked on the level of fear as measured by subjective units of distress (SUDS). SUDS are usually measured on a 1-10 or 1-100 scale in which 1 is equal to little or no subjective distress and 10 or 100 is equal to sig-

Table 40.3
Sample exposure hierarchy for bodily fluid contamination.

Exposure behaviour	Subjective units of distress
Touch public door handle	40
Use a vending machine	45
Shake hands with a friend	50
Touch the bottom of your shoe	55
Shake hands with a stranger	60
Use public transportation	65
Touch bathroom door handle	70
Touch faucet handle	75
Touch bathroom floor	80
Touch toilet paper dispenser	85
Touch floor near toilet	90
Touch toilet seat	95
Touch toilet water	100

nificant subjective distress. Table 40.3 provides an example of an exposure hierarchy that might be used to treat the contamination obsessions from the case presentation earlier in the chapter. It is recommended that the exposure work begins with mild to moderately challenging situations instead of starting with the lowest or easiest experiences as these gains may be dismissed as minimal later as the individual faces more difficult exposures.

Trigger exposure

Exposure to the intended trigger can be presented *in vivo* (confrontations with the actual trigger) or *imaginal* (intentional thinking about or imagined confrontation with the trigger). Imaginal exposures can be used where it is not feasible to do an exposure to the actual trigger (e.g., fear of aggressive impulses to harm someone), or they can be used in preparation for an in vivo exposure (e.g., imagining touching a dirty floor without washing your hands). Imaginal and in

vivo exposures are often used concurrently. For example, the individual will directly confront a trigger and then use imaginal exposure to confront the thoughts and images resulting from the in vivo exposure. Because it can be difficult to intentionally focus thinking, imaginal exposure can be organized by having the individual write out a scripted scenario that can be read repeatedly. This can be amplified by the use of technology with which the individual can record a verbal account of the script and listen to it repeatedly.

Habituation

Each exposure is followed by response prevention in which the individual does not complete the compulsion or ritual. Theoretically, the patient learns that the anxiety generated by the trigger will gradually decrease without performing the compulsion or avoidance behaviour. This learning process is referred to as habituation. Habituation occurs as the presented stimuli results in a reduced anxiety response to the trigger, and a decreased urge to engage in the compulsive response. Both exposure and response prevention are necessary for effective treatment of OCD symptoms. It is common to measure habituation during an exposure with repeated assessment of SUDS. As the SUDS reach 50% of their highest level, it is assumed that some habituation has occurred. As habituation occurs, the individual then moves to the next step in the exposure hierarchy until habituation has occurred with all of the targeted symptoms. ERP is more effective when it occurs frequently and repetitively, and gains are maintained when the treatment is intensive (i.e., multiple times a week) (46). It is also important that habituation occurs during the session practice with the therapist and then again as the individual performs self-directed exposures between therapy sessions.

ERP is widely recognized to be an effective treatment for OCD, but it can be an intimidating and difficult experience. Many patients decline recommendations for ERP treatment or drop out after starting it. It is also underutilized by treatment providers, often as a result of misconceptions about the treatment and its effects on the therapeutic relationship and the individual's ability to cope with the distress. There is some debate as to the nature of habituation and the most effective manner in which to administer exposures (47), but it is clear that ERP is an effective treatment when administered correctly.

Cognitive behavioural interventions

In addition to ERP, cognitive therapy (48) and acceptance and commitment therapy (49) have shown promise in treating OCD, both as stand-alone treatments and in combination with ERP. These approaches provide additional tools for the therapist and client to address underlying thoughts and emotions related to OCD. Cognitive therapy for OCD provides strategies for identifying and correcting dysfunctional beliefs and appraisals of OCD stimuli. Acceptance and commitment therapy provide guidance on how to change the functional response to private events (i.e., obsessions, anxiety, physiological response) with a focus on valued living and decreasing the influence of private events. Both approaches have shown an encouraging increase in treatment acceptability and reductions in treatment dropout.

Pharmacotherapeutical / Neurosurgical interventions

To complement the behavioural treatment of OCD, there is evidence for the effective use of medication to treat OCD. OCD symptoms have been linked to difficulty regulating the brain neurotransmitter, serotonin. The exact problems are not well understood, but there is good evidence that serotonin reuptake inhibitors are effective in reducing OCD symptoms as approximately 40- 60% of patients show significant improvement to SRI treatment (50). Clomipramine was the first SRI shown to be effective for treating OCD and received US Food and Drug Ad-

ministration approval for this. Accordingly, the first-line medication treatment for OCD is serial trials of clomipramine and at least two selective serotonin reuptake inhibitors (SSRIs) such as fluoxetine, sertraline, fluvoxamine, paroxetine, citalopram, or escitalopram (50). If the combination of behaviour therapy and SRI/SSRI trials does not produce a satisfactory response, SRI augmentation with clonazepam or buspirone can be the next alternative. There are also indications that conventional and atypical neuroleptics can be used to augment SRI/SSRI treatment including pimozide, haloperidol, risperidone, and olanzapine. In some cases of severe, treatment-refractory OCD after failing the array of treatment options, neurosurgical treatments or deep brain stimulation procedures have shown some evidence of treatment response.

Prognosis

In general, response rates for behavioural treatment range from 60% to 80%, and response rates for pharmacological treatment range from 40% to 60%. These estimates are for successful treatment completion and may not reflect severe or treatment-refractory cases. Long-term follow-up studies with individuals after treatment are lacking, but several retrospective and longitudinal studies provide insight into the course of the disorder. In a survey of early retrospective follow-up studies ranging from 6 months to 22 years after onset of the disorder, the percentage of individuals who were classified as 'much improved' or 'well' ranged from 24% to 77% (51). While the methodology, population, and assessment methods in these studies vary widely, more recent studies have found similar estimates of symptom improvement in retrospective or longitudinal follow-up. Most individuals with OCD will experience a chronic course that waxes and wanes, with about 15% experiencing deterioration in social and occupational functioning while about 5% experience an episodic course with minimal symptoms between episodes (1).

References

1 American Psychiatric Association. Diagnostic and statistical manual of mental disorders. Washington, DC: American Psychiatric Association 2000.

2 Franklin ME, Foa EB. Cognitive behavioral treatment of obsessive-compulsive disorder. In: Nathan PE, Gorman JM, eds. A guide to treatments that work. New York: Oxford, 2007:431-446.

3 Pitman, R. Obsessive-compulsive disorder in Western history. In: Hollander E, Zohar J, Marazziti D, Olivier B, eds. Current insights in obsessive compulsive disorder. New York: Wiley,1994:3-10.

4 Leckman JF, Grice DE, Boardman J, et al. Symptoms of obsessive-compulsive disorder. Am J Psychiatry 1997;154:911-917.

5 Foa EB, Kozak MJ, Goodman WK, Hollander E, Jenike M, Rasmussen S. DSM-IV field trial: obsessive-compulsive disorder. Am J Psychiatry 1995;152:90-94.

6 Hollander E, Friedberg JP, Wasserman S, Yeh C, Iyengar R. The case for the OCD spectrum. In: Abramowitz JS, Houts, AC, eds. Concepts and controversies in obsessive-compulsive disorder. New York: Springer 2005:95-113.

7 Karno M, Golding JM, Sorenson SB, Burnam MA. The epidemiology of obsessive-compulsive disorder in five US communities. Arch Gen Psychiatry 1988;45:1094-1099.

8 Myers JK, Weissman MM, Tischler GL, Holzer CE, Leaf PJ, Orvaschel H. Six-month prevalence of psychiatric disorders in three communities 1980 to 1982. Arch Gen Psychiatry 1984;41:949-958.

9 Robins LN, Helzer JE, Weissman MM, Orvaschel H, Gruenberg E, Burke JD, Regier DA. Lifetime prevalence of specific psychiatric disorders in three sites. Arch Gen Psychiatry 1984;41:958-967.

10 Weissman MM, Bland RC, Canino GJ, et al. The cross national epidemiology of obsessive-compulsive disorder. J Clin Psychiatry 1994;55:5-10.

11 Valleni-Basile LA, Garrison CZ, Jackson KL, et al. Frequency of obsessive-compulsive disorder in a community sample of young adolescents. J Am Acad Child Adolesc Psychiatry 1994;33:782-791.

12 Douglass HM, Moffitt TE, Dar R, McGee R, Silva P. Obsessive-compulsive disorder in a birth cohort of 18-year-olds: prevalence and predictors. J Am Acad Child Adolesc Psychiatry 1995;34:1424-1431.

13 Eisen JL, Rasmussen SA. Obsessive-compulsive disorder with psychotic features. J Clin Psychiatry 1993;54:373-379.

14 Leonard HL, Swedo SE, Rapoport JL, et al. Treatment of obsessive-compulsive disorder with clomipramine and desipramine in children and adolescents. A double-blind crossover comparison. Arch Gen Psychiatry 1989;46:1088-1092.

15 Rasmussen SA, Eisen JL. Epidemiology of obsessive compulsive disorder. J Clin Psychiatry 1990;51:10-13.

16 Antony MM, Downie F, Swinson RP. Diagnostic issues and epidemilogy in obsessive-compulsive disorder. In: Swinson RP, Antony MM, Rachman S, Richter MA, eds. Obsessive-compulsive disorder: theory, research, and treatment. New York: Guilford Press, 1998:3-32.

17 Dollard J, Miller NE. Personality and psychotherapy: An analysis in terms of learning, thinking and culture. New York: McGraw-Hill,1950.

18 Rachman SJ, Wilson GT. The effects of psychological therapy. Oxford, UK: Pergamon Press,1980.

19 Rachman S. A cognitive theory of obsessions. Behav Res Ther 1997;35:793–802.

20 Clark DA, Rhyno A. Unwanted intrusive thoughts in nonclinical individuals. In: Clark DA, editor. Intrusive thoughts in clinical disorders: theory, research, and treatment. Guilford Press, NY, USA; 2004 :1-29.

21 Salkovskis PM. Obsessional-compulsive problems: a cognitive-behavioral analysis. Behav Res Ther 1985;23:571–583.

22 Wells A. Emotional disorders and metacognitions: innovative cognitive therapy. Hoboken, NJ: Wiley, 2002.

23 Cromer KR, Schmidt NB, Murphy DL. An investigation of traumatic life events and obsessive-compulsive disorder. Behav Res Ther 2007;45:1683-1691.

24 Abramowitz JS, Nelson CA, Rygwall R, Khandker M. The cognitive mediation of obsessive-compulsive symptoms: A longitudinal study. J Anxiety Disord 2007;21:91-104.

25 Yoshida T, Taga C, Matsumoto Y, Fukui K. Paternal overprotection in obsessive-compulsive disorder and depression with obsessive traits. Psychiatry Clin Neurosci 2005;59:533–538.

26 van Grootheest DS, Cath DC, Beekman AT, Boomsma, DI. Twin studies on obsessive-compulsive disorder: a review. Twin Res Hum Genet 2005;8:450-458.

27 Grados MA, Walkup J, Walford S. Genetics of obsessive compulsive disorders: new findings and challenges. Brain Dev 2003;25:55–61.

28 Stewart SE, Yu D, Scharf JM, Neale BM, Fagerness JA, Matthews CA et al. Genome-wide association study of obsessive-compulsive disorder. Mol Psychiatry 2013;18:788-98.

29 Saxena S, Rauch SL. Functional neuroimaging and the neuroanatomy of obsessive-compulsive disorder. Psychiatr Clin North Am 2000;23:563-586.

30 Brennan BP, Rauch SL, Jensen JE, Pope HG. A critical review of magnetic resonance spectroscopy studies of obsessive-compulsive disorder. Biol Psychiatry 2013;73:24-31.

31 van den Heuvel OA, Veltman DJ, Groenewegen HJ, et al. Amygdala activity in obsessive-compulsive disorder with contamination fear: a study with oxygen-15 water positron emission tomography. Psychiatry Res 2004;132:225-237.

32 Kwon JS, Kim JJ, Lee DW, et al. Neural correlates of clinical symptoms and cognitive dysfunctions in obsessive-compulsive disorder. Psychiatry Res 2003;122:37-47.

33 Murphy TK, Kurlan R, Leckman J. The immunobiology of tourette's disorder, pediatric autoimmune neuropsychiatric disorders associated with streptococcus, and related disorders: a way forward J Child Adolesc Psychopharmacol 2010;20:317-331.

34 Swedo SE, Leckman JF, Rose NR. From research subgroup to clinical syndrome: modifying the PANDAS criteria to describe PANS (pediatric accute-onset neuropsychiatric syndrome). Pediatr Therapeut 2012;2:1113.

35 Kozak MJ, Foa EB. Obsessions, overvalued ideas, and delusions in obsessive-compulsive disorder. Behav Res Ther 1994;32:343-353.

36 Brown TA, Di Nardo PA, Barlow DH. Anxiety disorders interview schedule for DSM-IV (ADIS-IV). San Antonio, TX: Psychological Corporation/Graywind Publications Incorporated, 1994.

37 First MB, Spitzer RL, Williams JBW, Gibbon M. Structured clinical interview for DSM-IV (SCID). Washington, DC: American Psychiatric Association, 1996.

38 Goodman WK, Price LH, Rasmussen SA, et al. The Yale-Brown obsessive compulsive scale: pt. I. development, use, and reliability. Arch Gen Psychiatry 1989;46:1006–1011.

39 Eisen JL, Phillips KA, Baer L, Beer DA, Atala KD, Rasmussen SA. The Brown assessment of beliefs scale: reliability and validity. Am J Psychiatry 1998;155:102–108.

40 Foa EB, Huppert JD, Leiberg S, et al. The obsessive-compulsive inventory: development and validation of a short version. Psychol Assess 2002;14:485–496.

41 Obsessive Compulsive Cognitions Working Group. Psychometric validation of the obsessive beliefs questionnaire and the interpretation of intrusions inventory: part I. Behav Res Ther 2003;41:1245–1264.

42 Szymansky J, Bourne C. OCD and related disorders in the new *DSM* and what it means for you. International OCD Foundation Newsletter 2013;27:1-9.

43 Stein DJ, Fineberg NA, Bienvenu OJ, Denys A, Lochner C, Nestadt G, et al. Should OCD be classified as an anxiety disorders in DSM-5? Depress Anxiety 2010;27:495-506.

44 Pallanti S, Quercioli L. Treatment-refractory obsessive-compulsive disorder: methodological issues, operational definitions and therapeutic lines. Prog Neuropsychopharmacol Biol Psychiatry 2006;30:400–412.

45 Abramowitz JS. Effectiveness of psychological and pharmacological treatments for obsessive-compulsive disorder: A quantitative review. J Consult Clin Psychol 1997;65:44–52.

46 Abramowitz JS, Foa EB, Franklin ME. Exposure and ritual prevention for obsessive-compulsive disorder: Effects of intensive versus twice-weekly sessions. J Consult Clin Psychol 2003;71:394–398.

47 Baker A, Mystkowski J, Culver N, Yi R, Mortazavi A, Craske MG. Does habituation matter? Emotional processing theory and exposure therapy for acrophobia. Behav Res Ther 2010;48:1139-1143.

48 Clark DA. Cognitive-behavioral therapy for OCD. New York: Guilford Press, 2004.

49 Twohig MP, Hayes SC, Plumb JC, Pruitt LD, Collins AB, Hazlett-Stevens H, Woidneck MR. A randomized clinical trial of acceptance and commitment therapy versus progressive relaxation training for obsessive-compulsive disorder. J Consult Clin Psychol 2010;78:705–716.

50 Dougherty DD, Rauch SL, Jenike, MA. Pharmacological treatments for obsessive-compulsive disorder. In Nathan PE, Gorman JM, eds. A guide to treatments that work. New York: Oxford, 2007:447-473.

51 Eisen JL, Rasmussen SA. Phenomenology of obsessive-compulsive disorder. In: Stein DJ, Hollander A, eds. Textbook of anxiety disorders. Washington, DC: American Psychiatric, 200:173-189.

41

Impulse Control Disorders

Valerie Voon

Impulse control disorders (ICDs) or behavioural addictions in Parkinson's disease are commonly associated with dopaminergic medications and can potentially have marked consequences. They can be broadly defined as repeated urges and compulsive actions with associated negative consequences. These behaviours include pathological gambling (PG), hypersexuality, binge eating, compulsive shopping, punding and excessive dopaminergic medication use. Diagnostic criteria for these behaviours have been described previously (1) (see Table 41.1). Other behaviours have been more recently reported, including hoarding (2), kleptomania (3) and impulsive smoking (4).

The disorder of PG has now been classified in the newly published DSM-5 under the category of 'Substance-Related and Addictive Disorders' and will be renamed as 'Gambling Disorder'. The reclassification is based on epidemiological, clinical and neurobiological factors suggesting overlapping similarities with substance use disorders (5). The DSM-5 criteria for 'Gambling Disorder' has several modifications, including the following: the criterion 'has committed illegal acts such as forgery, fraud theft or embezzlement to finance gambling' has been removed, and the number of criteria required for diagnosis has been decreased to 4 with a time period specified as within 12 months.

Epidemiology

The largest epidemiological study is the multi-centre, cross-sectional, North American DO-MINION study (N = 3090 patients) reporting an ICD prevalence of 13.6% (6). PG was identified in 5.0%, compulsive sexual behaviour in 3.5%, compulsive buying in 5.7%, and binge eating disorder in 4.3%. Single ICDs were more common, with multiple ICDs present in >25%. ICDs were more common with dopamine agonists (17.1% versus 6.9%), with an odds ratio of developing an ICD on dopamine agonists of 2.72 (95% CI 2.08-3.54). The frequencies of ICDs on pramipexole and ropinirole (17.7% versus 15.5%, odds ratio 1.22; 95% CI 0.94-1.57) were compared, with no differences demonstrated between the two dopamine agonist drug types. An important question is whether ICDs occur more frequently in PD and/or restless legs syndrome (RLS) subjects on dopaminergic medications than in the general population. In a study assessing 'new onset heightened interest or drive' of 203 PD patients compared with 190 healthy controls, 14% of PD patients had a 'heightened interest' in ICD behaviours, with 3% interested in gambling, whereas 0% was reported in healthy volunteers (7). In another Italian sample of 98 PD patients and 392 general hospital control patients, 6.1% versus 0.25%, respectively, were identified with PG (8). However, in a comparison of 115 PD patients with 115 matched healthy controls, there were no differences in the frequencies of PG (0.85% versus 0.85%) (9). Larger sample sizes and appropriate screening tools are required to compare groups adequately. The frequencies of these disorders are also sensitive to the setting screened. For instance, the populations of PD screened for ICDs are commonly assessed in tertiary, subspecialized, movement disorder centres to which more complex cases and younger populations may be referred. Given this, the frequency of PG in PD (PG 2.9% and problem gambling 2.1% in North America) identified in the DOMINION study (6) based on movement disorder centre settings may not be fully comparable to population-based frequencies of PG (PG 1.14% and problem gambling 2.8% based on a meta-analysis of North American reports published in 1999) (10).

The influence of setting is a well-recognized issue in determining the prevalence of other psychiatric disorders associated with PD. For instance, in a meta-analysis of 36 well-designed studies, the prevalence rate of major depression in PD (which is understood to be both secondary to the neurobiology of PD and underlying individual susceptibility along with psychosocial factors) is 24.0% in outpatient clinics (11 studies) but markedly lower in population-based community studies (8.1%, 4 studies) (11). Thus, the prevalence rates of ICDs in community studies in the PD population may possibly be lower and more comparable to the prevalence rates of population-based community surveys of PG in the general population. An important issue may be the comparison of incidence rates as that of new onset ICDs without any previous history of the same age group in the general population may indeed be lower.

ICDs also occur in a diverse range of non-PD patients treated with dopaminergic medication, such as restless legs syndrome (12), progressive supranuclear palsy (13) and multiple sclerosis (14). Furthermore, the fact that PD patients display a greater frequency of pathological gambling than patients with amyotrophic lateral sclerosis suggests that ICDs are unlikely to be caused by a chronic neurological condition (15).

Pathophysiology

The observation that ICDs only occur in a subset of PD patients argues for a role for an interaction between other factors and dopaminergic

medication (6), suggesting that dopamine agonists play only a partial or interactive role and are not sufficient by themselves to result in the onset of ICDs (1,16,17). Thus, other factors are likely to play a role in mediating and influencing the association between dopamine agonists and ICDs. Factors that might interact with dopamine agonists can be subdivided into (i) the agonist preparation, the dose and/or co-administered medications, (ii) a possible role for PD itself and (iii) individual susceptibility (1,16) as discussed below. This issue of interacting factors addresses the question of why one person with PD given the same medication type or dose might develop an ICD while others might not.

Medication effects

The role of medication effects can be divided into the following factors: dopamine agonist dose, co-administered medications such as levodopa or amantadine, and the dopamine agonist preparation.

Dopamine agonist dose
Multiple studies suggest an association between higher dopamine agonist dose and an increased risk of ICD in subjects with PD and restless legs syndrome (RLS) (18-20). The multicentre DOMINION study is somewhat equivocal: 'on univariate analysis the median dopamine agonist LEDD (levodopa-dose equivalent daily dose) in ICD and non-ICD patients was numerically the same (300 mg) but the interquartile range was higher for ICD patients (200–450 mg vs 150–400 mg, overall $P = 0.002$)' (6). Subjects were included if dopamine agonists had not been initiated or stopped 6 months prior to study onset, but the dose of dopamine agonists could be adjusted during this period. Once they recognise an ICD, most neurologists would attempt to decrease the dose of dopamine agonists, thus possibly introducing a bias. That a decrease in dopamine agonist dose appears to be effective in improving ICDs in many subjects also suggests a role for

dose effects (21). To address the issue of the role of dopamine agonists dose adequately, longitudinal studies are needed, many of which are currently underway.

Co-administered medications

The majority of PD patients are commonly on multiple co-medications, including levodopa (6) or amantadine (22), both of which have been shown in the DOMINION study to be independently associated with an increased risk of ICDs. Both dopamine agonist (odds ratio 2.72 (95% CI: 2.07-3.57), P<0.001) and levodopa use (odds ratio 1.51 (95%CI: 1.09-2.09), P = 0.01) were independently associated with ICDs, with a higher odds ratio for dopamine agonists (6). Co-administration of dopamine agonist and levodopa has also been shown to increase the risk of ICDs as compared to dopamine agonist monotherapy. A higher levodopa dose has also been found to be associated with a greater risk of ICDs (6).

The association with amantadine, which has a weak antagonist effect on NMDA glutamate receptors and dopamine release, is less clear. An 8-week, crossover, randomized, double-blind, placebo-controlled trial of amantadine in 17 PD patients with PG demonstrated efficacy on symptom resolution (23). However, amantadine was more likely to be associated with ICDs (17.6% vs. 4.2%, p<0.001) in the DOMINION study (22). Similarly, another study also demonstrated a higher association of PG with amantadine users than non-users (2.4% versus 0.6%, p = 0.006) in their assessment of PG frequency in 1167 PD patients using the Minnesota Impulsive Disorders Interview (24).

Dopamine agonist preparation

In a recent congress, the comparative frequencies of long-acting and continuous stimulation dopamine agonists and ICDs were presented (25). In total, 52/373 (13.9%) of ICD cases were documented with a lower frequency on rotigotine delivered as a transdermal patch (5.3%) and long-acting pramipexole (6.3%) compared to that of short-acting pramipexole (13.4%) and ropinorole (14.9%). The long-acting nature of the formulation may be less likely to act in a non-physiological manner or result in sensitization effects and hence be associated with a lower risk of ICDs. Rotigotine acts as an agonist at dopamine receptors, with binding affinities at D3 and D2 receptors 2600 and 53 times higher than dopamine (D3>D2>D1) (26) but is administered as a transdermal patch in a continuous delivery system (CDS) suggesting that the predominant issue is the continuous delivery formulation rather than D3 receptor mechanisms. However, the results are not completely clear as long-acting ropinorole (14.7%) had a similarly elevated risk. Whether the CDS nature of rotigotine is less likely to be associated with ICDs requires further confirmatory studies.

Facilitating role of PD

The role of PD in the onset of ICDs is not yet completely established. There are two possibly conflicting theories underlying a role PD might play as either facilitating or protective (1). That ICDs occur in non-PD disorders treated with dopaminergic medications such as restless legs syndrome (12,27,28) suggests that PD is not absolutely necessary to initiate PG. One study that directly compared the frequency of ICDs in RLS and PD suggested the frequency of reward-seeking behaviours was higher in PD, an effect that was no longer significant after controlling for dose differences (29). This was suggested to be a function of the higher dopaminergic medication dose in PD and the pattern of administration. Furthermore, two studies investigating the frequency of ICD in new onset PD did not demonstrate any differences in frequency from the general population, suggesting that PD by itself does not increase the frequency of ICDs (30, 31). These observations do not rule out a potential role for PD in facilitating or interacting with dopaminergic medications in the onset of ICDs. For instance, a recent rodent study demonstrated that a parkinsonian rodent model had greater sensitivity to rewarding effects but not motor effects of pramipexole (32). Thus, although PD by itself is not associated with an increased expression of ICD, a factor related to PD might still interact with dopamine agonists to result in an enhanced expression of ICD. The following are examples of possible mechanisms in which PD may play a role in influencing the relationship between dopamine agonists and PD.

Overdose hypothesis

In PD, neurodegeneration of the substantia nigra pars compacta dopaminergic cells projecting to dorsal striatal or motor regions can affect up to 70% of dopaminergic cell bodies prior to the onset of parkinsonian motor symptoms. The neurodegeneration of the more mesial dopaminergic cells, the ventral tegmental area (VTA), projecting to the ventral striatum or nucleus accumbens and ventromedial prefrontal cortex (regions implicated in limbic processes such as reward and motivation), is much more variable in PD. Thus, in PD subjects who may have greater preservation of dopaminergic cells projecting to limbic regions (ventral striatal and ventromedial prefrontal) or associative cognitive regions (caudate, orbitofrontal or dorsolateral prefrontal cortex), treatment with dopaminergic medications targeting degenerated motor striatal regions may result in an 'overdose' of otherwise intact limbic and associative regions. This 'overdosing' may result in impairment of cognitive and behavioural functioning (1,33). The 'overdose' hypothesis has been well described and supported by experimental evidence suggesting that functioning of cognition or behaviour follows a U-shaped curve. Optimal functioning occurs at an optimal dopamine level with either higher or lower dopamine levels resulting in impairments in functioning.

Lewy body deposition

Another possible role for the neurobiology of PD might include the deposition of Lewy bodies in specific neural regions related to ICDs. The issue of visual hallucinations in PD gives a very relevant analogy. For instance, visual hallucinations are common in PD, occurring in 17%-40% of patients. Although they are clearly associated with the presence of dopaminergic medications, PD is now believed to play a clear role in the onset of hallucinations. For instance, hallucinations are associated with greater Lewy body deposition in the limbic regions (amygdala, hippocampus, medial temporal) (34,35). Similarly, postmortem studies in PD patients with ICDs may similarly reveal a greater deposition of Lewy bodies in limbic regions, thus predisposing the individual to a greater risk of an interaction with dopamine agonists, resulting in ICD symptoms.

PD subtypes

Specific subtypes of PD may be more likely to be at risk for the development of ICDs. That PG is associated with early-onset PD also suggests that specific subtypes of PD may have a differential pattern of neurodegeneration or neurobiology (6).

Dyskinesia

There is a unifying view that a common mechanism of action exists in the motor and non-motor domains of the corticostriatal circuitry, as evidenced by similarities between ICDs and levodopa-induced dyskinesias (36). ICDs in PD are associated with an oscillatory theta-alpha activity in the ventral subthalamic nucleus along with electroencephalographic coherence with non-motor prefrontal regions. In contrast, in dyskinesias, theta-alpha activity is associated with a dorsal localisation and a coherence with motor regions (37). PD patients with punding (38) or multiple ICDs (39) also have severer dyskinesias relative to PD controls. Taken together, this evidence supports potentially unifying neurophysiological mechanisms linking the motor and behavioural side-effects of dopaminergic treatment.

Apathy

A relationship to apathy (decreased motivation, interest and emotional response to external and internal stimuli) secondary to PD has been observed with ICDs (40). Apathy is commonly observed in PD, occurring in 17%-41% of patients and is understood to be related to its neurobiology (41). In a prospective study of subthalamic stimulation in PD patients, 17 of whom had ICDs, the discontinuation of the dopamine agonist and marked lowering of the dopaminergic medication dose was associated with an improvement in ICD in all subjects (40). However, half of the subjects developed apathy symptoms. The authors suggest a possible relationship between those who develop ICDs on dopaminergic medications and those suffering apathy off dopaminergic medications, implicating abnormalities in ventral striatal dopaminergic functioning. It was striking that apathy in PD outside of the context of subthalamic stimulation is likely to be much more complex and involve other neurotransmitters including acetylcholine and norepinephrine.

Cognitive deficits

Cognitive deficits in PD may facilitate the onset of ICDs (42,43). PD patients without ICDs were shown to have elevated delay discounting scores (tendency to select immediate smaller rewards over delayed larger rewards) both on and off medication (43). Elevated delay discounting is associated with ICDs in the general population (44,45), and three studies of PD patients with ICDs, particularly PG or compulsive shopping, demonstrated elevated delay discounting compared to PD controls without ICDs (39,46,47). Delay discounting is a known predictive risk factor for cocaine dependence in rodents. Rodents who have higher delay discounting scores at baseline are more likely to escalate into cocaine acquisition and compulsive drug-seeking behaviours than those with lower scores (48,49). Thus, the facts that elevated delay discounting (i) is a known predictor for substance dependence; (ii) is increased in ICDs in the general population and in ICDs in PD; and (iii) is increased in PD patients at baseline might suggest a potential interaction between a cognitive deficit in PD and dopamine agonists in the development of ICDs (42).

Protective role of PD

An alternate consideration is whether the neurobiology of PD itself may be protective prior to the onset of dopaminergic medications. For instance, an individual with a high susceptibility towards ICDs such as a family history of ICDs may not express the behaviour prior to the interaction with dopaminergic medications as a result of the neurobiology of PD (1). Multiple studies have demonstrated lower novelty-seeking as measured using Cloninger's temperament and character inventory (TCI) in cross-sectional studies on PD patients without ICDs (50). Novelty-seeking is a temperamental trait associated with the tendency towards exploratory behaviours, excitability in response to novel stimulation, greater extravagance, impulsive decision-making, being more quick-tempered and likely to break rules, and has been associated with dopaminergic activity (51). This observation of lower novelty-seeking in PD is believed to be related to the dopaminergic neurodegeneration affecting the mesolimbic system, influencing the sensitivity to reward and motivation (50). Multiple studies have demonstrated that PD patients are less likely to smoke and drink less alcohol prior to the onset of PD, an observation that has been suggested to reflect underlying differences in premorbid personality traits (52). Thus, premorbid decreases in novelty- or sensation-seeking related to the neurobiology of PD may moderate the expression of the individual susceptibility towards ICDs. To put it another way, if an individual with a premorbid susceptibility towards ICDs develops PD, the expression of the behaviour may be modified and the susceptibility may not express itself until it interacts with dopaminergic medications. PD patients with PG or compulsive shopping, but not binge eating or hypersexuality, have higher novelty-seeking traits compared to those without ICDs (39). Furthermore, novelty-seeking scores are elevated in both active and remitted PD patients with PG, whereas impulsivity was lower in those remitted compared to those with active symptoms. This suggests that novelty-seeking but not impulsivity may be a premorbid susceptibility trait (53).

Individual susceptibility factors

There are multiple known factors that contribute to the pathophysiology of PG in the general population that have also been demonstrated to be associated with PG in the PD population. The papers reporting associated factors with PG in the general population have been systematically assessed and ranked for level of evidence in a review by Johansson et al. (54). In this review, associated factors for PG in the general population are ranked by level of evidence (well-established: more than two studies to support conclusions; probable: 1-2 studies). The following sections discuss the identified factors associated with PG in the general population found in this review and compare evidence from the literature on factors associated with PG in the PD population. That the associated factors are similar between PG in the general population and in PD suggests a similar underlying individual vulnerability.

Age and gender

PG in the general population is associated with younger age and male gender (2:1 male to female ratio) based on Level 1 supportive evidence (54). Similarly, PG in PD is associated with younger age in multiple studies and definitively demonstrated as an independent associated factor for PG in PD in the DOMINION study (6). Although there were no gender differences for PG in PD in the DOMINION study, men were more likely

to express hypersexuality and women to express binge eating and compulsive shopping (6).

Depression

Depression is identified as a probable risk factor for PG in the general population (54), with a genetic link postulated between the two disorders (55). In a survey of 7869 individuals from the Vietnam era twin registry (middle-aged men), the odds ratio for major depression was elevated for PG (OR 4.06). Some 34% of the genetic variance for each disorder contributed to that of the other, with the best-fitting model estimating that 100% of the overlap between PG and MD was genetic (55). Furthermore, the likelihood of major depression predicting the onset of PG has been reported as 6.6 based on data from the US National Comorbidity Survey Replication study (56). Similarly, the DOMINION study identified higher depression scores in both the cross-sectional and case-control study as an independent risk factor in the association of ICDs in PD patients (6,39).

Substance use disorders

Alcohol and other substance use disorders have Level 1 evidence to support an association with PG in the general population (54), with a genetic link postulated between alcohol use disorders and PG (57). Substance use disorders such as alcohol or drug abuse, alcohol or drug dependence, or nicotine dependence have an odds ratio predicting the onset of PG of 5.4, 8.8 and 1.9, respectively, based on the US National Comorbidity Survey Replication study (56). In a twin study of genetics, 12%-20% of the genetic variation and 3%-8% of the non-shared environmental risk for PG was accounted for by the risk of alcohol dependence (57). Although the DOMINION cross-sectional study identified an increased association with a family history of alcohol use disorder with PG, this factor was not identified as an independent risk factor following multivariate analysis, suggesting that it is closely linked to another associated factor (e.g. current smoking or family history of gambling) (6,16). In a smaller study of 21 PD and PG patients compared to 42 PD controls, a personal or immediate family history of alcohol use disorders (rather than current alcohol use) was assessed. This factor along with novelty-seeking and younger age of PD onset predicted PG as 83.7% and accounted for 62% of the variance (53). Current alcohol use as measured using the AUDIT was not associated with PG in either the cross-sectional or case-control arms of the DOMINION study. In contrast, current cigarette smoking was identified as an independent factor associated in PG in both arms of the DOMINION study (6, 16). In a study of restless legs syndrome and ICDs, a premorbid history of experimental drug use was also highlighted as an independent associated factor (27).

Family history of gambling

Twin studies suggest possible genetic factors underlying PG. In PG-affected subjects, 8% of first-degree relatives had a lifetime history of PG compared to 2% of first-degree relatives in unaffected controls (58). In the Vietnam era twin registry study, 23% of monozygotic co-twins and 10% of dizogotic male co-twins had a lifetime history of PG (59), which modelling suggested was attributed to shared genetic rather than environmental factors (57). In the recent, community-based, Australian twin registry study, the variation in the risk for disordered gambling due to genetic influences was 49.2%, while no evidence for shared environmental influences contributed to the variation in risk (60).

PG in PD patients is also associated with a greater likelihood of a family history of gambling problems as an independent factor predicting the onset of PG in the DOMINION study (6). Similarly, in a study of RLS and ICDs, a family history of gambling problems was identified as an independent associated factor (27). These studies highlight the role of genetic and environmental factors in mediating the relationship between dopamine agonists and PG.

Personality and temperamental traits

PG in the general population is associated with greater impulsivity and novelty- and sensation-seeking as probable risk factors (54). PG is also associated with more personality disorders, specifically antisocial personality disorder, as a probable risk factor (54). For instance, in a study by Slutske et al. of the Vietnam era twin registry data, subjects with a history of PG had higher prevalence rates of antisocial personality disorder (odds ratio = 6.4), which precedes the onset of PG symptoms (61). PG is also significantly associated with delinquency, criminal and illegal activity with Level 1 supportive evidence (54). Similarly, PG and compulsive shopping subjects in the PD population have higher scores on novelty-seeking and impulsivity questionnaires as demonstrated in the case-control arm of the DOMINION study (39).

Social factors

The relationship between marital status and PG in the general population is less clear, with both being married and being single identified as associated factors (54). Proximity and availability of gambling are identified as associated factors for PG in the general population with Level 1 supportive evidence (54). In the cross-sectional arm of the DOMINION study, ICDs were independently associated with being unmarried and living in the United States as compared to Canada (6). The latter association may be mediated by the greater availability of casinos in the USA or by differences in medication practices. Thus, these individual susceptibility factors may modify the relationship between dopamine agonists and the expression of ICDs in PD.

Neural mechanisms

The following section discusses possible cognitive, neural and molecular mechanisms that underlie the expression of ICDs in PD.

Reward processing

Dopamine mediates reward-related processing, playing a role in the initial acquisition and the subsequent craving and compulsive use in substance use disorders. Phasic ventral striatal dopamine is triggered by the unexpected receipt of reward and shifts to the cue predicting reward after associative learning (62) and, along with glutamate, underlies the formation of conditioned responses. Converging human and primate studies have demonstrated that phasic dopamine encodes discrepancies between rewards received and those predicted, thus acting as a teaching signal signifying a prediction error (62).

In rodents, pramipexole acts similarly to methamphetamine, but not saline control, to promote conditioned place preference or learning to associate a context with a reward (32). Higher doses of pramipexole were required to achieve the same rewarding effect in sham rodents as compared to the lower doses required in parkinsonian rodents, but there were no differences in locomotor responses. The authors suggested that PD may play a role in enhancing responsiveness to the rewarding but not the motor effects of pramipexole.

Dopamine replacement therapy may influence physiological function via either exogenous tonic dopaminergic stimulation or interference with the endogenous, physiological, phasic pattern of striatal dopamine release. In response to conditioned cues or to a gambling task, PD+ICD patients demonstrate increased ventral striatal dopamine release as measured using (^{11}C)raclopride. Similarly, in response to conditioned cues or to unexpected and anticipated rewards, PD+ICD patients demonstrated increased ventral striatal activity (63-65).

DAs in PD patients with either problem gambling or compulsive shopping were shown to enhance the rate of learning from gain-specific outcomes (63), although not all studies demonstrated this effect (66). Using a reinforcement learning computational approach that models reward prediction error activity to assess the fMRI blood oxygen level-dependent (BOLD) response and indirectly phasic dopaminergic activity, DAs were shown to increase ventral striatal activity to prediction error in ICD, signifying a 'better-than-expected outcome' and enhanced reward prediction. These results are most consistent with the early acquisition stage and are relevant to forming learned associations with cues.

Incentive salience

The incentive motivation theory hypothesises that dopamine alters the nucleus accumbens sensitivity to incentive processing, such that motivational value is assigned to cues associated with rewards, making them desirable in their own right (67). Using (^{11}C)raclopride PET imaging, PD patients with mixed ICDs were shown to have a heightened striatal dopamine release to heterogenous reward-related visual cues as compared to levodopa or neutral cues (65). Similarly, using fMRI, PD patients with hypersexuality were shown to have greater ventral striatal activity to sexual cues compared to those without hypersexuality, an effect that correlated with an index of subjective sexual desire or wanting but not liking (68). These findings were suggested to be in support of an incentive salience process. Similarly, activation of the ventral striatum in response to gambling-related cues was demonstrated in a small fMRI study in PD patients with ICDs (69). These studies are consistent with studies in cocaine dependence demonstrating greater striatal dopamine release in response to cocaine cues (70).

Risk and uncertainty

Pathological behavioural choices are associated with both positive and negative financial, social and occupational outcomes, thus consistent with definitions of risky (with known probabilities) or uncertain (with unknown probabilities) choices. In rodent studies, pramipexole increases probabilistic discounting or the preference for the risky choice. This increase in risk-taking occurs irrespective of the presence of the parkinsonian model of 6-OHDA injected in the dorsolateral striatum (71). Similarly, d-amphetamine impaired task performance on a rodent gambling task modelled on the Iowa gambling task which measures risk-taking under uncertainty (72).

Two studies focusing on risk anticipation without outcome demonstrate that DAs increase risk-taking in PD patients with ICDs (66,73). This risk-taking bias appears to be unrelated to loss aversion and is accompanied by lower ventral striatal, orbitofrontal and anterior cingulate activity (73). The lower ventral striatal activity is consistent with an fMRI study of PD patients with ICDs using the balloon analogue risk task (BART) that examines uncertainty with feedback (74). Similarly, ICD subjects tested using the BART demonstrate greater risk-taking on medication as compared to off medication (75). A recent study has proposed that the findings of greater reflection impulsivity (or decisions under uncertainty without adequate information sampling) (76), delay discounting (selection of the immediate, salient, lower reward over the possibly more uncertain, delayed reward) (39,47), and novelty-seeking in the context of uncertainty (77) may reflect an underlying uncertainty about mapping future actions into rewards (78).

Behavioural regulation and impulsivity

Some evidence for impaired 'top-down' prefrontal regulation is beginning to emerge. Using H₂O PET on PD patients with pathological gambling engaged in a probabilistic gambling task, apomorphine challenge was associated with decreased activity in circuits involved in behavioural regulation, including the lateral orbitofrontal cortex and rostral cingulate cortex (79). Similarly, a resting state, single photon emission tomography (SPECT) study in PD patients with pathological gambling demonstrated decreased functional connectivity between the striatum and the anterior cingulate cortex, the latter being a region involved in negative feedback and conflict detection (80). Impulsivity, defined as a lack of behavioural inhibition, has motor and decisional subtypes. Impulsive choice is char-

acterised by a preference for small, immediate rewards, instead of larger, delayed rewards. Enhanced impulsive choice has been demonstrated in PD patients with ICDs using delay discounting tasks with hypothetical, long delayed, monetary rewards (39,47) and real-time, short delay, monetary rewards (39). In one study, impaired delay discounting with intact reward incentive performance in PD patients with ICDs was interpreted as evidence for a potential impairment in waiting for the delayed reward, rather than an enhanced incentive towards the immediate reward (47). Alternatively, impulsive choice normally demonstrates a magnitude effect, whereby lower impulsive choices accompany increasing reward magnitude. This magnitude effect in delay discounting is less pronounced in PD patients with ICDs, suggesting that dopamine agonists may be associated with greater subjective devaluation of the delayed, higher reward magnitude (39), resulting in greater impulsivity towards the smaller, immediate choice.

With respect to other forms of impulsivity, DAs in PD patients with ICDs appear to enhance the rapidity of decision-making, also known as reflection impulsivity, suggesting that the long-term negative consequences may not be as carefully considered as they otherwise would be (46). Impulsive PD patients do not perform differently to non impulsive PD patients on the Stroop colour word test (66) that probes inhibition of prepotent responses and response selection associated with anterior cingulate function.

Lateral prefrontal cortex function

Visuospatial working memory tested 'on' medication was impaired in medicated PD patients with ICD compared with those without (46). Similarly, PD patients with ICD both when 'on' and 'off' medication have a significantly reduced digit span compared with PD and control groups (66). These results suggest that dorsolateral cortico-striatal circuitry in PD with ICD might be similarly affected by 'overdose' from exogenous dopamine when 'on' medication and possibly from endogenous dopamine when 'off' medication.

Molecular mechanisms

Dopamine transporter levels

Two studies have demonstrated decreased striatal dopamine transporter (DaT) levels in PD patients with ICDs compared to those without (81,82). Dopamine reuptake via DaT, a membrane-spanning protein located in the axon terminals, is the primary mechanism by which striatal dopamine is removed from the synaptic cleft and dopamine neurotransmission regulated and terminated. These findings may help explain the observation of enhanced ventral striatal activity and enhanced dopamine release in PD+ICD patients in response to conditioned cues or to unexpected and anticipated rewards (63-65). Impaired clearance of dopamine may play a role in extending the physiological effect of dopamine at the synaptic terminal.

The binding levels of (^{123}I)FP-CIT may reflect either lower DaT levels or greater dopaminergic nerve terminal degeneration. However, there is no clear clinical evidence for a greater decrease in dopaminergic terminals in PD+ICD patients relative to PD controls (82), suggesting that the lower binding levels might reflect either greater sensitivity to medication-related DaT downregulation or baseline trait differences and hence higher dopaminergic activity. Lower DaT levels with similar nerve terminal density suggest that extracellular dopamine neurotransmission can be enhanced in distance from the synaptic cleft and duration of action.

Multiple substances of abuse, such as methamphetamine, cocaine and alcohol, can differentially affect the regulation of DaT. For instance, methamphetamine and alcohol are associated with decreased DaT density as measured using PET imaging and DaT ligands (83,84), particularly in early abstinence (<6 months) with some degree of recovery after prolonged abstinence (12-16 months) (85, 86). In contrast to the ef-

fects of substances of abuse, DaT regulation by levodopa or dopamine agonists appears to be modest, if it exists at all, and its effect might be dependent on its use in early versus late PD or as monotherapy versus co-therapy. Although any regulation of DaT by anti-parkinsonian medications appears to be modest (87-91), PD+ICD patients may be differentially sensitive to regulatory mechanisms of DaT expression (e.g. D2 autoreceptor, TAAR1, protein kinase A and C) (88) compared to PD controls. A mechanism implicating DaT downregulation would also suggest that symptom improvement following discontinuation of the dopamine agonist would have a delayed time course. This may also play a role in the observation of enhanced dopamine withdrawal symptoms (DAWS) observed following dopamine agonist discontinuation in PD patients with ICDs (89).

D2/D3 autoreceptor downregulation and increase in gain

Although acute dopamine agonist (pramipexole) administration in rodents has been shown to decrease the proportion of spontaneously firing dopaminergic neurons, chronic dopamine agonists normalize this proportion of firing neurons mediated via D2/D3 autoreceptor downregulation (90). Furthermore, chronic levodopa administration in a parkinsonian rodent model has been shown to increase the proportion of spontaneously firing dopaminergic neurons, secondary to D2/D3 autoreceptor downregulation (91). These spontaneously firing dopaminergic neurons are capable of phasic activity in response to a stimulus (e.g. the unconditioned rewarding stimulus, conditioned stimulus, a gambling task) (92). Thus, increasing the proportion of spontaneously firing neurons effectively increases the gain and proportion of dopamine neurons capable of phasically responding to a stimulus. There is preliminary evidence that PD patients with ICDs have a decreased sensitivity of the D2/D3 autoreceptor in the midbrain as measured using (^{11}C)FLB-457 PET (93). In this study, PD controls on dopamine agonists demonstrated decreased D2/D3 mid-brain autoreceptor binding to a gambling task as compared to a control task, consistent with the feedback regulation of endogenous dopamine released in the gambling task. In contrast, PD patients with ICDs on dopamine agonists failed to demonstrate a difference, suggesting decreased sensitivity of the D2/D3 autoreceptor. Thus, the enhanced dopamine levels observed in PD+ICD may be related to impaired regulatory feedback.

Dopamine receptor subtypes

Dopamine D3 receptors are predominantly expressed in the ventral striatum, and they mediate reward, emotional and cognitive processes. Pramipexole and ropinirole, two widely used, non-ergot DAs, have greater D2/D3 selectivity relative to D1. That concurrent levodopa use with a DA increases the odds of developing an ICD (6) is consistent with a primate study demonstrating that levodopa administration results in ectopic induction of dorsal striatal D3 receptors (94).

Genetic polymorphisms

Genetic polymorphisms may also contribute to ICD susceptibility. Evaluation of dopamine and glutamate receptors and serotonin transporter gene polymorphisms identified D3 dopamine receptor p.S9G and GRIN2B c.366C > G as a risk factor for ICDs in PD (95).

Diagnosis

Patients and caregivers should be warned about the risk of developing ICDs at treatment onset and actively questioned on follow-up. Patients with a premorbid history of substance or behavioural addiction may be at greater risk for the development of these disorders. The validated screening tool, questionnaire for impulsive-compulsive disorders in Parkinson's disease (QUIP), has >80% sensitivity and specificity and can be completed in 5 minutes (96). Given the low positive predictive value (21-59%), a clinical interview should follow a positive screening re-

sult. The QUIP is also valid when completed by the patient's informant (97). Table 41.1 provides some overview on current diagnostic criteria.

Treatment

Pharmacotherapy

Observational follow-up studies suggest that a decrease or discontinuation of the DA, if tolerated, may be efficacious for some patients. PD patients with ICDs will be more sensitive to dopamine agonist withdrawal symptoms (DAWS) (89). A recent, cross-over, randomised trial demonstrated the efficacy of amantadine (23); however, a contradictory report of increased risk of ICDs associated with amantadine (6) suggests its role is not yet established.

Cognitive behavioural therapy has been shown in a randomized waiting-list control with standard medical care to improve global symptom severity (98). Naltrexone, an opioid antagonist which has been shown to be effective in the management of PG in the general population, was effective in a case study involving 3 PD patients with PG (99). Other case reports have also reported preliminary efficacy with valproate (100) and clozapine (101).

Deep brain stimulation

There is as yet no clear consensus regarding the role of DBS for preoperative ICD and compulsive medication use. ICD behaviours have been reported to improve, remain unchanged, or worsen after surgery (102). De novo onset of ICDs has also been reported (103). In two retrospective case series, mixed ICD behaviours were reported primarily to remain unchanged or worsen following bilateral STN DBS or unilateral STN or GPi DBS. For instance, in one of the retrospective, bilateral STN and GPi DBS case series that included both ICDs and compulsive medication use, postoperative worsening of symptoms was associated with a lack of preoperative recognition of the disorder and high dopaminergic medication dose (102). In another ret-

Table 41.1
Diagnostic criteria for impulse control disorders.

Gambling Disorder (DSM 5): Substance-Related and Addictive Disorders
 	
Four criteria in a 12-month period
	A Persistent and recurrent, maladaptive gambling behaviour as indicated by 4 or more of the following:
	  1 Is often preoccupied with gambling
	  2 Need to gamble with increasing amounts of money to achieve desired excitement
	  3 Repeated, unsuccessful efforts to control, cut back or stop gambling
	  4 Feeling restless or irritable when attempting to cut down or stop gambling
	  5 Gambles when feeling distressed
	  6 'Chasing' losses
	  7 Lies to family members, therapists or others to conceal extent of involvement with gambling
	  8 Jeopardized or lost a significant relationship, job or educational or career opportunity because of gambling
	  9 Relies on others to provide money to relieve a desperate financial situation because of gambling

Hypersexuality (109)	**A** The sexual thoughts or behaviours are excessive or an atypical change from baseline marked by one or more of the following:
	  1 Maladaptive preoccupation with sexual thoughts
	  2 Inappropriately or excessively requesting sex from spouse or partner
	  3 Habitual promiscuity
	  4 Compulsive masturbation
	  5 Calls to telephone sex lines or viewing pornography
	  6 Paraphilias
	B The behaviour must have persisted for at least 1 month
	C The behaviour causes one or more of the following:
	  1 Marked distress
	  2 Attempts to control thoughts or behaviour that are successful or result in marked anxiety or distress
	  3 Becomes time-consuming
	  4 Significant interference with social or occupational functioning
	D The behaviour does not occur exclusively during periods of hypomania or mania
	E If all criteria except C are fulfilled, the disorder is subsyndromal

Compulsive shopping	**A** Maladaptive preoccupation with buying or shopping that is manifested as impulses or behaviours that
	  1 Are experienced as irresistible, intrusive or senseless
	  2 Result in frequent buying of more than can be afforded, items that are not needed or longer periods of time than intended
	B Causes marked distress, is time-consuming, significantly interferes with social or occupational functioning or result in financial problems.
	C The behaviours do not occur exclusively during periods of hypomania or mania.

Binge-eating (DSM 5)	A Recurrent and persistent episodes of binge-eating
	B Binge-eating episodes are associated with three or more of the following:
	1 Eating much more rapidly than normal
	2 Eating until feeling uncomfortably full
	3 Eating large amounts of food when not feeling physically hungry
	4 Eating alone because of being embarrassed by how much one is eating
	5 Feeling disgusted with oneself, depressed or very guilty after over-eating
	C Marked distress regarding binge-eating
	D Absence of regular compensatory behaviours (such as purging)

rospective unilateral STN DBS case series, only 2 of 7 subjects with preoperative ICD improved, with no clear relationship to medication dose (104). That there were no significant changes in medication dosage following the unilateral DBS may be an important limiting factor. Compulsive medication use in 5 patients persisted in the postoperative stage. In this same case series, 17 of 159 patients developed new-onset ICD behaviours, although the exact nature of these behaviours was not reported. In contrast, other small, retrospective studies have suggested that ICD can resolve after STN DBS and could become a new indication for surgery in this target (105,106). In a prospective study of 17 patients with preoperative ICDs treated with bilateral STN DBS, all ICD behaviours ceased according to systematic preoperative and postoperative evaluation of ICD and systematic discontinuation of dopamine agonists (40). In this study, however, preoperative overall appetitive behaviour changed into an overall more apathetic mode of functioning, which might mitigate the beneficial effect on ICD (40). Thus, careful preoperative behavioural assessment and management of postoperative medications are crucial. Overall, although ICDs can occur after surgery, the case reports suggest that their occurrence is rare, particularly pathological gambling or compulsive shopping. This may differ for the behaviours of binge eating and hypersexuality. The existing data suggest that with careful preoperative and postoperative assessment and management,

there is a role for STN DBS in the management of ICD in patients in whom medication changes are ineffective or poorly tolerated. Transient postoperative worsening might occur early in the postoperative stage. STN DBS allows a greater decrease in dopaminergic medication dose relative to GPi DBS, and enables a discontinuation of the dopamine agonist. However, patients may be reluctant to decrease their dopaminergic medication. Patients with ICD may also be at greater risk of DAWS, requiring careful titration of their medication (107), and of postoperative suicidal behaviour (108).

References

1 Voon V, Potenza MN, Thomsen T. Medication-related impulse control and repetitive behaviors in Parkinson's disease. Curr Opin Neurol 2007;20:484-492.

2 O'Sullivan SS, Djamshidian A, Evans AH, Loane CM, Lees AJ, Lawrence AD. Excessive hoarding in Parkinson's disease. Mov Disord 2010;25:1026-1033.

3 Bonfanti AB, Gatto EM. Kleptomania, an unusual impulsive control disorder in Parkinson's disease? Parkinsonism Relat Disord 2010;16:358-359.

4 Bienfait KL, Menza M, Mark MH, Dobkin RD. Impulsive smoking in a patient with Parkinson's disease treated with dopamine agonists. J Clin Neurosci 2010;17:539-540.

5 Leeman RF, Potenza MN. Similarities and differences between pathological gambling and

substance use disorders: a focus on impulsivity and compulsivity. Psychopharmacology (Berl) 2012;219:469-490.

6   Weintraub D, Koester J, Potenza MN, et al. Impulse control disorders in Parkinson disease: a cross-sectional study of 3090 patients. Arch Neurol 2010;67:589-595.

7   Giladi N, Weitzman N, Schreiber S, Shabtai H, Peretz C. New onset heightened interest or drive for gambling, shopping, eating or sexual activity in patients with Parkinson's disease: the role of dopamine agonist treatment and age at motor symptoms onset. J Psychopharmacol 2007;21:501-506.

8   Avanzi M, Baratti M, Cabrini S, Uber E, Brighetti G, Bonfa F. Prevalence of pathological gambling in patients with Parkinson's disease. Mov Disord 2006;21:2068-2072.

9   de Chazeron I, Llorca PM, Chereau-Boudet I, et al. Hypersexuality and pathological gambling in Parkinson's disease: A cross-sectional case-control study. Mov Disord 2011;26:2127-2130.

10 Shaffer HJ, Hall MN, Vander Bilt J. Estimating the prevalence of disordered gambling behavior in the United States and Canada: a research synthesis. Am J Public Health 1999;89:1369-1376.

11 Reijnders JS, Ehrt U, Weber WE, Aarsland D, Leentjens AF. A systematic review of prevalence studies of depression in Parkinson's disease. Mov Disord 2008;23:183-189.

12 Cornelius JR, Tippmann-Peikert M, Slocumb NL, Frerichs CF, Silber MH. Impulse control disorders with the use of dopaminergic agents in restless legs syndrome: a case-control study. Sleep 2010;33:81-87.

13 O'Sullivan SS, Djamshidian A, Ahmed Z, et al. Impulsive-compulsive spectrum behaviors in pathologically confirmed progressive supranuclear palsy. Mov Disord 2010;25:638-642.

14 Evans AH, Butzkueven H. Dopamine agonist-induced pathological gambling in restless legs syndrome due to multiple sclerosis. Mov Disord 2007;22:590-591.

15 Wicks P, MacPhee GJ. Pathological gambling amongst Parkinson's disease and ALS patients in an online community. Mov Disord 2009;24:1085-108.

16 Voon V, Mehta AR, Hallett M. Impulse control disorders in Parkinson's disease: recent advances. Curr Opin Neurol 2011;24:324-330.

17 Voon V, Fox SH. Medication-related impulse control and repetitive behaviors in Parkinson disease. Arch Neurol 2007;64:1089-1096.

18 Dodd ML, Klos KJ, Bower JH, Geda YE, Josephs KA, Ahlskog JE. Pathological gambling caused by drugs used to treat Parkinson disease. Arch Neurol 2005;62:1377-1381.

19 Driver-Dunckley E, Samanta J, Stacy M. Pathological gambling associated with dopamine agonist therapy in Parkinson's disease. Neurology. 2003;61:422-423.

20 Weintraub D, Siderowf AD, Potenza MN, et al. Association of dopamine agonist use with impulse control disorders in Parkinson disease. Arch Neurol 2006;63:969-973.

21 Mamikonyan E, Siderowf AD, Duda JE, et al. Long-term follow-up of impulse control disorders in Parkinson's disease. Mov Disord 2008;23:75-80.

22 Weintraub D, Sohr M, Potenza MN, et al. Amantadine use associated with impulse control disorders in Parkinson disease in cross-sectional study. Ann Neurol 2010;68:963-968.

23 Thomas A, Bonanni L, Gambi F, Di Iorio A, Onofrj M. Pathological gambling in Parkinson disease is reduced by amantadine. Ann Neurol 2010;68(3):400-4.

24 Lee JY, Kim HJ, Jeon BS. Is pathological gambling in Parkinson's disease reduced by amantadine? Ann Neurol 2011;69:213-414.

25 Rizos A, Kessel B, Henriksen T, et al., editors. Impulse control disorder/behaviour related to prolonged release oral and transdermal dopamine agonists: a comparative European multicenter survey 16th Int Congr PD and Mov Disord; 2012; Dublin.

26 Scheller D, Ullmer C, Berkels R, Gwarek M, Lubbert H. The in vitro receptor profile of rotigotine: a new agent for the treatment of Parkinson's disease. Naunyn-Schmiedeberg's archives of pharmacology 2009;379:73-86.

27 Voon V, Schoerling A, Wenzel S, Ekanayake V, Reiff J, Trenkwalder C, et al. Frequency of impulse control behaviours associated with dopaminergic

therapy in restless legs syndrome. BMC Neurol 2011;11:117.

28 Pourcher E, Remillard S, Cohen H. Compulsive habits in restless legs syndrome patients under dopaminergic treatment. J Neurol Sci 2010;290:52-56.

29 Ondo WG, Lai D. Predictors of impulsivity and reward seeking behavior with dopamine agonists. Parkinsonism Relat Disord 2008;14:28-32.

30 Weintraub D, Papay K, Siderowf A. Screening for impulse control symptoms in patients with de novo Parkinson disease: a case-control study. Neurology 2013;80:176-180.

31 Antonini A, Siri C, Santangelo G, Cilia R, Poletti M, Canesi M, et al. Impulsivity and compulsivity in drug-naive patients with Parkinson's disease. Mov Disord 2011;26:464-468.

32 Riddle JL, Rokosik SL, Napier TC. Pramipexole- and methamphetamine-induced reward-mediated behavior in a rodent model of Parkinson's disease and controls. Behav Brain Res 2012;233:15-23.

33 Cools R. Dopaminergic modulation of cognitive function-implications for L-DOPA treatment in Parkinson's disease. Neurosci Biobehav Rev 2006;30:1-23.

34 Harding AJ, Broe GA, Halliday GM. Visual hallucinations in Lewy body disease relate to Lewy bodies in the temporal lobe. Brain 2002;125:391-403.

35 Papapetropoulos S, McCorquodale DS, Gonzalez J, Jean-Gilles L, Mash DC. Cortical and amygdalar Lewy body burden in Parkinson's disease patients with visual hallucinations. Parkinsonism Relat Disord 2006;12:253-256.

36 Voon V, Fernagut PO, Wickens J, et al. Chronic dopaminergic stimulation in Parkinson's disease: from dyskinesias to impulse control disorders. Lancet Neurol 2009;8:1140-1149.

37 Rodriguez-Oroz MC, Lopez-Azcarate J, Garcia-Garcia D, et al. Involvement of the subthalamic nucleus in impulse control disorders associated with Parkinson's disease. Brain 2011;134(Pt 1):36-49.

38 Silveira-Moriyama L, Evans AH, Katzenschlager R, Lees AJ. Punding and dyskinesias. Mov Disord 2006;21:2214-2217.

39 Voon V, Sohr M, Lang AE, et al. Impulse control disorders in Parkinson disease: a multicenter case-control study. Ann Neurol 2011;69:986-996.

40 Lhommee E, Klinger H, Thobois S, et al. Subthalamic stimulation in Parkinson's disease: restoring the balance of motivated behaviours. Brain 2012;135:1463-1477.

41 Dujardin K, Defebvre L. Apathy in Parkinson disease: What are the underlying mechanisms? Neurology 2012;79:1082-1083.

42 Voon V, Dalley JW. Parkinson disease: impulsive choice-Parkinson disease and dopaminergic therapy. Nat Rev Neurol 2011;7:541-542.

43 Milenkova M, Mohammadi B, Kollewe K, et al. Intertemporal choice in Parkinson's disease. Mov Disord 2011;26:2004-2010.

44 Andrade LF, Petry NM. Delay and probability discounting in pathological gamblers with and without a history of substance use problems. Psychopharmacology (Berl) 2012;219:491-499.

45 Petry NM. Pathological gamblers, with and without substance use disorders, discount delayed rewards at high rates. J Abnorm Psychol 2001;110:482-487.

46 Voon V, Reynolds B, Brezing C, et al. Impulsive choice and response in dopamine agonist-related impulse control behaviors. Psychopharmacology (Berl) 2010;207:645-659.

47 Housden CR, O'Sullivan SS, Joyce EM, Lees AJ, Roiser JP. Intact reward learning but elevated delay discounting in Parkinson's disease patients with impulsive-compulsive spectrum behaviors. Neuropsychopharmacology 2010;35:2155-2164.

48 Belin D, Mar AC, Dalley JW, Robbins TW, Everitt BJ. High impulsivity predicts the switch to compulsive cocaine-taking. Science 2008;320:1352-1355.

49 Anker JJ, Perry JL, Gliddon LA, Carroll ME. Impulsivity predicts the escalation of cocaine self-administration in rats. Pharmacol Biochem Behav 2009;93:343-348.

50 Menza MA, Golbe LI, Cody RA, Forman NE. Dopamine-related personality traits in Parkinson's disease. Neurology 1993;43:505-508.

51 Cloninger CR. A unified biosocial theory of personality and its role in the development of anxiety states. Psych Develop 1986;4:167-226.

52 Evans AH, Lawrence AD, Potts J, et al. Relationship between impulsive sensation seeking traits, smoking, alcohol and caffeine intake, and Parkinson's disease. J Neurol Neurosurg Psychiatry 2006;77:317-321.

53 Voon V, Thomsen T, Miyasaki JM, det al. Factors associated with dopaminergic drug-related pathological gambling in Parkinson disease. Arch Neurol 2007;64:212-216.

54 Johansson A, Grant JE, Kim SW, Odlaug BL, Gotestam KG. Risk factors for problematic gambling: a critical literature review. J Gambl Studies 2009;25:67-92.

55 Potenza MN, Xian H, Shah K, Scherrer JF, Eisen SA. Shared genetic contributions to pathological gambling and major depression in men. Arch Gen Psychiatry 2005;62:1015-1021.

56 Kessler RC, Hwang I, LaBrie R, et al. DSM-IV pathological gambling in the National Comorbidity Survey Replication. Psychol Med 2008;38(9):1351-60.

57 Slutske WS, Eisen S, True WR, Lyons MJ, Goldberg J, Tsuang M. Common genetic vulnerability for pathological gambling and alcohol dependence in men. Arch Gen Psychiatry 2000;57:666-673.

58 Black DW, Monahan PO, Temkit M, Shaw M. A family study of pathological gambling. Psych Res 2006;141:295-303.

59 Eisen SA, Lin N, Lyons MJ, Scherrer JF, Griffith K, True WR, et al. Familial influences on gambling behavior: an analysis of 3359 twin pairs. Addiction 1998;93:1375-1384.

60 Slutske WS, Zhu G, Meier MH, Martin NG. Genetic and environmental influences on disordered gambling in men and women. Arch Gen Psychiatry 2010;67:624-630.

61 Waldman ID, Slutske WS. Antisocial behavior and alcoholism: a behavioral genetic perspective on comorbidity. Clin Psychol Rev 2000;20(2):255-87.

62 Schultz W, Dayan P, Montague PR. A neural substrate of prediction and reward. Science 1997;275:1593-1599.

63 Voon V, Pessiglione M, Brezing C, et al. Mechanisms underlying dopamine-mediated reward bias in compulsive behaviors. Neuron 2010;65(1):135-42.

64 Steeves TD, Ko JH, Kideckel DM, et al. Extrastriatal dopaminergic dysfunction in tourette syndrome. Ann Neurol 2010;67:170-181.

65 O'Sullivan SS, Wu K, Politis M, et al. Cue-induced striatal dopamine release in Parkinson's disease-associated impulsive-compulsive behaviours. Brain 2011;134:969-978.

66 Djamshidian A, Jha A, O'Sullivan SS, et al. Risk and learning in impulsive and nonimpulsive patients with Parkinson's disease. Mov Disord 2010;25:2203-2210.

67 Robinson TE, Berridge KC. The neural basis of drug craving: an incentive-sensitization theory of addiction. Brain Res Brain Res Rev 1993;18:247-291.

68 Politis M, Loane C, Wu K, et al. Neural response to visual sexual cues in dopamine treatment-linked hypersexuality in Parkinson's disease. Brain 2013;136:400-411.

69 Frosini D, Pesaresi I, Cosottini M, Belmonte G, Rossi C, Dell'Osso L, et al. Parkinson's disease and pathological gambling: results from a functional MRI study. Mov Disord 2010;25:2449-2453.

70 Volkow ND, Wang GJ, Telang F, Fowler JS, Logan J, Childress AR, et al. Cocaine cues and dopamine in dorsal striatum: mechanism of craving in cocaine addiction. J Neurosci 2006;26:6583-6588.

71 Rokosik SL, Napier TC. Pramipexole-induced increased probabilistic discounting: comparison between a rodent model of Parkinson's disease and controls. Neuropsychopharmacology 2012;37:1397-1408.

72 Zeeb FD, Robbins TW, Winstanley CA. Serotonergic and dopaminergic modulation of gambling behavior as assessed using a novel rat gambling task. Neuropsychopharmacology 2009;34:2329-2343.

73 Voon V, Gao J, Brezing C, et al. Dopamine agonists and risk: impulse control disorders in Parkinson's disease. Brain 2011;134:1438-1446.

74 Rao H, Mamikonyan E, Detre JA, et al. Decreased ventral striatal activity with impulse control disorders in Parkinson's disease. Mov Disord 2010;25:1660-1669.

75 Claassen DO, van den Wildenberg WP, Ridderinkhof KR, et al. The risky business of dopamine

agonists in Parkinson disease and impulse control disorders. Behav Neurosci 2011;125:492-500.

76 Djamshidian A, Sanotsky Y, Matviyenko Y, et al. Increased reflection impulsivity in patients with ephedrone-induced Parkinsonism. Addiction 2013;108:771-779.

77 Djamshidian A, O'Sullivan SS, Wittmann BC, Lees AJ, Averbeck BB. Novelty seeking behaviour in Parkinson's disease. Neuropsych 2011;49(9):2483-2488.

78 Averbeck BB, Djamshidian A, O'Sullivan SS, Housden CR, Roiser JP, Lees AJ. Uncertainty about mapping future actions into rewards may underlie performance on multiple measures of impulsivity in behavioral addiction: evidence from Parkinson's disease. Behav Neurosci 2013;127:245-255.

79 van Eimeren T, Pellecchia G, Cilia R, et al. Drug-induced deactivation of inhibitory networks predicts pathological gambling in PD. Neurology 2010;75:1711-1716.

80 Cilia R, Cho SS, van Eimeren T, et al. Pathological gambling in patients with Parkinson's disease is associated with fronto-striatal disconnection: a path modeling analysis. Mov Disord 2011;26:225-233.

81 Cilia R, Ko JH, Cho SS, et al. Reduced dopamine transporter density in the ventral striatum of patients with Parkinson's disease and pathological gambling. Neurobiol Dis 2010;39:98-104.

82 Voon V, Rizos A, Chakravartty R, Mulholland N, Robinson S, Howell NA, et al. Impulse control disorders in Parkinson's disease: decreased striatal dopamine transporter levels. J Neurol Neurosurg Psychiatry 2013 doi: 10.1136/jnnp-2013-305395

83 Sekine Y, Iyo M, Ouchi Y, et al. Methamphetamine-related psychiatric symptoms and reduced brain dopamine transporters studied with PET. Am J Psychiatry 2001;158:1206-1214.

84 McCann UD, Wong DF, Yokoi F, Villemagne V, Dannals RF, Ricaurte GA. Reduced striatal dopamine transporter density in abstinent methamphetamine and methcathinone users: evidence from positron emission tomography studies with [11C]WIN-35,428. J Neurosci 1998;18:8417-8422.

85 Volkow ND, Chang L, Wang GJ, et al. Loss of dopamine transporters in methamphetamine abusers recovers with protracted abstinence. J Neurosci 2001;21:9414-9418.

86 Laine TP, Ahonen A, Torniainen P, et al. Dopamine transporters increase in human brain after alcohol withdrawal. Mol Psych 1999;4:189-191.

87 Guttman M, Stewart D, Hussey D, Wilson A, Houle S, Kish S. Influence of L-dopa and pramipexole on striatal dopamine transporter in early PD. Neurology 2001;56:1559-1564.

88 Schmitt KC, Reith ME. Regulation of the dopamine transporter: aspects relevant to psychostimulant drugs of abuse. Ann N Y Acad Sci 2010;1187:316-340.

89 Rabinak CA, Nirenberg MJ. Dopamine agonist withdrawal syndrome in Parkinson disease. Arch Neurol 2010;67:58-63.

90 Chernoloz O, El Mansari M, Blier P. Sustained administration of pramipexole modifies the spontaneous firing of dopamine, norepinephrine, and serotonin neurons in the rat brain. Neuropsychopharmacology 2009;34:651-661.

91 Harden DG, Grace AA. Activation of dopamine cell firing by repeated L-DOPA administration to dopamine-depleted rats: its potential role in mediating the therapeutic response to L-DOPA treatment. J Neurosci 1995;15:6157-6166.

92 Grace AA. Dopamine system dysregulation by the hippocampus: implications for the pathophysiology and treatment of schizophrenia. Neuropharmacology 2012;62:1342-1348.

93 Ray NJ, Miyasaki JM, Zurowski M, et al. Extrastriatal dopaminergic abnormalities of DA homeostasis in Parkinson's patients with medication-induced pathological gambling: a [11C] FLB-457 and PET study. Neurobiol Dis 2012;48:519-525.

94 Bordet R, Ridray S, Carboni S, Diaz J, Sokoloff P, Schwartz JC. Induction of dopamine D3 receptor expression as a mechanism of behavioral sensitization to levodopa. Proc Natl Acad Sci U S A 1997;94:3363-3367.

95 Lee JY, Lee EK, Park SS, et al. Association of DRD3 and GRIN2B with impulse control and related behaviors in Parkinson's disease. Mov Disord 2009;24:1803-1810.

96 Weintraub D, Hoops S, Shea JA, et al. Validation of the questionnaire for impulsive-compulsive disorders in Parkinson's disease. Mov Disord 2009;24:1461-1467.

97 Papay K, Mamikonyan E, Siderowf AD, et al. Patient versus informant reporting of ICD symptoms in Parkinson's disease using the QUIP: validity and variability. Parkinsonism Relat Disord 2011;17:153-155.

98 Okai D, Askey-Jones S, Samuel M, et al. Trial of CBT for impulse control behaviors affecting Parkinson patients and their caregivers. Neurology 2013;80:792-799.

99 Bosco D, Plastino M, Colica C, et al. Opioid antagonist naltrexone for the treatment of pathological gambling in Parkinson disease. Clin Neuropharmacol 2012;35:118-120.

100 Sriram A, Ward HE, Hassan A, et al. Valproate as a treatment for dopamine dysregulation syndrome (DDS) in Parkinson's disease. J Neurol 2013;260:521-527.

101 Hardwick A, Ward H, Hassan A, Romrell J, Okun MS. Clozapine as a potential treatment for refractory impulsive, compulsive, and punding behaviors in Parkinson's disease. Neurocase 2012 [Epub ahead of print].

102 Lim SY, O'Sullivan SS, Kotschet K, et al. Dopamine dysregulation syndrome, impulse control disorders and punding after deep brain stimulation surgery for Parkinson's disease. J Clin Neurosci 2009;16:1148-1152.

103 Smeding HM, Goudriaan AE, Foncke EM, Schuurman PR, Speelman JD, Schmand B. Pathological gambling after bilateral subthalamic nucleus stimulation in Parkinson disease. J Neurol Neurosurg Psychiatry 2007;78:517-519.

104 Moum SJ, Price CC, Limotai N, et al. Effects of STN and GPi deep brain stimulation on impulse control disorders and dopamine dysregulation syndrome. PloS One. 2012;7:e29768.

105 Ardouin C, Voon V, Worbe Y, et al. Pathological gambling in Parkinson's disease improves on chronic subthalamic nucleus stimulation. Mov Disord 2006;21:1941-1946.

106 Witjas T, Baunez C, Henry JM, et al. Addiction in Parkinson's disease: impact of subthalamic nucleus deep brain stimulation. Mov Disord 2005;20:1052-1055.

107 Nirenberg MJ. Dopamine agonist withdrawal syndrome and non-motor symptoms after Parkinson's disease surgery. Brain 2010;133:155.

108 Voon V, Krack P, Lang AE, et al. A multicentre study on suicide outcomes following subthalamic stimulation for Parkinson's disease. Brain 2008;131:2720-2728.

109 Voon V, Hassan K, Zurowski M, et al. Prevalence of repetitive and reward-seeking behaviors in Parkinson disease. Neurology 2006;67:1254-1257.

PART VI

Phenomenology

42

The Art of Phenotyping in Movement Disorders

Daniel Waldvogel

The brain is the organ that defines each one of us as an individual human being. There is arguably only one voluntary output from the brain, i.e. the motor system. Any disturbance of the motor system is therefore a disturbance that cuts very close to our core as a human being since it disrupts our only output mechanism. This might explain why many of us, certainly the readers of this book, consider the study of movement disorders the most fascinating, important and intriguing subspeciality of neurology.

Another motivation may be that in times of an impressive increase in diagnostic procedures, from neuroimaging to genotyping, it is reassuring to know that bedside clinical assessment may still yield the best results, which is nowhere truer than in movement disorders. Any reasonable approach to a patient with a movement disorder starts with one and only one question: what type of movement disorder are we dealing with? (1) Some of the giants of the field, among them the late Charles David Marsden as well as his numerous famous disciples, have taught us that this is done best in a highly structured way, which is practised and appreciated in neurological practices and clinics as well as at video sessions of basal ganglia enthusiasts around the globe.

Structured clinical examination in movement disorders

A structured clinical examination with ancillary examinations of patients with movement disorders is the only way to analyze the clinical presentation and to answer the essential questions dealing with localization (what body parts are involved), phenomenology (what type of movement disorder is observed), pathophysiology (which physiological mechanisms are involved), aetiology (what is the cause of the disorder) and therapy (how to treat) (see Table 42.1).

The impact of the appreciation of a careful clinical assessment can best be seen in the steep learning curve of diagnosing Parkinson's disease. In 1992, Hughes, Daniel, Kilford and Lees published a paper on the accuracy of the clinical diagnosis of PD, which was a rather shockingly low 76% (2). Ten years later, in a follow-up paper, Hughes, Daniel and Lees found that the accuracy had risen to 90% (3) – a quite remarkable improvement. In their paper, the authors remark that 'this might suggest that clinicians looked at the overall picture and did not negate the diagnosis even in the presence of accepted exclusion criteria'. Looking at the overall picture is clinical assessment at its best and easily explains the enthusiasm that movement disorders specialists share for their speciality.

Regarding phenomenology, the first distinction made is between a hypokinetic and a hyperkinetic movement disorder. The hypokinetic movement disorders are the parkinsonian syndromes, while the hyperkinetic movement disorders are further subdivided into dystonia, tremor, myoclonus, chorea, tics, and ballism.

Table 42.1
Clinical examination (with ancillary examinations) of patients with movement disorders.

Questions	Techniques	Answers
Localization	Clinical examination	Focal Segmental Multifocal Unilateral Generalized
Phenomenology	Clinical examination	Rhythmic versus Non-rhythmic Spontaneous versus Evoked Position-evoked versus Action-evoked Hypokinesia versus Hyperkinesia
Pathophysiology	Clinical neurophysiology EEG +/- back averaging, EMG, SEP, MEP, tremor registration, coherence analysis Neuroimaging CT, MRI	Cortical Subcortical Brainstem Spinal cord Peripheral nervous system
Etiology	Laboratory tests Pharmacological tests Clinical neurophysiology Functional neuroimaging	Physiological Primary, Idiopathic, Essential Secondary, Symptomatic, Acquired Psychogenic

Phenotyping in movement disorders

Hypokinetic movement disorders

The hallmark of hypokinetic movement disorders is 'bradykinesia'. The literal translation, slowness of movement, does not capture the breadth of what clinicians mean when applying the term. On the one hand, it is used to describe the loss of automated movements like facial expression, gesture, arm swing or reduced rate of swallowing with the accumulation of saliva (all of which are better referred to as 'hypokinesia' or 'akinesia'). On the other hand, it is used to describe the progressive decrease in amplitude and frequency of repeated movements that is most characteristic of the parkinsonian syndromes. In other words, many patients may be slow because they are old, depressed, in pain or even dystonic, or have a lesion of their pyramidal tract, but only patients with a parkinsonian syndrome show what is often called 'true bradykinesia', i.e. the progressive decrease of amplitude and frequency of a movement with repetition. Of course, when testing for 'true

bradykinesia', the examiner should not simultaneously perform the movement himself, because he is otherwise offering an external clue which may mask the patient's impediment (please distinguish between externally and internally triggered movements, the latter being mostly affected in Parkinson's disease).

When facing a patient with a parkinsonian syndrome, a careful screen for the so-called 'red flags' is of course mandatory (4). From a purely phenomenological point of view, one may want to consider that the patient suffers from multiple system atrophy if he shows a disproportionate antecollis, lilac hands, a rather jerky tremor or even a polyminimyoclonus instead of a more regular resting or re-emerging postural tremor. The early occurrence of facial dyskinesias is a rather telling sign of an atypical parkinsonism, while ocular dyskinesias are seen in Parkinson's disease.

An unusually erect patient with a surprised expression or a so-called bad smell face who turns the head first with the eyes following when looking from you to his spouse should prompt the careful consideration of a progressive supranuclear palsy (5), while extremely unilateral symptoms with dystonia and myoclonus may suggest cortico-basal degeneration even in the absence of an alien limb phenomenon. Of course, these are only hints, but you may notice them at first sight, and they may motivate you to look particularly carefully for apraxia, cortical sensory loss or cognitive problems. If a patient's gait is shuffling with frequent festinations and relatively wide base, and if the arm swing is rather pronounced instead of reduced, vascular parkinsonism seems a likely differential diagnosis.

Hyperkinetic movement disorders
As mentioned above, the most important hyperkinetic movement disorders are dystonia, tremor, myoclonus, chorea, tics, and ballism.

Dystonia
Dystonia is defined as the pathological co-contraction of an agonist and an antagonist that leads to an unphysiological posture. Dystonia is not fixed and worsens with action. In children, it usually starts in the lower limbs and later ascends; in adults, dystonia is most commonly focal or segmental, involving the head, neck or upper extremities. If you see action-induced foot dystonia in an adult, you may want to search carefully for signs of Parkinson's disease (6). A severe unilateral dystonia of the upper limb may be the presenting sign of a cortico-basal degeneration, and therefore the search for stimulus-sensitive myoclonus, cortical sensory loss, apraxia, an alien limb phenomenon, aphasia or frontal executive dysfunction may be worthwhile. If the patient with dystonia shows marked oromandibular dyskinesia, even a 'fly catching tongue', your history-taking concerning neuroleptics should be particularly thorough, even more so when the patient has a retrocollis. A retrocollis and extension of the elbows with internal rotation of the shoulders and flexion of the wrists is most likely a tardive dystonia (7).

The one dystonia that should never be missed (except for Wilson's disease, of course) is dopa-responsive dystonia. The phenomenological presentation may change with age. In children, when it mostly becomes manifest, it may present as a spastic gait disorder resembling cerebral palsy, while in adults it may present as parkinsonism or focal dystonia (8).

Tremor
Tremor is defined as an involuntary movement disorder with rhythmic and sinusoidal, alternating movements of one or more body parts. Organic tremors are invariably rhythmic and invariable concerning their frequency, while the amplitude may change quite drastically from one moment to the other. The first important distinction for the clinician to make is the differentiation between a resting and an action tremor, the former being the hallmark of a parkinsonian tremor.

A resting tremor is defined as a tremor that occurs when the affected body part is supported against gravity. A hand that rests on the lap of the patient and trembles is easily classified as affected by 'resting' tremor. Less well appreciated is sometimes that a hand that shows a tremor when the arms are hanging qualifies as having a resting (dependent) tremor since the involved muscles are not actively contracted. A resting tremor can also reoccur when the arms are outstretched, i.e. the so called 're-emerging' tremor, which is different from the immediately occurring postural tremor associated with essential tremor. Thus, re-emerging tremor is a strong indicator for Parkinson's disease-related tremor. Action tremors are further subdivided into postural, kinetic and intention tremors. From a phenomenological point of view, it is worthwhile mentioning that most kinetic tremors show an increase in amplitude when approaching the target, i.e. are invariably associated with an 'intention tremor'.

A rather unhelpful criterion to distinguish between different forms of tremors is frequency. It is hard to assess frequency clinically, and there is considerable overlap between the different tremor syndromes. The only truly 'useful' tremor frequency, i.e. the 16 Hz tremor of orthostatic tremor, cannot be seen but only felt and heard. Most of us prefer to look for it with EMG when it is suspected from the typical history of a patient who can walk but not stand (9).

While frequency is often unhelpful, the location of tremor may be more telling. A tremor of the tongue, lip, chin or foot is most likely a parkinsonian tremor (albeit not exclusively) (10). A one-sided tremor is most likely a parkinsonian tremor; an essential tremor may be asymmetric but is hardly ever just one-sided. A voice tremor is most likely an essential tremor, as is a head tremor. On the other hand, a neck tremor in the 'no-no' direction, slightly jerky, and changing in amplitude depending on the head position deserves a careful consideration of dystonia, as does any task-specific tremor.

Whether a patient with an essential tremor can show some dystonic elements, as we see in other movement disorders, or whether a patient with tremor and some dystonia should essentially be classified as 'dystonic' is a matter of an ongoing debate and therefore beyond the scope of the present chapter (11). To make matters worse, a group has identified patients who manifest with resting tremor and bradykinesia resembling Parkinson's disease, but no signs of dopaminergic deficiency on SPECT scans (scans without evidence of dopaminergic deficit, SWEDDS). These patients were then (re)classified as dystonic. Phenomenologically, the most distinguishing hallmark in these patients might be the absence of 'true' bradykinesia, i.e. a decrease of amplitude and frequency with repeated movements, as discussed above (12). Sometimes, a difficult differentiation from tremor is rhythmic myoclonus.

Myoclonus

Myoclonus is sometimes difficult to differentiate from tremor. It is defined as brief, shock-like, in-

voluntary movements. A positive myoclonus is due to a muscle contraction, while a negative myoclonus (asterixis) is due to sudden loss of muscle tone, the latter mostly in conditions associated with metabolic encephalopathy. When the myoclonus is rhythmic, it can be mistaken for tremor, like in hereditary cortical myoclonus, making electrophysiology a helpful tool to improve the distinction. A rhythmical movement that must be highlighted is oculofaciomasticatory myorhythmia (13), not because of its rarity but because of its distinctiveness, allowing the clinician to make an etiopathological diagnosis purely based on a phenomenological observation. Oculofaciomasticatory myorhythmia is a slow, rhythmical movement of the jaw and face along with horizontal, pendular, ocular oscillations and is described in patients with cerebral Whipple's disease. Semirhythmical bulbar movements sometimes accompanied by semirhythmic limb movements and gaze deviation are another rare movement disorder which may hint to aetiology since it is described in patients with NMDA-antibody-associated encephalitis (14).

Chorea and ballism

Chorea is defined as an involuntary, excessive movement that flows randomly from one part of the body to another. It involves the distal extremities, the face and the neck as well as the trunk. If the excessive movements are more proximal and have a flinging character, the movements are referred to as ballism. If lip or tongue biting (15) or brief episodes of head drop (16) are observed in a patient with chorea, the diagnosis of neuroacanthocytosis should be pursued even in the absence of a typical blood smear.

Involuntary movements that may be mistaken for chorea are movements associated with loss of proprioception or movements associated with parietal lesions, which for the most part are more stereotyped than true chorea and of course should not be missed after a careful neurological examination. Involuntary movements due to a sensory afferent deficit are referred to as pseudoathetosis. Other excessive distal movements of the extremities that can be seen are the ones associated with restless limbs, either as rather stereotypical distal movements or even as proximal movements occurring at regular intervals with flexions of the hips and knees as well as upward flexion of the toes as seen in the sleep lab recordings of periodic leg movements during sleep (PLMS) (during daytime, PLM-like movements are sometimes referred to as 'dyskinesias while awake'). The painful legs and moving toes syndrome which indicates a nerve root or peripheral nerve lesion manifests with continuous stereotypical, sometimes almost ondulating movements (17), which are very different from the randomly flowing choreatic movements.

Tics

Brief jerky movements can be seen in patients with tics. Tics are stereotyped, and the examiner may feel a certain urge to mimic them after a brief period of observation. Mimicking tics is rather straightforward, unlike mimicking the randomly flowing movements of chorea. The defining feature of tics is that they can be voluntarily suppressed, but the patient feels an increasing urge to move while suppressing the tic.

Ancilliary measures

One of the most helpful ancilliary measures to assess movement disorders is a videocamera. It offers not only the advantage of being able to discuss a particular patient with colleagues, but also helps to identify patterns as it can be repeatedly reviewed without the stress of a time constraint consult. The use of a tripod usually facilitates the distinction between the shaking of the videographer and a true myoclonus of the patient and is therefore highly encouraged!

Table 42.2 gives some overview on distinct clinical signs that may lead to a diagnosis.

Table 42.2
Clinical signs that may guide to a diagnosis.

if you see the following at first glance...	you may want to consider...
disproportionate antecollis	MSA
polyminimyoclonus	MSA
facial dyskinesias	MSA, PSP
lilac hands	MSA
surprised look, 'bad smell face'	PSP
unusually erect posture	PSP
extraordinarily unilateral symptoms	CBD
shuffling gait but normal arm swing	Vascular parkinsonism
foot dystonia in an adult	PD
retrocollis	tardive dyskinesia
oromandibular dyskinesias	tardive dyskinesia
spastic gait in a child	dopa-responsive dystonia
re-emerging tremor	PD
tongue, lip, chin or foot tremor	PD
head or voice tremor	ET
semi-rhythmical bulbar movements in a comatose patient	NMDA-associated encephalitis
'pseudo'-athetosis	loss of proprioceptive feedback, parietal lesion
lip, tongue biting in a patient with chorea	neuroacanthocytosis
brief episodes of head drop	neuroacanthocytosis
rhythmical slow bulbar and ocular movements	Whipple

PD = Parkinson's disease; ET = Essential tremor; PSP = Progressive supranuclear palsy; CBD = Corticobasal degeneration.

References

1 Abdo WF, van de Warrenburg BPC, Burn DJ, Quinn NP, Bloem BR. The clinical approach to movement disorders. Nat Rev Neurol 2010;6:29-37.

2 Hughes AJ, Daniel SE, Kilford L, Lees AJ. Accuracy of clinical diagnosis of idiopathic Parkinson's disease: a clinico-pathological study of 100 cases. J. Neurol. Neurosurg. Psychiatr 1992;55:181-184.

3 Hughes AJ, Daniel SE, Lees AJ. Improved accuracy of clinical diagnosis of Lewy body Parkinson's disease. Neurology 2001;57:1497-1499.

4 Köllensperger M, Geser F, Seppi K, et al. Red flags for multiple system atrophy. Mov Disord 2008;23:1093-1099.

5 Williams DR, Lees AJ. Progressive supranuclear palsy: clinicopathological concepts and diagnostic challenges. Lancet Neurol 2009;8:270-279.

6 Lees AJ, Hardie RJ, Stern GM. Kinesigenic foot dystonia as a presenting feature of Parkinson's disease. J Neurol Neurosurg Psychiatry 1984;47:885.

7 Kang UJ, Burke RE, Fahn S. Natural history and treatment of tardive dystonia. Mov Disord 1986;1:193-208.

8 Tadic V, Kasten M, Brüggemann N, Stiller S, Hagenah J, Klein C. Dopa-Responsive Dystonia Revisited: Diagnostic Delay, Residual Signs, and Nonmotor Signs. Arch Neurol 2012;17:1-5.

9 Heilman KM. Orthostatic tremor. Arch Neurol 1984;41:880-881.

10 Silverdale MA, Schneider SA, Bhatia KP, Lang AE. The spectrum of orolingual tremor – a proposed classification system. Mov Disord 2008;23:159-167.

11 Quinn NP, Schneider SA, Schwingenschuh P, Bhatia KP. Tremor – some controversial aspects. Mov Disord 2011;26:18-23.

12 Schwingenschuh P, Ruge D, Edwards MJ, et al. Distinguishing SWEDDs patients with asymmetric resting tremor from Parkinson's disease: a clinical and electrophysiological study. Mov Disord 2010;25:560-569.

13 Schwartz MA, Selhorst JB, Ochs AL, Beck RW, Campbell WW, Harris JK, et al. Oculomasticatory myorhythmia: a unique movement disorder occurring in Whipple's disease. Ann Neurol 1986;20:677-683.

14 Kleinig TJ, Thompson PD, Matar W, et al. The distinctive movement disorder of ovarian teratoma-associated encephalitis. Mov Disord 2008;23:1256-1261.

15 Hardie RJ, Pullon HW, Harding AE, et al. Neuroacanthocytosis. A clinical, haematological and pathological study of 19 cases. Brain 1991;114:13-49.

16 Schneider SA, Lang AE, Moro E, Bader B, Danek A, Bhatia KP. Characteristic head drops and axial extension in advanced chorea-acanthocytosis. Mov Disord 2010;25:1487-1491.

17 Mhoon JT, Nandigam K, Juel VC. Teaching video NeuroImages: painful legs and moving toes syndrome. Neurology 2010;75:6.

43
Scales and Tests in Movement Disorders

Pablo Martínez-Martín, Carmen Rodríguez-Blázquez & Mónica M. Kurtis

Measurement, or determining the quantity of something by comparison with a given unit, is essential in science. When applied to clinical practice and research, measurement allows us to collect and record data and makes possible the use of statistical methods for description, comparison, association, prediction, etc.

In neurology, measures can be either objective (biological markers, functional tests) or subjective (rating scales, questionnaires). Many neurological and psychological phenomena are abstract concepts or 'constructs' which are not directly observable and must be estimated through measurable indicators related to the construct.

Rating scales and questionnaires are basic tools for evaluation with an inferential subjective component. They provide data on signs and symptoms (disability, pain, depression, etc.) that cannot be accessed through objective methods in a simple and quick way. Their characteristics (simplicity, quality and quantity of information at a low cost) make scales and questionnaires widely used in clinical and research settings. Rating scales should be developed and tested following a standardized methodology to guarantee their quality and usefulness.

Choosing the adequate measurement instrument is critical in research and in clinical practice. The available information on the psychometric properties of a rating scale should be taken into account and must guide the selection process. Rating scales are validated or tested in specific populations and settings, and they should not be applied in others without re-test-ing their psychometric characteristics. Thus, validation is a dynamic process, and each validation study enriches and expands the information on the attributes of a scale.

Design and validation of rating scales

Design

The design of a rating scale must follow several steps (3,4):
1 Specifying or identifying the construct to be measured and the target population;
2 Establishing the purpose or the intention of the instrument (discriminative, evaluative or predictive);
3 Determining the format and mode of application (interview, computerized, etc.);
4 Selecting the components (items and domains) of the instrument;
5 Choosing the type and number of questions and answers, time frame, score range and response options;
6 Undertaking a pilot study to test the scale's feasibility and to identify ambiguities, redundancies, shortcomings, etc.;
7 Validating the definitive version.

Validation

The validation process was developed according to two theories: the classical test theory (CTT) and the latent trait theories (LTT) – the item response theory (IRT) and the Rasch measurement theory (1,2). Although the CTT is the most widely known and used one, it has several disadvantages, which can be overcome by the

LTT. Whatever the selected approach may be, designing and validating a rating scale have to pass through several phases. Validating implies testing several attributes of the scale (3). According to the principles of the CTT, the fundamental psychometric attributes of a scale are:

Acceptability: the extent to which the measure is applicable to the target population. It is verified through the quality of data (completeness) and distribution of scores in the sample (floor and ceiling effect, skewness).

Scaling assumptions: the correct grouping of items in the scales and the extent to which a total score can be calculated from the direct sum of items' scores. The item-total corrected correlation and the multitrait-scaling methods are ways to check the scaling assumptions.

Reliability: the extent to which an instrument is free from random error. Aspects of reliability are: Internal consistency, extent to which the items of a scale are measuring the same construct, and reproducibility or stability at a point in time (inter-rater) or over time (test-retest, intra-rater).

Validity: it determines whether the test is measuring what it is intended to measure. Validity adopts several forms: face, content, criterion and construct validity. Face validity refers to the extent to which a scale gives the impression that it measures what it is intended to measure. Content validity refers to judgments about whether the important parts of the domain to be measured are covered by the scale components. Criterion validity denotes the relationship of the scale to the 'gold standard' of the construct. Construct validity (the degree to which an instrument is related to other constructs in a way that is consistent with underlying hypotheses on the concepts being measured) is commonly classified into three types: convergent validity (the correlation of the scale with other measures used to evaluate the same construct), divergent validity (the relationship of the scale to measures

assessing different constructs), and known-groups or discriminative validity (the ability of the scale to detect differences among groups).

Precision: it refers to the ability of a scale to detect small differences. It is established, for example, through the error variance or the standard error of measurement (SEM), which is related to the reliability of the scale.

Responsiveness: or sensitivity to change refers to the ability of the scale to detect changes. Other definitions refer to the ability for detecting a clinically important change or a real change, but these are aspects in the interface between responsiveness and interpretability of outcomes.

Interpretability: the extent to which the scale's scores are meaningful; that is to say, the extent to which a qualitative meaning can be assigned to a score.

Other aspects: administrative burden (time, effort and demands involved in the instrument application), cross-cultural adaptations (translation and adaptation to obtain an equivalent linguistic and conceptual version to be used in a different language or culture than the original), and alternative forms (different modes of administration: phone, interview, self-assessment) are other aspects to be taken into account when developing a new scale.

Scales and tests for movement disorders

The purpose of this chapter, a revised and updated version of the one published in 2010 (5), is to offer a review of the most relevant and widely used rating scales for movement disorders. It does not include information on instruments for assessing non-motor symptoms or health-related quality of life related to these disorders, whose complex nature surpasses the aim of this chapter. In order to guide the choice of a rating scale, the most frequent movement disorder syndromes are listed alphabetically with their most representative measuring instruments presented in order of relevance in clinical and research settings. Information is presented in a practical and summarized way with appropriate and selected references to allow readers to quickly capture the main features, psychometric properties and clinical applications of each scale. Scales for PD that achieved the qualification of 'recommended' by the Movement Disorder Society task force (6) are noted since they have been used in PD populations by different researchers and found to be clinimetrically sound (valid, reliable, and responsive).

Table 43.1 offers some overview on further scales and tests that are not discussed in detail.

Akathisia

Barnes akathisia rating scale, BAS, BARS (7)

The BARS is the most widely used scale for assessing the presence and severity of drug-induced akathisia. It is composed of 4 items (objective and subjective), rated from 0 to 3, with a total sum score. It shows adequate reliability, validity and sensitivity, and it has been objectively validated with movement measuring by actimetry.

Ataxia

Scale for the assessment and rating of ataxia, SARA (8)

This is a scale aiming at measuring the severity of ataxia. The 8 items (maximum total score: 40 points) that compose it are: gait (scored from 0 to 8), stance (0-6), sitting (0-4), speech disturbance (0-6), finger chase (0-4), nose-finger test (0-4), alternating hand movements (0-4), heel-shin slide (0-4). The movements of the last four items are rated for each side and averaged to provide a score. Time required for administration is about 5 minutes (one-third of the time necessary for the international cooperative ataxia rating scale ICARS). The scale has shown good internal consistency and intra-/inter-rater reliability for both spinocerebellar and non-spinocerebellar atax-

ia patients. It is apparently unidimensional and has a high correlation with other movement and disability scales.

International cooperative ataxia rating scale, ICARS (9)

The ICARS is a semi-quantitative assessment tool of cerebellar symptoms and impairment, with 4 subscales: posture and gait disturbances (7 items, maximum 34 points), kinetic functions (7 items, 52 points), speech disorders (2 items, 8 points), and oculomotor disorders (3 items, 6 points). The scale has been criticized for being long and cumbersome, and thus not practical in a clinical setting. Inter-rater and test-retest reliability and internal consistency have been tested in several movement disorders and are satisfactory, but factorial analysis has not confirmed the scale structure, and several items are redundant and overlapping.

Chorea

Huntington's disease (HD)

Unified Huntington's disease rating scale, UHDRS (10)

This complex scale assesses clinical and functional manifestations of HD in four domains: motor function, cognitive function, behavioural abnormalities and functional capacity. The motor section includes 15 items, scored from 0 to 4 and divided into six subdomains: oculomotor function, dysarthria, chorea, dystonia, gait, and postural stability. The cognitive function domain includes a phonetic verbal fluency test, the symbol digit modalities test (SDMT), and the Stroop interference test (SIT). The behavioural abnormalities domain rates frequency and severity of symptoms related to affectivity, thought content and confrontation styles from 0 to 4. The functional capacity domain includes a functional capacity scale with five items, scored on a 2- or 3-point scale; an independence scale, scored from 10 (totally dependent) to 100 (to-

Table 43.1
Other scales for movement disorders.

Movement disorder	Scale name	Reference
Akathisia	Akathisia Ratings of Movement Scale (ARMS)	Bodfish et al. Am J Ment Retard 1997;101:413-423.
Ataxia	Brief Ataxia Rating Scale (BARS)	Schmahmann et al. Mov Disord 2009;24:1820-1828.
	Modified ICARS (MICARS)	Schmahmann et al. Mov Disord 2009;24:1820-1828.
	Friedreich's Ataxia Impact Scale	Cano et al. Mov Disord 2009;24:984-992.
	Cerebellar Ataxia Scale	Klockgether et al. J Neurol Neurosurg Psychiatry. 1990;53:297-305.
	Nobile-Orazio Ataxia scale	Nobile-Orazio et al. Ann Neurol 1988;24:93-97.
Drug-induced movement disorders	St. Hans Rating Scale for Extrapyramidal Syndromes	Gerlach et al. Acta Psychiatr Scand 1993;87:244-252.
	Schedule for the Assessment of Drug-Induced Movement Disorders	Loonen et al. Int J Neuropsychopharmacol. 2000;3:285-296.
	Abnormal Involuntary Movement Scale, AIMS	Guy W. 1976 (49).
Dystonia	Barry-Albright Dystonia (BAD) Scale	Barry et al. Dev Med Child Neuro. 1999;41:404-411.
Myoclonus	Opsoclonus Myoclonus Syndrome Evaluation Scale	Pranzatelli et al. Clin Neuropharmacol 2001;24:352-357.
	Myoclonus Evaluation Scale	Chadwick et al. Brain 1977;100:455-487.
Parkinson's disease	Rapid Assessment of Disability Scale (RADS)	Martinez-Martin et al. Gac Sanit 2005;19(S1):68; J Neurol 2013;260:228–236
	Short Parkinson's Evaluation Scale (SPES)	Rabey et al. Clin Neuropharmacol 1997;20:322-337.
	Columbia University Rating Scale (CURS)	Yahr et al. Arch Neurol 1969; 21:343-354.
	Clinical Gait and Balance Scale (GABS)	Thomas et al. J Neurol Sci 2004;217:89-99.
	Clinical Dyskinesia Rating Scale (CDRS)	Hagell & Widner. Mov Disord 1999,14:448-455.
Restless legs syndrome	RLS-6 Severity Scales	Kohnen et al. Sleep 2003;26:A342.
	Augmentation Severity Rating Scale (ASRS)	García-Borregero et al. Sleep Med 2007;8:455-463.

Tics	Rush Video-Based Tic Rating Scale	Goetz et al. Mov Disord 1999;14:502-506.
	Hopkins Motor and Vocal Tic Scale (HMVTS)	Walkup et al. J Am Acad Child Adolesc Psychiatry 1992;31:472-477
	The Tourette's Disorder Scale (TODS)	Shytle et al. Assessment 2003;10:273-287.
	Tourette Syndrome Questionnaire (TSQ)	Jagger et al. Schizophr Bull 1982;8:267-278.
	Motor tic, Obsessions and compulsions, Vocal tic Evaluation Survey (MOVES)	Gaffney et al. J Child Adolesc Psychopharmacol 1994;4:269-280.
Essential tremor	Bain Findley Tremor Scale	Bain et al. J Neurol Neurosurg Psychiatry 1993;56:868-873
	Fahn-Tolosa-Marin Tremor Rating Scale (TRS)	Fahn et al. Parkinson's Disease and Movement Disorders, 2nd edit. . Baltimore-Munich: William & Wilkins, 1993:271-280.
	Essential Tremor Screening Questionnaire	Lorenz et al. Mov Disord 2008;23:1006-1012.

tally independent); and a checklist of common activities of daily living rated by means of yes/no response options. Higher scores mean better functional state. The UHDRS has shown satisfactory responsiveness in follow-up studies and clinical trials. Although its psychometric properties including internal consistency, inter-rater reliability and sensitivity to change are satisfactory, its length and administrative load have been criticized. A shortened version of the motor section of the UHDRS has been subsequently developed and validated (11).

Shoulson and Fahn functional disability scale for Huntington's disease (12)
The purpose of this scale is assessing occupation, handling financial affairs, coping with activities of daily living, managing domestic responsibilities, and required care in Huntington's disease. It has five items, scored from 0 to 3 (the first three) and from 0 to 2 (the last two), that can be converted into a five-stage disease classification. It has not been formally validated.

Huntington's disease activities of daily living scale, HD-ADL (13)
The HD-ADL is a rating scale for assessing a patient's adaptive functioning administered by

proxy. It consists of 17 items, each one scored from 0 to 3, with a maximum possible score of 51 points. The original study reported satisfactory internal consistency, test-retest reliability, and convergent validity, but there are no other validation data.

Behaviour observation scale Huntington, BOSH (14)
Aimed at describing the behavioural manifestations in later stages of HD, this scale is administered by nursing staff. It contains 32 items grouped in three subscales: activities of daily living (ADL); social-cognitive functioning; and mental rigidity and aggression. Inter-rater reliability and internal consistency are adequate, and the scale shows significant differences in HD manifestations as the disease progresses.

Sydenham's Chorea

UFMG Sydenham's chorea rating scale, USCRS (15)
The USCRS, designed to assess activities of daily living, behavioural problems and motor functioning in Sydenham's Chorea patients, contains 27 items scored from 0 (no symptom or sign) to 4 (severe disability). Test-retest and inter-rater

reliability have proved satisfactory. It is a scale owned and licensed by the Movement Disorder Society (MDS) (6).

Drug-induced movement disorders

Parkinsonism

Simpson-Angus scale, SAS (16)

This quick and easy scale, with 10 items scored from 1 to 5, is designed to assess the presence and severity of rigidity and bradykinesia induced by antipsychotics. It is the most widely used scale for extrapyramidal symptoms in clinical assays and has demonstrated internal consistency and inter-rater reliability in different populations. It is also suitable for clinical practice. Shortened versions with one and four items have been also developed

Global

Extrapyramidal symptom rating scale, ESRS (17)

It assesses the most frequent drug-induced movement disorders: parkinsonism, akathisia, dystonia, and tardive dyskinesia. It consists of 12 items that rate both frequency and movement amplitude using a 7-point response option for each item. The ESRS has shown satisfactory inter-rater reliability, convergent validity and sensitivity to change for antipsychotic-induced movement disorders and idiopathic Parkinson's disease (PD).

Dystonia

Generalized dystonia

Fahn-Marsden dystonia rating scale, F-M Scale (18)

This scale is divided into two parts: a movement evaluation that assesses the severity of dystonia and a patient-reported questionnaire assessing functional implications in activities of daily liv-

ing. The motor examination includes nine body regions (eyes, mouth, language/swallowing, arms, legs, and trunk). For each region, the rater evaluates: severity by five levels (0 = normal and 4 = severe); precipitating factors (provocation) by five levels (0 = no dystonia and 4 = dystonia at rest); and adds a weighting factor (0.5 for eyes, mouth and neck and 1.0 for the other body regions). The total score is the product of these three factors, with a maximum score of 120. The disability subscale evaluates the impact of dystonia on basic activities such as talking, writing, eating, swallowing, hygiene, dressing and walking, from the patient's perspective. Each item is also rated with up to five points (from 0 = normal to 4 = severe) except walking which is rated from 0 to 6, thus giving a maximum score of 30. The F-M scale is the standard instrument for assessing dystonia in clinical studies. It has shown adequate internal consistency, convergent validity and inter-rater (except for some body regions) and test-retest reliability. However, its sensitivity to change has still to be tested (19).

Unified dystonia rating scale, UDRS (20)

This scale was developed by expert consensus to overcome the limitations of the F-M Scale and includes a more detailed rating of 14 body regions and a dystonia duration factor, eliminating patients' perception of dystonia and the weighting factor. Maximum score is 112 and is the sum of two factors: severity and duration. Severity is scored from 0 (without dystonia) to 4 (extreme dystonia), and duration is also rated from 0 to 4, evaluating if dystonia occurs at rest or with action at maximal or submaximal intensity. The UDRS has been used as a measure of efficacy following surgical interventions and has shown better internal consistency than the F-M scale, satisfactory inter-rater reliability, and convergent validity with the F-M scale and global dystonia severity rating scale (GDS). However, its responsiveness has not been tested (20). It is a scale owned and licensed by the MDS (6).

Global Dystonia Rating Scale, GDS (20)

This rates dystonia severity in the same 14 regions evaluated by the UDRS, in a scale scored from 0 to 10 (0 = no dystonia, 1 = minimal dystonia, 5 = moderate dystonia, 10 = severe dystonia). The tested clinimetric properties (internal consistency, inter-rater reliability, and convergent validity) are excellent. It has been found to be easier to administer than the F-M and the UDRS. It is one of the scales owned and licensed by the MDS (6).

Blepharospasm

Blepharospasm rating scale, BRS (21)

This is a scale that rates the severity and disability caused by blepharospasm. It contains two sections: a movement scale (including severity of eyelid closure, frequency, location and precipitating factors for involuntary movements) and a disability scale. Only the disability section has been validated, with adequate internal consistency, convergent and discriminative validity, and responsiveness.

Blepharospasm disability scale, BDS (22)

Derived from the disability subscale of the BDS, it is a patient-reported, 8-item questionnaire regarding various activities of daily living (driving, reading, walking, etc.) with a varying score range (1 to 5 points) reaching a maximum score of 26. It is suitable for daily clinical practice since completion of the questionnaire is easy and takes only a few minutes. It has demonstrated satisfactory reliability, construct validity and sensitivity to change.

Cervical dystonia (CD)

Toronto Western spasmodic torticollis rating scale, TWSTRS (23)

The TWSTRS is a complex but very widely used scale for assessing CD in clinical practice and research. It consists of 3 subscales evaluating motor severity, disability and pain. Dystonia severity is rated by 10 items evaluating head posture in various axes, the effect of sensory tricks, range of motion and duration. It is scored heterogeneously with a maximum score of 35, and a teaching video is available. The disability subscale consists of 6 items assessing difficulties with several activities, scored from 0 to 5, with a maximum score of 30. The pain subscale measures intensity, duration, and disability due to pain, with a maximum score of 20. The total maximum scale score is 85. The TWSTRS is a validated scale, showing satisfactory inter-rater reliability and validity, but it has several disadvantages, such as the absence of items assessing dystonic tremor, no scientific evidence supporting the weighting of duration, underestimation of subtypes of CD, and the lack of information about its responsiveness (19).

Cervical dystonia severity scale, CDSS (24)

This scale is an objective measurement of head position in 5-degree intervals, using a wall chart and a protractor. The patient sits at rest, in a relaxed position, with eyes closed, without head support or sensory tricks. Head rotation deviation, laterocollis and anterocollis/retrocollis scores are measured in degrees of deviation (from 0 to 90°) and are transformed into a severity scale. Maximum score is 54. Good inter-rater and test-retest reliability was found in the original study, but validity and sensitivity studies are still required.

Spasmodic torticollis rating scale, STRS (25)

It is a brief and relatively simple scale with four subscales (movement amplitude, duration, shoulder elevation, and tremor) specifically designed to measure cervical dystonia severity in clinical trials. Only inter-rater reliability has been tested with satisfactory results, and it shows sensitivity to changes due to treatment, but some studies have detected significant differences between the scores and the patient's subjective report of therapeutic response and lack of standardized administration (19).

Torticollis rating scale, TRS (21)

This scale is aimed at evaluating both movement and disability of torticollis. The movement domain assesses direction of muscle pulling, influencing factors, severity of deformity and pain, and presence of jerking movements, with heterogeneous item scoring. The activities of daily living domain is scored on a scale from 1 to 2, 3 or 5 points (maximum score: 27). It has not yet been validated.

Limb dystonia

Arm dystonia disability scale, ADDS (21)

The ADDS assesses the functional impairment of the dystonic hand. It consists of 7 items scored from 0 to 3. It has been used as a treatment efficacy measure and shows adequate convergent validity with other rating scales.

Writer's cramp rating scale, WCRS (26)

This is an objective measure designed to quantify task-specific writer's dystonia severity and treatment response. It is divided into two parts: dystonic signs during writing with three items (dystonic posturing, latency and tremor) and writing speed (one item). Item scores range from 0 (none) to 2 (marked/severe). This scale has been mainly used to assess treatment efficacy, with good results. Inter-rater reliability was also satisfactory, though correlation with other writer's cramp measures (ADDS, kinematic patterns analysis) was low.

Frequency of abnormal movements scale, FAM Scale (27)

This was developed to assess musician's dystonia. The FAM score is the number of abnormal movements per second when playing an instrument. Internal consistency, test-retest and inter-rater reliability, convergent validity, and sensitivity are satisfactory and better than the F-M Scale and ADDS in assessing musician's dystonia.

Leg dystonia disability scale, LDRS (21)

It assesses functional impairment caused by dystonia of a lower limb when standing, walking, and other activities. It consists of 7 items, with the final total score expressed as a percentage. It has not been validated.

Oromandibular Dystonia

Oromandibular dystonia rating scale, ODRS (21)

It consists of a severity (severity, frequency, location, and influencing factors) and a disability scale for oromandibular dystonia. It has not been validated.

Myoclonus

Martí & Tolosa scale, MT scale (28)

Designed for the assessment of treatment efficacy in hemifacial spasm, a peripheral myoclonus, it rates severity, frequency and functional impairment. Severity is rated on a scale from 0 (no spasm) to 4 (severe). Frequency is scored from 0 (absent) to 5 (>75% of the time). Functional impairment, with 7 items (reading, sleep, social life, movies/television, concentration, eating, and conversation), is scored from 0 (no impairment) to 3 (severe). The maximum score is 21. Test-retest and inter-rater reliability have been analyzed, with good results.

Unified myoclonus rating scale, UMRS (29)

The UMRS assesses the characteristics and severity of myoclonus as well as functional implications. It contains 73 items, grouped into 5 sections: patient's questionnaire (12 items, scored from 1 to 5); myoclonus at rest (8 items, scored from 0 to 4, rating frequency and amplitude); stimulus sensitivity (17 items, dichotomous); myoclonus with action (10 items, scored for frequency and amplitude on a 5-point scale); and functional tests (5 items, scored from 0 to 4). It has also an item on global disability, ranging from 0 (normal) to 4 (severe disability, invalid) and two items on negative myoclonus, rating presence (yes/no) and severity (from 0, not present, to 3, severe). The UMRS displays good internal consistency and inter-rater reliability, as well as adequate sensitivity to change.

Parkinson's disease (PD)

Multi-domain scales

Unified Parkinson's disease rating scale (UPDRS) (30)

The UPDRS has until recently been the most widely used scale for assessing Parkinson's disease severity, both in clinical practice and in research settings. It is composed of four subscales: Section I, mentation, behaviour and mood; Section II, activities of daily living (ADL); Section III, motor examination; and Section IV, complications. In Sections I to III, items are scored on a 5-point scale, from 0 (no problems or normal) to 4 (severe problems). In Section IV, items are scored for presence (yes/no) and duration or severity of the problem (5-point scale, from 0 to 4). The UPDRS also includes the Hoehn and Yahr staging system and the Schwab and England scale, which are described below in this chapter.

The clinimetric properties of the UPDRS have been extensively tested (31), showing good internal consistency, adequate inter-rater and test-retest reliability and satisfactory validity. Its sensitivity to change has made it a reference measure for regulatory agencies. However, some shortcomings such as lack of symptoms addressing non-motor manifestations, redundancies in Sections II and III, inconsistent allocation of items, and cultural bias have been identified.

Movement disorders society-sponsored version of the UPDRS (MDS-UPDRS) (32)

This is the revised version of the UPDRS, designed to overcome its limitations. It maintains the UPDRS structure in four sections, although they have been renamed: Part I, non-motor experiences of daily living, with 6 rater-based items

and 7 for self-assessment; Part II, motor experiences of daily living, with 13 patient-based items; Part III, motor examination, 18 items (33 scores); and Part IV, motor complications, with 6 items. Items in Parts I to III are scored from 0 (normal) to 4 (severe). For Part IV, items are scored for presence (yes/no), frequency and severity of symptoms (from 0 to 4). Formulas for converting UPDRS scores into MDS-UPDRS scores (and vice versa) have been calculated.

The MDS-UPDRS has been carefully designed to be applicable to PD patients across all levels of severity and disability, avoiding medical jargon and with a vocabulary adapted to a seventh-grade level. Its psychometric properties are satisfactory (33), and it seems to be responsive, although its use in clinical trials is still scarce. Translations and certified raters training are available through the MDS (6).

Global severity

Hoehn and Yahr staging (HY) (34)

This is the most widely used system to classify the evolutionary course of PD. The original HY consists of a 5-point scale-scored single item (from 1 to 5) based on the patient's global functional and clinical status. A modification with 7 stages is also often used. It shows satisfactory inter-rater reliability and association with measures of quality of life, objective motor performance and disability. However, there is no data on its test-retest reliability, and its responsiveness is low, especially in the early stages. A revision of its clinimetric properties, advantages and disadvantages has been published (35).

Clinical impression of severity index (CISI-PD) (36)

This is a global severity index formed of 4 items: motor signs, disability, cognitive status and motor complications. All items are rated from 0 (not at all) to 6 (very severe or very disabled). The CISI-PD displays satisfactory internal consistency and test-retest reliability. It is highly correlated with the UPDRS, the HY and other clinical and psychosocial measures of PD. However, there is no information about responsiveness and inter-rater reliability.

Motor impairment and disability

Scales for outcomes in Parkinson's disease (SCOPA)-motor (37)

This is a scale developed for assessing motor signs (10 items), impairments in activities of daily living (7 items) and motor complications (4 items). Items are scored in a 4-point scale ranging from 0 (normal) to 3 (severe). The SCOPA-motor, with translations available in several languages, shows adequate internal consistency, inter-rater reliability and construct validity, with higher scores for more advanced disease stages. Although it has been used in several studies, there is no information on test-retest reliability and responsiveness.

Intermediate scale for assessment of Parkinson's disease (ISAPD) (38)

The ISAPD is a short scale composed of two sections, one on functional aspects (13 items) and the other on dyskinesias and fluctuations (4 items). All items are scored on a 4-point scale, from 0 to 3. The clinimetric properties, only assessed by the scale developers, are satisfactory, with good internal consistency and inter-rater-reliability, and moderate to high correlations with HY, UPDRS and Schwab and England Scale.

Schwab and England scale (SES) (39)

The SES has become a standard measure for the assessment of disability in clinical trials and research due to its simplicity, and it is included in the UPDRS. It consists of a single item scored from 100% (completely independent) to 0% (bedridden and in a vegetative state). However, it was not specifically designed for PD patients, and the information on its reliability and validity in this population is still limited. It displays convergent validity with other clinical and disability scales and responsiveness.

Rating scale for gait evaluation (RSGE) (40)

This is a scale for the global assessment of gait in PD patients, with two versions: the original one with 23 items, and a second version (2.0) that excludes two items on dyskinesia and axial rigidity. The RSGE is composed of four sections: socio-economic, functional, examination, and complications, with items scored from 0 to 3. Both versions showed adequate internal consistency, good inter-rater reliability and high correlation coefficients with other disability and clinical measures. The version 2.0 significantly distinguished among patients grouped by HY stages and showed good precision. There is no information on its responsiveness.

Motor complications and fluctuations

Unified dyskinesia rating scale (UDysRS) (41)

Intended to capture the essential features of dyskinesia in PD, the UDysRS is a scale with two sections: historical (on-dyskinesia and off-dystonia) and objective (impairment and disability). Good clinimetric properties have been demonstrated, with high internal consistency and acceptable inter-rater and test-retest reliability. The UDysRS is superior to other dyskinesia scales for detecting treatment effects. A standardized training program has been developed. It is one of the scales for dyskinesia recommended by the MDS (42).

Rush dyskinesia rating scale (RDysRS) (43)

This scale is aimed at assessing dyskinesia during three standardized motor tasks: walking, drinking from a cup and dressing. Severity of dyskinesia is rated from 0 (absent) to 4 (violent dyskinesia, incompatible with any normal motor task). Its clinimetric properties have been reviewed by the MDS, and it meets the criteria for being deemed recommended (43), despite some limitations.

Wearing-off questionnaires (WOQ) (44-47)

The set of wearing-off questionnaires were designed as self-completed screening tools for wearing-off. There are four versions, with 9 (WOQ-9), 10 (Q10), 19 (WOQ-19, or patient card questionnaire or the QUICK questionnaire), or 32 items (WOQ-32 or patient questionnaire). The 19-item version has shown good internal consistency and test-retest reliability, and it has an established cutoff of two symptoms. WOQ-19 and WOQ-9 are recommended by the MDS Task Force, whereas WOQ-32 is suggested for screening of wearing-off in PD (48).

Abnormal involuntary movement scale (AIMS) (49)

The AIMS assesses the severity of abnormal movements in different parts of the body with 10 items rated in a 5-point scale, from 0 to 4 (absent, minimal, mild, moderate, severe). It also includes three global assessments: overall severity, disability and patient's awareness of dyskinesias. Its satisfactory inter-rater and test-retest reliability, good convergent validity with other dyskinesia measures, wide use in clinical trials, and sensitivity to change made it a recommended scale (42).

Parkinsonisms

Multiple system atrophy (MSA)

Unified multiple system atrophy rating scale (UMSARS) (50)

This is a global scale designed to assess motor and autonomic manifestations and disability, composed of 4 subscales. Part I (historical review) includes 12 items and Part II (motor examination) has 14 items, with items scored from 0 to 4. Part III (autonomic examination) assesses cardiovascular parameters and orthostatic symptoms. Part IV (global disability scale) rates overall disability in a scale ranging from 1 (completely independent) to 5 (totally dependent). The development of the scale was based on the revision of other ex-

isting scales, previous literature on MSA and the principles set up by the European MSA-Study Group task force. Psychometric properties are adequate: high internal consistency in Parts I and II, good inter-rater reliability for Parts I, II and III, and satisfactory convergent, internal and discriminative validity. The UMSARS seems to capture disease progression and changes over time, and thus, it can be used as an outcome measure in clinical trials. However, there is a need for further validation and responsiveness studies. It is owned and licensed by the MDS (6).

Progressive supranuclear palsy (PSP)

Progressive supranuclear palsy rating scale (PSPRS) (51)

The PSPRS is a comprehensive disability measure for PSP composed of six dimensions: daily activities, behaviour, bulbar, ocular motor, limb motor and gait/midline examinations. It has 28 items scored 0-2 (6 items) and 0-4, providing a total score of 0-100. The scale has predictive validity in relation to subsequent survival.

Natural history and neuroprotection in Parkinson plus syndromes scale (NNIPPS) (52)

The NNIPPS scale was designed with the objective of developing a comprehensive rating scale for both PSP and MSA that can be applied in the early stages of disease. It has 83 items grouped in 15 dimensions assessing activity of daily living/mobility, axial bradykinesia, limb bradykinesia, rigidity, oculomotor, cerebellar, bulbar/pseudo-bulbar, mental, orthostatic, urinary, limb dystonia, axial dystonia, pyramidal, myoclonus and tremor. It has good internal consistency and inter-rater reliability in total scores and most dimensions, and it correlates with other clinical and severity measures. Responsiveness was higher for PSP than for MSA.

Psychogenic movement disorders

Rating scale for psychogenic movement disorders, PMD scale (53)

This is the most widely used scale to assess the complex phenomenology seen in psychogenic patients. The scale rates 10 types of manifestations (rest tremor, action tremor, dystonia, chorea, bradykinesia, myoclonus, tics, athetosis, ballism, and cerebellar ataxia), two functions (gait, speech) and 14 body regions. Items are scored for severity (from 0 = none, to 4 = severe), duration (from 0 = none, to 4 = >75% of the time) and incapacitation (from 0 = none, to 4 = severe). A total phenomenology and total function score and a total scale score can be calculated. Some clinimetric properties (inter-rater reliability, construct validity and responsiveness) have been studied, with satisfactory results.

Restless legs syndrome (RLS)

International restless legs syndrome study group (IRLS) rating scale (54)

The IRLS scale has been widely used in clinical trials and epidemiological studies to measure the severity and impact of RLS. It is a 10-item, self-administered scale with items scored from 0 (none) to 4 (very severe). Clinimetric properties have been extensively analyzed, using both CTT and IRT approaches: internal consistency, test-retest and inter-rater reliability, and the convergent and criterion validity have been found adequate. Factor analysis has revealed two factors: symptoms and symptom impact.

Johns Hopkins restless legs syndrome severity scale, JHRLSS (55)

This is a single-item scale that asks about the usual time of day when RLS symptoms start, rating severity from 0 (never, no symptoms) to 4 (severe, symptoms may start in the afternoon or may be present all day long). The scale correlates well with other RLS and sleep measures, and shows good inter-rater reliability. A telephone-based interview version has been derived from the JHRLSS (Johns Hopkins telephone diagnostic interview, TDI), with good clinimetric properties.

Tics and Gilles de la Tourette syndrome

Yale global tic severity scale, YGTSS (56)

The YGTSS is a complex global scale of the clinician's overall impression of the symptoms. It is made up of a semi-structured interview for the evaluation of motor and phonic symptom severity, including a tic inventory, as well as items on the number, frequency, intensity, complexity, and interference of motor and phonic tics, scored from 0 (none/absent) to 5 (severe/always). Total motor and phonic scores, an overall impairment rating, and a global severity score (the sum of motor, phonic, and impairment scores) can be calculated. Satisfactory results in terms of internal consistency, test-retest reliability and validity have been found. It is also sensitive to changes due to treatment.

Tourette syndrome global scale, TSGS (57)

The TSGS is a complex multidimensional scale with two parts: symptoms (4 dimensions, scored for frequency from 0 to 5, and degree of disruption, from 1 to 5) and social functioning (3 dimensions, rated on a continuous scale from 0, no impairment, to 25, severe impairment). Subscores and a total global score can be obtained. Despite its weaknesses (e.g., complexity, failure to assess tic types, lack of full validation studies), the TSGS has been used as a primary outcome variable in clinical trials, with good inter-rater reliability.

Shapiro tourette syndrome severity scale, STSSS (58)

It is a simple to use, valid, and reliable global severity rating of Tourette syndrome and its associated social disability. It contains 5 items: degree to which tics are noticeable to others; whether they elicit comments of curiosity; whether other individuals consider the patient odd or bizarre; whether tics interfere with functioning; and whether the patient is incapacitated, homebound or hospitalized, with a total score which provides a global severity index. It has been used to measure treatment results but does not include any assessment of tic characteristics.

Tremor

Washington Heights-Inwood genetic study of essential tremor rating scale, WHIGET (59)

This scale aims to evaluate the intensity, amplitude, oscillation prevalence, and persistence of essential tremor in a variety of tasks, distinguishing between rest, kinetic and postural tremors. The scale is made up of 26 items scored on a scale from 0 (no tremor) to 3 (large amplitude tremors that interfere severely with task). A revised version adds a score of 4 (very large amplitude tremor that renders the task impossible), with a teaching videotape, to ensure the scale's sensitivity and reliability in clinical trials. The scale displays good test-retest and inter-rater reliability and convergent validity with other measures of tremor.

Conclusions

The use of rating scales for the assessment of patients with movement disorders is necessary for sharing information, quantifying health status, and reporting research outcomes. When more than one scale is available, selection of the most suitable measure should be based on the designated study objectives, the target population and knowledge of the scales' characteristics and quality of psychometric attributes (namely, reliability, validity, and sensitivity to capture change). Other factors may also play an important role in scale selection, such as experience applying the scale, time of administration, use in similar studies, regulatory agency rules, payment for rights of use, and availability of statistical programs to analyze the results.

The rating scales revisions performed by the MDS task force are an important source of information (6). We recommend following the activity of this collaboration, which is actively incorporating new reviews on scales used for PD and also for a diversity of movement disorders. Many of the scales cited here can be obtained from the internet, in the 'We move' webpage (www.mdvu.org/library/ratingscales/) and through the MDS webpage (www.movementdisorders.org/publications/rating_scales/) (6).

References

1 Nunnally JC, Bernstein IH. Psychometric theory. New York: McGraw Hill; 1994.

2 Hobart JC, Cano SJ, Zajicek JP, Thompson AJ. Rating scales as outcome measures for clinical trials in neurology: problems, solutions, and recommendations. Lancet Neurol. 2007;6:1094-1105.

3 Terwee CB, Bot SDM, de Boer MR, van der Windt DAWM, Knol DL, Dekker J, et al. Quality criteria were proposed for measurement properties of health status questionnaires. J. Clin. Epidemiol. 2007;60:34-42.

4 Streiner DL, Norman GR. Health measurement scales. A practical guide to their development and use. 4th ed. Oxford: Oxford University Press; 2008.

5 Martinez-Martin P, Rodríguez-Blázquez C, Forjaz MJ. Rating scales in movement disorders. In: Kompoliti K, Verhagen Metman L, eds. Encyclopedia of Movement Disorders. Oxford: Academic Press. 2010; 8-16.

6 Movement Disorders Society. Rating Scales. (April 22, 2013). Retrieved from: www.movementdisorders.org/publications/rating_scales/

7 Barnes TR. A rating scale for drug-induced akathisia. Br. J. Psychiatry. 1989;154:672-676.

8 Schmitz-Hübsch T, du Montcel ST, Baliko L, et al. Scale for the assessment and rating of ataxia: development of a new clinical scale. Neurology. 2006;66:1717-1720.

9 Trouillas P, Takayanagi T, Hallett M, et al. International Cooperative Ataxia Rating Scale for pharmacological assessment of the cerebellar syndrome. The Ataxia Neuropharmacology Committee of

the World Federation of Neurology J Neurol Sci 1997;145:205-211.

10 Unified Huntington's Disease Rating Scale: reliability and consistency. Huntington Study Group. Mov Disord 1996;11:136-42.

11 Siesling S, Zwinderman AH, van Vugt JP, Kieburtz K, Roos RA. A shortened version of the motor section of the Unified Huntington's Disease Rating Scale. Mov Disord 1997;12:229-234.

12 Shoulson I, Fahn S. Huntington disease: clinical care and evaluation. Neurology 1979;29:1-3.

13 Bylsma FW, Rothlind J, Hall MR, Folstein SE, Brandt J. Assessment of adaptive functioning in Huntington's disease. Mov Disord 1993;8(2):183-90.

14 Timman R, Claus H, Slingerland H, et al. Nature and development of Huntington disease in a nursing home population: The Behavior Observation Scale Huntington (BOSH). Cogn Behav Neurol 2005;18:215-222.

15 Teixeira AL Jr, Maia DP, Cardoso F. UFMG Sydenham's chorea rating scale (USCRS): reliability and consistency. Mov Disord 2005;20:585-591.

16 Simpson GM, Angus JW. A rating scale for extrapyramidal side effects. Acta Psychiatr Scand 1970;212S:11-19.

17 Chouinard G, Margolese HC. Manual for the Extrapyramidal Symptom Rating Scale (ESRS). Schizophr Res 2005;76:247-265.

18 Burke RE, Fahn S, Marsden CD, Bressman SB, Moskowitz C, Friedman J. Validity and reliability of a rating scale for the primary torsion dystonias. Neurology 1985;35:73-77.

19 Jost WH, Hefter H, Stenner A, Reichel G. Rating scales for cervical dystonia: a critical evaluation of tools for outcome assessment of botulinum toxin therapy. J Neural Transm 2013;120:487-496.

20 Comella CL, Leurgans S, Wuu J, Stebbins GT, Chmura T. Rating scales for dystonia: a multicenter assessment. Mov Disord 2003;18:303-312.

21 Fahn S. Assessment of primary dystonias. In: Munsat T, ed. Quantification of neurological deficit. Boston: Butterworths1989;241-270.

22 Lindeboom R, De Haan R, Aramideh M, Speelman JD. The blepharospasm disability scale: an instrument for the assessment of functional health in blepharospasm. Mov Disord 1995;10:444-449.

23 Consky ES, Lang AE. Clinical assessments of patients with cervical dystonia. In: Jankovic J, Hallett M, eds. Therapy with Botulinum Toxin. New York: Marcel Dekker, Inc.;1994;211-237.

24 O'Brien C, Brashear A, Cullis P, et al. Cervical dystonia severity scale reliability study. Mov Disord 2001;16:1086-1090.

25 Tsui JK, Eisen A, Stoessl AJ, Calne S, Calne DB. Double-blind study of botulinum toxin in spasmodic torticollis. Lancet 1986;2:245-247.

26 Wissel J, Kabus C, Wenzel R, et al. Botulinum toxin in writer's cramp: objective response evaluation in 31 patients. J Neurol Neurosurg Psychiatry 1996;61:172-175.

27 Spector JT, Brandfonbrener AG. A new method for quantification of musician's dystonia: The frequency of abnormal movements scale. Med Probl Perform Art 2005;20:157-162.

28 Martí MJ, Tolosa E, Alom J. Botulinum toxin in hemifacial spasm: A double-blind controlled trial. In: Bartko D, editor. New Trends in Clinical Neuropharmacology: Calcium Antagonists, Acute Neurology, Headache and Movement Disorders. London: John Libbey & Co. 1988;304-307.

29 Frucht SJ, Leurgans SE, Hallett M, Fahn S. The Unified Myoclonus Rating Scale. Adv Neurol 2002;89:361-376.

30 Fahn S, Elton R, UPDRS program members. Unified Parkinson's disease rating scale. In: Fahn S, Marsden C, Goldstein M, Calne D, eds. Recent Developments in Parkinson's Disease. Florham Park, NJ: Macmillan Healthcare Information 1987;153-163.

31 The Unified Parkinson's Disease Rating Scale (UPDRS): status and recommendations. Mov Disord 2003;18:738-750.

32 Goetz CG, Fahn S, Martinez-Martin P, et al. Movement Disorder Society-sponsored revision of the Unified Parkinson's Disease Rating Scale (MDS-UPDRS): Process, format, and clinimetric testing plan. Mov Disord 2007;22:41-47.

32 Goetz CG, Tilly BC, Shaftman SR, et al. Movement Disorder Society-sponsored revision of the Unified Parkinson's Disease Rating Scale (MDS-UPDRS):

Scale presentation and clinimetric testing results Mov Disord 2008;23:2169-2170.

34 Hoehn MM, Yahr MD. Parkinsonism: onset, progression and mortality. Neurology 1967;17:427-442.

35 Goetz CG, Poewe W, Rascol O, et al. Movement Disorder Society Task Force report on the Hoehn and Yahr staging scale: status and recommendations. Mov Disord 2004;19:1020-1028.

36 Martínez-Martín P, Rodríguez-Blázquez C, Forjaz MJ, de Pedro J. The Clinical Impression of Severity Index for Parkinson's Disease: international validation study. Mov Disord 2009;24:211-217.

37 Marinus J, Visser M, Stiggelbout AM, et al. A short scale for the assessment of motor impairments and disabilities in Parkinson's disease: the SPES/SCOPA. J Neurol Neurosurg Psychiatry 2004;75:388-395.

38 Martínez-Martín P, Gil-Nagel A, Morlán Gracia L, et al. Intermediate scale for assessment of Parkinson's disease. Characteristics and structure. Parkinsonism Relat Disord 1995;1:97-102.

39 Schwab R, England A. Projection technique for evaluating surgery in Parkinson's disease. In: Gillingham FJ, Donaldson IML, eds. Third symposium for Parkinson's disease. Edingburg: Livingstone1969;152-157.

40 Martínez-Martín P, García Urra D, del Ser Quijano T, et al. A new clinical tool for gait evaluation in Parkinson's disease. Clin Neuropharmacol 1997;20:183-194.

41 Goetz CG, Nutt JG, Stebbins GT. The Unified Dyskinesia Rating Scale: presentation and clinimetric profile. Mov Disord 2008;23:2398-2403.

42 Colosimo C, Martínez-Martín P, Fabbrini G, et al. Task force report on scales to assess dyskinesia in Parkinson's disease: critique and recommendations. Mov Disord 2010;25:1131-1142.

43 Goetz CG, Stebbins GT, Shale HM, et al. Utility of an objective dyskinesia rating scale for Parkinson's disease: inter- and intrarater reliability assessment. Mov Disord 1994;9:390-394.

44 Stacy M, Bowron A, Guttman M, et al. Identification of motor and nonmotor wearing-off in Parkinson's disease: Comparison of a patient questionnaire versus a clinician assessment. Mov Disord 2005;20:726-733.

45 Stacy M, Hauser R. Development of a Patient Questionnaire to facilitate recognition of motor and non-motor wearing-off in Parkinson's disease. J Neural Transm 2007;114:211-217.

46 Stacy MA, Murphy JM, Greeley DR, Stewart RM, Murck H, Meng X. The sensitivity and specificity of the 9-item Wearing-off Questionnaire. Parkinsonism Relat Disord 2008;14:205-212.

47 Martinez-Martin P, Hernandez B. The Q10 questionnaire for detection of wearing-off phenomena in Parkinson's disease. Parkinsonism Relat Disord 2012;18:382-385.

48 Antonini A, Martinez-Martin P, Chaudhuri RK, et al. Wearing-off scales in Parkinson's disease: Critique and recommendations. Mov Disord 2011;26:2169-2175.

49 Guy W. Abnormal Involuntary Movement Scale. ECDEU Assessment manual for psychopharmacology. Washington DC: US Government Printing Office; 1976.

50 Wenning GK, Tison F, Seppi K, et al. Development and validation of the Unified Multiple System Atrophy Rating Scale (UMSARS). Mov Disord 2004;19:1391-1402.

51 Golbe LI, Ohman-Strickland PA. A clinical rating scale for progressive supranuclear palsy. Brain 2007;130:1552-1565.

52 Rolland Y, Vérin M, Payan CA, et al. A new MRI rating scale for progressive supranuclear palsy and multiple system atrophy: validity and reliability. J Neurol Neurosurg Psychiatry 2011;82:1025-1032.

53 Hinson VK, Cubo E, Comella CL, Goetz CG, Leurgans S. Rating scale for psychogenic movement disorders: scale development and clinimetric testing. Mov Disord 2005;20:1592-1597.

54 Walters AS, LeBrocq C, Dhar A, et al. Validation of the International Restless Legs Syndrome Study Group rating scale for restless legs syndrome. Sleep Med 2003;4:121-132.

55 Allen RP, Earley CJ. Validation of the Johns Hopkins restless legs severity scale. Sleep Med 2001;2:239-242.

56 Leckman JF, Riddle MA, Hardin MT, et al. The Yale Global Tic Severity Scale: initial testing of a clinician-rated scale of tic severity. J Am Acad Child Adolesc Psychiatry 1989;28:566-573.

57 Harcherik DF, Leckman JF, Detlor J, Cohen DJ. A
    new instrument for clinical studies of Tourette's syn-
    drome. J Am Acad Child Psychiatry 1984;23:153-160.

58 Shapiro AK, Shapiro E. Controlled study of pi-
    mozide vs. placebo in Tourette's syndrome. J Am
    Acad Child Psychiatry 1984;23:161-173.

59 Louis ED, Ottman R, Ford B, et al. The Washington
    Heights-Inwood Genetic Study of Essential Tremor:
    methodologic issues in essential-tremor research.
    Neuroepidemiology 1997;16:124-133.

44

Clinical Neurophysiology in Movement Disorders

John N. Caviness

There have been many significant discoveries about the molecular pathogenesis of various movement disorders in the last two decades. It is not yet clear in most instances how genetic and other biochemical abnormalities alter the movement circuitry of the central nervous system (CNS). We do know that these mechanisms create abnormal movement physiology within the CNS. These movement circuit abnormalities are transmitted via projecting motor pathways to produce the electrophysiological activation of the muscles which result in the various phenotypes. Clinical neurophysiology evaluates the abnormal electrophysiological activation of muscles as well as the involved parts of the CNS circuitry when possible.

Both hypokinetic/parkinsonism and hyperkinetic movement disorders exhibit multiple types of neurophysiological abnormalities. This manuscript will focus on electrophysiological abnormalities that are recorded with non-invasive techniques such as conventional scalp electro-encephalography (EEG) and surface electromyography (EMG), collectively called 'clinical neurophysiology'. Classic abnormalities may be observed during rest or with postural/kinetic activation tasks, while others must be elicited with sensory stimuli or more complex task or behavioural paradigms.

Careful clinical visual inspection is and must necessarily remain the primary method of movement disorder phenotypic classification. This chapter will discuss the movement disor-

der phenotypes of parkinsonism, tremor, myoclonus, periodic limb movements, dystonia, chorea, and tics. There are other phenotypes that will not be discussed that either are derivatives of them or are rare. Despite the acknowledged value of careful visual observation, there are limits to what even movement disorder experts can discern. The accurate classification of a movement disorder may depend on information that can only be accurately ascertained by clinical neurophysiology. For example, does the movement occur in a body part that is fully relaxed? Also, rhythmicity is not absolute in being present or not present. Mild irregularity may be evident only on the neurophysiology recordings. If a myoclonus is small and repetitive with muscle activation, it may appear to be a fast, mildly irregular tremor, but the surface EMG will show short duration hypersynchronous myoclonus EMG discharges. The ability to discern between these movement disorder phenotypes is critical for the diagnosis and treatment strategy. Thus, clinical neurophysiology techniques represent a true extension of the clinical examination (1). Besides adding information to the inspection of abnormal movement, clinical neurophysiology increases the sensitivity of detection and, in some instances, identifies pattern specificity that visual inspection does not provide.

Basic neurophysiology techniques for movement disorders

It is strongly recommended that those who perform neurophysiological examination of movement disorders should be trained in the basic principles of bioelectric signals. This includes routine clinical EEG and EMG recording and their clinical diagnostic uses. Safety considerations and artifact recognition cannot be covered here in detail, but training in these aspects is necessary. Surface EMG is the most important technique for movement disorders, but other useful tests include EEG, EEG-EMG polygraphy with back-averaging, elicited responses that include evoked potentials, and certain other reflex responses and task paradigms. Polygraphic EMG recording can define the temporal resolution on the order of milliseconds. Furthermore, the surface EMG reflects not only alpha motor neuron activity but more importantly the resultant normal or abnormal modulation patterns from the CNS. The patterns of abnormal and normal findings for certain movement disorders have been well described, and these characteristics can be used as supportive evidence for a more specific movement disorder diagnosis and/or origin.

Surface EMG

Surface EMG studies are non-invasive and are within the capability of most clinical neurophysiology laboratories. It can be performed with disk electrodes. Disposable adhesive Ag/AgCl EKG electrodes are often more convenient because they can be applied faster, which may be important when multiple muscles need to be recorded. The patient should be asked about any type of adhesive/tape allergies. After the skin has been cleaned and mildly abraded, the electrodes are placed 3-5 cm apart over the muscle belly, parallel to the direction of the muscle fibers. Special care should be taken with older individuals with thin skin and those who are anti-coagulated. If EEG is also to be recorded, the EEG ground may also suffice for the surface EMG electrodes. If only surface EMG is recorded, the iliac crest or another relatively inactive site will work for the ground electrode. Electrode impedances should be below 5 kilo-ohm for a high-quality recording, but more modern and advanced amplifiers may produce an EMG signal that lacks artifact (e.g. 60 Hz) with higher impedances.

A technical limitation of surface EMG studies is the lack of muscle selectivity. Unlike needle EMG, adjacent muscles inevitably contribute 'crosstalk' to the signal through volume conduction. This effect is minimized by the use of short interelectrode distances and by recording from relatively superficial and isolated muscles, such as the biceps, deltoid, quadriceps, tibialis anterior, or first dorsal interosseus. When recording from a group of muscles cannot be avoided, such as the wrist flexors or extensors, the group label should be used. For some movement disorders (e.g. tremor), an accelerometer is useful in addition to EMG recording for frequency measurements.

Ideally, a trained individual should monitor the surface EMG signal as it is being recorded. In this way, the correctness of that task can be ensured. In addition, it is important that monitoring for artifacts be done as the recording is happening. Such artifacts can often be corrected before the patient or subject leaves the laboratory. The quality of the surface EMG signal must also be assessed offline during analysis. Deep muscles, such as the gluteus maximus or any muscle in an obese person, may produce a signal that is too degraded for analysis. The frequency spectrum of the signal contains power throughout the range between 1 and 1000 Hz, with maximal power at approximately 100 Hz. In practice, a low-frequency filter cut-off of 1-30 Hz is used to eliminate the unwanted effects of DC (direct current) potential and low-frequency movement artifact. A high-frequency filter setting of 200-3kHz passes the high-frequency components of the signal. After the surface EMG signal has been collected, it may be displayed as recorded or it may be preferable to filter and/or digitally process the signal to display a full-wave rectified signal. In addition to correlating abnormal movements with surface EMG activity, it is important to note discharge duration, variability, and timing relationships between muscles.

Recording samples should be taken during rest, postural activation (e.g. arms outstretched), kinetic activation (e.g. finger to nose), functional tasks (e.g. drinking from a cup, handwriting), mental activation (e.g. counting backwards), and while performing associated movements (e.g. contralateral repetitive hand movements). The condition or state(s) that are known to bring out the movement disorder should be emphasized. This may include sleep. Of course, it is important to allow enough time to sample the movement disorder that is troubling the patient.

EEG

EEG recordings are made from electrodes in the standard 10-20 positions. Full-head coverage is useful for localization, particularly when using EEG mapping software. Important EEG electrode locations include frontal, central, parietal, and midline positions since they are usually the most active ones in movement disorders. EEG is very useful for correlating the state of consciousness with abnormal movement. Any EEG abnormality seen may have important diagnostic implications for the movement disorder, but paroxysmal abnormalities (e.g. epileptiform) are particularly relevant.

EEG-EMG polygraphy with back-averaging

The neurophysiologic evaluation of movement disorders is enhanced by simultaneous recording of EEG, surface EMG, and other modalities. This allows the potential detection of specific relationships between different types of physiological activity. Reflex activation by touch, deep tendon reflex, mixed nerve stimulation (median, tibial), light, sound, and digital nerve stimulation can be examined in this way. It is useful to add a channel to monitor the stimulus production. Back-averaging with computer assistance can be performed by marking the beginning of an EMG event or stimulus. This may be done online or offline. Epochs are then defined with time included both before and after the event marker (or trigger). Computer averaging of epochs increases the signal-to-noise ratio and allows the detection of time-locked relationships between waveforms of the same or different modalities. The larger the number of epochs used in the calculation, the more likely a smaller waveform will be discernible from the background EEG activity. A minimum of 100 epochs to show a time-locked relationship between EEG, EMG and other events is usually adequate, but more may be required. If an absence of a back-average movement-associated EEG transient is expected, then at least 200 epochs should be processed. More epochs may be needed if there is increased noise. Waveform averaging should be critically evaluated for its reproducibility, signal-to-noise ratio, and its ability to produce physiologically significant waves that are able to be interpreted logically.

Elicited or Reflex Responses

Evoked potentials and surface EMG responses to stimulation may be performed by standard techniques. If the movement disorder being examined is elicited by certain stimuli, then those stimuli should be part of the examination. The choice of what type of elicited response to test for is dictated by the known abnormalities in various movement disorders. The somatosensory evoked potential and long latency surface EMG reflexes are useful for the detection of cortical hyperexcitability in cases of myoclonus. Certain epilepsy syndromes respond to photic stimulation. Startle disorders typically show non-fatigable surface EMG responses of axial and proximal limb muscles. Other examples also exist. Proper grounding and other safety principles for electrical stimulation must be followed.

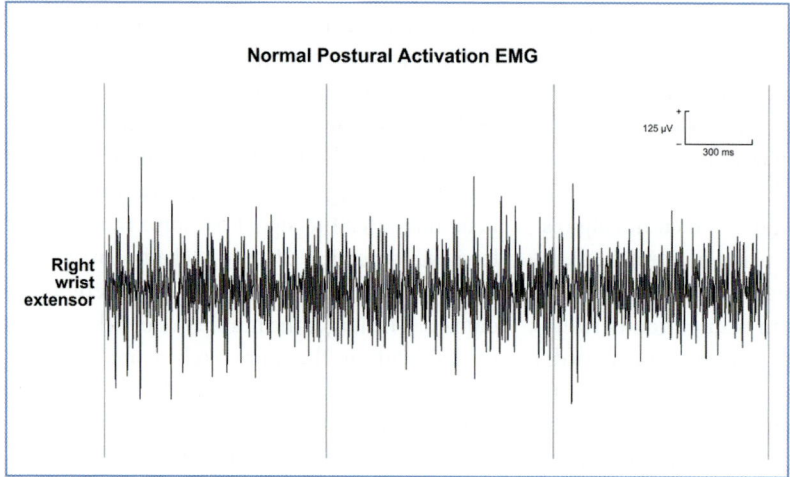

Figure 44.1
Surface EMG pattern during postural wrist extensor muscle contraction. There is a normal 'interference' signal pattern reflecting nearly continuous muscle electrical activation.

Clinical neurophysiology in movement disorders

Normal movements

A surface EMG records activation of multiple motor units. When an individual holds a body part in a constant posture against gravity, a tonic pattern of motor units is seen. The visual appearance is that of an 'interference pattern' of high-frequency EMG components without obvious modulation of frequency or amplitude (see Figure 44.1).

Such a posture elicits a broad frequency band of EMG activation that is mostly above 25 Hz (see Figure 44.2).

Most normal movement of the limbs during the day represents modulation of the tonic pattern, which produces relatively slow changes in amplitude of the tonic discharge. Tonic activity provides stiffness to the limbs and trunk which serves to stabilize posture and movements. When a large amount of stiffness is required for a movement, the agonist and antagonist muscles will co-contract. At the other end of the movement speed spectrum, there are ballistic patterns that produce phasic movements (2). A ballis-

tic pattern demonstrates a biphasic or triphasic pattern in which there are relatively short bursts of 50-100 msec in a reciprocal activation of agonist-antagonist or agonist-antagonist-agonist. The second burst in a ballistic EMG discharge sequence is thought to provide braking of the initial agonist burst. In everyday activity, most normal movements are a combination of tonic and ballistic components across space and time. Thus, tonic and ballistic movements are two ends of a spectrum of normal movements. The third type of surface EMG discharge is the reflex pattern, which is a normal, involuntary discharge in response to stimulation. Monosynaptic reflex activation of segmental motorneuron pools is the classic example. Such discharges are very brief (30-50 msec) and may occur as agonist only or co-activation of agonist and antagonist muscles. When studying the neurophysiology patterns of movement disorders, it is important to be acquainted with the patterns seen in healthy individuals during the postural, kinetic, and task activation of limbs as well as the stabilizing core muscles.

Motor Parkinsonism

Parkinson's disease (PD) is the classic hypokinetic ('less movement') movement disorder. The primary motor symptoms (motor parkinsonism) of PD are rest tremor, bradykinesia ('slow movement'), and rigidity. Bradykinesia and rigidity that may be due to many causes is often referred to as 'parkinsonism' (see also Chapter

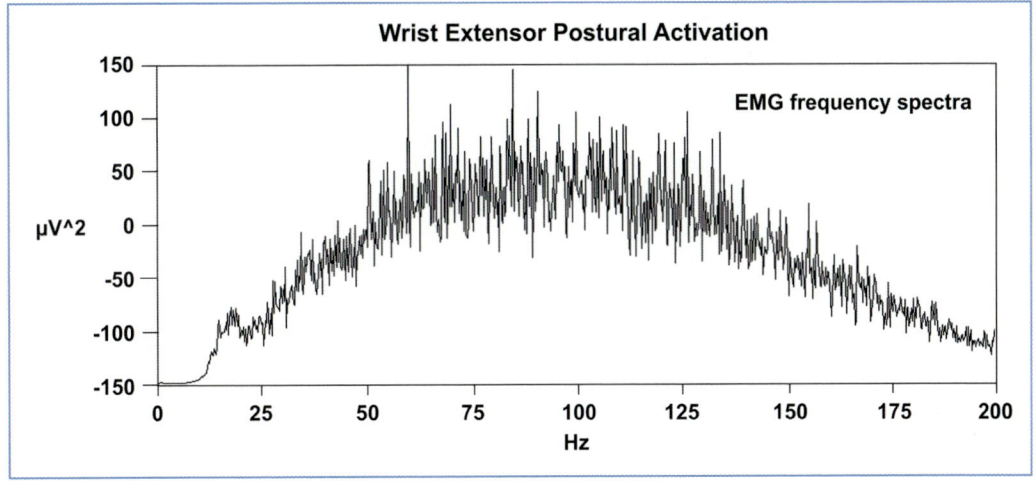

Figure 44.2
Frequency spectra from normal wrist muscle activation by surface EMG showing broad band of frequencies from 15 to 200 Hz. Band filters were set at 1-200 Hz.

5). Rest tremor will be covered in the section below on tremor.

Bradykinesia

Multiple reasons for bradykinesia have been suggested by different studies. The ballistic movements in PD are characterized by a low amplitude of the initial agonist burst (3). This results in a small-amplitude movement that the patient compensates for by making sequential, small, triphasic bursts. When PD patients are given a simple reaction time task, most studies reveal a small delay (4). If the movement is more complex, the abnormality is more significant. Simultaneous and sequential movements are also abnormal and improve with levodopa (5-7). Rigidity per se is not believed to contribute to bradykinesia. Finally, Brown et al. determined that abnormal synchronization prevents the normal fusion of muscle activation, leading to 'weakness' (8,9).

Cognitive decline

Parkinson's disease is associated with cognitive decline (10). Multiple mechanisms have been postulated and include cortical pathology, abnormal basal ganglia input, and disruption of acetylcholine, norepinephrine, serotonin, and dopamine systems that project to cortical areas. Whatever the mechanism, EEG frequencies are slower for both PD-related dementia and mild cognitive impairment (11). It is possible that some changes predict the eventual development of cognitive impairment in PD (12). Cortical myoclonus occurs in diffuse Lewy body disease, alpha-synuclein triplication, and with small amplitude in idiopathic PD (13). This myoclonus is evidence for cortical dysfunction and may have relevance to PD-related cognitive decline due to cortical dysfunction. Increased alpha-synuclein accumulation has been reported in the motor cortex of PD patients with small-amplitude cortical myoclonus (14).

Tremor

Tremor is the oscillation of one body part in relation to another body part and is approximately sinusoidal and rhythmic. In tremor, surface EMG discharges reflect the oscillating positive and negative influences on the intended voluntary activation or resting state. It records the grouping of motor unit potentials as discrete bursts of activity (15). Analysis of these EMG bursts helps to establish whether a movement is truly tremor, with a modulation envelope that appears sinusoidal and rhythmic. Disorders such as phasic dystonia may appear regular on visual inspection but are shown to be irregular when measured on an EMG recording. Conversely, a low-frequency tremor with some irregularity may appear to exhibit movement more like jerking (see also Chapter 25).

Practical considerations

Electrodes are placed over the agonist and antagonist pairs of muscles including and just beyond the tremor distribution. The amplitude of the tremor bursts should be evaluated during different tasks such as rest, postural activation, kinetic activation, and task-specific. A useful classification is to group them into those occurring at rest and those occurring with action. Action tremors are further subdivided into postural tremors (a body part maintains its position against gravity), isometric tremors (muscle contraction against a stationary object), simple kinetic tremor (non-target-directed voluntary movement), and intention tremor (at the termination of a target-directed movement) (16). Task-specific tremors are those seen during a defined activity such as handwriting. The frequency should be noted for every distribution and activation state. Another observation in tremor analysis is the pattern of agonist–antagonist firing. One muscle may fire while the other is silent, in a 'reciprocal' pattern. In other tremors, the pair may fire simultaneously in a synchronous or co-contracting pattern. Occasionally, the EMG pattern may shift from one pattern to another during the period of recording.

Frequency measurement is important for tremor assessment (15). Even though the surface EMG discharges will have an apparent frequency, the frequency of the movement oscillation is more easily assessed with an accelerometer. Different causes of tremor have fairly well-defined frequency ranges. However, there is much overlap between these frequency ranges, so their diagnostic usefulness is limited (15). Even so, the frequency may be measured in specific patients so as to allow monitoring of the tremor.

Physiological tremor

'Physiological tremor' occurs in all healthy individuals. This tremor may not be visually perceptible, but very small rhythmic movements may be detected by sensitive methods. Since body parts have mass, they have a mechanical resonance frequency particularly when force is applied to them during muscle activation. This 'mechanical component' can be detected with an accelerometer but normally does not have a grossly identifiable surface EMG modulation component. Adding weights to the body part will change the frequency of the mechanical component, and this provides a method for detecting the mechanical component of tremor. However, in some individuals, a 6-12 Hz CNS 'physiologic' modulation is exerted through modulation of the EMG discharge. If the displacements are large enough with either central or mechanical isolation, a reflex component through peripheral nerve reflex loops can add to tremor activity. Thus, these three components, mechanical, reflex, and central oscillator, can play a role in physiological tremor. The same components comprise the components of pathological tremor, with abnormal central oscillators playing a major role.

Exaggerated physiological tremor

There are certain disorders in which physiological tremor becomes pathologically exaggerated. In these instances, the amplitude of the tremor becomes symptomatic and readily detectable visually. This condition is called exaggerated physiologic tremor. The abnormal surface EMG activity emerges through increased reflex activation. Synchronous bursts of 50-100 msec duration and a frequency of 8-12 Hz are seen most prominently in the distal arms during their postural activation. Sometimes, this pattern may affect axial and lower extremity muscles also. One common cause is a drug that stimulates beta receptors. Other possible conditions include hyperthyroidism, anxiety, increased levels of catecholamines in the blood, and others.

Essential tremor

Essential tremor is the most common movement disorder. It is usually a bilateral, symmetrical, postural or kinetic tremor involving the upper extremities. Other locations such as the head and voice are common. The CNS oscillator may be located in the brainstem-cerebellar circuits (see also Chapter 25). The surface EMG usually shows bursts of activity that are synchronous in agonist and antagonist muscles, with possible frequency ranges of 4-12 Hz and 5-8 Hz being the most common ones. Figure 44.3 shows the EMG polygraphy of a moderate-amplitude, low-frequency wrist essential tremor during postural activation.

When the tremor is severe, rest tremor may be evident, but care should be taken to make sure the subject is fully relaxed. A reciprocal or co-contraction pattern between agonist and antagonist may be observed in postural activation for patients with essential tremor (17,18). The surface EMG characteristics in neuropathic tremor are identical to those in essential tremor.

Parkinsonian tremor

Parkinson's disease is classically associated with a rest tremor that attenuates with muscle activation. The dominant frequency is 4-7 Hz. Surface EMG studies of PD rest tremors classically demonstrate a reciprocal contraction pattern. However, a more co-contracting pattern may also be seen and may change depending on the position of the limbs. Burst durations are typically in the range of 50-100 msec. Figure 44.4 shows the EMG polygraphy of a left arm rest tremor from a PD patient.

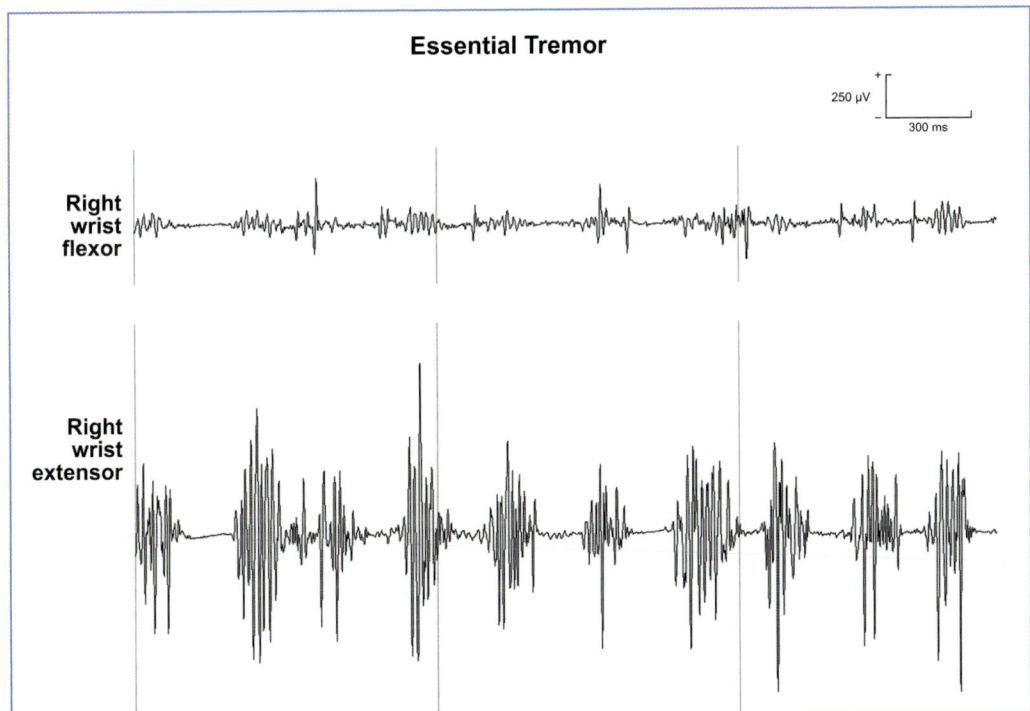

Figure 44.3
Essential tremor. Surface EMG pattern shows rhythmic oscillating muscle activation during attempted arm postural activation. Co-contraction of agonist and antagonist muscle activation is seen.

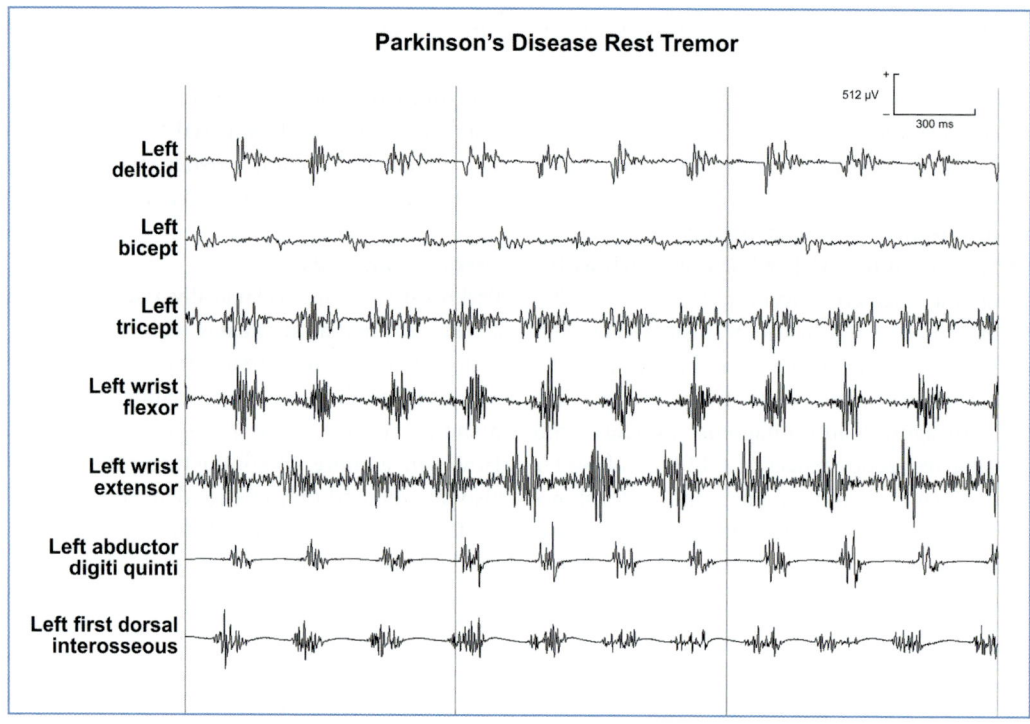

Parkinson's Disease Rest Tremor

512 µV

300 ms

Left deltoid

Left bicept

Left tricept

Left wrist flexor

Left wrist extensor

Left abductor digiti quinti

Left first dorsal interosseous

Figure 44.4

Parkinson's disease resting tremor. Reciprocal contraction of agonist and antagonist is seen.

Evidence favors basal ganglia dysfunction in the genesis of parkinsonian rest tremor. In incidental Lewy body disease (ILB) cases with subclinical rest tremor discharges, Lewy-type synucleinopathy was more prominent in their brainstem (19). Patients may demonstrate 're-emergent tremor', which is a reappearance during postural activation of the tremor form seen during rest. The frequency of the postural 're-emergent tremor' is the rest tremor frequency or up to 1.5 Hz higher. Small postural hand tremors are common in PD and are probably different from 're-emergent tremor'. The postural hand tremor frequency range is the same as for essential tremor, although it is controversial as to whether this constitutes an association between PD and essential tremor. Similar rest and muscle activation tremors may occur in other conditions that exhibit parkinsonism.

Cerebellar tremor

Limb cerebellar tremor is most prominent during limb movement ('kinetic') and as the target is being reached. The tremor frequency is usually less than 5 Hz, and the distribution may be distal, proximal, or both. Postural tremor may also be present. Serial dysmetria should not be confused with kinetic tremor. In dysmetria, surface EMG studies indicate that the terminal movements are not the regular oscillations of tremor but rather a series of inaccurate, irregular, ballistic movements. Trunk and other midline tremors may also affect patients with cerebellar disorders, and their frequency can be quite slow (3-5 Hz).

Midbrain tremor

Midbrain tremor (also known as rubral tremor, or Holmes tremor) (see Chapter 25) increases when changing from rest to postural activation and increases further from postural activation to kinetic or intention movement. This tremor occasionally has an irregular presentation. The tremor frequency is usually less than 4.5 Hz and often associated with a lesion that can be acute or precede the tremor onset by up to 1-2 years.

Task- and position-specific tremor

Several tremors occur only with specific tasks or positions. The classic example is primary writing tremor. Although this tremor is predominant during writing, it often spills over into other activities such as eating. The surface EMG correlate consists of 75-125 msec duration bursts that occur maximally in the forearm muscles. The pattern may be synchronous or reciprocal. Isolated voice tremor and tremor when playing a musical instrument are other examples. It is not known whether these tremors represent a form of essential tremor or an entirely different entity.

Orthostatic tremor

Heilman described orthostatic tremor. Patients complain of tremor, vibration, or shaking in their legs shortly after they stand (20). This may cause a sense of instability so severe that walking becomes difficult (see Chapter 25). The surface EMG pattern is distinctive and displays high-amplitude, 13-18 Hz tremor bursts. The bursts are recorded in the legs and paraspinal muscles, with the patient standing. Figure 44.5 shows the EMG polygraphy of orthostatic tremor. The agonist–antagonist relationship may vary during the recording.

At rest, the legs are electrically silent. The rapid discharge frequency can be difficult to detect clinically. A surface EMG study is highly recommended to make the definitive orthostatic tremor syndrome diagnosis. The differential diagnosis for this movement disorder includes slower tremors, myoclonus, and sometimes etiologies

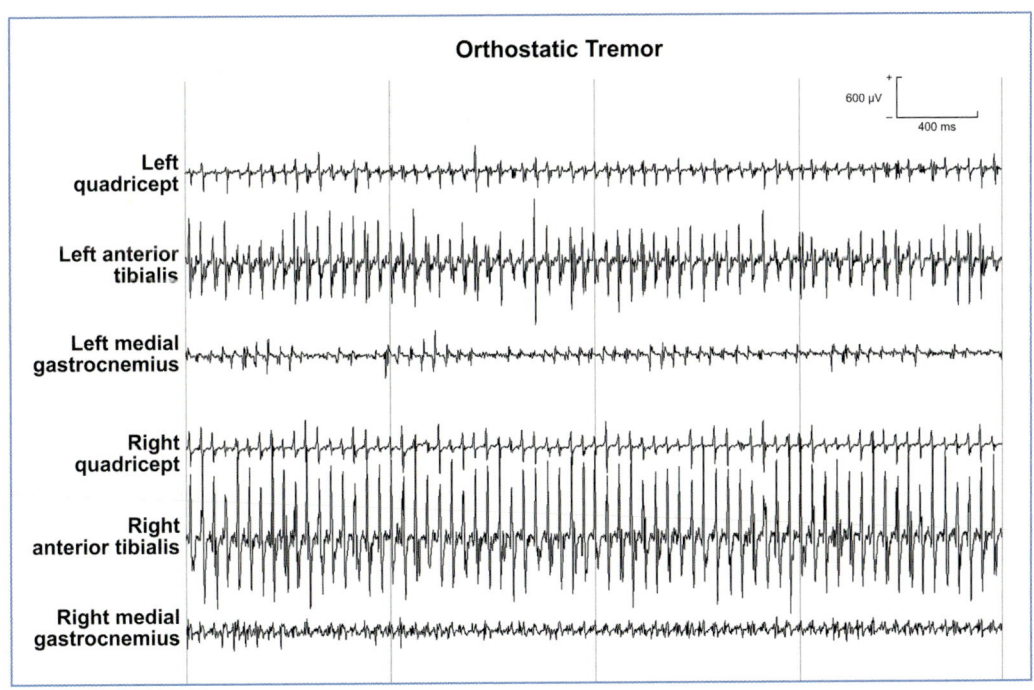

Figure 44.5

Orthostatic tremor. 13-16 Hz high frequency surface EMG discharges in lower extremities of a patient with orthostatic tremor.

of imbalance not associated with involuntary movements.

Psychogenic tremor

Tremors may be seen in conversion disorder or malingering disorders. A surface EMG can provide supportive evidence only by demonstrating a pattern that does not correspond to a typical tremor pattern. Psychogenic tremors tend to be paroxysmal, have inconsistent activation, and seldom display a dominant frequency throughout a prolonged recording. Indeed, the tremor frequency and amplitude tend to vary widely with time, with change of position, or with distraction. However, diagnostic proof for a psychogenic or voluntary origin for a tremor cannot be offered. Surface EMG does not detect psychogenicity or malingering. The utility of surface EMG or any movement disorder testing in these circumstances is often to detect classical patterns that are being questioned on the basis of phenotypic appearance (see also Chapter 38).

Myoclonus

Myoclonus is defined as sudden, brief, shock-like, involuntary movements caused by muscular contractions or inhibitions (21). Muscular contractions produce 'positive myoclonus' while muscular inhibitions produce 'negative myoclonus' or asterixis. Myoclonus has different possible etiologies, anatomical sources, and pathophysiology mechanisms. It can be classified by examination findings, presentation, aetiology, and clinical neurophysiology testing. The most commonly accepted method to organize the possible clinical presentations and etiologies of myoclonus is the well-known major clinical syndrome categories of Marsden et al. and their corresponding lists of known etiologies (22) (see also Chapter 28).

Myoclonus neurophysiology principles

Information about the neurophysiology of myoclonus is of critical importance. Neurophysiological examination characterizes to some extent the location and nature of the aberrant neuronal circuits that generate the myoclonus. Certain neurophysiology patterns can correlate with a diagnostic classification as well as predict which treatments may work effectively. Both exam characteristics and clinical neurophysiology testing are used to determine the physiological classification of the myoclonus for a particular patient. Common techniques used in this testing include EEG, surface EMG, EEG-EMG polygraphy with back-averaging, evoked potentials, long-latency EMG responses, and coherence analysis (21,23). Major categories of the physiological classification refer to the neuroanatomical source and provide some information about the nature of the aberrant neuronal circuits. The main physiological classification categories for myoclonus are:

- Cortical
- Cortical-subcortical
- Subcortical-nonsegmental
- Segmental
- Peripheral

Further subdivision is based on other physiological properties as well as the clinical syndrome and/or the specific disease in which the myoclonus occurs. In this chapter, because of their clinical overlap with myoclonus, psychogenic myoclonus, abnormal startle disorders and periodic limb movements of sleep will also be discussed. In practical terms, the classification of a particular example of myoclonus is derived from the results of the clinical neurophysiological testing as well as of an appreciation of the clinical context in which they occur. Multiple myoclonus physiology types might occur in the same patient.

Cortical

The cerebral cortex is the most common origin for myoclonus. The jerks are most often multifocal, but focal, segmental, and generalized myoclonus can also occur. Action myoclonus is very common in these patients and provides most of the disability. Cortical myoclonus is defined by the demonstration of a focal, time-locked, cortical transient that precedes the myoclonus in a given muscle by a short latency (<40 msec for arm). This may be associated with enlarged, cortical, somatosensory evoked potentials (SEP) waves and/or enhanced, long-latency EMG responses to electrical nerve stimulation.

Myoclonus EMG discharges are often very brief, with a range of 25-75 msec. These discharges are characteristically co-contractions between agonists and antagonists. Corticomuscular conduction occurs quickly via corticospinal pyramidal pathways. Sometimes spikes and/or sharp waves can be seen in the gross EEG. However, EEG-EMG polygraphy or jerk-locking with back-averaging are more reliable methods for demonstrating time-locked, cortical, transient, preceding myoclonus EMG discharges or jerks. Such patients may have reflex jerks, but it is usually easier to collect many myoclonus events by muscle activation of the limb. The back-averaged transient in cortical myoclonus is a fo-

cal, biphasic or triphasic spike beginning with a positive deflection that precedes the onset of the myoclonic discharge by 6-22 msec in the upper extremity (24). The duration of the transient is 15-40 msec. The conduction of the spike to motorneuron pools is presumed to occur through corticospinal (pyramidal) pathways. The maximum of the transient is usually located over the sensorimotor cortex at the central or centro-parietal electrode according to anatomical somatotopic mapping, contralateral to the myoclonus EMG discharge. Figure 44.6 shows the raw EMG and EEG tracings during myoclonic jerking from a patient with cortical myoclonus. Also shown is the back-averaging of the myoclonus EMG and pre-myoclonus cortical transient.

In cases of *cortical reflex myoclonus*, the cortical SEP P25-N33 parietal wave from median nerve stimulation is enlarged. The establishment of normal values for a particular laboratory is encouraged (23). Another phenomenon seen in such cases is abnormal, long-latency EMG dis-

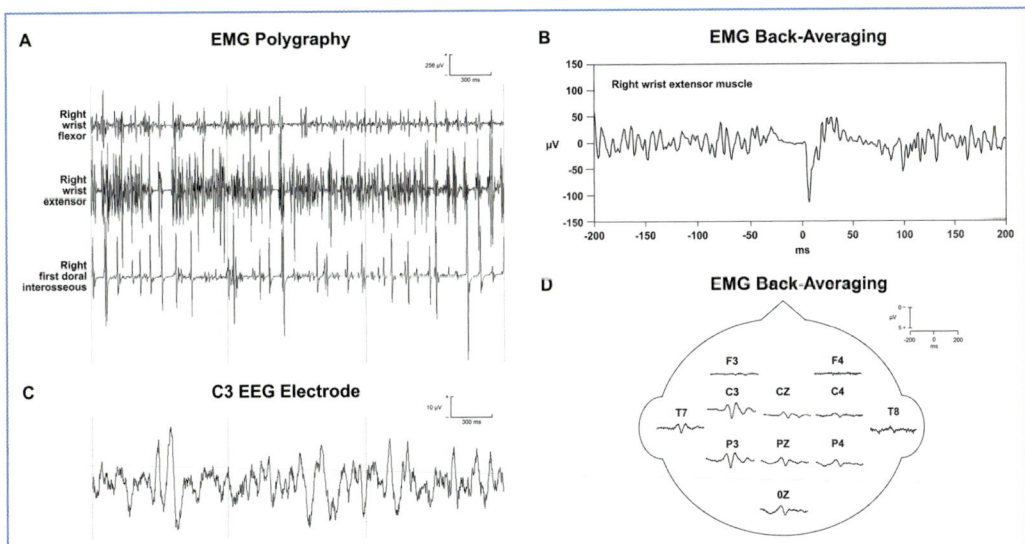

Figure 44.5

Electrophysiological analysis of cortical myoclonus. A: Surface EMG polygraphy during myoclonus showing multiple short-duration myoclonus EMG discharges. B: Back-averaging of multiple myoclonus EMG discharges with trigger set at discharge beginning. C: Raw EEG tracing at central EEG electrode contralateral to the averaged myoclonus EMG discharges. Time epoch is the same as that for surface EMG polygraphy in "A". D: Back-averaging of EEG to the myoclonus EMG discharge beginning trigger as in "B". A focal EEG transient is shown preceding the myoclonus.

charges that are elicited by median nerve stimulation. At rest, in a normal individual, no response should be present. These EMG discharges have a 50 msec latency or greater (range 40-60 msec) from the stimulus artifact trigger mark (25). Repetitive discharges may be seen, at intervals of 20-40 msec.

Asterixis is a synonym for negative myoclonus and refers to a decrease in tonic EMG activity. Negative myoclonus correlates with an average EMG silence duration of 50-200 msec. Negative myoclonus is believed to be generated from cortical or subcortical circuits. The EMG silences of negative myoclonus usually have a multifocal distribution.

Cortical-subcortical

The term 'cortical-subcortical' myoclonus refers to myoclonus arising from an abnormal interaction between the cortical and subcortical networks (26). For these entities, one location is not primarily responsible by itself for the excessive excitation of motor pathways leading to the jerk. There is strong evidence that some generalized seizure phenomena arise from paroxysmal abnormal and excessive oscillation in bidirectional connections between cortical and subcortical sites. The term 'cortical-subcortical' myoclonus refers to myoclonus arising from this type of physiology to produce myoclonic seizures and related phenomena. Despite the subcortical involvement, the cortical discharge (e.g. spike or spike and wave) precedes and drives the myoclonus event. This myoclonus usually occurs as paroxysms from rest and can be associated with other seizure phenomena that may even be more clinically significant than the myoclonus itself. The myoclonus is often generalized or bilaterally synchronous, but focal or multifocal distributions also occur. This neurophysiology classification includes the myoclonus that is seen during myoclonic and absence seizures and other phenomena.

Myoclonic seizures

Myoclonic seizures are epileptic seizures for which the movement manifestation is myoclonus. The myoclonus is usually generalized and thus has a different appearance than in partial motor seizures or a single jerk of classical cortical myoclonus. The movements may be confused with other seizures that result in jerks (e.g. atonic and tonic seizures). 'True' myoclonic seizures result in brief positive myoclonus (27). The myoclonus is accompanied by a generalized (primary or secondary), ictal, epileptiform EEG discharge. 'Fragments' of the generalized epileptiform EEG discharge often occur. Likewise, the myoclonus is usually generalized, but it can be segmental or occasionally focal. Thus, 'fragments' of both the epileptiform discharge as well as the myoclonus are seen. Myoclonic epilepsy syndromes commonly manifest other seizure types besides myoclonic seizures. Juvenile myoclonic epilepsy manifests muscle jerks associated with spike and wave EEG discharges. This myoclonus is the classic example of cortical-subcortical myoclonus in which both cortical and subcortical networks are hyperactive (26).

Subcortical-nonsegmental

The clinical and neurophysiological characteristics of subcortical myoclonus are more variable than those of cortical or cortical-subcortical myoclonus. The myoclonus EMG duration may be longer than in cortical or cortical-subcortical myoclonus. Simultaneous rostral and caudal recruitment of the myoclonus in the EMG channels supports a subcortical generator. There is no evidence for abnormal cortical excitability (e.g. EEG spikes, back-averaged transients, enlarged cortical SEP waves) in subcortical myoclonus that is tightly correlated to the myoclonus. Assignment of a case to the subcortical category can be problematic if it is based largely on the absence of evidence for abnormal cortical excitability or circumstantial findings rather than direct evidence. Unfortunately, this often happens since it is difficult to show altered subcortical circuit activation directly by non-invasive techniques. A distinction must be made between subcortical and segmental myoclonus (discussed below), and therefore the term 'subcortical-nonsegmental' myoclonus. Four major examples of subcortical-nonsegmental myoclonus are essential myoclonus, reticular reflex myoclonus, opsoclonus-myoclonus syndrome, and propriospinal myoclonus.

Essential myoclonus
In most cases, the myoclonus EMG discharge duration is 50-200 msec. However, longer discharge duration values have been described, especially in those cases with dystonia. The co-appearance of dystonia has led some to use the term 'myoclonus-dystonia' syndrome. The EMG patterns can be agonist-only or co-contracting agonist-antagonist. Often, the discharges are irregular with respect to amplitude, duration, and timing between agonist and antagonist. The SEP and long-latency EMG responses are normal. The routine EEG is normal. No focal EEG correlates have been reported, and most EEG-EMG back-averaging has been unrevealing. Roze et al. have provided a clinical neurophysiological description of several epsilon-sarcoglycan mutation-positive cases (28).

Reticular reflex myoclonus
This myoclonus manifests as stimulus-sensitive, generalized jerks that involve axial and proximal limb muscles. The post-hypoxic state and uremia are known causes. The EMG discharges are brief at 25-75 msec (29). The key neurophysiology characteristic is the EMG discharge sequence that reflects a simultaneous, bilateral, rostral and caudal recruitment that originates from brain-stem-innervated muscles. It is believed that it originates from the area of the medullary reticular formation. The EEG may show epileptiform discharges, but they follow rather than precede the first EMG activation, vary from jerk to jerk, and do not show a time-locked relationship to the myoclonus. Therefore, the EEG discharges may reflect the cortical response to increased ascending activity. The SEP is normal.

Opsoclonus-myoclonus syndrome
The opsoclonus-myoclonus syndrome consists of opsoclonus, myoclonus, and variably other manifestations such as ataxia, tremor, and behaviour problems (30). The myoclonus presents as multifocal muscle action jerks. The EMG discharges are less than 100 msec, often occur in trains, and can show agonist-only or agonist-antagonist co-contraction. The EEG is usually normal, and if abnormalities do exist, they have no relationship to the myoclonus per se. There is no EEG transient on back-averaging of the myoclonus (31). The cortical SEP and long-latency EMG responses are normal.

Propriospinal myoclonus
This myoclonus was described by Peter Brown and colleagues (32). The movements occur as trunk flexion or extension with axial muscle activation. The proximal limb muscles are often involved in the jerk bilaterally, but the predominant action is in the axial muscles. Myoclonus occurs from rest and/or is activated by stimuli such as touch, deep tendon reflex, or muscle stretch. Single or repetitive jerks may occur. Both reciprocal and co-contracting agonist-antagonist patterns are seen. The EMG discharge lasts typically 50-300 msec but sometimes longer. A major characteristic of the EMG discharge is a simultaneous, bilateral, rostral and caudal recruitment originating from the area of the spinal cord origin. Propriospinal pathways are proposed to be responsible for the relatively slow activation speed of muscle recruitment. One study has shown defects in spinal white-matter tracts by diffusion tensor imaging (33). No EEG abnormalities in the routine recording or with back-averaging have been reported. Cortical SEP is normal.

Segmental
Segmental myoclonus has its generator in a particular segment or contiguous segments of the

brainstem and/or spinal cord (34). This segmental generator produces movements for circumscribed segments or contiguous muscle segments. Palatal and spinal types of segmental myoclonus are the two classic varieties of segmental myoclonus. Other examples include diaphragmatic and abdominal myoclonus. Surface EMG usually shows synchronous activation of the affected muscles (34). The typical frequency is in the range of 0.5-3 Hz, and the typical EMG discharge duration varies widely between 50 and 500 msec. The EEG and SEP are normal.

Palatal myoclonus
Palatal myoclonus demonstrates characteristics of a segmental myoclonus physiology (34). It has been divided into essential (EPM) and symptomatic (SPM) cases. The EEG and SEP are normal. Brainstem auditory evoked potentials (BAEP) have shown abnormal findings in some individuals with palatal myoclonus (35). These inconsistent BAEP abnormalities probably represent the same lesion type, but not the same exact location, as that responsible for the palatal myoclonus pathophysiology. Some differences in neurophysiological testing have been found between EPM and SPM (36). EPM shows a complete suppression with sleep, but sleep only produces mild variations in rate with SPM. In studies examining brainstem reflexes, EPM had only polysynaptic brainstem reflex abnormalities, whereas SPM patients can have abnormalities of monosynaptic, oligosynaptic, and polysynaptic brainstem reflexes.

Spinal myoclonus
Spinal segmental myoclonus neurophysiology is more easily studied than palatal myoclonus. EEG abnormalities are not detected, back-averaging never elicits a cortical transient, and cortical SEP is normal. The surface EMG shows synchronous, rhythmic or semi-rhythmic discharges in muscles supplied by the corresponding spinal segmental generator. The polygraphic surface EMG study usually shows synchronous activation of the affected muscles. The typical frequency is in the range of 1-3 Hz with a broad reported range of 0.2 - 8 Hz. The typical surface EMG discharge duration varies widely between 50 and 500 msec (37). However, some responses to sensory stimulation are abnormal and may show insight into the segmental physiological defect. Somatosensory evoked spinal potential recovery curves were abnormal in a case of segmental myoclonus involving the L2-L4 myotomes. This finding may suggest that dorsal horn interneurons are abnormally hyperactive and can contribute to the generation of spinal segmental myoclonus (34).

Peripheral
Peripheral myoclonus refers to myoclonic jerks whose generation is related to a lesion of a peripheral nervous system site. The classic example is hemifacial spasm. Such EMG discharges are characterized by marked variability in duration from discharge to discharge (23). The appearance and timing of EMG discharges at a given time, which are supplied by the same nerve, are similar. The spectrum of EMG discharge duration may merge continuously with those EMG discharges that are responsible for movements that are longer lasting, such as in the prolonged spasms of hemifacial spasm.

Psychogenic jerks
Jerks that arise from a psychogenic mechanism may appear quick enough to overlap with myoclonus. Most often, however, such jerks more closely resemble 'spasms' because they are not brief enough to be called myoclonus. Caution should be emphasized when using clinical neurophysiology to evaluate these patients. It is unwise to employ these techniques alone to 'prove' or 'rule out' a psychogenic basis for myoclonus. Possible pitfalls should be realized. A psychogenic myoclonus EMG discharge may show the voluntary, reciprocal, biphasic/triphasic agonist-antagonist/agonist pattern with the duration of each burst being 50-100 msec. Stimulus-evoked jerks or 'jumps' with a mean latency in excess of

100 msec may suggest voluntary or psychogenic jerks (38). A bereitschaftspotential (BP) is a back-averaged, negative EEG cortical potential that occurs before self-paced, voluntary, phasic movements. Some have found that the presence of a BP preceding psychogenic myoclonus to be supportive evidence for a psychogenic aetiology (38). However, because recording movements from a psychogenic individual may be technically challenging or inadequate, the absence of the BP should not be used to indicate that voluntary mechanisms have been ruled out.

Startle disorders

The normal startle reflex is a whole-body jerk that commonly occurs in response to a sudden, unexpected noise or touch. Its phenotype is often associated with myoclonus. Orbicularis oculi leading muscle sequence occurs at 30–40 msec and the sternocleidomastoid follows at 55–85 msec. Limb muscles are less consistently active, with the biceps activated at 85–100 msec and leg muscles at 100–140 msec (39). Burst durations range from 50 to 400 msec. The reflex habituates rapidly. Normal startle represents a form of physiologic myoclonus.

Exaggerated startle arising from pathology has numerous etiologies, such as inflammatory brainstem lesions, anoxic injuries, psychiatric illnesses, and drug intoxication. Hereditary hyperekplexia is an autosomal dominant condition characterized by exaggerated startle to unexpected stimuli. The audiogenic myoclonic jerks in hyperekplexia clearly correspond to the normal startle pattern (40). However, the startle reflex is increased in magnitude and is poorly habituating in this disorder (see also Chapter 28).

Periodic limb movements of sleep

Periodic jerks of the legs may interrupt sleep and cause insomnia or excessive daytime somnolence. Once light sleep is obtained, the movements occur with some regularity every 30 and 45 seconds. The movements do not resemble myoclonus, so the previous designation of nocturnal myoclonus has been abandoned. Most often, the burst durations last from 500 msec to a few seconds. The earliest and most actively involved muscle is often the anterior tibialis muscle. Although the jerks may appear unilateral, bilateral asynchronous EMG activation is the common occurrence. Such periodic limb movements of sleep commonly accompany restless legs syndrome or are 'idiopathic'. Trauma of the spinal cord or vascular injury may also be a cause, implicating damage to descending inhibitory pathways (see also Chapter 36).

Dystonia

Dystonia is a syndrome of involuntary, sustained muscle contractions that produce abnormal postures, twisting and repetitive movements. It may be focal or generalized. The most common focal dystonia is cervical dystonia, or 'torticollis'. Blepharospasm, oromandibular dystonia, and writers' or occupational cramps are other common focal dystonias. Generalized dystonia is usually a manifestation of hereditary torsion dystonia. Generally, neurophysiologic studies are most helpful in evaluating a focal dystonia. Often the information can be used to guide therapeutic injections of botulinum toxin (see also Chapter 24). The physiologic hallmark of dystonia is abnormal co-contraction of agonist and antagonist muscles, producing a marked increase in stiffness across the joint with abnormal postures. Thus, muscles acting across the postured joint should be studied to look for synchronous activation. The EMG discharges may be tonic or with repetitive, rhythmic (like tremor) or irregular discharges (phasic dystonic movements). This latter pattern may distinguish itself from tremor by the variability of the burst durations. One study found that a dominant bursting EMG pattern in dystonic conditions predicted an early response to pallidal stimulation (41). It must be realized that agonist-antagonist co-contraction is not specific for dystonia. Normal voluntary movement as well as nonspecific spasms can produce similar EMG patterns.

Spasmodic torticollis

Deuschl and colleagues have described the patterns of EMG discharge in spasmodic torticollis (42). With rotational torticollis, the contralateral sternocleidomastoid and the ipsilateral splenius capitus are most often active. In retrocollis, all posterior neck muscles are active, and in laterocollis, the ipsilateral splenius capitus and sternocleidomastoid muscles are active. Variations in a particular pattern of muscle activity are common. Thus, performing multichannel EMG recording with intramuscular electrodes before injecting botulinum toxin may be useful in some patients (43).

Chorea and Tics

Surface EMG recordings in chorea parallel the clinical appearance of the movement disorder. Marked variations in surface EMG discharge duration and sequence are seen. Some EMG discharges may be quite brief (of the order of 100 msec) while other discharges may last a second or more. Tics show brief surface EMG discharge durations. Both patterns for chorea and tics may resemble normal movement patterns.

References

1 Caviness JN. Movement Disorders. In: Clinical Neurophysiology. Daube and Rubin (eds), Oxford University press, third ed. 2009:551-573.

2 Hallett M, Shahani BT, Young RR. EMG analysis of stereotyped voluntary movements in man. J Neurol Neurosurg Psychiatry 1975;38:1154-1162.

3 Berardelli A, Dick JP, Rothwell JC, Day BL, Marsden CD. Scaling of the size of the first agonist EMG burst during rapid wrist movements in patients with Parkinson's disease. J Neurol Neurosurg Psychiatry 1986;49:1273-1279.

4 Jahanshahi M, Brown RG, Marsen CD. A comparative study of simple and choice reaction time in Parkinson's, Huntington's and cerebellar disease. J Neurol Neurosurg Psychiatry 1993;56:1169-1177.

5 Benecke R, Rothwell JC, Dick JP, Day BL, and Marsden CD. Performance of simultaneous movements in patients with Parkinson's disease. Brain 1986;109:739-757.

6 Benecke R, Rothwell JC, Dick JP, Day BL, and Marsden CD. Disturbance of sequential movements in patients with Parkinson's disease. Brain 1987;110:361-379.

7 Benecke R, Rothwell JC, Dick JP, Day BL, and Marsen CD. Simple and complex movements off and on treatment in patients with Parkinson's disease. J Neurol Neurosurg Psychiatry 1987;50:296-303.

8 Brown P, Corscos DM, and Rothwell JC. Does parkinsonian action tremor contribute to muscle weakness in Parkinson's disease? Brain 1997;120:401-408.

9 Brown P, Corscos DM, and Rothwell JC. Action tremor and weakness in Parkinson's disease: a study of the elbow extensors. Mov Disord 1998;13:56-60.

10 Caviness JN, Lue L, Adler CH, Walker DG. Parkinson's disease dementia and potential therapeutic strategies. CNS Neurosci Ther 2011;17:32-44.

11 Caviness JN, Hentz JG, Evidente VGH, et al. Both early and late cognitive dysfunction affects the electroencephalogram in Parkinson's disease. Parkinsonism Rel Disord 2007;13:348-354.

12 Klassen B, Hentz J, Shill H, et al. Quantitative Electroencephalography as a Predictor for Parkinson's Disease Dementia. Neurology 2011;77:118-124.

13 Caviness JN, Adler C.H., Beach T, Wetjen K, Caselli RJ. Myoclonus in Lewy Body Disorders. Adv Neurol 2002;89:23-30.

14 Caviness JN, Lue LF, Beach TG, et al. Parkinson's Disease, Cortical Dysfunction, and Alpha-Synuclein. Mov Disord 2001;26:1436-1442.

15 Mansur PHG, Cury LKP, Andrade CAO, et al. A Review on Techniques for Tremor Recording and Quantification. Critical Reviews in Biomedical Engineering 2007;35:343-362.

16 Deuschl G, Bain P, Brin M. Consensus statement of the Movement Disorder Society on Tremor. Ad Hoc Scientific Committee. Mov Disord 1998;13(S3):2-23.

17 Sabra AF, Hallett M. Action tremor with alternating activity in antagonist muscles. Neurology 1984;34:151–156.

18 Milanov I. Clinical and electromyographic examinations of patients with essential tremor. Can J Neurol Sci 2000;27:65–70.

19 Caviness, JN, Adler CH, Hentz JG, et al. Electrophysiological Biomarkers of Incidental Lewy Body Disease. Clinical Neurophysiology 2011;122:2426-2432.

20 Heilman KM. Orthostatic tremor. Arch Neurol 1984;41:880–881.

21 Caviness JN, Brown P. Myoclonus: current concepts and recent advances. Lancet Neurology 2004;3:598-607.

22 Marsden CD, Hallett M, Fahn S. The nosology and pathophysiology of myoclonus. In: Movement Disorders. Marsden, CD, Fahn, S (eds), Butterworths. 1982:196-248.

23 Caviness JN. Clinical Neurophysiology of Myoclonus. In: Movement Disorders. M. Hallett (ed.), Handbook of Clinical Neurophysiology 2003;1:521-548.

24 Shibasaki H. Electrophysiologic studies of myoclonus. AAEE Minimonograph 30. Muscle & Nerve 2000;23:321-335.

25 Caviness JN, Kurth M. Cortical Myoclonus in Huntington's Disease Associated With an Enlarged Somatosensory Evoked Potential. Mov Disord 1997;12:1046-1051.

26 Caviness JN. Epileptic myoclonus. In: Atlas of video-EEG monitoring. Sirven JI, Stern JM (eds). McGraw-Hill Medical. 2011;309-328.

27 Guerrini, R, Bonanni, P, Parmeggiani, L, et al. Pathophysiology of Myoclonic Epilepsies. Adv Neurol 2005;95:23-46.

28 Roze F, Apartis E, Clot F, et al. Myoclonus-dystonia: clinical and electrophysiologic pattern related to SGCE mutations. Neurology 2008;70:1010-1016.

29 Hallett M, Chadwick D, Adam J, Marsden CD. Reticular reflex myoclonus: A physiological type of human post-hypoxic myoclonus. J Neurol Neurosurg Psychiatry 1977;40:253-264.

30 Caviness JN, Forsyth PJ, McPhee T, Layton DD. The movement disorder syndrome of adult opsoclonus. Mov Disord 1995;10:22-27.

31 Gwinn KA, Caviness JN. Electrophysiological Observations in Idiopathic Opsoclonus-Myoclonus Syndrome. Mov Disord 1997;12:438-442.

32 Brown P, Thompson PD, Rothwell JC, Day BL, Marsden CD. Axial myoclonus of propriospinal origin. Brain 1991;114:197–214.

33 Roze E, Bounolleau P, Ducreux D, et al. Propriospinal myoclonus revisited: Clinical, neurophysiologic, and neuroradiologic findings. Neurology 2009;72:1301-1309.

34 Caviness JN. Segmental myoclonus. In: Hyperkinetic movement disorders: differential diagnosis and treatment. Albanese A, Jankovic J (eds), Wiley-Blackwell. 2012;221-35.

35 Westmoreland BF, Sharbrough FW, Stockard JJ, et al. Brainstem auditory evoked potentials in 20 patients with palatal myoclonus. Arch Neurol 1983;40:155-158.

36 Deuschl G, Toro C, Valls-Sole J, et al. Symptomatic and essential palatal tremor. 1. Clinical, physiological and MRI analysis. Brain 1994;117:775-788.

37 Calancie B. Spinal myoclonus after spinal cord injury. J Spinal Cord Med 2006;29:413-424.

38 Brown P, Thompson PD. Electrophysiological Aids to the Diagnosis of Psychogenic Jerks, Spasms, and Tremor. Mov Disord 2001;16: 595-599.

39 Brown P, Rothwell JC, Thompson PD, Britton TC, Day BL, Marsden CD. New observations on the normal auditory startle reflex in man. Brain 1991;114;1891-1902.

40 Wilkins DE, Hallett M, Wess MM. Audiogenic startle reflex of man and its relationship to startle syndromes. A review. Brain 1986;109:561–573.

41 Yianni J, Yan Wang S, Liu X, et al. A dominant bursting electromyography pattern in dystonic conditions predicts an early response to pallidal stimulation. J Clin Neurosci 2006;13:38-746.

42 Deuschl G, Heinen F, Kleedorfer B, Wagner M, Lucking CH, Poewe W. Clinical and polymyographic investigation of spasmodic torticollis. J Neurology 1992; 239:9–15.

43 Van Gerpen JA, Matsumoto JY, Ahlskog JE, Maraganore DM, McManis PG. Utility of an EMG mapping study in treating cervical dystonia. Muscle Nerve 2000;23:1752–1756.

45

Neuroimaging in Movement Disorders

David J. Brooks

Structural and functional imaging both have a role in the diagnosis, understanding, and management of movement disorders and their complications. The ways in which magnetic resonance imaging (MRI), transcranial sonography (TS), positron emission tomography (PET) and single photon emission computed tomography (SPECT) can contribute are discussed in this chapter. Imaging biomarkers can help discriminate the different parkinsonian disorders from one another and provide a rationale for the use of dopaminergic medications. Imaging can also detect subclinical disease activity in subjects at risk for Parkinson's disease and involuntary movement disorders such as dystonia and Huntington's chorea, and monitor the functional efficacy of putative neuroprotective and restorative therapies.

Structural imaging in hypokinetic disorders

Parkinsonism (a combination of bradykinesia, rigidity, tremor) can result when the nigrostriatal dopaminergic projections or the outflow tracts from the striatum and pallidum are interrupted. In Parkinson's disease (PD) the neurons of the substantia nigra compacta (SNc) are targeted by Lewy body inclusions containing aggregated α-synuclein. Multiple system atrophy (MSA) and progressive supranuclear palsy (PSP) are atypical forms of degenerative parkinsonism. MSA-P is associated with autonomic failure and ataxia and argyrophilic inclusions containing aggregated α-synuclein are found in

the SNc and striatum. PSP is associated with an impaired control of volitional eye movements, axial rigidity, early bulbar symptoms and falls. Here, neurofibrillary tau tangles are present in the SNc, basal ganglia, superior colliculi, brainstem and oculomotor nuclei, and the periaqueductal gray matter (see Chapter 4).

Magnetic resonance imaging (MRI)

Secondary parkinsonisms
Conventional T1- and T2-weighted MRI sequences can exclude secondary structural causes of parkinsonism with great sensitivity, such as basal ganglia tumors, toxic necrosis following exposure to agents such as manganese ores or after methcathinone (ephedrone) ingestion, small vessel ischaemic disease, and calcification (see Chapter 18). Volumetric MRI can detect patterns of cortical atrophy and hydrocephalus with great sensitivity.

Parkinson's disease
In PD, conventional 1-3 tesla MRI shows a normal nigral signal, but with 7 tesla magnets, signal change can be detected in the lateral nigra where the cell loss is pathologically greatest (Bajaj N; personal communication). Volumetric MRI has so far failed to demonstrate consistent reductions in SNc volume in PD, probably because of the difficulty in defining the borders of this structure by MRI due to its high iron content. However, using voxel-based morphometry, frontal, temporal and parietal atrophy can be detected in PD patients who have cognitive problems, mild cognitive im-

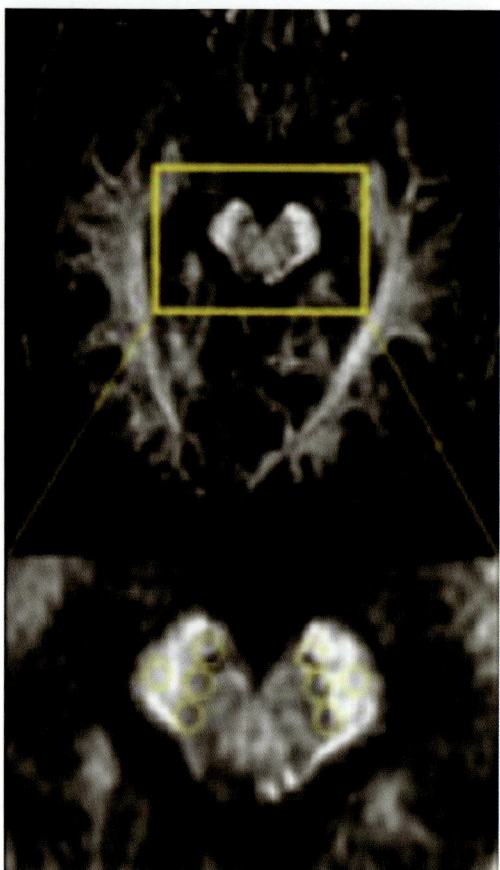

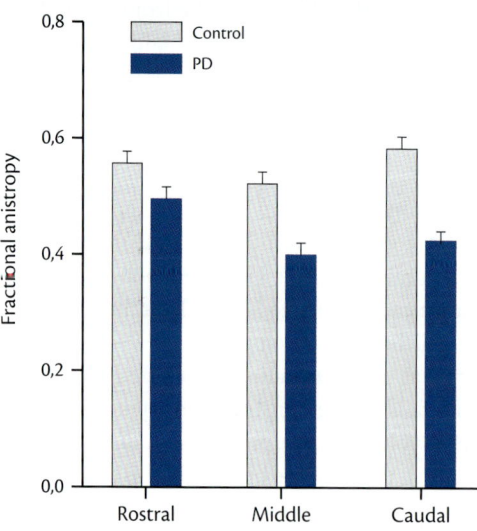

Figure 45.1

Fractional anisotropy (FA) of the midbrain. Nigral FA is reduced in a rostral caudal gradient in PD (51).

pairment or frank dementia (1). Diffusion tensor imaging (DTI) uses field gradient sequences which allows MRI to detect the directionality (anisotropy) and amplitude (diffusivity) of water movement along fibre tracts. DTI detects reduced fractional anisotropy (FA) of SNc water diffusion in de novo PD cases, changes again being the greatest in the lateral nigra where the pathology is known to be most severe (see Figure 45.1) (2). Susceptibility (R2*) imaging uses sequences sensitive to levels of iron deposition. Nigral R2* signals are increased in PD, and their levels correlate with the degree of disability rated with the unified Parkinson's disease rating scale (UPDRS) (3). It is known that the olfactory tracts of PD patients can be affected by Lewy body pathology in Braak stage 1 of the disorder. Recently, it has been reported that increased water diffusivity can be detected with DTI in the olfactory tracts of hyposmic PD cases (4).

Atypical parkinsonisms

While MRI shows a normal putamen signal in PD, a reduced lateral putamen signal can be seen with T_2-weighted MRI in established MSA due to the cell loss and iron deposition present (see Figure 45.2). This signal loss may be accompanied by a lateral rim of increased signal due to accompanying gliosis. Degeneration of the pons leads to lateral as well as longitudinal pontine fibers becoming evident on MRI as a high signal, and this has been termed the 'hot cross bun' sign (5). In advanced MSA, cerebellar and pontine atrophy becomes visually evident, and obvious and altered signal can be detected in the middle cerebellar peduncles. PSP patients do not show putamen signal changes on MRI, but sagittal views in established cases show third ventricular widening and midbrain atrophy, known as the 'humming bird' sign. While MSA targets the middle cerebellar peduncle, it is the superior cerebellar peduncle that atrophies in PSP.

While the above patterns of MRI change are specific for the different atypical parkinsonian syndromes, they are not sensitive markers of these

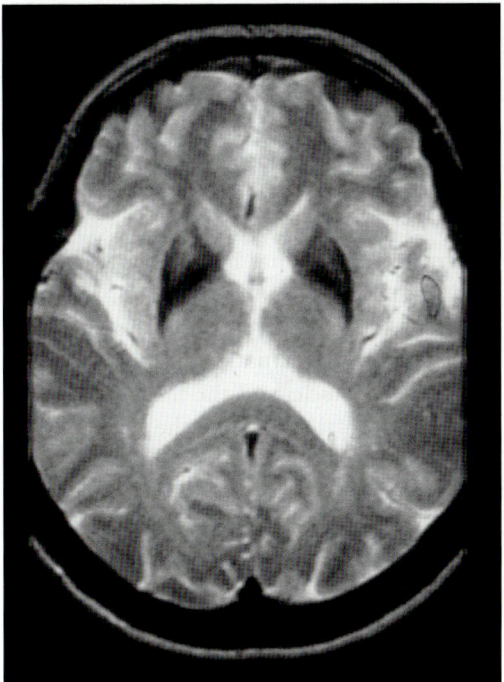

Figure 45.2a
T2-weighted MRI showing low lateral putamen signal at the same level as the pallidum in MSA.

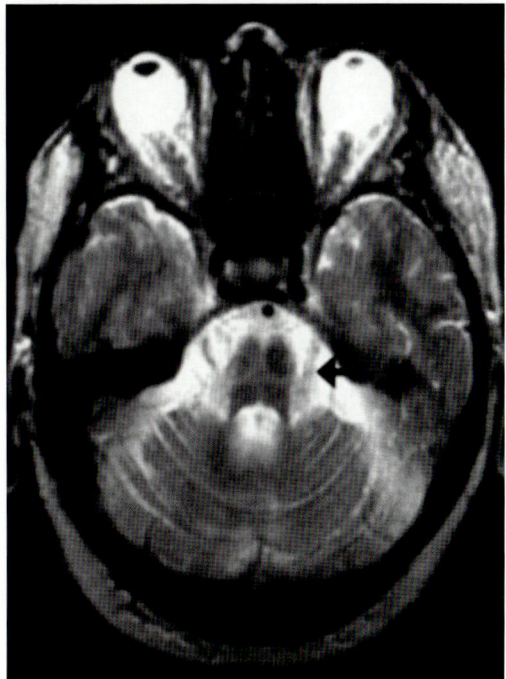

Figure 45.2b
T2-weighted MRI showing the pontine hot-cross-bun sign in MSA.

disorders as they are only seen in more advanced cases. Diffusion-weighted MRI provides a more sensitive modality for discriminating atypical from typical parkinsonian disorders. DTI of the striatum is normal in PD, but putamen water diffusivity is increased and FA reduced in MSA and PSP (2). MSA and PSP can be discriminated from each another by the pattern of increased diffusivity in the cerebellar peduncles, the middle cerebellar peduncles being abnormal in MSA and the superior cerebellar peduncles in PSP.

Transcranial sonography

Transcranial sonography (TCS) detects reflection of ultrasound waves and can reveal structural midbrain and striatal changes in parkinsonian disorders as a hyperechogenic signal. Over 90% of PD cases show increased midbrain echogenicity with TCS (see Figure 45.3), but this can also be seen in 10% of normal elderly people and 15% of essential tremor cases, so the specificity

for PD is not optimal (6). In a blinded series of patients with uncertain PD, the nigral hyperechogenicity detected with TCS showed a high sensitivity of 91% and a positive predictive value of 93% for detecting idiopathic PD. The specificity, however, was lower at 82%, and the negative predictive value was only 78%, suggesting TCS is susceptible to false positive diagnoses (7). The intensity of midbrain hyperechogenicity detected with TCS does not correlate with locomotor disability in PD nor progress with disease duration. It has been suggested that its presence is more a trait marker of susceptibility to PD rather than a state marker. In support of this, abnormal nigral hyperechogenicity can be detected in subjects at risk for PD, such as carriers of α-synuclein, LRRK2, parkin, and DJ1 gene mutations or subjects with late-onset hyposmia (8,9). Nigral hyperechogenicity is not seen in the atypical parkinsonian disorders despite the presence of dopamine cell loss at postmortem.

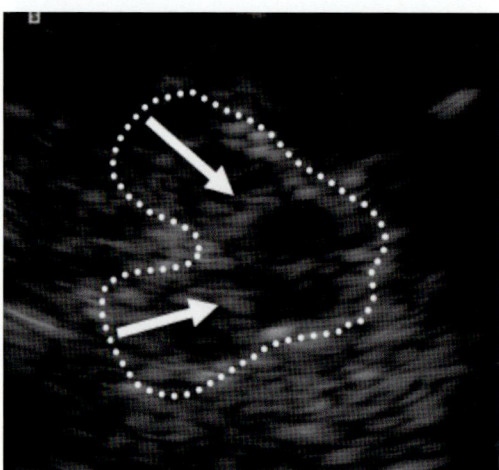

Figure 45.3
Transcranial sonography showing hyperechogenicity from the lateral midbrain (substantia nigra) in PD (6).

In contrast, hyperechogenic lentiform signal can be detected with TCS in MSA patients, and this, when combined with normal midbrain signals, can help discriminate MSA from PD with high sensitivity (10).

Structural imaging in hyperkinetic disorders

Dystonia

DYT1 is the most common familial form of generalized dystonia. It shows autosomal-dominant inheritance with around 40% penetrance and is usually early onset, starting in a lower limb, but adult-onset forms can be segmental. The DYT1 mutation is a GAG deletion within the coding region of the gene on chromosome 9q34 which codes for torsin A, an adenosine 5'-triphosphate (ATP)-binding protein of unknown function. DYT6 is the second most common generalized dystonia arising due to mutations of the Thanatos-associated, domain-containing, apoptosis-associated protein 1 (THAP1) gene on chromosome 8p. THAP1 binds to and modulates the torsin A promotor, and affected individuals tend to show adult onset, presenting with craniocervical or focal dystonic symptoms.

Conventional MRI is normal in the idiopathic and genetic dystonias, though in acquired dystonia cases due to stroke, tumors, or toxic damage, it may show structural lesions in the lentiform nucleus or posterior thalamus. Wilson's disease patients characteristically show cystic lesions in their basal ganglia. With the development of DTI and tractography, it has now become clear that brain connectivity is not normal in the genetic dystonias (11). DYT1 and DYT6 dystonia cases show abnormal structural connectivity between the cerebellar nuclei and the thalamus and between the frontal cortex and the striatum. DTI abnormalities have also been reported in focal dystonias such as torticollis, writer's cramp, and spasmodic dysphonia involving white-matter connections of pathways between the basal ganglia, cortex, and cerebellum. It seems likely that idiopathic and genetic dystonias are associated with the abnormal development of subcortical–cortical connections.

Huntington's disease (HD)

HD is an autosomally dominantly transmitted disorder associated with an excess of CAG triplet repeats (>38) in the huntingtin (HTT) gene on chromosome 4. The function of this gene is still uncertain, but the pathology of HD involves abnormal aggregation of huntingtin protein associated with its elongated polyglutamine chain and targetting the medium spiny projection neurons in the striatum which contain intranuclear and cytoplasmic inclusions. MRI shows increased, striatal, T_2-weighted signal and caudate atrophy in more advanced cases of established Huntington's disease, while MR volumetry can reveal subclinical caudate and putamen atrophy in premanifest gene carriers along with cortical grey matter loss and whole-brain atrophy in more advanced cases (12). Caudate volume abnormalities have been correlated with cognitive function, repeat length, and age of manifestation of clinical symptoms. DTI can reveal widespread brain abnormalities of water diffusivity which correlate with locomotor and cognitive disability. In tractography studies of pre-symptomatic HD patients, a reduction of frontal-caudate connectivity has been demonstrated (13).

Functional imaging in movement disorders

The changes in regional cerebral function that characterize different movement disorders can be examined in two main ways. First, focal changes in resting levels of regional cerebral metabolism, blood flow, and neuroreceptor availability can be measured. Second, abnormal patterns of regional brain activation evidenced as changes in blood flow or levels of neurotransmitter release can be detected when patients with movement disorders perform motor and cognitive tasks or are exposed to drug challenges.

Parkinson's disease

The presynaptic dopaminergic system

Dopamine terminal function in PD can be examined in vivo in three main ways (14): terminal dopa decarboxylase activity can be measured with ^{18}F-dopa PET; vesicle monoamine transporter (VMAT2) density can be studied with ^{11}C- or ^{18}F-dihydro-tetrabenazine (DTBZ) PET; and the availability of dopamine transporters (DaT) can be assessed with ^{11}C-methylphenidate (MP) and ^{11}C-nomifensine PET or tropane-based PET and SPECT markers such as ^{11}C-CFT, ^{18}F-FP-CIT, ^{123}I-altropane, ^{123}I-beta-CIT and ^{123}I-FP-CIT (see Figure 45.4).

In PD patients with early Hoehn and Yahr stage 1 disease lateralised to one side, bilaterally reduced putamen tracer uptake can be seen, the activity being most depressed in the putamen contralateral to the clinically affected limb (15). In the head of the caudate, dopamine terminal function remains relatively preserved until later in the condition. Onset of symptoms has been estimated to occur after a 30-50% loss of putamen dopamine terminal function. Unlike nigral hyperechogenicity, levels of putamen dopamine terminal function correlate well with the severity of limb rigidity and bradykinesia though not with the severity of tremor. In essential and dystonic tremor patients, dopamine function is normal, and PET and SPECT can thus differentiate these tremors from clinically probable PD with a sensitivity and specifici-

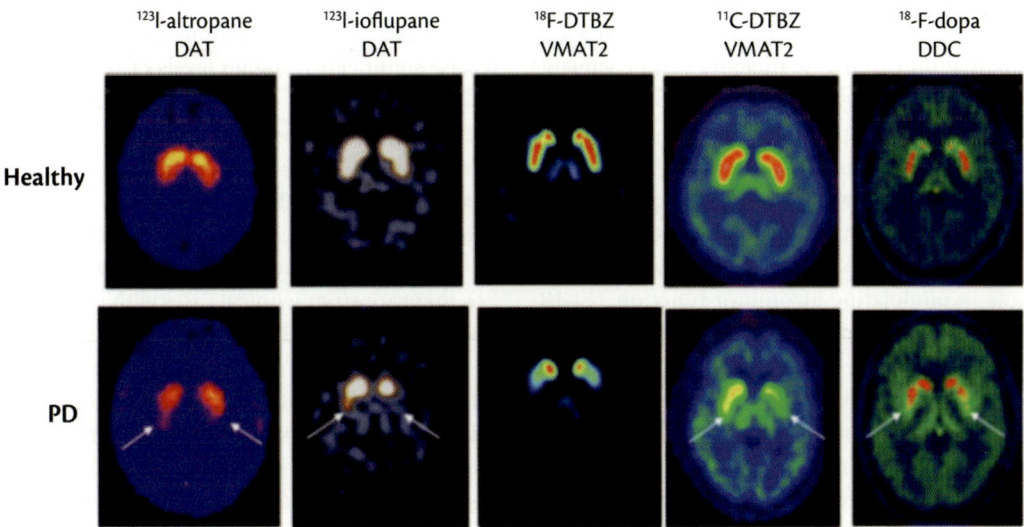

| ^{123}I-altropane DAT | ^{123}I-ioflupane DAT | ^{18}F-DTBZ VMAT2 | ^{11}C-DTBZ VMAT2 | ^{18}-F-dopa DDC |

Healthy

PD

Figure 45.4
SPECT and PET images of dopamine terminal function in normal subjects and early PD patients.

ty greater than 90% (16). An abnormal PET or SPECT scan provides support for a diagnosis of a dopamine-deficient parkinsonian syndrome and a rationale for treating with dopaminergic agents while a normal scan effectively excludes this diagnosis. Several studies have examined the utility of using DaT imaging to support or refute a diagnosis of dopamine-deficient parkinsonism. Using long-term clinical follow-up by experts as the gold standard, these trials have suggested that the baseline specificity of DaT imaging for correctly classifying PD is 90-100%, while clinicians tend to overdiagnose PD when uncertain (17). In the clinically uncertain parkinsonian syndromes (CUPS) trial, the diagnosis of dopamine-deficient parkinsonian syndrome was revised in 52% of the 118 cases and the management strategy changed in 72% of cases when FP-CIT SPECT findings were revealed to clinicians (18). Adult-onset dystonic tremor, drug-associated and psychogenic parkinsonism can all mimic PD. Marshall and co-workers presented 11 patients who initially fulfilled diagnostic criteria for PD and were treated with dopaminergic agents but in whom emerging diagnostic doubts led to DaT imaging with FP-CIT SPECT (19). This was negative, and subsequent antiparkinsonian therapy withdrawal was achieved without clinical deterioration, suggesting that dopaminergic imaging can be valuable where an inappropriate use of anti-parkinsonian medication is suspected.

Post-synaptic dopaminergic receptors

The striatum contains primarily dopamine D1 and D2 receptor subtypes, and they both play a role in modulating locomotor function. ^{123}I-IBZM (iodobenzamide) SPECT studies have reported normal levels of striatal D2 binding in untreated PD, while ^{11}C-raclopride PET detects a 10-20% increase in putamen D2 availability (14). As ^{11}C-raclopride competes with endogenous dopamine for D2 binding, this raised receptor availability probably reflects the dopamine depletion present rather than an adaptive

rise in receptor numbers. In chronically levodopa-exposed PD cases, levels of putamen D2 binding normalise as the synaptic levels of dopamine are restored.

Striatal dopamine level

As ^{11}C-raclopride competes with synaptic dopamine to bind to D2 receptors, its uptake is sensitive to changes in the synaptic levels of striatal dopamine so PET can be used to detect changes in dopamine induced by drugs or behaviours. Microdialysis studies in animals suggest that a 10% reduction in striatal ^{11}C-raclopride binding reflects a fivefold increase in synaptic dopamine levels. When PD patients take oral L-dopa, transient rises in synaptic dopamine result. ^{11}C-raclopride PET has shown that improvements in disability after L-dopa correlate with the estimated rises in putamen dopamine (20). Some PD patients compulsively take far larger doses of levodopa than are clinically required; this has been termed the dopamine dysregulation syndrome (DDS). Compared with PD patients who are not compulsively taking excess medication, DDS patients show enhanced levodopa-induced dopamine generation in the ventral striatum (21). In agreement, PD cases who develop impulse control disorders such as compulsive gambling when taking dopamine agonist therapy release significantly higher levels of ventral striatal dopamine when exposed to relevant stimuli such as betting on games of chance (22).

Premotor Parkinson's disease

It has been estimated from postmortem studies that for every patient who develops clinical PD, there are 10 subclinical cases with incidental brainstem Lewy body disease in the community. The greatest risk factors for PD are age and a family history. Late-onset, idiopathic hyposmia and REM behaviour sleep disorder (RBD) are also associated with later onset of Lewy body disorders. ^{18}F-dopa PET has detected subclinically reduced dopaminergic function in asymptomatic, adult, identical co-twins and relatives of idiopathic PD cases as well as parkin and LRRK2 gene carriers (14). Reduced striatal DaT binding can be detected in around 10% of late-onset hyposmic subjects (23) and a majority of patients with idiopathic RBD (24). The detection of reduced putamen dopaminergic function in asymptomatic, adult, identical co-twins of apparently sporadic PD cases emphasises that, even here, there is a likely role of inheritance.

Levodopa-induced dyskinesias

PD patients with early disease and sustained therapeutic responses to L-dopa show a reduction in striatal ^{11}C-raclopride binding after oral levodopa that is maintained for several hours, compatible with a sustained increase in synaptic dopamine levels. In contrast, dyskinetic cases show larger, but short-lived, falls in ^{11}C-raclopride binding, implying that pulsatile swings in dopamine levels are occurring (25). As the loss of dopamine terminals in PD becomes severe, the striatum fails to store dopamine and buffer synaptic levels when exogenous L-dopa is taken. This is magnified by a relatively greater loss of dopamine transporters from terminals, the mechanism for dopamine uptake from the synapse, compared with intra-terminal dopa decarboxylase activity (26). Pulsatile swings in synaptic dopamine levels will promote internalisation of dopamine receptors, which then become inactivated and unavailable, so unpredictable, fluctuating treatment responses can result. The severity of peak dose dyskinesias following oral L-dopa administration to PD patients has been shown to correlate with the induced rises of synaptic dopamine, as reflected by levels of reductions in putaminal ^{11}C-raclopride binding (20). The striatum contains high densities of adenosine A2A sites, which are found on the soma of striatal neurons of the indirect pathway and regulate its activity. Uptake of ^{11}C-SCH442416 and ^{11}C-TSMX, both markers of A2A binding, is normal in the striatum of non-dyskinetic PD patients but becomes raised in dyskinetic cases (27,28). N-methyl-D-aspartate (NMDA) receptors are a subclass of glutamate receptors that contain a voltage-gated ion channel which is opened during learning and memory tasks. ^{11}C-CNS5161 PET is a use-dependent marker of NMDA ion channel activity, and recently, striatal uptake of ^{11}C-CNS5161 has been shown to be increased when PD patients are actively experiencing L-dopa-induced limb dyskinesias (29). Increased NMDA ion channel activation during dyskinesias could help to explain the beneficial mode of action of amantadine, an NMDA antagonist.

Parkinson's disease-related depression

A majority of PD patients experience depressive symptoms. It has been suggested that serotonergic loss might contribute to depression in PD, but to date the results from neuroimaging studies have not supported this view. Midbrain uptake of [123]I- ß-CIT reflects serotonin transporter availability, and while it is reduced in PD, levels do not differ between PD patients with and without depression or correlate with Hamilton depression rating scale (HDRS) scores (30). Remy and co-workers used ^{11}C-RT132 PET, a marker of dopamine and noradrenaline transporters, to assess PD patients with and without depression (31). The depressed PD patients had lower ^{11}C-RT132 binding in the locus ceruleus and areas of the limbic system than non-depressed PD patients. This finding suggests that loss of limbic dopamine and noradrenaline rather than serotonin deficiency may be more relevant to the pathogenesis of depression in patients with PD.

Parkinson's disease-related cognitive dysfunction

Some 80% of PD patients will develop dementia if they survive for 20 years with their illness. This can reflect the presence of cortical Lewy body disease, Alzheimer pathology, cerebral small-vessel disease, and the degeneration of dopaminergic and cholinergic projections to cortical areas. Cholinergic terminal function can be assessed with ^{11}C-N-methylpyrrolidon (NMP)4A and [11]C- polymethylpentene (PMP)

PET, markers of acetylcholine esterase activity (32). Non-demented PD patients show focally reduced cholinergic function in the parietal and occipital cortex. When overt dementia is present in PD cases, they manifest a global and severe reduction of cortical ^{11}C-NMP4A binding. Levels of cortical acetylcholinesterase activity in PD correlate with MMSE scores and performance on executive tests such as card sorting and trail-making. These results suggest that progressive cognitive impairment in PD is in part a consequence of a cholinergic deficit.

Levels of [18]FDG (^{18}F-2-fluoro-2-deoxyglucose) uptake reflect neuronal synaptic activity. In non-demented PD patients, cortical FDG uptake is generally within normal limits, but covariance analysis reveals an abnormal profile of a relatively increased lentiform nucleus and reduced fronto-parietal metabolism (33). This has been labelled the PD-related profile (PDRP), and its degree of expression correlates with the degree of motor disability. The PDRP normalises after successful treatment with both dopaminergic drugs or deep brain stimulation. Frankly demented PD patients show an Alzheimer's disease pattern of impaired brain glucose utilization, with posterior cingulate, parietal and temporal association areas being affected the most (34). PD patients with mild cognitive impairment (MCI) show a similar pattern of glucose hypometabolism, though to a lesser extent (35). This pattern of glucose hypo-

metabolism in demented PD patients may reflect cortical Lewy body disease, coincidental AD, or some other degenerative process. In cases pathologically proven later on to have cortical Lewy body disease, there tends to be greater hypometabolism of the primary occipital cortex than that seen in Alzheimer's patients (36). This could explain the tendency of these cases to develop illusions and hallucinations. The PET ligand ^{11}C-PIB, a neutral thioflavin-T analogue developed to image ß-amyloid plaques in AD, has recently been employed to study PD patients with dementia, and at risk of it. Only a minority of these cases showed significantly increased ^{11}C-PIB uptake, suggesting that amyloid pathology is not a major contributor to the cognitive problems in PD cases with late-onset, PD-related dementia (PDD) (37).

Parkinson's disease-related cardiac sympathetic dysfunction

^{123}I-MIBG SPECT is a marker of adrenergic terminal function and can be used to study the functional integrity of cardiac sympathetic innervation in PD. The mediastinal ^{123}I-MIBG (iodine-131-meta-iodobenzylguanidine) signal is reduced in a majority of PD cases, even in the absence of overt impairment of cardiovascular reflexes (see Figure 45.5). However, 50% Hoehn and Yahr stage 1 PD cases still show normal levels of cardiac MIBG uptake, so this modality is not as sensitive a marker as DaT imaging, where

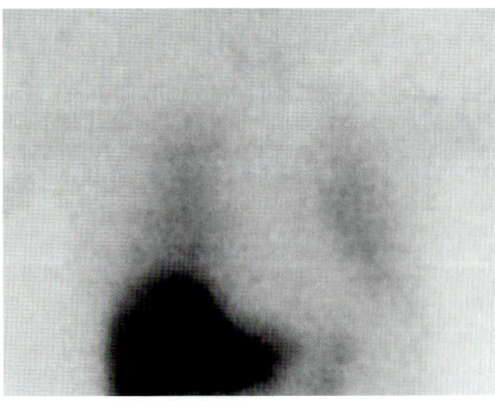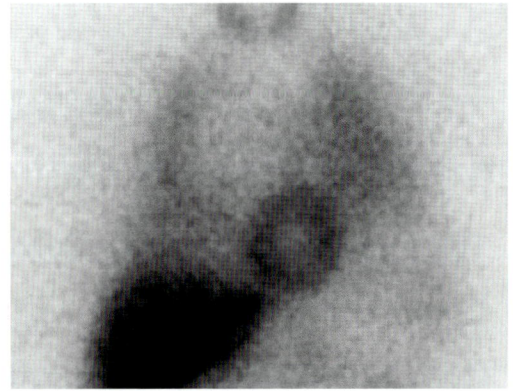

Figure 45.5
^{123}I-MIBG images of cardiac sympathetic function in PD and MSA (52).

putamen DaT binding is reduced by at least 30% (38).

Atypical Parkinsonisms

Multiple System Atrophy (MSA)

Loss of pre-synaptic dopaminergic function has an overlapping pattern in PD and MSA, both conditions showing asymmetric loss of putamen function, though the head of the caudate may be more targeted in MSA. So, while striatal ^{18}F-dopa, VMAT2, and DaT imaging can separate these parkinsonian conditions from healthy patients and benign tremors, it cannot reliably discriminate MSA and PD from each another (39). [18]FDG PET studies in MSA do show reduced levels of striatal, brainstem, and cerebellar glucose metabolism, while they are preserved or raised in PD, allowing 90% of MSA-P cases to be discriminated from PD (40). MSA is also associated with a loss of putamen dopamine D2 site binding, while this is preserved in PD (see Figure 45.6). However, these reductions are mild in MSA and do not provide a sensitive discrimination of this condition from PD. In one series, ^{123}I-IBZM SPECT detected reduced striatal D2 binding in two-thirds of de novo parkinsonian patients who had a negative apomorphine response and were thought to have early MSA-P (41).

^{123}I-MIBG SPECT, a marker of cardiac adrenergic terminal function, is normal in MSA as the autonomic dysfunction results from a loss of pre- rather than post-synaptic innervation (see Figure 45.5) (42). This differentiates MSA from PD where the sympathetic loss is post-synaptic and provides another means of discriminating these two conditions.

Progressive supranuclear palsy (PSP)

PSP is also associated with a striatal loss of pre-synaptic dopaminergic function but, in contrast to PD and MSA, this tends to be symmetrical, and the head of the caudate and putamen are uniformly targeted (14). Corticobasal degeneration and small-vessel disease can also target the head of the caudate, but the reductions in ^{18}F-dopa, VMAT2, and DaT imaging are usually also asymmetrical. FDG PET reveals depressed frontal cortex, basal ganglia, cerebellar, and thalamic glucose metabolism in PSP, which correlates with disease duration and performance on psychometric tests of frontal function. The presence of reduced striatal metabolism sensitively discriminates 90% of PSP cases from PD, but as striatal hypometabolism is also a feature of MSA, FDG PET cannot reliably discriminate these two atypical parkinsonian conditions. Striatal D2 binding is reduced in a majority of PSP

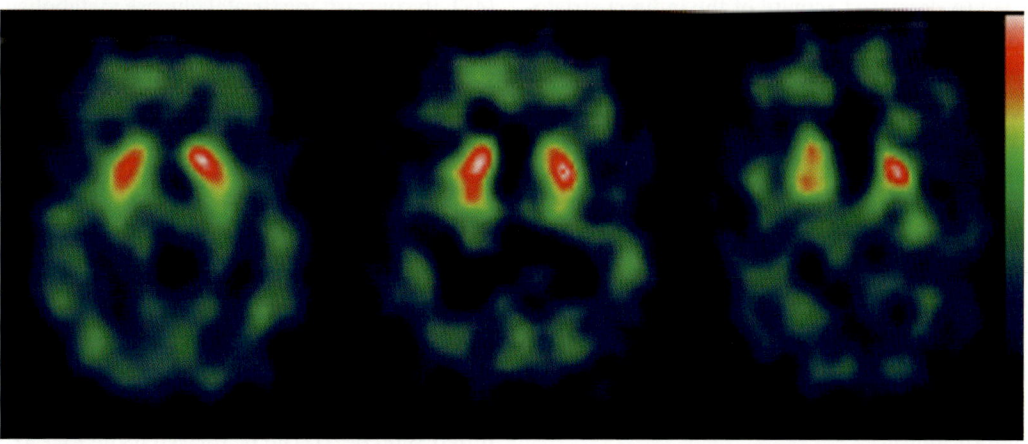

Figure 45.6
^{123}I-IBZM SPECT images of dopamine D2 receptor binding in a normal subject, PD, and MSA cases. Striatal D2 binding is reduced in MSA case (courtesy of Gregor Wenning).

cases, and this can be detected with ^{11}C-raclopride PET or IBZM SPECT.

Involuntary Movement Disorders

Dystonia

FDG PET shows normal levels of resting glucose metabolism in DYT1 carriers, but covariance analysis reveals an abnormal resting metabolic profile where the levels of lentiform nucleus glucose metabolism are relatively reduced and the frontal metabolism raised (43). This pattern, almost the reverse of that reported for Parkinson's disease, shows whether DYT1 gene carriers are clinically affected or asymptomatic. A PET study of DYT1 dystonic patients performed while they slept also showed this abnormal profile of resting glucose metabolism, confirming that it is not movement-related. A similar profile has been reported in DYT6 dystonia and in essential blepharospasm. These findings suggest that resting dysfunction of a common network involving the basal ganglia and frontal cortex may underlie the clinical expression in all genetic dystonias. ^{18}F-dopa PET and ^{123}I-beta-CIT SPECT studies have shown normal dopamine storage in a majority of idiopathic torsion dystonia (ITD) cases. In contrast, PET and SPECT have shown that striatal D2 binding is reduced (44). This could conceivably lead to decreased activity of the indirect striatopallidal pathway, which normally acts to inhibit unwanted movements or actions. Recently, it has been reported that the uptake of ^{11}C-flumazenil, a PET marker of benzodiazepine receptor binding on the GABA$_A$ complex, is reduced in motor and premotor areas in a group of DYT1 and sporadic dystonics (45). Such a deficit in GABAergic function could result in a failure of normal cortical inhibitory circuits, also allowing involuntary muscle contractions to occur.

Dopa-responsive dystonia and/or dystonia-parkinsonism

Dominantly inherited dopa-responsive dystonia (DRD) is related to a mutation in the DYT5 gene coding for GTP cyclohydrolase 1. This enzyme constitutes part of the tetrahydrobiopterin synthetic pathway, the cofactor for tyrosine hydroxylase. Patients are unable to manufacture endogenous levodopa, and hence dopamine, from tyrosine but can still convert exogenous levodopa to dopamine. DRD cases generally present in childhood with diurnally fluctuating, lower-limb dystonia and later develop generalized background parkinsonism. Occasionally, the condition presents as pure parkinsonism in adulthood. ^{18}F-dopa PET and ^{123}I-beta-CIT SPECT findings are normal in DRD patients, which distinguishes this condition from early-onset dystonia-parkinsonism where severely reduced putamen ^{18}F-dopa and ^{123}I-beta-CIT uptake is found (46).

Huntington's disease (HD) and other choreas

Degenerative disorders associated with chorea include HD, neuroacanthocytosis (NA), dentatorubro-pallidoluysian atrophy (DRPLA), and benign familial chorea (BFC). The inflammatory disorders systemic lupus erythematosus (SLE) and Sydenham's chorea are also associated with chorea, as is chronic neuroleptic exposure (see Chapter 29). Clinically affected HD, NA, DRPLA, and occasional BFC cases show reduced striatal levels of the resting glucose metabolism (47). In contrast, the striatal glucose metabolism is normal or raised in inflammatory or tardive choreas. The medium spiny striatal neurons that degenerate in HD express D2 receptors. ^{11}C-raclopride PET studies show striatal D2 binding is reduced by at least 30% when HD patients manifest symptoms (48). Reduced striatal ^{11}C-raclopride binding is also seen in NA, but the binding is normal in SLE and tardive choreas.

Around 50% of premanifesting adult HD gene carriers show reduced levels of striatal glucose metabolism and D2 binding, indicating that active subclinical disease is present. The rate of progression of HD can be tracked using PET as a biomarker. The caudate glucose metabolism has been reported to decline by 3% per annum, while striatal D2 binding declines by 3-6% (48). These findings suggest that functional imaging could provide an objective means of following HD progression in the event of effective neuroprotective or restorative interventions being found.

Microglia constitute 10–20% of white cells in the brain and form its natural defence mechanism. They are normally in a resting state, but local injury causes them to activate and swell, expressing HLA antigens on the cell surface and releasing cytokines such as IL1 and TNFα. The mitochondria of activated microglia express the translocator protein (TSPO), which is a steroid transporter previously known as the peripheral benzodiazepine site. ^{11}C-PK11195 is an isoquinoline which binds selectively to the TSPO and so provides an in vivo PET marker of microglial activation.

Post-mortem studies of HD brains have shown a significant accumulation of activated microglia in the basal ganglia and the frontal cortex. HD patients show significant increases in striatal ^{11}C-PK11195 binding, which correlate with clinical disease severity as measured with the unified Huntington's disease rating scale (UHDRS), with striatal reductions in ^{11}C-raclopride binding, and with the size of the patients' CAG triplet expansion (49). Increased striatal and cortical ^{11}C-PK11195 binding can also be seen in many adult, premanifest, HD gene carriers, suggesting microglial activation is an early event (see Figure 45.7) (50). Taken together, the findings from postmortem and neuroimaging studies support the view that activated microglia contribute to the ongoing neuronal degeneration in HD.

Conclusions

Structural imaging

- Structural changes in PD nigra can now be detected with 7 tesla high-field MRI, 3 tesla

| Normal | Huntington gene carrier |

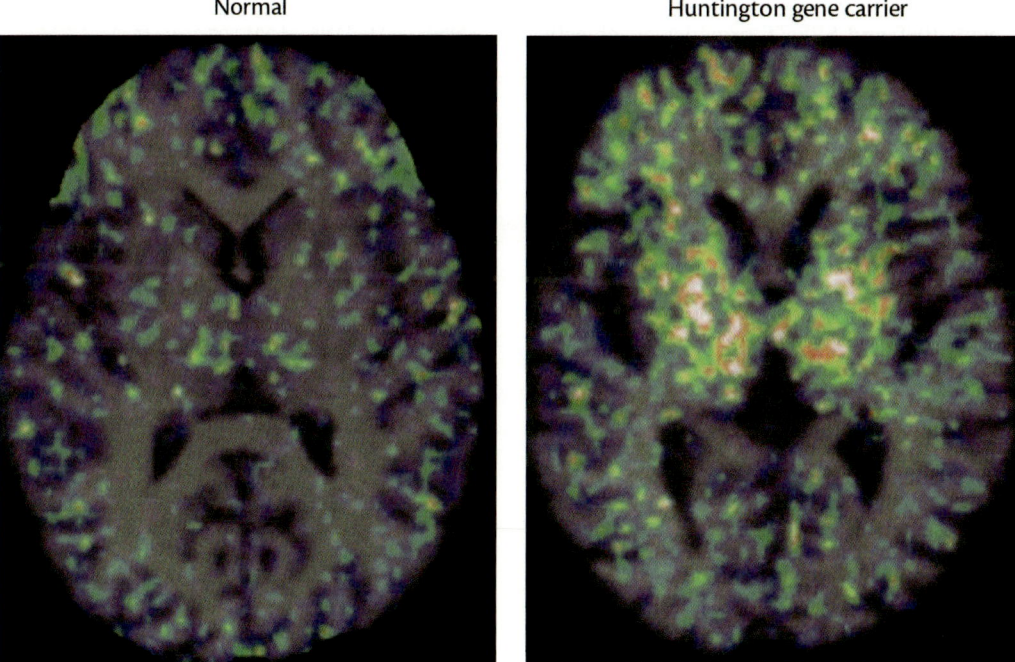

Figure 45.7

Figure 45.7: ^{11}C-PK11195 PET scans of a healthy subject and HD gene carrier. Mild microglial activation is seen in the thalamus of the healthy control whereas significantly raised activation is evident in the frontal cortex and striata of the HD patient (courtesy of Nicola Pavese).

diffusion tensor imaging, and transcranial sonography.

- The presence of midbrain hyperechogenicity reveals a susceptibility trait to PD but does not correlate with severity of disease or change as the disease progresses.
- Atypical parkinsonian syndromes can be discriminated from typical PD by the presence of abnormal lentiform nucleus signals detectable with both diffusion-weighted MRI and TCS and an absence of midbrain hyperechogenicity.
- In MSA the middle cerebellar peduncle is targeted, showing DTI signal changes, while the superior cerebellar peduncle is targeted in PSP.
- DTI with tractography reveals abnormal cerebellar-thalamic and fronto-striatal connectivity in the genetic dystonias.

Functional imaging

- Detecting dopamine terminal dysfunction with PET and SPECT provides an objective means of supporting a diagnosis of dopamine-deficient parkinsonism where clinical doubt exists. It can provide a rationale for a trial of dopaminergic medication.
- FDG PET sensitively detects striatal hypometabolism in suspected atypical PD variants, thus discriminating them from PD.
- PET and SPECT can detect subclinical dopamine terminal dysfunction in subjects at risk for PD. This could help identify cases for neuroprotective approaches if a successful therapy is identified.
- Dyskinesias in PD are associated with excessively raised synaptic levels of dopamine after levodopa and altered opioid, adenosine, and glutamate transmission.
- Impulse control disorders in PD are associated with an excessive ventral striatal production of dopamine when exposed to relevant stimuli.

- FDG PET reveals a common abnormal profile of resting glucose metabolism in genetic and sporadic dystonias.
- PET can detect reduced striatal D2 binding and striatal inflammation (microglial activation) in premanifesting HD gene carriers, providing evidence of disease activity and a rationale for testing anti-inflammatory neuroprotective strategies.

References

1 Song SK, Lee JE, Park HJ, Sohn YH, Lee JD, Lee PH. The pattern of cortical atrophy in patients with Parkinson's disease according to cognitive status. Mov Disord 2011;26:289-296.

2 Prodoehl J, Li H, Planetta PJ, et al. Diffusion tensor imaging of Parkinson's disease, atypical parkinsonism, and essential tremor. Mov Disord 2013; doi: 10.1002/mds.25491.

3 Du G, Lewis MM, Sen S, et al. Imaging nigral pathology and clinical progression in Parkinson's disease. Mov Disord 2012;27:1636-1643.

4 Scherfler C, Schocke MF, Seppi K, et al. Voxel-wise analysis of diffusion weighted imaging reveals disruption of the olfactory tract in Parkinson's disease. Brain 2006;129:538-542.

5 Schrag A, Good CD, Miszkiel K, et al. Differentiation of atypical parkinsonian syndromes with routine MRI. Neurology 2000;54:697-702.

6 Berg D, Siefker C, Becker G. Echogenicity of the substantia nigra in Parkinson's disease and its relation to clinical findings. J Neurol 2001;248:684-689.

7 Gaenslen A, Unmuth B, Godau J, et al. The specificity and sensitivity of transcranial ultrasound in the differential diagnosis of Parkinson's disease: a prospective blinded study. Lancet Neurol 2008;7:417-424.

8 Walter U, Klein C, Hilker R, Benecke R, Pramstaller PP, Dressler D. Brain parenchyma sonography detects preclinical parkinsonism. Mov Disord 2004;19:1445-1449.

9 Sommer U, Hummel T, Cormann K, et al. Detection of presymptomatic Parkinson's disease: combining smell tests, transcranial sonography, and SPECT. Mov Disord 2004;19:1196-1202.

10 Behnke S, Berg D, Naumann M, Becker G. Differentiation of Parkinson's disease and atypical parkinsonian syndromes by transcranial ultrasound. J Neurol Neurosurg Psychiatry 2005;76:423-425.

11 Carbon M, Argyelan M, Eidelberg D. Functional imaging in hereditary dystonia. Eur J Neurol 2010;17S1:58-64.

12 Georgiou-Karistianis N, Scahill R, Tabrizi SJ, Squitieri F, Aylward E. Structural MRI in Huntington's disease and recommendations for its potential use in clinical trials. Neuroscience and biobehavioral reviews 2013;37:480-490.

13 Della Nave R, Ginestroni A, Tessa C, et al. Regional distribution and clinical correlates of white matter structural damage in Huntington disease: a tract-based spatial statistics study. AJNR Am J Neuroradiol 2010;31:1675-1681.

14 Brooks DJ. Imaging approaches to Parkinson disease. J Nucl Med 2010;51:596-609.

15 Morrish PK, Sawle GV, Brooks DJ. Clinical and [18F]dopa PET findings in early Parkinson's disease. JNeurolNeurosurgPsychiat 1995;59:597-600.

16 Benamer TS, Patterson J, Grosset DG, et al. Accurate differentiation of parkinsonism and essential tremor using visual assessment of [123I]-FP-CIT imaging: The [123I]-FP-CIT Study Group. Mov Disord 2000;15:503-510.

17 Jennings DL, Seibyl JP, Oakes D, Eberly S, Murphy J, Marek K. (123I) beta-CIT and single-photon emission computed tomographic imaging vs clinical evaluation in Parkinsonian syndrome: unmasking an early diagnosis. Arch Neurol 2004;61:1224-1229.

18 Catafau AM, Tolosa E. Impact of dopamine transporter SPECT using 123I-Ioflupane on diagnosis and management of patients with clinically uncertain Parkinsonian syndromes. Mov Disord 2004;19:1175-1182.

19 Marshall VL, Patterson J, Hadley DM, Grosset KA, Grosset DG. Successful antiparkinsonian medication withdrawal in patients with Parkinsonism and normal FP-CIT SPECT. Mov Disord 2006;21:2247-2250.

20 Pavese N, Evans AH, Tai YF, et al. Clinical correlates of levodopa-induced dopamine release in Parkinson disease: a PET study. Neurology 2006;67:1612-1617.

21 Evans AH, Pavese N, Lawrence AD, et al. Compulsive drug use linked to sensitized ventral striatal dopamine transmission. Ann Neurol 2006;59:852-858.

22 Steeves TD, Miyasaki J, Zurowski M, et al. Increased striatal dopamine release in Parkinsonian patients with pathological gambling: a [11C] raclopride PET study. Brain 2009;132:1376-1385.

23 Ponsen MM, Stoffers D, Wolters E, Booij J, Berendse HW. Olfactory testing combined with dopamine transporter imaging as a method to detect prodromal Parkinson's disease. J Neurol Neurosurg Psychiatry 2010;81:396-399.

24 Eisensehr I, Linke R, Noachtar S, Schwarz J, Gildehaus FJ, Tatsch K. Reduced striatal dopamine transporters in idiopathic rapid eye movement sleep behaviour disorder - comparison with Parkinson's disease and controls. Brain 2000 Jun;123:1155-1160.

25 de la Fuente-Fernandez R, Sossi V, Huang Z, et al. Levodopa-induced changes in synaptic dopamine levels increase with progression of Parkinson's disease: implications for dyskinesias. Brain 2004;127:2747-2754.

26 Troiano AR, de la Fuente-Fernandez R, Sossi V, et al. PET demonstrates reduced dopamine transporter expression in PD with dyskinesias. Neurology 2009;72:1211-1216.

27 Ramlackhansingh AF, Bose SK, Ahmed I, Turkheimer FE, Pavese N, Brooks DJ. Adenosine 2A receptor availability in dyskinetic and nondyskinetic patients with Parkinson disease. Neurology 2011;76:1811-1816.

28 Mishina M, Ishiwata K, Naganawa M, et al. Adenosine A(2A) receptors measured with [C]TMSX PET in the striata of Parkinson's disease patients. PLoS One 2011;6:e17338.

29 Ahmed I, Bose SK, Pavese N, et al. Glutamate NMDA receptor dysregulation in Parkinson's disease with dyskinesias. Brain 2011;134:979-986.

30 Kim SE, Choi JY, Choe YS, Choi Y, Lee WY. Serotonin transporters in the midbrain of Parkinson's disease patients: a study with 123I-beta-CIT SPECT. J Nucl Med 2003;44:870-876.

31 Remy P, Doder, M., Lees, A.J., Turjanski, N., Brooks, D.J. Depression in Parkinson's disease: loss of dopa-

mine and noradrenaline innervation in the limbic system. Brain 2005;128:1314 - 1322.

32 Bohnen NI, Albin RL. The cholinergic system and Parkinson disease. Behavioural brain research 2011;221:564-573.

33 Eidelberg D. Metabolic brain networks in neurodegenerative disorders: a functional imaging approach. Trends Neurosci 2009;32:548-557.

34 Kuhl DE, Metter EJ, Benson DF. Similarities of cerebral glucose metabolism in Alzheimer's and Parkinsonian dementia. JCerebBlood Flow Metab 1985;5:S169-S170.

35 Pappata S, Santangelo G, Aarsland D, et al. Mild cognitive impairment in drug-naive patients with PD is associated with cerebral hypometabolism. Neurology 2011;77:1357-1362.

36 Bohnen NI, Koeppe RA, Minoshima S, et al. Cerebral Glucose Metabolic Features of Parkinson Disease and Incident Dementia: Longitudinal Study. J Nucl Med 2011.

37 Edison P, Rowe CC, Rinne JO, et al. Amyloid load in Parkinson's disease dementia and Lewy body dementia measured with [11C]PIB positron emission tomography. J Neurol Neurosurg Psychiatry 2008;79:1331-1338.

38 Nagayama H, Hamamoto M, Ueda M, Nagashima J, Katayama Y. Reliability of MIBG myocardial scintigraphy in the diagnosis of Parkinson's disease. J Neurol Neurosurg Psychiatry 2005;76:249-251.

39 Brooks DJ. Can imaging separate multiple system atrophy from Parkinson's disease? Mov Disord 2012;27:3-5.

40 Spetsieris PG, Ma Y, Dhawan V, Eidelberg D. Differential diagnosis of parkinsonian syndromes using PCA-based functional imaging features. Neuroimage 2009;45:1241-1252.

41 Schwarz J, Tatsch K, Arnold G, et al. 123I-iodobenzamide-SPECT predicts dopaminergic responsiveness in patients with de-novo parkinsonism. Neurology 1992;42:556-561.

42 Druschky A, Hilz MJ, Platsch G, et al. Differentiation of Parkinson's disease and multiple system atrophy in early disease stages by means of I-123-MIBG-SPECT. J Neurol Sci 2000;175:3-12.

43 Asanuma K, Carbon-Correll M, Eidelberg D. Neuroimaging in human dystonia. J Med Invest 2005;52 Suppl:272-279.

44 Perlmutter JS, Stambuk MK, Markham J, et al. Decreased [F-18] spiperone binding in putamen in idiopathic focal dystonia. JNeurosci 1997;17:843-850.

45 Garibotto V, Romito LM, Elia AE, et al. In vivo evidence for GABA(A) receptor changes in the sensorimotor system in primary dystonia. Mov Disord 2011;26:852-857.

46 Turjanski N, Bhatia K, Burn DJ, Sawle GV, Marsden CD, Brooks DJ. Comparison of striatal 18F-dopa uptake in adult-onset dystonia-parkinsonism, Parkinson's disease, and dopa-responsive dystonia. Neurology 1993;43:1563-1568.

47 Hosokawa S, Ichiya Y, Kuwabara Y, et al. Positron emission tomography in cases of chorea with different underlying diseases. JNeurolNeurosurgPsychiat 1987;50:1284-1287.

48 Andrews TC, Weeks RA, Turjanski N, et al. Huntington's disease progression PET and clinical observations. Brain 1999 Dec;122:2353-2363.

49 Pavese N, Gerhard A, Tai YF, et al. Microglial activation correlates with severity in Huntington disease: a clinical and PET study. Neurology 2006;66:1638-1643.

50 Tai YF, Pavese N, Gerhard A, et al. Microglial activation in presymptomatic Huntington's disease gene carriers. Brain 2007;130:1759-1766.

51 Vaillancourt DE, Spraker MB, Prodoehl J, et cl. High-resolution diffusion tensor imaging in the substantia nigra of the novo Parkinson disease. Neurology 2009;72:1378-1384.

52 Braune S, Reinhardt M, Schnitzer R, Riedel A, Lücking CH. Cardiac uptake of [123]IMIBG seperates Parkinson's disease from multiple system athophy. Neurology 1999;53:1020-1025.

Addenda

Video Fragments

PLAY

Video fragments on Dropbox:
www.dropbox.com/sh/bj1qt1yy1qum2bd/WkT2T1yrP-

Fragment 5.1
Parkinsonism (Segments 1-10)
The clinical hallmarks of (motor) parkinsonism are shown in this video fragment.
Segments 1-3 display bradykinesia, segment 4 hypokinesia, segment 5 the typical parkinsonian rest tremor, and segment 6 rigidity with the cogwheel phenomenon in various patients suffering from motor parkinsonism. Segment 7 shows the loss of postural reflexes with instability, the phenomena of propulsion (segment 8) and retropulsion (segment 9), and stooped posture (segment 10) in motor parkinsonism (courtesy Erik Wolters).

Fragment 5.2
Parkinson's disease (Segments 1-5)
This fragment shows a 60-year-old woman suffering from right > left-sided Parkinson's disease, with hypokinesia (masked face: segment 1), reduced arm swing (segment 2), tremor (segment 3), and bradykinesia in the right body-half (segments 4 and 5) (courtesy Teus van Laar).

Fragment 9.1
REM sleep behaviour disorder (1)
Nocturnal video-polysomnography of a 78-year-old male patient with idiopathic Parkinson's disease and REM sleep behaviour disorder (RBD).

In this patient with severe comorbid depression, RBD manifests with expression of joy and laughter (courtesy Christian Baumann).

Fragment 9.2
REM sleep behaviour disorder (2)
Nocturnal video-polysomnography of a 71-year-old female patient with idiopathic Parkinson's disease. On the left side, sleep electro-encephalogram (bottom), electro-oculogram (top) and electro-myogram are visible. The patient is in rapid eye movement (REM) sleep. REM sleep behaviour in this patient manifests primarily with expression of fear and screaming, but not with motor activity (courtesy Christian Baumann).

Fragment 11.1
Allied health strategies in PD (Segments 1-2)
Patients suffering Parkinson's disease with progressive instability and/or freezings, limiting their activities of daily living, might be helped by external cues. Two examples are given: the first segment shows an elderly man, passing sliding doors without and later with acoustic cues (rhythmic ticks with his cane). The second segment shows the impact of visual cues on a late-stage PD patient with severe walking problems in the home situation (with lines on the floor) (courtesy Erik Wolters).

Fragment 12.1
Motor fluctuations in PD (Segments 1-4)
Earlier or later, PD patients will develop levodopa-induced and to a lesser extent dopamine agonists-induced complications, such as hyperkinesias (segment 1), off-related dystonia (segment 2), unpredictable 'on-off' fluctuations (segment

3) and/or diphasic dyskinesias (segment 4), which were induced in this patient by threshold concentrations of L-dopa, related to a discontinuous medication schedule (courtesy Erik Wolters).

Fragment 12.2
Peak-dose chorea
Videofragment showing typical levodopa-induced, peak-dose, choreatic hyperkinesia (courtesy Erik Wolters).

Fragment 12.3
Dopamine dysregulation syndrome
In this video, note the disabling clinical expression of the consequences of a disorder associated with the abuse (overuse) of levodopa in a young PD patient (dopamine dysregulation syndrome) (courtesy Erik Wolters).

Fragment 14.1
CDS-LCIG (1) (segments 1-4).
This video shows a 34-year-old man, suffering since the age of 24 from right-sided, subtle motor parkinsonism, diagnosed three years later as idiopathic PD, and treated with levodopa (segment 1: off-medication). After 1.5 years of treatment, he developed motor fluctuations and dyskinesias, necessitating continuous dopaminergic stimulation; two years later, the effects of the medication became unpredictable, with alternating, short-lived 'on' with dyskinesias (UPDRS III: 15) and akinetic 'off' (UPDRS III: 40) periods (segment 2: 'on' with dyskinesias). In segments 3 and 4 the effects of LCIG (levodopa-carbidopa intestinal gel) 700 mg/day (without bothersome dyskinesia) are evident 6 months and 3 years, respectively, after application (courtesy Angelo Antonini).

Fragment 14.2
CDS-CLIG (2) (segments 1-2)
Here you see a young man suffering from idiopathic PD since the age of 11, treated with PEG-J-applied continuous (levodopa-carbidopa intestinal gel) CLIG before (segment 1) and after

(segment 2) discontinuation of this application (courtesy Erik Wolters).

Fragment 17.1
Vascular parkinsonism
Typical walking pattern of a hypertensive man, with small steps, difficulty with turning, freezing episodes, and a well preserved arm swing (lower body-half parkinsonism) (courtesy Erik Wolters).

Fragment 18.1
Ephedrine-induced parkinsonism (Segments 1-3)
This videotape displays the clinical presentation of an ephedrine-induced encephalopathy manifesting with bradykinesia and hypokinesia (segment 1), the typical cock gait (segment 2) and the specific dysarthria (segment 3) (courtesy Andrzej Friedmann).

Fragment 20.1
Progressive supranuclear palsy (1)
(segments 1-5)
Patient suffering PSP with typical, vertical, supranuclear, downward gaze paralysis (segment 1), bradykinesia (segment 2), pseudobulbar speech (segment 3), micrography (segment 4) and postural instability with falls (segment 5) (courtesy Andrew Lees).

Fragment 20.2
Progressive supranuclear palsy (2)
(segments 1-5)
71-year-old patient with progressive supranuclear palsy. Segment 1 shows the patient's hypophonia, segment 2 the bilateral bradykinesia. In segment 3 and 4, the patient's postural instability and bradykinetic gait might be appreciated. Typical slow vertical saccades are shown in segment 5 (courtesy Christian Baumann).

Fragment 22.1
DYT1 dystonia
Young man with a DYT1 mutation (early-onset torsion dystonia), showing a generalized torsion dystonia (courtesy Erik Wolters).

Fragment 22.2
Secondary dystonia (Segments 1-2)
The first patient suffers from a pantothenate kinase-associated neurodegeneration (PKAN), formerly called Hallervorden-Spatz disease (segment 1). The second patient suffers from the X-linked dystonia-deafness syndrome (Mohr-Tranebjaerg syndrome) (segment 2) (courtesy Erik Wolters).

Fragment 22.3
Focal/segmental dystonia (Segments1-4)
The first patient shows mainly focal blepharospasms with a slight dystonia of the perioral muscles (segment 1), the second patient suffers from a severe, segmental Meige syndrome with overflow to the trapezius muscles (segment 2), the third patient suffers from a focal torticollis spasmodica (segment 3), and the fourth patient from a focal spasmodic dysphonia. This last segment shows this patient's initially normal breathing, followed by supraglottic hyper-adduction during phonation, resulting in a typical dysphonic speech. The final part of this segment evidences the significant improvement after injection with botulinum toxin in the thyro-arythenoid muscles, producing reduced supraglottic adduction (segment 4) (courtesy Martin Horstink).

Fragment 23.1
Wilson's disease (Segments 1-6)
Mild signs of parkinsonism can be appreciated in this video fragment of a young woman suffering Wilson's disease: hypokinesia (segment 1), resting tremor (segment 2), intention tremor (segment 3), bradykinesia (segment 4), instability and loss of postural reflexes with retropulsion (segment 5) as well as the typical corneal Kayser-Fleischer rings (segment 6) (courtesy Erik Wolters).

Fragment 26.1
Essential tremor
Here you might appreciate the clinical expression of a patient suffering a mild, (asymmetric postural and accompanying action) tremor of both hands (courtesy Erik Wolters).

Fragment 26.2
Parkinson tremor
Unilateral resting tremor with a shortlasting suppression of the tremor amplitude after positioning of the hands (courtesy Erik Wolters).

Fragment 26.3
Enhanced physiological tremor
This patient shows a distal, high-frequency tremor with small amplitude, especially in the left hand/thumb (courtesy Erik Wolters).

Fragment 26.4
Tremor associated with dystonia (TAWD)
Young woman suffering from cervical dystonia and torticollis, with an irregular, jerky, postural tremor of the head with a directional preponderance, using a sensory trick to reduce the tremor amplitude (courtesy Erik Wolters).

Fragment 26.5
Cerebellar tremor
Woman diagnosed with MS, showing titubation of the head, cerebellar ataxia, and an intention tremor of both hands (courtesy Erik Wolters).

Fragment 26.6
Task-specific tremor
Patient with a task-specific tremor of the right hand, only when writing (primary writing tremor) (courtesy Erik Wolters).

Fragment 26.7
Orthostatic tremor
Patient without tremor in the sitting position, showing continuous movements of both legs, starting directly after rising. EMG showed a high-frequency tremor (17 Hz) in the standing position, which disappeared immediately upon sitting (courtesy Erik Wolters).

Fragment 26.8
Midbrain ('Holmes' or 'rubral' tremor)
Young man with a posttraumatic midbrain tremor, consisting of a low-frequency position, rest

and intention tremor of his left arm (courtesy Erik Wolters).

Fragment 26.9
Essential palatal tremor
Young-onset, rhythmic, low-frequency contractions of the tensor veli palatine resulting in elevations of the roof of the soft palate, with opening/closing of the Eustachian tube and the symptom of ear-clicking (which, unfortunately, cannot be appreciated in this video) (courtesy Erik Wolters).

Fragment 27.1
Psychogenic tremor
Inconsistent distal tremor of the right hand, with variable frequency and amplitude. This tremor originally had the characteristics of a position tremor, but later on, there were also aspects of a resting tremor. The tremor is suppressed by entrainment (courtesy Erik Wolters).

Fragment 27.2
Bilateral Vim-DBS in essential tremor PD (2)
(segments 1-2)
In this video you might see the significant effects of bilateral thalamic Vim-DBS in a 70 yr old lady with a disabling essential tremor before (segment 1) and after (segment 2) Vim-DBS (courtesy Christian Baumann).

Fragment 27.3
STN-DBS in tremor-dominant PD (1)
In this video you might appreciate the quick response of rest tremor to STN-DBS macrostimulation during operative implantation of bilateral subthalamic electrodes in a 68-year-old patient with tremor-dominant idiopathic Parkinson's disease (courtesy Christian Baumann).

Fragment 28.1
Negative myoclonus
This video fragment shows a patient with renal failure. While keeping his wrists actively extended, negative myoclonus (asterixis) can be seen due to muscular inhibition (courtesy Marina de Koning-Tijssen).

Fragment 28.2
Cortical myoclonus
This 7-year-old patient suffers from cortical myoclonus and ataxia. Genetic analysis revealed a mutation in the GOSR2 gene. The video shows multifocal myoclonus of muscles in the head, face and distal upper limbs. Myoclonus is provoked by somasthetic stimulus (reflex myoclonus) (courtesy Marina de Koning-Tijssen).

Fragment 28.3
Subcortical myoclonus
The video shows a patient with myoclonus dystonia (with a mutation in the SGCE gene). Myoclonic jerks are seen in the upper part of the body. During action the myoclonus is exacerbated and also appears in the upper limbs. The patient suffers from a mild dystonia of the neck. Writer's cramp is shown on the video (courtesy Marina de Koning-Tijssen).

Fragment 28.4
Spinal myoclonus
The video shows a patient with propriospinal myoclonus. The bilaterally synchronised jerks are mainly located in the axial muscles. Electromyographic examination shows the fixed pattern of muscle activation on left side, starting in the lumbar spinal muscles and travelling cranially. A 'bereitschaft potential' (BP) was absent (courtesy Marina de Koning-Tijssen).

Fragment 28.5
Peripheral myoclonus
This patient suffers from peripheral nerve damage due to HMSN type II. Notice the atrophy of the hand muscles. Myoclonus is absent at rest, but during posture, peripheral minipolymyoclonus is seen (courtesy Marina de Koning-Tijssen).

Fragment 29.1
Chorea (Segments 1-4)
This videotape shows a senile chorea (segment 1), followed by hemichorea (ballism) after a striatal haemorrhage (segment 2) and hemichorea after stenting the left medial carotid artery (segment 3), and posttraumatic dystonic hemichorea (segment 4) (courtesy Jan Roth).

Fragment 29.2
Chorea (Huntington's disease) (Segments 1-5)
Here are two patients suffering Huntington's disease (segments 1 and 2), followed by the tongue protrusion test in an HD patient (segment 3), the typical choreatic gait in HD patients (segment 4), and the impaired voluntary movements in these patients (segment 5) (courtesy Jan Roth).

Fragment 29.3
Chorea (young-onset Huntington's disease) (Segments 1-3)
This tape demonstrates a parkinsonian phenotype in a young-onset HD patient (segment 1), as well as a bradykinetic dystonic phenotype (segment 2) and a clinical manifestation of a young-onset HD with myoclonus, tics, and stereotypies (segment 3) (courtesy Jan Roth).

Fragment 30.1 (24.1)
Hemiballism
This elderly woman shows continuous, irregular, flinging movements over the left side of her body, induced by a cerebral infarction involving the subthalamic nucleus (courtesy Erik Wolters).

Fragment 31.1 (21.1)
Gilles de la Tourette syndrome (Segments 1-2)
The first segment shows a mentally handicapped man with several stereotypic motor tics. The second segment shows a patient with a mild multiple tic syndrome, consisting of facial and phonic tics, with a good response on tetrabenazine (courtesy Erik Wolters).

Fragment 32.1
Kearns-Sayre syndrome
This patient suffers from Kearns-Sayre syndrome, with generalized cerebellar ataxia and progressive ophthalmoplegia due to a mitochondrial DNA mutation (courtesy Teus van Laar).

Fragment 33.1
Non-degenerative cerebellar ataxia
This videotape shows an MS patient with an atactic gait, axial titubation, and incoordinated volitional movements (courtesy Erik Wolters).

Fragment 33.2
Sporadic cerebellar atrophy
A case with SCA17 with Huntington phenotype (courtesy Jan Roth).

Fragment 34.1
Nystagmus in cerebellar disorders (segments 1-3)
In segment 1, a gaze-evoked nystagmus in a female patient presenting with cerebellar degeneration secondary to superficial siderosis is shown. Holding her eyes in an eccentric position (30 degrees to the left), her eyes drift slowly back to the primary position, which is then centrally compensated by an outwardly directed correction saccade. Note the absence of any downbeat nystagmus when looking eccentrically, and of any downbeat or rebound nystagmus after returning to the primary position. Segment 2 demonstrates a downbeat nystagmus in a young patient (aged 27 years) with presumably hereditary cerebellar degeneration. In the primary position his eyes drift slowly upwards, which is then followed by a downward correction saccades. The last fragment, segment 3, shows a rebound nystagmus in the same patient, elicited after a prolonged (20 seconds) eccentric gaze. During this eccentric gaze (in darkness, looking at a briefly flashing red dot at 30 degrees eccentricity), a gaze-evoked nystagmus can be seen, although it lessens over time. Upon returning to the primary position, a strong drift towards the previous eccentric eye position followed by centripetal correction saccades (a

so-called rebound nystagmus) can be appreciated. This phenomenon is thought to be the consequence of central compensation for the gaze-evoked nystagmus (courtesy Alexander Tarnutzer).

Fragment 36.1
PMLS in RLS
52-year-old patient with restless legs syndrome. Nocturnal polysomnography with (from top to bottom) electro-oculography, chin electromyography, electro-encephalography, electrocardiography, and tibial electromyography (EMG) reveals periodic limb movements of sleep (PLMS) which can be seen both clinically and in EMG recordings (courtesy Christian Baumann).

Fragment 37.1
Somatoform Disorders (Segments 1-4)
In this fragment some somatoform movement disorders are shown: a pseudo-paresis of the non-dominant body-half in a young woman (segment 1), a rather inconsistent tremor in the left arm of a right-handed young man (segment 2) (courtesy Erik Wolters), a generalized, bizarre, hyperkinetic disorder, probably to be diagnosed as malingering (segment 3), and a man with bizarre posturing (segment 4) (courtesy Teus van Laar).

Fragment 38.1
Catatonia
This video displays an akinetic-mutistic young man with typical posturing (note his catalepsy: the tonic maintenance for a long period of time of a limb in a potentially uncomfortable posture, where it has been placed by the examiner) and staring. His catatonia was diagnosed as manifestation of an acute psychotic condition, and he responded well to treatment with neuroleptics (courtesy Erik Wolters).

Fragment 38.2
Iatrogenic acute dystonia (Segments 1-2)
The dramatic presentation of a young man with a frightening, obviously painful, generalized dystonic storm (segment 1). Dystonic features include characteristic orofacial and axial dystonia with cervical and/or thoracic hyperextension, lateroflexion, and torsion. After intravenous application of anticholinergics, this dystonic storm disappeared within minutes (segment 2) (courtesy Erik Wolters).

Fragment 38.3
Tardive tremor
A patient with a tardive tremor (courtesy Erik Wolters).

Fragment 38.4
Tardive dyskinesia
A patient with haloperidol-induced, tardive blepharospasm and typical perioral dyskinesia (stereotypies) (courtesy Jan Roth).

Fragment 38.5
Tardive chorea
A patient with lamotrigine-induced tardive chorea with stereotypies (courtesy Jan Roth).

Index